a **LANGE** clinical manual

Family Medicine

Ambulatory Care & Prevention

fifth edition

Edited by

Mark B. Mengel, MD, MPH
Vice-Chancellor, Regional Programs
University of Arkansas for Medical Sciences
Little Rock, Arkansas

L. Peter Schwiebert, MD
Professor, Residency Program
Department of Family and Preventive Medicine
University of Oklahoma Health Sciences Center
Oklahoma City, Oklahoma

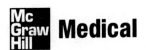 **Medical**

New York Chicago San Francisco Lisbon London Madrid Mexico City Milan
New Delhi San Juan Seoul Singapore Sydney Toronto

The McGraw·Hill Companies

Family Medicine: Ambulatory Care & Prevention, Fifth Edition

1 2 3 4 5 6 7 8 9 0 DOC/DOC 12 11 10 9

Set ISBN 978-0-07-149456-4; Set MHID 0-07-149456-1
Book ISBN 978-0-07-149457-1; Book MHID 0-07-149457-X
Card ISBN 978-0-07-149458-8; Card MHID 0-07-149458-8

ISSN 1066-2715

This book was set in Helvetica by Aptara®, Inc.
The editors were James Shanahan and Christie Naglieri.
The production supervisor was Catherine Saggese.
Project Management was provided by Sumbul Jafri, Aptara®, Inc.
The index was prepared by by Aptara®, Inc.
The cover designer was Mary McKeon.
Photo: doctor examines patient © LWA-Stephen Welstead/CORBIS.
RR Donnelley was printer and binder.

This book is printed on acid-free paper.

Contents

Color insert appears between pages 462 and 463

Contributors

Marc Jay Altshuler, MD
Assistant Professor, Assistant Residency Director, Department of Family and Community Medicine, Jefferson Medical College, Thomas Jefferson University Hospital, Philadelphia, Pennsylvania

Heather Anne Bartoli, PA-C
Physician Assistant, Oklahoma City, Oklahoma

James R. Barrett, MD, CAQSM
Professor, Family and Preventive Medicine, University of Oklahoma Health Sciences Center, Oklahoma City, Oklahoma

David Berkson, MD, FAAFP
Program Director, Family Medicine Residency, Assistant Professor, Department of Family, Community, and Preventive Medicine, Drexel University College of Medicine, Philadelphia, Pennsylvania

Shawn H. Blanchard, MD
Assistant Professor, Department of Family Medicine, Associate Director, Predoctoral Education, Oregon Health & Science University, Portland, Oregon

Ted Boehm, MD
Volunteer Faculty, Primary Care Sports Medicine Fellowship, Department of Family Medicine, University of Oklahoma Health Sciences Center, Oklahoma City, Oklahoma; Primary Care Sports Medicine Physician, Oklahoma Sports and Orthopedics Institute, Norman, Oklahoma

Douglas G. Browning, MD, ATC-L
Wake Forest Family Practice, Winston Salem, North Carolina

Bryan Cairns, MD
Resident Physician, Family Medicine, University of Cincinnati, Cincinnati, Ohio

William Edward Cayley, Jr., MD, MDiv
Associate Professor, Eau Claire Family Medicine Residency, Department of Family Medicine, University of Wisconsin, Eau Claire, Wisconsin

Jason Chao, MD, MS
Professor, Family Medicine, Case Western Reserve University, Family Medicine, University Hospitals Case Medical Center, Cleveland, Ohio

James C. Chesnutt, MD
Assistant Professor of Family Medicine, Oregon Health Sciences University, Portland, Oregon

Neal Clemenson, MD
Great Plains Family Practice, Oklahoma City, Oklahoma

Stephen W. Cobb, MD
Exempla Larkridge Family and Occupational Medicine, Thornton, Colorado

Jennifer Cocohoba, PharmD
Assistant Clinical Professor, Department of Clinical Pharmacy, University of California—San Francsco, San Francisco, California

Brian R. Coleman, MD
Director, Primary Care Sports Fellowship, Family and Preventive Medicine, Oklahoma University, Oklahoma City, Oklahoma

Amy Crawford-Faucher, MD
Associate Program Director, Crozer-Keystone Family Medicine Residency Program, Springfield, Pennsylvania

Dan F. Criswell, MD
Associate Professor, Family and Preventive Medicine Health Sciences Center, University of Oklahoma, Oklahoma City, Oklahoma; Program Director, Southwest Oklahoma Family Medicine Residency, Lawton, Oklahoma

Michael A. Crouch, MD, MSPH
Associate Professor, Family and Community Medicine, Baylor College of Medicine, Houston, Texas

Andrea Darby-Stewart, MD
Assistant Professor, Mayo Clinic College of Medicine, Scottsdale, Arizona

Kent W. Davidson, MD
Arkansas Specialty Orthopedics, Little Rock, Arkansas

D. Todd Detar, DO
Associate Professor, Department of Family Medicine, Medical University of South Carolina, Charleston, South Carolina

Vanessa A. Diaz, MD, MS
Assistant Professor, Department of Family Medicine, Medical University of South Carolina, Charleston, South Carolina

Victor A. Diaz, Jr., MD
Assistant Professor, Family and Community Medicine, Jefferson Medical College, Assistant Medical Director, Jefferson Family Medicine Associates, Thomas Jefferson University Hospital, Philadelphia, Pennsylvania

Larry L. Dickey, MD, MSW, MPH
Associate Adjunct Professor, Family and Community Medicine, University of California—San Francisco, Sacramento, California

Philip M. Diller, MD, PhD
Associate Professor and Program Director, The Christ Hospital, University of Cincinnati, Cincinnati, Ohio

Carmelo DiSalvo, MD
Mid Atlantic Family Practice, Lewes, Delaware

Charles Eaton, MD, MS
Professor, Family Medicine, Department of Family Medicine, Director, Heart Disease Prevention Center, Brown University School of Medicine, Pawtucket, Rhode Island

Sarah R. Edmonson, MD, MS
Instructor, Family and Community Medicine, Baylor College of Medicine, Houston, Texas

Mari Egan, MD, MHPE
Clinical Associate, Department of Family Medicine, The University of Chicago Pritzker School of Medicine, Chicago, Illinois

Robert Ellis, MD
Assistant Professor, Department of Family Medicine, University of Cincinnati, Assistant Professor, Department of Family Medicine, The Christ Hospital, Cincinnati, Ohio

Stephanie L. Evans, PharmD, BCPS
Pharmacist, Wal-Mart Pharmacy, Benton, Kentucky

Brooke Farley, PharmD, BCPS
Clinical Pharmacist and Assistant Professor, Pharmacy Practice, Mercy Family Medicine, Saint John's Mercy Family Medicine Residency Program and the Saint Louis College of Pharmacy, St. Louis, Missouri

Rhonda Faulkner, PhD
Assistant Professor, Department of Family Medicine, University of Illinois at Chicago College of Medicine, Chicago, Illinois

Jonathan D. Ference, PharmD, BCPS
Assistant Professor, Department of Pharmacy Practice, Nesbitt College of Pharmacy and Nursing, Wilkes-Barre, Pennsylvania; Clinical Pharmacist, Wyoming Valley Family Medicine Residency Program, Wyoming Valley Health Care System, Kingston, Pennsylvania

Jeanne M. Ferrante, MD, MPH
Associate Professor, Family Medicine, UMDNJ-Robert Wood Johnson Medical School, Somerset, New Jersey

Scott A. Fields, MD
Vice Chair, Family Medicine, Oregon Health Sciences University, Portland, Oregon

Laura Frankenstein, MD
Clinical Assistant Professor, Department of Community and Family Medicine, Saint Louis University, St. Louis, Missouri

Judith Kerber Frazier, MD
Family Medicine Physician, Mustang, Oklahoma

Keith A. Frey, MD, MBA
Professor, Mayo thunderbird, Family Medicine, Mayo Clinic-Scottsdale, Scottsdale, Arizona

Jennifer Gafford, PhD
Consulting Psychologist, The Family Care Health Centers, St. Louis, Missouri, MO

Ronald H. Goldschmidt, MD
Professor, Family and Community Medicine, University of California, San Francisco, California

Meredith Ann Goodwin, MD
Assistant Professor, Family Medicine and Rural Health, Florida State University College of Medicine, Resource Staff Physician, Tallahassee Memorial Hospital, Tallahassee, Florida

Marjorie Guthrie, MD
Assistant Professor, SLU Family Medicine Residency Program, Saint Louis University, Belleville, Illinois

Gregg M. Hallbauer, DO, MCG (Clinical Gerontology)
Associate Program Director for Curriculum, Conroe Family Medicine Residency, Conroe, Texas

Brian H. Halstater, MD
Assistant Clinical Professor, Department of Family Medicine Residency Program, Department of Family and Community Medicine, Duke University School of Medicine, Durham, North Carolina

John G. Halvorsen, MD, MS
Professor and Chair, Department of Family and Community Medicine, University of Illinois, Peoria, Illinois

Richard J. Ham, MD
Director and Professor, Geriatric Medicine and Psychiatry, Center on Aging, University of West Virginia, Morgantown, West Virginia

Mike D. Hardin, Jr., MD
Faculty Member, Department of Family Medicine, McLennan County Medical Education and Research Foundation, University of Texas Southwestern Medical School, Waco, Texas

Laura Hargro, MD, MBA
Assistant Professor, Dept. of Family Medicine, UMDNJ-New Jersey Medical School, Newark, New Jersey

Radhika R. Hariharan, MRCP(UK)
Assistant Professor, Family and Community Medicine, Baylor College of Medicine, Houston, Texas

Suzanne Leonard Harrison, MD
Assistant Professor, Department of Family Medicine & Rural Health, Florida State University College of Medicine, Tallahassee, Florida

John A. Heydt, MD
President and CEO, University Physicians & Surgeons, Senior Associate Dean of Clinical Affairs, University of California, Irvine

Allen L. Hixon, MD
Associate Professor and Vice Chairman, Department of Family Medicine and Community Health,
John A. Burns School of Medicine, University of Hawaii, Mililani, Hawaii

David Holmes, MD
Clinical Associate Professor, Family Medicine, University at Buffalo, State University of New York,
Family Physician, Family Medicine, Kaleida Health, Buffalo, New York

Felix Horng, MD, MBA
Woodbury Medical Group, Irvine, California

Mark K. Huntington, MD, PhD
Associate Professor, Sanford School of Medicine, The University of South Dakota; Assistant Director,
Sioux Falls Family Medicine Residency Program, Sioux Falls, South Dakota

May S. Jennings, MD
Assistant Professor, Department of Medicine, University of Alabama at Birmingham, Birmingham,
Alabama

Andrew D. Jones, MD
Assistant Professor, Department of Family and Preventive Medicine, Associate Program Director,
Family Medicine Residency Program, University of Oklahoma Health Sciences Center, Oklahoma
City, Oklahoma

Cathy Kamens, MD
Lecturer, Department of Family and Community Medicine, University of Toronto, Family Physician,
Women's College Hospital, Toronto, Ontario, Canada

Mitchell A. Kaminski, MD, MBA
Chairman, Department of Family Medicine, Clinical Associate Professor, Temple School of Medicine,
Crozer-Chester Medical Center, Upland, Pennsylvania

Amanda J. Kaufman, MD
Assistant Professor, Department of Family Medicine, University of Michigan, Ann Arbor, Michigan

Nancy D. Kellogg, MD
Professor and Division Chief, Department of Pediatrics, University of Texas,
San Antonio, Texas

Sanford R. Kimmel, MD
Professor and Vice-Chair, Department of Family Medicine, University of Toledo College of Medicine,
Chief of Staff, University of Toledo Medical Center, Toledo, Ohio

Fred Kobylarz, MD, MPH
Associate Professor, Center for Healthy Aging, Department of Family Medicine, UMDNJ—Robert
Wood Johnson Medical School, Department of Family Medicine, Robert Wood Johnson University
Hospital, New Brunswick, New Jersey

Charles M. Kodner, MD
Associate Professor, Family and Geriatric Medicine, University of Louisville School of Medicine,
Louisville, Kentucky

Geoffrey S. Kuhlman, MD, CAQSM, FAAFP
Director of Sports Medicine, Hinsdale Family Medicine Residency, Hinsdale, Illinois

David C. Lanier, MD
Associate Director, Center for Primary Care, Prevention and Clinical Partnerships, Agency for
Healthcare Research and Quality, Rockville, Maryland

Allen Robert Last, MD, MPH
Assistant Professor, Family and Community Medicine, Medical College of Wisconsin, Family
Medicine, Wheaton Franciscan Healthcare—All Saints, Racine, Wisconsin

Damon F. Lee, MD
Assistant Professor, Family Medicine and Community Health, University of Hawaii John A. Burns
School of Medicine, Mililani, Hawaii

Paul E. Lewis, MD, MPH
Assistant Professor, SLU Family Medicine Residency Program, Saint Louis University, Belleville, Illinois

Tammy J. Lindsay, MD
Flight Commander; Interim Associate Program Director, SLU Family Medicine Residency Program, 375th MDOS and Saint Louis University, Belleville, Illinois

Martin Stephen Lipsky, MD
Professor, Department of Family Medicine, Dean, University of Illinois College of Medicine, Rockford, Illinois

Jonathan MacClements, MD
Associate Professor, Residency Program Director, Family Medicine, University of Texas, Tyler, Texas

Diane J. Madlon-Kay, MD, MS
Associate Professor, Department of Family Medicine and Community Health, University of Minnesota Medical School, Minneapolis, Minnesota

Megan Mahoney, MD
Assistant Clinical Professor, Family and Community Medicine, UCSF-SFGH FPR, San Francisco, California

Arch G. Mainous III, PhD
Professor, Department of Family Medicine, Medical University of South Carolina, Charleston, South Carolina

Robert Mallin, MD
Associate Professor, Family Medicine, Medical University of South Carolina, Charleston, South Carolina

William T. Manard, MD
Clinical Instructor, Department of Community and Family Medicine, Saint Louis University School of Medicine, Primary Care Physician, Alexian Brothers Community Services PACE Program, St. Louis, Missouri

James P. McKenna, MD
Residency Director, Family Medicine Residency, Hentage Valley Beaver, Beaver, Pennsylvania

Mark B. Mengel, MD, MPH
Vice Chancellor, Regional Programs, University of Arkansas for Medical Sciences, Professor, Family and Preventive Medicine, University of Arkansas for Medical Sciences, Little Rock, Arkansas

Michael Michener, MD
Associate Professor, SLU Family Medicine Residency Program, 375th MDOS and Saint Louis University, Belleville, Illinois

Julie A. Murphy, PharmD, BCPS
Clinical Pharmacist and Associate Professor of Pharmacy Practice, Mercy Family Medicine, Saint John's Mercy Family Medicine Residency Program and the Saint Louis College of Pharmacy, St. Louis, Missouri

Ryan M. Niemiec, PsyD
Assistant Clinical Professor, Community and Family Medicine, Saint Louis University School of Medicine, Psychologist, Saint Louis Behavioral Medicine Institute, St. Louis, Missouri

Karen D. Novielli, MD
Senior Associate Dean for Faculty Affairs and Professional Development, Jefferson Medical College, Philadelphia, Pennsylvania

Tomás P. Owens, Jr, MD
Chair, Department of Family Medicine-Integris Baptist Medical Center, Associate Director, Great Plains Family Medicine Residency, Clinical Professor, Departments of Internal Medicine, Geriatric Medicine and Family and Preventive Medicine, University of Oklahoma Health Sciences Center, Oklahoma City, Oklahoma

Philip R. Palmer, MD
Faculty, Great Plains Family Medicine Residency, Chief, Family Medicine, Deaconess Hospital, Oklahoma City, Oklahoma

William G. Phillips, MD
Family Practice, Atlanta, Georgia

Marjorie Shaw Phillips, MS, RPh, FASHP
Clinical Research Pharmacist and Medication Safety Coordinator, Medical College of Georgia Health System and Clinical Professor, University of Georgia College of Pharmacy, Augusta, Georgia

Heather Pickett, DO
Associate Professor and Deputy Military Program Director, SLU Family Medicine Residency Program, 375th MDOS and Saint Louis University, Belleville, Illinois

David C. Pole, MPH
Deputy Director, Predoctoral and AHEC Programs, Community and Family Medicine, Saint Louis University, St. Louis, Missouri

Michael Polizzotto, MD
Associate Program Director, Department of Family Medicine, University of Illinois College of Medicine Rockford, Rockford, Illinois

Mark C. Potter, MD
Assistant Professor and Residency Director, Department of Family Medicine, University of Illinois at Chicago, Chicago, Illinois

Brenda Powell, MD
Staff, Cleveland Clinic, Family Medicine, Women's Health, Travel Medicine, Beachwood, Ohio

Robert Glenn Quattlebaum, MD
Trident Medical Center/Medical University of South Carolina, Family Medicine Residency Program, Charleston, South Carolina

Kalyanakrishnan Ramakrishnan, MD
Professor, Department of Family and Preventive Medicine, OUHSC, Family Medicine Center, Oklahoma City, Oklahoma

Goutham Rao, MD
Clinical Director, Weight Management and Wellness Center, Associate Professor of Pediatrics and Family Medicine, University of Pittsburgh School of Medicine, Pittsburgh, Pennsylvania

Brian C. Reed, MD
Assistant Professor, Department of Family and Community Medicine, Baylor College of Medicine, Houston, Texas

Jeri R. Reid, MD
Associate Professor, Department of Family and Geriatric Medicine, University of Louisville, Louisville, Kentucky

Kathryn Reilly, MD, MPH
Professor and Associate Residency Director, Department of Family and Community medicine, University of Oklahoma Health Science Center, Oklahoma City, Oklahoma

Jose E. Rodríguez, MD
Associate Professor, Department of Family Medicine and Rural Health, Florida State University College of Medicine, Florida

John C. Rogers, MD, MPH, MEd
Professor of Family and Community Medicine, Professor-in-Residency, Office of Undergraduate Medical Education, Baylor College of Medicine, Houston, Texas

Montiel T. Rosenthal, MD
Associate Clinical Professor and Director of Maternity Services, Family Medicine, College of Medicine, University of Cincinnati, Director, Prenatal Clinic and Residency Faculty, Family Medicine, The Christ Hospital, University of Cincinnati, Family Medicine Residency Program, Cincinnati, Ohio

Michael P. Rowane, DO, MS, FAAFP, FAAO
Associate Clinical Professor of Family Medicine and Psychiatry, Case Western Reserve University, Director of Medical Education, University Hospitals Richmond Medical Center Director of Osteopathic Medical Education, University Hospitals Case Medical Center, Richmond Heights, Ohio

George P.N. Samraj, MD
Associate Professor, Family Medicine, University of Florida, Gainesville, Florida

Ted C. Schaffer, MD
Clinical Associate Professor, Department of Family Medicine, University of Pittsburgh School of Medicine, Pittsburgh, Pennsylvania

Richard Schamp, MD
Associate Clinical Professor and Medical Director, Alexian Brothers Community Services (PACE Program), Saint Louis University, St. Louis, Missouri

F. David Schneider, MD, MSPH
Professor and Vice Chair, Department of Family and Community Medicine, University of Texas, San Antonio, Texas

L. Peter Schwiebert, MD
Professor, Residency Program, Department of Family and Preventive Medicine, University of Oklahoma Health Sciences Center, Oklahoma City, Oklahoma

H. Russell Searight, PhD, MPH
Associate Professor, Psychology, Lake Superior State University, Sault Sainte Marie, Michigan

Aamir Siddiqi, MD
Associate Professor, Family Medicine, Associate Director, St. Luke's Family Medicine Residency, Medical Director, Aurora Family Care Center, President Medical Staff, Aurora Sinai Medical Center

Jeannette E. South-Paul, MD
Professor and Chair, Department of Family Medicine, University of Pittsburgh, Pittsburgh, Pennsylvania

Mark R. Stephan, MD
Family Practice, Phoenix, Arizona

Nicole G. Stern, MD
Campus Health Service, Tucson, Arizona

Carol Stewart, MD, FAAFP
Assistant Professor, Department of Family Medicine, David Geffen School of Medicine at UCLA, Les Kelley Family Health Center, Attending Physician, Department of Family Medicine, Santa Monica UCLA Medical Center and Orthopaedic Hospital, Santa Monica, California

Daniel Stulberg, MD, FAAFP
Associate Professor, Department of Family and Community Medicine, University of New Mexico, Albuquerque, New Mexico

Jeff Susman, MD
Professor and Chair, Department of Family Medicine, University of Cincinnati, Section Head, Family Medicine, University Hospital, Cincinnati, Ohio

Melissa A. Talamantes, MS
Faculty, Department of Family Practice, University of Texas HSC, San Antonio, San Antonio, Texas

Michael Temporal, MD
Associate Professor, SLU Family Medicine Residency Program, Saint Louis University, Belleville, Illinois

William L. Toffler, MD
Professor, Department of Family Medicine, Director, Predoctoral Education, Oregon Health & Science University, Portland, Oregon

Terrence T. Truong, MD
Faculty, Great Plains Family Medicine Residency Program, Oklahoma City, Oklahoma

Nancy Tyre, MD
Associate Physician Diplomate, Family Medicine, David Geffen School of Medicine, at UCLA Los Angeles, California

Anthony Valdini, MD, MS
Associate Professor, Family Medicine and Community Health, University of Massachusetts Medical School, Worcester, Massachusetts, Attending Physician, Family Medicine and Internal Medicine, Lawrence General Hospital, Lawrence, Massachusetts

Kirsten R. Vitrikas, MD
Assistant Professor, Department of Community and Family Medicine, SLU Family Medicine Residency Program, Belleville, Illinois

H. Bruce Vogt, MD
Professor and Chair, Department of Family Medicine, Sanford School of Medicine, The University of South Dakota, Sioux Falls, South Dakota

Cynthia M. Waickus, MD, PhD
Associate Chair for Educational Programs Department of Family Medicine, Rush Medical College Chicago, Illinois

Linda L. Walker, MD, FAAFP
Associate Director, Family Medicine Program, The Medical Center, Columbus Georgia

Jie Wang, MD
Clinical Assistant Professor, Department of Family Medicine, University of Wisconsin—Madison, Madison, Wisconsin

Lara Carson Weinstein, MD
Assistant Professor, Family and Community Medicine, Jefferson Medical College of Thomas Jefferson University, Attending Physician, Family and Community Medicine, Thomas Jefferson University Hospital, Philadelphia, Pennsylvania

Barry D. Weiss, MD
Professor of Family and Community Medicine, University of Arizona College of Medicine, Tucson, Arizona

Stephen F. Wheeler, MD
Associate Professor, Department of Family and Geriatric Medicine, Director, Residency Education, University of Louisville, Louisville, Kentucky

LeRoy C. White, MD, JD
Family Medicine—Enid, Oklahoma University Health Sciences Center, Oklahoma City, Oklahoma

Lesley D. Wilkinson, MD
Associate Clinical Professor, Family Medicine, David Geffen School of Medicine, at UCLA Los Angeles, California

George R. Wilson, MD
Professor and Chair, Community Health/Family Medicine, UF COM—Jacksonville, Jacksonville, Florida, Chief of Service, Family Medicine/Occupational Medicine, Shands Jacksonville Medical Center, Jacksanville, Florida

Deborah Kay Witt, MD
Assistant Professor, Department of Family and Community Medicine, Jefferson Medical College, Thomas Jefferson University, Philadelphia, Pennsylvania

Aylin Yaman, MD
Specialist of Neurology, Department of Neurology, Antalya State Teaching and Training Hospital, Antalya, Turkey

Hakan Yaman, MD, MS
Assistant Professor, Department of Family Practice, Akdeniz University Faculty of Medicine, Antalya, Turkey, Head, Department of Family Practice, Akdeniz University Hospital, Antalya, Turkey

Aleksandra Zgierska, MD, PhD
Clinical Instructor, Department of Family Medicine, University of Wisconsin School of Medicine and Public Health, Madison, Wisconsin

PURPOSE

This manual presents information on the most common complaints, problems, conditions, and diseases encountered by family medicine physicians and other primary care providers who practice in the ambulatory settings. These common conditions, which have been selected from surveys taken from family medicine, internal medicine, and pediatrics, are arranged alphabetically in five sections. Evidence-based information, including strength of recommendation ratings, is presented in such a way that busy practitioners can access information rapidly. Practical, specific treatment information, including starting doses of medication, is offered. This manual also addresses evidence-based preventive interventions commonly used in primary care settings.

ORGANIZATION SCOPE

Although most medical books are organized by organ system, we have structured this manual according to typical patient presentations in primary care settings, for example, common symptoms and signs, follow-up needs for chronic physical or mental illness, and reproductive health concerns. In addition, we provide information on preventive health care recommendations.

Section I contains information on the most commonly encountered acute/undifferentiated problems in the primary care setting. Information is presented in such a way that a busy practitioner can quickly form a list of diagnostic possibilities, perform a cost-effective evidence-based diagnostic workup, and prescribe evidence-based treatment for the most common causes of these complaints.

Section II offers information on the treatment of patients with common chronic illnesses. Each chapter provides practical follow-up strategies for such patients, integrating cost-effective evidence-based clinical management with important psychosocial issues.

Section III is important because many patients seen in the primary care clinics have either a primary psychiatric disorder or a psychiatric disorder complicating the management of preexisting medical conditions. Strategies that effectively identify and treat patients with psychiatric disorders are presented clearly and succinctly.

Section IV addresses common reproductive woman's health issues that present in the primary care setting including contraception, infertility, and prenatal and postnatal care.

Section V will assist primary care clinicians in the prevention of important diseases in their patients. Authors of these chapters recommend interventions that can be easily applied in primary care practices including counseling, immunizations, screening tests, and chemoprophylaxis. Chapters on travel medicine and the preoperative evaluation complete this section.

In all chapters, authors have integrated principles of clinical decision making, evidence-based medicine, and cost-effective clinical management and have considered psychosocial and contextual issues; where applicable, areas of controversy are identified. Where appropriate, complimentary and alternative medical interventions are discussed.

Other useful features of this manual include the following:

- A convenient outline format and selective use of boldface type to afford quick, easy access to key aspects of diagnosis and treatment.
- Flowcharts facilitating the diagnostic workup and common management strategies for specific conditions.

- Emphasis on cost-effective evidence-based strategies, with strength of recommendation ratings clearly visible.
- Each chapter is introduced by key point section that summarizes main issues.
- Sidebars in chapters highlight more than 70 specific conditions.
- Streamline organizational framework makes it easy to find sections on diagnosis, symptoms and signs, evaluation and management strategies.

STRENGTH OF RECOMMENDATION TAXONOMIES

For this fifth edition, we have asked all the authors to use the strength of recommendation taxonomy used by major family medicine journals. Recommendations are graded as A, B, or C based on the quality and quantity of evidence as shown in the table below.

Strength of Recommendation	Basis for Recommendation
A	Consistent or good quality of patient-oriented evidence.
B	Inconsistent or limited quality of patient-oriented evidence.
C	Consensus, disease-oriented evidence, usual practice, expert opinion, or case series.

Patient-oriented evidence measures outcomes that matter to patients, such as morbidity, mortality, symptom improvement, cost reduction, and quality of life. Disease-oriented evidence measures intermediate physiologic or surrogate endpoints that may or may not reflect improvement in patient outcomes.

ACKNOWLEDGMENTS

First, we thank those of you who have used this manual. We have received very positive feedback from medical students, residents, and practitioners who found the previous editions of *Family Medicine* to be a quick, practical reference text. We particularly appreciate those comments that have enabled us to strengthen many chapters in this handbook.

Second, we thank our authors of this fifth edition, many of whom were willing to come back and update their previous work. We were pleasantly surprised to discover that most of our authors were enthusiastic about updating their chapters with strength of recommendation ratings.

Third, we thank the editors and their staff at McGraw Hill for their encouragement and support. We are now updating *Family Medicine* approximately every 3 years; feeling this more rapid revision cycle is necessary due to the growth in medical knowledge.

Lastly, but far from least, we thank our spouses, Laura and Kathy, and our children, Sally, Kristin, and Matt, for their support and patience throughout this rapid editorial process. We both have had to take a great deal of work home and our families deserve special thanks and gratitude.

Mark B. Mengel, MD, MPH
L. Peter Schwiebert, MD
Little Rock, Arkansas, and
Oklahoma City, Oklahoma
December 2008

SECTION I. Common Complaints

1   Abdominal Pain

Kalyanakrishnan Ramakrishnan, MD

KEY POINTS

- Most patients presenting with abdominal pain have minor, nonsurgical causes. Nonspecific abdominal pain (NSAP) is most common and accounts for 90% of pain in children. Chronic abdominal pain is most often gastrointestinal in origin.
- Proper history taking and a stepwise physical examination enable a diagnosis to be made in most patients.
- Any woman of childbearing age presenting with abdominal pain should have a pregnancy test. Management in pregnancy should focus on both mother and fetus.
- Presentation of abdominal pain in the elderly is modified by comorbid illness and medications. Classical history and physical findings may be absent.

I. **Definition.** Abdominal pain is defined as a subjective feeling of discomfort in the abdomen. When the duration is less than 6 hours, it is referred to as acute. Abdominal pain may be caused by luminal obstruction (appendicitis, cholecystitis, renal or ureteral colic, diverticulitis), an inflamed organ (pancreatitis, hepatitis), ischemia (mesenteric ischemia, ischemic colitis), or bowel motility disorders/multifactorial causes (irritable bowel syndrome [IBS], NSAP).

II. **Common Diagnoses.** Abdominal pain accounts for 2.5 million office visits and 8 million emergency-department visits every year in the United States. It is the most frequent cause for gastroenterology consultation. Most patients have minor problems, such as dyspepsia, although 20% to 25% are found to have a more serious condition requiring hospitalization. Table 1–1 lists the common causes of acute abdominal pain in adults and the elderly. In children, urinary tract disease, peptic ulcer, inflammatory bowel disease (IBD), and gastroesophageal reflux disease may present acutely; constipation, lactose intolerance, mid-cycle pain, and psychological (secondary gain, sexual abuse, school phobia) causes of abdominal pain are more chronic.

   A. **NSAP.** NSAP occurs in approximately one-third (35%) of patients presenting with acute abdominal pain. More than 90% of children who have abdominal pain have NSAP. IBS rarely presents initially in the elderly.

   B. **Appendicitis.** Appendicitis occurs in 7% of the US population (3% of women and 2% of men older than 50 years), with an incidence of 1.1/1000 people per year. It is the most common nonobstetric cause of surgical emergency during pregnancy and is more common in the second trimester. Perforation rates are higher in patients younger than 18 and older than 50 years.

   C. **Gallstones.** Approximately 10% to 20% of adults aged 20 to 50 years have gallstones; people in their advancing age, Native Americans, and younger women (where it is 2–6 times more frequent than in men) are at increased risk. Other risk factors include pregnancy, oral contraceptive use, hormone replacement therapy, obesity, rapid weight loss, diabetes mellitus, liver cirrhosis, Crohn's disease, and sedentary lifestyle.

   D. **Pancreatitis.** The annual incidence of acute pancreatitis in the United States is approximately 10 new cases per 100,000. The most common causes include cholelithiasis (40%), alcohol abuse (40%), drugs (steroids, azathioprine, estrogens, diuretics), trauma, viral infections, and hypercalcemia.

   E. **Diverticular disease.** The prevalence of diverticular disease is age dependent, increasing in the United States from <5% at age 40 to 65% by age 85; males and females are equally affected. Most cases (70%) are discovered incidentally, in 15% to 25% diverticulitis develops, and 5% to 15% bleed. Risk factors, besides age, include low fiber intake; increased consumption of red meat, fat, alcohol and caffeine; sedentary lifestyle; and obesity.

   F. **Mesenteric vascular occlusion.** Risk factors for mesenteric vascular occlusion include age (>60 years) and atherosclerosis (embolic events in 50% and also thrombotic or

TABLE 1–1. DISTRIBUTION OF ACUTE ABDOMINAL PATHOLOGY

Diagnosis	>50 years	<50 years
Intestinal obstruction	15%–30%	2%–6%
Biliary tract	15%–30%	2%–6%
Malignancy	4%–13%	1%
Peptic ulcer	5%–10%	2%–8%
Diverticulitis	5%–10%	<1%
Perforated viscus	4%–6%	1%
Appendicitis	3%–10%	15%–30%
Hernia	3%–4%	1%–2%
Vascular emergencies	2%–3%	<1%
Nonspecific abdominal pain	15%–30%	40%–50%

From Landry F. Evaluation of abdominal pain. In: *Emergency Clinical Guide.* http://www.anisman.com/ecg/index.asp.

low-flow state with associated vasoconstriction). Hypercoagulable states, intra-abdominal sepsis, portal hypertension, and cancer increase risk for **mesenteric vein thrombosis,** although the cause in 5% to 10% of patients remains idiopathic. In the elderly, arteriosclerosis, shock, congestive heart failure, and aortoiliac surgery cause **ischemic colitis;** in younger patients, oral contraceptive use, vasculitis, and hypercoagulable states are risk factors.

G. **Bowel obstruction.** Obstruction of the large or small bowel is a major health problem in the elderly, accounting for approximately 12% of cases of abdominal pain. Risk factors for small-bowel obstruction are adhesions as a result of previous abdominal surgery, neoplasms, or hernia. For large-bowel obstruction, risk factors include colon carcinoma, diverticulitis, and sigmoid volvulus.

H. **Other causes.** Other common causes of abdominal pain not discussed here include dyspepsia (see Chapter 19), peptic ulcer disease (see Chapter 82), and pelvic inflammatory disease (see Chapter 51).

III. **Symptoms.** Proper history taking is the foundation for a correct diagnosis and should address a variety of features (Table 1–2). Knowing about a history of ulcer disease, biliary colic, or diverticulitis is helpful. Alcohol and drug use should be addressed. Alcohol abuse contributes to pancreatitis, hematemesis, esophageal rupture, and spontaneous bacterial peritonitis. Nonsteroidal anti-inflammatory drugs (NSAIDs), prednisone, and immunosuppressants cause bleeding and perforation; aspirin, NSAIDs, and anticoagulants increase risk of bleeding. Drugs in the elderly induce nausea, vomiting, anorexia, and constipation and affect vital signs. Menstrual history is also important. Nausea, vomiting, constipation, urinary frequency, and pelvic or abdominal discomfort may all be experienced in normal pregnancy. Accuracy of history taking in the elderly may be affected by cognitive impairment, decreased auditory and visual acuity, and atypical symptoms.

A. **NSAP and IBS.** Pain may be colicky or persistent, and aggravated by meals. Most patients have a long history of recurrent abdominal pain relieved by defecation, a change in the frequency or consistency of the stool, abdominal bloating, and passage of excessive mucus (Manning criteria). There is no weight loss, constitutional symptoms (fever, anorexia, nausea, arthralgia), or intestinal bleeding.

B. **Appendicitis.** Anorexia and periumbilical pain followed by nausea, right lower quadrant (RLQ) pain, and vomiting occur in 50% of cases. Migration of pain has high sensitivity and specificity (approaching 80%). During pregnancy, the site of pain shifts progressively upward with increasing gestational age. Changes in bowel habits and hematuria/pyuria (pelvic appendicitis in 20%) may also be seen. Perforation results in generalized abdominal pain, fever, and tachycardia.

C. **Cholelithiasis.** More than 50% of patients with gallstones remain asymptomatic. Recurrent right upper quadrant or epigastric pain, radiating to the back or right shoulder blade, peaking over hours and resolving completely, suggests **biliary colic.** Upper abdominal pain in **cholecystitis** is severe, persistent, associated with constitutional symptoms and possibly jaundice. Perforation leading to **biliary peritonitis** causes spreading abdominal pain and worsening constitutional symptoms. Stone in the common bile duct may cause deepening jaundice, associated with fever, chills, and pain—**Charcot's triad. Gallstone ileus** presents with pain, distention, and vomiting—features of small-bowel obstruction.

TABLE 1–2. CORRELATION OF ABDOMINAL PAIN AND PATHOLOGY

Nature of Pain	Organ/Pathology
Acute or chronic (lasting weeks, months, years)	*Acute:* Biliary colic, renal colic, intestinal obstruction, perforated peptic ulcer, ruptured aneurysm, ruptured ectopic gestation *Chronic:* Peptic ulcer disease, chronic pancreatitis, diverticulosis
Onset of pain	*Sudden:* Sudden severe pain—perforated peptic ulcer, acute pancreatitis, ruptured aneurysm, ruptured ectopic gestation, renal/ureteric colic
Migration of pain	Appendicitis: Periumbilical, migrating to right iliac fossa Ureteric colic: From loin to groin
Referred pain	Biliary colic: Pain referred to the back and shoulder blades Pancreatitis: Referred to the back
Character of pain	*Burning pain:* Peptic ulcer *Colicky pain:* Biliary, renal, ureteric, intestinal colic (hollow organs) *Dull, continuous ache:* Solid organs (liver, spleen, kidneys)
Site of pain	*Epigastrium:* Stomach, liver, pancreas *Right hypochondrium:* Liver, biliary tree, hepatic flexure of colon *Left hypochondrium:* Spleen, tail of pancreas, splenic flexure of colon *Umbilicus:* Pancreas, transverse colon, small bowel *Right iliac fossa:* Appendix, cecum, ascending colon, terminal ileum, right tube, ovary, right ureter *Left iliac fossa:* Left tube and ovary, sigmoid colon, left ureter *Hypogastrium:* Urinary bladder, uterus *Back (renal angle):* Right/left kidney
Relieving factors	Antacids, food: Duodenal ulcer Sitting up, leaning forward: Pancreatitis Vomiting, antacids: Gastric ulcer
Associated symptoms	*Anorexia:* Gastric ulcer, appendicitis, peritonitis *Jaundice:* Biliary colic, cholecystitis, pancreatitis *Fever:* Appendicitis, cholecystitis *Vomiting:* Intestinal obstruction, pancreatitis, renal colic, ureteric colic, biliary colic, gastroenteritis *Hematemesis/melena:* Peptic ulcer disease *Diarrhea:* Gastroenteritis, colitis *Constipation:* Intestinal obstruction, appendicitis *Amenorrhea:* Pregnancy-related causes *Dysuria:* Urinary infection *Hematuria/smoky urine:* Renal/ureteric colic

  D. **Mid-epigastric or diffuse abdominal pain**—relieved by bending forward; associated with gall stones, recent surgery, or invasive procedures; or occurring 1 to 3 days after a binge or cessation of drinking—suggests **pancreatitis.** Nausea, vomiting, restlessness, and agitation accompany the pain. Chronic pancreatitis causes pain, malabsorption, diarrhea (steatorrhea), weight loss, or diabetes mellitus.
  E. **Diverticular disease.** Most diverticula are asymptomatic. **Diverticulitis** causes severe, abrupt, worsening left lower abdominal pain, fever, anorexia, nausea, vomiting, and constipation.
  F. **Ischemic bowel disease** presents with severe localized or diffuse abdominal pain (out of proportion to physical findings), unexplained abdominal distention, or gastrointestinal bleeding (bloody diarrhea, hematemesis) indicating bowel infarction (Evidence rating C). Elderly individuals with chronic mesenteric ischemia (**intestinal angina**) experience recurrent upper abdominal cramps 10 to 15 minutes after meals that subside over 1 to 3 hours. Bloating, flatulence, episodic vomiting, constipation, or diarrhea and severe weight loss may occur. Steatorrhea develops in half of affected persons. A history of angina, claudication, or transient ischemic attacks may be present.
  G. **Bowel obstruction.** Obstruction causes colicky pain, vomiting, abdominal distention, and constipation. In acute (small-bowel) obstruction, pain appears first followed by vomiting,

TABLE 1–3. PHYSICAL EXAMINATION IN ABDOMINAL PAIN

Inspection	Palpation	Percussion	Auscultation
Shape of the abdomen (scaphoid)	Guarding Rigidity	Tenderness Free fluid (ascites)	Bowel sounds
Whether all quadrants move equally with respiration	Of solid organs (liver, spleen, kidney, uterus, abdominal aorta, other palpable masses)	Organomegaly (liver, spleen, kidney, other masses)	Bruits (renal)
Engorged veins, visible abdominal pulsations, visible peristalsis	Testes, appendages (epididymis, spermatic cord)		
Hernial orifices (umbilical, inguinal, femoral)	Rectal/vaginal examination		
Scars of prior surgery			
Scrotum (testes, spermatic cord)			

distention, and constipation. In chronic (large-bowel) obstruction, constipation, followed by distention, pain, and vomiting, is seen (Evidence rating C).

IV. **Signs** (Table 1–3). Clinical stability of the patient (pulse, respiration, blood pressure, oxygen saturation, level of consciousness) should be assessed initially. Shock, pallor, sweating, or syncope indicates serious abdominal pathology. Rebound tenderness, guarding, and rigidity suggest a surgical cause. Operative scars suggest adhesions and bowel obstruction; abnormal orifices can be sites of hernias. Rectal and vaginal examinations assess pelvic or intraluminal pathologic findings. Guarding and rigidity may be absent during pregnancy, because of stretching of the abdominal wall, and the enlarged uterus prevents direct contact between an underlying inflamed organ and the parietal peritoneum. To distinguish uterine from extrauterine tenderness, patients should be examined in the right or left decubitus position.

A. In **NSAP,** bowel sounds may be increased; a fecal mass may present in either iliac fossa.
B. **Helpful findings in appendicitis** include guarding, RLQ tenderness, rebound tenderness, pain on percussion, and rigidity. Nonspecific findings include a positive Rovsing sign (pain elicited by compression of the left iliac fossa), positive iliopsoas sign (pain precipitated by extension of the ipsilateral hip), and a positive Cope obturator test (pain on internal rotation of the right hip).
C. **Biliary colic** is characterized by right upper quadrant tenderness worse on deep inspiration (Murphy sign), when the inflamed gallbladder comes in contact with the examiner's hand.
D. **Patients with pancreatitis** have epigastric or periumbilical guarding, abdominal distention, and ileus. Those with **hemorrhagic pancreatitis** may develop shock, coma, and signs of retroperitoneal bleeding may be present, as indicated by ecchymoses in the flanks (Grey Turner sign) or around the umbilicus (Cullen sign).
E. **Localized peritonitis in diverticulitis** may result in abdominal distention and ileus; rebound tenderness may be elicited in the left iliac fossa.
F. **Mesenteric ischemia** produces few significant abdominal signs in the early stages. A systolic upper abdominal bruit is heard in half of patients with intestinal angina. Mild tenderness and guarding in the left flank or iliac fossa is usual in ischemic colitis.
G. **Bowel obstruction** produces abdominal distention with hyperperistaltic bowel sounds. Guarding and rigidity suggest strangulation, as do the features of sepsis or shock. Hernial orifices and scars should be palpated for a mass, suggesting a hernia.

V. **Laboratory Tests.** The following approach relates to patients with **acute abdominal pain.** In **chronic abdominal pain** (see sidebars), testing must be individualized.

ABDOMINAL WALL PAIN

Abdominal wall pain occurs in the young secondary to trauma, overexertion, or epigastric or incisional hernias. In the elderly, it may be secondary to herpes zoster and postherpetic neuralgia, or soft tissue tumors (neurofibroma). The pain often has an insidious onset, being sharp initially and becoming dull over time. Straining, as in sneezing, coughing, or lifting heavy objects, aggravates it; changing positions or applying heat may relieve it. A positive Carnett sign (tenderness reproduced by tensing the abdominal wall) may be present.

Useful measures include NSAIDs (e.g., oral ibuprofen 400–600 mg 3 times daily), muscle relaxants (e.g., cyclobenzaprine 10 mg 3 times daily, methocarbamol 1000 mg 4 times daily), antidepressants (e.g., amitriptyline), local application of ethyl chloride or capsaicin cream 0.025%, and trigger point injections of bupivacaine hydrochloride 0.35% plus triamcinolone 10 to 40 mg (most effective).

INFLAMMATORY BOWEL DISEASE

Chronic abdominal pain is more common in **Crohn's disease** than in **ulcerative colitis** and is located in the RLQ. Fever, weight loss, arthralgia, and chronic diarrhea (with blood and mucus in stool) may be present, as are extraintestinal manifestations (arthralgias, skin ulcers, visual disturbances). Skin changes (pyoderma gangrenosum, erythema nodosum) and eye changes (iritis) may be present. A mass (thickened terminal ileum and cecum) may be palpable in the RLQ in **Crohn's disease.** Anemia, low serum albumin, elevated C-reactive protein level, and sedimentation rate are often present. Barium contrast studies and colonoscopy are diagnostic. Treatment involves long-term medications, including 5-aminosalicylic acid, steroids, and immunosuppressants such as azathioprine or 6-mercaptopurine. Ablative surgery (right hemicolectomy) may be necessary in the presence of obstruction, fistula formation, or nonresponse to medical management.

CHRONIC ABDOMINAL PAIN

Chronic pain implies persistence for 3 to 6 months and impact on the patient's activities of daily living. Evaluation begins with ruling out gastrointestinal causes. A blood count, sedimentation rate, chemistry, plain abdominal x-rays, abdominal ultrasound, and colonoscopy rule out most serious causes. When the initial evaluation suggests the presence of a specific pathology, specialized tests (e.g., endoscopic retrograde cholangiopancreatogram, angiography) can be considered. In children, sonography of the abdomen and pelvis is usually performed first to exclude nonintestinal causes.

Optimal treatment incorporates acknowledging the reality of the pain, reassuring the patient that an underlying serious abnormality is unlikely to be missed, setting appropriate goals to minimize the impact of the pain on daily patient functioning, minimizing testing, and treating pain early using a multidisciplinary approach. Psychological evaluation and treatment, biofeedback and relaxation therapy, use of oral antidepressants (e.g., amitriptyline 25–50 mg at bedtime) as analgesic adjuncts, and referral to a pain management specialist may be indicated.

Recurrent abdominal pain syndrome in children is vague, unrelated to meals, activity, or stool pattern, and does not awaken patients. An epigastric location is sometimes reported. Pallor, nausea, dizziness, headache, and fatigue may be present. Family history is often positive for functional bowel disease. Indicators of serious disease in children include vomiting, localized pain away from midline, altered bowel habits, growth disturbance, nocturnal episodes, radiation of pain, incontinence, presence of systemic symptoms, and family history of peptic ulcer and IBD. Response to empiric intervention (trial of lactose elimination, reduction of excessive juice intake, addition of a fiber supplement in constipation) and behavior and psychological management are valuable, as is educating the child and parents about diagnosis and treatment options. A symptom diary allows the child to play an active role in the diagnostic process. It is important for the child to maintain a normal routine, including school activities and diet.

A. **Hematologic tests.** Initial laboratory tests in acute abdominal pain should include a complete blood count with differential, serum chemistries (electrolytes, serum glucose, liver and kidney function tests, amylase and lipase), urinalysis, coagulation panel in the elderly or if the drug history indicates it, and a pregnancy test in women of childbearing age. In children, investigations other than a complete blood count, urinalysis, urine culture, and stool hemoccult are selected based on clinical suspicion of specific pathology (sonography in pelvic pain or appendicitis, endoscopic evaluation with pain suspected of gastrointestinal origin). Blood may need to be typed and crossmatched before surgery or in patients with suspected bleeding. Blood cultures may be drawn, if the patient is febrile. An electrocardiogram may be ordered in the elderly before surgery or if a cardiac origin for the pain is considered.

1. **Blood count.** Anemia is a feature of bleeding peptic ulcers, ruptured aneurysm, IBD (along with raised sedimentation rate), and malignancies. Thrombocytopenia (platelets <50,000) may be seen in Henoch–Schönlein purpura in children. Leukocytosis, white cell count >12,000, is seen in appendicitis (sensitivity 91%, specificity 21%), cholecystitis (sensitivity 78%, specificity 11%), diverticulitis, and bowel ischemia. Leukocytosis is typical in the second and third trimesters of pregnancy and in early labor.

2. **Serum chemistry**
   a. Hypocalcemia and elevations in serum amylase (sensitivity 74%, specificity 50%) and lipase may be seen in pancreatitis. Amylase is elevated early (within 24 hours) in pancreatitis and lipase within a few days after symptom onset.
   b. Metabolic acidosis (in 50% of patients) and elevations of serum and peritoneal fluid amylase, alkaline phosphatase, and inorganic phosphate are seen in mesenteric ischemia.
   c. C-reactive protein may be elevated in appendicitis; normal levels in patients with symptoms more than 24 hours rule out appendicitis.

B. **Radiologic tests**
   1. **X-rays** in acute abdominal pain should include a flat plate and upright view of the abdomen, and an erect chest x-ray. X-rays have poor specificity (<15%), and in most instances do not change the clinical diagnosis.
      a. **Chest x-ray** is useful in detecting pneumoperitoneum and cardiopulmonary pathology.
      b. **Abdominal films** also identify subdiaphragmatic or retroperitoneal gas associated with perforation, features of bowel obstruction (distended bowel, air-fluid levels), air in the biliary tree (gallstone ileus), calcium deposits (e.g., gallstones [10%–20% sensitivity], renal or ureteral stones, appendicoliths, calcification in chronic pancreatitis, aortic aneurysm), foreign bodies, and pneumatosis (i.e., air in the bowel wall suggesting possible ischemia).
   2. **Ultrasound** detects gallstones (sensitivity 85%–90%), sludge, gallbladder wall thickening (>5 mm is diagnostic), pericholecystic fluid (in cholecystitis), and intrahepatic or extrahepatic bile duct dilatation, associated with biliary obstruction (Evidence rating C).
      a. Ultrasound can also identify pancreatitis, pseudocysts and tumors, ascites, chronic liver disease (e.g., fatty liver or cirrhosis), gynecologic abnormalities, renal or adrenal pathologic findings, and acute appendicitis (sensitivity 85%–90%, specificity 92%–96%).
      b. **Duplex ultrasonography** is highly specific (92%–100%) for mesenteric arterial stenosis or occlusion.
   3. **Computerized tomography** is the most sensitive study in evaluating patients with acute abdominal pain, particularly obese patients. It has high sensitivities (pancreatitis, 65%–100%; appendicitis, 96%–98%; pancreatic tumors, 95%; high-grade bowel obstruction, 86%–100%) (Evidence rating C). It detects smaller volumes of free air, as compared to plain x-rays, can detect loculated air, and is the diagnostic modality of choice in intraperitoneal and retroperitoneal abscess, in diverticulitis, and in determining the presence and extent of diverticular complications, such as fistulas or sinus tracts.

C. **Radionuclide scanning**
   1. In acute cholecystitis, the cystic duct is obstructed; a technetium-labeled hepatic iminodiacetic acid scan showing nonvisualization of the gallbladder is 95% accurate in diagnosing acute cholecystitis. Poor fractional excretion of hepatic iminodiacetic acid (<15%) is characteristic of biliary dyskinesia (Evidence rating C).
   2. Preferential uptake of sodium Tc-pertechnetate by ectopic gastric tissue in a Meckel diverticulum (sensitivity 85% and specificity 95% in children) enables diagnosis of pathology related to the diverticulum (diverticulitis, bleeding).

D. **Miscellaneous tests**
   1. **Magnetic resonance angiography,** with and without gadolinium, detects severe narrowing or occlusion of the celiac axis and superior mesenteric artery. **Mesenteric**

angiography can show the presence and site of emboli and thrombi and mesenteric vasoconstriction as well as the adequacy of the splanchnic circulation. The angiographic catheter also provides a route for the administration of intra-arterial vasodilators or thrombolytic agents.

2. **Barium enema or colonoscopy** is diagnostic in IBD and ischemic colitis, outlining ulcerations, thickened bowel, pseudopolyps, and strictures. **Water-soluble contrast medium** (meglumine diatrizoate [Gastrografin]) is preferred if contrast enema is to be performed in diverticulitis; it shows the diverticula and leakage and may outline a fistulous tract.

3. **Endoscopic retrograde cholangiopancreatogram** is diagnostic in chronic pancreatitis, shows associated pseudocysts and glandular and ductal pathology (strictures, calculi), and helps rule out malignancy.

VI. **Treatment.** Once the patient's condition is stabilized, the physician can obtain a detailed history, perform a clinical examination and investigations, and formulate a treatment plan. Providing pain relief should not await a definitive diagnosis, because unrelieved acute pain produces adverse consequences and there is no evidence that immediate pain relief delays diagnosis or treatment.

A. **NSAP.** Watchful waiting with close follow-up is recommended, because most patients have a benign, self-limited illness. Providing reassurance, having patients avoid foods that precipitate the pain, and prescribing oral antispasmodics such as dicyclomine hydrochloride (e.g., Bentyl), 20 mg 4 times daily, or propantheline bromide (e.g., Pro-Banthine), 15 mg before meals and at bedtime, are useful. Narcotic analgesics should be avoided.

B. **IBS.** Treatment is directed at reducing anxiety and stress, increasing dietary fiber with bulk agents such as oral psyllium (e.g., Metamucil), avoiding foods that exacerbate or trigger IBS, and using antispasmodics such as dicyclomine hydrochloride. Psychotherapy may be useful. In patients with diarrhea, oral loperamide hydrochloride (e.g., Imodium) 2 to 4 mg, or diphenoxylate hydrochloride with atropine (e.g., Lomotil), 10 to 20 mg 4 times a day, is useful. Frequent follow-up may be needed until symptoms stabilize. Alosetron (Lotronex) 1 mg once or twice daily and tegaserod (Zelnorm) 6 mg twice daily are useful in diarrhea-predominant and constipation-predominant IBS, respectively, in women. (Evidence rating B).

C. **Appendicitis.** Diagnostic scoring systems (Table 1–4) used to predict the likelihood of appendicitis offer sensitivity and specificity >90% and reduce rates of perforation and negative laparotomy by 50%. Appendectomy is the treatment of choice with early diagnosis, if an abscess develops, or in recurrent appendicitis. A laparoscopic approach is less traumatic and has fewer complications (bleeding, wound infection, intra-abdominal sepsis) than open appendectomy. Other treatment measures include analgesics, intravenous (IV) fluids, and antibiotics. If an appendicular mass (inflamed appendix walled off by omentum) is noticed, nonoperative treatment (bowel rest, analgesics, IV fluids, and antibiotics) is continued until symptoms improve and the mass resolves.

D. **Biliary disease**

1. Most patients with **biliary colic** respond to oral analgesics (hydrocodone/acetaminophen 5–7.5/500 mg, e.g., Lortab, every 4–6 hours) and clear liquids for 2 to 3 days.

TABLE 1–4. THE ALVARADO SCORING SYSTEM FOR LIKELIHOOD OF ACUTE APPENDICITIS

Features	Score
Migratory right iliac fossa pain	1
Nausea/vomiting	1
Anorexia	1
Right iliac fossa tenderness	2
Fever >37.3°C	1
Rebound tenderness in right iliac fossa	1
Leukocytosis >10,000/mm^3	2
Neutrophilic shift to the left >75%	1
Total score	**10**

Score < 4 indicates no appendicitis, 5 or 6 indicates compatible with acute appendicitis, 7 or 8 indicates probable acute appendicitis, 9 or 10 indicates very probable acute appendicitis.

2. **Cholecystitis** responds to IV hydration, bowel rest, and broad-spectrum IV antibiotics (e.g., cefotaxime 2 g 3 times daily) for 2 to 3 days. Interval elective laparoscopic cholecystectomy (6 weeks later) is curative.

3. Chemical dissolution of gallstones using ursodiol 600 mg daily given in divided doses is reserved for patients refusing surgery or in whom it is contraindicated and is successful in 55% of patients older than 12 months. An oral cholecystogram is performed initially to confirm normal gallbladder function, a prerequisite for dissolution.

E. Pancreatitis

1. Most patients improve on bowel rest, IV hydration, and pain relief for 2 to 3 days. Morphine sulfate 5 to 10 mg IV every 3 hours may be used in both biliary pathologic findings and pancreatitis; recent studies do not link morphine with causing or aggravating pancreatitis or cholecystitis.

2. Once pancreatitis resolves, biliary stones should be removed and cholecystectomy performed. Alcohol intake should be avoided.

3. Local complications include abscess formation, pseudocyst, bowel necrosis, pancreatic ascites, and splenic vein thrombosis. Shock or respiratory or renal failure is more likely in hemorrhagic pancreatitis. Initial leukocytosis ($>16,000/mm^3$), hyperglycemia (>200 mg%), elevated liver enzymes (lactate dehydrogenase >350 IU/L, aspartate aminotransferase >250 IU/L), and age >55 years are associated with a poorer prognosis (**Ranson criteria**).

4. Large pseudocysts may need surgical consultation for percutaneous or internal drainage. Medication intake (e.g., steroids, azathioprine) may need to be modified, and metabolic abnormalities (e.g., hypercalcemia) corrected to avoid recurrence and development of chronicity.

5. Pain management in **chronic pancreatitis** is difficult and may require long-term narcotics (despite the strong predilection in alcoholics for addiction), or celiac plexus block with phenol or alcohol by a radiologist. Steatorrhea should be treated with fat restriction (20 g/day) and Viokase (3 tablets with meals). Diabetes mellitus, if occurs is treated (see Chapter 74).

F. Diverticulitis

1. Mild cases respond to a 7- to 10-day course of oral ciprofloxacin, 500 mg twice daily, and metronidazole (e.g., Flagyl) 250 mg 3 times a day.

2. Patients with vomiting, sepsis, or peritonitis require hospitalization for bowel rest, IV hydration, and antibiotics. Laparotomy and bowel resection is indicated in bowel perforation or obstruction, fistula, suspected cancer, massive hematochezia, or failed medical treatment. Percutaneous drainage of localized abdominal or pelvic abscesses by a radiologist under ultrasound or computerized tomography guidance is feasible.

G. Ischemic bowel disease requires hospitalization; patient stabilization; nasogastric aspiration; broad-spectrum antibiotics; interventional radiologist consultation for selective mesenteric arterial catheterization; possible vasodilator or thrombolytic infusion; and possible surgical consultation for embolectomy, bowel resection, or revascularization. Surgical resection is indicated in ischemic colitis if abdominal findings, fever, and leukocytosis suggest deterioration, or if the patient has diarrhea or bleeding for more than 2 weeks.

H. Patients with obstruction of the large or small bowel require hospitalization for IV hydration, correction of fluid and electrolyte imbalance, bowel rest, decompression through nasogastric aspiration, and administration of enemas to induce evacuation. Small-bowel obstruction caused by adhesions and incomplete large-bowel obstructions respond to this treatment. Endoscopic decompression relieves a sigmoid volvulus. Surgical consultation is indicated in patients not responding to conservative treatment, with guarding and rigidity indicating bowel ischemia or irreducible hernia.

REFERENCES

Chan MYP et al. Alvarado score: An admission criterion in patients with right iliac fossa pain. *Surg J R Coll Surg Edinb Irel.* 2003;1:39-41.

Dominitz JA, Sekijima JH, Watts M. Abdominal pain. http://www.uwgi.org/cme/cmeCourseCD/ch_06/CH06TXT.HTM.

Fishman MB, Aronson MD. History and physical examination in adults with abdominal pain. UpToDate 2006. http://www.utdol.com/utd/content/topic.do?topicKey=pri_gast/5211&type=A&selectedTitle=3~197.

Graff LG IV, Robinson D. Abdominal pain and emergency department evaluation. *Emerg Med Clin North Am.* 2001;19:123-136.

Kizer KW, Vassar MJ. Emergency department diagnosis of abdominal disorders in the elderly. *Am J Emerg Med.* 1998;16:357-362.

Penner RM, Majumdar SR. Diagnostic approach to abdominal pain in adults. Up To Date 2006. http://www.utdol.com/utd/content/topic.do?topicKey=pri_gast/4946&type=A&selectedTitle=1~197.

Perry R. Acute abdomen in pregnancy. *eMedicine Journal.* 2002;3(5). http://www.emedicine.com/med/topic3522.htm

Portis AJ, Sundaram CP. Diagnosis and initial management of kidney stones. *Am Fam Physician.* 2001;63:1329-1338.

2   The Abnormal Pap Smear

Kathryn Reilly, MD, & Neal D. Clemenson, MD

KEY POINTS

- Human papilloma virus (HPV) infection causes most abnormal Pap smears and virtually all cervical dysplasia.
- Many abnormal Pap smears resolve spontaneously as the underlying HPV infection clears.
- HPV testing is now widely available and can assist with decision making in some situations.

I. **Definition.** The Pap smear, a cytologic examination of exfoliated cervical and endocervical cells, was developed in the 1930s by Papanicolaou and is currently used as a screening tool for cervical neoplasia and carcinoma. Largely because of the use of the Pap smear, deaths in the United States from cervical cancer fell 74% between 1955 and 1992; in 2005 approximately 10,500 new cases of cervical cancer were diagnosed and 3900 deaths from cervical cancer occurred.

Advances in our understanding of cervical disease, new reporting systems, and new diagnostic and treatment modalities make a systematic approach to the abnormal Pap smear very important. Recommendations for the frequency and method of the Pap smear may be found in Chapter 102.

Several systems are used for reporting the results of the Pap smear. The Bethesda system provides the most complete information and has been widely adopted; its classification scheme, updated in 2001, is used in this chapter. Equivalent classifications in the World Health Organization and cervical intraepithelial neoplasia (CIN) systems are provided. Since the systems are not interchangeable, it is essential that clinicians become familiar with the system used by their particular laboratory.

HPV infection is extremely common. At least 50% of sexually active men and women become infected by age 50. Most of them will clear the infection over time. Persistent infection with high-risk subtypes, especially 16 and 18, has been linked to development of cervical cancer (OR as high as 45). However, a large majority of those with persistent infection with high-risk types do not develop high-grade dysplasia.

II. **Common Diagnoses.** Many types of cervical and vaginal abnormalities can be detected by the Pap smear, including the following:

A. **Atypical squamous cells (ASC).** These cells are further classified as "of uncertain significance" (ASC-US) or "cannot exclude HSIL" (ASC-H). (HSIL refers to high-grade squamous intraepithelial lesions.) ASC may be caused by infection (see Section II.E), including HPV infection (Section II.C), but may also occur in the absence of infection; in many cases this is caused by atrophic changes in the vaginal epithelium. Under the Bethesda system, up to 5% of Pap smears can be read as ASC.

B. **Low-grade squamous intraepithelial lesions** (LSIL, mild dysplasia, or CIN 1). These are generally caused by a transient **HPV** infection. HPV is a small DNA virus that replicates in the nuclei of epithelial cells; some types of HPV, which are termed "high risk," can cause malignant transformation by incorporation into the host DNA in chronic infections.

Infection with HPV may be subclinical or may cause condylomata (by "low-risk" subtypes such as 6 or 11) or other lesions on the vulva, vagina, or cervix. HPV infection is generally contracted by sexual contact with an infected partner, who may be asymptomatic, although infection from nongenital lesions may occur as well. As with other sexually transmitted diseases, the risk increases with the number and risk status of sexual partners and may be reduced by the use of barrier contraception (e.g., condoms). In adolescents, 90% of LSIL regressed after 3 years. Even when teens were infected with high-risk HPV, their rate of regression to normal was 81%; only 6% progressed to high-grade lesions. The regression rate in adult women is 50% to 80%.

- **C. High-grade squamous intraepithelial lesions.** These include moderate and severe dysplasia (CIN 2 and 3) and carcinoma in situ (CIN 3). They represent chronic HPV infection and are more likely to progress to more severe dysplasia or cancer. Twenty-two percent of CIN 2 and 14% of CIN 3 will progress to carcinoma in situ or invasive cancer; 43% of untreated CIN 2 will regress as will 32% of untreated CIN 3.
- **D. Atypical glandular cells (AGC).** These may be caused by inflammation or neoplasia in the endocervix, endometrium or, rarely, in the fallopian tubes or ovary. They may be characterized as endocervical, endometrial, or not otherwise specified.
- **E. Frank cervical carcinomas.** These include squamous cell carcinomas and adenocarcinomas, as well as noncervical carcinomas, including endocervical carcinoma and vaginal carcinoma. Cervical carcinomas are discussed in Section V.E; the other carcinomas are beyond the scope of this chapter.
- **F. Organisms,** including **bacteria** (e.g., *Chlamydia* or *Gardnerella*), **fungi** (e.g., *Candida*), or **protozoa** (e.g., *Trichomonas*), can colonize or infect the vaginal or cervical epithelium. This may occur without altering the mucosa, or the infectious agent may elicit an inflammatory response and resultant cellular changes. *Chlamydia* and *Trichomonas* infections are sexually transmitted, and multiple sexually transmitted diseases may coexist. *Candida* infections are probably caused by alterations in the usual vaginal flora and may be triggered by antibiotics, altered host defenses, or other poorly understood causes. Frequent or severe *Candida* infections may occur in women with human immunodeficiency virus (HIV) infection or diabetes mellitus. Bacterial vaginosis is also caused by altered flora, but the cause of the alteration is not clear; it is generally believed not to be transmitted sexually.

III. Symptoms

- **A. ASC** and **inflammation** are usually asymptomatic unless associated with an infection (see Section II.F), although bleeding, especially after intercourse, may occur. Upon examination, the cervix may appear normal or may show redness, erosions, or friability, especially with some infections.
- **B. LSILs** are usually asymptomatic. The cervix may appear normal or may show redness, erosions, friability, or gross lesions. Acetic acid application (see Section IV.B.1) may identify lesions that are not grossly visible.
- **C. HSILs** are usually asymptomatic but may be associated with bleeding; large lesions may cause vaginal discharge. The cervix may appear normal or may show redness, erosions, friability, or gross lesions. Acetic acid application (see Section IV.B.1) may identify lesions that are not grossly visible.
- **D. AGC** may be asymptomatic or may have symptoms related to the underlying disease (e.g., irregular bleeding with endometrial neoplasia).
- **E. Carcinomas** may be asymptomatic or may cause bleeding or vaginal discharge. Metastatic disease may be associated with abdominal fullness, weight loss, or other symptoms related to the sites and nature of the metastases.
- **F. Infections** may be asymptomatic or may be associated with vaginal discharge, odor, or itching. Signs may include vaginal or cervical discharge or inflammation.

IV. Laboratory Tests

- **A.** The **Pap smear** report should include the following information:
  - **1. Specimen adequacy.** An unsatisfactory smear should be repeated; a less than optimal smear may warrant repeat treatment or follow-up, depending on the specific findings and clinical situation. Many authorities no longer consider the absence of endocervical cells alone to be an indication of an inadequate smear, and the need to repeat smears without endocervical cells is a clinical judgment.
  - **2.** The report should specify any **epithelial cell abnormalities** using the terminology of the particular reporting system. Other findings may include organisms or other

evidence of infection, reactive cellular changes (e.g., inflammation), or endometrial cells.

3. The report may include **educational notes and suggestions** regarding treatment, follow-up, or both. This information may be helpful, but the clinicians should determine the plans for the patient, depending on the situation and their own clinical judgment.

B. Additional tests

1. **Acetic acid application.** Applying 5% acetic acid solution to the cervix for 1 minute will cause many condylomata or dysplastic areas to turn white (acetowhite lesions). These lesions should be evaluated by colposcopy and biopsy (see Section IV.B.3).

2. **Biopsy.** Prior to the widespread use of colposcopy, cervical biopsies of suspicious areas, or random biopsies of visually normal areas, were used to evaluate abnormal smears. With the availability of colposcopy, biopsy should be done only in conjunction with colposcopy.

3. **Colposcopy,** cervical examination under stereoscopic magnification by an experienced examiner, along with endometrial sampling and biopsy of abnormal areas is the definitive procedure for assessing Pap smear abnormalities.

4. **HPV testing** can be done to determine whether one of the types likely to cause malignancy is present. This technology is now widely available and is a useful option in the management of ASC-US (see Section V.A.3). Reflex testing can be performed if the Pap result is ASC-US when liquid-based Pap testing is done. Alternatively, many laboratories will hold the sample for a short period, which would allow HPV testing to be ordered if the Pap smear is abnormal. A third option is to have the patient return for HPV testing when the Pap result is ASC-US and the Pap was performed using conventional slide technology.

V. Treatment. Many strategies have been proposed for the treatment of abnormal Pap smears, especially ASC-US. The following strategies are based primarily on the 2001 Consensus Guidelines developed under the sponsorship of the American Society for Colposcopy and Cervical Pathology.

A. ASC-US. Any of the following options is appropriate, depending on patient and clinician preferences and available resources:

1. **Repeat cytologic testing.** Repeat Pap smears at 4- to 6-month intervals until two consecutive negative smears are obtained, after which the Pap smear should be repeated in 12 months. If a repeat smear shows ASC-US or a higher-grade abnormality, colposcopy should be performed. If the woman is postmenopausal and is not receiving estrogen replacement, the smear can be repeated 1 week after a course of vaginal estrogen (e.g., conjugated estrogen cream, 2 g every other day for 4 weeks). If the smear remains abnormal, colposcopy should be considered. (SOR **A**)

2. **Colposcopy.** Colposcopy is performed; if no CIN is found, the Pap smear should be repeated in 12 months. (SOR **A**)

3. **HPV testing.** If negative for high-risk HPV, the Pap smear should be repeated in 12 months. If positive for high-risk HPV, colposcopy should be performed. (SOR **A**)

B. ASC-H. Colposcopy should be performed on women with ASC-H results.

C. LSIL. Colposcopy is currently recommended for most women with LSIL. In adolescents, ACOG recommends that either repeat Pap smears at 6 and 12 months (with colposcopy if ASC-US or greater) or HPV testing at 12 months (with colposcopy if positive for high-risk types) be performed, rather than immediate colposcopy. (SOR **C**)

D. HSIL. Colposcopy should be performed for HSIL. (SOR **C**)

E. AGC. Colposcopy should be performed for AGC specified as endocervical or not otherwise specified. Endometrial sampling should be performed initially for AGC specified as endometrial cells. Women older than 35 years or with unexplained vaginal bleeding should have endometrial sampling and colposcopy. (SOR **C**)

F. Carcinomas. The treatment of carcinomas is generally surgical; referral to a physician experienced in gynecologic oncology is indicated.

G. Specific **vaginal infections,** with confirmation as clinically appropriate, should be treated as described in Chapters 31 and 64. If the infection is sexually transmitted, the patient's partner(s) should be treated in order to prevent reinfection. If reactive cellular changes, inflammation, or both are noted, reexamination of the patient may be appropriate to rule out infection. Empiric therapy with topical or systemic antimicrobial agents is not recommended.

H. Endometrial cells may be found on a Pap smear taken during or shortly after menstruation, but if they are found in the second-half of the menstrual cycle or in a postmenopausal woman, endometrial biopsy or other endometrial sampling should be considered.

I. HIV. Since women with HIV are at higher risk for cervical neoplasia, some clinicians perform more frequent Pap smears. Annual colposcopy in place of Pap smears has also been recommended, but the practicality and cost-effectiveness of this approach are unclear. (SOR **C**)

J. Pregnancy. The management of ASC-US and LSIL in pregnancy is the same as discussed in Section V.A, except that colposcopy should either be delayed until after delivery or performed without endocervical sampling. ASC-H and HSIL results should prompt colposcopy without endocervical curettage. If colposcopy is to be performed, the optimal time is probably the mid-second trimester.

K. Adolescents. Infection with HPV occurs in most adolescents within the first few years of sexual activity. The majority of these infections are transient, resolving on their own within 2 years. Active infection with both high-risk and low-risk HPV causes changes in cervical cytology, which are read as LSIL. ACOG recommends that teens whose Pap smear is read as either ASC-US or LSIL be monitored (see V.A and V.C above). ACOG also recommends that destruction of normal cervical tissue should be minimized when possible in treating adolescents with more advanced lesions. (SOR **C**)

REFERENCES

ACOG Committee Opinion No. 330. Evaluation and management of abnormal cervical cytology and histology in the adolescent. *Obstet Gynecol.* 2006;107:963-968.

ACOG Practice Bulletin No. 66. Management of abnormal cytology and histology. *Obstet Gynecol.* 2005;106:665-666.

Apgar BS. Management of cervical cytologic abnormalities. *Am Fam Physician.* 2004;70(10):1905-1916.

Cohen DE. Primary care issues for HIV-infected patients. *Infect Dis Clin North Am.* 2007;21(1):49-70.

Guido R. Guidelines for screening and treatment of cervical disease in the adolescent. *J Pediatr Adolesc Gynecol.* 2004;17(5):303-311.

Walter LC. Screening for colorectal, breast and cervical cancer in the elderly; a review of the evidence. *Am J Med.* 2005;118(10):1078-1086.

---

3   Amenorrhea

Amanda Kaufman, MD

KEY POINTS

- **Primary amenorrhea** should be investigated at age 13 if there are no secondary sexual characteristics or at age 15 with otherwise normal secondary sexual development. (SOR **C**)
- **Secondary amenorrhea** is commonly caused by pregnancy, polycystic ovarian syndrome (PCOS), and stress such as calorie deficit or traumatic psychosocial events.
- In prolonged amenorrhea, osteoporosis should be screened for and treated if present. (SOR **A**)

I. Definition. Amenorrhea is the absence of menses for 3 months in a woman with previously normal menses, no menses by age 15 in an adolescent with normal sexual development, or no menses by age 13 in an adolescent without normal sexual development. **Primary amenorrhea** refers to women who have never menstruated, while **secondary amenorrhea** refers to cessation of menses in a previously menstruating female. Oligomenorrhea of less than nine cycles a year should also be evaluated. (SOR **C**) The ages defining primary amenorrhea have changed as the average age of thelarche and menarche have decreased; the ages of 13 and 15 are two standard deviations above the current average ages for thelarche and menarche in North America. Normal menstruation depends on integrated hypothalamic, pituitary, ovarian follicular and endometrial function, and a patent outflow tract. Any hormonal disruption or anatomic blockage will prevent normal menstruation.

II. **Common Diagnoses.** Amenorrhea not because of pregnancy, lactation, or menopause occurs in 3% to 4% of women. Although the list of aberrations that cause amenorrhea is long, the majority are caused by PCOS, hypothalamic amenorrhea, hyperprolactinemia, and ovarian failure.

  A. **Polycystic ovarian syndrome** is the most common cause of **normogonadotropic amenorrhea,** an endocrinopathy affecting 5% to7% of premenopausal women and associated with obesity in 75% of North American patients. PCOS patients are more likely to present with oligomenorrhea (76%) than amenorrhea (24%).

  B. **Hypogonadotropic amenorrhea (also known as hypothalamic amenorrhea)** has many causes. Among those with primary amenorrhea, the most common cause is constitutional delay of growth and puberty. Secondary amenorrhea is commonly caused by **psychosocial and physical stress** including excessive strenuous **exercise or eating disorders associated with calorie deficit states and weight loss.** Chronic debilitating diseases, such as uncontrolled juvenile diabetes, end-stage kidney disease, malignancy, and AIDS are uncommon causes.

  C. **Hyperprolactinemia has many causes** (see Table 3–1). **Pregnancy and lactation** elevate prolactin causing GnRH suppression and are the most common cause of amenorrhea in women of childbearing age. **Medications,** prolonged **hypothyroidism,** or prolactin-secreting tumors can elevate prolactin. In women with hyperprolactinemia, the prevalence of a pituitary tumor is 50% to 60%. The likelihood of a pituitary tumor is unrelated to the level of prolactin. (SOR **Ⓑ**) Usually, however, patients with amenorrhea have larger tumors than patients with oligomenorrhea. The poor correlation between tumor presence and prolactin level indicates that magnetic resonance imaging (MRI) should be performed whenever prolactin levels are persistently elevated. (SOR **Ⓑ**)

  D. **Hypergonadotropic amenorrhea** is most commonly seen in premature ovarian failure (POF). POF affects 1% to 5% of women younger than 40. Forty percent are found to have autoimmune conditions, most commonly autoimmune thyroiditis. Iatrogenic POF from chemotherapy or radiation have the potential for recovery. Women younger than 30 with POF should undergo karyotyping, as many genetic conditions can cause POF including carriers of Fragile X. (SOR **Ⓒ**) Turner syndrome (XO karyotype) can present with primary amenorrhea because of failure of ovarian development.

  E. **Anatomic defects.** The outflow tract may be blocked from **imperforate hymen, transverse vaginal septa, or a stenotic cervix.** Among those with primary amenorrhea, 10% are found to have Müllerian agenesis, with absence or partial development of the uterus or vagina. Five percent with primary amenorrhea are found to have androgen insensitivity, also called testicular feminization (46XY karyotype). **Asherman syndrome** is occasionally seen after postpartum endometritis or curettage of the uterus causing intrauterine synechiae formation blocking menstrual flow.

III. **Symptoms.** A careful history is essential for narrowing the differential diagnosis and should include the following:

  A. A detailed **menstrual and puberty history,** including dates of last menstrual period, age at menarche, pubic hair growth, and breast development. **Oligomenorrhea progressing gradually to amenorrhea** characterizes PCOS, hypogonadotropic, or hyperprolactinemic amenorrhea.

  B. Gynecologic and obstetric history, especially infections and procedures.

  C. **Medication history** (Table 3–2) for medication-induced hyperprolactinemia. After discontinuation of oral contraceptives, amenorrhea may occur for up to 6 months.

  D. Family history including menarche of mother and sisters and genetic conditions.

  E. Dietary history, excessive activity level, and fluctuations in weight as evidence of an eating disorder.

  F. Psychosocial stressors. Women exposed to the violence of war as soldiers or civilians commonly have amenorrhea.

  G. **Symptoms of pregnancy** including sudden missed menses, nausea, fatigue, and breast tenderness.

  H. **Galactorrhea** (milky discharge from the breasts) indicating hyperprolactinemia.

  I. **Hyperandrogenism** (acne, hirsutism) and infertility increase likelihood of PCOS.

TABLE 3–1. ETIOLOGY OF HYPERPROLACTINEMIA

Physiologic	Pathologic	Pharmacologic
Pregnancy	*Hypothalamic-pituitary stalk damage*	*Neuropeptides*
Lactation	Tumors	Thyrotropin-releasing hormone
Stress	Granulomas	PRL-releasing peptide
Sleep	Infiltrations	*Drug-induced hypersecretion*
Coitus	Rathke cyst	Dopamine receptor blockers
Exercise	Irradiation	Phenothiazines: chlorpromazine, perphenazine
	Trauma	Butyrophenones: haloperidol
	Pituitary	Thioxanthenes
	Prolactinoma	Metoclopramide
	Acromegaly	Dopamine synthesis inhibitors
	Macroadenoma (compressive)	α-Methyldopa
	Idiopathic	Catecholamine depletors
	Plurihormonal adenoma	Reserpine
	Lymphocytic hypophysitis or parasellar mass	*Cholinergic agonists*
	Macroprolactinemia	Physostigmine
	Surgery	*Antihypertensives*
	Trauma	Labetolol
	Systemic disorders	Reserpine
	Chronic renal failure	Verapamil
	Polycystic ovarian disease	*H_2 antihistamines*
	Cirrhosis	Cimetidine
	Pseudocyesis	Ranitidine
	Epileptic seizures	*Estrogens*
	Cranial radiation	*Oral contraceptives*
	Chest—neurogenic chest wall trauma,	*Oral contraceptive withdrawal*
	surgery, herpes zoster	
		Anticonvulsants
		Phenytoin
		Anesthetics
		Neuroleptics
		Chlorpromazine
		Promazine
		Promethazine
		Trifluoperazine
		Fluphenazine
		Butaperazine
		Perphenazine
		Thiethylperazine
		Thioridazine
		Haloperidol
		Pimozide
		Thiothixene
		Molindone
		Opiates and opiate antagonists
		Heroin
		Methadone
		Apomorphine
		Morphine
		Antidepressants
		Tricyclic antidepressants
		Chlorimipramine
		Amitriptyline
		Selective serotononin re-uptake inhibitors
		Fluoxetine

TABLE 3-2. MEDICATION CAUSES OF HYPERPROLACTINEMIA

Psychotropic drugs
Benzodiazepines
Selective serotonin reuptake inhibitors (SSRIs)
Tricyclic antidepressants
Phenothiazines
Buspirone
Monoamine oxidase (MAO) inhibitors
Neurologic drugs
Sumatriptan
Valproic acid
Dihydroergotamine
Hormonal medications
Danazol
Estrogen
Depo-Provera
Oral contraceptives
Drugs that work on the gastrointestinal tract
H$_2$ blockers
Cardiovascular drugs
Atenolol
Verapamil
Reserpine
Methyldopa
Herbal preparations
Fenugreek seed
Fennel
Anise
Illicit drugs
Amphetamines
Cannabis (marijuana)

   J. Symptoms of **hypoestrogenic state** such as hot flashes, vaginal dryness, or decreased libido, which may indicate POF or menopause. POF occurs in 1% to 5% of women.
   K. Any history of **brain injury** (trauma, tumor, tuberculosis, syphilis, meningitis, sarcoidosis)**, pelvic radiation, or autoimmune disease can affect central or ovarian hormone production and cause POF.** HIV has been associated with amenorrhea by an unknown mechanism, though a central mechanism has been proposed. POF is more common in type 1 diabetes, autoimmune thyroiditis, and myasthenia gravis.

FEMALE ATHLETE TRIAD

The **female athlete triad consists** of amenorrhea, eating disorder, and osteoporosis. The prevalence of eating disorders and amenorrhea in athletes is reported as high as 62%. Aesthetic sports (gymnastics, figure skating, ballet) and endurance sports (distance running) share increased risk of the female athlete triad. Other risk factors include self-esteem focused on athletic pursuits solely, presence of stress fractures, and social isolation caused by intensive involvement in sports. The negative caloric state of not ingesting enough calories for the exercise performed causes luteinizing hormone (LH) suppression or disorganization of its pulsatile release and results in amenorrhea. Resolution focuses on correcting this deficit.

 IV. Signs. Although usually normal, a focused examination guided by history should address the following:
   A. The genital examination will be abnormal in 15% with primary amenorrhea. If the patient or parent declines an examination, a transabdominal ultrasound will be useful to confirm the presence or absence of a uterus. (SOR **C**)
       1. Atrophic vaginal changes and **vaginal dryness** suggest a hypoestrogenic state.
       2. Absent pubic hair and inguinal masses (testes) are signs of androgen insensitivity.

   3. **Clitoromegaly** is suggestive of androgen excess as is temporal balding and deepening voice.
   4. If cervical stenosis is suspected, gentle penetration may be attempted with a uterine sound. (SOR **C**) Further investigation requires referral for hysteroscopy.
   B. Breast examination: Normal breast development requires estrogen. **Galactorrhea** indicates **hyperprolactinemic** state.
   C. Thyroid examination for masses, enlargement, or tenderness.
   D. Obesity, **hirsutism,** acne, or acanthosis nigricans may be present in PCOS.
   E. Signs of emotional distress (depression, agitation) or of any severe chronic illness.
   F. **Visual field defect** on confrontation suggesting pituitary adenoma.
   G. **Short stature, widely spaced nipples, and neck webbing** characterize Turner syndrome.
   H. Striae, buffalo hump, significant central obesity, easy bruising, hypertension, and proximal muscle weakness as signs of Cushing disease.
V. **Laboratory Tests.** Unless the diagnosis is obvious from the history and physical examination, testing will be necessary. The work-up can be done in a stepwise fashion (Figure 3–1) to avoid unnecessary testing.
   A. A **pregnancy test** is always indicated. (SOR **C**)
   B. **Thyroid-stimulating hormone** level. Only 4.2% of amenorrheic adult women in a recent study had an abnormal thyroid-stimulating hormone; however, given the ease of treatment and the impact of thyroid dysfunction on prolactin levels, testing is recommended. (SOR **B**)
   C. **Serum prolactin level** should be tested, because 7.5% of cases of amenorrhea are associated with hyperprolactinemia. (SOR **B**)
   D. Hyperprolactinemia warrants an **MRI of the brain** to evaluate for pituitary adenoma. (SOR **B**) If amenorrhea because of hypothalamic causes persists despite long-term correction of stressors or calorie deficits, MRI should be considered to evaluate for possible hypothalamic or pituitary disease.
   E. **Gonadotropin levels.** An FSH persistently greater than 40 mIU/mL suggests POF or menopause. Because of the gravity of the diagnosis of POF, experts recommend checking FSH level on initial evaluation. (SOR **C**) An LH level could be useful if PCOS is suspected, as the LH:FSH ratio can be >2:1.
   F. **Androgen testing** (testosterone, androstenedione, dehydroepiandrosterone sulfate [DHEA-S], 17-hydroxyprogesterone) should be done in amenorrheic women with signs of androgen excess (virilization, hirsutism, acne). (SOR **C**) Testosterone levels >200 ng/dL and DHEA-S levels >700 ng/dL necessitate CT scan of the adrenals and ultrasound testing of the ovaries to rule out neoplasm. (SOR **A**) Elevated 17-hydroxyprogesterone can help diagnose adult-onset congenital adrenal hyperplasia. A testosterone level can differentiate between genital abnormalities caused by Müllerian agenesis (normal female range) or androgen insensitivity (normal male range or elevated).

1. History and Physical
2. Rule out pregnancy
3. TSH, FSH, & Prolactin

Abnormal Exam	Elevated TSH	Elevated FSH	Low or Normal FSH	Elevated Prolactin
Pelvic US, testosterone level, or karyotype as appropriate for suspected diagnosis	Treat thyroid dysfunction	Evaluate for POF, karyotype if <30 or other stigmata	Consider PCOS or hypothalamic cause	Correct underlying cause or obtain MRI for possible adenoma

FSH/LH, follicle-stimulating hormone/luteinizing hormone; MRI, magnetic resonance imaging; PCOS, polycystic ovarian syndrome; TSH, thyroid-stimulating hormone.

FIGURE 3–1. Suggested evaluation of women with amenorrhea.

G. Fasting **serum insulin levels** may be elevated in women with PCOS.

H. **Karyotyping** should be performed in women with POF before age 30 or with stigmata of Turner syndrome. (SOR **C**)

I. The **progestin challenge test** is performed by giving medroxyprogesterone acetate (Provera), 10 mg daily for 7 days. Any bleeding during the week following the final dose is a positive test. Recent consensus states that the test correlates poorly with estrogen status and the test imposes a delay in the diagnostic process. (SOR **A**) The false-positive rate is high: up to 20% of women with oligomenorrhea or amenorrhea in whom estrogen is present have no withdrawal bleeding. The false negative rate is also high; withdrawal bleeding occurs in up to 40% of women with amenorrhea caused by stress, weight loss, exercise, or hyperprolactinemia (where estrogen production is usually reduced) and in up to 50% of women with ovarian failure.

J. The **estrogen–progestin challenge test** is performed by giving estrogen (Estradiol 1 mg) for 21 to 25 days and a progestational agent (Provera 10 mg) for the final 5 to 7 days of estrogen therapy to stimulate withdrawal bleeding. If no bleeding occurs, an anatomic abnormality exists.

K. Referral for **hysteroscopy** may be needed to evaluate anatomic defects.

L. **Bone densitometry** is indicated in any women with amenorrhea >6 to 12 months. (SOR)

M. **Consider HIV testing** (see Section III.J) if no other etiologies can be determined.

VI. Treatment must be based on a firm diagnosis and must attempt to resolve **underlying problems** while restoring menses, treating symptoms associated with estrogen deficiency, and addressing fertility when applicable.

A. Hyperprolactinemic amenorrhea

1. If medications, thyroid abnormality, or other etiology listed in Table 3–1 is suspected, the underlying cause should be corrected and prolactin level repeated in 2 to 3 months.

2. **Pituitary macroadenoma:** If a pituitary adenoma is identified, the goals of treatment are to suppress prolactin, decrease tumor size, prevent recurrence, and induce ovulation. In the absence of another organic condition, dopamine agonists are the preferred treatment of hyperprolactinemia with or without a pituitary tumor.

   a. **Bromocriptine** is the drug most often used for first-line therapy for hyperprolactinemia because it inhibits the secretion of prolactin, shrinks prolactinomas, eliminates galactorrhea, and reestablishes menses and fertility. (SOR **A**) Menses usually return 6 to 12 weeks after prolactin levels are normalized.

   b. **Medroxyprogesterone acetate** (Provera), 10 mg/d taken for 10 days each month, is useful to induce menses if a woman does not desire fertility, does not have galactorrhea, or cannot tolerate bromocriptine. Provera does not affect prolactinoma size or prolactin levels.

   c. In the past, treatment of pituitary adenoma was commonly **transsphenoidal resection.** However, recurrence of these tumors is common and therefore bromocriptine is the usual first-line therapy for both microadenomas and macroadenomas. (SOR **A**) Microadenomas grow slowly; prolactin levels should be monitored yearly and neuroimaging should be done every 2 to 3 years. (SOR **C**)

B. **Hypogonadotropic amenorrhea (also known as hypothalamic amenorrhea)** is resolved when the stress causing the decreased GnRH secretion is lessened. In the meantime, other interventions are important.

1. **Dietary modification** to reverse a calorie deficit and maintain at least 90% of ideal body weight is critical. (SOR **B**) Eighty-six percent who maintain their ideal body weight will see resumption of menses within 6 months.

2. To protect the patient from bone loss, **estrogen supplementation** with oral contraceptives should be provided until normal menstruation is established. (SOR **A**) Several studies have found that oral contraceptives prevent further bone loss, improve spine bone density measurements, but do not improve hip bone density measurements. Use of 25 μg ethinyl estradiol pills is as effective as 35 μg pills. (SOR **A**)

3. **Smoking should be discouraged** and **adequate calcium intake** (1.5 g/day) and vitamin D (800 IU/day) encouraged to **prevent bone loss. (**SOR **C**)

4. Antiresorptive therapy (e.g., alendronate, 10 mg orally daily or 70 mg orally weekly) should be initiated if osteoporosis is identified. (SOR **A**) Bisphosphonates are all pregnancy category C drugs.

C. **Hypergonadotropic amenorrhea** with diagnosed POF requires a hormone replacement therapy regimen that maintains bone mass. (SOR **A**) A higher **daily dose of estrogen** than what is generally administered in hormone replacement therapy is required in younger women with POF to prevent bone loss. (SOR **A**) **Calcium and vitamin D supplementation** should be initiated and bisphosphonates discussed for prevention or treatment of **osteoporosis.** (SOR **C**) If a genetic abnormality is found (Fragile X), referral for genetic counseling should be considered. (SOR **C**)

D. Normogonadotropic amenorrhea manifested as PCOS may require multifaceted therapy including the following:

1. **Reduction of insulin resistance.** Insulin-sensitizing agents such as metformin have been shown to reduce hyperinsulinemia and restore ovulation. Oral metformin (up to 2550 mg daily) has been shown to enhance ovulation. (SOR **A**) Weight loss is recommended. (SOR **A**)

2. If pregnancy is desired, patients with PCOS are candidates for **induction of ovulation** with medications such as clomiphene citrate (Clomid).

3. If pregnancy is not desired, therapy should be directed at **interruption of the unopposed estrogen** and its effects. Use of oral contraceptives suppresses ovarian androgens and thus minimizes hirsutism, as well as providing a progestational agent to oppose estrogen and provide withdrawal bleeding.

4. Women with PCOS should be screened for diabetes mellitus with a fasting glucose. (SOR **B**)

5. Spironolactone, an aldosterone antagonist, is an androgen blocker used for the **treatment of hirsutism.** Oral doses of 100 mg, daily or twice daily are usually effective. (SOR **B**) Spironolactone works through a different mechanism than oral contraceptives and, therefore, using these agents concomitantly improves their effectiveness.

REFERENCES

Apgar B. Diagnosis and management of amenorrhea. *Clin Fam Pract.* 2002;4(3):643-666.

Barbieri R. Metformin for the treatment of polycystic ovary syndrome. *Obstet Gynecol.* 2003;101:785-793.

Helen C et al. Effects of human immunodeficiency virus on protracted amenorrhea and ovarian dysfunction. *Obstet Gynecol.* 2006;108:1423-1431.

Larsen PR. *Williams Textbook of Endocrinology.* 10th ed. Philadelphia, PA: Saunders; 2003.

Martin V, Reid R. Amenorrhea. In: Rakel & Bope, eds. *Conn's Current Therapy.* 60th ed. Philadelphia, PA: Saunders; 2008:1046-1049.

Rotterdam ESHRE/ASRM Sponsored PCOS consensus workshop group consensus on diagnostic criteria and long-term health risks related to PCOS. *Fertil Steril.* 2004;81:19-25.

Speroff L & Fritz M. *Clinical Gynecological Endocrinology and Infertility.* 7th ed. Philadelphia: Williams & Wilkins; 2004.

The Practice Committee of the American Society for Reproductive Medicine. Current evaluation of amenorrhea. *Fertil Steril.* 2006;86(5 suppl):S148-S155.

4   Anemia

Gregg M. Hallbauer, DO, & Andrew D. Jones, MD

KEY POINTS

- Anemia is one of the major signs of disease and is never normal. Its cause should always be sought.
- Iron deficiency anemia is the most common cause.
- Anemia is usually asymptomatic, although some syndromes are associated with specific signs and symptoms.
- Anemia can usually be diagnosed accurately with simple laboratory tests such as serum hemoglobin, RBC indices, ferritin, and reticulocyte count.
- Testing for fecal occult blood should be routinely done when evaluating anemias in adults. Screening colonoscopy is recommended for all adults starting at age 50.

I. Definition. Anemia is an abnormally low hemoglobin (Hb) or hematocrit (Hct) value compared to age-matched norms. In general, anemia is defined in adult males as Hb <13 g/dL and in adult females as Hb <12 g/dL. Anemia of pregnancy occurs at Hb <10 g/dL. Anemia of childhood occurs at Hb <10.5 g/dL. Hb is considered a better measure of anemia than Hct.

II. **Common Diagnoses**
  A. **Iron deficiency**
    1. **Nutritional/absorption.** Iron deficiency secondary to reduced intake is the most common cause of nutritional anemia worldwide. However, iron deficiency anemia from nutritional deficiencies is uncommon in adults in developed countries, because such deficiencies must occur for at least 5 years to produce iron deficiency anemia in the presence of normal iron physiology. **Newborn infants** who are breast-fed or who are taking non–iron-enriched formulas are an exception and may become iron deficient in the first year of life. **Children aged 12 to 24 months** may also become iron deficient as they transition from iron-fortified formula to cow's milk and solid foods. (See the sidebar on anemia from cow's milk in children.) **Malabsorption** resulting from disease, resection of the small bowel, or partial gastric resection accounts for a small percentage of iron deficiency.

ANEMIA FROM COW'S MILK IN CHILDREN

One particular cause of anemia in children is iron deficiency anemia caused by early initiation of cow's milk feedings. To prevent this, the American Academy of Pediatrics recommends: (1) breast-feeding for 6 to 12 months, (2) using only iron-fortified formulas, (3) avoiding cow's milk during the first year of life, and (4) eating iron-enriched cereals with the initiation of solid foods. High-risk infants (poverty, black, Native American, Alaskan Native, immigrant from a developing country, preterm or LBW, or if primary dietary intake is unfortified cow's milk) aged 6 to 12 months should be given routine iron supplementation. (SOR **B**)

2. **Blood loss.** In the absence of malnutrition or malabsorption, iron deficiency results from bleeding. **In young women,** most cases are caused by menstrual blood loss and increased iron requirements of pregnancy.

Gastrointestinal (GI) bleeding is another common source of blood loss; this is often because of the erosive effects of nonsteroidal anti-inflammatory drugs. In elderly patients, colonic carcinomas, diverticular disease, and vascular malformations are other major causes of GI bleeding. **Rare causes of blood loss** include chronic hemolysis, hemoptysis, and bleeding disorders. (Also see the sidebar on acute hemorrhage.)

ACUTE HEMORRHAGE

Acute hemorrhage is a potentially life-threatening cause of anemia. Acute severe blood loss is as much a problem of low circulating blood volume as it is of low Hb or Hct. Acute blood loss may present with minimal to no reduction in Hb/Hct yet still be clinically significant. Acute hemorrhage may be asymptomatic or may present with severe shock including fatigue, lightheadedness, or alteration in level of consciousness, possibly accompanied by menorrhagia, melena, hematochezia, hematemesis, or hemoptysis. Acute hemorrhage is associated with orthostasis (positive tilt test) and is treated with hospitalization for fluid resuscitation, transfusion, and identification and management of underlying causes.

B. **Vitamin B$_{12}$ deficiency** causes anemia in 5% to 10% of elderly patients. (See the sidebar on anemia in the elderly.)

ANEMIA IN THE ELDERLY

Anemia is common and present in 8% to 44% of those older than 65 years; 9% of adults older than 65 years with iron deficiency anemia have a GI malignancy. Symptoms and signs of anemia may be difficult to detect in the elderly and may present as a worsening of underlying medical conditions. Therefore, a high index of suspicion is necessary in the evaluation of anemia in the elderly. Although the evaluation of anemia in the elderly is very similar to that described in this chapter, it must be remembered that low Hb or Hct values are not a normal consequence of aging, and a cause for anemia must be sought.

   1. **Malabsorption.** Vitamin B_{12} deficiency is almost always caused by malabsorption related to atrophic gastritis. **Pernicious anemia (PA),** or failure to absorb vitamin B_{12} because of reduced production or secretion of intrinsic factor, occurs commonly; chronic histamine blockers, proton pump inhibitor treatment, and *Helicobacter pylori* gastritis may also play a role in development of PA. Other **less common causes of vitamin B_{12} malabsorption** include small-bowel overgrowth; ileal malfunction; acidification of the small intestine; pancreatic disease; and certain drugs (*p*-aminosalicylic acid, neomycin, and potassium chloride). Vitamin B_{12} deficiency increases the likelihood of subsequent development of gastric cancer or polyps, which is thought to be related to the gastritis associated with vitamin B_{12} malabsorption.
   2. **Diet.** The only source of cobalamin is animal products; thus, vegans who eat no meat, eggs, or cheese for a number of years may develop a nutritional deficiency state.
C. **Folate deficiency** occurs because average dietary folic acid intake does not greatly exceed nutritional requirements and body folate reserves are relatively small, depleting in 4 months. Deficiency thus occurs in patients who either do not consume or absorb enough folic acid or who have some condition that depletes their body reserves.
   1. **Decreased folate intake. Decreased intake** can occur when the diet is deficient in fresh green vegetables, nuts, yeast, and liver. Decreased intake may occur in the elderly, in alcoholics, and because of loss of food folate through excessive cooking.
   2. **Decreased absorption/effectiveness. Folate malabsorption** can be caused by GI conditions such as jejunal atrophy from celiac disease and drugs such as phenytoin or sulfasalazine. **Folate antagonists** include certain chemotherapeutic agents, antiviral drugs (e.g., azidothymidine [AZT] and zidovudine), folate antagonists (e.g., methotrexate), trimethoprim, nitrous oxide, primidone, and phenobarbital. Individuals on methotrexate should be supplemented with 1 mg of folic acid daily.
   3. **Increased demand.** The increased nutritional demands of pregnancy and the increased requirements of chronic hemolytic anemia and exfoliative psoriasis may deplete folic acid reserves.
D. **Anemia of chronic disease (ACD)** is present in up to 6% of adults hospitalized by family physicians and is caused by reduced ability to incorporate stored iron into Hb, despite adequate iron stores. ACD may also be exacerbated by features of the underlying disease, including blood loss, hemolysis, malabsorption, malnutrition, or bone marrow replacement or suppression by infection or drugs. (Also see the autoimmune hemolytic anemia sidebar.)

AUTOIMMUNE HEMOLYTIC ANEMIA

Autoimmune hemolytic anemia is rare and may occur idiopathically or secondary to other disorders, such as systemic lupus erythematosus, chronic lymphocytic leukemia, non-Hodgkin lymphoma, Hodgkin disease, and cancer. Drugs such as α-methyldopa, penicillin, rifampin, sulfonamides, quinidine, and chlorpropamide may induce an immune hemolysis, clinically indistinguishable from immune hemolytic anemia. Autoimmune hemolytic anemia may have a dramatic clinical presentation. The anemia may occur rapidly and be life-threatening, and patients may present with angina or congestive heart failure associated with jaundice developing over a 1- to 3-day period. Patients with thrombotic thrombocytopenic purpura, a type of autoimmune hemolytic anemia, may present with petechiae, fever, altered mental status, or focal neurologic findings.

E. **Hemolytic processes**
   1. **Sickle cell disease** is inherited as an autosomal trait; it occurs in the heterozygous state as **sickle trait** in 8% to 10% of blacks in the United States. Sickle trait rarely occurs in Eastern Mediterranean people or people of Indian or Saudi Arabian ancestry. **Sickle cell disease** develops in persons who are homozygous for the sickle gene (*HbSS*) and affects approximately 2% of blacks in the United States. Other sickle

syndromes, such as sickle-β-thalassemia and sickle C disease, are uncommon in the United States.

2. **Thalassemia** is most common in Mediterranean and Asian populations. Sporadic cases of thalassemia are found among Africans and American blacks.

3. **Hereditary elliptocytosis and spherocytosis** are autosomal dominant disorders affecting approximately 200 to 300 million people worldwide, although these conditions are uncommon in the United States. These membrane defects cause intravascular hemolysis of red blood cells (RBCs).

4. **Glucose-6-phosphate dehydrogenase (G6PD)** deficiency is one of the most common disorders causing hemolysis worldwide, affecting 10% of black males in the United States. The gene for G6PD is carried on the X chromosome, and female carriers are rarely affected.

5. **Pyruvate kinase deficiency** is another common RBC enzyme deficiency. The intravascular hemolysis caused by these conditions is particularly worsened by illness, stress, and, with G6PD, some medications.

F. **Bone marrow deficits**

1. **Aplastic anemia** occurs because of a marrow disturbance resulting in defective RBC synthesis. This may be caused by marrow infiltration by tumor or fibrosis; dose-related, idiosyncratic, or hypersensitivity effects of drugs (e.g., antithyroid medications, gold, chemotherapeutic agents, AZT, phenytoin, and phenylbutazone); radiation; autoimmune suppression (e.g., with systemic lupus erythematosus); and infections such as tuberculosis, atypical mycobacterial infections, brucellosis, hepatitis A and B, and, rarely, mumps, rubella, infectious mononucleosis, influenza, human immunodeficiency virus, parvovirus, and fungal and parasitic infections.

2. **Myelodysplastic syndromes (MDSs)** are diagnosed in 1 to 10 per 100,000 people every year, and are more common in elderly males. MDSs are stem-cell disorders resulting in abnormal hematopoietic precursors causing disturbances of RBCs, white blood cells, and platelets. Previous treatment with radiation or mutagenic chemicals may result in MDSs.

G. **Anemia of pregnancy can have the same etiologies seen in the nonpregnant state. Iron deficiency anemia during pregnancy is the consequence primarily of expansion of plasma volume without normal expansion of maternal Hb mass.**

III. **Symptoms and Signs.** In anemia, these may be nonexistent or vague. Some symptoms are more common in particular age groups and some syndromes do have characteristic symptoms and signs (Table 4–1).

IV. **Laboratory Tests.** One approach to the diagnosis of anemia using Hb, RBC indices, and reticulocyte count is presented here (Figure 4–1). Peripheral smear should be obtained if thalassemia or bone marrow disturbance is suspected.

A. **Iron deficiency anemia.** Essential diagnostic features include low serum ferritin (<20 ng/mL reflects deficient iron stores), low serum iron, and high iron-binding capacity; microcytic and hypochromic peripheral RBCs occur later with absent marrow iron stores. Hb and ferritin are the best tests for diagnosis of iron deficiency anemia. (SOR **C**) In adults with anemia, a serum ferritin <15 ng/mL (or 15 μg/L) has a likelihood ratio of 51.8, which suggests a very high probability of being iron deficient. Values >100 ng/mL indicate adequate iron stores and a low likelihood of an iron deficient state. A normal RBC distribution width (RDW) effectively eliminates iron deficiency as a cause of microcytic anemia. Men or women older than 65 years with iron deficiency require GI endoscopy to

TABLE 4–1. FINDINGS IN COMMON ANEMIAS

Diagnosis	Abnormal Findings
Iron deficiency	Pica; esophageal webs (Plummer–Vinson syndrome); pallor of mucosa and nail beds; atrophic glossitis, angular stomatitis, cheilosis
B$_{12}$ deficiency	Tongue burning/soreness; numbness/paresthesias; yellow skin; vitiligo; glossitis; hepatomegaly; splenomegaly; mental status changes
Hemolytic anemia	Fever, pain; jaundice; hepatomegaly; cardiomegaly; murmur
Folate deficiency	Malnourishment; diarrhea, glossitis, cheilosis; no neurologic abnormalities but mild mental status changes
Thalassemia	Bony deformities; growth failure; hepatosplenomegaly

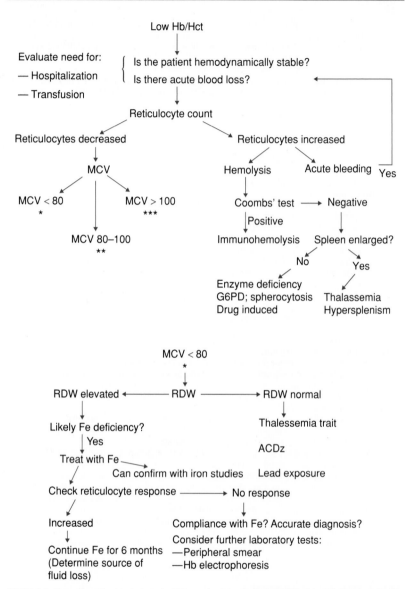

FIGURE 4–1. Diagnosis and treatment of anemia. ACD, anemia of chronic disease; G6PD, glucose-6-phosphate dehydrogenase; Hb/Hct, hemoglobin/hematocrit; MCV, mean corpuscular volume; MMA, methylmalonic acid; RDW, red blood cell distribution width. (*Continued*)

screen for malignancy, (SOR **B**) as do men and nonmenstruating women younger than 65 years with unexplained iron deficiency. (SOR **B**) The differential diagnosis of microcytic anemia includes thalassemia, sideroblastic anemias, some types of ACD, and lead poisoning.

B. Vitamin B$_{12}$ and folate deficiencies. These deficiencies cause megaloblastic anemia (macrocytosis and hypersegmented granulocytes in the peripheral blood smear); mean

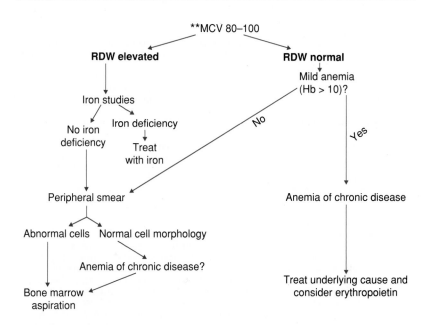

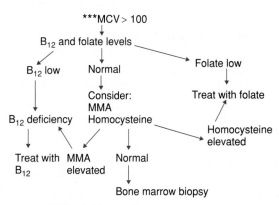

FIGURE 4–1. (*Continued*).

corpuscular volume elevation (frequently >110 fL but may be normal with coexisting thalassemia); indirect hyperbilirubinemia; elevated lactate dehydrogenase levels; normal mean corpuscular Hb concentration (range, 31–35 g/dL); low reticulocyte count; and possibly decreased leukocyte and platelet counts. With macrocytosis, serum B_{12} and folate levels should be obtained and, if these are normal, measuring levels of cobalamin metabolites (methylmalonic acid and homocysteine) should be considered. Normal levels rule out a vitamin B_{12} or folate deficiency. In patients who are vitamin B_{12} deficient, serum folate is usually normal or elevated unless there is a coexisting folate deficiency. Serum homocysteine levels are markedly increased in folate deficiency. **Bone marrow biopsy** may be necessary to rule out MDSs and malignancy if levels of vitamin B_{12}, folate, and metabolites are normal, since these disorders may present with peripheral megaloblastosis.

C. ACD is usually mild in degree and not progressive, with the Hct rarely falling below 25%, except in renal failure. Common findings in ACD are normochromic, normocytic RBCs; low reticulocyte production; low or normal serum iron; low total iron-binding capacity; and usually normal RDW. Reticuloendothelial iron stores are usually adequate, serum ferritin levels are >50 ng/mL, and bone marrow iron is normal or increased. Serum erythropoietin levels are reduced in inflammatory disorders. The marrow is usually hypocellular, with decreased myeloid precursors.

D. Hemolytic anemia. The cardinal diagnostic feature of hemolytic anemia is significant reticulocytosis.

    1. Immunohemolysis is diagnosed based on Coombs testing, with a positive direct Coombs test indicating surface RBC antibodies and a positive indirect Coombs test indicating circulating RBC antibodies. Cold agglutinins will be found in patients with immune hemolysis caused by cold-reactive antibodies.

    2. In **extravascular hemolysis,** serum indirect bilirubin and lactate dehydrogenase levels rise, while haptoglobin decreases. In sustained and severe hemolytic anemia, nucleated RBCs may enter the circulation.

E. Hemoglobinopathies

    1. Sickle cell anemia

        a. Hb levels commonly range between 5 and 10 g/dL, neutrophil and platelet counts are frequently elevated, and the blood smear shows sickle cells, Howell–Jolly bodies, reticulocytosis, and usually high white blood cell and platelet counts.

        b. Hb electrophoresis shows RBCs containing 85% to 95% Hb S and, in homozygous S disease, no Hb A. Elevated levels of Hb A_2 on Hb electrophoresis and a positive family history of thalassemia are characteristic of sickle-β-thalassemia.

    2. The peripheral smear in **thalassemias** shows hypochromia and microcytosis with basophilic stippling, potentially confusing them with iron deficiency anemia; however, findings with iron deficiency also include a reduced RBC count, an elevated RDW, and reduced serum iron, whereas patients with β-thalassemia minor have normal or minimally reduced RBC counts, profound microcytosis, normal serum iron, and normal RDW. Hb electrophoreses in patients with β-thalassemia shows increased levels of Hb A_2 and Hb F.

F. Anemia of chronic kidney disease

    1. Anemia increases in prevalence and severity as glomerular filtration rate reaches 60 mL/min or less.

    2. Deficiency of erythropoietin is the primary cause of anemia in chronic kidney disease. A minimal work-up is necessary to rule out iron deficiency and other cell-line abnormalities.

    3. An anemia work-up should be initiated in patients with chronic kidney disease when Hb <11 g/dL in premenopausal females and prepubertal patients or <12 g/dL in adult males and postmenopausal females. The recommended evaluation should include Hb, RBC indices, reticulocyte count, iron studies, and testing for stool occult blood.

V. Treatment. The treatment of anemia generally involves addressing underlying etiology.

A. Iron deficiency anemia. A trial of iron is a reasonable approach in children, adolescents, and women of reproductive age if the history, review of systems, and physical examination are negative.

    1. Iron preparations such as ferrous sulfate, ferrous gluconate, ferrous fumarate, or polysaccharide-iron complexes (ferric polymaltose) can replenish iron deficiency. The usual dose is 100 to 200 mg of elemental iron daily (e.g., ferrous sulfate, 325 mg, 3 times a day). Reticulocytosis follows within a few days. An increase in the Hb of 1 g/dL should be expected every 2 to 3 weeks with iron therapy. Once the Hb has corrected, it may take up to 4 months for iron stores to return to normal. If a rise of 1 to 2 g of Hb is not seen within 4 weeks, possibilities include iron malabsorption, bleeding, or an unknown lesion. Therapy should continue for 4 to 6 months to replenish iron stores. Transfusion should be considered in symptomatic patients and in asymptomatic cardiac patients with an Hb level <10 g/dL.

    2. Prenatal vitamins with iron are recommended during pregnancy. Supplemental iron therapy is recommended at Hb <10 g/dL.

    3. In children, iron is replaced with once-daily dosing of 3 mg/kg/d of elemental iron for 3 months. Cramping, nausea, constipation, and diarrhea can be side effects of iron therapy. Rinsing the mouth is suggested to prevent tooth staining from liquid preparations.

4. **To minimize GI side effects,** iron therapy should begin with one tablet a day with meals, and the dose should be gradually increased. Ferrous gluconate, ferrous fumarate, and ferric polymaltose are less likely to cause GI side effects but are more expensive than ferrous sulfate.

5. **Nonresponse to iron therapy** is usually owing to noncompliance, but may be caused by incorrect diagnosis (e.g., ACD or thalassemia), ongoing GI blood loss, or, rarely, poor absorption.

6. **Intravenous iron therapy** may be indicated in patients with chronic bleeding, malabsorption, intolerance to oral iron, noncompliance, or an Hb level <6 g/dL.

B. **Vitamin B_{12} deficiency.** Patients with confirmed vitamin B_{12} deficiency from PA must receive vitamin B_{12} therapy for the duration of their lives. Intramuscular dosing is 1000 μg/d for the first week, then 1000 μg weekly until hematologic values normalize or for at least 6 months if neurologic complications exist, then 1000 μg monthly for life. Oral treatment with 1000 to 2000 μg daily is as effective but requires much greater patient compliance. Intranasal gel preparations also exist but are not first-line therapy.

C. **Folate deficiency.** This deficiency is treated with oral folic acid, 1 mg/d.

D. **ACD.** There is no specific treatment other than for the underlying illness. Recombinant erythropoietin should be considered for all patients with anemia of renal failure or patients undergoing chemotherapy. An additive deficiency state worsens the anemia; however, unless a specific deficiency exists, treatment with iron, vitamin B_{12}, and folic acid is useless.

E. **Hemolytic processes**

1. Patients with **sickle cell disease** should be immunized against *Streptococcus pneumoniae, Haemophilus influenzae,* hepatitis B, and influenza according to Centers for Disease Control and Prevention recommendations. Infections should be treated early and aggressively. **Antibiotic prophylaxis** with penicillin should be given to children between the ages of 2 months and 5 years because of the high risk of pneumococcal infection. A typical regimen is oral penicillin, 125 mg twice daily until age 2 to 3, then 250 mg twice daily. **Regular ophthalmologic examination** should be done every 1 to 2 years beginning at age 10 years because of a high incidence of retinopathy. Patients should be maintained chronically on folic acid supplements.

2. The most common hemolytic condition requiring treatment is **sickle cell crisis.** Treatment of sickle cell crises consists of rest, hydration, and analgesia. Transfusions should be reserved for aplastic or hemolytic crises and for patients in the third trimester of pregnancy. No treatment is required for patients with sickle trait.

F. **Chronic kidney disease.** Recombinant erythropoiesis-stimulating agents may be considered. Patients receiving these agents should also receive supplemental iron, probably parenterally. However, owing to increased clotting risks, Hb levels should be monitored very frequently to ensure they do not exceed 12 g/dL.

REFERENCES

Dhaliwal G, Cornett PA, Tierney LM. Hemolytic anemia. *Am Fam Physician.* 2004;69(11):2599-2606.

Gunn VL, Nechyba C, Eds. *Harriet Lane Handbook.* 16th ed. Mosby; St. Louis, Baltimore, Boston, Chicago, 2002:284-285.

Irwin JJ, Kirchner JT. Anemia in children. *Am Fam Physician.* 2001;64(8):1379-1386.

Killip S, Bennett JM, Chambers MD. Iron deficiency anemia. *Am Fam Physician.* 2007;75(5):671-678.

Nurko S. Anemia in chronic kidney disease: causes, diagnosis, treatment. *Cleve Clin J Med.* 2006;73(3):289-297.

Zlotkin S, Arthur P, Antwi KY, Yeung G. Randomized, controlled trial of single versus 3-times-daily ferrous sulfate drops for treatment of anemia. *Pediatrics.* 2001;108:613-616.

5   Ankle Injuries

Philip R. Palmer, MD

KEY POINTS

- Ankle sprains are among the most common injuries in sports and recreational activities.
- Forty percent of sprains have significant morbidity associated with them.
- Radiographic high-yield criteria can reliably identify fractures.
- Other problems, such as Achilles tendon ruptures, fractures of the proximal fifth metatarsal, and navicular fractures, may present as suspected ankle sprains.

I. **Definition.** Ankle injuries are very common among active individuals although evaluating pain about the ankle can be a challenging undertaking. In order to develop a proper differential, it is important to have an understanding of the major bones, ligaments, and tendons comprising and surrounding the ankle joint (Figure 5–1). Range of motion occurs primarily in one plane: plantar flexion and dorsiflexion. Dorsiflexion is somewhat restricted as a result of the anterior widening of the talar dome. There is minimal inversion and eversion at the true ankle joint with most of this motion occurring at the subtalar joint. The subtalar joint of the foot allows for the full range of inversion, eversion, supination, and pronation. The medial malleolus (distal tibia) and the longer lateral malleolus (distal fibula) provide a significant amount of bony stability to the ankle joint through their downward extension along the talar dome.

Ligaments provide medial and lateral stability (resisting eversion and inversion). The tibiofibular ligament syndesmosis, which runs between the tibia and fibula, maintains mortise stability, and a variety of tendons traversing the joint serve as secondary stabilizers.

Ankle injuries involve trauma to the bony or soft tissue structures of the ankle. **Sprains** involve tears to the ligaments, whereas **strains** involve tears of the muscle–tendon unit.

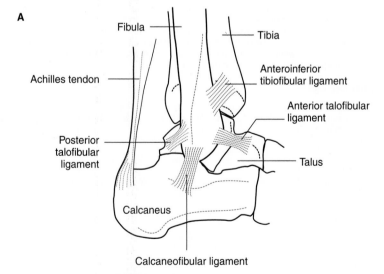

FIGURE 5–1. Ankle ligaments: (**A**) lateral views.

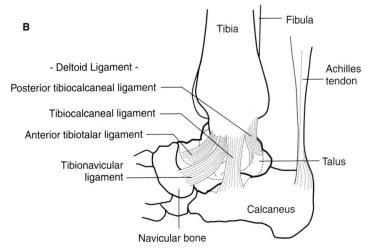

FIGURE 5-1. (*Continued*) (**B**) medial views.

Contusions are bruises; **tenosynovitis** is the inflammation of the tendon and its sheath. **Fractures** are disruptions of the bony anatomy.

II. **Common Diagnoses.** Ankle injuries represent approximately 20% of all sports injuries.

    A. Sprains (85% of all ankle injuries). Sprains are particularly common in individuals who participate in basketball, volleyball, ice-skating, or soccer. Most ankle sprains involve the ligaments of the lateral compartment. Less than 10% of ankle sprains involve the medial compartment, and this is usually a more serious injury than a lateral sprain.

    B. Strains (5% of all ankle injuries). Strains are common in persons who engage in ballistic activities, such as track and field events. These injuries can also result from overuse of the muscle–tendon unit, particularly in endurance running, dancing, or gymnastics.

    C. Tenosynovitis (5% of all ankle injuries). Tenosynovitis most often occurs in individuals who are running, jumping, or dancing. This condition results from either a direct blow or overuse with repetitive overloads and faulty technique.

    D. Fractures (<5% of all ankle injuries). Fractures are more common than sprains in prepubertal children because the ligamentous structures are typically stronger than the bones, especially at the growth plates. Fractures occur most frequently in persons who engage in high-velocity, high-impact sports (e.g., football, soccer, skiing, hockey, or skateboarding).

        1. Stress fractures occur most frequently in running, gymnastics, or dancing.

        2. Salter type I and II fractures of the distal fibula are the most common ankle injuries in children. (For discussion of the Salter classification, see Chapter 29.)

    E. Contusions (<5% of all ankle injuries). Contusions involving the ankle are significantly underreported and often occur in persons who participate in contact sports. Such injuries may also result from faulty footwear and poor field conditions. Contusions are primarily a diagnosis of exclusion and will not be discussed further.

III. **Symptoms and Signs**

    A. Sprains: Sprains present with varying degrees of pain, swelling, disability, and joint laxity depending upon how severely the ligaments have been damaged.

        1. Grade 1 sprains are mild injuries with minimal pain and usually no impairment of weight bearing. These injuries are minimally tender over the involved ligament and present with minimal swelling. There is no associated joint laxity.

        2. Grade 2 sprains are a more significant injury. Individuals experience moderate pain, and weight bearing will be impaired causing them to walk with a limp. There is moderate tenderness and swelling present, and swelling may extend beyond the area of the injured ligaments. Ecchymosis may be present and joint laxity will be demonstrated with anterior drawer testing and perhaps talar tilt testing as well.

3. Grade 3 sprains are the most significant injury. Affected athletes will not be able to bear weight because of extreme pain. There will be marked, diffuse swelling and significant tenderness. Ecchymosis will typically be present. Anterior drawer testing and talar tilt testing will demonstrate laxity although many individuals will not tolerate such stress tests initially because of extremes of pain and swelling (Table 5–1).

4. Syndesmotic ankle sprains typically present much as a grade 2 or 3 lateral ankle sprain. Pain and swelling may be pronounced and weight bearing is very limited, if not impossible. A squeeze test (compressing the distal thirds of the tibia and fibula together) will produce pain at the ankle.

B. Strains: Strains also present with pain and swelling, although the pain is typically noticed only with activity and swelling is usually minimal. The location of pain provides a clue to the diagnosis of strains.

1. Posterior pain on ambulation indicates a strain of the Achilles tendon.

2. Pain posterior and inferior to the medial malleolus suggests a strain of the tibialis posterior tendon.

3. A painful anterior tibia and ankle and medial foot indicate a strain of the tibialis anterior tendon.

4. Pain posterior and inferior to the lateral malleolus suggests a strain of the peroneal tendons.

5. Chronic inflammation of a tendon can result in rupture. Classic findings are an inability to actively move in the plane controlled by that muscle–tendon unit. For example, individuals with a ruptured Achilles tendon cannot plantar flex their foot against resistance. These patients would also demonstrate a positive Thompson test where compression of the calf musculature does not produce plantar flexion of the foot (Table 5–1).

C. Tenosynovitis: Pain and swelling over an affected tendon suggests tenosynovitis. Additional signs include tenderness with palpation, a thickening of the tendon, and weakness of involved muscle groups. Crepitus (described as a "packed snow" sensation) over the involved tendon is a classic finding, though it is often not present.

D. Fractures: Fractures are frequently associated with immediate disability and a patient report of an audible "pop" or crack. Abrupt moderate to severe pain and swelling, localized bony tenderness, and possible crepitus and ecchymosis are signs of an **acute** fracture. An avulsion fracture of the base of the fifth metatarsal typically presents with symptoms and a mechanism of injury identical to an ankle sprain. **Occult** fractures typically present with a history of a "sprained" ankle that resists all treatment, dull ache with slight swelling after excessive walking, increased pain with activity, and complete relief with rest. With occult fractures, the physical examination findings are usually negative, except for point tenderness over the distal fibula (stress fracture) or on the talar dome with ankle plantar flexion (osteochondral fracture).

IV. Laboratory Tests. Routine studies need not be performed. Imaging may be warranted in the following circumstances:

A. X-rays (The Ottawa ankle and foot rules) (Figure 5–2)

1. **X-rays** are indicated if there is an **inability to bear weight** both immediately after injury and in the emergency department (four steps) and any of the following findings:

a. **Ankle:** Pain near the malleoli and **bone tenderness** in the posterior half of the lower 6 cm of the tibia or fibula or at the tip of either malleolus.

b. **Foot:** Pain in the midfoot and **bone tenderness** at the navicular or the base of the fifth metatarsal.

TABLE 5–1. MANEUVERS IMPORTANT IN EXAMINING THE INJURED ANKLE

Maneuver	Findings
Anterior drawer test, which involves drawing the calcaneus and talus anteriorly while stabilizing the tibia	3–14 mm indicates grade 2 sprain; >15 mm indicates grade 3 sprain
Talar tilt test, which involves stressing the ankle laterally (inversion) and medially (eversion) while stabilizing the patient's leg	5- to 10-degree difference between ankles indicates grade 2 sprain; >10-degree difference indicates grade 3 sprain
Thompson squeeze test, which involves squeezing the mid-third of the calf with the knee flexed 90 degrees	Loss of plantar flexion with Achilles tendon rupture

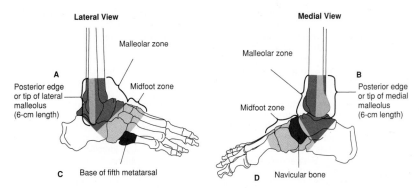

Lateral View

Malleolar zone

A
Posterior edge or tip of lateral malleolus (6-cm length)

Midfoot zone

C Base of fifth metatarsal

Medial View

Malleolar zone

Midfoot zone

B
Posterior edge or tip of medial malleolus (6-cm length)

D Navicular bone

FIGURE 5–2. The Ottawa ankle and foot rules.

    c. Studies indicate that if a patient does not meet these criteria, radiographs are unnecessary. (SOR **A**)
  2. **Appropriate** x-rays to evaluate the bony anatomy include an anteroposterior, a lateral and a mortise view. A mortise view is obtained by adducting the foot 15 degrees from its position for the anteroposterior view. Oblique views can be a useful addition when investigating for osteochondral defects or fractures of the talar dome.
  3. Comparing anteroposterior, lateral, and mortise views between affected and uninjured ankles helps demonstrate fracture fragments and is useful in identifying Salter–Harris fractures in children. **Mortise** and **oblique views** are useful for detecting **osteochondral fragments.** Routine films will not show stress fractures for the first 2 to 3 weeks following injury.
  4. **Stress films** (i.e., x-raying the ankle while performing an anterior drawer and/or a talar tilt test) may be indicated when there is marked joint laxity present on examination but it is unclear as to how severe to grade the sprain. Stress films are best done with local anesthesia and must be compared with stress views of the uninjured ankle. An anterior subluxation of more than 3 mm suggests anterior talofibular ligament disruption and an increased talar tilt of >10 degrees when compared with the uninjured ankle is linked to marked problems with ankle instability. These films are somewhat controversial, as degree of laxity by x-ray does not necessarily correlate with clinical instability.
 B. **Arthrography**
  1. Arthrography may be indicated with certain patients in order to define the extent of damage. This technique is diagnostic for calcaneofibular tears (shown by extravasation of dye).
  2. **Disadvantages** of arthrography include expense, invasiveness, allergic reactions to dye, and false-negative results several days after the injury. This procedure is usually not necessary with the availability of magnetic resonance imaging (MRI).
 C. **Computerized tomography and MRI** are >80% sensitive and specific in detecting soft tissue damage. These tests are recommended for locating fragments and determining the percentage of joint surface involved in osteochondral fractures. Compared to arthrography, computerized tomography and MRI have a greater predictive value and better patient acceptance.
 D. **Bone scans** are helpful in detecting **stress fractures** in individuals with suggestive symptoms and normal plain films.
V. **Treatment**
 A. **Sprains**
  1. **Acute management**
    a. **Protection, rest, ice, compression, elevation, modalities, and medications (PRICEMM)** are the keys for treating any ankle injury. Ice reduces edema and works better than heat to speed recovery to activity in moderate to severe sprains. (SOR **B**) Functional compression with a semi-rigid brace (Aircast) or a soft, lace-up brace helps manage swelling. These braces protect against inversion and eversion

while allowing dorsiflexion and plantar flexion. This type of functional treatment for acute sprains is recommended over immobilization. (SOR **Ⓐ**)

b. Nonsteroidal anti-inflammatory drugs (NSAIDs) (e.g., naproxen 440 mg twice daily with food) and analgesics (e.g., acetaminophen, 500–650 mg every 4–6 hours) should be given until edema and pain subside. NSAIDs not only reduce swelling and pain, but they may decrease the time it takes to return to usual activities. (SOR **Ⓑ**)

2. Rehabilitation

  a. Range of motion (ROM) exercises should begin within 48 hours of injury and weight bearing should progress as tolerated while wearing a functional brace. ROM includes controlled stretching of the Achilles tendon to help regain full dorsiflexion.

  b. Strengthening. Isometric exercises are started when pain and swelling have subsided and ROM is progressing. All four planes of motion (dorsiflexion, plantar flexion, inversion, and eversion) are worked against an immovable object. Progressive resistive exercises (PRE) in the same planes of motion follow and are readily accomplished by the use of elastic tubing. Toe raises and heel and toe walking are introduced as well.

  c. Proprioceptive exercises (balance/wobble board) are started when the patient can walk pain free. Walking on a variety of surfaces (flat floor to level ground to uneven terrain) in a progressive fashion and single leg balancing can also be used to help develop proprioception.

  d. Functional training. The next phase involves exercises that are more dynamic. The exercises are a mix of walking and jogging in both a straight line (forward and backward) and in patterns such as a figure of eight. Athletic individuals would then progress on to these exercises with a mix of jogging and running, and finally incorporate sport-specific drills to further strengthen the ankle prior to a return to competition.

3. Prevention of sprains.

  a. Functional drills, proprioceptive training, and strengthening of the ankle all play a role in reducing the occurrence or reoccurrence of an ankle sprain. Attention to the peroneal muscles (everters) is one of the keys to preventing a lateral ankle sprain. Progressive exercise programs, especially when proprioceptive training is incorporated, will help reduce the risk of an ankle sprain. (SOR **Ⓑ**)

  b. The use of a semirigid ankle brace during high-risk sports will reduce the risk of a recurrent sprain in a previously injured ankle. (SOR **Ⓐ**) There is also some evidence that the use of braces will reduce the risk of a sprain in uninjured ankles as well. (SOR **Ⓑ**)

B. Strains should be managed as described above for sprains (see Section V.A).

C. Tenosynovitis

  1. Initial treatment includes **PRICEMM, NSAIDs, and analgesics** as needed. **Injection of a corticosteroid** (e.g., methylprednisolone acetate, 4 mg, with an equal volume of 1%–2% lidocaine [Xylocaine]) may be helpful. This treatment is contraindicated in Achilles tendinitis, in the presence of infection, or if the patient has received a similar injection within the past 4 weeks or has a history of more than three such injections.

  2. Long-term management includes application of a **short leg, non–weight-bearing cast for 1 to 3 weeks.** ROM and PRE should be used for 1 to 3 weeks after cast removal (see Section V.A.2).

  3. Surgical consultation is indicated in cases of refractory pain and disability that are unresponsive to conservative therapy. Tenolysis and debridement may prove helpful in such cases.

D. Fractures

  1. Initial management of all fractures includes **PRICEMM, NSAIDs, and analgesics** as needed. A **posterior splint** should be used, and no weight bearing should be permitted unless certain that the fracture is stable. Consultation is advised for unstable, epiphyseal, and osteochondral fractures.

  2. Long-term management of most stable fractures includes a neutral positioned **walking cast for 4 to 6 weeks.** Rehabilitation after immobilization includes 2 to 4 weeks of ROM, PRE, and proprioceptive and functional exercises, as already described for ankle sprains (see Section V.A.2).

3. Avulsion fractures of the base of the fifth metatarsal and small avulsion fractures of the distal fibula heal very well and can often be managed similar to an ankle sprain with the understanding that the recovery will be somewhat slower.

REFERENCES

Birrer RB. Ankle Injuries. In: Mengel, MD and Schwiebert, LP (eds): *Family Medicine Ambulatory Care and Prevention*, 4th ed, McGraw-Hill; 2005:24-30.

Gravlee JR, Van Durme DJ. Braces and splints for musculoskeletal conditions. *Am Fam Physician.* 2007;75(3):342-348.

Ivins D. Acute ankle sprain: An Update. *Am Fam Physician.* 2006;74(10):1714-1720.

Nugent PJ. Ottawa ankle rules accurately assess injuries and reduce reliance on radiographs. *J Fam Practice.* 2004;53(10):785-788.

Safran MR et al. Lateral ankle sprains: A comprehensive review. *Med Sci Sports Exerc.* 1999;31(7S):429-437.

Stiell IG et al. Implementation of the ottawa ankle rules. *JAMA.* 1994;271:827-832.

Thompson C et al. Heat or ice for acute ankle sprain? *J Fam Practice.* 2003;52(8):642-643.

Veenema KR. Ankle sprain: Primary care evaluation and rehabilitation. *J Musculoskel Med.* 2000;17:563-576.

Wolfe MW et al. Management of ankle sprains. *Am Fam Physician.* 2001;63(1):93-104.

---

6   Arm & Shoulder Complaints

Brian R. Coleman, MD

KEY POINTS

- Knowledge of arm and shoulder anatomy is vital to proper diagnosis of arm and shoulder complaints.
- Overuse syndromes cause many shoulder complaints.
- Appropriate focused history and physical examination allows diagnosis of most arm and shoulder complaints and guides further testing.

I. Definition. The shoulder consists of four joints (glenohumeral, acromioclavicular, sternoclavicular, and scapulothoracic), which allow for movement in multiple planes. Unlike the hip, which is a stable joint having a deep acetabular socket, the shoulder is a mobile joint with a shallow glenoid fossa. The humerus has only minimal osseous support and is suspended from the glenoid by soft tissue, muscles, ligaments, and a joint capsule.

Glenohumeral stability is owing to a combination of ligamentous and capsular constraints, musculature, and the glenoid labrum. **Static shoulder stability** is owing to the joint surfaces and the capsulolabral complex. **Dynamic shoulder stability** results from rotator cuff muscles and the scapular rotators (trapezius, serratus anterior, rhomboids, and levator scapulae).

The **rotator cuff** is composed of four muscles, which assist in motion and depress the humeral head in the glenoid. The subscapularis assists internal rotation, the supraspinatus facilitates abduction, and the infraspinatus and teres minor assist in external rotation.

Arm and shoulder complaints comprise generalized or localized discomfort in the upper extremity. These may result from **direct trauma** (e.g., acromioclavicular injuries, shoulder dislocation/subluxation, olecranon bursitis) or from **overuse** (e.g., rotator cuff impingement/subacromial bursitis, olecranon bursitis, medial/lateral epicondylitis). Overuse of the musculotendinous unit evolves through several stages, beginning with inflammation (pain, swelling, erythema, warmth), followed by reparation (proliferative and maturation stages) and often, with continued overuse, fibrosis, which features histologically disorganized restructuring of the musculotendinous unit predisposing to degeneration, stenosing

TABLE 6–1. DIFFERENTIAL DIAGNOSIS OF COMMON ARM/SHOULDER COMPLAINTS

Condition	Risk Factors	Symptoms	Signs	Testing
AC injuries	Male:female, 5:1; 16–30 years old Direct blow to tip of shoulder (e.g., football, lacrosse, wrestling)	Pain with shoulder forward flexion/adduction	AC joint tenderness without gross deformity and with abnormal cross-arm test (Table 6–2) in grade I or II dislocation; clavicular displacement (mildly and superiorly with grade III and markedly superiorly or inferiorly or posteriorly accompanied by neurovascular or muscle compromise with grades IV–VI)	Plain AP/lateral shoulder radiographs; stress radiographs are not recommended because they do not affect treatment
Glenohumeral instability	History of previous dislocation; adolescent female athletes; repetitive overhead activity (e.g., gymnasts, swimmers, tennis, baseball pitching)	Vague pain referred to deltoid; feeling of impending dislocation or worse pain with overhead/abducted/extended rotated shoulder; "dead arm" after repetitive motion (e.g., pitching)	Abnormal apprehension/sulcus tests (Table 6–2)	Results from AP/lateral shoulder radiographs are usually negative, but may show anteroinferior glenoid rim fracture (Bankart lesion)
Dislocation/subluxation	Contact sports (e.g., football, lacrosse, rugby); fall on outstretched arm (e.g., skaters, skiers, motorcyclists)	Pain; inability to abduct arm; possible arm paresthesias	Asymmetry compared to unaffected shoulder (prominent humeral head, sulcus between acromion and humerus)	Results from AP/transscapular lateral Y and axillary lateral views should be obtained; postreduction x-rays indicated to detect Bankart lesion
Impingement/bursitis continuum	Repetitive overhead motion (e.g., throwing, racquet sports, swimming); overuse (e.g., carpenters, painters, plumbers); age >40	Pain with overhead activities, worse at night; anterolateral shoulder pain, possibly radiating to elbow	Abnormal Apley scratch, Neer, Hawkin, "empty can," or drop-arm tests (Table 6–2)	AP and transscapular lateral plain radiographs for degenerative changes; outlet or Alexander view visualizes subacromial space to grade acromial impingement; MRI 95% sensitive/specific detecting partial/complete tears, cuff degeneration, and chronic tendinitis
Adhesive capsulitis	Highest incidence in 40- to 50-year-olds; shoulder immobilization; involves nondominant arm more often and women >men	Painful loss of motion progressing to relatively pain-free restricted motion	Deltoid atrophy; decreased ROM, especially external rotation	AP/lateral radiographs useful to detect alternate diagnoses (fracture or calcification); arthrography may be helpful in diagnosis but is still controversial because of associated risks; MRI currently diagnostic test of choice
Olecranon bursitis	Direct contusion (e.g., skaters, skateboarders, football players)	Swollen/fluctuant elbow extensor surface with or without pain	Fluctuant/tender or nontender mass over olecranon	Plain lateral radiograph may demonstrate bone spur or fracture with history of trauma or in recurrent, poorly responsive cases
Medial epicondylitis ("golfer's elbow")	Golfers; Little League pitchers	Pain medial elbow/forearm; decreased pitch control	Tender medial epicondyle	No testing, unless atypical presentation; plain radiographs can show fracture, OA, intra-articular loose bodies; EMG can document radiculopathy/neuropathy; MRI helpful in documenting soft tissue fraying or tear if surgical referral is considered.
Lateral epicondylitis ("tennis elbow")	Age 40–60; 7 times as common as medial epicondylitis, 75% involve dominant arm; found in carpenters/painters/tennis players, or persons using poor equipment (wrong grip sizes, weight of racquet)	Pain lateral elbow/forearm (e.g., holding a telephone, opening a door, or picking up a coffee cup); decreased grip	Tender lateral epicondyle, worse with resisted extension of middle digit	

AC, acromioclavicular; AP, anteroposterior; EMG, electromyography; MRI, magnetic resonance imaging; OA, osteoarthritis; ROM, range of motion.

tenosynovitis, and even rupture. Aging also predisposes to these degenerative musculo-tendinous changes.

II. **Common Diagnoses** (Table 6–1). Arm and shoulder complaints are very common in family practice. Causes of these complaints are based on patient age and activity level. (See sidebars for information on burners/stingers, thoracic outlet syndrome, and acute brachial plexus neuritis.)

BURNERS/STINGERS

Burners/stingers are stretching/compression brachial plexus injuries caused by a blow to the patient's extended or flexed neck while in rotation. These injuries are most common in contact sports (e.g., football, hockey, and lacrosse), are more common in males, and may also result from bicycling or motorcycle accidents.

Patients typically complain of burning/paresthesias of the arm and may experience some arm weakness hours to days after the injury, but should not have neck pain. Patients should have a thorough but brief neurologic examination of the affected extremity, as well as a cervical spine examination. Patients complaining of neck pain should be managed as if they have potential cervical spine injuries, with immobilization and emergency department evaluation. For uncomplicated stingers, radiographs are typically not required, and electromyography is required only if symptoms persist for 2 to 3 weeks (which occurs in <5%–10% of patients). Stingers usually resolve on their own; in athletic play situations, the patient may return to play once burning resolves, provided there is no neck pain, weakness, or concussion.

THORACIC OUTLET SYNDROME

Thoracic outlet syndrome results from the compression of the neurovascular supply to the upper limb in the supraclavicular area and shoulder girdle. It tends to occur in young adults, particularly women, and has been associated with cervical ribs, diabetes, thyroid disease, alcoholism, and obesity. Patients may complain of pain in the neck or shoulder with numbness involving the entire upper extremity or forearm and hand; symptoms may be exacerbated by overhead activity. Nocturnal pain and paresthesias are common and should be distinguished from carpal tunnel syndrome. Thoracic outlet symptoms can often be reproduced and the condition diagnosed using the following maneuvers: Adson maneuver (with the arm at the side and the neck hyperextended and turned to the affected side) and Wright maneuver (with the arm abducted and externally rotated). Rib films will rule out cervical ribs or long transverse processes; if clinical evaluation is suggestive, cervical magnetic resonance imaging scan may help to rule out discogenic disease, and chest radiographs can evaluate for apical lung masses. Treatment for thoracic outlet syndrome involves management of underlying causes (e.g., thoracic surgery consultation for cervical rib).

ACUTE BRACHIAL PLEXUS NEURITIS

Acute brachial plexus neuritis is an uncommon disorder, which can be confused with more common causes of shoulder pain. Brachial plexus neuritis most often affects those between ages 20 and 60 years, with a male-to-female ratio ranging from 2:1 to 11.5:1. A viral or other infectious cause has been suggested. Patients present with severe acute burning shoulder/upper arm pain without a known precipitant; the pain usually diminishes over days to weeks, replaced by upper arm weakness. Neck or arm movements typically do not affect pain. Brachial plexus neuritis must also be differentiated from cervical radiculopathy (Chapter 48), which radiates from the neck down the arm, may be related to trauma or exertion, and is exacerbated by neck movements. In brachial plexus neuritis, electromyography and nerve conduction studies 3 to 4 weeks after symptom onset reveal abnormalities in more than one nerve (i.e., the brachial plexus); in contrast, cervical radiculopathy may feature osteophytes and interspace narrowing on cervical spine radiography and neuroforamenal disk impingement on magnetic resonance imaging scan. Treatment for acute brachial plexus neuritis is supportive, with physical therapy to maintain shoulder strength/mobility, analgesics as needed for pain, and reassurance that the condition generally will improve, albeit slowly.

A. Acromioclavicular (AC) injuries are rare in skeletally immature individuals.

B. Glenohumeral instability is an increase in translation of the glenohumeral joint and may occur in one or multiple directions. Generalized ligamentous laxity can also contribute to instability, especially in young athletic females and individuals with Marfan syndrome.

C. Dislocations and subluxations of the shoulder are common and account for 45% of all dislocations. Anterior dislocations account for approximately 90% of glenohumeral dislocations. Active patients younger than age 25 with a history of previous dislocation have an 85% risk of recurrence.

D. Rotator cuff impingement and **subacromial bursitis** form a continuum, beginning with impingement with arm elevation, resulting in soft tissue edema/inflammation. **Before the age of 25,** ligamentous laxity predisposes to impingement; **beyond 25 years of age,** impingement is usually related to overuse and frequently results in partial- or full-thickness rotator cuff tears after age 40.

E. Adhesive capsulitis is thickening and contraction of the capsule around the glenohumeral joint.

F. Olecranon bursitis is inflammation of the superficial olecranon bursa caused by acute or chronic elbow trauma.

G. Medial epicondylitis is inflammation of tendons and ligaments attaching to that structure.

H. Lateral epicondylitis is pain over the lateral elbow precipitated by repetitive forearm dorsiflexion, supination, and radial deviation.

III. **Symptoms** (Table 6–1). Important elements include a careful history of the mechanism of acute injury, the patient's occupational/recreational activities, as well as location, precipitants, and any symptoms associated with the patient's shoulder/arm complaint.

   A. Location
   1. Vague pain radiating to the deltoid insertion occurs in patients with **glenohumeral instability.**
   2. Anterolateral shoulder pain possibly radiating to the elbow is consistent with **rotator cuff impingement/subacromial bursitis.**
   3. Lateral elbow pain characterizes **lateral epicondylitis;** medial elbow pain characterizes **medial epicondylitis.**

   B. Precipitants
   1. Pain with shoulder forward flexion/adduction characterizes AC **joint injury.**
   2. Pain with the shoulder overhead, abducted, and externally rotated occurs with **glenohumeral instability.**
   3. Shoulder pain with overhead activities and worsening at night is a clue to **rotator cuff impingement/subacromial bursitis.**
   4. Pain following a direct blow to the elbow may indicate **olecranon bursitis.**

   C. Associated symptoms
   1. A feeling of impending dislocation with the shoulder overhead, abducted, and externally rotated points toward **glenohumeral instability,** as does "dead arm" after repetitive shoulder motion.
   2. Painful decreased range of motion (ROM), developing over time into relatively pain-free restricted ROM, is consistent with **adhesive capsulitis.**
   3. Extensor elbow swelling indicates **olecranon bursitis.**
   4. Patients with lateral epicondylitis complain of decreased/weakened grip.

IV. **Signs** (Table 6–1). Examination of the patient with arm/shoulder complaints should always include inspection (for asymmetry in AC or shoulder dislocations), palpation (for localized tenderness), and ROM/special maneuvers (Table 6–2).

V. **Laboratory Tests** (Table 6–1). In most patients with arm and shoulder complaints, a careful history and physical examination should clarify the diagnosis. Further testing should be undertaken on a case-by-case basis.

VI. **Treatment** of arm and shoulder complaints is directed at the underlying condition, which can be established through a careful focused history, examination, and selective testing.

   A. Grade I–II **AC joint injuries** are often treated with several days' rest and a shoulder sling for comfort. Ice and analgesics for pain and early range-of-motion exercises are important. Grade III–VI (severe) AC sprains or dislocations warrant orthopedic consultation for possible surgical consideration. (SOR **A**)

   B. Glenohumeral instability is treated primarily with physical therapy consultation for rotator cuff strengthening exercises. Nonsteroidal anti-inflammatory medications (NSAIDs) (e.g., oral ibuprofen 600–800 mg 3 times daily with meals, or naproxen 550 mg twice daily with meals) may decrease pain and inflammation, but are not necessary. A history

TABLE 6–2. MANEUVERS USED IN EVALUATING COMMON ARM/SHOULDER COMPLAINTS

Test Name	Description of Maneuver	Testing for . . .
Apley scratch test	Patient reaches (a) above/behind the head, then (b) behind the back, attempting to touch contralateral scapula	Rotator cuff (a) abduction/external rotation (b) adduction/internal rotation
Neer sign	Forced shoulder flexion with forearm extended/pronated (scapula stabilized)	Subacromid impingement
Hawkin test	Forced shoulder internal rotation with arm forward elevated to 90 degrees	Subacromial impingement/rotator cuff tendinitis
"Empty can" test	With elbows extended, thumbs pointing downward and arms abducted to 90 degrees in forward flexion, patient attempts to elevate arms against examiner resistance	Rotator cuff (supraspinatus) weakness
Drop-arm test	After passive arm abduction, patient attempts to slowly lower arm to side	Rotator cuff tear/supraspinatus dysfunction (arm drops after 90 degrees)
Cross-arm test	Patient raises arm to 90 degrees, then actively adducts, attempting to touch opposite shoulder	AC joint dysfunction
Sulcus test	With arm extended and resting at patient side, examiner exerts downward traction on humerus, watching for sulcus or depression lateral/inferior to acromion	Glenohumeral instability
Anterior/posterior apprehension test	With patient's arm abducted to 90 degrees and elbow bent, examiner externally rotates arm and exerts (a) anterior or (b) posterior pressure on humeral head	(a) Anterior and (b) posterior glenohumeral instability
Yergason test	With patient's arm at side, elbow flexed to 90 degrees and thumb pointing up, examiner resists patient's attempts to supinate forearm and flex elbow	Biceps tendinitis (may be concomitant or confused with rotator cuff tendinitis)
Spurling test	Patient extends neck; examiner axially compresses head and rotates it toward side of shoulder/arm complaint	Cervical nerve root compression

of recurrent dislocation warrants orthopedic consultation for consideration of surgical reconstruction. (SOR **B**)

C. **Rotator cuff injuries** may be very difficult to treat. Initial therapy consists of rest, ice, and NSAIDs. Early physical therapy consultation is recommended for range-of-motion and strengthening exercises. A sling may provide some comfort, but could lead to decreased ROM. **If a complete tear is noted,** then surgical intervention is necessary, but surgery is necessary in partial tears only after physical therapy has failed. (SOR **B**)

D. **Subacromial bursitis** is treated with relative rest, ice, range-of-motion exercises, and possible injection in the bursa (see sidebar).

SUBACROMIAL BURSA INJECTION

Informed consent should be obtained.

Equipment: 0.5 to 1 cc Aristocort 40 mg/mL and 3 to 4 cc lidocaine 1% combined in 5-cc syringe with 25G, 112? needle.

Technique: Injection can be done using either a posterolateral (just inferior to the posterior tip of the acromion into the space between the acromion and humeral head and directed anteriorly toward the coracoid process) or lateral approach; the lateral approach is described here. The patient should be seated with the arm hanging by the side to distract the humerus from the acromion. The edge of the acromion should be identified and marked. After cleansing the injection site with appropriate antiseptic rinse (e.g., Betadine), the needle should be inserted with a slight upward angle at the midpoint of the acromion into the space between the humeral head and acromion. The needle is then slowly withdrawn while injecting the fluid in a bolus, ensuring there is no resistance. Occasionally, the fluid will cause a visible swelling around the edge of the acromion. If needed, a "Band-Aid" dressing can be applied.

E. Adhesive capsulitis often resolves spontaneously, and treatment should focus on symptom relief. Gentle range-of-motion exercises, stretching, and **graded resistance training** have been shown effective. **Manipulation under anesthesia** requires orthopedic referral and is a very controversial treatment of capsulitis; it should be reserved for cases refractory to the foregoing measures. Corticosteroid injections (subacromial and intra-articular) may reduce pain, but have not been shown to affect recovery. (SOR **B**)

F. Olecranon bursitis is treated with ice, NSAIDs, and close monitoring. Aspiration is performed only when swelling causes significant pain and loss of motion. Aspirated fluid should be analyzed for cell count, crystals, and Gram stain (see Chapter 39). Steroid injections have been used with mixed results and should only be performed if no infection is present.

G. Medial epicondylitis is most easily treated conservatively with rest, ice, NSAIDs, and gradual increase in stretching-and-strengthening exercises. (SOR **B**) Local steroid injections (see Section VI.H) should be considered if there is a poor response to 2 to 3 weeks' conservative therapy.

H. For **lateral epicondylitis,** conservative initial management involves NSAIDs, ice after activities or 3 times daily, emphasis on proper technique for work or sports activities, forearm or counterforce bracing, and physical therapy referral for stretching-and-strengthening exercises with a goal of pain-free ROM. Steroid injection (1 mL of betamethasone mixed with 3–5 mL bupivacaine into point of maximum tenderness in a spoke-and-wheel fashion) should be considered after poor response to 2 to 3 weeks' conservative management. Poor response to 6 to 12 months' treatment warrants consideration of orthopedic referral for possible debridement and tenotomy.

REFERENCES

Chumbly EM, O'Connor FG, Nirschl RP. Evaluation of overuse elbow injuries. *Am Fam Physician.* 2000;61:691.

Ejnisman B, Andreoli CV, Soares BGO, et al. Interventions for tears of the rotator cuff in adults. *Cochrane Database Syst Rev.* 2004.

Miller JD, Pruitt S, McDonald TJ. Acute brachial plexus neuritis: an uncommon cause of shoulder pain. *Am Fam Physician.* 2000;62:2067.

Spencer EE Jr. Treatment of grade iii acromioclavicular joint injuries: a systematic review. *Clin Orthop Relat Res.* 2007;455:38.

Tallia AF, Cardone DA. Diagnostic and therapeutic injection of the shoulder region. *Am Fam Physician.* 2003;67:1271.

Woodward TW, Best TM. The painful shoulder: part I. Clinical evaluation. *Am Fam Physician.* 2000;61:3079.

Woodward TW, Best TM. The painful shoulder: part II. Acute and chronic disorders. *Am Fam Physician.* 2000;61:3291.

---

7   Bites & Stings

Brenda Powell, MD

KEY POINTS

- Mammalian bites cause morbidity from tissue destruction and introduction of pathogens.
- Insect and arachnid bites cause morbidity from hypersensitivity reactions, toxins, and introduction of pathogens.
- Treatment is based on the reaction type and the introduced infectious agent.

I. Definition. A mammalian bite is a skin wound caused by the teeth of a human or other mammal. Mammalian bites cause morbidity both from mechanical disruption and introduction of pathogens, which include oral aerobic and anaerobic flora and viruses such as hepatitis B and rabies, a fatal viral encephalitis.

Insect and arachnid bites and stings involve penetration of the victim's skin by some part of the animal, with host reaction depending on the type of bite. Hypersensitivity to the organism itself occurs with lice, mosquito saliva, scabies, and hymenoptera stings. Spider bites cause neurotoxicity and local necrosis with hemorrhage and thrombosis. Bites can transmit other diseases (e.g., malaria and encephalitis from mosquitoes, Lyme disease and Rocky Mountain spotted fever from ticks, plague, and typhus from fleas).

II. **Common Diagnoses.** Approximately 1 million animal bites require medical attention each year in the United States. Lice and scabies are increasing in prevalence. Tick-borne diseases are the most common vector-borne illness in the United States. Hymenoptera stings cause more deaths than any other venomous animal (6 deaths per 100,000 people per year).

The following inflict the majority of bite and sting injuries to humans in the United States.

A. **Mammals,** including humans and other mammals, both domestic and wild. Approximately 90% of these bites are from dogs.

1. **Bite injuries from humans** are common in fights; these injuries involve primarily teenagers and alcohol-intoxicated males aged from 30 to 35 years. Abused children, children who live in shelters for the homeless, and residents and staff of institutions for the mentally retarded are at especially high-risk for human bites.

2. Seventy-five percent of **animal bites** are considered "unprovoked." Sixty percent of dog bites involve neighborhood pets; 40% of these bites are superficial. Half of dog bite victims are children younger than 15 years. In the United States, rabies is found in unvaccinated domestic animals and wild animals such as skunks, raccoons, and bats.

B. **Insects,** encompass diptera (mosquitoes, flies, and gnats); fleas and bedbugs; hymenoptera (bees, wasps, hornets, yellow jackets, and ants); and pubic, head, and body lice. **Mosquitoes** breed in stagnant water during the warm season. **Fleas** can be found in grass, rugs, upholstery, floor cracks, and pet bedding, especially during warm, humid months; the majority of flea bites usually result from contact with dogs or cats. **Bedbugs** feed nocturnally on mammals and birds and may survive in clothing, furniture, and bedding for 6 to 8 weeks without a blood meal. **Bee and wasp stings** are common in suburbs and rural areas. The bites of **fire ants** are a significant problem in the southeastern United States. **Pubic lice** are usually transmitted by close body contact and are rarely spread by fomites. **Head lice,** which are commonly transmitted by the exchange of hats, combs, and brushes, may also be spread by close personal contact. Epidemics occur in schools. **Body lice,** associated with poor hygiene, are rare.

C. **Arachnids,** include mites that cause scabies, chiggers, hard and soft ticks, brown recluse, and black widow spiders. **Scabies** (adult mites or eggs) are readily transmitted by personal contact, especially within families or in crowded living situations. These parasitic mites burrow into the epidermis and lay eggs. **Chiggers (harvest mites)** are prevalent in the southern and Midwestern United States and bite gardeners, hikers, and campers. **Ticks** can be acquired by contact with pets, vegetation, or the burrows of host animals such as mice. Several human diseases are transmitted by ticks. Rocky Mountain spotted fever and tick-borne relapsing fever are endemic to the western mountain states. Tularemia from tick bites occurs mainly in western states. Lyme disease, which is endemic to semiwooded areas in New England, New York, and Wisconsin, occurs sporadically in the Midwest and the West. The bites of **brown recluse-*Loxosceles*** and **black widow spiders-*Lactrodectus*** cause serious morbidity and result in approximately 5% of all deaths from venomous animals. **Brown recluse spiders** are endemic to the south central United States. These spiders, which are active nocturnally, hide both indoors and outdoors. They bite humans only when they are disturbed. **Black widow spiders** are found throughout the United States and Canada. They nest outdoors in crevices near the ground, especially where flies are present (e.g., outhouses).

D. Less common bites and stings not discussed in this chapter include **marine envenomations** and **snakebites.**

III. **Symptoms and Signs**

A. **Mammalian bite wounds.** These bites may be **superficial abrasions; puncture wounds that are sometimes arcinate; lacerations, often with crushed and macerated edges,** or **wounds that may involve avulsion of tissue.** The wound should be examined for a visible evidence of damage to underlying structures; diminished circulation or excessive bleeding; and decreased sensation, weakness, limited movement, or pain with movement. Signs of infection may become evident within hours of a bite. **Rabies** begins with pain and numbness in the area of the bite, followed by fever, dysphagia, pharyngeal spasms ("hydrophobia,") paralysis, convulsions, and death.

B. Insect bite wounds. Itching is a symptom of **mosquito, flea, bedbug, lice, mite, and tick bites.**

1. The bites of **mosquitoes** are **pruritic, red papules, or vesicles.**
2. The bites of **fleas and bedbugs** are **pruritic, red papules, or vesicles.** They often occur in clusters or in a linear pattern on exposed areas, especially the wrists, ankles, and legs (fleas), and the hands, face, and neck (bedbugs).
3. The normal local reaction to **hymenoptera venom** is heat, redness, and tenderness. A **local allergic reaction** consists of a red papule surrounded by a pale zone of edema with varying amounts of local swelling. More severe **immediate hypersensitivity reactions** manifest the signs of generalized urticaria (see Chapter 62), redness, swelling, and anaphylaxis. A **delayed hypersensitivity reaction (serum sickness)** with fever, arthralgias, and malaise may occur 10 to 14 days after the sting. **Fire ants** cause multiple papules, which become necrotic pustules within several hours.
4. The bites of **lice** are **pruritic, red papules, or vesicles.** The itching from lice begins approximately 21 days after infestation. **Pubic lice** live in pubic and axillary hair and skin, but move all over the body and may be found in eyelashes, eyebrows, and the hairline, especially in children. **Head lice** live on the scalp. The seams of clothing and folds of bedding should be searched for **body lice.** Nits of pubic and head lice attach to hairs at the skin level; since hairs grow 1 mm every 3 days, one can determine how recently nits were deposited by their distance from the skin on the hair shaft. This information is particularly helpful in deciding whether nits represent a new infestation following a course of treatment.

C. Arachnid bite wounds

1. **Mites**
   a. The female mite's burrow in **scabies** typically takes the form of a short, serpiginous lesion on wrists, elbows, finger webs, or intertriginous areas. Myriad other skin lesions, including erythematous papules, nodules, scaly patches, excoriations, and secondary impetigo, can occur. Except in infants, scabies does not infest the scalp or the face. Scabies mites can live for 4 days off of the host.
   b. The bites of **chiggers** are **pruritic, red papules, or vesicles.** They often occur in clusters or in a linear pattern on the exposed areas, especially the wrists, ankles, and legs. The bites of chiggers and flies have central puncta or vesicles, which may become hemorrhagic.
2. After a **hard tick** has been attached for several days, its neurotoxin can cause an ascending, progressive paralysis, similar to Guillain-Barré syndrome, with hyporeflexia.
   a. **Lyme disease, caused by the spirochete *Borelia burgdorferi*,** is the most common vector-borne illness in the United States. Illness usually begins with a slowly spreading, annular skin lesion—erythema chronicum migrans—accompanied by regional lymphadenopathy and minor constitutional symptoms, fatigue, myalgias, arthralgias headache, and fever. Early disseminated disease consists of multiple system involvement, lymphadenopathy, musculoskeletal pain, attacks of arthritis, cranial nerve palsies, meningitis, cardiac conduction defects or pericarditis, and myocarditis. Late Lyme disease is most often seen as a chronic arthritis involving a large joint. The neurologic system may be involved.
   b. **Rocky Mountain spotted fever is caused by *Rickettsia rickettsii*. Patients present with fever, headache, malaise, and myalgias.** A rash, typically of red macules begins on the extremities and becomes purpuric, spreading to the trunk, palms, and soles.
   c. **Tularemia, Francisella tularensis,** is characterized by pain and ulceration at the bite site, with acutely inflamed, sometimes draining lymph nodes, or occasionally by severe pharyngeal inflammation with exudate, conjunctivitis, hepatosplenomegaly, or pneumonia.
3. **Spiders**
   a. A **brown recluse spider bite** is often unnoticed until local pain and itching begin; it becomes a hemorrhagic bulla surrounded by induration and erythema after 6 to 12 hours. The area of skin and subcutaneous necrosis may progress over a few days, forming an ulcer, which heals slowly over 2 to 4 months. Systemic symptoms include headache, fever, chills, malaise, weakness, nausea, vomiting, and joint pains. Signs of systemic intoxication, including morbilliform rash, tachycardia, hypotension, intravascular coagulopathy (petechiae, purpura, and bleeding diathesis), and hemolysis, may appear 1 to 3 days after the bite and is termed loxoscelism.

Brown recluse spiders have a 3- to 5-cm leg span and a 1- to 2-cm brown, fuzzy body, with a violin-shaped dark band on the dorsum.

   b. The **black widow spider bite** is a mild prick, followed in 1 to 3 hours by severe, cramping pain at the bite site, spreading to adjacent parts of the body. Pain, abdominal wall rigidity, muscle cramps, anxiety, weakness, sweating, salivation, lacrimation, bronchorrhea, nausea, vomiting, and fever may occur in hours. Lactrodectism is severe muscle cramping, nausea, and vomiting. The skin lesion develops a pale center with a red-blue border. Muscle rigidity, with tremor and fibrillations, develops in body parts near the bite. Signs of **cholinergic excess** (fever, lacrimation, rhinorrhea, and bradycardia) and **sympathetic activation** (hypertension and tachyarrhythmias), intensify over the next several hours, but may recur for up to 3 days. Black widow spiders have 1- to 2-cm shiny, black bodies, with a red hourglass mark on the underside.

IV. Laboratory Tests

A. Mammalian bites

   1. Culture with sensitivity studies. More than one-third of deeper human bite wounds and a smaller proportion of animal bites become infected; abrasions seldom reach that stage. Even apparently insignificant bites on the hand are prone to infection. Therefore, **culture with sensitivity studies** is recommended for the following types of mammalian bite wounds: deep puncture wounds, all bite wounds that are sutured, wounds that are clinically infected or require hospital treatment, and full-thickness bites on the hand.

   2. Radiograph. A plain radiograph should be obtained when osteomyelitis is suspected. Forceful injuries, such as a hand bite from a blow to a tooth, require an x-ray to look for fractures and embedded tooth fragments.

   3. Fluorescent antibody staining. An **animal suspected of being rabid** should be killed and its head sent to a health department laboratory, where the brain will be examined for rabies antigens by fluorescent antibody staining.

B. Tests for possible scabies infestation.
Scabies mites, eggs, or feces may be found by scraping open a pruritic lesion (especially the end of a burrow) with a no. 15 scalpel blade dipped in mineral oil, and then examining this material microscopically under a coverslip.

C. Tests for suspected tick-borne diseases

   1. In the presence of **erythema chronicum migrans,** routine serologic testing for antibodies is not necessary and the patient should receive treatment with antibiotics. Otherwise, acute and convalescent titers of IgM and IgG to *Borrelia burgdorferi* can be drawn.

   2. Spirochetes can be seen in the blood smear in 70% of cases of **tick-borne relapsing fever.**

   3. Rocky Mountain spotted fever and **tularemia** are diagnosed by antibody titers to *Rickettsia rickettsii* and *Francisella tularensis,* respectively. Serology will be positive at 2 weeks. Treatment is begun based on signs and symptoms. In **Rocky Mountain spotted fever,** the initial laboratory tests may often demonstrate normal or slightly depressed WBC, thrombocytopenia, elevated transaminases, and hyponatremia. In **tularemia,** the WBC and erythrocyte sedimentation rate may be normal or slightly elevated. The organism can be cultured, but this is not often done, because of the risk of transmission to laboratory workers.

D. Tests for brown recluse spider bite with systemic involvement.
If this kind of bite is suspected, order blood type and screen, coagulation studies, complete blood cell count, electrolytes, blood urea nitrogen, creatinine, and urinalysis.

V. Treatment

A. Mammalian bites

   1. Wound care is similar for human and other mammalian bites.

      a. Thorough cleansing is necessary. At home, this means repeatedly flushing the wound with soap and water, 3% hydrogen peroxide, or iodine solution. In the office, this involves pressure irrigation or scrubbing with gauze sponges (under local anesthesia, if necessary) and 1% benzalkonium or povidone-iodine solution. The edges of a full-thickness wound should be debrided (see Chapter 41). Pressure irrigation should follow.

      b. Closure

         (1) Primary closure with sutures or wound tapes (Steri-Strips) may be considered for dog bites and for human and other animal bites on the face if the patient is treated within 3 to 6 hours after injury and if the wound appears to be uninfected. Subcutaneous sutures should be avoided. A pressure dressing should be applied for 24 hours, and the wound should be inspected for signs of infection after 48 hours.

A single layer of skin sutures may be replaced with Steri-Strips after 5 to 7 days.

(2) Bite wounds on the hands should never be closed primarily. A bitten hand should be immobilized, by splinting from the fingertips to the mid forearm, and elevated. Because of the risk of infection, the wound should be reexamined within 24 hours. After approximately 5 days, movement should be encouraged to minimize swelling and stiffness.

(3) Other bite wounds should be packed with gauze impregnated with an antibacterial agent and seen on day 2 and 4 to 7 days later. Revision and delayed primary closure may be considered at that time.

c. The reporting of animal bites (and of human bites in some locales) to the local health department is mandatory.

2. Antibiotic therapy

a. Indications

(1) Infected bite wounds require antibiotic therapy. Patients with such bites on the hand should be hospitalized to receive intravenous antibiotics.

(2) Prophylactic antibiotics should be considered for cat and human bites (SOR **Ⓒ**) and for dog bites that are >8-hours-old.

(3) It is reasonable to treat with antibiotics bite wounds that have been sutured or followed up for possible delayed closure, all bites on the hand, (SOR **Ⓒ**) bites causing deep puncture wounds, and all bites in diabetic patients or immunosuppressed patients.

b. Agents of choice and treatment regimens. Animal bites (especially cat bites) may become infected with *Pasteurella multocida*. Human bite infections are more likely to become infected than animal bites and be polymicrobial in nature. Commonly isolated are *S aureus*, *Streptococci*, *Eikenella corrodens* and *Bacteroides* spp *Staphylococci*, and other penicillinase-producing organisms are present in up to 41% of bite wound infections. First-generation cephalosporins are not effective as monotherapy because *E corrodens* and anerobes are often resistant.

(1) Amoxicillin with clavulanic acid (Augmentin) is the oral drug of choice for treatment (10-day course) or prevention (5-day course) of bite wound infection. The adult dose is 875 mg orally every 12 hours. Children should receive 30 to 50 mg/kg/d in 3 divided doses.

(2) Penicillin V, 250 mg orally every 6 hours (30–50 mg/kg/d for children), may be adequate initial therapy for animal but not human bites. Infection developing within the first 24 hours suggests *Pasteurella* infection and constitutes an indication for penicillin.

(3) Patients allergic to penicillin may receive the following antibiotics.

(a) For adults and children aged 8 years or older: **erythromycin** (e.g., **erythromycin ethylsuccinate,** 400 mg every 6–8 hours) *and* **tetracycline hydrochloride,** 250 mg orally every 6 hours, or **doxycycline,** 100 mg orally every 12 hours. Another regimen can be clindamycin plus either a floroquinolone or trimethoprim-sulfamethoxazole

(b) For children younger than 8 years, for whom tetracycline is contraindicated: **erythromycin** *alone,* 30 to 50 mg/kg/d in 3 divided doses.

3. Hospitalization is indicated in the following situations:

a. Bites to the hand, except those that are very superficial and do not appear to be infected.

b. Bites involving tendon, joint capsule, bone, or facial cartilage.

c. Signs of infection despite antibiotics or when treatment has been delayed.

d. Severe disfigurement, or tissue loss that may require plastic surgery or grafting.

e. Potential poor compliance with outpatient therapy.

4. Rabies postexposure prophylaxis

a. Indications (Table 7–1). Contact the local health department or the Rabies Investigation Unit, Centers for Disease Control and Prevention, Atlanta, Georgia, at (404) 639 to 3534 or (800) 311 to 3435 for additional information.

TABLE 7-1. RABIES POSTEXPOSURE PROPHYLAXIS

Animal	Animal Condition	Appropriate Treatment
Wild carnivores (e.g., skunks, bats, or raccoons)	Available	Obtain fluorescent rabies antibody (FRA) test on animal. Begin HRIG* and HDCV.[†] Discontinue HDCV, if FRA test is negative.
	Unknown	Assume rabid. Begin HRIG* and HDCV.[†]
Domestic dog or cat	Healthy/available	Observe animal for 10 d. If animal stays healthy, no treatment is necessary.
	Rabid/suspected rabid	Obtain FRA test on animal. Begin HRIG* and HDCV. [†] Discontinue HDCV, if FRA test is negative.
	Unknown	Low risk of rabies in most areas. Consult local health department.
Rodents	Generally unknown	Prophylaxis rarely indicated. Consult local health department.

*Human rabies immune globulin, 20 U/kg intramuscularly on day 0. Before HRIG is given, serum should be drawn for measurement of rabies antibody titer.
[†] Human diploid cell vaccine, 1 mL intramuscularly on days 0, 3, 7, 14, and 28.
(Adapted from the Centers for Disease Control and Prevention recommendations, 1991.)

   b. **Regimen.** Human rabies immune globulin, 20 immunizing units per kilogram is given, half-intramuscularly and half-infiltrated around the wound, up to 8 days after exposure. Active immunization with human diploid cell rabies vaccine, 1 mL intramuscularly, is given on days 0, 3, 7, 14, and 28. Pregnancy is not a contraindication. Immunosuppressive drugs such as corticosteroids should be avoided, if possible.
   5. **Tetanus prophylaxis.** Tetanus prophylaxis should be administered according to the indications outlined in Chapter 41.
B. **Insect bites. Symptomatic relief** is all that is needed for most bug bites, including those of mosquitoes, flies, fleas, and bedbugs. Topical lotions or creams such as **calamine** or **0.5% hydrocortisone** or applications of ice may relieve itching. Occasionally, an oral antihistamine, such as **diphenhydramine** (Benadryl), 25 mg 3 times a day for adults, ameliorates the urticarial reaction. Other, more specific treatments are discussed below.
   1. **For flea and mite infestations,** thorough **housecleaning,** including vacuuming, along with washing clothes and bedclothes, is indicated.
   2. **Eradication of fleas and bedbugs** is best performed by a professional exterminator. After **fumigation,** pets, children, and pregnant women should stay away for at least 4 hours.
   3. **Pets with fleas should be treated with insecticide** (e.g., pyrethrum or malathion) after consultation with a veterinarian.
   4. **Hymenoptera**
      a. The **stinger** (if present) **should be removed** by scraping sideways so as not to squeeze the attached venom sac.
      b. **Local pain and swelling** may be controlled by applying ice and a protease (e.g., a paste of meat tenderizer and water) to the site.
      c. **Local allergic reactions.** **Antihistamines,** such as **diphenhydramine,** 25 to 50 mg (up to 1–2 mg/kg for children) orally every 6 to 8 hours, and **prednisone,** 1 mg/kg/d for 3 days, may also be effective.
      d. If **cellulitis** is present, an antibiotic, such as erythromycin, should be added to the above regimen (see Chapter 9).
      e. **Immediate hypersensitivity reactions** must be treated promptly with **epinephrine,** 1:1000, 0.01 mL/kg, up to 0.5 mL, injected subcutaneously, and repeated, if necessary, in 5 to 10 minutes. A large-bore intravenous line should be started and the patient should be observed for at least 6 to 8 hours, since the vast majority of rebound or biphasic anaphylactic reactions will occur during this period. Additional measures for treatment of anaphylaxis should be available, if necessary. Intravenous diphenhydramine, 50 mg, is given to block H_1 receptor sites. Aerosolized bronchodilators such as albuterol, 2.5 mg (0.5 mL of 5 mg/mL solution) in 3 mL of normal saline, should be used for bronchospasm. Simultaneous use of H_2 blockers (e.g., ranitidine, 50 mg intravenously every 8 hours, or cimetidine, 300 mg intravenously every 6 hours) provides an additional benefit.

    f. For **serum sickness** that occurs 10 to 14 days after hymenoptera stings, **prednisone,** 1 to 2 mg/kg/d orally in divided doses, should be tapered over 2 weeks.

    g. Prophylaxis. Any individual who has had *any* systemic allergic symptoms or progressively severe local reactions from hymenoptera stings should carry a kit with injectable epinephrine (e.g., **Epi-Pen**), wear a medical identification bracelet, and avoid walking barefoot or wearing bright-colored clothing, flowers, or scent outdoors. Patients with allergic reactions may be evaluated by an allergist for desensitization treatment with venom extracts.

5. Lice

    a. Pediculosis capitis should be treated with a topical scabicide applied to dry hair and left on for 10 minutes before rinsing. (Permethrin 1% preferred, (SOR **A**) pyrethrum insecticides are pregnancy category B; lindane 1% is an option, but not in children younger than 2 years or pregnant women.) After treatment, nits may be loosened by wrapping the hair for 30 to 60 minutes with a towel soaked in vinegar or using a 50% water and vinegar rinse. Nits may be combed out with a fine-tooth comb. Parents should check for treatment failure (new nits visible close to the skin) at 12 hours and every 2 days for 2 weeks; if failure occurs, a second line medication should be used such as 0.5% malathion lotion. (SOR **A**) Insecticides should be kept away from the eyes; on eyelashes, a thick coating of petroleum jelly should be applied twice a day for 8 days.

    b. Pediculosis corporis responds to a hot shower and laundering clothing/bed linens in hot water (60°C) and heated drying. (SOR **A**)

    c. Pediculosis pubis responds to the same measures as pediculosis capitis (i.e., permethrin 1% as preferred agent, permethrin 5%, a second option, and lindane 1%, a third option). (SOR **A**) It is important to treat all contacts. Bedding and clothing should be washed and dried in a hot dryer, or dry cleaned or bagged in plastic for 72 hours. (SOR **C**)

6. Scabies. All household members should be treated simultaneously; bed linens and clothing used in the previous 4 days should be washed in hot water. Items that cannot be washed should be dry cleaned or sealed in a plastic bag for 5 days. (SOR **C**)

    a. Permethrin 5% (Elimite cream), 1 oz per person, is massaged into the skin from the neck to the toes (and also on the head in infants) and left on for 8 to 14 hours, then thoroughly washed off. (SOR **A**)

    b. A less expensive and equally effective treatment is **1% gamma-benzene hexachloride** (lindane [Kwell or Scabene]) **lotion,** applied to cool skin from the neck down for 8 to 12 hours, then washed off with soap and water. Since systemic absorption and neurotoxicity can occur, it should not be used on children younger than 2 years, pregnant or lactating women, patients with seizures or other neurologic disease, or those with extensively inflamed skin.

    c. Despite elimination of live mites, pruritus and existing skin lesions may persist for several weeks. Itching may be treated with **hydrocortisone** or **0.1% triamcinolone cream, with or without oral antihistamines.**

    d. Oral ivermectin (Stromectol), 200 μg/kg in a single dose is effective in eradicating scabies, but is not approved by the US Food and Drug Administration for routine use. It should probably be reserved for scabies crustosa (Norwegian scabies). (SOR **B**)

7. Ticks

    a. Hard ticks should be removed. The tick should be grasped very close to the skin with blunt forceps, and pulled with slow constant traction. If the tick is not completely removed, it should be excised (e.g., using a skin biopsy punch). Sometimes a diligent search is required to locate an attached tick.

    b. Skin infections should be treated with antibiotics (see Chapter 9).

    c. For **Lyme disease,** the length of treatment is dependent on the stage of the disease.

        (1) Early localized Lyme disease may be treated for 14 to 21 days with **doxycycline,** 100 mg twice a day, or **amoxicillin,** 250 to 500 mg 3 times a day (20–40 mg/kg/d for children).

        (2) Early disseminated disease is treated with intravenous therapy for 2 to 3 weeks. Options are ceftriaxone 2 g daily, cefotaxime 3 g twice a day, and chloramphenicol 50 mg/kg/d in 4 divided doses. The risk of transmission of the disease is low, less than 5%, even in areas where the disease is hyperendemic; it is therefore probably not cost-effective to treat prophylactically with antibiotics after a tick bite.

  d. For **Rocky Mountain spotted fever,** treatment should be started promptly with oral **tetracycline** (if the patient is older than 8 years), 25 to 30 mg/kg/d in 4 divided doses, or with 1 dose of **chloramphenicol,** 50 mg/kg, followed by 50 mg/kg/d in 4 divided doses. When the patient becomes afebrile, the dose should be halved, and then discontinued after 2 to 3 days. If untreated, death may occur in 8 to 15 days. Untreated RMSF has a fatality rate of 25% and 5% in treated cases.
  e. Adults with **tularemia** can be treated with **streptomycin,** 0.5 g intramuscularly twice a day for 1 week. (SOR **C**)
  f. **Tick-borne relapsing fever** in adults is treated with **tetracycline,** 500 mg orally 4 times daily for 10 days.
8. **Spider bites**
  a. **Hospitalization** is indicated for patients with black widow spider bites who are symptomatic, elderly, or very young. Hospital treatment may also be necessary for patients with brown recluse spider bites if they have systemic symptoms or if laboratory evidence of intravascular coagulation and hemolysis exists.
  b. For **local lesions caused by brown recluse spider bites,** good wound care is important. (SOR **C**) A bitten extremity should be splinted and elevated. Soaks and sterile dressings, and possibly topical antibacterial agents such as silver sulfadiazine, are applied to the necrotic ulcer. Systemic antibiotics such as **erythromycin ethylsuccinate,** 400 mg orally 4 times a day, have been used but are not routinely indicated. **Excision** of the bite wound is ineffective and **contraindicated.** Local and systemic corticosteroids are of no benefit. The following treatments are **experimental:** antivenom, hyperbaric oxygen, and dapsone, (SOR **B**) a polymorphonuclear cell inhibitor (dosage, 50–200 mg/d). The latter agent has potentially serious side effects.
  c. Tetanus prophylaxis should be given (see Chapter 41). (SOR **C**)
  d. Initial therapy for **black widow spider bites** consists of application of ice and extremity elevation. Calcium gluconate in a 10% solution (10 mL given by intravenous push over 5 minutes) may provide relief from muscle spasm. (SOR **A**) Narcotics and diazepam in standard doses can be initiated to relieve pain and muscle spasm.
  e. Antivenom is recommended for significant symptoms of widow bites. (SOR **B**) Before administering **black widow spider antivenom,** testing for sensitivity to horse serum should be done. The test packaged with the antivenom can be used. One 2.5mL ampule of black widow spider antivenom intramuscularly or intravenously in 10 to 15 mL of normal saline over 10 to 15 minutes can then be administered.
C. **Prevention**
  1. **Hepatitis B.** Persons at occupational risk for human bites, including health and dental workers and employees of institutions for the mentally retarded, should receive hepatitis B vaccine.
  2. **Rabies.** Veterinary workers occupationally exposed to animal bites and people traveling to areas where rabid dogs are common should be immunized with 1 mL of human diploid cell rabies vaccine intramuscularly on days 0, 7, 21, or 28.
  3. **Outdoor insect bites** can be prevented by avoiding their habitats, covering the skin with clothing, and using effective insect repellents that contain diethyltoluamide (DEET 30%). **Permethrin** (Permenone Tick Repellent) sprayed on clothing protects against mosquitoes and ticks.

REFERENCES

Blackman James. Spider bites. *J Am Board Fam Prac.* 1995;8:4.
Bunzli W, et al. Current management of human bites. *Pharmacotherapy.* 1998;18:227.
Depietropaola Danie,l et al. Diagnosis of lyme disease. *Am Fam Physician.* 2006;72:2.
Dire DJ. Emergency management of dog and cat bite wounds. *Emerg Med Clin North Am.* 1992;10:719.
Flinders David. Pediculosis and scabies. *Am Fam Physician.* 2004;69:2.
Hogan DJ, Schachner L, Tanglertsampan C. Diagnosis and treatment of childhood scabies and pediculosis. *Pediatr Clin North Am.* 1991;38:941.
Kelleher A, Gordon S. Management of bite wounds and infection in primary care. *Cleve Clin J Med.* 1997;54:137.
Kemp E. Bites and stings of the arthropod kind. *Postgrad Med.* 1998;103:88.
Norris R. Managing arthropod bites and stings. *Physician Sports Med.* 1998;26(7):47.

8   Breast Lumps & Other Breast Conditions

Diane J. Madlon-Kay, MD, MS

KEY POINTS
- Benign breast disease affects almost all women.
- Mammograms are not recommended for women younger than 30 years.
- Family physicians can do needle aspirations of breast masses to determine whether they are cystic or not.

I. **Definition.** Breast lumps are any areas of the breast that feel different from surrounding breast tissue. The normal breast is lumpy because of its cystlike architecture.

II. **Common Diagnoses**
- A. **Fibrocystic changes** are the most common benign condition of the breast. The incidence of this disorder increases with age; approximately 25% of premenopausal women and up to 50% of postmenopausal women have this condition. Cysts may range in size from 1 mm to large macrocysts >1 cm.
- B. **Breast cancer** will eventually develop in one of every nine women. Risk factors include age, genetic factors, and hormonal factors.
- C. **Fibroadenomas** are most prevalent in women younger than 25 years and in black women.
- D. **Mastitis** is almost always associated with lactation. This condition results from the entrance of *Staphylococcus aureus* or streptococci into the breast tissue through abraded skin or a cracked nipple. Streptococcal infection usually leads to cellulitis, whereas staphylococcal infection may lead to abscess formation.

GYNECOMASTIA

Gynecomastia is a benign enlargement of the male breast. It may be asymptomatic or painful, unilateral or bilateral. It commonly occurs during puberty. It also occurs in adults, with the highest prevalence among 50- to 80-year-old patients. Most patients seeing a physician for gynecomastia will have idiopathic gynecomastia (25%) or gynecomastia because of puberty (25%), drugs (10%–20%), cirrhosis or malnutrition (8%), or primary hypogonadism (8%).

Gynecomastia appearing during mid-to-late puberty requires only a history and physical examination, including careful palpation of the testicles and, if the results are normal, reassurance and periodic follow-up. In most boys, the condition resolves spontaneously within a year and no further evaluation is necessary. Since gynecomastia is so common in men, the presence of nontender, palpable breast tissue on a routine examination should not lead to a major laboratory evaluation. In most instances, taking a careful history is sufficient to uncover most of the conditions associated with gynecomastia. If no abnormalities are found on physical examination or after the assessment of hepatic, renal, and thyroid function by serum chemistry profiles, further specific evaluation is unlikely to be useful. The patient should be reexamined in 6 months. If a patient reports the recent onset of progressive breast enlargement and no underlying cause is apparent, measurements of serum beta-human chorionic gonadotropin, testosterone, estradiol, luteinizing hormone, follicle-stimulating hormone, and prolactin may help elucidate the cause.

Most patients require no therapy other than the removal of any identified inciting cause. Specific treatment is indicated if the gynecomastia causes sufficient pain or embarrassment. Several medical regimens have been tried, including dihydrotestosterone, danazol, clomiphene citrate, tamoxifen, and testolactone. Surgical removal is also an option.

III. **Symptoms**
- A. One common symptom is **breast lumps.** In approximately 70% to 80% of women in whom breast cancer develops, the first and only symptom is the incidental discovery of a mass by the patient.

B. Breast pain is the most common symptom of fibrocystic changes. The pain is usually bilateral and often in the upper outer quadrants. Characteristically, the pain begins 1 week before menstruation and diminishes with the onset of menstrual flow. The pain is caused by breast swelling; breast volume may increase up to 15%.

C. Nipple discharge of a yellow or greenish-brown color occurs in up to one-third of patients with mastitis. The second most frequent symptom of breast cancer, nipple discharge in women older than 50 years, is of more concern than it is in younger women. If the discharge is associated with a mass, the mass is the primary concern. Spontaneous, recurrent, or persistent discharge requires surgical exploration. The character of the discharge cannot be used to distinguish benign from malignant causes. However, bloody, serous, serosanguineous, or watery discharges should be regarded with suspicion.

MASTALGIA

Mastalgia is the most common breast symptom causing women to consult physicians. Although fibrocystic disease is often present in the biopsy specimens of women with breast pain, fibrocystic changes are also present in the breasts of 50% to 90% of asymptomatic women.

Most commonly, breast pain is associated with the menstrual cycle (cyclic), but it can be unrelated to the menstrual cycle or occur postmenopausally. Cyclic breast pain is usually bilateral and poorly localized. It is often described as a heaviness that radiates to the axilla and arm and is relieved with the onset of menses. Cyclic mastalgia occurs more often in younger women. Noncyclic mastalgia is most common in women 40 to 50 years of age. It is often unilateral and is described as a sharp, burning pain that appears to be localized in the breast.

In most women with breast pain, the physical examination and mammogram, if indicated, reveal no evidence of breast pathology. Patients can be reassured that breast pain has a spontaneous remission rate of 60% to 80%. Further treatment modalities are described in Section VI. A.

IV. **Signs**
  A. **Breast lumps.** Ideally, examination of the patient should take place 7 to 9 days after the onset of menstrual flow. In general, fibrocystic areas are slightly irregular, easily movable, bilateral, and in the upper outer quadrants. Compression often causes tenderness, especially premenstrually.

  On palpation, a cancerous lesion is usually solitary, irregular or stellate, hard, nontender, fixed, and not clearly delineated from surrounding tissues.

  Fibroadenomas are usually rubbery, smooth, well-circumscribed, nontender, and freely mobile.

  B. **Breast inflammation.** Mastitis is characterized by inflamed, edematous, erythematous, indurated tender areas of the breast.

  C. **Surface of the breast**
    1. **Retraction.** Breast cancer frequently causes fibrosis. Contraction of this fibrotic tissue may produce dimpling of the skin, alteration of the breast contours, and flattening or deviation of the nipple.
    2. **Edema of the skin.** Lymphatic blockage produces thickened skin with enlarged pores characteristic of the so-called pigskin or "orange peel" (*peau d'orange*) appearance in breast cancer.
    3. **Venous pattern.** This may be prominent unilaterally in breast cancer.

V. **Laboratory Tests.** Diagnostic testing is unnecessary in women with multiple, bilateral, diffuse, symmetric breast lumps without dominant masses.
  A. **Mammography**
    1. **Indication.** A woman older than 30 to 35 years with a solitary or dominant mass, or an area of asymmetric thickening in the breast should undergo mammography. A breast lump is described as a dominant mass when the breasts are diffusely nodular, but one mass is clearly larger, firmer, or asymmetric in location.
    2. **Contraindication.** Since breast tissue is very dense in young women, mammograms are *not* recommended in women younger than 30 years. In older women, some fatty displacement of breast tissue has occurred, and mammograms are more worthwhile.

    3. Efficacy. Although 85% of all breast cancers are documented by mammography, as many as 15% of women with breast cancers have a normal mammogram. Therefore, a palpable mass is of concern even if a mammographic report shows no evidence of malignancy. **A biopsy is the only test that definitively excludes cancer.**

    4. Interpretation. Mammograms are interpreted in the following ways:

       a. Additional imaging required.

       b. Negative.

       c. Benign finding.

       d. Probably benign finding. Short interval follow-up suggested.

       e. Suspicious abnormality. Biopsy should be considered.

       f. Highly suggestive of malignancy.

B. Other imaging techniques. Although ultrasonography is not useful as a screening tool for breast cancer, it is useful for discriminating solid from cystic lesions. Other imaging techniques considered experimental or of no proven benefit for evaluation of breast conditions include thermography, diaphanography, computerized tomography, magnetic resonance imaging, and digital imaging.

C. Aspiration of a suspected breast cyst. Needle aspiration may be used to define the cystic nature of any breast mass.

    A 20- or 22-gauge needle attached to a 10- or 20-mL syringe should be used. After the skin is cleaned with alcohol, the cyst is fixed between the fingers of one hand while the needle is directed into the cyst with the other. The aspirated fluid is usually amber to green in color. If the fluid is bloody or if the mass is still palpable or reappears within 1 month of observation, a biopsy is necessary. (SOR **C**) The fluid is usually discarded.

D. Breast biopsy. The cytologic or histologic characteristics of a clearly dominant breast mass should be confirmed by biopsy, regardless of other clinical or mammographic findings.

    1. Fine needle aspiration biopsy is used to determine the cytology of suspected breast cancer. Accurate interpretation requires proper smearing and fixation of the slides, as well as an experienced pathologist. In expert hands, the false-negative rate is 1.4% and the false-positive rate is near 0%.

    2. Excisional biopsy

       a. Excisional biopsy is indicated if the results of the physical examination or mammogram suggest cancer even when the cytologic findings of aspiration are benign, or if a breast mass may be cancerous and fine needle aspiration biopsy and cytologic evaluation are not available.

       b. The biopsy is usually performed as an outpatient procedure using local anesthesia. Removal of the entire mass is the objective.

    3. Incisional biopsy may be performed in the following circumstances:

       a. To confirm the diagnosis of advanced cancer. If the mass is strongly suspected of being malignant, a cutting-edge core needle can be used.

       b. To evaluate a breast mass that is too large to be excised easily and completely.

E. Genetic testing for breast cancer. Women at risk for genetic mutations should be identified by taking a thorough personal and family history for breast or ovarian cancer, or both. Women at low risk for a genetic mutation should not undergo genetic testing because of the risk of indeterminate or false-positive results and the psychologic and social risks associated with testing. A helpful tool to calculate breast cancer risk is the Breast Cancer Risk Assessment Tool developed by the National Cancer Institute, available at http://www.cancer.gov/bcrisktool/. For women in whom genetic testing is warranted, testing should be done only in the context of careful genetic counseling.

VI. Treatment

A. Fibrocystic changes

    1. General measures

       a. Supportive measures that may be helpful include the use of loose, light clothing, and a comfortable, supporting, well-padded bra.

       b. Dietary changes

          (1) Caffeine intake. Although studies of dietary restriction of **caffeine** and other methylxanthines are conflicting, some reports suggest that eliminating consumption of such substances may be efficacious.

          (2) Vitamin E. This vitamin has not been found to be beneficial in placebo-controlled studies. (SOR **B**)

(3) **Evening primrose oil** is often used because of its low incidence of side effects, and nonhormonal composition. Unfortunately, study results are conflicting regarding its effectiveness. The average dose is 3000 mg/d in divided doses for a minimum of 3 to 4 months. Evening primrose oil can be obtained without a prescription and costs less than $1 a day. (SOR **B**)

2. **Pharmacologic therapy** (Table 8–1). Before beginning treatment, the woman's symptoms should be carefully evaluated. Minimal symptoms for only a few days of the month do not require drug therapy. It may take 3 to 4 months for evidence of improvement with any treatment regimen.

   Although other drugs can be used for this purpose, **danazol** is the only pharmacologic agent approved by the US Food and Drug Administration for use in the treatment of fibrocystic changes. Since danazol therapy is associated with significant side effects, this agent should be administered only by a physician familiar with its use. (SOR **B**)

3. **Surgery.** A subcutaneous mastectomy with implants or bilateral reduction mastectomies may be considered in the following patients.

   a. In women with an extremely high-risk of breast cancer (e.g., a history of breast cancer in a mother and a sister).

   b. In women with ductal or lobular, atypical hyperplasia on biopsy. The risk of breast cancer is increased by a factor of approximately 5 in these women.

   c. In women with breast pain that is resistant to nonsurgical treatment.

B. **Breast cancer.** The objective of treatment is to provide the greatest chance for cure or long-term survival. Whether this objective can be met while preserving the major portion of the breast is controversial. Radical mastectomy is now performed rarely, since modified radical mastectomy results in comparable survival. Lumpectomy is an option for some women.

1. **Surgery.** The primary care physician is responsible for referring the patient to a surgeon, who should provide individualized counseling to the patient so that the appropriate option is selected. Breast cancers are staged at surgery, at which time tissue is obtained for estrogen and progesterone receptors.

   Most women can be fitted with a **prosthesis** within 3 to 6 weeks of surgery. The option of breast reconstruction should be discussed before surgery because it can often be performed at the same time.

2. **Chemotherapy, hormonal therapy, and radiation therapy** should be directed by an oncologist.

3. **Careful and frequent follow-up** is important. The history and the physical examination should be directed toward the breasts, bones, liver, chest wall, and nervous system. An annual mammogram of both breasts is recommended.

4. **Discussion of social and emotional issues is crucial.** The American Cancer Society's Reach to Recovery program is a valuable resource for patients.

C. **Fibroadenoma. Surgical excision,** preserving as much normal breast tissue as possible, is the preferred treatment. After excision, the patient should be reassured that she is at no increased risk of cancer.

D. **Mastitis.** Lactating women should be encouraged to continue nursing.

1. Ten days of an antibiotic effective against *S aureus* and streptococci should be sufficient.

   a. A penicillinase-resistant synthetic penicillin, such as dicloxacillin, 500 mg orally every 6 hours, should be used.

TABLE 8–1. PHARMACOLOGIC THERAPY FOR fiBROCYSTIC CHANGES

Drug	Dosage	Effectiveness (%)	Significant Side Effects
Danazol*	100–400 mg by mouth daily for 4–6 mo	60–90	Yes
Oral contraceptives (e.g., Loestrin 1/20)	1 tablet by mouth daily for 1–2 y	70–90	Some
Medroxyprogesterone acetate	10 mg by mouth on days 15–25 of the menstrual cycle for 9–12 mo	85	Some
Tamoxifen	10–20 mg by mouth daily for 4 mo	70–90	Yes
Bromocriptine	1.25–5.0 mg by mouth daily for 2–4 mo	50–80	Yes

*The only drug approved by the US Food and Drug Administration for the treatment of fibrocystic changes.

   b. For patients who are allergic to penicillin, erythromycin, 500 mg orally every 6 hours, is a reasonable alternative.
   2. Local heat is also of benefit.
   3. Failure of symptoms to respond to treatment in 48 hours or the development of a mass may indicate a breast abscess that requires incision and drainage. Inflammatory breast cancer must be considered in any mastitis that does not respond to treatment after 5 days or in non-nursing women with mastitis. A biopsy will establish the diagnosis.

REFERENCES

Bembo SA, Carlson HE. Gynecomastia. Its features, and when and how to treat it. *Cleve Clin J Med.* 2004;71:511.
Klein S. Evaluation of palpable breast masses. *Am Fam Physician.* 2005;71:1731.
Lucas JH, Cone DL. Breast cyst aspiration. *Am Fam Physician.* 2003;68:1983.
Santen RJ, Mansel R. Benign breast disorders. *N Engl J Med.* 2005;353:275.
Smith RL, Pruthi S, Fitzpatrick, LA. Evaluation and management of breast pain. *Mayo Clin Proc.* 2004;79:353.

---

9   Cellulitis & Other Bacterial Skin Infections

Donald B. Middleton, MD

KEY POINTS

- Most cellulitis and other skin infections are caused by *Staphylococcus aureus,* which is currently often methicillin resistant or to *Streptococcus pyogenes,* which remains sensitive to first-generation cephalosporins and penicillins.
- Skin infection with organisms such as *Pseudomonas aeruginosa* often suggests underlying bacteremia.
- Hospitalization is indicated for those who fail to respond to outpatient treatment, are toxic, or have high-risk medical conditions.

I. Definition. Bacterial infection of the superficial or deep layers or specialized structures of the dermis is common. Infection may be a primary process resulting from an often trivial breach of the skin's surface barrier allowing bacteria to penetrate or may reflect lymphatic or hematogenous spread from infection of another organ system. Factors facilitating infection include **primary skin diseases** (e.g., eczema or psoriasis); **trauma** (e.g., abrasions, burns, or bites); **immunologic defects** (e.g., AIDS, alcoholism, multiple myeloma, or diabetes mellitus); **contaminated wounds** (e.g., from dirty water, soil, or feces); concurrent or preexisting **viral or fungal infections** (e.g., herpes simplex cold sore or athlete's foot); **bacterial infection** in structures contiguous to the skin (e.g., osteomyelitis, tooth abscess, or sinusitis); **circulatory dysfunction** (e.g., edema or lymphedema); **bacteremia** (e.g., sexually transmitted diseases or subacute bacterial endocarditis); **pruritus** (uremia); and **psychologic distress** (neurodermatitis). Bacterial exotoxins enhance invasion and promote excretion of cytokines and lymphokines that cause inflammatory warmth and erythema. Out of more than 100 different bacterial pathogens reported to produce skin infection, by far the most common are *Staphylococcus aureus* or *Streptococcus pyogenes.* The likelihood of other organisms depends on host factors (e.g., age or immune status), source of inoculum (e.g., human or animal bite), and lesion morphology (e.g., erythema migrans in Lyme disease).

II. Common Diagnoses. In the primary care setting, bacterial skin infections account for at least 2% of ambulatory visits and are the 28th most common diagnosis in hospitalized persons, accounting for more than 30,000 admissions per year. Common bacterial skin infections are:

   A. Superficial infection (above or into the upper dermal papillae).
   1. Impetigo (Figure 9–1) is endemic in children, especially preschoolers. At least 20% of children have one or more bouts of this infection. The incidence peaks in late summer and early fall, when minor trauma from insect bites or abrasions promotes infection.

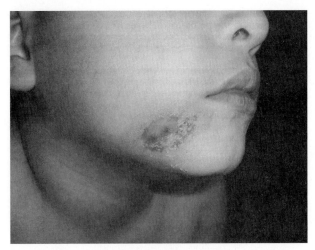

FIGURE 9–1. Erythrasma (see color insert). (Credit to Dr. Richard Usatine.)

Close person-to-person contact or scratching from winter dryness, hives, chickenpox, scabies, pediculosis, or tinea can initiate the infection and enhance spread. Epidemics of impetigo occur occasionally, for example, infecting a whole wrestling team. Underlying chronic disorders such as eczema or vascular stasis ulcers promote secondary infection. Impetigo can complicate surgical wounds.

2. **Erythrasma** (Figure 9–2) caused by *Corynebacterium* affects young men. In tropical climates, up to 20% of men develop this often chronic infection.

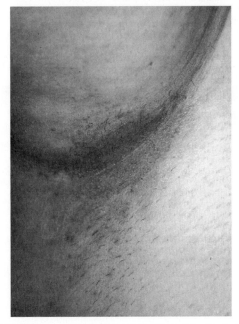

FIGURE 9–2. Impetigo (see color insert). (Credit to Dr. Richard Usatine.)

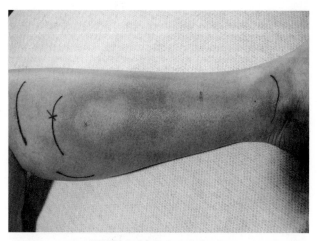

FIGURE 9–3. Cellulitis (see color insert).

B. Deep infection (epidermis and full dermal layer down into the subcutaneous fat).
  1. Cellulitis (Figure 9–3) follows trauma to the skin or occurs spontaneously in the young, elderly, diabetic, alcoholic, edematous, or immunocompromised patients. Recurrent cellulitis is common in those with an underlying chronic, dermatologic process such as lymphedema or eczema. Cases occur around year. Many subtypes are recognized. For example, **necrotizing fasciitis** occurs most commonly in the elderly patients, a minority of those who have diabetes mellitus or myxedema. Intravenous drug abusers and those with malignancy, anal fissure, hemorrhoids, peripheral vascular disease, or penetrating trauma are also at risk. Most cases are polymicrobial or caused by *S pyogenes* or *S aureus*. *S pyogenes* fasciitis often follows other illness such as chickenpox.
  2. A **furuncle (boil)** arises in an area prone to perspiration and friction and is most common in adults. Obesity, immunocompromise, and self-trauma, including squeezing a pimple, are important etiologic factors.
  3. A **carbuncle** (Figure 9–4) usually develops in those with immunodeficiencies owing to alcoholism or diabetes mellitus or those who self-traumatize a furuncle.

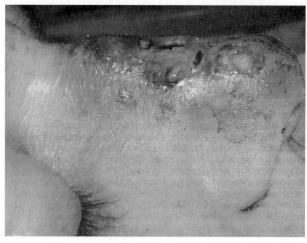

FIGURE 9–4. Carbuncle of the nose (see color insert).

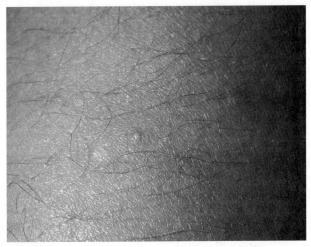

FIGURE 9-5. Folliculitis (see color insert). (Credit to Dr. Richard Usatine.)

4. **Ecthyma** is an ulcerated pyoderma that occurs in children or the neglected elderly patients, often after insect bites or skin excoriation.
5. **Erysipelas** is common in alcoholics, diabetics, or immunocompromised hosts but occasionally arises spontaneously in preschool children or older adults. Roughly 30% of patients have recurrences.

C. Specialized skin structure infection (initially localized to a hair follicle, sebaceous cyst, or sweat gland).
  1. **Folliculitis** (Figure 9–5) develops in moist areas with traumatized hair follicles. It often follows shaving, rubbing from tight clothing, or immersion in a hot tub and is usually caused by *Pseudomonas*.
  2. **Sebaceous gland abscess** occurs in those with repetitive sebaceous cyst trauma from squeezing or rubbing.

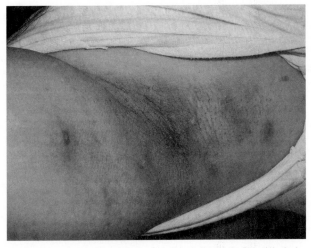

FIGURE 9-6. Hidradenitis suppurativa (see color insert). (Credit to Dr. Richard Usatine.)

TABLE 9–1. DIAGNOSING AND TREATING LESS COMMON BACTERIAL SKIN INFECTIONS

Condition	Findings	Treatment
Anthrax (*Bacillus anthracis*)	Painless papule progressing to vesicle to ulcer over 3–5 d Best diagnosed with punch biopsy of indurated plaque	Penicillin, ciprofloxacin, or doxycycline $\geq$ 10 d
Gangrene (*Clostridium perfringens* or mixed)	Gas in wound	Debride, oxygen, penicillin, or clindamycin
Erysipeloid (Erysipelothrix rhusiopathiae)	Contaminated animals or fish	Erythromycin or penicillin
Bacillary angiomatosis (*Rochalimaea henselae or R quintana*)	Typically AIDS/HIV patient with cherry angiomatous or pyogenic granuloma-like lesions	Erythromycin or doxycycline for 2 wks
Chancriform lesions (venereal [syphilis or chancroid or mycobacterial)	Ulcerative lesions (syphilitic are painless; chancroid are painful)	Based on cause
Lyme disease (*Borrelia burgdorferi*)	Red $\geq$ 5 cm circinate macule or target lesion at site of tick bite; similar distant lesions occur with hematogenous spread	Doxycycline or amoxicillin for 14–21 d
Paronychia or felon (*S aureus, S pyogenes*)	Red, swollen digit tip or nail bed	Warm soaks; I and D for felon; clindamycin or amoxicillin-clavulanate

3. **Hidradenitis suppurativa** (Figure 9–6), a sweat gland infection, does not occur prepubertally and usually follows axillary or groin shaving, particularly in the obese. Men are more likely to have perianal infection, and women are more likely to have axillary disease.

Some less common but important infections are listed in Table 9–1.

III. **Symptoms.** Most listed symptoms are common to all forms of infection.

A. **Pain** at the site of infection occurs with most infections, except perhaps impetigo, Lyme disease, and erythrasma.

B. **Pruritus** is common in impetigo, cellulitis, folliculitis, and erythrasma. Scratching often causes further trauma and promotes spread of infection.

C. **Feverishness, chills,** and **malaise** can develop acutely. These symptoms often reflect invasion of deeper tissues or the bloodstream, especially with cellulitis, erysipelas, or a carbuncle. Severely ill patients may either become septic or die. Erysipelas is especially prone to cause high fever.

IV. **Signs** (Table 9–2). The hallmarks of infection are tenderness, swelling, redness, and warmth. Most bacterial skin infections have a pathognomonic appearance, but some must be distinguished from allergic conditions (e.g., eczema), contact dermatitis (e.g., poison ivy), insect stings, trauma, and viral or fungal infections. A red streak emanating from the rash suggests lymphangitic spread from an infectious cellulitis. Scattered purple or red skin papules or macules may reflect underlying bacteremia with agents such as *Pseudomonas* or gonorrhea.

A. **Superficial infection**

1. Streptococcal **impetigo** presents as small vesicles with a red halo that gradually enlarge to 1 to 2 cm and develop central honey crusts. "Kissing" lesions occur where two skin surfaces touch. Autoinoculation and multiple lesions are common, particularly on the face. Classically, staphylococcus causes bullous lesions with little surrounding erythema, but it is often grown from nonbullous lesions. A varnishlike finish often coats ruptured bullae. Underlying viral or fungal infections can be distinguished from impetigo by the appearance of the primary lesions (the smaller vesicles of chickenpox or the circinate raised edge and central clearing of tinea corporis).

2. **Erysipelas** (Figure 9–7) is a fulminating cellulitis, with a raised, demarcated edge, and systemic fever. Seventy percent of cases are on the lower extremity, but it can occur on the forehead, face, and abdomen. A central *peau d'orange* ("orange peel") appearance is typical.

TABLE 9-2. DIAGNOSIS AND TREATMENT FOR COMMON SKIN INFECTIONS

Class	Condition	Findings	Treatment (Table 9-3)
Superficial infections	Impetigo	Small vesicles, enlarging to 1–2 cm with red halo and central "honey" crust (strep) versus bullous lesions with minimal surrounding erythema (staph)	Penicillinase-resistant penicillin, macrolide, or first generation cephalosporin; doxycycline, trimethaprim/sulfa, clindamycin, fluoroquinolone for MRSA; topical agents for small areas or nasal carriage; good hygiene (avoid scrubbing)
	Erythrasma	Finely scaled red-brown lesions, especially in genital folds	Erythromycin for 14–21 d
Deep infections	Cellulitis	Typically poorly demarcated Warmth/erythema/tenderness	Cephalosporin, fluoroquinolone, amoxicillin-clavulanate, azithromycin, clarithromycin, clindamycin; supportive care (limb elevation, warm soaks, and analgesics); hospitalization, if severely ill, immunocompromised, or gram-negative, or mixed aerobic/anaerobic cellulitis
	Erysipelas	Ill patient with well-demarcated erythema (70% involve lower extremity) with central *peau d'orange* appearance	Penicillin or erythromycin
	Preseptal orbital cellulitis	Red, swollen, tender eyelids	Amoxicillin-clavulanate, cefuroxime. Hospitalization, if ill-appearing
	Postseptal orbital cellulitis	Red, swollen, tender eyelids with proptosis, dysconjugate gaze, painful eye movement	Hospitalization for parenteral antibiotics
	Necrotizing fasciitis	Abrupt, painful onset; ill patient with initially only mildly abnormal skin	Multiple drug regimen.
	Furuncle	Hot/tender deep purulent boil.	Hospitalization for surgical debridement.
	Ecthyma	Typically neck, axilla, buttock, thigh	Moist heat, avoidance of squeezing, incision and drainage, if fluctuant
		Deep ulcerating lesions, especially in children or neglected elderly patients	Penicillin, cephalosporin; antipseudomonal, if testing warrants
Special skin structure	Carbuncle	Conglomeration of boils, with multiple purulent sites	Hospitalization for parenteral antistaphylococcal antibiotics and possible incision and drainage (I and D)
	Folliculitis	Red dome-shaped pustule(s) involving hair follicle(s)	Antistaphylococcal antibiotics (antipseudomonal with warm compresses and avoidance of cosmetics, if hot-tub folliculitis).
	Sebaceous cyst abscess	Painful, warm nodule with central black punctum	Office I and D, packing, 24 h follow-up; possibly antistaph antibiotics for 3–7 d
	Hidradenitis suppurativa	Carbuncle in axilla or groin, varying from acute/tender to chronically draining lesions	**Acute:** Antistrep or antistaph antibiotics, warm compress, topical isotretinoin, avoid shaving or deodorants, surgical referral **Chronic:** May respond to ≥3 mo of tetracycline

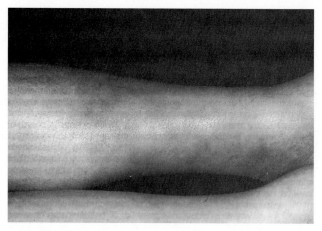

FIGURE 9–7. Erysipelas (see color insert). (Credit to Dr. Richard Usatine.)

   3. Erythrasma is usually located in intertriginous areas, especially the genitals or some-
      times the feet, is colored red-brown and is finely scaled. Secondary to *Corynebac-
      terium minutissimum* invasion, it is often mistaken for *Candida*.
B. Deep infection
   1. Cellulitis is acutely tender, red, and hot. The leading edge is not raised but can be
      well defined. Propagation from a central traumatic lesion is centripetal and rapid,
      often resulting in lymphangitis or lymphadenopathy. An allergic reaction is seldom as
      warm, tender, or well demarcated. Infection is occasionally indolent and can spread
      to regional lymph nodes, blood, fascia, or muscle, creating a life-threatening situation.
      Special situations are listed below.
      a. Cellulitis of the head. **Preseptal orbital cellulitis** (Figure 9–8), involving only the
         eyelids, and **postseptal orbital cellulitis,** including orbital structures, both make
         the eyelids red and swollen. Postseptal cellulitis presents with dysconjugate gaze,

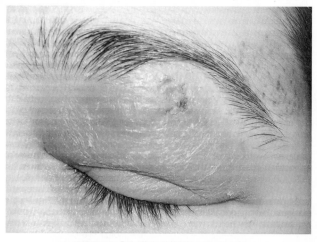

FIGURE 9–8. Periorbital cellulitis (see color insert).

proptosis, and painful eye movements. Cheeks that are marked by a bluish discoloration and woody consistency indicate facial or buccal cellulitis, often secondary to *Haemophilus influenzae* type b (Hib) or pneumococcus.
   b. Hand cellulitis often follows puncture wounds, such as animal bites or foreign body insertion. Cat or dog bites may often produce infection with *Pasteurella multocida.* **Cellulitis of the foot or the leg** often coexists with osteomyelitis in the immunocompromised or diabetic host.
   c. Cellulitis with a tense firm portion may indicate subcutaneous abscess formation.
   d. Infection caused by**necrotizing fasciitis** has an abrupt, exquisitely painful onset that evolves over 1 to 3 days from cyanosis and edema into necrosis, sometimes accompanied by subcutaneous crepitance indicating gas-forming agents.
   2. A **furuncle** is a localized, deep-seated, hot, tender pus-containing boil, commonly on the neck, axillae, buttock, or thigh.
   3. A **carbuncle** is a conglomeration of boils with suppuration and many pus-draining ports.
C. Special skin structure infection.
   1. Folliculitis produces small, red, domed-shaped pustules over the hair follicles that can be acute or chronic.
   2. Sebaceous cyst abscess is a raised, painful, hot boil in sebaceous cyst. A black dot in the center of the lesion is a pore indicative of sebaceous gland involvement.
   3. Hidradenitis suppurativa is a carbuncle of the axilla or groin involving the apocrine sweat glands. It has a highly variable clinical course from an acute, red, tender infection with multiple drainage sites to a chronic scarified slowly draining lesion.
V. Laboratory Tests. Most skin infections, such as impetigo or cellulitis, can be treated empirically based on morphology and likely causative agents. Cultures of the leading edge (10%–15% positive), central abrasions (15%–50% positive), or blood (a small % positive) are minimally beneficial. Cultures of skin biopsies also have marginal value.
A. Cultures are warranted in certain situations.
   1. Blood cultures are positive in 80% of patients with Hib and in approximately 20% of pneumococcal cellulitis of the eye or face. Blood cultures should be obtained from patients who are toxic or immunocompromised, who have preseptal or postseptal orbital cellulitis, necrotizing fasciitis, diabetes, facial cellulitis, or fever with scattered papules/macules, or who fail to respond to treatment.
   2. Needle aspiration of unruptured bullae or pus from incised abscesses provides reliable culture data, especially with **paronychia** or a **boil.** However, cultures are unnecessary in most cases. **Gram stain** and **culture** are often helpful, especially in severely ill patients.
   3. Conjunctival cultures may be useful in preseptal or postseptal cellulitis.
   4. Skin biopsy may help with atypical lesions. For example, anthrax is best diagnosed with a **punch biopsy** of the indurated plaque.
   5. Bone biopsy with culture is the definitive test to diagnose coexistent osteomyelitis. Orthopedic consultation is required for bone biopsy, although some neuropathic patients with open wounds may have protruding fractured bone fragments that can be removed for culture.
B. Special procedures are sometimes helpful.
   1. Plain radiographs may detect tissue gas or foreign bodies, as well as bone, tooth socket, or sinus infection.
   2. Sonograms have proven value to detect underlying abscess or pus collection.
   3. Magnetic resonance imaging (MRI) or **computerized tomography scans** can distinguish preseptal from postseptal cellulitis. MRI is useful to detect underlying osteomyelitis or abscess formation, especially in diabetics or immunocompromised hosts.
   4. Bone scans in selected cases (diabetics with foot infection, cases of extremity cellulitis that fail to improve, or trauma victims with crush injury) can detect concomitant osteomyelitis.
   5. Wood's lamp illumination is useful in erythrasma; the infected skin fluoresces coral red.
VI. Treatment (Tables 9–1 to 9–3). A 7- to 10-day course of antibiotics is required for nearly all bacterial skin infections, (SOR **A**) most of which can be managed as outpatient therapy. Ordinarily, complete resolution is achievable, but recurrences are common. Therapeutic decisions include whether to hospitalize or seek consultation. Toxic patients or those with mixed aerobic and anaerobic infections, postseptal cellulitis, necrotizing fasciitis, or gram-negative

TABLE 9–3. ANTIBIOTICS FOR SKIN INFECTIONS (USUAL COURSE 7–14 D)

Drug (Trade Name)	Route of Administration*	Pediatric Dose (mg/kg/d)[†,‡]	Adult Dose (g/d)[†]	Interval (dose/day)
Penicillins				
Penicillin G	IV	250,000–400,000 units	8–24 million units	4
Penicillin V	po	25–50	1–2	4
Amoxicillin	po	20–40	0.75–1.5	3
Ampicillin	po, IV, Im	25–200	1–12	4
Ampicillin-clavulanate (Augmentin)	po	20–40	0.75–1.5	3
Nafcillin	po, IV, Im	50–200	1–12	4
Oxacillin	po, IV, Im	50–200	1–12	4
Dicloxacillin	po	12.5–25	1–2	4
Piperacillin-tazobactam	IV	Dose based on piperacillin content; 100–300; safety not established under age 12 y	6–24	4–6
Cephalosporins				
For use against gram-positive cocci and some gram-negative agents				
Cefadroxil (Duricef)	po	30	1–2	1–2
Cephalexin (Keflex)	po	25–100	1–4	4
For use against above plus *Haemophilus influenzae*				
Cefaclor (Ceclor)	po	20–40	0.750–4	2–3
Cefprozil (Cefzil)	po	15–30	0.5–2	1–2
Ceftibuten (Cedax)	po	9	0.09–0.4	1
Cefuroxime axetil (Ceftin)	po	20–30 or 125 or 250 mg/dose	0.5–1	2
Loracarbef (Lorabid)	po	15–30	0.4–0.8	2
For use against primarily gram-negative agents and most gram-positive cocci				
Cefixime (Lupin)	po	8	0.4	1
Cefpodoxime (Vantin)	po	10	0.2–0.8	1–2
Ceftriaxone (Rocephin)	IV, IM	50–100	1–4	1–2
Other antibiotics				
Erythromycin (many)	po, IV	30–50	1–2	3–4
Clarithromycin (Biaxin)	po	15	0.5–1	2
Azithromycin (Zithromax)	po	5–10	0.5 initial, then 0.25	1
Doxycycline (many)	po	Over age 8 y	200	2
Clindamycin (Cleocin)	po, IV	10–40	0.6–2.7	3–4
Metronidazole (Flagyl)	po, IV	15–30	0.75–2	3
Vancomycin (Vancocin)	IV	10–15	0.5–2	1–4
Linezolid (Zyvox)	po, IV	30	800–1200	2–3
Trimethoprim/sulfamethoxazole (Bactrim)	po, IV	5 mL syrup/10 kg/dose (max 20 mL)	320/1600	2
Tigecycline (Tygacil)	IV	Not used	0.1 initial then 0.05	2
Fluoroquinolones (over age 18 y only)				
Ciprofloxacin (Cipro)	po, IV	Not used	0.5–1.5	2
Gatifloxacin (Tequin)	po, IV	Not used	0.4	1
Levofloxacin (Levaquin)	po, IV	Not used	0.25–0.75	1
Lomefloxacin (Maxaquin)	po	Not used	0.4	1
Moxifloxacin (Avelox)	po, IV	Not used	0.4	1
Ofloxacin (Floxin)	po, IV		0.4–0.8	2
Topical agents				
Mupirocin (Bactroban)	Topical			2–5
Bacitracin (many)	Topical			3–5
Retapamulin (Altabax)	Topical			2

*po, oral; IV, intravenous; IM, intramuscular.
[†] Dosage may require adjustment in renal failure.
[‡] Not to exceed the adult dose.

cellulitis, especially *Pseudomonas,* or inadequate social supports are best hospitalized. Unfamiliar lesions are best handled through consultation. Patients with preseptal cellulitis, cellulitis of the hand, or immunocompromised status have been successfully treated as outpatients.

A. Superficial infection

1. **Impetigo** is best treated with a penicillinase-resistant penicillin, macrolide, or first-generation cephalosporin. (SOR **Ⓐ**) Recent studies suggest that *S aureus,* usually phage group II, is a major culprit. **Cephalexin** seems ideal for all cases of **impetigo,** but alternatives include any agent that eradicates streptococci and staphylococci, such as **clindamycin, azithromycin, clarithromycin,** or **amoxicillin-clavulanate.** Streptococcus has been reported to be resistant to erythromycin. Unfortunately methicillin-resistant *S. aureus* (MRSA) is becoming much more common causing up to 50% of cellulitis and skin abscesses in some series. Persons who fail to respond to oral cephalosporins should be considered to have MRSA and treated appropriately (see below). Topical agents, especially **mupirocin** ointment (Bactroban) (SOR **Ⓐ**) applied 3 times a day, and perhaps **retapamulin** (Altabax), are effective for small areas. Agents such as **hexachlorophene** are not highly efficacious. With treatment, impetigo responds rapidly in more than 90% of cases; the spontaneous resolution rate is 60% in 10 days. Glomerulonephritis or, rarely, toxic shock, may complicate streptococcal impetigo. Scalded skin syndrome, or, rarely, toxic shock may follow staphylococcal disease. Parents and patients should be warned to look for hematuria and peeling skin in the week following treatment. Although good hygiene is helpful, scrubbing tends to spread infection. Eradication of nasal carriage of staphylococci or streptococci with topical **mupirocin** or oral **rifampin** may interrupt repetitive infections.

2. Topical **isotretinoin (Retin A)** applied to areas of recurrent infection once a day and doxycycline orally have proven prophylactic valve, especially for **hidradenitis suppurativa.**

3. **Erysipelas** is treated with penicillins or cephalosporins and usually defervesces within 24 to 48 hours of initiation of appropriate treatment but may recur in up to 30% of cases.

4. **Erythrasma** is treated with macrolide antibiotics (14–21 days of erythromycin) and topical econazole cream applied twice daily but can relapse into asymptomatic infection lasting for years.

B. Deep infection. Although the major pathogens in **cellulitis** are group A (rarely group C or G) *S pyogenes* and *S aureus,* numerous other bacteria are capable of producing cellulitis, including Hib (buccal cellulitis in young infants), *S pneumoniae* (preseptal or postseptal orbital cellulitis), mouth anaerobes such as peptostreptococcus (human bites), soil bacteria such as *Clostridia* (necrotizing fasciitis), *P multocida* (cat bites), and coliform organisms (decubitus ulcers).

1. In selecting an antibiotic for cellulitis, likely etiologic agents, cost, and side effect profile should be considered. Cellulitis responds well to **cephalosporins, fluoroquinolones, amoxicillin-clavulanate, azithromycin, clarithromycin,** and **clindamycin. Cephalexin, cefadroxil, cefaclor, cefuroxime,** and **cefixime** are the most often utilized cephalosporins, but cefixime is not effective for staphylococcus. MRSA responds to **sulfamethoxazole/trimethaprim** or **doxycycline.** Scattered reports of community-acquired MRSA resistance to other often used drugs (**clindamycin, fluoroquinolones, minocycline, and doxycycline**) exist. **Vancomycin** is warranted for systemically ill MRSA patients. (SOR **Ⓐ**) In streptococcal disease, penicillin or cephalexin are the drugs of choice, whereas synthetic penicillins such as oxacillin are highly effective for both staphylococcus and streptococcus. Severely ill or immuno-compromised patients should be broadly treated initially with a penicillin/β–lactam combination or a third-generation cephalosporin with vancomycin until culture results direct narrowing of the antibiotic regimen. Although no randomized controlled trials are available, a trial of intravenous **cefazolin** plus oral probenecid proved equal to intravenous **ceftriaxone** in adults with moderate to severe cellulitis. Oral cephalosporin or fluoroquinolone (contraindicated in children younger than 19 years) offers a satisfactory alternative to prolonged hospitalization.

a. **Necrotizing ("flesh-eating") fasciitis** usually reflects group A streptococcus infection alone or mixed with other, usually anaerobic, bacteria. If the infection is gas producing, *Clostridia* should be suspected. **Necrotizing fasciitis** requires hospitalization for surgical debridement and treatment with parental clindamycin and penicillin. (SOR **Ⓐ**)

2. **Supportive care** includes limb elevation, moist warm soaks, and analgesics (e.g., acetaminophen, aspirin, or ibuprofen in appropriate doses). However, some nonsteroidal anti-inflammatory drugs (NSAIDs) may actually delay recovery. Patients with underlying congestive heart failure, stasis ulceration, or diabetes mellitus frequently develop recurrent cellulitis of the legs. Support stockings or Unna boot therapy may help. Hyperbaric oxygen is of limited value for routine cellulitis but may benefit clostridial infections.

3. **Carbuncles** should be treated with systemic antibiotics directed against staphylococci (e.g.,**nafcillin, cefazolin, clindamycin, or vancomycin)**, incision and drainage, and hospitalization.

4. **Ecthyma** is treated with penicillin, a cephalosporin, or in appropriate instances an antipseudomonal antibiotic.

C. **Specialized skin structure infection**

1. Recurrent **folliculitis** may be treated prophylactically with chronic topical antibiotics. Normal saline compresses and avoidance of hot tubs or cosmetics help in some cases. **Sycosis barbae,** a deep folliculitis of the beard, is treated with saline compresses, topical mupirocin, or bacitracin and if recalcitrant, with oral cephalosporins for 7 to 10 days.

2. Incision, drainage, and packing alone may be adequate for **sebaceous cyst abscess**. Some advise antistaphylococcal antibiotics (e.g., cephalexin) for 3 to 7 days to reduce chance of spread.

3. **Hidradenitis suppurativa** is treated with antibiotics, warm compresses, referral for surgical excision, avoidance of shaving and deodorants, topical daily isotretinion, and occasionally prednisone, 40 to 60 mg orally daily for 5 to 10 days, to diminish scarring. Chronic infection may respond to a tetracycline (e.g., doxycycline) orally for ≥ 3 months.

REFERENCES

Cox NH. Management of lower leg cellulitis. *Clin Med*. 2002;2:23.

Stevens DL et al. IDSA practice guidelines for the diagnosis and management of skin and soft-tissue infections. *Clinical Infect Dis*. 2005;41:1373.

Stevens DL. Infections of the skin, muscle, and soft tissues. In: Kasper DL et al., eds. *Harrison's Principles of Internal Medicine*. 16th ed. McGraw-Hill; 2005:740.

Stulberg DL et al. Common bacterial skin infections. *AFP*. 2002;66:119.

Swartz MN, Pasternak MS. Cellulitis and subcutaneous tissue infections. In: Mandell GL, et al., eds. *Principles and Practice of Infectious Diseases*. 6th ed. New York: Churchill Livingstone; 2005:1172.

Swartz MN. Cellulitis. *NEJM*. 2004;350:904.

Tayal VS et al. The effect of soft-tissue ultrasound on the management of cellulitis in the emergency department. *Acad Emerg Med*. 2006;13:384.

---

10   Chest Pain

George P.N. Samraj, MD

KEY POINTS

- In most cases, the chest pain encountered in ambulatory primary care is not life-threatening and is related to chest wall or gastrointestinal in origin.
- Most causes of chest pain can be managed in the primary care ambulatory setting.
- Missed diagnosis of coronary artery disease (CAD) is common (~20%) in the emergency department (ED) and in primary care clinics
- A careful and comprehensive history and physical examination with risk factor assessment and focused testing (laboratory studies, imaging studies) uncover potentially serious conditions, including coronary ischemic disorders or pulmonary embolism (PE).

I. **Definition.** Chest pain (CP) is discomfort or pain that is experienced anywhere along the front of the body between neck and the upper abdomen. The chest pain can be acute (<72 hours), subacute (3 days to a month), chronic (more than a month), or chronic with an acute exacerbation and can be produced by a plethora of conditions, including cardiac, pulmonary, musculoskeletal , upper gastrointestinal (GI), and psychologic.

II. **Common Diagnoses.** CP is one of the most common symptoms for which patients seek medical attention. CP is because of myriad common and non-life-threatening conditions, as well as life-threatening conditions including myocardial infarction, aortic dissection, pneumothorax, pulmonary embolism, and esophageal rupture.

   A. Thirty-six to 38% of chest pain is **chest wall pain** (neuromusculoskeletal disorders); 20% is owing to muscle pain; 13% to costochondritis; 2% to broken ribs; and <1% each to fibrocystic breast disease, sickle cell crisis, herpes zoster, and chest wall bruising or trauma. Protracted cough or vomiting may contribute to chest wall syndromes. Chest wall pain is most common in active, young men and women, especially with a history of chest trauma or work/recreational activities involving repetitive upper extremity motion, lifting, or range of motion extremes.

   B. **GI sources** account for 20% to 30 % of chest pain, including gastroesophageal reflux disease (GERD) and esophagitis (13%), achalasia and esophageal spasm (4%), dyspepsia (1%–2%), peptic ulcer disease and gallbladder disease (1% each), and hiatal hernia, and other esophageal motility disorders (<1% each). Factors increasing the likelihood of a GI source of chest pain include past history of ulcers or dyspepsia, cigarette use, use of nonsteroidal anti-inflammatory drugs (NSAIDs), or use of other gastric irritants (e.g., ethanol, aspirin, erythromycin, tetracycline, or alendronate). It is wise for clinicians to specifically inquire about over-the-counter (OTC) NSAID and aspirin products, which patients often fail to recognize and which carry similar GI risk as prescription products.

   C. **Cardiovascular (CV) conditions** account for approximately 20% of all CP. The most common CV causes include angina (10%), myocardial infarction (2%–3%), unstable angina (1.5%), cardiac arrhythmia (1%), and mitral valve prolapse (2%); CP caused by aortic dissection or aortic aneurysm, pericarditis, and pericardial tamponade is substantially less frequent (each <1%). Heart disease is the leading cause of death for both women and men in the United States and accounts for 29% of all deaths. Each year over a million people in the United States suffer from myocardial infarction. The likelihood of CV causes of CP increases in older patients, those with previous history of CAD (coronary artery disease), and persons with a burden of CV risk factors, such as hypertension, dyslipidemia, smoking, and diabetes. Illicit substance use, particularly cocaine, is increasingly recognized as a contributor to acute chest pain, including MI, especially in younger persons, even in the absence of traditional CV risk factors. Within 1 hour of cocaine use, risk of MI is increased 24-fold compared to risk in nonusers.

THORACIC AORTIC DISSECTION/ANEURYSM

CP is the most common presentation of aortic dissection. Aortic dissection often presents suddenly with an abrupt onset of unremitting excruciating, ripping or tearing, and knifelike chest pain, radiating through to the back. Less commonly, dissection presents as less severe nagging midchest discomfort and occasionally painlessly. Aortic arch dissection may present with neck pain. Risk factors are hypertension, tobacco abuse, congenital aortic valvular or ascending aortic disease, atherosclerotic inflammatory/collagen aortic disease, pregnancy, cocaine use. Physical examination may reveal an anxious, dyspneic patient with hypo- or hypertension, differences between right and left arm blood pressures, absent arm or other pulses, a harsh/holosystolic heart murmur associated with aortic insufficiency, pulsus paradoxus, and less often, paralysis.

When dissection is suspected by clinical history, the patient should be hospitalized, with emergent cardiothoracic surgery consult and imaging studies (e.g., chest computerized tomography [CT] scan, echocardiography) to confirm the diagnosis.

PERICARDITIS

Pericarditis is because of inflammation of pericardium caused by various factors including infections (e.g., tuberculosis, HIV, or viral), inflammatory conditions (e.g., connective tissue disease), malignancy (e.g., leukemia, other cancers), endocrinologic disorders (e.g., hypothyroidism), renal disorders (e.g., kidney failure), postMI, and medications (e.g., procainamide, hydralazine, isoniazid). Pericarditis usually presents with substernal CP that is relieved by sitting up and leaning forward. The pain is typically pleuritic with a sharp and stabbing character, which may radiate to the neck, shoulder, back, or abdomen. Pericarditis pain often increases with deep breathing or lying flat, and may also increase with coughing and swallowing. Patients may experience dyspnea, including orthopnea, fever, fatigue, anxiety, and cough may be seen, and heart failure secondary to tamponade may lead to lower extremity edema.

CV examination may reveal a pericardial rub. Heart sounds may be heard as muffled or distant. Lung examination may reveal signs of pleural effusion. Appropriate evaluations include chest x-ray (which may reveal cardiomegaly, a bottle-shaped heart in myocarditis, but sometimes is completely normal.), EKG (manifesting abnormalities in voltage and ST-segment elevation in up to 90% of patients), CBC, cardiac enzymes, CRP (C-reactive protein), erythrocyte sedimentation rate (ESR), blood cultures. Echocardiogram is of great help in identification of pericardial effusion. Sometimes CT scan, magnetic resonance imaging (MRI), or radionuclide scanning assists to clarify etiology and therapy. Pericardiocentesis can be both diagnostic and therapeutic. Treatment is supportive with serial monitoring, use of oral anti-inflammatory drugs, and treatment of underlying disease processes.

D. **Psychosocial sources** account for **10% to 20%** of all chest pain; these include stress-related sources (8%) and panic disorder and somatization disorder (<1% each). Chest pain is a pain in which as many as 75% of patients with panic disorder present to the ED. Emotional stress may also exacerbate GERD, cardiac chest pain, and asthma.

E. Five to 10% of chest pain is **pulmonary,** including bronchitis (2%); pleurisy (1%–2%); pneumonia (1%); and pneumonitis, sarcoidosis, obstructive lung mass, pulmonary embolus, pulmonary abscess, ruptured bullae, pneumothorax, asthma, or viral upper respiratory infection (<1% each). Risk factors for **bronchitis/pneumonia** include chronic lung disease, altered consciousness/impaired gag reflex, immunodeficiency, neuromuscular disease, and thoracic cage deformity. **Pneumonitis** tends to occur with occupational or other exposure to chemical irritants (e.g., farming, factory/foundry work, cleaning). Teens who recreationally sniff chemicals are at high risk for pneumonitis. Risk factors for **deep venous thrombosis and pulmonary embolism (PE)** (see sidebar) include prolonged immobilization, pregnancy or recent delivery, pelvic or lower extremity trauma, hypercoagulability, estrogen use, and malignancy. (see also Chapters 23 and 42.)

PULMONARY EMBOLISM (PE)

PE presents with shortness of breath, (either active or at rest) and/or with CP worse with deep breathing and unrelieved by rest. CP can be sharp, stabbing, or dull aching. It may be associated with tachycardia, dyspnea, tachypnea, occasional hemoptysis, sweating, or lightheadedness.

Physical findings range from normal to tachypnea, isolated rales, and occasionally a pulmonary rub (an end-inspiratory rubbing sound). Pulmonary hypertension associated with PE may produce left heart failure (fine bibasilar lung rales) or will be restricted to echocardiographic or angiographic abnormalities. Clinical scoring systems (Table 10–1) can be helpful in determining the risk for PE and the need for further testing, which should be done in the hospital setting.

F. Although rare in the office setting, **major trauma** (e.g., cardiac tamponade, tension pneumothorax) also produces chest pain.

III. **Symptoms.** A careful history can narrow the differential diagnosis of chest pain and should address location and quality of pain, risk factors, exacerbating/alleviating factors, and associated symptoms.

A. **Location/quality of pain**

1. **Ischemic heart disease** patients complain of substernal tightness, pressure, or both, which may radiate to either arm or to the jaw, the back, or both. It may be associated with sob, nausea, vomiting, dizziness, syncope, and sweating.

TABLE 10–1. PREDICTION RULES FOR SUSPECTED PULMONARY EMBOLISM

Geneva Score	Points	Wells' Score	Points
Previous pulmonary embolism or deep vein thrombosis	+2	Previous pulmonary embolism or deep vein thrombosis	+1.5
Heart rate >100 beats per minute	+1	Heart rate >100 beats per minute	+1.5
Recent surgery	+3	Recent surgery or immobilization	+1.5
Age (y)		Clinical signs of deep vein thrombosis	+3
60–79	+1	Alternative diagnosis less likely than pulmonary embolism	+3
>80	+2	Hemoptysis	+1
P_aCo_2		Cancer	+1
<4.8 kPa (36 mm Hg)	+2		
4.8– 5.19 kPa (36–38.9 mm Hg)	+1		
<6.5 kPa (48.7 mm Hg)	+4		
Clinical probability		Clinical probability	
Low	0–4	Low	0–1
Intermediate	5–8	Intermediate	2–6
High	>9	High	>7

2. **Mitral valve prolapse (MVP)** produces an often sudden onset of chest discomfort/pain with palpitations.
3. **Pleuritic pain** is often sharp, stabbing, and localized within the left or right hemithorax and aggravated by breathing and coughing.
4. **Chest wall/muscle pain** is also a sharp to dull ache and may be localized anywhere on the chest wall.
5. **GI pain** may be substernal and burning (dyspepsia/GERD) or squeezing, substernal pressure (achalasia/esophageal spasm). Achalasia presents with pain behind the sternum or midchest. Peptic ulcer and pancreatitis may present with pain in the epigastrium and sometimes in the back.
6. **Some psychiatric conditions** present with precordial CP. **Hyperventilation presents with** precordial pain associated with dyspnea, tingling and numbness of the limbs, and dizziness, whereas depression may present with constant or intermittent heaviness unrelated to activity or meals.

B. **Risk factors** (see Section II.A–E.)

C. **Exacerbating/alleviating factors**
1. **Pain from ischemic heart disease** is worsened with activity or stress and alleviated by rest or by oxygen, nitrates, or both.
2. **Chest wall/muscle strain pain** is worsened with arm movements or deep inspiration. **Pleuritic chest pain** may also be produced or exacerbated by deep inspiration or cough.
3. **GI pain** is exacerbated by meals (particularly large meals) and supine position; antacids, protein pump inhibitors, or histamine-2 (H_2) blockers typically alleviate this pain. In particular, **gallbladder pain** is classically brought on by high-fat meals.

D. **Associated symptoms**
1. Nausea, dyspnea, diaphoresis, or sudden, severe overwhelming fatigue (particularly in women) may accompany **ischemic heart disease.**
2. **MVP** may be associated with **palpitations** (especially when supine), lightheadedness, dyspnea, anxiety, or headaches.
3. **Cough** frequently accompanies **pulmonary chest pain** or **heart failure;** fever with productive or nonproductive cough occurs in **pneumonia;** insidious-onset cough with dyspnea and occasionally fever characterizes **pneumonitis.**
4. **Syncope and hypotension** may be seen with myocardial ischemia, aortic dissection, or PE.
5. **Fatigue with CP** is a presentation of ischemia.
6. **Associated arrhythmia:** Palpitations (e.g., owing to ventricular ectopy, atrial fibrillation) may be associated with CAD. In a patient with new onset of atrial fibrillation and chest pain, **PE** should be considered as a diagnosis.
7. **GI chest pain** is often associated with nocturnal/morning cough, flatus, belching, hoarseness, halitosis, dysphagia, or odynophagia.

8. A sensation of dyspnea, an inability to breathe deeply, or frank hyperventilation often accompanies **psychogenic chest pain.** Such pain is frequently associated with other somatic pain (chronic headaches, abdominal or pelvic pain); panic disorder may feature the foregoing, along with paresthesias, dizziness, trembling, diaphoresis, and a sense of "impending doom."

E. **Patient characteristics:**

   Age, gender, ethnicity, culture, and comorbid medical conditions are pertinent in the evaluation of CP; e.g., younger patients are less likely to have underlying CAD; women and older individuals (>70 years) are more likely to have 'atypical' presentations. (SOR **Ⓐ**)

F. **Location and nature of pain**
   1. **Ischemic pain** tends to be nonlocalized, involves a larger area, and can be difficult to describe (diffused discomfort, ill-defined area), whereas **musculoskeletal and pleuritic pain** are easy to describe and localized (may point with one finger).
   2. **Referred pain** may follow nerve distribution and is sometimes difficult to localize.
   3. **Radiation to both arms** (left or right: left more than the right), neck, throat, lower jaw, teeth, upper extremity, shoulders are strong predictors of myocardial ischemic pain.

G. **Time of onset and duration of pain:**
   1. **Abrupt CP of great intensity** is more common with PE, aortic dissection, or pneumothorax; myocardial ischemic pain (and esophageal disease) is usually more gradual, with crescendo intensity over time.
   2. **Persistent pain of longer duration (days)** without progression is associated with functional disease.
   3. **Fleeting pain**, lasting only a few seconds is unlikely to be ischemic. Similarly, **enduring pain (weeks)** is probably not ischemic in origin Ischemic pain, although it may occur at any time, is disproportionately frequent in the **early morning hours.**
   4. **Cold weather, emotional stress, or sexual activities** are commonly recognized triggers for myocardial ischemia.

IV. **Signs.** Important aspects of the focused physical examination in all patients with chest pain include general appearance and vital signs, palpation (chest wall and epigastrium), and cardiopulmonary auscultation.

A. **General appearance/vital signs.** Those with **acute cardiac ischemia** (crescendo angina or MI) and those with **panic/anxiety** may appear anxious and dyspneic; **ischemic heart disease** may also cause hyper- or hypotension and diaphoresis; **panic/anxiety** may cause tremor.

B. **Palpation**
   1. In **chest wall pain,** opposed movement or palpation of affected muscles or ligaments reproduces pain, while palpation of the costochondral junction (especially of the third and fourth ribs) reproduces **costochondral chest wall pain.** Chest wall tenderness may be present in patients suffering from myocardial ischemia. Herpes zoster is associated with rash and **hyperalgesia**; pain may precede the rash of zoster; uncommonly, zoster pain may occur without rash.
   2. **GI pain** may be associated with midepigastric tenderness.

C. **Auscultation**
   1. **Cardiac auscultation** in **ischemic heart disease** may be normal or may reveal a new murmur or S_3 or S_4 gallop; in **MVP,** auscultation classically reveals a mid-to-late systolic click and a late systolic murmur.
   2. **Pulmonary auscultation**
      a. **Pleuritic pain** may feature a friction rub, an end-inspiratory sound consistent with the rubbing of one's hand against rubber.
      b. Findings in **pneumonia** include localized rales, egophony ("e" to "a" changes), and expiratory sounds such as wheezes or more course rhonchi, which may decrease or be brought out by coughing.
      c. **Pneumonitis** may be accompanied by fine bibasilar rales.

V. **Laboratory Testing** (Figure 10–1). When a common cause of chest pain is highly probable based on focused history and examination (e.g., chest wall pain or costochondritis), further testing is unnecessary and treatment can be initiated. Further testing is necessary when the etiology or severity of the chest pain remains unclear after focused history and examination, as is often the case with ischemic heart and pulmonary diseases.

A. **Hematologic tests**
   1. **Complete blood count** may show leukocytosis and left shift with bacterial pneumonia and lymphocytosis with viral pneumonia or reduced haemoglobin suggestive of anemia.

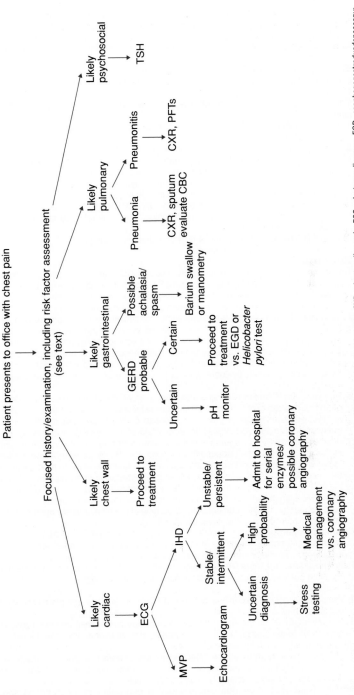

FIGURE 10-1. An approach to evaluation of common causes of chest pain. CBC, complete blood count; CXR, chest radiograph; ECG, electrocardiogram; EGD, esophagogastroduodenoscopy; GERD, gastroesophageal reflux disease; IHD, ischemic heart disease; MVP, mitral valve prolapse; PFTs, pulmonary function tests; TSH, thyroid-stimulating hormone.

2. **Metabolic panel** assesses kidney function (before imaging with contrast),
3. **Thyroid-stimulating hormone levels** may be low or undetectable in hyperthyroidism, which may contribute to anxiety states.
4. **Blood *Helicobacter pylori* testing** can evaluate for this potential cause of refractory dyspepsia.

B. **Electrocardiogram (ECG)** is often normal in ischemic heart disease (IHD); in a setting compatible with acute IHD, ST-segment elevation, or depression can assist the decision to hospitalize.

C. **Chest radiography** is helpful in both suspected cardiac and pulmonary causes of chest pain.
   1. **Cardiomegaly** may be seen in dilated cardiomyopathy because of chronic ischemic heart disease (IHD).
   2. **Infiltrates** may be apparent in pneumonia or pneumonitis.
      a. **Lobar consolidation** (bacterial pneumonia) or diffused infiltrates (atypical or early pneumonia) may occur, but they generally lag behind clinical symptoms by hours-to-days and may be better visualized after rehydration.
      b. **Diffused infiltrates** may also be seen in pneumonitis.
      c. **Pneumothorax.** In tension pneumothorax, CXR may show increased thoracic volume, ipsilateral heart border flattening, contralateral mediastinal deviation, depression of hemidiaphragm
      d. **In CHF, there may be** signs of fluid collection in the lungs.
      e. **Rib fractures may be evident.**

D. **Stress testing**
   1. **Exercise stress electrocardiography** detects ECG changes occurring during exercise and absent on resting ECG. Dramatic ST-segment changes (>2 mm), particularly at low workloads (i.e., <6 minutes on Bruce protocol or at <70% of age-predicted maximum heart rate) indicate severe IHD and the need for coronary angiography.
   2. **Exercise stress echocardiography** allows for similar evaluation as exercise stress ECG; however, echocardiography is preferred in certain patients, including women and those with obesity, pendulous breasts, left ventricular hypertrophy, or previous ECG changes (such as a bundle branch block, pacemaker, or previous MI) precluding evaluation for ischemia using ECG alone. In addition to ECG changes, stress echocardiography can evaluate wall motion abnormalities and ventricular ejection fraction.
   3. **Pharmacologic stress testing** is preferred in individuals unable to achieve adequate heart rate through exercise; this inability may be because of severe arthritis, neurologic or vascular disease, obesity, pulmonary disease, or simply severe deconditioning. Categorically, pharmacologic stress tests employ either coronary vasodilators (e.g., dipyridamole, adenosine), or agents which increase heart rate (e.g., dobutamine). Either stressor will accentuate inadequacies on coronary flow. Since vasodilators preferentially dilate the non-stenotic coronary circulation, adenosine/dipyridamole will magnify the circulatory deficit seen under exercise by preferentially shunting flow to the non-stenotic areas. By increasing heart rate, a pharmacologic agent (e.g., dobutamine) simulates exercise without the patient exercising. Intravenous administration of a radioisotope (e.g., thallium, technetium-sestamibi) at the time of stress testing provides additional information about myocardial perfusion.

E. **Coronary angiography,** which delineates coronary artery anatomy, is the gold standard for confirming abnormal stress testing and guiding therapy (i.e., medical versus surgical management, including stenting and coronary artery bypass grafting).

F. **Pulmonary function tests (PFTs)** can be helpful in patients with pulmonary chest pain in clarifying obstructive versus restrictive disease and its severity.

G. **GI studies**
   1. **Esophageal pH probe** can help confirm GERD in cases where symptoms are atypical or cardiac evaluation is normal.
   2. In known GERD, **esophagogastroduodenoscopy** can assess for complications or severity of disease (e.g., Barrett's esophagus, erosive esophagitis) and allow gastric biopsy to diagnose infection with *H pylori*.
   3. **Upper GI barium study** allows detection of fixed anatomic esophageal lesions (e.g., Schatzki's ring, tumors) and may also help detect motility disorders and hiatal hernia; manometry increases sensitivity in detecting motility disorders.

VI. **Treatment. Treatment of various cardio vascular and pulmonary conditions should include specific management, discussion about lifestyle changes** (smoking cessation, stressreduction, diet, sleep hygiene, lipid-lowering agents, and planned exercise discussed based on the disease), and follow-up.

A. Chest wall pain/muscle strains
1. Treatment includes rest initially, avoidance if possible of precipitating activities, warm moist compresses, and local ice packs after activity.
2. **Oral NSAIDs** (e.g., ibuprofen, 600–800 mg with meals) may provide relief.
3. Pain that is localized (e.g., trigger point or costochondral), disabling, and resistant to the foregoing measures may be alleviated with an injection (e.g., wheel-and-spoke administration of a local anesthetic, such as 0.5–1 cc of bupivacaine or 1%–2% lidocaine, into a trigger point, or a mixture of 0.5–1 cc local anesthetic and 0.5 cc of Aristocort to 40 into a costochondral joint). Particularly with intercostal trigger point injection, care must be taken to avoid pleural penetration.

B. GI (see Chapters 19 and 82).

C. Cardiovascular
1. **Acute angina** or **escalating unstable or crescendo angina** or **suspected MI** is a medical emergency demanding immediate hospitalization for close monitoring, serial cardiac enzymes, oxygen, nitrates, pain management, aspirin, or other anticoagulation. Mortality has also been shown to be decreased through risk factor identification/modification (e.g., lipid panel assessment and statin administration) and early beta blockade, if not contraindicated. For myocardial ischemia management refer to AHA 2007 guidelines. SOR **Ⓐ**
2. **Chronic stable angina** (see Chapter 77).
3. **MVP**
   a. Explanation of the diagnosis and **reassurance** may be sufficient in those with minimal symptoms.
   b. **Those bothered with palpitations,** anxiety, or chest pain may be helped by counseling to minimize caffeine/ethanol intake and use of a beta-blocker (e.g., atenolol, 25–50 mg orally daily, with a gradual upward titration of dose based on symptoms and heart rate).
   c. **Endocarditis prophylaxis** is not indicated in MVP. (SOR **Ⓐ**)

D. Treatment of chest pain from **psychiatric disease** involves addressing underlying disorders (see Chapters 89, 92, and 94).

E. Pulmonary
1. **Pneumonia** (see Chapter 13).
2. **Pleurisy** may benefit from NSAIDs (see Section VI.A.2). Incentive spirometry or deep breathing 10 to 20 times every few hours helps prevent atelectasis or secondary pneumonia from the splinting occurring with pleuritic pain.
3. **Pneumonitis**
   a. With normal PFTs, pneumonitis requires avoidance of precipitants and periodic monitoring of symptoms/PFTs.
   b. Symptomatic pneumonitis with abnormal PFTs generally should be evaluated and initially managed by a pulmonologist, who may initiate oral steroids (e.g., prednisone, 40–100 mg daily).

REFERENCES

Lee TH, Goldman L. Evaluation of the patient with acute chest pain. *New Engl J Med.* 2000; 342(16):1187-1195.

Nilsson S, Scheike M, Engblom D, et al. Chest pain and ischemic heart disease in primary care. *Br J Gen Pract.* 2003;53:378-382.

Swap C, Nagurney J. Value and limitations of chest pain history in the evaluation of patients with suspected acute coronary syndromes. *JAMA.* 2005;294:2623.

Chagnon I et al. Comparison of two clinical prediction rules and implicit assessment among patients with suspected pulmonary embolism. *Am J Med.* 2002;113(4):269.

Kroenke K, Mangelsdorff AD. Common symptoms in ambulatory care: incidence, evaluation, therapy and outcome. *Am J Med.* 1989;86(3):262.

Mark DB. Risk stratification in patients with chest pain. *Prim Care.* 2001;28(1):99.

Schmermund A. Assessment of clinically silent atherosclerotic disease and established and novel risk factors for predicting myocardial infarction and cardiac death in healthy middle-aged subjects: rationale and design of the Heinz Nixdorf RECALL Study. Risk factors, evaluation of coronary calcium and lifestyle. *Am Heart J.* 2002;144(2):212.

Anderson et al. ACC/AHA 2007 Guidelines for the Management of Patients With Unstable Angina/Non ST-Elevation Myocardial Infarction Executive Summary. *J Am Coll Cardiol.* 2007;50:652-726.

11   Confusion

Robert C. Salinas, MD, & Heather Bartoli, PA-C

KEY POINTS

- Delirium or acute confusional state is a syndrome for which an underlying cause must be found; it represents a true medical emergency.
- Delirium may be caused by a medical condition, drug abuse, prescription medication, toxin, or a combination thereof.
- The elderly and those with underlying dementia are most susceptible to developing delirium.

I. **Definition.** Confusion is a general term that is used to describe some aspect of global cognitive impairment, characterized by disorientation or inappropriate reaction to environmental stimuli. Confusion can develop suddenly (acute) or insidiously (chronic). Dementia and other chronic confusional states are discussed in Chapter 73. This chapter focuses on the evaluation and management of **delirium (acute confusional state),** which is a medical term used to describe a constellation of clinical symptoms characterized by acute onset, disturbance in consciousness, reduced ability to focus, and impaired cognition that is often precipitated by one or more underlying medical-related causes (Table 11–1).

II. **Common Diagnoses.** It is thought that up to 35% of elderly patients age 65 years and older and who are admitted to the hospital from the emergency department meet the criteria for delirium. In addition, all postoperative patients and hospitalized elderly patients are also at risk of developing delirium. Delirium increases length of hospital stay, increase morbidity and mortality, and likelihood of being discharged to a long-term institution. (SOR **B**) Table 11–2 highlights risk factors for development of delirium; vulnerable populations particularly at risk include (1) the **elderly,** because of sensory/cognitive impairment, underlying chronic illness, polypharmacy, and possibly changes in the synthesis of neurotransmitters (e.g., acetylcholine and dopamine) felt vital to attention, learning, and memory; (2) **abusers of ethanol and illicit drugs** (e.g., cocaine and hallucinogens), because of drug-induced imbalances in neurotransmitters, such as acetylcholine, serotonin, and gamma-aminobutyric acid; (3) those with **underlying structural brain disease** (dementia, Parkinson's disease); and (4) the **terminally ill,** because of medications (e.g., opiates) and anxiety/depression/sleep disturbance associated with disease progression. Figure 11–1 illustrates the complex interplay between different patient predisposing vulnerabilities and environmental insults (iatrogenic) causing delirium, particularly in the hospital setting.

A. **Specific conditions predisposing to delirium**
  1. **General medical conditions** (Table 11–3).
  2. **Drug intoxication,** most often from cannabis, cocaine, or hallucinogens, is the most common cause of acute confusional state in older adolescents and young adults.
     a. **Substance withdrawal delirium** is most often caused by high doses of ethanol, sedative hypnotics, or anxiolytic agents.
     b. **Substance-induced delirium** is caused by exposure to toxins (e.g., carbon monoxide, insecticides, industrial solvents).
     c. **Prescription medications** (Table 11–4). Delirium from prescription medication should always be considered in the elderly, who account for approximately 36% of all prescribed medications, some of which have centrally acting anticholinergic properties.
  3. **Change in environmental** setting (e.g., transfer to hospital or a new place of residence following acute hospitalization).
  4. **Structural brain disease** (Alzheimer's disease, vascular dementia, Lewy body dementia, Parkinson's disease).
  5. **Depression.** Depression coexists in more than one-third of outpatients diagnosed with dementia and even more so in nursing home residents with dementia.
B. **Conditions that often mimic delirium** include dementia (Chapter 73), depression (Chapter 92), other psychiatric disturbances, age-associated memory disorder (minimal cognitive impairment), malingering, and factitious disorder.

TABLE 11–1. DSM-IV CRITERIA FOR DELIRIUM

- Disturbance of consciousness (i.e., reduced clarity of awareness of the environment) with reduced ability to focus, sustain, or shift attention
- Change in cognition (such as memory deficit, disorientation, language disturbance) or the development of a perceptual disturbance that is not better accounted for by a preexisting, established, or evolving dementia
- Disturbance that develops over a short period of time (usually hours to days) and tends to fluctuate over the course of the day
- Evidence from the history, physical examination, or laboratory findings that the disturbance is caused by the direct physiologic consequences of a specific medical condition, substance intoxication, substance withdrawal, multiple causes, causes not otherwise specified: insufficient evidence to establish a specific cause, or from other reasons such as sensory deprivation.

III. **Symptoms.** In delirium, obtaining a careful history from a caregiver familiar with the patient's underlying medical problems, medication use including those that are prescribed, herbal or natural products, and purchased over-the-counter, and functional independence baseline may shed light on likely reversible causes. History details should include the following:
   A. **Onset and course** of the confusional state (Tables 11–5 and 11–6), which clarify whether delirium is present and its severity.
   B. **Risk factors** (Table 11–2).
   C. **Chronic illnesses** (Table 11–3).
   D. **Drug use** (Table 11–4). Specifically, commonly prescribed medications with known anti-cholinergic activity or those that cause electrolyte disturbance.
IV. **Signs.** A systematic physical examination often provides clues to underlying causes of delirium and in addition should include the following:
   A. **Evaluation of mental status**
      1. The **Mini-Mental State Examination (MMSE)** (Table 11–7) has high sensitivity and specificity in evaluating memory loss and cognitive impairment; using a cutoff score of 23 or less, the MMSE has a sensitivity of 87% and a specificity of 82%. The MMSE cannot itself diagnose dementia or delirium, and results should be considered in the context of hearing, vision problems, physical disabilities, age, educational level, and cultural influences.
      2. The Confusion Assessment Method (**CAM**) instrument (Table 11–5) has been used to evaluate hospitalized patients with suspected delirium and has a sensitivity of 94%

TABLE 11–2. RISK FACTORS FOR DELIRIUM

Age	• Reduced capacity for homeostasis • Impairments in vision/hearing • Age-related changes in pharmacokinetics and pharmacodynamics • Chronic diseases • Psychosocial precipitants such as sleep loss, sensory deprivation, sensory overload, bereavement, or relocation • Structural brain disease
Preexisting dementia	• Imbalance of noradrenergic/cholinergic neurotransmission • Inflammatory mechanisms • HPA axis abnormalities • Disrupted circadian rhythm
Hospitalization	• Relocation • Euthyroid sick syndrome • Severe illness • Disrupted sleep–wake cycle • Physical restraints • Bladder catheterization • Addition of new medications
Polypharmacy	• Drug interactions • Additive effects
Surgical factors	• Significant intraoperative blood loss • Hemodynamic instability • Emergent versus elective surgery • History of noncardiac thoracic surgery or AAA repair
History of drug abuse	• Especially alcohol, cannibis, cocaine, hallucinogens

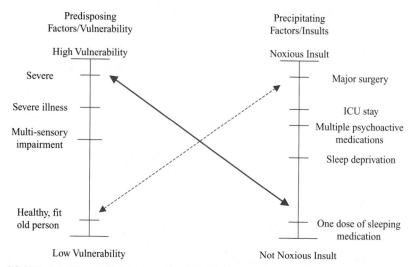

FIGURE 11–1. Multifactorial model for delirium. In a patient with high vulnerability (e.g., severe dementia, severe underlying illness, multisensory impairment), delirium may develop with a relatively benign insult (*black arrow*). Conversely, a patient with low vulnerability would be relatively resistant and require multiple noxious insults before delirium would develop (*dotted arrow*). (Taken from Inouye SK, Carpenter PA. Precipitating factors for delirium in hospitalized elderly person: predictive model and inter-relationship with baseline vulnerabilities. *JAMA.* 1996;275:852-857.)

to 100% and specificity of 90% to 95%. The tool itself takes approximately 5 minutes to administer and a positive diagnosis requires that both Features 1 and 2 be present, along with either Feature 3 or Feature 4. (SOR **A**)

3. An **agitated confusional state without focal signs** may occur following head trauma. Hyperalert confusion may result from alcohol withdrawal. A person who is excited, hyperalert, and hallucinating may be experiencing toxicity from amphetamine, lysergic acid diethylamide (LSD), cocaine, or phencyclidine (PCP).

B. Vital signs

1. If **diastolic blood pressure is >120 mm Hg,** hypertensive encephalopathy should be considered.
2. If **systolic blood pressure is <90 mm Hg,** confusion may be from impaired cerebral perfusion secondary to shock. Drug overdose, adrenal insufficiency, and hyponatremia should also be considered.
3. **Tachycardia** suggests sepsis, delirium tremens, hyperthyroidism, hypoglycemia, or an agitated, anxious patient.
4. **Fever** may indicate infection, delirium tremens, cerebral vasculitis, or fat embolism syndrome. **Hypothermia** is defined as a core temperature (rectal or esophageal) below 35°C (95°F) and may cause confusion.

TABLE 11–3. GENERAL MEDICAL CONDITIONS OFTEN CAUSING DELIRIUM

Metabolic disturbances	Hyponatremia, hypo-/hyperkalemia, hypo-/hyperthyroidism, anemia, hypercarbia, hypo-/hyperglycemia, dehydration, malnutrition, hypothermia, heat stroke
Neurologic	Head trauma, CVA, normal pressure hydrocephalus, subdural hematoma, meningitis, encephalitis, brain abscess, neurosyphilis, seizure disorders (ictal and postictal states)
Neoplastic	Primary intracranial neoplasm, metastatic disease to the brain
Cardiovascular	MI, CHF, arrhythmia, severe aortic stenosis, hypertensive encephalopathy
Pulmonary	Pneumonia, COPD exacerbation, respiratory failure
Gastrointestinal	Fecal impaction, intra-abdominal infection, liver failure
Urinary	Urinary tract infection, urinary retention

TABLE 11–4. DRUGS WITH ANTICHOLINERGIC PROPERTIES

Classical anticholinergics
  Atropine
  Scopolamine
Antidepressants
  Tricyclic, i.e., Elavil, Sinequan
Antiemetics
Antihistamines
  Benadryl
Antiparkinsonian
Antipsychotics
Antispasmodics
  Gastrointestinal, i.e., Bentyl, Levsin
  Urinary tract, i.e., Ditropan
Muscle relaxants
Prednisolone
Cimetidine

TABLE 11–5. THE CONFUSION ASSESSMENT METHOD (CAM) DIAGNOSTIC ALGORITHM*

Feature 1	*Acute onset and fluctuating course* This feature is usually obtained from a family member or a nurse and is shown by positive responses to the following questions: Is there evidence of an acute change in mental status from the patient's baseline? Did the (abnormal) behavior fluctuate during the day, that is, tend to come and go, or increase and decrease in severity?
Feature 2	*Inattention* This feature is shown by a positive response to the following questions: Did the patient have difficulty focusing attention, for example, being easily distractible, or having difficulty keeping track of what was being said?
Feature 3	*Disorganized thinking* This feature is shown by a positive response to the following question: Was the patient's thinking disorganized or incoherent, such as rambling or irrelevant conversation, unclear or illogical flow of ideas, or unpredictable switching form subject to subject?
Feature 4	*Altered level of consciousness* This feature is shown by any answer other than "alert" to the following question: Overall, how would you rate this patient's level of consciousness? (Alert [normal], vigilant [hyperalert], lethargic [drowsy, easily aroused], stupor [difficult to arouse], or coma [unarousable])

*The diagnosis of delirium by CAM requires the presence of features 1 and 2 and either 3 or 4.
Reproduced with permission from Inouye SK, Van Dyck CH, Alessi CA, et al. Clarifying confusion: the confusion assessment method. *Ann Intern Med*. 1990;113(12):947.

TABLE 11–6. FEATURES OF DELIRIUM AND DEMENTIA

Feature	Delirium	Dementia
Onset	Abrupt	Insidious
Duration	Acute illness, generally days to weeks	Chronic illness, characteristically progressing over years
Reversibility	Usually reversible	Usually irreversible, often chronically progressive
Orientation	Disorientation early	Disorientation later in the illness, often after months or years
Stability	Variability from moment to moment, hour to hour, throughout the day	Much more stable day to day (unless superimposed delirium develops)
Physiologic changes	Prominent physiologic changes	Less prominent physiologic changes
Consciousness	Clouded, altered, and changing level of consciousness	Consciousness not clouded until terminal
Attention span	Strikingly short attention span	Attention span not characteristically reduced
Sleep–wake cycle	Disturbed sleep–wake cycle with hour-to-hour variation	Disturbed sleep–wake cycle with day–night reversal, but not hour-to-hour variation
Psychomotor changes	Marked psychomotor changes (hyperactive or hypoactive)	Psychomotor changes characteristically late (unless superimposed depression)

TABLE 11–7. MINI-MENTAL STATE EXAMINATION (MMSE) SAMPLE ITEMS

Orientation to Time
"What is the date?"
Registration
"Listen carefully. I am going to say three words. You say them back after I stop.
Ready? Here they are...
APPLE (pause), PENNY (pause), TABLE (pause). Now repeat those words back to me." [Repeat up to 5 times, but
score only the first trial.]
Naming
"What is this?" [Point to a pencil or pen.]
Reading
"Please read this and do what it says." [Show examinee the words on the stimulus form.]
CLOSE YOUR EYES

5. **Tachypnea** suggests hypoxia. A patient with chronic obstructive lung disease receiving fractional inspiratory oxygen >0.28, may be confused from hypercarbia.

C. **Eye examination**
   1. **Papilledema** suggests hypertensive encephalopathy or an intracranial mass.
   2. **Dilated pupils** suggest sympathetic outflow, which is common with delirium tremens. **Pinpoint pupils** suggest narcotic excess or constricting eye drops.

D. **Other findings**
   1. **Bibasilar crackles** on lung auscultation indicate pulmonary edema with potential accompanying hypoxia secondary to heart or lung disease.
   2. **Acute confusion, ataxia, bilateral sixth-nerve palsy, and diarrhea** suggest Wernicke-Korsakoff encephalitis.

V. **Laboratory Tests.** Unless the cause of the acute confusional state is obvious from the history and physical examination, further diagnostic testing is important.

A. **Initial workup** may include complete blood cell count with differential; erythrocyte sedimentation rate; serum chemistry profile, magnesium, and calcium; toxicologic screen of urine, blood, or both; urine analysis; chest x-ray; electrocardiogram; and serum drug levels of prescribed medication as indicated.

B. A **lumbar puncture** should be considered in any delirious patient for whom the possibility of bacterial or viral meningitis is entertained. Relative contraindications include rapid improvement in the patient's clinical status and concerns about increased intracranial pressure from a mass lesion.

C. An **electroencephalogram** may identify partial complex seizures disorder, metabolic encephalopathy, or sedative use and should be considered in patients suspected of these disorders.

D. **Computerized tomography (CT)** of the head is the method of choice for the initial evaluation of confused obtunded patients to rule out subdural hematoma, epidural hematoma, stroke, cerebral abscess, or neoplasm. Repeat CT after 24 to 48 hours should be done if acute infarct is suspected. Magnetic resonance imaging with magnetic resonance arteriography may be useful to rule out chronic subdural hematoma, regional blood flow abnormalities, or aneurysm.

E. **Additional tests** to consider are arterial blood gas analysis, blood cultures, serum ammonia levels, liver function studies, thyroid function tests, cortisone levels, antinuclear antibodies, serum protein electrophoresis, serum B_{12} and folate levels, syphilis test (VDRL), serum and urine osmolality, HIV titer, and urine tests for heavy metals and metanephrines.

VI. **Treatment**

A. **General principles.** Patients with delirium should usually be hospitalized for identification and management of underlying causes. Terminally ill hospice patients with delirium may be managed at home or an inpatient hospice setting, depending on patient and family desires. Principles of management include the following:

   1. **Supportive care.** Supportive care while workup progresses includes a quiet private room with familiar objects, presence of a family member, and maintenance of a normal sleep–wake pattern.

2. **Drug therapy.** Agitation and behavioral problems posing harm to the patient or others may require the use of neuroleptic agents for sedation. When considering such medication, the goal should be control of dangerous behavior, while avoiding excessive sedation.

   a. **Haloperidol.** A recent Cochrane review suggests that low-dose haloperidol (0.25–2 mg) given intramuscularly may be helpful in the urgent setting. Occasionally, maintenance doses of haloperidol (0.25–0.5 mg orally 2 or 3 times daily) may be used to control agitation while the underlying cause of delirium is determined and treated. (SOR **A**)

   b. Some of the newer atypical neuroleptic agents may be reasonable options and can also be used for maintenance purposes. In such cases, **risperidone** (0.5 mg orally twice daily up to 4–6 mg daily) can be used for agitation.

   c. **Paradoxical physiologic reactions** can occur with any of these medications through anticholinergic properties and can worsen extrapyramidal symptoms.

   d. **Benzodiazepines** may be useful in delirium from ethanol withdrawal. If a benzodiazepine is used, **lorazepam (Ativan)** is usually the drug of choice because of its relatively short half-life. However, this too can paradoxically worsen agitation in patients with preexisting dementia.

   e. **In hospice patients,** the foregoing medications may be of benefit in treating confusion; treatment of pain, anxiety, and depression may also be indicated. However, forgoing a search for a reversible underlying cause of the delirium may be appropriate in the terminally ill.

3. **Open communication.** Open communication with family members about suspected causes and prognosis of the delirium is essential as caregivers may experience great distress in observing behavioral changes associated with cognitive impairment.

B. **Treatment of specific conditions** (see Chapters 73 and 92).

C. **Prevention.** Understanding that intrinsic and extrinsic factors may predispose patients in certain age groups to delirium will help develop preventive strategies. The incidence of delirium may be decreased by limiting polypharmacy in the elderly, closely monitoring drug usage by the elderly, and recognizing prodromal symptoms of insomnia, nightmares, fleeting hallucinations, and anxiety. (SOR **B**)

REFERENCES

Inouye SK. Delirium in older people. *N Engl J Med.* 2006;354(11):1157-1165.

Lonergan E, Britton AM, Luxenberg J, Wyller T. Antipsychotics for delirium. Art. No:CD005594. doi:10.1002/14651858.CD0005594.pub2.

Lundstrom M, Edlund A, Karlsson S, et al. A multifactorial intervention program reduces the duration of delirium, length, of hospitalization, and mortality in delirious patients. *J Am Geriatr Soc.* 2005;53(4):622-628.

Potter J,George J. The prevention, diagnosis, and management of delirium in older people: concise guidelines. *Clin Med.* 2006;6(3):303-308.

Weber JB, Coverdale JH, Kunik ME, et al. Delirium:current trends in prevention and treatment. *Intern Med J.* 2004;34(3):115-121.

---

12   Constipation

Allen R. Last, MD, MPH, & Jonathan D. Ference, PharmD, BCPS

KEY POINTS

- Constipation can represent many things to different patients but generally is defined as infrequent bowel movements or straining to achieve a bowel movement.
- The presence of hematochezia, family history of colon cancer or inflammatory bowel disease, anemia, positive fecal occult blood testing, weight loss, persistent constipation

unresponsive to treatment, and new onset constipation in patients older than 50 years of age requires a diagnostic evaluation.
- Those without warning symptoms can be treated empirically with lifestyle modification such as dietary fiber, exercise and hydration, and medications when necessary.

I. **Definition.** Constipation is either the actual or perceived difficulty with defecation. This can be from infrequent stools or difficult passage of stool or both. Classically, constipation has been defined as having three or fewer bowel movements per week. Often patients report being constipated in spite of having more than three bowel movements and usually have some problem with the passage of stool. The American College of Gastroenterology Chronic Constipation Task Force defines constipation as "unsatisfactory defecation characterized by infrequent stools, difficult stool passage or both. Difficult stool passage includes straining, a sense of difficulty passing stool, incomplete evacuation, hard/lumpy stools, prolonged time to stool, or need for manual maneuvers to pass stool." Chronic constipation should include some combination of these symptoms for at least 3 of the previous 12 months.
II. **Common Diagnosis.** Constipation is a common problem in Western cultures with 15% of the population reporting these symptoms at any given time. It is reported more commonly among women, elderly, non-caucasian ethnicity, individuals from lower socioeconomic groups and those living in northern states and rural areas. It results in 2.5 million office visits to physicians and 92,000 hospital admissions annually in the United States. Nearly 5% of all pediatric office visits are for constipation.

Constipation can be categorized as normal-transit constipation, slow-transit constipation, and pelvic floor dysfunction constipation.
- A. **Normal-transit constipation** (also called "functional constipation") is the most common form. These patients have normal stooling frequency but perceive constipation because of symptoms of bloating, abdominal pain, and hard stools. Causes include poor fiber intake, dehydration, physical inactivity, motility disorders such as irritable bowel syndrome, and suppressing the defecation reflex, as sometimes seen in children who have had previous painful experiences with bowel movements.
- B. **Slow-transit constipation** is typically seen in young women, often beginning with the onset of puberty. These patients often have fewer high-amplitude peristaltic waves than patients without constipation, resulting in colonic contents not being advanced effectively.
- C. **Pelvic floor dysfunction constipation** results from abnormal anal sphincter tone or pelvic floor muscle tension and contraction. Stool accumulates in the distal colon normally, but patients are unable to relax the perineum and anal sphincter to allow for the passage of stool normally. Risk factors include multiparity, perineal surgeries and a prolonged history of straining to stool.
- D. **Secondary causes** should be considered in the diagnosis of constipation (Table 12–1). Included among the secondary causes are medications (Table 12–2), mechanical or anatomical obstruction (rectoceles, cancers, and postsurgical scarring), metabolic derangements (hypothyroidism, diabetes mellitus, and hypercalcemia), myopathies (amyloidosis and scleroderma), neuropathies (Parkinson's, multiple sclerosis, cerebrovascular events), and other conditions.

    Hirschsprung's disease should be considered in any neonate that does not have a bowel movement within 48 hours of birth. It is typically diagnosed in newborns, but if not identified until infancy often presents with abdominal bloating, pencil-thin stools, failure to thrive, and bilious vomiting. The rectum will be empty on examination. A delay in diagnosis can lead to enterocolitis (fever, bloody diarrhea, and abdominal distension) in the second or third month of life.
- E. **Fecal impaction** is the presence of stool that cannot be evacuated by the patient. Prolonged and chronic constipation can lead to impaction. The majority occur in the rectum and should be removed by manual disimpaction (scooping or scissoring motion of the fingers in the rectum). Higher impactions should be loosened with enemas. Avoid oral laxatives agents until after an impaction has been resolved. Endoscopy is sometimes needed to remove higher impactions.
III. **Symptoms**

A thorough history is needed to rule out secondary causes and define the underlying process when constipation does not respond to initial therapy. Symptoms suggesting constipation include abdominal bloating and/or pain, infrequent bowel movements, straining to defecate,

TABLE 12–1. SECONDARY CAUSES OF CONSTIPATION

Drug effects	See Table 12–2
Mechanical obstruction	
	Colon cancer
	External compression from malignancy
	Strictures
	Rectocele
	Postsurgical changes
	Megacolon
	Anal fissure
	Inflammatory bowel disease
Metabolic conditions	
	Diabetes mellitus
	Hypothyroidism
	Hypercalcemia
	Hypokalemia
	Hypomagnesemia
	Uremia
	Cystic fibrosis
	Heavy metal poisoning
Myopathies	
	Amyloidosis
	Myotonic dystrophy
	Scleroderma
Neuropathies	
	Parkinson's disease
	Spinal cord injury or tumor
	Cerebrovascular accident
	Autonomic neuropathy
	Hirschsprung's disease
	Multiple sclerosis
Other conditions	
	Anxiety
	Depression
	Somatization
	Cognitive impairment
	Immobility
	Pregnancy

hard stools, infrequent defecation, inability to defecate at will, and sometimes nausea. The history should elicit details about the problem such as the frequency and consistency of bowel movements, whether straining or external manipulation is necessary to induce a bowel movement, what attempts at treatment have been made, and the effectiveness of these attempts. A review of systems to rule out the presence of secondary causes should be performed. The presence of any alarm symptoms (Table12–3) should prompt a thorough evaluation.

IV. **Signs**

    A. Abdominal examination. Normal or hypoactive bowel sounds may be auscultated. Palpation may reveal an abdominal mass, typically in the left lower quadrant, which represents a stool bolus or more rarely a tumor or intussusception. Serial examinations should be performed to rule out a fixed mass.

    B. Rectal examination. A careful rectal examination is often the most helpful portion of the clinical evaluation. The perianal skin should be assessed for scars, fissures, hemorrhoids, and fistulas. The perineum should be observed at rest and during straining to evaluate the degree of perineal descent (1–3.5 cm is normal). A digital rectal examination should be performed to determine sphincter tone and rule out impaction, anal strictures, and masses. Women should be evaluated for a rectocele as a potential cause of constipation.

V. **Laboratory tests.**

    A. Laboratory tests. Laboratory testing is only indicated if alarm symptoms are present, including lack of response to initial therapy or if specific medical disorders are identified

TABLE 12–2. MEDICATIONS ASSOCIATED WITH CONSTIPATION

	Examples
Nonprescription medications	
Sympathomimetics	Ephedrine
Nonsteroidal anti-inflammatory drugs	Ibuprofen, naproxen
Antacids	Aluminum hydroxide, calcium carbonate
Calcium supplements	Calcium carbonate/citrate
Iron supplements	Ferrous sulfate/gluconate
Antidiarrheals	Loperamide, bismuth salicylate
Prescription medications	
Anticholinergics	Benztropine, trihexylphenidate
Antihistamines	Diphenhydramine
Antidepressants	Tricyclics, amitriptyline
Antiparkinson agents	Levodopa
Calcium channel blockers	Verapamil
Antispasmodics	Dicyclomine
Antipsychotics	Chlorpromazine
Diuretics	Furosemide
Opioids	Codeine, morphine, oxycodone, hydrocodone

from the history and physical examination. Thyroid-stimulating hormone, serum electrolytes, calcium, glucose, complete blood count, and urinalysis may be useful in patients with constipation. (SOR Ⓒ)

B. **Stool guaiac testing.** Fecal occult blood testing is a quick, inexpensive screening test for colon cancer, but suffers from a relatively high rate of false positives and negatives.

C. **Colonic imaging.** Plain film radiographs will reliably diagnose fecal impactions, but are less useful for routine constipation. Colonoscopy or barium enema should be pursued in patients older than 50 years of age or in whom alarm symptoms are present. (SOR Ⓒ)

D. **Specialized testing.** Colonic-transit testing can be measured in those with normal laboratory evaluation and without structural abnormalities on colonic imaging. Normal transit time is less than 72 hours. Anorectal manometry can measure the pressures generated in the rectum to diagnose pelvic floor dysfunction and Hirschsprung's disease. Balloon expulsion testing (a balloon filled with 50cc of air or water) can reveal a defecatory disorder. Defecography (an expulsion of a barium enema under fluoroscopy) can evaluate the emptying mechanism of the rectum. (SOR Ⓒ)

VI. **Treatment.** Treatment of constipation should be directed by history, physical examination, and diagnostic testing. Treatment of underlying disorders or discontinuation of offending agents may improve constipation. When no warning symptoms are present, empiric treatment should be tried initially. The basis of therapy includes nonpharmacologic therapy, such as lifestyle modification and pharmacologic therapy if needed.

A. **Lifestyle modifications** may be employed alone or in addition to pharmacologic therapy. Appropriate lifestyle modifications are the basis of maintenance of normal bowel function. Increasing fiber, fitness, and fluids ("The 3 Fs") are simple measures to improve bowel function.

1. **Bowel training** may be a simple first-line approach. Patients should be instructed to attempt to move their bowels at the same time each day. Optimal times to have a bowel movement are typically after waking, eating, or physical activity. Colonic activity is the greatest during these times. A stool diary may be helpful to record frequency, consistency, size, and degree of straining. (SOR Ⓒ)

2. Increasing **dietary fiber bulk** is considered a mainstay of nonpharmacologic therapy. Adding dietary or supplemental fiber is easy and inexpensive. The daily recommended fiber intake is 20 to 30 g, but most Americans consume 5 to 10 g. Patients should increase fiber by 5 g/d each week until reaching the daily recommended intake. (SOR Ⓒ)

3. Patients should be encouraged to be as **physically active** as possible as a low activity level is associated with a twofold increased risk of constipation. (SOR Ⓒ)

4. Adequate **fluid** intake is considered important to maintain normal bowel motility. A general recommendation of 32 oz of water daily may help maintain normal stool frequency. (SOR Ⓒ)

TABLE 12–3. **ALARM SYMPTOMS/SIGNS REQUIRING DIAGNOSTIC EVALUATION**

1. Hematochezia
2. Family history of colon cancer
3. Family history of inflammatory bowel disease
4. Anemia
5. Positive fecal occult blood test
6. Weight loss
7. Severe, persistent constipation that is not responsive to treatment
8. New onset constipation in people older than 50 y.

   B. Pharmacologic therapy (Table 12–4) may be employed when nonpharmacologic measures fail. Aggressive laxative use can obscure underlying pathology; if constipation is refractory to medical treatment, referral for further evaluation is warranted.

      1. Bulk-forming agents including psyllium (natural), calcium polycarbophil, and methylcellulose (synthetic) increase stool mass and soften stool consistency by absorbing water from the intestinal lumen. Generally these agents are well tolerated, but synthetic agents may cause less bloating and flatulence because they are indigestible. However, psyllium may be more effective in increasing stool frequency than synthetic agents. Patients should be instructed to increase daily fluid intake (up to 2–3 quarts of water) to maintain adequate hydration. (SOR **B**)

      2. Surfactants (stool softeners) lower surface tension and allow more water to be incorporated into stool. Although these agents are well tolerated, they may not be as effective as psyllium in increasing stool frequency and are ineffective as monotherapy in the treatment of opioid-induced constipation. Mineral oil is not routinely recommended because of the potential risk of aspiration or depletion of fat soluble vitamins A,D,E,K. (SOR **B**)

      3. Osmotic laxatives cause secretion of water into the intestinal lumen by osmotic activity. These agents may be **saline laxatives** (magnesium hydroxide [milk of magnesia] or magnesium citrate and sodium biphosphate) or **hyperosmolar** agents (lactulose, sorbitol, polyethylene glycol [PEG]).

         a. Saline laxatives work within the lumen and are not systemically absorbed, but may cause electrolyte disturbances within the lumen resulting in hypokalemia and salt overload. Hypermagnesemia can result from chronic use of magnesium products, especially in patients with renal insufficiency. There are insufficient data to make a recommendation about the effectiveness of milk of magnesia for chronic constipation (SOR **B**).

TABLE 12–4. **COMMON LAXATIVES**

Laxative	Generic Name	Brand Name	Adult Dosing	Onset (h)
Bulk forming	Bran	—	25 g/d	12–72
	Psyllium	Metamucil	12 g qd to tid	12–72
	Methylcellulose	Citrucel	19 g qd–tid	12–72
	Polycarbophil	FiberCon, Konsyl	500 mg/d	12–72
Stool softener	Docusate sodium	Colace	100–200 mg/d	24–72
	Docusate calcium	Surfak	240 mg/d	24–72
	Docusate potassium	Dialose Plus	100 mg qd–tid	24–72
Salines	Magnesium sulfate	Epsom salt	1–2 tsp qd–bid	0.5–3
	Magnesium hydroxide	Milk of Magnesia	30–60 mL/d	0.5–3
	Magnesium citrate	Citrate of Magnesia	200 mL/d	0.5–3
	Sodium phosphate	Fleets phospho–soda	up to 45 mL/d	0.5–3
Hyperosmolar agents	Sorbitol	—	30–60 mL/d	24–48
	Lactulose	Chronulac	30–60 g/d	24–48
	Polyethylene glycol	GoLYTELY, Miralax	17 g/d	0.5–4
Stimulants	Bisacodyl	Dulcolax, Correctol	5 mg qd–tid	6–10
	Senna	Senokot	8.6 mg qd–bid	6–10
Chloride channel activators	lubiprostone	Amitiza	24 mcg BID w/ food	—

   b. Lactulose and polyethylene glycol (PEG) are available as prescription and sorbitol as a nonprescription product. Poor systemic absorption of these agents often causes flatulence and abdominal pain. Large doses of hyperosmolar agents are frequently used to evacuate the bowel for endoscopy or surgery. Glycerin suppositories are locally active when inserted in the rectum. Lactulose and PEG are effective in improving stool frequency and consistency in patients with chronic constipation. (SOR **Ⓐ**)
   4. Stimulant laxatives are the most common products used for acute symptomatic relief. Senna and bisacodyl exhibit their effects within hours by stimulating the colonic myenteric plexus, increasing motility. Bedtime administration may be beneficial in producing a morning bowel movement. Stimulant laxatives should not be used in patients with suspected intestinal obstruction, and research is not available to support their routine use for the treatment of chronic constipation. (SOR **Ⓑ**)
   5. Enemas are useful for evacuating the distal colon and rectum. Various agents are used, but plain warm water suffices in most cases. Enemas are usually the treatment of choice for fecal impactions.
   6. Tegaserod (Zelnorm) is effective in improving stool frequency and consistently in patients with chronic constipation. However, the FDA requested Zelnorm's manufacturer to withdraw the drug from the market because of a relationship between Zelnorm prescriptions and increased risks of heart attack and stroke.
   7. Lubiprostone (Amitiza) may be beneficial in the treatment of adults with chronic constipation refractory to other treatments. Amitiza activates small intestine chloride channels resulting in increased intestinal secretion. Amitiza use may increase bowel movement frequency while decreasing symptoms of bloating. Nausea occurs in one-third of users, but no electrolyte disturbances have been observed. Administering Amitiza with food may reduce risk of nausea. (SOR **Ⓑ**)

REFERENCES

American College of Gastroenterology Chronic Constipation Task Force. An evidence-based approach to the management of chronic constipation in North America. *Am J Gastro.* 2005;100:S1-S22.
Biggs WS, Drey WH. Evaluation and treatment of constipation in infants and children. *Am Fam Physician.* 2006;73:469-477.
Hsieh C. Treatment of constipation in older adults. *Am Fam Physician.* 2005;72:2277-2284.
Lembo A, Camilleri M. Chronic constipation. *N Engl J Med.* 2003;349:1360-1368.

---

13   Cough

David Holmes, MD

KEY POINTS

- The most common cause of acute cough is viral upper respiratory illness.
- The most common causes of chronic cough are postnasal drainage in nonsmokers and tobacco irritants/chronic bronchitis in smokers. Other common causes are asthma and gastroesophageal reflux disease.
- Treatment of cough is directed at underlying disease. Antibiotics are not indicated for viral infections.

I. Definition. A **cough** is a sudden explosive forcing of air through the glottis, occurring immediately on opening the previously closed glottis. It is initiated by airway inflammation, mechanical/chemical irritation of airways, or pressure from adjacent structures.

It takes 7 weeks for bronchial hyperreactivity to return to normal following viral upper respiratory illness (URI). Therefore, the following classification of cough is used: **acute cough** lasts <3 weeks, **subacute cough** lasts 3 to 8 weeks, and **chronic cough** lasts >8 weeks.

II. Common Diagnoses. Cough is the fifth most common presenting complaint in primary care, accounting for approximately 30 million office visits each year in the United States. At any given time approximately 18% of people have a cough.

A. Acute cough. Common causes of acute cough are reflected in the mnemonic **AAA VIRUS**—that is, **A**sthma exacerbation, **A**cute Bronchitis (almost always viral), **A**spiration, **V**iral URI (most common cause), **I**rritants (i.e., tobacco and marijuana smoke, allergens, air pollution, dust, sulfur dioxide, nitrogen oxide, ammonia, and ozone), **R**hinitis (allergic), **U**ncomplicated pneumonia, **S**inusitis/postnasal drainage (PND).

1. **Asthma exacerbation.** Nine to twelve million people in the United States have asthma and 4000 to 5000 die each year of it. Risk factors for asthma exacerbation include allergen exposure (i.e., mold, pollen, dust, animal danders, cosmetics); respiratory infection; exposure to irritants (i.e., smoke); certain medications (i.e., beta-blockers, aspirin); and psychological stress.

2. **Acute bronchitis.** Acute bronchitis is one of the most common diagnoses in primary care. Up to 95% is viral—influenza (types A and B), respiratory syncytial virus, parainfluenza, coronavirus, and adenovirus; less common causes include *Mycobacterium pneumoniae, Bordetella pertussis,* and *Chlamydia pneumoniae.* Risk factors for acute bronchitis include exposure to viral URI, cigarette smoke and other irritants, and history of chronic obstructive pulmonary disease (COPD) or lupus.

3. **Aspiration.** Virtually everyone aspirates what they are eating or drinking at some point in their lives, but subsequent cough reflex protects the airway. Risk factors for more serious aspiration include being very old or very young (younger than 3 years) or having impaired gag or swallowing reflex.

4. **Viral** upper respiratory illnesses (**URIs**). Viral URIs are the most frequent illnesses in humans, with a prevalence as high as 35% worldwide. Thirty to fifty percent of all common colds are caused by rhinovirus; other causative organisms include echovirus, coxsackievirus, influenza virus, respiratory syncytial virus, parainfluenza virus, coronavirus, and adenovirus. Risk factors for development of URIs include exposure to URI, cigarette smoke, and other irritants.

5. **Irritants.** Cigarette smoke is the most common offending irritant; the 20% to 25% of Americans who smoke and those breathing their smoke are at risk for this cause of coughing. Other irritants include pollutants and allergens.

6. **Allergic rhinitis.** Allergies to dust mites, molds, animals, and pollen occur in 7% of North Americans, predominantly children and adolescents. Risk factors for allergic rhinitis include asthma, eczema, urticaria, and a family history of related symptoms.

7. **Uncomplicated pneumonia.** Each year there are four million cases of pneumonia in the United States, 600,000 hospitalizations, and 75,000 deaths, making pneumonia the sixth most common cause of death in the United States. Persons at highest risk for pneumonia include smokers; those with chronic lung disease; the elderly; the immunocompromised; those with renal or hepatic failure, diabetes, or malignancy; and those in nursing homes or hospitals. A patient's age helps determine likely causative organisms, i.e., <**6 months:** *Chlamydia trachomatis,* respiratory syncytial virus; **6 months to 5 years:** *Haemophilus influenzae;* **young adults:** *Streptococcus pneumoniae, Mycoplasma pneumoniae,* and *C pneumoniae;* **elderly:** *S pneumoniae, H influenzae, Mycoplasma catarrhalis,* and *Legionella pneumophila.*

8. **Sinusitis/postnasal drainage (PND).** Sinusitis/PND is very common in the United States, resulting in 25 million office visits annually. Fifteen percent of sinusitis is viral; other identified organisms include *S pneumoniae* (most common bacterial etiology), *H influenzae, M catarrhalis,* Grp A streptococci, *Staphylococcus aureus,* and anaerobes. Risk factors for sinusitis include history of URI, allergic rhinitis, nasotracheal or nasogastric intubation, dental infections, barotrauma (deep-sea diving, air travel), cystic fibrosis, irritants, nasal polyps, and tumors (cause ostia obstruction).

B. Subacute and chronic cough (Table 13–1). Airway hyperresponsiveness following URI is a common cause of **subacute cough,** usually resolving by 7 weeks after the URI. The prevalence of **chronic cough** in the United States is 14% to 23% in nonsmoking adults and children and much higher in smokers. Chronic cough is more common in the elderly, school-aged children, and people exposed to air pollution in urban areas. In more than 90% of persons, chronic cough (>8 weeks) is caused by PND, asthma, smoking/chronic bronchitis, and gastroesophageal reflux disease (GERD). Often chronic cough is caused by a combination of diagnoses. The differential diagnosis of subacute/chronic cough is incorporated in the mnemonic **GASP YE & HACK IT UP (see Table 13–1).**

TABLE 13-1. DIFFERENTIAL DIAGNOSIS OF SUBACUTE AND CHRONIC COUGH: GASP YE & HACK IT UP

Differential Diagnosis	Etiology/Mechanism of Action	Risk Factors/History	Signs per Physical Examination	Testing
Gastroesophageal reflux disease (GERD)	Transient loss of LES tone → increase in acid reflux and aspiration of gastric contents → irritation and airway inflammation	Chronic cough is sole symptom in up to 75%; heartburn, sour taste in back of throat, sore throat, regurgitation, laryngitis, dysphonia, symptoms worse with lying down, exercise, caffeine, alcohol, acidic foods. GERD causes chronic cough in up to 41% of adults	Usually absent, possible epigastric tenderness	24-h pH monitoring (consider if symptoms do not resolve after 3–6 mo of therapy); upper GI series and upper endoscopy in those chronically symptomatic to assess complications of GERD
Asthma	Inflammation (mast cells infiltrate the smooth muscle cells in the airways) and hyperresponsiveness of airways resulting in airflow obstruction	Nonproductive cough is sole symptom in 50%; history of allergies and atopy, family history, wheezing, dyspnea, chest tightness, disturbed sleep. Symptoms exacerbated by exercise, cold air, nighttime, allergens, and respiratory infection.	Bilateral expiratory wheezing and prolonged expiratory phase; respiratory distress, dyspnea, tachypnea, use of accessory respiratory muscles	PFTs (pre- and postbronchodilator therapy); consider methacholine challenge test, pulse oximetry, sputum for eosinophils (should be high), sinus CT for concomitant sinusitis
Smoking and other environmental irritants	Irritation of airways	Smoker or exposure to secondhand smoke or other irritants, cough worse in specific environments such as work or home; cough >3 weeks occurs in 14%–23% of nonsmokers	Often absent; possible wheezing	CXR
Postnasal drainage (or "upper airway cough syndrome")	Rhinitis (allergic and nonallergic) and sinusitis cause PND, which is aspirated. Bacterial causes of chronic sinusitis include *Haemophilus influenzae, Streptococcus pneumoniae,* and oral anaerobes	Most common cause of chronic cough in nonsmokers; persistent URI symptoms, history of seasonal allergies, feeling something dripping/tickling in back of throat, frequently clearing throat, hoarseness, facial pain, tooth pain. **Allergic:** Red, itchy eyes, tearing, itching roof of mouth, otherwise unexplained cough, symptoms made worse by rhinitis or sinusitis, lying down, allergens, temperature changes, pregnancy	Erythematous and swollen nasal mucosa and turbinates, nasal polyps, deviated nasal septum, purulent nasal discharge, sinus tenderness; pharyngeal cobblestoning/postnasal drainage. **Allergic:** boggy nasal mucosa, conjunctivitis, tearing	Sinus CT
Youth—Infants and children	Vascular anomalies most common in infants, asthma is most common in children. Also common are GERD, respiratory infections, psychogenic, Less common is cystic fibrosis, immunologic and fungal disorders, Tourette's Syndrome, and primary ciliary dyskinesia	Wheezing, respiratory distress, persistent URI symptoms	Wheezing, dyspnea, tachypnea	CXR (all ages), barium swallow (infants), PFTs (children ≥5 y), consider sinus CT, 24 h pH probe, Sweat Chloride test, HIV/CD4, sputum cultures, ciliary function tests

Condition	Pathophysiology	History/Presentation	Physical Exam	Diagnostic Tests
Eosinophilic Bronchitis (nonasthmatic)	Eosinophilic airway inflammation, similar to asthma, but with no airflow obstruction or airway hyperreactivity. Mast cells localize within airway epithelium, unlike in asthma where the mast cells infiltrate airway smooth muscle cells.	Cough, but no wheeze. Exposure to allergens and occupational chemicals	Often absent, Lung sounds are clear	Sputum for eosinophils (should be high), CXR (should be negative), PFTs (should be normal)
Hyper-responsiveness of airways after URI (or "postinfectious cough")	URI → extensive inflammation → airway epithelial damage → hypersensitivity of the airway receptors to inhaled irritants	Recent URI; cough usually resolves in 3 wk but may persist up to 7 wk	Usually absent, possible wheezing	None
ACE inhibitors (ACEIs) and other medications	ACEI: unclear mechanism, but accumulation of bradykinin and prostaglandins that sensitize cough receptors is implicated. Beta-blockers → bronchospasm. Nitrofurantoin → pulmonary fibrosis	5% of those taking ACEI develop cough. Onset of cough is usually within 2 wk of starting suspect medication but may be delayed up to 6 mo.	Usually absent	None
Chronic bronchitis and COPD	Bronchial inflammation, excessive mucous production, and decreased ability of mucociliary system to clear secretions	Most common cause of chronic cough in smokers; history of smoking, ↑ sputum production, worse in morning, shortness of breath, dyspnea on exertion, wheezing. Chronic bronchitis is diagnosed with productive cough for at least 3 mo/y for 2 consecutive years.	Scattered rhonchi, wheezes (especially forced expiration), crackles, prolonged expiration or distant breath sounds, thought lungs may be clear, no evidence of pulmonary consolidation	CXR, pulse oximetry, PFTs (pre- and postbronchodilator therapy), ABG
Killer cancer (primary pulmonary, Hodgkin's lymphoma, metastatic)	Mechanical compression of airways	Rarely presents solely with cough; weight loss, dyspnea, hemoptysis, history of smoking	Weight loss, cachexia, fever, dyspnea	CXR, CT scan, MRI, bronchoscopy with biopsy, sputum cytology
Idiopathic (or "Unexplained")	It is important to make sure that the diagnostic workup and the treatment attempts have been comprehensive before declaring that a cough is unexplainable			
Tuberculosis (TB)	*Mycobacterium tuberculosis* infection transmitted by inhaling airborne bacilli from a person with active TB	History of TB exposure, HIV, immigration from countries with high prevalence, homelessness, substance abuse, in prison or nursing home; fatigue; fever, night sweats, weight loss, anorexia, dyspnea, hemoptysis, pleuritic chest pain	Fever, crackles near lung apices, septic appearing extrapulmonary TB may involve almost any organ and produce signs related to the specific site (such as recurrent UTIs, adenopathy, and meningitis)	PPD, CXR, acid-fast stain, and sputum culture (takes 2–6 wk to be positive). Testing for extrapulmonary TB as directed by history and examination.

(Continued)

TABLE 13-1. (Continued)

Differential Diagnosis	Etiology/Mechanism of Action	Risk Factors/History	Signs per Physical Examination	Testing
Uncommon causes	"A CHEST BIZ" (see text)			One or more of the following (based on clinical suspicion): echocardiogram, BNP (CHF), HIV testing (AIDS), fungal antibody titers (suspected fungal infection)
Pertussis	Inflammation of larynx, trachea, and bronchi caused by *Bordetella pertussis*	Occurs in 5.5% of pts ≥16 y with persistent (average 6.5 wk) cough. Initially: URI symptoms. 10–14 d after infected: paroxysmal cough (bursts of coughing during single inhalation) often ,but not necessarily, followed by an inspiratory "whooping") sound posttussive vomiting. 2–12 wk: paroxysms gradually improved	Afebrile or slightly febrile, weight loss, lung consolidation (in 20%–25% of cases), post-tussive cyanosis	PCR testing of a nasopharyngeal specimen and serologic assays [LOR: C]; WBC count (usually 15–20,000 and lymphocytosis >70%)
Persistent Pneumonia	Typical: *Strep pneumoniae*, *Staph aureus* Atypical: mycoplasma, influenza, Chlamydia, legionella, adenovirus	Elderly and very young are at risk for typical pneumonia. Young adults are at risk for atypical. Other risks: immunocompromised, recent antibiotics use, comorbidities (i.e., asthma, COPD, CHF, DM, cancer, liver and kidney disease, etc.). Symptoms: fever, pleuritic chest pain, myalgia, dyspnea, fatigue, wheezing,	Fever >38°C (100.4°F), tachypnea, crackles, rhonchi, wheezing, ergophony, bronchial breath sounds, dullness to percussion.	Sputum Gram stain, culture and sensitivity, CBC, CXR, consider chest CT scan, HIV/CD4
Psychogenic (or "Habit Cough")		Children ages 6–16 y, history of school phobia, cough is absent during sleep	Normal examination, or signs of anxiety/depression	No testing, but cough should improve with psychological therapy. If it does not, then the Dx should be "unexplained"

ABG, arterial blood gases; BNP, B-type natriuretic peptide; CHF, congestive heart failure; COPD, chronic obstructive pulmonary disease; CT, computerized tomography; CXR, chest x-ray; GERD, gastroesophageal reflux disease; HIV, human immunodeficiency virus; LES, lower esophageal sphincter; MRI, magnetic resonance imaging; PCR, polymerase chain reaction; PFTs, pulmonary function tests; PPD, purified protein derivative; pts, patients; URI, upper respiratory infection; UTI, urinary tract infection.

1. Approximately 10 million people in the United States are infected with **tuberculosis (TB):** the risk of infection increases with history of travel to or immigration from countries where TB is prevalent (most countries in Latin America and the Caribbean, Africa, Asia, Eastern Europe, and Russia); African Americans and Hispanic Americans are also at increased risk.

2. **Uncommon causes** are reflected in the mnemonic: cough is "A CHEST BIZ," i.e., **A**bscess (pulmonary), **C**HF (congestive heart failure), **H**yperthyroidism, **E**xternal Auditory Canal Irritation (i.e., Arnold's reflex—cerumen or hair on the tympanic membrane stimulating cough receptors), **S**arcoidosis, **S**uture (retained), **T**racheobronchial collapse, Tourette's Syndrome (with a cough tic), **B**ronchiectasis (irreversible dilation of bronchi/bronchioles because of inflammation or obstruction), **I**mmunodeficiency and fungal disorders, **I**rritable larynx (i.e., cancer, laryngotracheomalacia), and **Z**enker's (hypopharyngeal) diverticulum.

III. **Symptoms.** Diagnosis can be made by history alone in 70% to 80% of individuals with cough. Characteristics of cough, such as paroxysmal, barking, honking, brassy, self-propagating, and productiveness and timing during the day, have not proved reliable in determining diagnosis.

A. **Acute cough**

1. **Asthma exacerbation** (see Table 13–1).

2. **Acute bronchitis/COPD exacerbation.** Following URI symptoms, a nonproductive cough, becomes productive. This occurs in 90% of patients with acute bronchitis. Cough persists ≤3 weeks in 50% of patients, but more than a month in 25%. Other symptoms include wheezing, fatigue, hemoptysis, and mild dyspnea.

3. In **aspiration,** there is sudden intractable cough, which may be accompanied by choking, vomiting, wheezing, shortness of breath, dysphagia, and acute anxiety.

4. **Viral URI.** Viral URI features coryza, malaise, chills, rhinorrhea, fever, sore throat, sneezing, and nasal congestion (see Chapter 55).

5. With **irritants,** there may be few symptoms, other than cough. Chemical gas irritant exposure may in addition cause headache, lightheadedness, or confusion.

6. **Rhinitis (allergic)** (see Table 13–1).

7. **Uncomplicated pneumonia.** Symptoms include fever, chills, pleuritic chest pain, dyspnea, and myalgia; the elderly may also or predominantly present with confusion or delirium.

8. **Sinusitis/PND.** Sinusitis/PND is suggested by URI symptoms lasting >10 days, nasal congestion, PND, maxillary or frontal headaches and purulent rhinorrhea. Fever is uncommon.

B. **Subacute/chronic cough** (Table 13–1) may cause chest pain (chest wall, rib fracture), abdominal wall pain, insomnia, hemoptysis, urinary incontinence, syncope, bloodshot eyes (subconjunctival hemorrhage), shortness of breath (pneumothorax), headache, social isolation, anxiety, fatigue, myalgia, and dysphonia.

IV. **Signs.** The physical examination in patients with acute or chronic cough should focus on **temperature** (higher temperature tends to indicate bacterial infection); **ear canals** (for hairs/cerumen on tympanic membrane [Arnold's reflex]); **nares** (for edema, drainage, polyps, erythema); **sinuses** (for tenderness, possibly indicative of underlying sinusitis); **oropharynx** (for cobblestoning, indicative of PND); **neck** (for masses/lymphadenopathy, possibly indicative of infection or cancer); **lungs** (for localized inspiratory wheeze [foreign body or masses], diffused expiratory wheeze [bronchospasm], basilar fine crackles [pulmonary edema], percussion dullness, egophony, decreased breath sounds [pneumonia], or rhonchi [nonspecific], though absence of these findings does not exclude lung disease); **heart** (for S3 [CHF], or murmur [valvular disease]).

A. **Acute cough**

1. **Asthma exacerbation** (Table 13–1).

2. **Acute bronchitis/COPD** exacerbation may feature crackles, rhonchi, or wheezing (especially with forced expiration), but often lungs are clear. Fever, injected pharynx, or cervical lymphadenopathy may also occur. Acute bronchitis should not be diagnosed till viral URI, asthma, and an acute exacerbation of chronic bronchitis have been ruled out. [SOR **C**]

3. Findings with **aspiration** may range from minimal to localized wheezing to severe dyspnea.

4. **Viral URI** often features normal examination, but may present with clear rhinorrhea, pharyngeal erythema, cervical adenopathy, low-grade fever, and clear lungs.

5. **Irritants** (see Table 13–1).
6. **Rhinitis (allergic)** (see Table 13–1).
7. **Uncomplicated pneumonia** may present with fever, tachypnea, hypoxia, cyanosis, and evidence of pulmonary consolidation, or localized crackles or rhonchi. Atypical pneumonia may have minimal or no lung findings. The elderly may show mental status changes.
8. **Sinusitis/PND** (see Table 13–1).

B. **Subacute/chronic cough** (see Table 13–1).

V. **Laboratory Tests.** Tests are directed by history and examination findings (see Table 13–1). In patients with acute cough, where a cause is clear, treatment can generally be initiated without further testing. Further testing in acute cough is generally reserved for the very ill, atypical presentations, or poor response to standard treatment (see below).

A. **Hematologic tests**
1. **White blood cell (WBC) count** assists in febrile patients to support a diagnosis of bacterial infection (increased neutrophils) or viral infection (increased lymphocytes).
2. **Antibody titers** may be helpful in suspected fungal infection (aspergillosis, histoplasmosis, or coccidioidomycosis).
3. **Arterial blood gases** can assist assessment of hypoxemia in patients with severe asthma, pneumonia, COPD, or other pulmonary disease.
4. **Serologic testing (e.g., enzyme-linked immunosorbent assay [ELISA])** helps confirm suspected human immunodeficiency virus (HIV) infection.
5. **B-type natriuretic peptide (BNP),** a cardiac neurohormone produced by the ventricles in response to ventricular volume expansion and pressure overload, may assist in differentiating a cardiac from a pulmonary origin of cough. Levels > 100 pg/mL indicate CHF and those > 480 pg/mL correlate with a nearly 30-fold increase in cardiac events over the next 6 months. Since samples remain viable < 4 hours, this test is usually performed in the emergency department or inpatient setting.

B. **Pulmonary function tests (PFTs)** can differentiate obstructive from restrictive disease (asthma, COPD from sarcoid, pneumoconiosis, cystic fibrosis, respectively).
1. **Pre- and postbronchodilator testing** clarifies fixed compared with reversible disease (e.g., asthma).
2. **Bronchoprovocative testing** with methacholine inhalation uncovers subtle reversible airways obstruction in suspected asthmatic patients with normal or near-normal basic PFTs. Methacholine challenge is not widely available; its specificity approaches 100% in ruling out asthma, but its sensitivity is 60% to 80%, so positive testing does not conclusively rule asthma in.
3. PFTs are difficult to perform in children younger than 5 years, so diagnosis in these patients is based on history, examination, and response to treatment.
4. **Peak expiratory flow rate (PEFR)** testing is an office procedure helpful in quantifying severity of airflow obstruction and response to treatment in acute asthma exacerbations.

C. **Radiography/special imaging**
1. **Chest x-ray (CXR)** is helpful in evaluating for pneumonia or complicated aspiration (localized infiltrates), bronchiectasis, COPD (hyperinflation/flat diaphragms), TB (fibronodular upper lobe infiltrates, cavitary lesions, hilar adenopathy, pleural effusion), sarcoid (hilar adenopathy), pulmonary edema/congestive heart failure (vascular congestion, Kerley B-lines, perihilar infiltrates, pleural effusion, cardiomegaly). This testing is readily available and, depending on clinical presentation/level of pretest diagnostic certainty, should be ordered early in the evaluation of cough.
2. **Barium swallow** is helpful in young children with chronic cough to assess for vascular anomalies, such as aberrant innominate artery.
3. **Upper GI series** assists in evaluating those with chronic cough and poorly responsive GERD (for hiatal hernia or complications, such as ulceration and stricture).
4. **Computerized tomographic (CT) or magnetic resonance imaging (MRI) scanning** of the chest assists in evaluating for mass lesions of sarcoid or neoplasms in patients whose clinical evaluation raises suspicion for these problems. CXR should precede CT or MRI imaging. **Sinus CT** is the gold standard for diagnosing chronic sinusitis and should be considered with chronic PND, recurrent episodes of sinusitis, or pediatric asthma. Approximately 50% of children with asthma have radiographic evidence of sinusitis, and studies have shown that treatment of sinusitis decreases

bronchial hyperresponsiveness. Therefore, all children with asthma should be evaluated for concurrent sinusitis.

5. **2D echocardiogram** assesses left ventricular function and ejection fraction in suspected CHF. Multigated acquisition scan (**MUGA**) provides a more accurate ejection fraction than 2D Echo, but is more expensive and may not be as readily available.

D. Endoscopy

1. Referral for **bronchoscopy** is indicated in patients with (1) recurrent hemoptysis, (2) CT/MRI suggesting malignancy, or (3) chronic cough and negative results on basic clinical and testing evaluation.

2. **Nasopharyngoscopy** can be helpful in visualizing the turbinates/sinus ostia, pharynx, and larynx in individuals suspected of having cough originating in these structures (e.g., those with chronic sinusitis).

3. **Esophagogastroduodenoscopy (EGD)** is used to evaluate for GERD complications (such as esophagitis, ulceration and stricture, Barrett's esophagus, and adenocarcinoma).

E. Other tests

1. **Sputum cytology** may be helpful if history or CT/MRI suggest malignancy.

2. **Sputum Gram stain, culture, and smears** may also be used. Many eosinophils suggest eosinophilic bronchitis. Gram stains of induced sputum may be useful in determining a likely cause of pneumonia. Although not useful in identifying gram-positive organisms, cultures are helpful in identifying gram-negative bacteria, penicillin-resistant *S pneumoniae, Mycobacterium* species (acid-fast stain), and fungi.

3. **24-hour esophageal pH monitoring** is 92% sensitive for GERD but is invasive. It should therefore be performed only after failure of empiric GERD treatment and a negative evaluation for asthma and sinusitis.

4. **Pulse oximetry** allows easy, noninvasive assessment of arterial oxygen saturation and is helpful in monitoring severity or response to therapy in patients with asthma or COPD.

5. **Purified protein derivative (PPD)** skin testing is a useful screen for pulmonary TB and should be considered in all patients with chronic cough, especially those at high risk. PPD needs to be read within 48 to 72 hours of placement. A test is considered positive if the diameter of the reaction measures ≥ 5 mm for HIV-infected and other immunocompromised individuals, ≥ 10 mm for those at high risk and ≥ 15 mm for all others. If a PPD test is positive, a CXR should be ordered. Symptomatic patients should be placed in respiratory isolation, pending results of a sputum smear with acid-fast stain and mycobacterium culture. The Centers for Disease Control and Prevention no longer recommends routine anergy testing in conjunction with PPD skin testing among HIV-infected individuals.

6. **Nasal smear** may be helpful in differentiating allergic from infectious rhinitis (showing eosinophils and white blood cells, respectively).

7. **Skin testing** for allergies may be helpful in clarifying the role of allergens in cough and in evaluating severe, poorly controlled perennial allergic symptoms for possible benefit from desensitization.

8. **Polymerase chain reaction** testing of a nasopharyngeal specimen is helpful in diagnosing pertussis in individuals with suggestive clinical findings.

9. **Sweat chloride testing** is necessary in evaluating children with cough and other features suggestive of cystic fibrosis (failure to thrive, gastrointestinal abnormalities, and recurrent infections).

VI. **Treatment** directed at the underlying disease is reported to be successful 80% to 95% of the time. For most conditions, management should include hydration, humidification, and rest. [SOR **C**] If the diagnosis is initially unclear, empiric treatment for the most likely cause may be preferable to extensive investigation, because such treatment may provide relief as well as diagnosis (Figure 13–1). Adequate treatment is important. In one study, many patients were correctly diagnosed by their primary care physician before pulmonology referral, but treatment was not aggressive enough to stop the cough. There is no evidence for the use of beta-2 agonists (i.e., albuterol), leukotriene inhibitors, or inhaled steroids in treating nonspecific cough in children or adults who do not have airflow obstruction. (SOR **A**)

There are no randomized, controlled studies assessing the efficacy of prescription benzonatate (Tessalon Perles) compared with placebo.

Most nonprescription medications for cough of presumed viral origin are no better than placebo. [SOR **A**] However, there is some evidence that the older, sedating

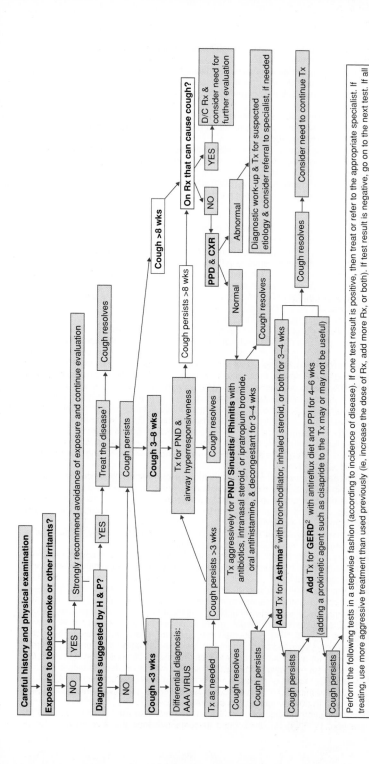

FIGURE 13–1. Cough management algorithm. [1] or discontinue medication, such as ACEI, if that is thought to be the cause of cough. [2] Tx for asthma and GERD are added, not substituted, based on the fairly high prevalence of patients having two (23%–42%) or even three (3%–15%) causes of chronic cough. ACEI, angiotensin converting enzyme inhibitor; CT, computerized tomography; CXR, chest x-ray; GERD, gastroesophageal reflux disease; PND, postnasal drainage; PPI, proton pump inhibitor; PPD, purified protein derivative; Rx, prescription; Tx, therapy.

The algorithm contains the following flow elements:

Careful history and physical examination

Exposure to tobacco smoke or other irritants?
- YES → Strongly recommend avoidance of exposure and continue evaluation
- NO → Diagnosis suggested by H & P?
  - YES → Treat the disease[1]
    - Cough resolves
    - Cough persists
  - NO → Cough <3 wks

Differential diagnosis: AAA VIRUS
- Tx as needed
  - Cough resolves
  - Cough persists >3 wks

Cough persists

Cough 3–8 wks → Tx for PND & airway hyperresponsiveness

Tx aggressively for **PND/ Sinusitis/ Rhinitis** with antibiotics, intranasal steroid, or ipratropium bromide, oral antihistamine, & decongestant for 3–4 wks
- Cough resolves
- Cough persists

Add Tx for **Asthma**[2] with bronchodilator, inhaled steroid, or both for 3–4 wks
- Cough resolves
- Cough persists

Add Tx for **GERD**[2] with antireflux diet and PPI for 4–6 wks (adding a prokinetic agent such as cisapride to the Tx may or may not be useful)
- Cough resolves
- Cough persists

Cough >8 wks

Cough persists >8 wks

On Rx that can cause cough?
- YES → D/C Rx & consider need for further evaluation
- NO → **PPD & CXR**
  - Normal
  - Abnormal → Diagnostic work-up & Tx for suspected etiology & consider referral to specialist, if needed

Cough resolves → Consider need to continue Tx

Perform the following tests in a stepwise fashion (according to incidence of disease). If one test result is positive, then treat or refer to the appropriate specialist. If treating, use more aggressive treatment than used previously (ie, increase the dose of Rx, add more Rx, or both). If test result is negative, go on to the next test. If all test results are negative, then refer to a pulmonologist for evaluation (including bronchoscopy) and treatment. **Test sequence:** Sinus CT, Pulmonary function tests, Methacholine challenge test, 24-hr esophageal pH monitoring. Other testing to rule out less common causes of chronic cough. Refer to pulmonologist.

antihistamine–decongestant combination medications are useful in treating cough in adults, but not in children. [SOR **B**] Treatment should take effect within 1 week. The newer, nonsedating antihistamines have not been shown to be efficacious in adults or children.

Several over-the-counter products are associated with side effects, particularly in children younger than 6 years, where some adverse effects of over-the-counter medications may be life-threatening. Reported adverse reactions of common medications include hypertension, tachycardia, central nervous system (CNS) stimulation (agitation, psychosis, seizures, insomnia), dysrhythmias and myocardial infarction (**pseudoephedrine**); CNS depression and anticholinergic symptoms, tachycardia, blurred vision, agitation, hyperactivity, seizures, torsades de pointes (**chlorpheniramine and brompheniramine**); and lethargy, stupor, hyperexcitability, abnormal limb movements, and coma (**dextromethorphan**).

If patients want to try an over-the-counter cough suppressant or expectorant (and are older than 6 years), they can, as there may be a beneficial placebo effect. Sucking on hard candies may have a similar effect.

A. Acute cough
1. **Asthma exacerbation** (see Chapter 68).
2. **Acute bronchitis/COPD exacerbation** (see Chapter 70). Supportive treatment for acute bronchitis includes rest, fluids (3 to 4 L/d, especially with fever), and albuterol inhaler if there is evidence of bronchospasm. Beta-2 agonists (i.e., Albuterol) are not effective, if there is no bronchospasm. [SOR **A**] Patients should expect to have a cough for 10 to 14 days. Patient satisfaction with the office visit does not depend on receiving an antibiotic, but instead on effective physician–patient communication. Patients should be advised that antibiotics are probably not going to be beneficial and that antibiotic treatment is associated with significant risks and side effects. To help patients understand the viral nature of their illness, it is helpful to refer to acute bronchitis as a "chest cold." Initial antibiotic prescription may be considered in patients with significant COPD, immunocompromised patients, patients with CHF, the elderly, and those appearing very ill or with high fever. [SOR **C**] The American College of Chest Physicians recommends considering an antibiotic if there is not at least some improvement of the cough by day 7. [SOR **B**]
3. **Aspiration.** Most swallowed foreign bodies are coughed up or passed through the gastrointestinal tract without difficulty. Ten to twenty percent (especially swallowed button batteries) need intervention (laryngoscopy, bronchoscopy, esophagogastroscopy), and 1% need surgery. Surgical removal should be considered for a foreign body distal to the pylorus that serial abdominal plain films reveal to be unchanged in position for >5 days.
4. **Viral URI** (see Chapter 55). Central cough suppressants, such as codeine and dextromethorphan, are not recommended for cough caused by URI, [SOR **B**] neither is zinc. [SOR **B**] However, there is some evidence that the older sedating antihistamine–decongestant combination medications (not the newer ones) and naproxen are useful in treating cough in adults, but not in children. [SOR **B**] Antibiotics are not indicated. If the cough does not start to improve after 1 week then another diagnosis, such as sinusitis, should be considered. [SOR **C**]
5. **Irritant-related cough.** Avoidance of the offending agent and smoking cessation should be encouraged. Approximately 75% of people stop coughing within a month of eliminating offensive exposures. (See Chapter 100 for suggestions on effective smoking cessation techniques.)
6. **Rhinitis (allergic)** (see Chapter 55).
7. **Uncomplicated pneumonia**
   a. **Antibiotics** for outpatient treatment of community-acquired pneumonia include a macrolide [LOR: A] (e.g., erythromycin, azithromycin, or clarithromycin) for suspected *M pneumoniae* or trimethoprim-sulfamethoxazole or amoxicillin clavulanate for other causes. [SOR **A**] Treatment should generally continue for 10 to 14 days, and symptomatic improvement should occur within 2 to 3 days.
   b. **Supportive treatment** includes antipyretics/analgesia and hydration.
   c. **Hospitalization** may be necessary, depending on comorbidities, support at home, and severity of illness. Indicators of severe illness include age older than 65 years with multiple medical problems, altered mental status, hypoxia (O_2 saturation <90% or PaO_2 <60 mm Hg on room air), hypercapnia ($PaCO_2$ >45 mm Hg), acidosis

(arterial pH <7.35), hypotension, sepsis, multiorgan dysfunction, anemia (Hb <9 g/dL), significant leukopenia or leukocytosis (<4000 WBC/mm^3 or >30,000 WBC/mm^3, respectively), or multilobe densities or large pleural effusion on CXR.

8. **Sinusitis/**postnasal drainage (see Chapter 55).

B. Subacute/chronic cough

1. **Gastroesophageal reflux disease (GERD)** (see Chapter 19). Four to six weeks of treatment with a proton pump inhibitor successfully diagnoses and treats the vast majority of patients with GERD-related cough. [SOR **A**]

2. **Asthma** (see Chapter 68).

3. **Smoking and other environmental irritants** (see Section VI.A.5).

4. **Postnasal drainage (PND)** (see Chapter 55). Treatment with antihistamine and decongestant combination alone is successful in >50% of nonsmokers with PND and chronic cough. [SOR **B**]

5. **Youth** Underlying disease should be treated. If the cough is thought to be psychogenic, a referral of the child and family for counseling should be considered. Children with vascular anomalies should be referred to a vascular surgeon. In general, medications to treat nonspecific cough in children (<15 years old) have not been shown to be effective and are therefore not recommended. [SOR **B**] However, a little improvement has been demonstrated in children with chronic nocturnal cough who were treated with high-dose inhaled steroids. [SOR **B**] Also, a Cochrane review of two studies supported the use of antibiotics in children <7 years old with chronic cough. [SOR **B**] It is important to discuss with parents their expectations and fears regarding their child's condition. Education and reassurance may be valuable in the management of cough. [SOR **C**]

6. **Eosinophilic bronchitis (nonasthmatic).** If an allergen or specific occupational exposure is identified as the cause, it should be avoided. [SOR **C**] Inhaled corticosteroids have been shown to be effective. [SOR **B**] If they are not effective, oral steroids should be given. [SOR **C**]

7. **Hyperresponsiveness of airways.** Hyperresponsiveness of airways persists for up to 8 weeks after URI and resolves without treatment. Significant cough warrants trial of a bronchodilator and an antihistamine, with addition of an inhaled steroid. [SOR **B**] If cough persists ,oral steroids [SOR **B**] and/or inhaled ipratropium bromide [SOR **B**] should be used.

8. **Angiotensin converting enzyme (ACE) inhibitors and other medicines.** ACE inhibitors and other medicines causing cough should be eliminated or changed (e.g., substituting an angiotensin receptor blocker for an ACE). Cough should resolve within 4 weeks after these changes.

9. **Chronic bronchitis/COPD** (see Chapter 70). According to a Cochrane review of patients with COPD exacerbations, antibiotic therapy significantly reduced short-term mortality by 77%, treatment failure by 53%, and sputum purulence by 44%, regardless of the specific antibiotic used. Antibiotics did not affect arterial blood gasses and peak flows. Antibiotics are recommended to treat moderately or severely ill patients with COPD exacerbations and a cough with purulent sputum. [LOR A] Salmeterol has been shown to decrease symptoms of cough, sputum and shortness of breath in patients with COPD. [SOR **B**] Codeine and dextromethorphan are recommended for short-term symptomatic relief of cough. [SOR **B**]

10. **Killer cancer.** Referral to an oncologist is indicated.

11. **I**diopathic (or "unexplained")—if no etiology can be determined, then options for adults are limited to nonspecific therapies such as dextromethorphan, [SOR **B**] inhaled ipratropium [SOR **B**] and/or codeine. [SOR **B**] It is important to periodically reevaluate the patient for new signs and symptoms, which may suggest an underlying illness.

12. **Tuberculosis**

    a. **Latent TB** (positive PPD and normal CXR) is treated with oral isoniazid, 300 mg daily for 9 months, with addition of oral pyridoxine (Vitamin B$_6$), 25 mg daily to prevent neuropathy in those older than 35 years.

    b. **Active TB** (positive PPD test and abnormal CXR or positive acid-fast bacilli culture/smear) requires reporting to the local health department, respiratory isolation and multidrug therapy (e.g., oral isoniazid combined with rifampin, pyrazinamide, streptomycin, or ethambutol). Because of variable resistance, consultation with an infectious disease specialist for assistance in drug selection and monitoring is prudent. During therapy, liver function tests should be monitored in those older than 35 years or with a history of drug/alcohol abuse or liver disease.

    c. To ensure compliance and effective treatment and to minimize the emergence of resistant strains, **directly observed therapy** should be implemented throughout treatment.

13. Uncommon causes. Treat according to etiology.

14. Pertussis

    a. Antibiotics. Antibiotics do not alter the course of the illness, unless initiated early in its course; however, antibiotics do prevent transmission and decrease the need for respiratory isolation from 4 weeks to 1 week.

    b. Suggested regimens

        (1) Macrolide antibiotics. Macrolide antibiotics are the treatment of choice; [SOR **A**] oral **erythromycin,** 500 mg 4 times a day in adults (40–50 mg/kg/d divided into 4 doses in pediatric patients, with maximum of 2 g/d) for 14 days, or oral. Side effects include nausea, vomiting, diarrhea and, in infants, pyloric stenosis. **Azithromycin,** 500 mg on day 1 and 250 g on days 2 to 5 for adults (10 mg/kg/d for 5 days in pediatric patients) are effective. It is the safest therapy for infants younger than 1 month. [SOR **B**] Clarithromycin 500 mg bid for 7 days (15 mg/kg divided bid in pediatric patients) is also effective.

        (2) Alternative regimen. Oral trimethoprim-sulfamethoxazole-DS twice daily in adults (8 mg TMP + 40 mg SMX/kg/d divided into twice-daily doses in pediatric patients) for 14 days is also effective. [SOR **A**] It should be used only in patients who are allergic to macrolides or have an intolerance to them. It is contraindicated in women who have a term pregnancy or are breast feeding, and in infants <2 months old.

        (3) Hospitalization. Hospitalization is recommended for seriously ill patients, especially infants. [SOR **C**]

    c. Close household contacts should be treated with antibiotics to prevent transmission of the disease. [SOR **B**]

    d. Vaccine. Adolescents should receive Tdap instead of the Td booster. [SOR **C**] Adults should receive a Tdap booster one time instead of Td. [SOR **C**]

15. Persistent Pneumonia (see Chapter 20). Respiratory fluoroquinolones should be given when first-line treatments (i.e., macrolides, trimethoprim/sulfamethoxazole, doxycycline) have failed. [LOR C]

16. Psychogenic (habit cough). Providing reassurance of normal test results can alleviate patient anxiety, increase patient acceptance of diagnosis, and decrease cough symptoms. Persistent psychogenic cough warrants psychological therapy such as counseling, behavior modification, and biofeedback. [SOC C]

REFERENCES

Bolser D. Cough suppressant and pharmacologic protussive therapy, ACCP evidence-based clinical practice guidelines. *Chest.* 2006;129:238S-249S.

D'Urzo A, Jugovic P. Chronic cough: three most common causes. *Can Fam Physician.* 2002;48:1311.

Holmes R, Fadden C. Evaluation of the patient with chronic cough. *Am Fam Physician.* 2004;69:2159-2166.

Irwin R, et al. Diagnosis and management of cough executive summary – ACCP evidence-based clinical practice guidelines. *Chest.* 2006;129:1S-23S.

Poe RH, Kallay MC. Chronic cough and gastroesophageal reflux disease: experience with specific therapy for diagnosis and treatment. *Chest.* 2003;123:679.

Ram FS, Rodriquez-Roisin R, Granados-Navarrete A, Garcia-Aymerich J, Barnes N. Antibiotics for exacerbations of chronic obstructive pulmonary disease. *Cochrane Database Syst Rev.* 2006;(2):CD004403.

Schroeder K, Fahey T. Systematic review of randomized controlled trials of over the counter cough medicines for acute cough in adults. *BMJ.* 2002;324:329.

14   Dermatitis & Other Pruritic Dermatoses

Jie Wang, MD, Aleksandra Zgierska, MD, PhD, William G. Phillips, MD,
& Marjorie Shaw Phillips, MS, RPh, FASHP

KEY POINTS

- Generalized pruritus requires as specific a diagnosis and treatment plan as possible.
- Many serious systemic diseases produce generalized pruritus without skin manifestations.
- Chronic pruritus has a variety of psychological explanations and consequences.

I. **Definition. Pruritus** is a sensation that causes one to itch, which is a peculiar irritating sensation in the skin that arouses the desire to scratch. **Dermatitis** is inflammation of the skin, whereas **dermatosis** is defined as any disease of the skin in which inflammation is not necessarily a feature.

For the purposes of this chapter, dermatitis and pruritic dermatoses will be considered in terms of the following: (1) primary dermatoses, (2) symptoms of significant internal medical or surgical illness, and (3) primary psychological disturbances.

II. **Common Diagnoses.** Approximately 15% of all patients presenting to primary care providers do so for care of a skin disease or lesion, and pruritic dermatoses are a significant proportion of these. Severe and chronic pruritus may significantly affect quality of life, including causing insomnia/daytime drowsiness, anxiety, distraction from one's daily social functioning, and personal embarrassment.

A. **Pruritic dermatoses**

1. **Atopic eczema** (Figure 14–1) a chronic inflammatory pruritic skin disease, is found in approximately 7 to 24 individuals per 1000 in the United States. It affects children and adults; however, it is more common in infancy and childhood. In 50% of affected children, the condition persists into adulthood. According to the PRACTALL Consensus Report, risk factors for developing and predicting the severity of the atopic dermatitis are parental atopy, exposure to aeroallergens (pets, mites, and pollens), sensitization to food allergens, and severity of disease in infancy.

2. **Contact dermatitis** (Figure 14–2) affects one in 1000 workers annually and accounts for 50% of occupational illness. Those particularly at risk include workers in manufacturing, food production, construction, machine tool operation, printing, metal plating, and leather processing. The majority of occupational contact dermatitis is irritant-related; however, approximately 40% of cases are believed to be **allergic.** Allergic contact dermatitis is uncommon in young children and less common in deeply pigmented individuals.

3. **Scabies** (Figure 14–3) caused by the mite *Sarcoptes scabiei,* is an extremely common pruritic infestation, with estimated global prevalence of 300 million. It occurs in both genders and across all ages; it is transmitted by close skin-to-skin contact. Scabies should always be considered when multiple family members develop an intense pruritic rash at the same time.

4. **Head lice (pediculosis capitis)** affect 6 to 12 million people in the United States annually, occur most frequently in school or day care settings, and require significant head-to-head contact for transmission. Head lice infest all levels of societal and ethnic groups. **Pediculosis pubis** is usually transmitted sexually; it is often seen in the context of venereal disease clinics and student health services. **Body lice (pediculosis humanus)** are much less common than pediculosis pubis or capitis and are usually seen in a setting of poor hygiene, homelessness, and crowded conditions.

5. **Lichen simplex chronicus** (Figure 14–4) is more common in adults than in children; it preferentially affects middle-aged women, atopic individuals, and those experiencing substantial stress.

6. **Lichen planus** (Figure 14–5) typically begins in the fourth decade. It is associated with a positive family history in approximately 10% of cases. It has also been linked to

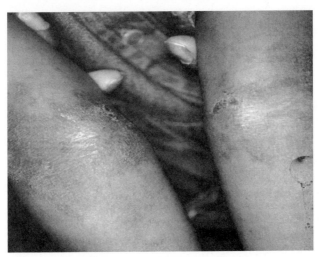

FIGURE 14–1. Atopic dermatitis (see color insert). (This photograph has been taken by and is the property of Dick Anstett, MD, MPH. Faculty, Family Medicine Residency of Idaho, Boise, Idaho.)

liver disease (e.g., hepatitis C) and use of certain medications, especially thiazides, captopril, and antimalarials. It is rare in children younger than 5 years.

7. **Xerosis (dry skin)** is common in northern climates, particularly during the winter months with indoor heating and low relative humidity. It is a common problem in the elderly, but can also affect younger individuals and children. It is seen particularly in atopic individuals, who bathe frequently (especially using soap), chemical or solvent exposure, as well as with hypothyroidism, antiandrogen or diuretic therapy.

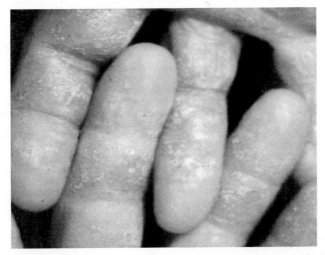

FIGURE 14–2. Contact dermatitis from dishwasher water (see color insert). (This photograph has been taken by and is the property of Dick Anstett, MD, MPH. Faculty, Family Medicine Residency of Idaho, Boise, Idaho.)

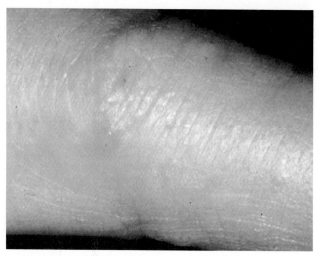

FIGURE 14–3. Scabies (see color insert). (This photograph has been taken by and is the property of Dick Anstett, MD, MPH. Faculty, Family Medicine Residency of Idaho, Boise, Idaho.)

8. **Dyshidrosis** (Figure 14–6) accounts for 5% to 20% of all hand dermatitis, is more common during spring and summer in warmer climates, and may be associated with stress.

9. **Pityriasis rosea** (Figure 14–7) is seen more frequently in women than in men, and mostly in persons 10 to 35 years old. The incidence of the disease is higher during the colder months, and some patients have a recent history of viral upper respiratory infection associated with fatigue, headache, sore throat, and fever.

10. **Psoriasis** (Figure 14–8) affects 2% of people of European ancestry. It has a presumed autoimmune etiology and 40% of patients have a positive family history. Summer season, sunlight, and relaxation can improve psoritic lesions, while upper respiratory and streptococcal infections, trauma to the skin, stress, and certain medications (lithium, beta-blockers, angiotensin converting enzyme inhibitors, and indomethacin) can exacerbate psoriasis. Approximately 15% of affected patients develop a seronegative inflammatory arthritis that clinically resembles rheumatoid arthritis. **Guttate psoriasis** occurs in 2% of patients with psoriasis, typically begins before age 30 and affects all races.

11. **Dermatophyte infection** is common, with 10% to 20% estimated lifetime risk of acquisition. **Tinea capitis** is most common in 3- to 8-year-old boys and may occur in epidemics. **Tinea corporis** is frequently seen in farmers and people who have pets. **Tinea cruris** is 4 times more common in young adults and males than in other groups. Obesity, heat, humidity, perspiration, and chafing predispose individuals to this condition. **Tinea pedis** affects mostly adults (children are rarely infected) and more males than females. Acquisition of the disease appears to depend on a susceptibility factor.

11. **Seborrhea, a chronic inflammatory skin disease** (Figure 14–9) is often familial and most commonly occurs in adult men. It can be associated with hyperandrogenicity (e.g., polycystic ovarian syndrome, hirsutism), diabetes mellitus, sprue, Parkinson disease, and epilepsy; seborrhea may be a symptom of human immunodeficiency virus (HIV) infection before other more specific symptoms of this illness occur.

12. **Nummular** (Figure 14–10) **eczema** typically occurs in young adults and, less commonly, in children. Its etiology is unknown, although the history is often positive for asthma or seasonal allergies, and, in the elderly, a low-protein diet.

B. **Pruritus in systemic disease**

1. **Pruritus can be a presenting symptom of systemic disease** in 10% to 50% of elderly patients. Systemic diseases associated with pruritus include hyperthyroidism,

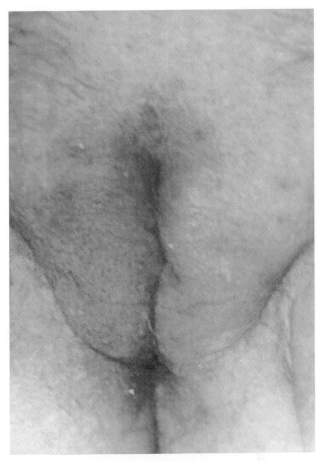

FIGURE 14–4. Lichen simplex chronicus (see color insert). (This photograph has been taken by and is the property of Dick Anstett, MD, MPH. Faculty, Family Medicine Residency of Idaho, Boise, Idaho.)

hypothyroidism, polycythemia vera, iron deficiency, obstructive biliary disease, multiple myeloma, HIV, lymphoma, Hodgkin disease (up to 30% of Hodgkin disease patients present with generalized pruritus), and end-stage renal failure (severe pruritus affects up to 25% of patients with chronic renal failure).

2. **Puritic urticarial papules and plaques of pregnancy** (Figure 14–11) (PUPP) is the most common skin condition of pregnancy, usually appearing in the late third trimester.

C. **Pruritus with a prominent psychogenic component**

1. **Delusions of parasitosis** (Figure 14–12) are an example of a primary psychiatric disorder with dermatologic manifestations. Those affected by this disorder experience delusions of being infested by bugs, mites, worms or other creatures, and experience a severe itching as a result of "infestation." Delusions of parasitosis can be symptoms of a primary mental health disorder (schizophrenia, psychotic depression, hypochondriasis, or some of the addictive disorders, such as alcohol withdrawal, amphetamine or cocaine effects); they can also be associated with medical conditions (vitamin B_{12} deficiency, cerebrovascular disease, neurosyphilis, multiple sclerosis) or caused by medication side effects (glucocorticoids) or medication-related allergic reactions.

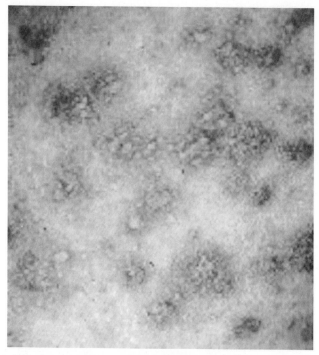

FIGURE 14–5. Lichen planus (see color insert). (This photograph has been taken by and is the property of Dick Anstett, MD, MPH. Faculty, Family Medicine Residency of Idaho, Boise, Idaho.)

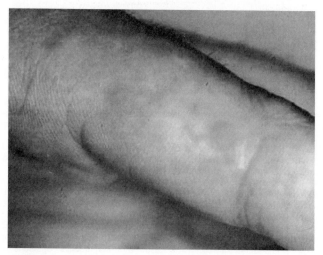

FIGURE 14–6. Dyshidrotic eczema (see color insert). (This photograph has been taken by and is the property of Dick Anstett, MD, MPH. Faculty, Family Medicine Residency of Idaho, Boise, Idaho.)

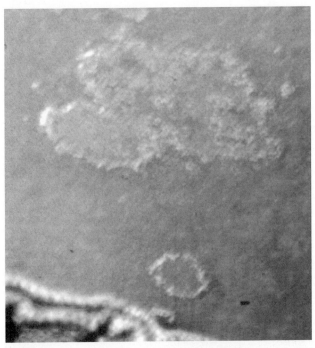

FIGURE 14–7. Herald patch, pityriasis rosea (see color insert). (This photograph has been taken by and is the property of Dick Anstett, MD, MPH. Faculty, Family Medicine Residency of Idaho, Boise, Idaho.)

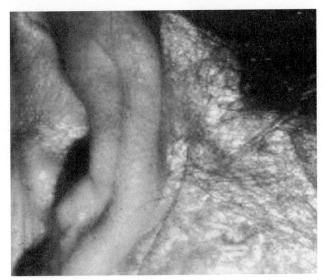

FIGURE 14–8. Psoriasis (see color insert). (This photograph has been taken by and is the property of Dick Anstett, MD, MPH. Faculty, Family Medicine Residency of Idaho, Boise, Idaho.)

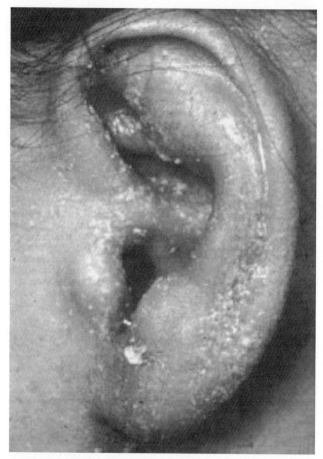

FIGURE 14–9. Seborrhea dermatitis (see color insert). (This photograph has been taken by and is the property of Dick Anstett, MD, MPH. Faculty, Family Medicine Residency of Idaho, Boise, Idaho.)

    2. Localized psychogenic pruritus or localized itchiness with subsequent scratching, without identifiable organic pathology, occurs in 9% of patients with pruritus. It typically begins between ages 30 and 45, and is more prevalent in women (52%–92% of patients). Depression, anxiety, and other mental health disorders can play a significant role in the etiology of the behavior.

III. Symptoms. The intensity of pruritus in the pruritic dermatoses may vary from mild and annoying to intense. All patients presenting with pruritus, especially when it is chronic and without characteristic features of common dermatoses (Table 14–1), should be assessed for systemic disease or psychiatric disorders (e.g., anxiety/depression, obsessive–compulsive disorder, or somatoform disorder).

IV. Signs (Table 14–1)

    A. Pruritic dermatoses. As with many dermatologic conditions, the diagnosis of most pruritic dermatoses is made on the basis of pattern recognition of skin lesions. **Pattern recognition** is the ability to identify a skin condition by its basic morphology, shape, size, color, distribution and presence or absence of secondary features, such as pruritus. At times, a particular feature of a lesion or the history of the lesion may be extremely helpful

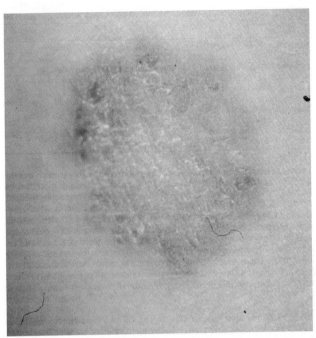

FIGURE 14–10. Nummular eczema (see color insert). (This photograph has been taken by and is the property of Dick Anstett, MD, MPH. Faculty, Family Medicine Residency of Idaho, Boise, Idaho.)

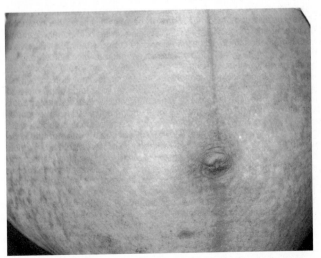

FIGURE 14–11. PUPP (see color insert). (This photograph has been taken by and is the property of Dick Anstett, MD, MPH. Faculty, Family Medicine Residency of Idaho, Boise, Idaho.)

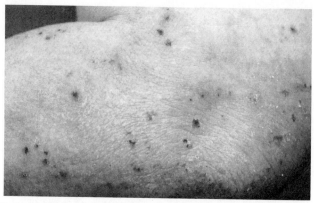

FIGURE 14–12. Delusion of parasitosis (see color insert). (This photograph has been taken by and is the property of Dick Anstett, MD, MPH. Faculty, Family Medicine Residency of Idaho, Boise, Idaho.)

in forming a diagnosis. Examples include: (1) the presence of a "herald patch" in pityriasis rosea, (2) the classic distribution of lichen simplex chronicus on the back of the neck, (3) the presence of lice or nits in pediculosis, (4) the presence of mite eggs or feces in scabies, and (5) the linear vesicles or symmetric lesions of contact dermatitis.

1. **Dyshidrosis** presents with many deep-seated, small, intense pruritic vesicles, most commonly occurring on the hands and feet. These acute lesions usually last for 3 to 4 weeks and spontaneously resolve, often with associated scaling. Dyshidrosis can recur or progress into chronic lesions that include lichenification and fissuring.

2. **Pityriasis rosea** generally starts as a single large patch (herald patch) followed several days later by more lesions that often follow cleavage lines or appear in a "Christmas tree" pattern. These oval lesions, usually with some scaling at the edges, may take 6 to 12 weeks to spontaneously resolve. Instead of characteristic truncal lesions, African Americans may have facial or extremity lesions.

3. **PUPP** presents with intensely pruritic papules that usually develop on the gravid abdomen near the umbilical area and spreads to the thighs and extremities, sparing the face, palms, and soles. The lesions usually resolve spontaneously within 1 week of parturition.

B. In patients whose lesions lack the morphology of primary dermatoses (Table 14–1), especially in the elderly, signs of underlying systemic disease (e.g., cholestasis, chronic renal failure, lymphoma, HIV, multiple myeloma, etc.) should be carefully sought.

C. Primary psychiatric disorders. Patients with **delusions of parasitosis** often have a positive "matchbox" sign: The patient brings in a matchbox or other container with bits of excoriated skin, debris, or "insect parts" as a "proof" of infestation.

V. Laboratory Tests

A. The history and the physical examination are generally all that is necessary to correctly diagnose common primary dermatoses. The tests listed below can be useful to confirm a particular diagnosis.

1. **Microscopic examination**

    a. With **mineral oil.** In suspected scabies, scrapings of suspected mite burrows should be microscopically examined (with mineral oil); findings of mites, their eggs or feces confirm the diagnosis.

    b. With **potassium hydroxide (KOH).** In tinea, microscopic examination with KOH is the classic test. Skin scrapings are placed on a glass slide, one or two drops of 10% to 20% KOH are added, and the slide is heated gently to dissolve cellular material. Hyphae or spores are characteristic of tinea.

2. **Wood's light examination** is useful in the differential diagnosis of tinea capitis from other conditions. Some forms of tinea capitis fluorensce bright yellow–green in the Wood's lamp light. Erythrasma, a skin condition resembling tinea and caused by *Corynebacterium minutissimum*, will fluoresce red.

TABLE 14–1. DIFFERENTIAL DIAGNOSES OF COMMON PRURITIC DERMATOSES

Diagnosis	Locations(s) Affected	Usual Morphology
Atopic eczema	Symmetrical—cheeks/scalp/chest/ extensor (infants); lichenified flexural/eyelids/perioral (children) flexural hands/forearms/wrists/feet (teen/adult)	Thickened dry plaques
Contact dermatitis	At sites of irritant exposure; shape of irritant (e.g., watchband)	Vesicles (acute) Crusty, lichenification (chronic)
Scabies	Web spaces of fingers, hands, wrists, axillae, buttocks, groin; facial/scalp (infants)	Linear vesicles, erythematous papules Lichenified, excoriated
Lice	Scalp, pelvic, pubic	Nits on hairs $1/4''$ from skin (capitis/pubis) Excoriation (body lice)
Lichen simplex chronicus	Back of neck, shoulders, forearms, lower legs, cheeks, perianal	Liner excoriations, scabs, scars
Lichen planus	Flexural wrists, scalp, trunk, ankles, genital, buccal mucosa	Violaceous flat-topped polygonal plaques White streaks on buccal mucosa (Wickham striae)
Xerosis	Especially lower legs	Exaggerated skin lines, plaques with superficial fissures
Dyshidrosis	Palms/web spaces (80% of patients) Feet (10%) Feet and hands (10%)	Burning or itching, followed by deep ("tapioca-like") vesicles
Pityriasis rosea	Chest and trunk	Initially papulosquamous oval scaly 2- to 10-cm diameter pink "herald patch" followed by "Christmas tree" pink, scaly oval, salmon-colored macules on back
Psoriasis	Symmetrical—elbows/knees/ears/ scalp/ umbilicus/gluteal cleft/ genitalia/nails	Sharply demarcated erythematous plaque covered with grayish-white or silver–white scale; pitting/thickened nails 1- to 10-mm pink/red papules with fine scale (guttate)
Tinea corporis	Extremities, face, trunk	Flat scaly papules spreading radially into circinate lesion with raised scaly edge and central clearing
Tinea pedis	Interdigital; plantar	Interdigital scale/fissures Scaling plantar surface ("moccasin") Vesiculobullous
Tinea cruris	Groin folds	Radially expanding raised edge with central clearing, slight scale
Seborrhea	Scalp, nasolabial folds, upper chest, postauricular creases, brows, eyelashes	Occasional dry flakes to thick greasy scale Diffuse erythema to oozing cracks
Nummular eczema	Extremities	Coin-red plaques 1–5 cm diameter with minimal scaling
Primary psychological disorders	Face/scalp/trunk/arms/legs	Bitane excoriations because of scratching or self-inflicted damage from cigarettes, chemicals or sharp instruments without evidence of underlying skin disorder
Localized psychogenic pruritus	Localized lesions (neck, trunk, extremities)	Linear excoriations, scab, scar

3. **Patch testing** is the classic test for allergic contact dermatitis. A patch containing the suspected allergen is applied to the skin for 48 hours and then removed. The skin is observed 20 minutes later for skin reaction in the "patched" area.
4. **Biopsy**
   a. If an eczema-like lesion involves the nipple and does not subside with simple treatment, biopsy should be performed to evaluate for Paget disease: More than 95% of people with Paget disease of the nipple also have breast cancer.

    b. In cases of pityriasis, the physician should consider a serologic test or a biopsy to rule out syphilis.

    c. When the diagnosis is in doubt, a biopsy should always be considered.

B. When the diagnosis of a common primary pruritic dermatosis is questionable and the above tests fail to confirm it, additional tests should be considered. Further testing is especially indicated in the absence of reassuring factors (e.g., localized lesions, recent travel, contacts with a person displaying similar lesions, occupational exposure), in elderly patients or in those with suspected underlying systemic disease. Additional tests include thyroid-stimulating hormone, bilirubin, alkaline phosphatase, blood urea nitrogen, creatinine, complete blood count, HIV testing and chest radiographs.

VI. Treatment. Treatment goals include (1) appropriate management of diseases causing pruritus, (2) symptomatic relief, and (3) cosmetic improvement, if indicated.

A. General measures

  1. Nonmedication measures (SOR **C**) include some or all of the following:

    a. Bathing no more frequently than daily, for 5 to 10 minutes, using warm (not hot) water.

    b. Using mild soap (e.g., Alpha-Keri, Cetaphil, Dove, Nivea Cream, Oilatum, Purpose, Basis) or soap-free cleansers (e.g., Cetaphil lotion, Aquanil lotion, SFC lotion, Lowila, Aveeno cleansing), and limiting soap use to specific body areas only (e.g., axillae, genitals, feet, etc.).

    c. Patting (not rubbing) the skin during drying.

    d. Applying emollients within a few minutes of bathing. Emollients range from lotions (least occlusive) to creams (most cosmetically acceptable) to ointments (most occlusive, but also greasy). Additives such as urea (e.g., Carmol, Aqua Care, and Ureacin) or lactic acid (e.g., Lac-Hydrin, Penecare) may be indicated to decrease dryness and promote skin hydration.

    e. Using a humidifier during cold months.

    f. Soaking dry, pruritic areas in cool solution of colloidal oatmeal (Aveeno) or baking soda.

    g. Cutting fingernails and wearing cotton gloves during sleep (for individuals who have difficulty controlling scratching).

    h. Avoiding known irritants, for example, alcohol, caffeine, rubber shoes, dyed socks, cosmetics, hairspray, or jewelry.

  2. Medications. In individuals with more severe symptoms or lesions that have been refractory to nonmedication measures (Section VI.A.1), one or a combination of the following medications may be beneficial.

    a. Topical medications

      (1) Corticosteroids (SOR **C**) (Table 14–2)

        (a) The efficacy and side effects of topical corticosteroids depend on several factors, including steroid **potency** (ranging from group 1 to 7, where 1 indicates most potent), **vehicle** potency (ointment > cream > lotions), **anatomic area** (for a given agent, the greatest penetration occurs on the face and groin, the lowest on palms and soles), and lesion **thickness** (thickened plaques are more resistant to treatment than thinner lesions).

        (b) As a general rule, the least potent effective medication and vehicle should be chosen first to treat the lesion; this preparation should be used for as short a time as necessary. For example, in pediatric patients or those with intertriginous lesions, a group 6 or 7 (the least potent) topical corticosteroid should be prescribed; group 1 or 2 (the most potent) agents are appropriate for thickened lesions on the palm or sole.

        (c) Side effects associated with use of topical corticosteroids are mainly localized to the area of application and include skin atrophy, telangiectasia, striae, hypopigmentation, rosacea, acne, or perioral dermatitis. The risk of systemic side effects (e.g., cataracts, glaucoma, growth suppression in children, Cushing syndrome, hypothalamic-pituitary-adrenal suppression, osteoporosis, etc.) increases with the percentage of treated body surface, duration of treatment, and potency of the steroid.

      (2) Topical antihistamines (e.g., diphenhydramine) or **topical doxepin** (a trycyclic antidepressant), applied to affected areas 3 to 4 times daily (doxepin for maximum of 8 days), may be used to relieve pruritus. However, they may cause allergic contact dermatitis.

TABLE 14–2. TOPICAL STEROIDS FOR DERMATOSES

Generic Name of Product	Dosing*	Trade Name(s)	Cost[†]
Lowest potency			
Hydrocortisone (cream, ointment, lotion) 0.5%–2.5%	qd–qid	Generic	$–$$
2.5% cream		Hytone, Synacort, etc.	$$–$$$
0.5%–1% available without prescription			
Dexamethasone (topical aerosol) 0.01%	bid–qid	Aeroseb-Dex[‡]	$$$$
Low potency			
Betamethasone valerate (cream) 0.01%	qd–tid	Valisone Reduced Strength	$$$$
Fluocinolone acetonide (cream, ointment) 0.01%	bid–qid	Generic, Flurosyn	$–$$
		Synalar	$$
Flurandrenolide (cream,[‡] ointment,[‡] lotion) 0.025%	bid–tid	Cordran, Cordran SP	$$$$
Triamcinolone acetonide (cream, ointment, lotion, aerosol) 0.025%	tid–qid	Generic	$
		Aristocort, Aristocort A, Kenalog	$$$
High potency (for acute, self-limited dermatosis; avoid on face)			
Fluocinolone acetonide (cream) 0.2%	bid–qid	Synalar-HP	$$$$
Fluocinonide (cream, gel, ointment, solution) 0.05%	bid–qid	Generic	$$$
		Lidex, Lidex-E	$$$$
Halcinonide (cream, ointment, solution) 0.1%	qd, bid–tid	Halog, Halog-E	$$$$
Triamcinolone acetonide (cream, ointment) 0.5%	bid–qid	Generic	$
		Aristocort, Aristocort A, Kenalog	$$$$$

*Usual adult doses. Patients should be instructed to apply sparingly to skin in a light film and rub in gently.
[†]Average wholesale cost to the pharmacist for 15 g of ointment or cream: $, <$2; $$, $2–5; $$$, $5–10; $$$$, $10–20; $$$$$, >$20.
[‡]Available as a 58-g spray.

b. Oral medications

    (1) Antihistamines The value of antihistamines in the treatment of pruritus is mainly because of their sedative properties. (SOR **C**) They may be useful as a short-term, adjuvant therapy added to topical treatment. The newer second-generation antihistamines are less sedating, but also less effective in controlling pruritus when compared to older sedating agents.

        (a) **First-generation antihistamines** are sedating and associated with decreased alertness and worsening of psychomotor performance. Examples of first-generation antihistamines include: **hydroxyzine** (adults: 25–100 mg orally [po] every 6–8 hours; children older than 12 years: adult dosing, but start with lower doses; children 6–12 years old: 12.5–25 mg po every 6–8 hours; children younger than 6 years: 2 mg/kg/d po in 3–4 divided doses) and **diphenhydramine** (over-the-counter *Benadryl*; administer as needed, adults: 25–50 mg po every 4–6 hours, maximum 400 mg/d; children older than 12 years: adult dosing, but start with lower doses, maximum 300 mg/d; children 6–12 years old: 12.5–25 mg po every 4–6 hours, maximum 150 mg/d; children 2–6 years old: 6.25–12.5 mg po every 4–6 hours, maximum 37.5 mg/d; not recommended in infants or neonates).

        (b) **Second-generation antihistamines** are less sedating, but generally less effective in controlling pruritus than older agents. Examples of second-generation antihistamines include **loratadine** (*Claritin OTC*; adults and children older than 6 years: 10 mg po once daily; children 2–6 years old: 5 mg po once daily), **fexofenadine** (adults and children older than 12 years: 180 mg po once daily or 60 mg po twice a day; children 6–11 years old: 30 mg po twice a day; children 6 months to 5 years old: 15–30 mg po twice a day), **cetirizine** (adults and children older than 6 years: 5–10 mg po once daily; children 2–6 years old: 2.5–5 mg po daily; children 12–24 months old: 2.5 mg po once–twice daily, maximum 5 mg/d; children 6–12 months old: 2.5 mg po once daily).

      (c) Tricyclic antidepressants have antihistaminic and sedative effects and may be beneficial in reducing pruritus, as well as promoting sleep (e.g., **doxepin,** adults: 10 mg po once daily at bedtime, may gradually increase to 25 mg at bedtime; it is not approved to use in the pediatric patients). Tricyclic antidepressants should be used with caution in persons receiving other sedative medications, in the elderly, and in patients with cardiac conduction defects or prostatic hypertrophy.

    (2) Oral corticosteroids (SOR **C**) may be beneficial for acute flare-ups or pruritic lesions that have been refractory to other therapies (described above). Prednisone can be prescribed as a short "burst"(4–5 days, 40–60 mg/d on average, this dosing can be stopped without tapering) or longer therapy, if needed (e.g., starting with 60 mg/d for 1–3 days, followed by tapering). "Burst" therapy minimizes side effects complicating long-term oral steroid therapy, which can include growth disturbance, osteoporosis, cataracts, and immunosuppression. Systemic corticosteroid therapy should be particularly cautious in children.

B. Therapies for specific dermatoses

  1. Atopic dermatitis (atopic eczema)

    a. The foundation of treatment is regular use of emollients and conscientious **skin hydration** (see Section VI.A.1), as well as avoidance of irritants and specific triggers. (SOR **C**)

    b. For mild breakthrough symptoms despite the foregoing treatment, a **low-tomoderate-potency steroid** can be added; (SOR **C**) for persistent or more severe breakthrough symptoms, a higher-potency topical steroid can be used (see Table 14–2).

    c. Oral antihistamines, especially the first-generation sedating agents, may be beneficial as a short-term, adjuvant therapy in relieving pruritus, in conjunction with topical therapy.

    d. Topical immunosuppressant, tacrolimus and **pimecrolimus,** are approximately as effective as medium-potency topical corticosteroids. They can be used when glucocorticoids are ineffective or contraindicated, and are considered a second-line therapy for moderate to severe atopic dermatitis. (SOR **C**) Common side effects associated with use of these medications include skin burning, erythema, and pruritus that are usually minor, self-limited, resolving after a few days of therapy. Tacrolimus and pimecrolimus do not cause skin atrophy, but have received a "black box warning" owing to possibility of being linked to rare cases of malignancies (e.g., skin cancer and lymphoma). Therefore, current recommendations (SOR **C**) include avoiding continuous long-term use of topical tacrolimus and pimecrolimus, and their use should be limited to areas affected by atopic dermatitis. **Dosage of tacrolimus:** adults can apply thin layer of 0.03% or 0.1% ointment topically to affected areas twice a day; children older than 2 years can apply a thin layer of 0.03% ointment twice a day; of **pimecrolimus:** adults can apply 1% cream topically to affected areas twice daily; children 2 years and older can use 1% cream twice daily. Tacrolimus and pimecrolimus are not approved for topical use in children younger than 2 years.

    e. Patients who are compliant with prescribed treatment, but respond poorly, should generally be evaluated by a dermatologist for consideration of ultraviolet phototherapy or oral immunosuppressant therapy (e.g., cyclosporine).

  2. Contact dermatitis is best treated by identifying and removing the offending agent. Existing evidence supports use of barrier creams containing dimethicone, short-term use of high-lipid content moisturizers, and use of cotton liners if occlusive gloves are worn for prevention and treatment of irritant contact dermatitis. (SOR **B**) Barrier creams with aluminum chlorohydrate seem to be ineffective. (SOR **B**) **Acute** contact dermatitis (weepy, edematous, vesicular lesions) is best treated with cotton dressings soaked in Burrow solution (aluminum acetate diluted 1:40 with cool water), applied 4 to 6 times daily. **Chronic** contact dermatitis (dry, scaly, thickened lesions) can be treated with emollients (Section VI.A.1) and topical corticosteroids (Section VI.A.2.a.(1) and Table 14–2).

  3. Scabies and **lice**—for treatment details see Chapter 7.

  4. Lichen simplex chronicus. Treatment involves managing underlying mood disorders (Chapters 89, 92, and 94), and educating patients about the itch–scratch cycle and ways to control it (see Section VI.A). In addition, topical and systemic antipruritic medications and general measures can be used to alleviate symptoms.

5. **Lichen planus** should be treated with general measures (Section VI.A) and topical corticosteroids (Section VI.A.2.a.(1) and Table 14–2). Steroid gels (e.g., 0.05% fluocinonide applied 2 times daily) can be effective for intraoral lesions.

6. **Dry skin (xerosis).** Elimination of aggravating factors (e.g., certain medications) is an essential aspect of treatment. Good skin hydration and lubrication (as outlined in Section VI.A.1) alleviate symptoms.

7. **Dyshidrosis.** Nonpharmacologic management includes use of mild cleansers and soap substitutes, wearing protective gloves, and avoiding known hand irritants. Burrow solution (Section VI.B.2) can help improve bullous lesions. Medium- and high-potency topical corticosteroids can be used for flare-ups (Section VI.A.2.a.(1) and Table 14–2). Oral steroids (Section VI.A.2.b.(2)) may benefit more severe or acute symptoms. Those with persistent or refractory dyshidrosis should be referred to a dermatologist for psoralen plus ultraviolet A or low-dose methotrexate therapy.

8. **Pityriasis rosea** does not have a specific treatment. Oral antihistamines as well as Aveeno baths may reduce pruritus. Patients should be reassured that the condition is benign, self-limited, and usually lasts for 6 to 8 weeks.

9. **Psoriasis.** Treatment of psoriatic lesions aims at the reduction of epidermal cell turnover and consists of topical, systemic, and phototherapy.
   a. **Topical therapy**
      (1) Emollients (e.g., Desitin ointment or A and D ointment, applied 3 times a day) should be applied chronically to affected areas.
      (2) Keratolytic agents, such as salicylic acid (e.g., salicylic acid soap), applied daily, can bring limited improvement, but also irritate inflamed skin.
      (3) Topical steroid ointments, mild to moderate potency, (see Table 14–2) are one of the mainstays of treatment, (SOR **Ⓒ**) but can cause localized skin atrophy with prolonged use.
      (4) Tar preparations (e.g., Estar applied at bedtime to affected areas, allowing the gel to remain for 5 min and then removing any excess by patting with tissues) can also be used. (SOR **Ⓒ**)
      (5) Calcipotriene (Dovonex), a topical treatment for psoriasis of mild to moderate severity, (SOR **Ⓒ**) is a vitamin D derivative that inhibits epidermal cell proliferation in vitro. Calcipotriene should be applied twice daily to psoriatic plaques on the trunk or the extremities. Application should be avoided with occlusion, or to the face and the groin where it may cause irritation. Topical calcipotriene is approximately as effective as moderate to high potency topical steroids, but may require 6 to 8 weeks of use before lesion improvement is noted. Absorption of calcipotriene is a problem only if large quantities (>100 g/week) are applied. Calcipotriene should not be used by patients with hypercalcemia or evidence of vitamin D toxicity.
   b. Patients with generalized psoriasis, psoriatic arthritis, and who are acutely ill or requiring specialized treatment should be referred to a dermatologist. Dermatology consultation should also be considered for localized psoriasis requiring specialized treatment, or uncontrolled with topical corticosteroids, calcipotriene, or coal tar products.

10. **Dermatophyte infection**
    a. **Tinea capitis** and **barbae**—for treatment see Chapter 32.
    b. **Tinea corporis.** Superficial and localized lesions respond well to topical antifungal agents (SOR **Ⓒ**) applied once or twice daily for 1 to 2 weeks beyond when clinical response is first noted. These agents include topical clotrimazole, econazole, ketoconazole, miconazole, and terbinafine. More extensive lesions or lesions unresponsive to a topical therapy should be treated for 2 to 4 weeks with an oral agent (e.g., griseofulvin ultramicrosize, adults: 375 mg daily; children 2 years old and older: 5–10 mg/kg/d divided into 1 or 2 doses). (SOR **Ⓒ**)
    c. **Tinea pedis.** Tinea pedis can be treated with topical antifungal preparations, although sometimes it may require 4 to 8 weeks of concomitant oral antifungal treatment (e.g., griseofulvin ultramicrosize, adults: 250 mg 3 times daily; children 2 years and older: 5–10 mg/kg/d divided into 1 or 2 doses). (SOR **Ⓒ**)

11. Seborrhea

    a. In adults, conventional therapy for **seborrheic dermatitis** of the scalp is a shampoo containing one of the following compounds: **salicylic acid** (e.g., X-Seb T or Sebulex), **selenium sulfide** (e.g., Selsun or Excel), **coal tar** (e.g., DHS Tar, Neutrogena T-Gel, or Polytar), or **pyrithione zinc** (e.g., DHS Zinc, Danex, or Sebulon). (SOR **C**) Each of these shampoos can be used 2 or 3 times a week. After application, shampoos should be left on the hair and scalp for at least 5 minutes to ensure that the medication reaches the skin. In more severe cases, adults may massage topical steroid lotions such as **2.5% hydrocortisone** lotion into the scalp once or twice daily.

    b. **Flares or more resistant cases** may respond to antifungal preparations (e.g., 2% ketoconazole shampoo used daily on affected scalp or beard for at least a month; 2% ketoconazole cream used topically to affected area twice a day for 4 weeks or until clinical clearing; 2% ketoconazole gel topically to affected area once daily for 2 weeks). Scalp scaling may be treated with 2% salicylic acid shampoo. A peanut oil/mineral oil/corticosteroid preparation (Derma Smoothe/FS) is helpful in individuals with dry scalp who are unable to tolerate daily shampooing with other products.

    c. **Facial seborrheic dermatitis** often responds well to 1% metronidazole gel. (SOR **C**) One percent pimecrolimus cream can also be effective in treating moderate to severe facial seborrhea and is usually well tolerated (see Section B.1.d for description of FDA "black-box warning").

    d. **Infantile seborrheic dermatitis.** The usual treatment approach is conservative, with the use of a mild, nonmedicated shampoo first (e.g., baby shampoo twice a week), followed by the use of a shampoo with coal tar in resistant cases. Topical steroids should be avoided in infants if possible, because of significant percutaneous absorption.

12. Nummular eczema may respond to the same measures as **atopic dermatitis.**

REFERENCES

Akdis CA, Akdis M, Bieber T, et al. Diagnosis and treatment of atopic dermatitis in children and adults: European Academy of Allergology and Clinical Immunology/American Academy of Allergy, Asthma and Immunology/PRACTALL consensus report. *Allergy.* 2006;61(8):969-987.

Fleischer AB, Jr. Black box warning for topical calcineurin inhibitors and the death of common sense. *Dermatol Online J.* 2006;12(6):2.

Saary J, Qureshi R, Palda V, et al. A systematic review of contact dermatitis treatment and prevention. *J Am Acad Dermatol.* 2005;53(5):845.

Wollina U, Hansel G, Koch A, Abdel-Naser MB. Topical pimecrolimus for skin disease other than atopic dermatitis. *Expert Opin Pharmacother.* 2006;7(14):1967-1975.

---

15   Dermatologic Neoplasms

Daniel L. Stulberg, MD, & Douglas G. Browning, MD, ATC-L

KEY POINTS

- For any lesion exhibiting uncertain behavior, a biopsy should be done to rule out malignancy.
- The primary preventable cause of skin malignancies is chronic sun exposure.
- A person with a history of a skin malignancy should have regular skin examinations to evaluate any suspicious lesions.
- Actinic keratoses are squamous cell carcinoma in situ, and are seen in association with basal and squamous cell cancers elsewhere.
- Malignant melanoma can readily metastasize and is the skin malignancy with the poorest prognosis.

I. **Definition. Neoplasm** means new growth. A **dermatologic neoplasm** occurs when skin or subcutaneous cells begin to abnormally proliferate. Such new growths are extremely common and may be benign, premalignant, or malignant. They may arise in the **epidermis** (e.g., acrochordon, keratoacanthoma, seborrheic keratoses, basal and squamous cell carcinomas, malignant melanoma, nevi, actinic keratoses), the **dermis** (e.g., sebaceous hyperplasia, dermatofibromas, pyogenic granulomas, cherry angiomas, epidermoid cyst), or **subcutaneous** (e.g., lipomas).

II. **Common Diagnoses.** Of patients who consult primary care physicians for skin problems, ~20% are diagnosed as having skin neoplasm or tumor.

   A. **Macular lesions**

      1. **Nevi** (moles) are aberrant collections of melanocytes in the epidermis, dermis, or dermo-epidermal junction. Approximately 1% of infants have one or more nevi at birth. They can be flat (macular) or raised and be benign, atypical, dysplastic, or develop into malignant melanoma. The number of nevi increases during adolescence to an average of 20 to 40 lesions by the third decade. These lesions are more prevalent in whites, and sun exposure increases their number.

      2. **Ephelides ("freckles") and lentigines** are hyperpigmented macular lesions that increase with sun exposure. Ephelides are found most commonly in children or young adults with light complexions. In elderly individuals, lentigines become more prevalent in sun-exposed areas, where they are recognized as age or liver spots.

      3. **Congenital nevi** occur in approximately 1% of the population.

      4. **Familial atypical mole and melanoma syndrome (FAMMS)**, previously known as dysplastic nevus syndrome or **atypical mole syndrome,** is a familial autosomal dominant syndrome in which individuals have multiple nevi (macular or papular) increasing in size and number with age. (Figure 15–1) The risk for having cutaneous melanoma develop is 15% if there is one first-degree relative and is nearly 100% if there are two first-degree relatives with melanomas.

      5. **Malignant melanomas** account for 2% to 3% of all skin cancers, but more than two-thirds of skin cancer mortality. Melanoma rates are highest in developed countries and areas closer to the equator. Greater ultraviolet light exposure through depletion of the ozone layer may contribute to the increasing incidence of melanoma; however, correlation with sun exposure is less frequent for melanoma than for basal and squamous cell cancers. Rather than duration, *intensity* of sun exposure is more relevant (i.e., a history of blistering sunburn before age 20 doubles the risk of melanoma) Other risk factors include congenital nevi, FAMMS, and personal history of previous melanoma. The relative incidence of the four histologic subtypes of melanoma is as follows:

          Superficial spreading (70% of melanomas).
          Lentigo maligna (12% of melanomas).
          Nodular (10% of melanomas).
          Acral lentiginous (8% of melanomas).

   B. **Papular lesions**

      1. **Nevi** may be macular or papular, see discussion above.

      2. **Cherry angiomas,** dilated capillaries and postcapillary venules, occur in up to 50% of adults, beginning in adulthood and increasing with age (Figure 15–2).

      3. **Seborrheic keratoses** (seborrheic or senile warts) are common in middle-aged and older individuals, occurring equally in men and women (Figure 15–2).

      4. **Verrucae (warts)** can occur at any age, but are more common in children and young adults. Their incidence, severity, and prevalence are greater in the immunocompromised patient.

      5. **Keratoacanthoma** previously thought to be a form of squamous cell cancer is benign, tends to occur in older individuals, and may be related to sun exposure (Figure 15–3).

      6. **Pyogenic granulomas** are related to skin irritation, damage or pregnancy. They are a proliferation of fragile vascular and epithelial tissues that are commonly seen at the newborn umbilicus and the gums of pregnant women (Figure 15–4).

      7. **Actinic keratoses** were formerly considered premalignant skin lesions. They are now considered squamous carcinoma in situ. They are mostly found on sun-exposed areas in middle-aged and older persons with light complexions and a history of chronic sun exposure. The lifetime risk of a cutaneous squamous cell carcinoma developing in an individual with actinic keratoses is approximately 20% (Figure 15–5).

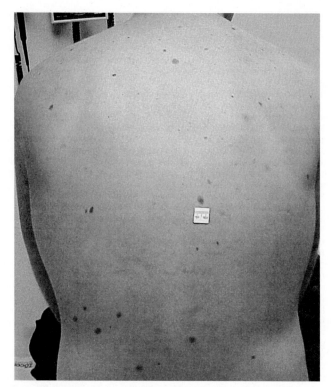

FIGURE 15–1. FAMMS; note multiple macular to papular lesions with variable coloring and size (see color insert).

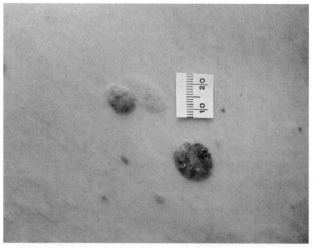

FIGURE 15–2. Multiple macular cherry angiomas. More advanced lesions may be raised or even polypoid. Note several verrucous irregularly pigmented seborrheic keratoses which are also age related (see color insert).

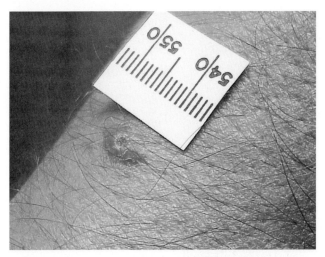

FIGURE 15-3. Keratoacanthoma with raised borders and central keratin plug (see color insert).

8. **Basal cell carcinoma** is the most common skin cancer occurring mostly but not exclusively on sun-exposed skin. According to the American Cancer Society one million cases of basal and squamous cell cancers were diagnosed in the United States in 2007 (Figure 15–6).

9. **Squamous cell carcinoma** usually develops in sun-exposed areas of the body. The incidence of squamous cell cancer is higher in individuals with fair skin, immune disorders, outdoor occupations, and exposure to hydrocarbons such as soot, coal tar, and lubricating oils (Figure 15–5).

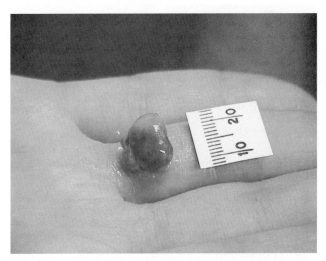

FIGURE 15-4. Pyogenic granuloma with glistening fragile overgrowth of capillaries and epithelium (see color insert).

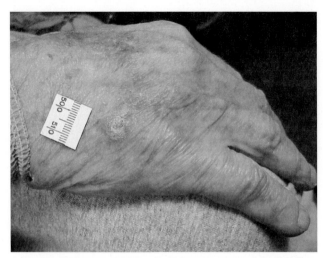

FIGURE 15–5. Actinic keratosis which has reached the raised actinic horn stage and also note the diffuse raised erythematous base of progression to squamous cell cancer (see color insert).

      10. Acrochordon, or skin tags, can occur as single or multiple lesions. They are found in 25% of individuals, increase with age, and obesity and frequently occur on the neck, axillae, and under the breasts.
  C. Nodular lesions
      1. Lipomas, subcutaneous encapsulated tumors of adipose cells, occur in 1 of 1000 individuals. They are solitary in 80% of cases, but may be multiple, especially in young men (Figure 15–7).

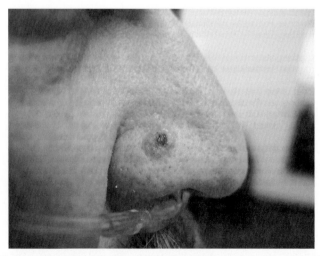

FIGURE 15–6. Basal cell cancer. Note similar appearance to keratoacanthoma with raised borders, but has telangiectasias and central ulceration (see color insert).

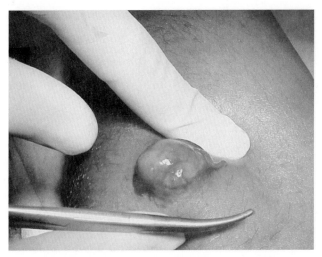

FIGURE 15–7. Lipoma with capsule being expressed after blunt dissection from a relatively small incision (see color insert).

2. **Dermatofibromas,** subcutaneous scar tissue, may occur in reaction to trauma, insect sting, or folliculitis; multiple lesions may be associated with autoimmune disease (Figure 15–8).
3. **Epidermal cysts** are smooth, pearl-colored cysts akin to very large comedones. Multiple epidermal cysts are associated with Gardner's syndrome of adenomatous polyposis.
4. **Sebaceous hyperplasia,** enlarged sebaceous glands, is most common in middle-aged and older individuals (Figure 15–9).

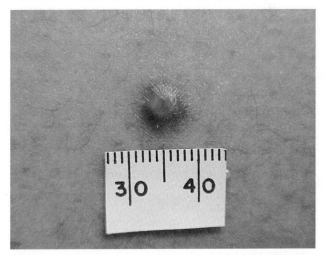

FIGURE 15–8. Dermatofibroma typically pigmented and sometimes raised (see color insert).

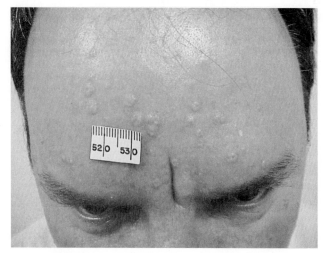

FIGURE 15–9. Sebaceous hyperplasia, common on the forehead and face looks similar to early BCCs, but is often seen as multiple lesions (see color insert).

III. **Symptoms.** Dermatologic neoplasms are often asymptomatic. When symptoms occur, they may include the following:
   A. **Cosmetic change** or disfigurement.
   B. **Local irritation** with friction from clothing (collars, bras, belts), jewelry, skin folds, or trauma with shaving.
   C. **Anxiety over changes** in size or number of lesions, local discomfort, bleeding, discharge, or ulceration.
IV. **Signs**
   A. Common types of **verrucae (warts),** which can occur as single or grouped lesions:
      1. **Flat warts** (verruca plana), 1- to 3-mm lesions with smooth, flesh-colored surfaces, generally found on the face, neck, hands, and lower legs in a linear distribution.
      2. **Periungual warts,** rough-surfaced lesions found adjacent to and sometimes extending beneath the nails.
      3. **Plantar warts,** thick, coalescing lesions typically on the heels or balls of the feet revealing pinpoint-sized bleeding points when pared.
      4. **Genital warts (condylomata acuminata or venereal warts),** velvety, moist, slightly raised, cauliflower-like lesions occurring singularly or in clusters genitally or perianally.
   B. **Melanomas** can arise from moles that have been present or appear as a new lesion. The American Cancer Society ABCD guidelines (see Table 15–1) for suspicious characteristics are useful for the general public and as a starting point for practitioners' evaluations. (SOR **Ⓒ**) Familial atypical mole and melanoma syndrome (FAMMS) **nevi** differ from common nevi in size (5–10 mm compared to <6 mm for common nevi), shape and contour (irregular borders with poor margination compared to symmetric, uniform borders for

TABLE 15–1. AMERICAN CANCER SOCIETY ABCD GUIDELINES FOR SUSPICIOUS LESION CHARACTERISTICS PROMPTING FURTHER EVALUATION

A—Asymmetry	Lesions with one portion looking different than the rest
B—Border	Borders that are ill defined or spreading in appearance
C—Color	The colors of the US flag (Red White and Blue) plus black
D—Diameter	Greater than 6 mm (approximately the size of a pencil's eraser)
E (NOT part of the American Cancer Society guidelines, but used by others)—Enlarging or evolution	Lesion growing in size or changing over time

TABLE 15–2. CONGENITAL NEVI

	Size	Malignant Potential	Treatment
Small	<1.5 cm	Low and rare before puberty	Follow clinically. If desired prophylactic excision before puberty
Medium	1.5–19.9 cm	Varies by depth of lesion epidermal versus deeper	Can biopsy: If epidermal follow clinically or excise. If dermal then excise as cannot accurately follow clinically.
Large	>20 cm or >5% of body surface area	Up to 7%	Excise prophylactically as early as possible. Half of melanomas develop by age 3–5 y old and cannot accurately follow clinically.

common nevi), and color (intra- and interlesional variations of brown, black, or red compared to more homogenous variations of tan, brown, or black for common nevi).

Congenital nevi are classified according to size into small, medium, and large with varying degrees of malignant potential. See Table 15–2.

    C. Epidermoid cysts may become fluctuant and tender if inflamed (Figure 15–10).

V. Laboratory Tests. In most cases, where physical examination clarifies the nature of a lesion, no further testing is necessary. Dermoscopy by an experienced clinician using a hand-held magnifier can increase the accuracy delineating between benign and malignant nevi. (SOR Ⓐ) Biopsies of suspicious lesions should be done. (See Chapter 41 for details of shave and punch biopsies, and excision of lesions.) These lesions include the following:

    A. Any lesion that the clinician is suspicious about based on clinical appearance or history.

    B. Lesions with **unexplained** tenderness, itching, bleeding, or ulceration.

    C. Lesions with **recent growth, ulceration,** or characteristics suggestive of basal cell carcinoma, squamous cell carcinoma, or melanoma.

VI. Treatment

    A. Benign neoplasms

        1. Nevi usually require no treatment except for cosmetic or diagnostic purposes. Most are easily removed by shave, punch, or excisional biopsy (see Chapter 41).

            a. Shave excision is useful for elevated lesions and those in which depth of excision is unimportant.

            b. Punch biopsy is an easy way to obtain a full-thickness diagnostic specimen, although irregular, large, or cystic lesions may be better off excised.

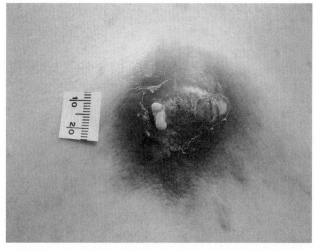

FIGURE 15–10. Epidermal cyst which has become infected, inflamed, and painful which requires incision and drainage (see color insert).

    c. Excisional biopsy allows for a complete, full-thickness excision of a worrisome skin lesion.

2. Removal of **seborrheic keratoses** may be achieved by cryosurgery or by shave excision after anesthetizing the skin with a local anesthetic.

3. **Warts**

    a. Common warts can be treated by many different methods. Starting with over-the-counter salicylic acid liquids or "wart stick" applicators (daily) or tapes (every 2–3 days) is prudent and approximately 60% effective. It may take weeks to months, but is one of the most benign and inexpensive therapies available other than watchful waiting. (SOR **Ⓐ**) Soaking the wart for 10 to 15 minutes before application, debriding any dead or peeling skin from the lesion and occluding the application of acid may all help with treatment success. Office-based cryotherapy with liquid nitrogen or, compressed nitrous oxide, or liquid refrigerants have similar efficacy. Home-based over-the-counter cryotherapy (Wartner) may be 50% effective. Candida antigen mixed 10% in lidocaine and injected into the base of the wart may induce an immune response and resolution of the wart(s.) Weekly applications of bi- or tri-chloroacetic acid in the office may be used as well as sensitization with dinitrochlorobenzene via consultation with a specialist. More aggressive destruction can be achieved with electrodesiccation and curettage or laser, but there is no guarantee of an increased rate of resolution of the wart and there are associated surgical side effects. Even weekly occlusion of the lesion with **duct tape**, with removal of the devitalized skin between applications, proved to be 85% effective in eradicating warts within 2 months, according to one small study in a pediatric population.

        Flat warts tend to be numerous and often on the face or forehead making treatment with **cryosurgery, bichloroacetic acid,** or over-the-counter **salicylic acid** more difficult because of the amount of inflammation and potential for noticeable pigmentation changes. Imiquimod 5% cream (Aldara) applied daily or every other day for several weeks can be useful. Alternatively, **tretinoin (retinoic acid)** cream or lotion (0.025%, 0.05%, or 0.1%) can be applied once or twice daily to produce mild inflammation and subsequent regression (may require several weeks). **Fluorouracil** (Efudex) cream, 5%, applied once or twice a day for 3 to 5 weeks, is also effective.

    b. Periungual warts should be treated cautiously because of the proximity of the nail bed. **Cryosurgery** can be done, taking care to avoid injury to the nail matrix and superficial nerves. Alternatively, **topical keratolytics** as listed above for common warts may be applied until the wart regresses. Occasionally, eradication can only be achieved by blunt dissection.

    c. Plantar warts may cause foot pain. Topical keratolytic agents as listed above for common warts may be used, but treatment usually requires several weeks. Paring down the lesion can reduce the painful sensation of "walking on a rock in my shoe." See the recommendations above for treatment of common warts as they are treated the same but, **cryosurgery** or **excision** of these warts tends to temporarily cause pain and loss of mobility.

    d. Treatment of **anogenital warts** (**condylomata acuminata** or venereal warts) is discussed in Chapter 31.

4. **Lentigines** pose no health threat. Removal by topical or surgical techniques is unnecessary, and lesions tend to recur. Routine use of sunscreens can reduce the rate of additional lesions. Creams containing hydroquinone to bleach the skin may make these lesions less noticeable, and gentle cryotherapy can selectively damage melanocytes in relation to keratinocytes, decreasing pigmentation, hopefully without much destruction to other tissue.

5. **Cherry angiomas** may be electrocauterized or removed by shave excision after local anesthesia, if necessary, but are usually left alone.

6. **Sebaceous hyperplasia** does not require treatment except for cosmetic purposes. Individual lesions may be removed by curetting or light cauterization, but at the risk of leaving a pit or indentation. When they are severe, extensive, or disfiguring, oral isotretinoin (or in females, antiandrogens) may help improve their appearance at least temporarily.

7. **Acrochordon** ("skin tags") may be removed by cryosurgery with liquid nitrogen, electrosurgery, or by snip excision with sharp iris scissors.

8. **Dermatofibromas** require no treatment unless the diagnosis is uncertain, the lesion is symptomatic from repeated trauma or is undesirable from a cosmetic standpoint. Pigmentation and the raised portion can be reduced with cryotherapy. If excision is desired, dermatofibromas require a full-thickness approach because of the depth of the lesion.

9. Although **keratoacanthoma** are benign and most will eventually spontaneously resolve, excision or destruction is recommended to prevent the long duration of disease and the ultimate usual scarring. Electrodesiccation and curettage can be used for small lesions. Larger lesions may be surgically excised or the patient may be referred for topical 5-fluorouracil, or imiquimod, or intralesional 5-fluorouracil, methotrexate, interferon alfa 2a, or isotretinoin.

10. **For pyogenic granuloma,** shave excision is considered for diagnosis or to rule out amelanotic melanoma. Treatment is with electrodesiccation and thorough curettage or topical application of silver nitrate.

11. **Epidermal (sebaceous) cysts** can recur if there are adjacent cysts or they are not completely excised. Traditionally, if desired, these are excised via an incision down to the capsule and blunt dissection around the capsule to remove the cyst intact. A newer technique uses a smaller incision into the cyst, expressing the contents and then inverting and removing the cyst wall. If the lesion is friable and intact removal is not possible, the cyst wall can be curetted out or removed with forceps. If the cyst becomes infected then it should be sharply incised, drained, and packed using gauze strip with appropriate follow-up care.

12. **Lipomas** generally require no treatment, unless they interfere with the movement of adjacent muscles, in which case they may be removed by simple surgical excision or liposuction.

B. **Premalignant lesions** should be treated to prevent malignant degeneration. Patients with these lesions should be educated regarding **sun protection** (i.e., covering exposed areas), **use of sunscreens** with a sun protection factor of 15 or more, **avoidance of sun exposure** between 10 AM and 4 PM, performance of regular **skin self-examination,** and avoidance of tanning salons.

1. **Actinic keratoses.** Untreated actinic keratoses may progress from the in situ phase to squamous cell carcinomas. **Cryotherapy, or electrodesiccation with curettage,** is practical if there are a limited number of lesions. For areas with extensive lesions, **5% topical 5-fluorouracil** (Efudex) is used twice daily until marked inflammation occurs. Treatment for the face and lips is approximately 2 weeks. Treatment for thicker skin may require 4 or more weeks. Imiquimod 5% cream (Aldara) applied topically for 8 hours twice weekly for 16 weeks (SOR **Ⓐ**) is also effective for the majority of lesions, and the remaining lesions can be treated as above. Topical steroids may be used to decrease posttreatment inflammation as needed.

   Tretinoin (0.05% or 0.1%) **cream,** applied daily, may be used in patients with mild actinic damage. **Dermabrasion** and **chemical peel** are also effective, but should be performed only by physicians trained and experienced in these techniques.

2. **FAMMS.** This syndrome requires frequent examinations, a low threshold for biopsy of suspicious lesions and consideration for body mapping (serial photographs.)

C. **Malignant lesions**

1. **Basal cell cancers (BCCs).** Untreated basal cell carcinoma grows slowly, but if left untreated can invade contiguous soft tissue, bone, and cartilage. The method of removal depends on lesion size, location, and physician preference. Treatment technique for small lesions usually involves **excision** or **electrodesiccation and curettage (ED&C).** Cryosurgery or topical 5% imiquimod (Aldara) can be used for superficial lesions with a slightly lower cure rate. **Radiation** therapy can be used for rare cases where a patient cannot tolerate these other treatments. Shave biopsy is the simplest way to confirm the diagnosis. **Small BCCs** may be removed by a primary care physician using **ED&C,** a punch or an elliptical excision to obtain clear margins around the lesion. If excised, clear margins surrounding the lesion in all directions should be verified by pathology. **ED&C** is usually performed after confirming the diagnosis by a shave biopsy, and its technique of curetting in all directions helps to detect and remove subclinical spread at the margins of the lesion. Larger BCCs, recurrent BCCs, and those located on sensitive structures including the **eyes or ears** should be referred for expert surgical removal. This might include excision by a dermatologist trained in **Moh's micrographic surgery** or excision by a plastic surgeon.

2. **Squamous cell carcinomas.** Spread most commonly occurs by local extension and, less commonly, by metastasis. Superficial squamous cell carcinomas may be treated with electrodesiccation and curettage. Excisional treatment is recommended for most lesions and Moh's micrographic surgery should be used for large lesions or those near sensitive structures. Squamous cell lesions arising within chronic ulcers, burns, or scar tissue or in mucous membranes have a high metastatic potential, and patients with such lesions should be referred to a specialist.

3. **Malignant melanomas.** Malignant melanomas have a tendency to spread rapidly and metastasize early. Prognosis, margin for re-excision, and recommendations for further treatment are based on Breslow's method of measuring the depth of tumor on initial excision. Tumors greater than 1 mm in depth warrant a 2-cm margin with re-excision, sentinel lymph node biopsy by an experienced surgeon, and regular follow-up for recurrent disease. (SOR **A**)

4. **Congenital nevi.** Congenital nevi have malignant potential based on their size and composition. See Table 15–2 for treatment recommendations. For large congenital lesions referral to a plastic surgeon experienced in this area is important.

REFERENCES

American Cancer Society Web site. www.Cancer.org.

Bafounta ML. Is dermoscopy (epiluminescence microscopy) useful for the diagnosis of melanoma? Results of a meta-analysis using techniques adapted to the evaluation of diagnostic tests. *Arch Dermatol.* 2001;137(10):1343-1350.

Habif TP *Clinical Dermatology: A Color Guide to Diagnosis and Therapy.* 4th ed. St Louis, MO: Mosby; 2004.

Johnson TM, Sondak VK, Bichakjian CK, Sabel MS. The role of sentinel lymph node biopsy for melanoma: Evidence assessment. *J Am Acad Dermatol.* 2006;54(1);19-27.

Luba MC, Bangs SA, Mohler AM, Stulberg DL. Common benign skin tumors. *Am Fam Physician.* 2003;67:729.

Szeimies RM, Gerritsen MJ, Ortonne JP, et al. Imiquimod 5% cream for the treatment of actinic keratosis: Results from a phase III, randomized, double-blind, vehicle-controlled clinical trial with histology. *J Am Acad Dermatol.* 2004;51(4);547-555.

Townsend CM. *Sabiston Textbook of Surgery.* 17th ed. Philadelphia, PA: Saunders; 2004.

---

16   Diarrhea

Laura Hargro, MD, & Jeanne M. Ferrante, MD

KEY POINTS

- Most episodes of acute diarrhea are self-limited.
- A thorough history is crucial to accurate patient assessment.
- Supportive care is usually the only required treatment.

I. **Definition. Diarrhea** is an increased number (three or more) or decreased consistency of stools (soft or liquid) during a 24-hour period.

A. Duration of symptoms of 14 days or less is **acute diarrhea.** Causes include (Table 16–1):

1. **Viral infections** (e.g., rotavirus, enteric adenovirus, Norovirus/Norwalk virus).

2. **Bacterial infections** characterized as **enterotoxigenic** (*Escherichia coli/Staphylococcus aureus/Bacillus cereus/Clostridium perfringens/Clostridium difficile*) or **inflammatory** (*Salmonella* spp/*Shigella* spp/*Campylobacter* spp/*Yersinia enterocolitica/Shiga toxin producing E coli* 0157:H7 [*STEC*]).

3. **Parasitic infections** (e.g., *Giardia lamblia, Cryptosporidium*).

4. **Drugs** (e.g., caffeine, alcohol, other prescription and over-the-counter drugs).

5. **Chemical contamination of water (e.g., copper, ethylene glycol, ethyl benzene)**

TABLE 16–1. CAUSES OF ACUTE INFECTIOUS DIARRHEA

Bacteria	Viruses	Parasites/Protozoa
E coli (enterotoxigenic, enteroinvasive, enterohemorrhagic)	Enteric adenovirus (types 40, 41)	Entamoeba histolytica
Campylobacter spp	Rotavirus	Giardia lamblia
Salmonella spp	Norwalk agent	Cryptosporidium parvum
Shigella spp	Calicivirus	Microsporidium
Vibrio cholera and other vibrios	Astrovirus	Isospora belli
Clostridium difficile	Cytomegalovirus	Cyclospora cayetanensis
Aeromonas spp		
Pleisiomonas spp		
Yersinia spp		

Reproduced with permission from Gadewar S, Fasano A. Current concepts in the evaluation, diagnosis, and management of acute infectious diarrhea. *Curr Opin Pharmacol.* 2005;5:559–565.

6. **Miscellaneous noninfectious causes** (e.g., irritable bowel syndrome; fecal impaction with paradoxical diarrhea; inflammatory bowel disease; or ingestions of large amounts of lactose, fructose, or artificial sweeteners).
   B. Symptoms lasting for more than 14 days define **persistent diarrhea,** and symptoms lasting for more than 1 month constitute **chronic diarrhea.**
      1. **Chronic diarrhea** may be classified as:
         a. **Watery—because of** the following:
            (1) **Osmotic factors** (osmotic gap of stool >50 mOsm/kg; large volume decreased with fasting, e.g., magnesium laxatives, lactase deficiency).
            (2) **Secretory factors** (osmotic gap of stool <50 mOsm/kg; endogenous—large volume not decreased with fasting, e.g., carcinoid, gastrinoma; exogenous—large volume decreased with removal of offending agent, e.g., stimulant laxatives, medications, toxins).
            (3) **Dysmotility** (e.g., irritable bowel syndrome, diabetes, thyrotoxicosis, scleroderma).
         b. **Inflammatory—because of infections** (possibly with fever, eosinophilia, e.g., parasitic, helminthic); **inflammatory bowel disease** (with fever, hematochezia, e.g., ulcerative colitis); **neoplasia; ischemia;** or **radiation.**
         c. **Fatty—because of malabsorption** (e.g., celiac disease) or **maldigestion** (e.g., pancreatic insufficiency).
II. **Common Diagnoses.** Diarrhea is one of the most common symptoms for which patients visit their physician. In the United States, there are estimated 211 to 375 million annual episodes of diarrheal illnesses, resulting in 73 million physician visits, >900,000 hospitalizations, and 6000 deaths. Up to 55% of travelers to less developed areas of the world (e.g., Mexico, Latin America, Africa, the Middle East, and Asia) will have travelers' diarrhea (see Chapter 104). The prevalence of chronic diarrhea is estimated to be 5% with direct costs from medical care predicted at $524 million per year and the indirect costs from disability and lost productivity exceeding $136 million per year.
   For other causes of diarrhea, see the sidebars on sexually transmitted proctitis and colon ischemia.
   A. **Acute diarrhea.** Most acute diarrhea is caused by infections and usually occurs after the ingestion of contaminated food or water, or by direct person-to-person contact. **Underlying medical conditions** predisposing to infections include extremes of age, recent hospitalization, impaired immune system, human immunodeficiency virus, immunosuppressive therapy for organ transplant, long-term prednisone therapy, cancer chemotherapy, immunoglobulin A deficiency, or prior gastrectomy. **Other risk factors** include recent travel to developing countries, day care attendance, residence at an institution (nursing home, psychiatric facility, prison), lowered gastric acidity (patients taking H2 blockers or proton pump inhibitors), and certain occupations (farmer, food handler, health care, or day care provider). The common causes include: (SOR **Ⓓ**)
      1. **Viral** (70%–80% of acute infectious diarrhea). **Rotavirus,** the most frequent cause, typically presents in winter and may be transmitted by aerosol spread as well as through the fecal–oral route. Most cases occur between the ages of 3 months and

2 years. **Enteric adenoviruses** are the second most common type. Contaminated water, salads, and shellfish may transmit **Norwalk virus, one of the Noroviruses, which are the most common causes of outbreaks especially on cruise ships.**

2. **Bacterial** (10%–20% of acute cases). Risk factors include consumption of cooked foods that are later refrigerated, such as custard, pastries, and processed meats (*S aureus*); raw or undercooked meat (*Salmonella, Yersinia, STEC*) or seafood (*Vibrio, Plesiomonas*); improperly refrigerated foods (*B cereus, C perfringens*); or unpasteurized milk, juice, soft cheese, or unheated deli meats (*Listeria monocytogenes*). *C difficile* causes approximately 20% of antibiotic-associated diarrhea. The most common antibiotics to cause *C difficile* infection are clindamycin, cephalosporins, and penicillin derivatives taken in the past 8 weeks.

3. **Parasitic** (<10% of acute diarrhea). Parasitic infections (*G lamblia, Cryptosporidium, Entamoeba histolytica*) are uncommon in the general population, but may be more prevalent in children in day care centers, residents of mental institutions or nursing homes, immunocompromised persons, or persons exposed to untreated water from a lake or stream. *E histolytica* may be found in up to 30% of homosexual men.

4. **Drugs.** Common causes include laxatives, antiulcer drugs, antibiotics, cardiovascular drugs, nonsteroidal anti-inflammatory drugs, antiparkinson drugs, colchicine, and excessive caffeine or alcohol. Any new drug or recent dosage change may result in diarrhea.

5. **Seafood ingestion syndromes** can also cause diarrhea in travelers and include diarrhetic shellfish poisoining, ciguatera poisoning, and scrombroid poisoning.

SEXUALLY TRANSMITTED PROCTITIS

Sexually transmitted proctitis can cause rectal pain, small-volume bloody diarrhea, and tenesmus. **Herpesvirus, gonorrhea, chlamydia,** and **syphilis** are likely causes. Those at risk are homosexual men and receptive partners during anal intercourse. Diagnosis is by proctoscopy with rectal swabs sent for polymerase chain reaction (PCR) testing or cultures. Treatment consists of antiviral drugs or antibiotics for the sexually transmitted disease.

COLON ISCHEMIA

Colon ischemia is a rare cause of diarrhea, but it can be life-threatening. The diarrhea may be associated with mild-to-moderate abdominal pain or lower intestinal bleeding. Risk factors include history of cornary artery disease/hypertension/chronic renal failure/arrthymias, recent aortic or cardiac bypass surgery, vasculitides (e.g., systemic lupus erythematosus), infections (e.g., **STEC, cytomegalovirus**), coagulopathies (e.g., protein C and S deficiencies), medications (e.g., vasoactive meds, oral contraceptives), drugs (e.g., cocaine), long-distance running, preceding major cardiovascular episode with hypotension, and obstructing lesions of the colon (e.g., carcinoma). Diagnosis is by colonoscopy or arteriography. Most cases resolve spontaneously within 48 hours and do not require specific therapy. Patients with severe or continuing symptoms should be hospitalized and placed on bowel rest (nothing by mouth for 48–72 hours), intravenous fluids, and broad-spectrum antibiotics. Surgery is required for patients with peritoneal signs or those unresponsive to medical therapy.

B. The differential diagnosis of **chronic diarrhea** is very extensive (Table 16–2).

1. Most chronic diarrheas in **adults** are caused by:

a. **Irritable bowel syndrome (IBS),** a complex of abnormal gastrointestinal motility, altered visceral sensation, and psychologic factors, occurs in 20% of the US population, but only 10% to 20% of people with irritable bowel syndrome seek medical care. In more than 50% symptoms develop before age 35, and women are twice as likely to have irritable bowel syndrome as developed in men.

b. **Lactose intolerance,** which is genetically controlled and occurs because of a normal decline in the intestinal lactase activity after childhood. It is present in 75% to 90% of US blacks, Asians, American Indians, persons of Mediterranean origin, and Jews, compared to less than 5% of descendants of Northern and Central Europeans. Secondary lactose intolerance can develop from injury to the intestinal

TABLE 16-2. DIFFERENTIAL DIAGNOSIS OF CHRONIC DIARRHEA CLASSIFIED BY TYPICAL STOOL CHARACTERISTICS

Watery Diarrhea	Fatty Diarrhea	Inflammatory Diarrhea
Osmotic diarrhea	*Malabsorption syndromes*	*Inflammatory bowel disease*
Mg^{2+}, po_4^{-3}, SO_4^{-2} ingestion	Mucosal diseases	Ulcerative colitis
Carbohydrate malabsorption	Short-bowel syndrome	Crohn's disease
Secretory diarrhea	Postresection diarrhea	Diverticulitis
Laxative abuse (nonsomotic laxatives)	Mesenteric ischemia	Ulcerative jejunoileitis
Congenital syndromes	*Maldigestion*	*Infectious diseases*
Bacterial toxins	Pancreatic insufficiency	Ulcerating viral infections
Ileal bile acid malabsorption	Bile acid deficiency	Cytomegalovirus
Inflammatory bowel disease		Herpes simplex
Ulcerative colitis		*Ischemic colitis*
Crohn's disease		*Radiation colitis*
Microscopic (lymphocytic and		*Neoplasia*
collagenous) colitis		Colon cancer
Diverticulitis		Lymphoma
Vasculitis		
Drugs and poisons		
Disordered motility		
Postvagotomy diarrhea		
Postsympathectomy diarrhea		
Diabetic autonomic neuropathy		
Hyperthyroidism		
Irritable bowel syndrome		
Neuroendocrine tumors		
Gastrinoma		
VIPoma		
Somatostatinoma		
Mastocytosis		
Carcinoid syndrome		
Medullary carcinoma of Thyroid		
Neoplasia		
Colon carcinoma		
Lymphoma		
Villous adenoma		
Addison's disease		
Epidemic secretory diarrhea		
Idiopathic secretory diarrhea		

Reproduced with permission from Schiller LR. Chronic diarrhea. *Gastroenterology*. 2004;127:287–293.

mucosa (e.g., infectious diarrhea, celiac disease) or a decrease in mucosal surface (e.g., resection), and is transient with successful treatment of the underlying disease.

c. **Idiopathic inflammatory bowel disease. Crohn's disease,** characterized by transmural, focal, and asymmetric inflammation of any part of the gastrointestinal tract, occurs in 5 to 10 per 10,000 individuals and occurs most frequently in people of European descent, particularly Jews. The onset is usually in adolescence and young adulthood. **Ulcerative colitis** is a diffused, continuous, superficial inflammation of the rectum and colon, occurring in 2 to 7 per 10,000 individuals. Its onset is between ages 15 and 35 years, with a second and smaller peak in the seventh decade. Ulcerative colitis is also more common in Jews, and there is a positive family history in approximately 10%. Occasionally, it develops after an acute infection.

d. **Malabsorption syndrome.** Celiac disease, an autoimmune inflammatory disease of the small intestine precipitated by gluten ingestion, is more common than previously thought, at approximately 1 case per 120 to 300 persons. Approximately 75% of new adult cases are in women. Celiac disease should be considered in patients at genetic risk (i.e., family history of celiac disease or personal history of type I diabetes) and in patients with unexplained chronic diarrhea, anemia, fatigue, or weight loss.

    e. Chronic infections (usually parasitic infections). Risk factors include travel to endemic areas, including Russia (*Giardia*), Peru, Haiti (*Cyclospora*), Thailand (Campylobacter), Nepal (Cyclospora and Campylobacter), or any developing country (*E histolytica*), and drinking from lakes or streams (*Giardia*). Immunosuppressed individuals and the elderly may have persistent diarrhea from *Campylobacter* and *Salmonella*. Risk factors for relapse of *C difficile* infection (20% of patients) include intercurrent antibiotics, renal failure, and female sex. Other uncommon bacterial causes include *Aeromonas* (untreated water), *Plesiomonas* (foreign travel, raw shellfish, untreated water), *Yersinia* (contaminated stream and lake water, milk, or ice cream), *Mycobacterium tuberculosis* (travel to undeveloped country), Brainerd diarrhea agent (unpasteurized milk and water). (SOR **C**)

  2. In **children,** most chronic diarrheas are caused by the following factors:

    a. Postinfectious diarrhea (Intractable diarrhea of infancy). Postinfectious diarrhea is characterized by the persistence of diarrhea and failure to gain weight more than 7 days after hospital admission for gastroenteritis. Risk factors include being a neonate or very young; being nonwhite; using antibiotics or antidiarrheal agents before admission; or having a previous history of diarrhea, a longer duration of diarrhea before hospitalization, severe diarrhea during the initial enteritis, weight below the tenth percentile, low-blood urea nitrogen, and bacterial etiology of the initial enteritis.

    b. Primary lactase deficiency. This deficiency starts between ages 3 and 5 years. Secondary lactose intolerance develops in 50% or more of infants with an acute or chronic diarrhea (especially with rotavirus) and is also fairly common with giardiasis, inflammatory bowel disease, and the AIDS malabsorption syndrome.

    c. Cow's milk and soy protein hypersensitivity. Cow's milk hypersensitivity is the most common sensitivity in infancy, with an incidence between 0.3% and 7.0%. Thirty to fifty percent of infants with cow's milk protein sensitivity may also have soy protein hypersensitivity. Most patients achieve tolerance during their second year of life.

    d. Celiac disease (see Section II.B.1.d).

    e. Chronic nonspecific diarrhea. Chronic nonspecific diarrhea (irritable bowel syndrome of children or toddler's diarrhea) appears between 6 months and 2 years of age. The cause is unknown but may follow an acute infection or gastroenteritis. It is self-limited, usually resolving spontaneously before age 4.

    Infrequent causes of chronic diarrhea in children include immune deficiencies, AIDS, endocrine disorders (e.g., hyperthyroidism, adrenal insufficiency, diabetes), IBS, cystic fibrosis, and anatomic lesions (e.g., Hirschsprung's disease). Pseudomembranous enterocolitis with *C difficile* is rare, but it is severe and sometimes fatal. It is precipitated by antibiotics and causes profuse diarrhea, dehydration, abdominal pain, fever, electrolyte imbalance, hypoproteinemia, and leukocytosis.

III. Symptoms. A thorough history is a key in guiding the evaluation and management of patients with diarrhea. Important questions include **when and how the illness began** (abrupt or gradual onset, duration of diarrhea), **stool characteristics** (frequency; quantity; watery, bloody, mucus-filled, purulent, greasy), symptoms of **dehydration** (thirst, lethargy, postural lightheadedness, decreased urination), presence of **dysentery** (fever; tenesmus; blood, pus, or both), and **associated symptoms** (nausea, vomiting, abdominal cramps, bloating, constipation, flatus or belching, headache, myalgias). (SOR **A**)

    In **chronic diarrhea,** a history of **other medical conditions** may be helpful in diagnosis, such as seronegative spondyloarthropathies (inflammatory bowel disease), autoimmune diseases such as diabetes or thyroid disorders (chronic dysmotility diarrhea, celiac disease), and immune deficiencies (infections). Patients should be asked about **fecal incontinence,** especially with low-volume stools, because the evaluation for incontinence differs from that of diarrhea. **Previous surgery** to the gastrointestinal or biliary tracts may be the cause of chronic diarrhea. Use of all **current medications** including over-the-counter medicines, nutritional supplements, illicit drugs, alcohol, and caffeine should be elicited. Questions on antibiotic use in the past 8 weeks, a new or increased dose in medication, and laxative use should be specifically asked.

  A. Viral diarrheas are usually self-limited, large volume, and watery, without blood, lasting from 1 to 2 days to 1 week. There may be nausea, vomiting, headache, low-grade fever, cramping, and malaise. Dehydration, especially in children, can occur.

B. Bacterial diarrhea

1. **Food poisoning** by *S aureus* and *B cereus* cause symptoms from preformed toxins within 1 to 6 hours of exposure. *C perfringens* causes symptoms within 8 to 16 hours. These symptoms are of a sudden onset and generally last 2 to 24 hours. Nausea and vomiting are variable with some abdominal cramping. There is usually no fever, severe abdominal pain, headache, malaise, myalgia, prolonged nausea, and vomiting.

2. Most **bacterial diarrheas** are more gradual in an onset, causing symptoms after 16 hours and lasting 1 to 7 days. Traveler's diarrhea typically begins 3 to 7 days after the arrival in a foreign location (see Chapter 104). With invasive disease fever, tenesmus, and gross blood, pus, or both are usually present. STEC causes bloody diarrhea without high fever or leukocytes. Severe cases may lead to hemolytic-uremic syndrome (bloody diarrhea, thrombocytopenia, hemolytic anemia, and renal failure). Reiter syndrome (arthritis, conjunctivitis, and urethritis or cervicitis) is a known complication of infections with Campylobacter, Salmonella, Shigella, and Yersenia, especially in persons who are HLA-B27 positive. Campylobacter has also been associated with Guillan-Barre (group of demyelinating diseases of peripheral nerves causing ascending progressive weakness). There is an increasing body of literature linking infectious, invasive gastroenteritis, and traveler's diarrhea with chronic gastrointestinal complaints and the onset of postinfectious IBS. Infection with *C difficile* can occur several days to 8 weeks after use of antibiotics. Watery diarrhea and abdominal cramps are typical. In severe cases, bloody diarrhea, fever, and abdominal pain can be present. There is usually no nausea or vomiting.

C. Parasitic diarrhea

1. *G lamblia* causes watery diarrhea, sometimes with mucus. Nausea, anorexia, abdominal cramping, flatulence, steatorrhea, and weight loss may be present.

2. *Cryptosporidium* causes prolonged diarrhea, associated with fatigue, flatulence, and abdominal pain. Fever is usually not present.

3. Clinical symptoms of *E histolytica* vary from asymptomatic carriage to severe bloody diarrhea that can be indistinguishable from ulcerative colitis. Abdominal cramping, diarrhea with blood or mucus, and malaise are common. In severe cases, massive bleeding, obstruction, dilation, or perforation may occur. Liver abscesses may result from systemic spread.

D. Chronic diarrhea. Watery stools suggest osmotic or secretory diarrhea. **Gross blood in the stool** suggests inflammatory bowel or malignancy. The description of **foul-smelling,** light-colored, floating stool, or undigested foods in stool suggests malabsorption.

1. The Rome II criteria are helpful to differentiate **irritable bowel syndrome** from organic pathology. The diagnosis is likely with 12 weeks or more in past 12 months of abdominal bowel pain or discomfort that has two out of the three following symptoms: relief with defecation, onset associated with change in frequency of stool, or onset associated with change in form (appearance) of stool. In children old enough to provide an accurate history of pain, Rome II criteria can be applied. However, onset may be 6 to 18 months of age with 6 to12 loose, explosive bowel movements containing food particles. Growth and development are normal, and there is no structural or metabolic abnormality to explain symptoms.

2. The severity of symptoms in **lactose intolerance** varies with the lactose load and other foods consumed at the same time, and may include diarrhea, bloating, cramping, abdominal discomfort, flatulence, and rumbling (borborygmi). In children, vomiting is common and malnutrition can occur.

3. **Crohn's disease** typically presents with diarrhea, abdominal pain, and weight loss. The clinical picture of **ulcerative colitis** is variable, from occasional rectal bleeding to profuse watery and bloody diarrhea with crampy lower abdominal pain and weight loss.

4. **Celiac disease** may present with a range of symptoms including diarrhea, constipation, dyspepsia, gastroesophageal reflux, bloating, flatus, belching, fatigue, weight loss, depression, fibromyalgia-like symptoms, aphthous stomatitis, hair loss, and bone pain. Infants typically present with failure to thrive, diarrhea, abdominal distention, developmental delay, and occasionally, severe malnutrition. Older children may have constitutional short stature or dental enamel defects.

IV. **Signs.** The physical examination is most important in assessing volume status and nutrition. Other clinical signs may be important clues in differentiating chronic causes of diarrhea.

A. Vital signs. Fever greater than 101.3°F suggests an acute inflammatory diarrhea. Postural changes in systolic blood pressure (decrease of 10 mm Hg) and pulse rate (increase of 20 beats per minute) support dehydration. In children, acute body weight changes best assess dehydration; other helpful measurements include dry mucous membranes, decreased capillary refill time, absence of tears, and alteration in mental status. In chronic cases, weight loss and failure to thrive suggest malabsorption, inflammatory bowel disease, infection, and neoplasm.

B. Skin. Characteristic skin changes can be seen in less common causes of chronic diarrhea, such as carcinoid syndrome (flushing, telangiectasias), celiac disease (dermatitis herpetiformis), mastocytosis (urticaria, linear telangiectasias), and Addison's disease (hyperpigmentation).

C. Oral. Aphthous oral ulcers and stomatitis may be present in inflammatory bowel disease or celiac disease.

D. Thyroid. Nodules or mass may suggest medullary carcinoma of thyroid or thyroid adenoma.

E. Cardiac. Right-sided heart murmur may be present in carcinoid syndrome. Signs of severe atherosclerosis or peripheral vascular disease may be present with intestinal ischemia.

F. Abdominal examination. This examination should assess for distention (irritable bowel syndrome, infections), bruit (colon ischemia), tenderness (irritable bowel syndrome, inflammatory bowel disease, infections, ischemia), mass (neoplasia), and hepatosplenomegaly (amyloidosis).

G. Rectal examination. This examination should evaluate sphincter tone (fecal incontinence) and tenderness (proctitis). The presence of fistula, painless anal fissure, or a perirectal abscess may suggest Crohn's disease. Fecal impaction in pediatric or geriatric age groups may suggest overflow diarrhea.

H. Extremities. Edema and clubbing suggest malabsorption. Arthritis may be noted in inflammatory bowel disease, Whipple's disease, and some enteric infections.

I. Lymphadenopathy. Lymphadenopathy may suggest lymphoma or other neoplasm.

V. Laboratory Tests

A. Acute diarrhea (Figure 16–1). Testing is needed only in patients with dysentery, patients aged younger than 3 months or older than 70 years, immunocompromised patients, patients with persistent diarrhea, or those at risk of transmitting infections (e.g., food handlers in food service establishments, health care workers, attendees/residents, employees of day care, or an institutional facility such as a psychiatric hospital, prison, or nursing home). The modified 3-day rule rejects submitting routine stool cultures for low-risk patients hospitalized <3 days and dictates performing only Clostridium difficile toxin tests. (SOR **B**)

B. Chronic diarrhea (Figure 16–2). Findings from the history, examination, routine laboratory tests, and quantitative stool analysis should guide specific, confirmatory testing or a trial of empiric therapy.

   1. The **complete blood count** may show anemia (blood loss, malabsorption) or leukocytosis (infection).

   2. A **chemistry screen** may be helpful in assessing fluid/electrolyte balance and nutritional status (malabsorption).

   3. TSH and tissue transglutaminase antibodies (for celiac disease) may also be ordered.

   4. A **48-hour quantitative stool collection** on a regular diet of moderately high fat (80–100 g fat per day) can help classify diarrhea as osmotic, secretory, inflammatory, or fatty. The fecal analysis should include weight, electrolytes, calculation of osmotic gap $(290 - 2[Na^+ + K^+])$, pH, occult blood, stool leukocytes (or lactoferrin), quantitative fecal fat and concentration, and analysis for laxatives.

VI. Treatment for acute and chronic diarrheas should include supportive measures as well as measures directed at underlying causes determined through careful history, examination, and appropriate laboratory evaluation (Figures 16–1 and 16–2).

A. Maintenance of hydration and rehydration

   1. In the **healthy adult with mild-to-moderate acute diarrhea,** oral glucose or starch containing products, for example carbonated drinks, fruit juice, or sports drinks with saltine crackers, are adequate. (SOR **A**) These should not be used in infants and young children because of excessive carbohydrate content and inadequate sodium and potassium.

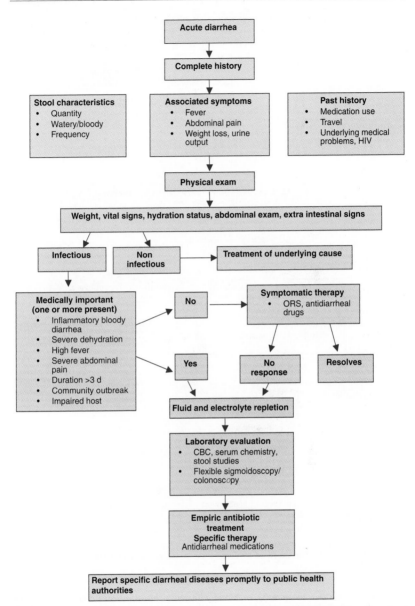

FIGURE 16–1. Diagnostic and management algorithm for patients presenting with acute infectious diarrhea. (Reproduced with permission from Gadewar S, Fasano A. Current concepts in the evaluation, diagnosis, and management of acute infectious diarrhea. *Curr Opin Pharmacol.* 2005;5:559–565.)

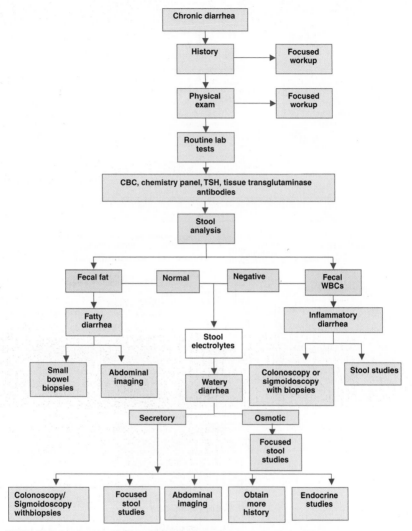

FIGURE 16–2. Guidelines from American Gastroenterology Association for evaluating patients w/chronic diarrhea. (Reproduced with permission from Headstrom PD, Surawicz CM. Chronic diarrhea. *Clin GastroenterolHepatol.* 2005;3: 734–737.)

2. For **children, the elderly, or those with moderate-to-severe diarrhea,** the World Health Organization (WHO) formula or commercial oral rehydration solutions (ORS) such as Pedialyte, Rehydralyte, Infalyte, Naturalyte, or Resol are recommended and are superior to intravenous fluids in resolving diarrhea and restoring weight. WHO's recently restructured formula reflects decreased osmolality from 311 to 245 in response to studies noted by Cochrane that showed reduced osmolarity ORS when compared to WHO standard ORS was associated with fewer unscheduled intravenous fluid infusions, lower stool volume postrandomization, and less vomiting with no additional risk of developing hyponatremia. (SOR Ⓐ) **Homemade ORS** can be prepared using 7 teaspoons of sugar and 1 teaspoon of salt to 1 L of bottled water. **Rice-based ORS**

decreases stool output compared to standard ORS and can be prepared by mixing half cup dry, precooked baby rice cereal with 2 cups water, and one-fourth tsp salt. With mild-to-moderate dehydration, 50 to 100 mL/kg should be given over 2 to 4 hours and an additional 50 to 100 mL after each stool to children younger than 2 years, 100 to 200 mL to 2 to 10-year-old child, and unlimited to children older than 10 years and adults.

3. In **severe dehydration** with obtunded mental status or when oral intake is not able to keep up with ongoing losses, intravenous fluids (0.9 N saline or Ringer's solution 20–40 mL/kg/h for children, D5 Ringer's lactate or D5 0.9 N saline 1 L every 1–2 hours for adults) should be given for 4 to 6 hours until adequate rehydration (determined by weight gain in children and clinical signs in adults) is established. The patient's usual diet supplemented with ORS can then be resumed.

B. Diet

1. **Children** should be continued on their preferred, usual, and age-appropriate diet. Frequent small feedings (every 10–60 minutes) of any tolerated foods or ORS may be helpful, if vomiting occurs. Breast-feeding should be continued. Formula-fed infants should continue with their usual formula immediately upon rehydration.

2. **Adults** should be encouraged to eat potatoes, rice, wheat, noodles, crackers, bananas, yogurt, boiled vegetables, and soup. Dairy products, caffeine, and alcohol should be avoided.

3. In **chronic diarrhea,** fasting can differentiate between osmotic diarrhea (which resolves with fasting) and some secretory diarrheas. Dietary measures beneficial in chronic diarrhea include eating a high-fiber diet for irritable bowel syndrome, avoiding lactose for lactose intolerance, and avoiding wheat, barley, and rye for celiac disease. In children with postinfectious diarrhea, management with a soy-based formula, lactose-free formula, or semielemental diet is indicated.

C. Symptomatic treatment

1. **Antimotility agents** may be considered in adult patients with watery, noninflammatory diarrhea. They should be avoided in young children and patients with dysentery. (SOR **B**) First-line therapies are usually opiate derivatives such as loperamide (Imodium) or diphenoxylate with atropine (Lomotil), used after each diarrheal movement, not to exceed 8 tablets per day. (SOR **A**)

2. In **chronic diarrhea,** bulk-forming agents (psyllium or methylcellulose) may be used to increase stool bulk and consistency, but they do not reduce stool weight. Opiates (e.g., tincture of opium, 6 drops every 4–6 hours, or codeine, 15–30 mg every 4–6 hours) may be necessary.

D. Antibiotic treatment (see Table 16–3).

1. **Empiric treatment**
   a. Treatment for **travelers' diarrhea** (see Chapter 104).
   b. Patients with **persistent diarrhea** may be empirically treated for presumed giardiasis, especially if there was a history of travel or exposure to untreated water (e.g., lake, stream, or well), and if other evaluations are negative.
   c. Empiric treatment can also be considered in those with **dysentery,** those who appear **septic or toxic,** and **high-risk patients** (infants younger than 3 months, persons older than 70 years, and immunocompromised patients) after a stool specimen is obtained.
   d. In **chronic diarrhea,** a therapeutic trial of broad-spectrum antibiotics may be considered for suspected small-bowel bacterial overgrowth (resulting from stasis of intestinal contents, e.g., in diabetics with slowed intestinal motility, postgastrectomy, or persons with partial intestinal obstruction from Crohn's disease).

2. **Specific antibiotic treatment.** Other infections should be treated based on the specific causative organism. Antibiotics or antimotility agents should not be used in enterohemorrhagic shiga toxin producing *E coli* 0157:H7 (*STEC*), as they may enhance toxin release and increase the risk of hemolytic-uremic syndrome.

E. Probiotics

1. Probiotics containing *Lactobacillus species* or *Saccharomyces boulardii* can decrease the likelihood of **antibiotic-induced diarrhea (but not traveler's diarrhea)** by 33% in children and adults. (SOR **A**) These products (e.g., Culturelle) are sold over the counter and can be found in the vitamin or diarrhea section of the pharmacy. A typical dosage is 5 to 10 billion viable organisms 3 to 4 times a day in adults (half the dosage in children) for the duration of antibiotic use.

TABLE 16–3. ANTIBIOTIC TREATMENT FOR SPECIfiC PATHOGENS

Pathogen	Antibiotic of Choice	Alternative
Aeromonas/Plesiomonas	Ciprofloxacin 500 mg po bid × 3 d	TMP-SMX DS po bid × 3 d
Campylobacter species	Azithromycin 500 mg po qd × 3 d or ciprofloxacin 500 mg po bid	Erythromycin stearate 500 mg qid po × 5 d
Clostridium difficile	Metronidazole 500 mg po tid or 250 mg qid × 10–14 d	Vancomycin 125 mg po qid × 10–14 d; Teicoplanin 400 mg po bid × 10 d
Cryptosporidium species‡	Nitazoxanide 500 mg po bid × 3 d	HIV w/immunodeficiency: antiretrovirals Nitazoxanide 500 mg po bid × 14 d
Cyclospora species	TMP-SMZ DS po bid × 7–10 d	AIDS pt: TMP-SMZ† qid × 10 d, then 1 tab po 3 × wk
Entamoeba histolytica	Metronidazole 500–750 mg po tid × 10 d or tinidazole 2 g po qd × 3 d, followed by either iodoquinol 650 mg po tid × 20 d or paromomycin 500 mg po tid × 7 d	Tinidazole 1 g po q12 h × 3 d or Ornidazole 500 mg po q12 h × 5 d, followed by either Iodoquinol 650 mg po tid × 20 d or paromomycin 500 mg tid × 7 d
Escherichia coli (except enterohemorrhagic)	Fluoroquinolone po bid × 3 d*	Azithromycin 500 mg × 1, then 250 mg qd × 4 d (peds 5–10 mg/kg/d in 1 dose); Rifaximin 200 mg tid × 3 d†
Giardia	Tinidazole 2 g po × 1 or Nitazoxanide 500 mg po bid × 3 d	Metronidazole 500–750 mg po tid × 5 d, Paromomycin 500 mg qid × 7 d
Isospora species	TMP-SMZ DS 1 po bid × 10 d; AIDS pt: TMP-SMZ DS qid × 10 d and then bid × 3 wks	(Pyrimethamine 75 mg po qd + folinic acid 10 mg po qd) × 14 d; Ciprofloxacin 500 mg bid × 7 d
Listeria monocytogenes	Ampicillin 50 mg/kg IV q6 h	TMP-SMZ 20 mg/kg/d IV divided q6–8 h
Microsporidium species‡	Albendazole 400 mg bid × 3 wks; peds dose: 15 mg/kg qd divided into 2 daily doses × 7 d	
Nontyphi species of Salmonella	Cipro 500 mg bid × 5–7 d	Azithromycin 1 g po × 1, then 500 mg qd × 6 d; Ceftriaxone 100 mg mg/kg/d
Shigella	Fluoroquinolone po bid × 3 d*	TMP-SMX bid × 3 d†; Azithromycin 500 mg × 1, then 250 mg × 4 d; Ceftriaxone 50–75 mg/kg/d × 2-5 d
Vibrio cholerae (primary treatment is hydration)	Azithromycin 1 g po × 1	Cipro 1 g po × 1
Yersenia (no treatment unless severe)	Doxy 100 mg bid IV + (Tobra or Genta 5 mg/kg/d qd)	TMP-SMX or FQs

*Ciprofloxacin 500 mg bid, ofloxacin 300 mg bid, levofloxacin 500 mg qd, or norfloxacin 400 mg bid. Peds and pregnancy avoid FQs.
† Bactrim/Septra and doxycycline are no longer recommended because of the development of widespread resistance. Rifaximin approved for age 12 years and older; does not treat Shigella.
‡ Only for septic/toxic, extremes of age, or immunocompromised patients.

2. They do, however, appear to be a useful adjunct to rehydration therapy in **treating acute, infectious diarrhea, decreasing the duration of illness by 30 to 48 hours**. (SOR **A**) Efficacy is most evident in viral diarrheas and less or absent in invasive, bacterial diarrheas. In children, Lactobacillus GG has been shown to reduce the duration of acute diarrhea by 1 day and duration of rotavirus shedding but are most effective when given during the first 2.5 days of illness. The dosage is at least 10 billion colony-forming units daily. (SOR **B**)

F. **Other agents for chronic diarrhea.** Empiric trials of cholestyramine (for bile acid diarrheas, after ileal resection, vagotomy, or cholecystectomy) and pancreatic enzymes (for pancreatic insufficiency) may be diagnostic and therapeutic. Lactase capsules can be helpful in lactose intolerance.

REFERENCES

Camilleri M. Chronic diarrhea: a review on pathophysiology and management for the clinical gastroenterologist. *Clin Gastroenterol Hepatol.* 2004;2:198-206.

Gadewar S, Fasano A. Current concepts in the evaluation, diagnosis and management of actue infectious diarrhea. *Curr Opin Pharmacol.* 2005;5:559-565.

Headstrom PD, Surawicz CM. Chronic diarrhea. *Clin Gastroenterol Hepatol.* 2005;3:734-737.

Juarez J, Abramo TJ. Diarrhea in the recent traveler. *Pediatr Emerg Care.* 2006;22:602-608.

Keating JP. Chronic diarrhea. *Pediatr Rev.* 2005;26:5-14.

Schiller LR. Chronic diarrhea. *Gastroenterology.* 2004;127:287-293.

Wilson ME. Diarrhea in nontravelers: risk and etiology. *Clin Infect Dis.* 2005;41:S541-S546.

Yates J. Traveler's diarrhea. *Am Fam Physician.* 2005;71:2095-2100.

17   Dizziness

Diane J. Madlon-Kay, MD, MS

KEY POINTS

- Peripheral vestibular disorders are the most common cause of dizziness.
- A directed history and physical examination can usually rule out the few serious causes of dizziness.
- Treatment options are limited, although symptoms resolve spontaneously in most patients.

I. **Definition.** *Dizziness* is an imprecise term commonly used by patients to describe symptoms such as faintness, giddiness, lightheadedness, or unsteadiness.

II. **Common Diagnoses.** In up to 19% of cases, a definitive cause of dizziness cannot be found. The various diagnoses of dizziness can be divided into three main categories.

   A. **Peripheral vestibular disorders,** which account for up to 44% of cases, include vestibular neuronitis, benign positional vertigo, Meniere disease, acoustic neuroma (see sidebar), and otitis media. These patients have a disorder at some point along the course of the vestibular nerve other than at its origin in the brain stem. Most often, the problem is at the termination of the nerve in the inner ear, known as the labyrinth.

ACOUSTIC NEUROMA

Acoustic neuroma typically presents as unilateral tinnitus and hearing loss. Few patients have vertigo initially. Symptoms are slowly progressive, and continued growth of the tumor is associated with facial weakness and ataxia.

   B. **Systemic diseases,** such as cardiac problems, diseases resulting from drug use, metabolic abnormalities, anemia, infection, and psychogenic causes, may result in dizziness. Twenty to thirty percent of all cases of dizziness are believed to be psychogenic. Disorders in almost any organ system can cause dizziness. Spatial orientation depends on the complex interaction of adequate sensation, central integration, and the proper motor response.

   C. **Central nervous system diseases,** such as stroke, transient ischemic attack, migraines, or multiple sclerosis, are responsible for dizziness in 5% of patients (see sidebar). Any disease that disrupts the pathway between the vestibular apparatus and the brain may result in dizziness. Normally, impulses from this apparatus proceed through the eighth cranial nerve to the vestibular nuclei of the brain stem. From the brain stem, they are transmitted to the cerebellum and the cerebral cortex.

CENTRAL NERVOUS SYSTEM DISEASES

Central nervous system diseases, such as strokes, can cause vertigo. However, the vertigo is almost always accompanied by other central nervous system symptoms, such as facial

TABLE 17–1. TYPES OF DIZZINESS

	Vertigo	Presyncope	Disequilibrium	Lightheadedness
Sensation	Rotational; spinning or whirling	Lightheaded, faint feeling	Unsteadiness; loss of balance on walking	Vague; may be floating sensation
Temporal characteristics	May be episodic or continuous	Typically episodes last seconds to hours	Usually present, although it may fluctuate in intensity	Usually present all or most of the time for days or weeks, sometimes years
Simulation tests	Dix–Hallpike maneuver	Orthostatic blood pressure measurement	Romberg test, tandem gait	Hyperventilation
Differential diagnosis	***Peripheral causes*** • Vestibular neuronitis • Benign positional vertigo • Meniere disease • Acoustic neuroma • Otitis media • Motion sickness • Drug use ***Central causes*** • Stroke • Transient ischemic attack • Multiple sclerosis • Basilar artery migraine • Temporal lobe seizure	• Arrhythmias • Vasovagal reflex • Orthostatic hypotension • Anemia • Aortic stenosis • Low cardiac output states • Carotid sinus hypersensitivity • Hypoglycemia • Hypoxemia	• Multiple sensory deficits • Altered visual input • Primary disequilibrium of aging • Parkinsonism • Cerebellar disease • Frontal lobe apraxia • Drug use	• Anxiety • Depression • Hyperventilation • Panic disorder

numbness, hemiparesis, or diplopia. Dysarthria, facial numbness, hemiparesis, or diplopia may be found on examination.

III. **Symptoms.** Dizziness can be divided into four basic types: vertigo, presyncope, disequilibrium, and lightheadedness. The symptoms of each type are described in this section. Further details about the types of dizziness are shown in Table 17–1.

   A. Complaints of **vertigo** (i.e., a sensation of turning or spinning) accompanied by **nausea, vomiting, diaphoresis,** and **difficulty with balance** suggest peripheral vestibular disorders. Patients may also have **auditory symptoms** such as decreased hearing, tinnitus, or ear pain. Symptoms of particular disorders are described below.

      1. **Vestibular neuronitis or acute labyrinthitis.** After an acute onset of severe vertigo lasting several days, gradual improvement follows for several weeks. Symptoms frequently follow a viral illness.

      2. **Benign positional vertigo.** Instances of vertigo related to position are extremely brief, can be associated with nausea, and often will wake the patient from sleep when turning over in bed. Although the disorder is generally self-limited, its course is variable.

      3. **Meniere disease.** Patients with this disease have discrete attacks of vertigo of abrupt onset. The attacks last for several hours, not days, and are often accompanied by nausea and vomiting. The interval between attacks may be weeks to months. Between attacks, the patient is asymptomatic. Fluctuating hearing loss, typically accompanied by tinnitus and a feeling of pressure in the ear, is usually present during attacks. Irreversible hearing loss and chronic tinnitus develop in the affected ear over time.

   B. **Presyncope** is dizziness associated with the feeling of an impending faint. Actual loss of consciousness does not occur. It is episodic.

   C. **Disequilibrium** is a problem with balance, usually associated with an unsteady gait. If patients are asked, "Is the dizziness in your head or in your feet?" those with disequilibrium respond with the latter choice.

TABLE 17–2. DISTINGUISHING PERIPHERAL FROM CENTRAL VERTIGO WITH POSITION TESTING

	Peripheral	Central
Latency (time to onset of vertigo or nystagmus)	3–10 s	None; begins immediately
Fatigability (lessening signs and symptoms with repetition)	Yes	No
Nystagmus direction	Fixed	Changing
Intensity of signs and symptoms	Severe	Mild

    D. Lightheadedness is a vague or floating sensation, often imprecisely described by the patient. Such dizziness is generally present much of the time. It is often accompanied by other somatic symptoms, such as headache and abdominal pain.

IV. Signs

    A. The Dix–Hallpike (Nylen–Barany) maneuver can be helpful in distinguishing peripheral from central vestibulopathy. The patient should sit on the edge of the examining table and lie down suddenly, with the head hanging 45 degrees backward and turned 45 degrees to one side. Then repeat the test twice, once with the head turned to the other side and once with the head in the middle position. The patient's eyes should be kept open to observe (1) the development of vertigo and (2) the time of onset, duration, and direction of nystagmus. This maneuver will reveal a central or peripheral pattern of vertigo, as shown in Table 17–2. (SOR **C**)

    B. Inspection of the eardrum may reveal otitis media or serous otitis.

    C. Orthostatic blood pressure determinations are helpful when the history suggests dizziness caused by hypovolemia from blood loss or dehydration. A drop in systolic blood pressure of as much as 20 mm Hg, a decline in diastolic pressure of up to 10 mm Hg, and a rise in pulse rate of up to 20 beats per minute can be normal findings with standing. If standing causes a greater blood pressure drop or pulse rise and reproduces the patient's symptoms, some form of hypovolemia is the most likely cause.

    D. If the history suggests disequilibrium, gait and stationary testing should be done. Static balance can be tested with the Romberg test. The gait may be tested by asking the patient to rise from a chair, without using their arms, walk 10 feet, and then turn around. In addition, evaluation of muscle strength, coordination, reflexes, and proprioception should be conducted. The posture should be inspected. Often patients with postural instability stand bent over, with their knees and hips flexed. A gentle tap on the chest (the nudge test) while standing behind the patient can give an indication of the patient's likelihood of falling backward. Testing visual fields and acuity may uncover visual impairment.

    E. If the history suggests a psychological cause, the patient should hyperventilate by blowing vigorously for 3 minutes on a paper towel held 6 inches from the mouth. This action may cause some circumoral and digital numbness, as well as reproduce the patient's dizziness.

V. Laboratory Tests

    A. Few patients with suspected peripheral vestibular disorders require laboratory testing. Patients whose symptoms are progressive or recurrent should have an **audiologic evaluation** that includes a pure tone audiogram, speech discrimination testing, and tympanometry. Such patients should also undergo vestibular examination by **electronystagmography.**

        Laboratory testing of patients whose dizziness may be caused by systemic diseases must be guided by the history and physical examination. Most "screening" laboratory tests, such as complete blood cell counts and electrolyte determinations, are rarely helpful.

    B. Magnetic resonance imaging with gadolinium enhancement is particularly useful in detecting acoustic neuromas, and is the current gold standard test. (SOR **C**)

VI. Treatment

    A. Peripheral vestibular disorders. The symptoms of vertigo are frightening to patients. The physician must be supportive and reassuring, since most causes of vertigo are not a serious health threat.

        1. Initial treatment of acutely vertiginous patients usually involves having them lie still in a darkened room and avoid head movement. It is important to have patients mobilized as soon as the most severe nausea and vertigo subside, to avoid protracted disability.

2. Drug therapy may provide symptomatic relief.
   a. Antihistamines, the most commonly prescribed drugs for vertigo, suppress the vestibular end organ receptors and inhibit activation of vagal responses. Patients should take the medication for a few weeks and then try discontinuing the drug. The major side effects are dry mouth and sedation. Commonly recommended drugs are meclizine, 25 mg orally every 4 to 6 hours, and diphenhydramine, 50 mg orally every 4 to 6 hours. (SOR **C**)
   b. Antiemetics can be tried when nausea and vomiting are pronounced. These agents suppress central vestibular pathways, which activate a vagal response. Their major side effect is sedation. Commonly recommended antiemetic drugs are prochlorperazine, 5 to 10 mg orally every 6 hours *or* 25-mg suppository by rectum twice daily, and trimethobenzamide, 250 mg orally every 6 hours *or* 200-mg suppository by rectum every 6 hours. Acute dystonic reactions may occur occasionally with prochlorperazine.
3. Vestibular exercises can reduce symptoms, disability, and handicap from movement provoked dizziness. (SOR **B**)
4. The **canalith repositioning maneuver** eliminates symptoms of benign positional vertigo in up to 80% of patients after one treatment. (SOR **A**)
5. Surgery may be indicated if other medical therapies fail to adequately relieve severe vertigo. Surgical procedures include sectioning of the vestibular nerve, repair of an inner ear fistula, labyrinthectomy, or placement of a lymphatic shunt. Unilateral deafness may result.
B. Systemic diseases. Systemic diseases causing dizziness require treatment that is specific to the particular cause.
C. Central nervous system diseases. Symptomatic treatment of vertigo as described above may be helpful. Treatment of the underlying central nervous system condition is crucial.

REFERENCES

Chawla N, Olshaker JS. Diagnosis and management of dizziness and vertigo. *Med Clin N Am.* 2006;90:291-304.
Kanagalingman J, Hajioff D, Bennett S. Vertigo. *BMJ.* 2005;330:523.
Labuguen RH. Initial evaluation of vertigo. *Am Fam Physician.* 2006;73:244-251.
Yardley L, Donovan-Hall M, Smith HE, Walsh BM, Mullee M, Bronstein AM. Effectiveness of primary care-based vestibular rehabilitation for chronic dizziness. *Ann Intern Med.* 2004;141:598-605.

---

18   Dysmenorrhea

Suzanne Leonard Harrison, MD

KEY POINTS

- Dysmenorrhea is the most commonly reported gynecologic symptom, with an estimated 90% of all women being affected at least once in life.
- Dysmenorrhea causes significant disruption in the quality of life. It is the leading cause of short-term school absenteeism in adolescents, and a common cause of missed work for adult women.
- If dysmenorrhea fails to respond to first-line treatment with nonsteroidal anti-inflammatory drugs (NSAIDs) or oral contraceptives (OCPs), an underlying cause should be considered (i.e., secondary dysmenorrhea).

I. Definition. Dysmenorrhea is painful menstruation, frequently described as crampy pelvic pain that may radiate to the low back and thighs. Discomfort usually begins just before or at the onset of menstrual bleeding and typically lasts 1 or 2 days. The distinction must be

TABLE 18–1. DIFFERENTIAL DIAGNOSIS OF PRIMARY AND SECONDARY DYSMENORRHEA

	Primary Dysmenorrhea	Secondary Dysmenorrhea
Onset	Onset 6–12 months after menarche	Onset usually after age 25 but can occur at any time
Timing	Pelvic pain with onset of menstruation, lasting 1–3 d	Pain may not be limited to menstruation, and may present with change in timing or intensity of preexisting primary dysmenorrhea
Associated Symptoms	May be associated with low back and thigh pain, diarrhea, headache, nausea and vomiting	May have other gynecologic symptoms such as dyspareunia, abnormal uterine bleeding, pelvic pressure, infertility
Physical Examination	Physical examination is typically normal	Pelvic abnormalities on examination, depending on cause of secondary dysmenorrhea

made between **primary dysmenorrhea,** which generally starts in adolescence and occurs in women with normal pelvic anatomy, and **secondary dysmenorrhea,** which is pain secondary to pelvic organ pathology (Table 18–1).

Increased levels of prostaglandins in menstrual fluid have been identified in women with dysmenorrhea, especially on the first 2 days of menses. Prostanoids cause uterine contractions and pain. Vasopressin is also elevated in women with dysmenorrhea, and causes increased uterine contractility and ischemic pain secondary to vasoconstriction. Women with painful menses have increased uterine basal tone and myometrial contractile pressure. Uterine contractions are more frequent and dysrhythmic in those women diagnosed with dysmenorrhea. Altered levels of leukotrienes, thromboxanes and prostacyclin have also been implicated, and may contribute to the uterine hypercontractility and vasoconstriction seen in severe dysmenorrhea.

II. **Common Diagnoses**

   A. **Primary dysmenorrhea** affects 40% to 70% of menstruating women. Prevalence is highest in teens, with estimates as high as 90%. Fifteen percent of adolescents report severe dysmenorrhea that causes significant disruption in activities, including school absence. Nulliparity and heavy menses are risk factors for dysmenorrhea. Behavioral risk factors include cigarette smoking and weight loss attempts (independent of body mass index). Mental health risk factors include depression, anxiety, and disruption of social support networks.

   B. **Secondary dysmenorrhea** has several underlying causes:

      1. **Endometriosis** occurs in less than 10% of women of reproductive age, and more often in women with chronic pelvic pain and infertility. The age at the time of diagnosis is typically 25 to 35 years. Endometriosis is caused by foci of endometrial tissue outside the endometrial cavity and uterine musculature.

      2. **Leiomyomas (fibroids)** are uterine smooth muscle tumors. They are the most common gynecologic tumors, and are more common in black women. Twenty percent of women develop fibroids by age 40, although most are asymptomatic.

      3. **Adenomyosis** is observed most frequently in women after age 35, and is caused by foci of endometrial tissue in the myometrium. Fifteen percent of women with adenomyosis have associated endometriosis.

      4. **Pelvic inflammatory disease (PID)** (see Chapter 51).

      5. **Nonhormonal intrauterine devices (IUDs).**

      6. **Endometrial polyps.**

      7. **Anatomical** causes of dysmenorrhea include congenital anomalies (bicornuate or septate uterus), cervical stenosis, and imperforate hymen.

III. **Symptoms**

   A. **Primary dysmenorrhea** usually begins approximately 6 to 12 months after menarche, with the onset of ovulatory cycles. Discomfort is strongly associated with menstruation and often accompanied by associated symptoms, including diarrhea, headache, fatigue, nausea, and vomiting. Pain starts just before or with the onset of bleeding and lasts from 8 to 72 hours, often radiating to low back and inner/anterior thighs on the first and second days of menstruation. Women with migraines have an increased incidence of headaches before or during menses.

   B. The pain of **secondary dysmenorrhea** is not always limited to the time of menstruation, and may present early after menarche (first or second cycle) or after age 25. It often presents later in a woman's reproductive life, or as a change in the timing or intensity of preexisting primary dysmenorrhea. Causes of secondary dysmenorrhea should be evaluated if a woman describes dyspareunia, menorrhagia, dyschezia, intermenstrual bleeding, postcoital bleeding, or irregular cycles.

1. **Endometriosis** is usually a deep aching pain that begins several days prior to menses, may last throughout the cycle, and may be associated with dyspareunia, infertility, hematuria, unilateral pain, or abnormal uterine bleeding. Not all women with endometriosis have dysmenorrhea or chronic pelvic pain.

2. Most **leiomyomas** (fibroids) are asymptomatic. Women may experience pelvic pressure, bloating, menorrhagia, or metrorrhagia, depending on the location and size of the tumor.

3. **Adenomyosis** is usually associated with severe dysmenorrhea and menorrhagia, although some patients are asymptomatic.

IV. **Signs**

A. **Primary dysmenorrhea.** Most commonly, the physical examination will be normal. Tenderness on uterine palpation may be present during menstruation.

B. **Secondary dysmenorrhea**

1. **Endometriosis** is classically associated with palpable nodules in the posterior cul-de-sac and anterior vaginal wall, and a tender fixed uterus on bimanual examination. The physical examination may be normal.

2. **Leiomyomas** are suspected if the uterus is irregularly enlarged or nodular.

3. **Adenomyosis** is associated with a symmetrically enlarged uterus.

4. **PID** (see Chapter 51).

V. **Laboratory Tests**

A. **Primary dysmenorrhea.** With a suggestive history and a normal physical examination, no laboratory evaluation is indicated. Pelvic examination is not necessary in all women, but is indicated in those with a history of sexual activity or symptoms inconsistent with primary dysmenorrhea. If menorrhagia is present, it may be prudent to check a hemoglobin to evaluate for microcytic anemia.

B. For **secondary dysmenorrhea,** workup may include the following:

1. **Gonococcal and chlamydia cultures** if signs or symptoms suggest pelvic inflammatory disease, or the patient is at risk for sexually transmitted diseases.

2. **Pelvic ultrasonography** to diagnose fibroids, mass lesions, endometriomas, or ovarian cysts. Stage three or four endometriosis can sometimes be identified with high-resolution ultrasonography.

3. **Hysterosalpingogram** if a uterine anomaly is suspected.

4. **Laparoscopy** for diagnosing endometriosis and if other tests do not reveal the cause of secondary dysmenorrhea.

5. **Urinalysis** is indicated if the patient gives a history consistent with endometriosis and reports hematuria.

VI. **Treatment** (Figure 18–1).

A. **Pharmacologic approaches (Table 18–2).**

1. **Prostaglandin synthetase inhibitors (i.e., NSAIDs)** are effective in relieving primary dysmenorrhea in 70% to 90% of cases, and should be considered first-line therapy unless there is a contraindication. NSAIDs inhibit endometrial prostaglandin production without affecting endometrial development but also have direct analgesic properties at the central nervous system level. They should be started a few hours before the onset of menstrual bleeding or with the onset of pain and continued for 1 to 3 days. NSAIDs appear to be equal in efficacy and so cost, convenience, and patient preference should be used to determine the best choice for a particular woman.

   Contraindications to NSAIDs include gastrointestinal symptoms, bronchospasm and fluid retention, but side effects are usually mild and occur in fewer than 5% of patients. SOR **🅐**.

2. **Cyclooxygenase II inhibitors (COX II inhibitors)** do not demonstrate improved efficacy when compared with traditional NSAIDs. Because of the concern for cardiovascular safety, some have been withdrawn from distribution. SOR **🅑**.

3. **Oral contraceptives** suppress both menstrual fluid volume and prostaglandin release, but not synthesis; this is achieved by causing endometrial hypoplasia. OCPs are effective in most patients, and are best suited for those also desiring hormonal contraception. Combination, extended-cycle, and progestin-only pills may be used. Contraceptive patches are less effective than oral contraceptive pills in treating dysmenorrhea. If severe dysmenorrhea is not improved with combined use of NSAIDs

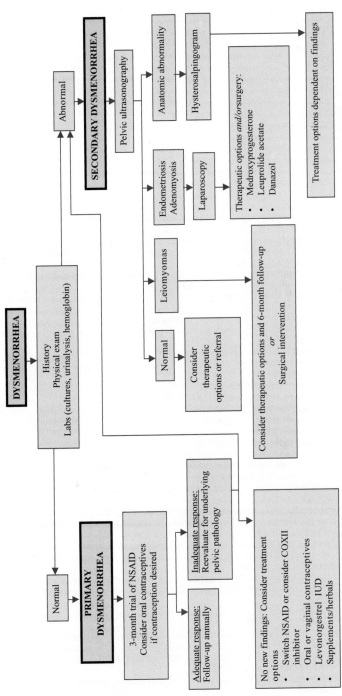

FIGURE 18–1. Evaluation and treatment of dysmenorrhea. NSAID, nonsteroidal anti-inflammatory drugs; COX, cyclooxygenase; IUD, intrauterine device.

TABLE 18–2. PHARMACOLOGIC TREATMENT OF DYSMENORRHEA

Medication*	Dose (mg)
NSAIDs	
Ibuprofen	400–600 mg every 6 h
Ketoprofen	50 mg every 8 h
Naproxen sodium	500–550 mg, followed by 275 mg every 6 h
Diclofenac	50 mg every 8 h
Indomethacin	25–50 mg every 8 h
Oral Contraceptives	1 tablet daily
Danazol	100–200 mg twice daily
Leuprolide	3.75 mg IM monthly
Supplements	
Thiamine	100 mg daily
Omega-3 fatty acids	2 g daily

*Consult full prescribing information before administering any of these drugs.

and oral contraceptives, reevaluation for underlying pelvic pathology should be pursued. SOR **B**.

4. **Levonorgestrel intrauterine devices** effectively cause amenorrhea after the first year and decrease the prevalence of dysmenorrhea by 50%; effective in treatment of endometriosis. SOR **B**.

5. **Depo-medroxyprogesterone acetate** induces anovulation and is often used in women with endometriosis. SOR **B**.

6. **Intravaginal administration** of combination contraceptives such as the etonogestrel and ethinyl estradiol vaginal ring or even standard oral contraceptives with levonorgestrel and ethinyl estradiol decreases dysmenorrhea. There seem to be fewer systemic side effects when compared to oral administration of combination contraceptives. SOR **B**.

7. **Danazol or leuprolide acetate** may be considered in refractory causes of secondary amenorrhea caused by endometriosis and chronic pelvic pain not limited to the time of menses SOR **B**.

8. **Calcium channel blockers** reduce myometrial activity and relieve dysmenorrhea by decreasing uterine contractions. SOR **C**.

9. **Glyceryl trinitrate** has been shown to be helpful with severe dysmenorrhea, especially when taken in the first 6 hours of menstruation. It is strongly associated with headache. SOR **C**.

10. **Supplements** such as thiamine, pyridoxine, vitamin E, and omega-3 fatty acids have all been used to effectively treat dysmenorrhea. SOR **B**.

11. **Herbal** preparations have been used for treatment of menstrual pain. Toki-shakuyakusan, a Japanese herb, has been shown to be effective, although the dose is unclear. Ovulatory function and thus fertility does not seem to be suppressed. SOR **B**.

B. **Nonpharmacologic** approaches to the treatment of dysmenorrhea.

1. **Low fat vegetarian diet** is associated with decreased duration and intensity of dysmenorrhea. SOR **B**.

2. **Exercise** may stimulate the release of endorphins, which can act as nonspecific analgesics, but the evidence is insufficient to support recommendation as a treatment for dysmenorrhea. SOR **C**.

3. **Physical treatments** for dysmenorrhea may be used in combination with pharmacologic treatments, and often provide relief for those women choosing not to use medications.

    a. **Heating pad or patch** diminishes menstrual pain, and seems to be as efficacious as NSAIDs. SOR **B**.

    b. **Acupuncture and acupressure** have been shown to be effective in some patients. Acupressure was shown to be as effective as ibuprofen in one study. SOR **B**.

    c. **Trancutaneous electrical nerve stimulation (TENS)** is effective for some refractory dysmenorrhea. SOR **B**.

    d. **Manipulation** has not been shown to be an efficacious treatment for dysmenorrhea. SOR **C**.

C. **Surgical therapies** should be reserved for those patients unresponsive to other treatment modalities.
   1. **Hysterectomy** is sometimes used for refractory dysmenorrhea, and is commonly used in the treatment of fibroids. SOR **B**.
   2. **Laparoscopic uterosacral nerve ablation (LUNA)** and **presacral neurectomy** are used only in the most severe cases. Presacral neurectomy has more adverse effects. SOR **C**.
   3. **Endometrial ablation** is sometimes used in women with severe dysmenorrhea and menorrhagia.

REFERENCES

Berek JS. *Berek & Novak's Gynecology*. 14th ed. Philadelphia, PA: Lippincott Williams & Wilkins; 2007.
Darwood MY. Primary dysmenorrhea. *Obstet Gynecol*. 2006;108(2):428-441.
French L. Dysmenorrhea. *Am Fam Physician*. 2005;71(2):285-291.
Proctor M, Farquhar C. Diagnosis and management of dysmenorrhoea. *BMJ*. 2006;332:1134-1138.
Scott J, Gibbs RS, Karlan BY, Haney AF. *Danforth's Obstetrics & Gynecology*. 9th ed. Philadelphia, PA: Lippincott Williams & Wilkins; 2003.

---

19   Dyspepsia

Kalyanakrishnan Ramakrishnan, MD

KEY POINTS

- The majority of patients with dyspepsia have no structural abnormality (nonulcer dyspepsia).
- Patients without alarm symptoms should be tested for *Helicobacter pylori* and treated if test results are positive ("test and treat" strategy).
- Patients with nonulcer dyspepsia may be treated with a proton pump inhibitor (PPI), histamine-2 receptor blocking agent (H_2 blocker), or a prokinetic agent.

I. **Definition.** Dyspepsia is defined as pain or discomfort felt to arise in the upper gastrointestinal (GI) tract with symptoms on greater than 25% of the days over the past 4 weeks. It may be characterized by epigastric discomfort or pain and can be associated with epigastric heaviness or fullness, belching or regurgitation, bloating, early satiety, heartburn, food intolerance, nausea, or vomiting. Lower bowel function is usually not affected.

II. **Common Diagnoses.** Dyspepsia is a common complaint, occurring in 20% to 30% of the general population. It accounts for approximately 2% to 5% of family practice consultations. Common causes include:

A. **Medications.** Aspirin, nonsteroidal anti-inflammatory drugs (NSAIDs), steroids, bisphosphonates, iron, erythromycin, tetracycline, alcohol, and potassium supplements can cause upper abdominal discomfort.

B. **Nonulcer dyspepsia (NUD).** This disorder is found in up to 60% of patients with dyspepsia. The incidence of NUD is age dependent; approximately 70% of patients younger than age 40 have NUD, as opposed to only 40% of those older than age 60. The exact cause of NUD is unknown. No definite link between NUD and *H pylori* has been established.

C. **Peptic ulcer disease (PUD).** PUD includes gastric and duodenal ulcers, gastritis, and duodenitis and is found in 20% to 30% of patients with dyspepsia. Together, NUD and PUD probably account for 50% to 80% of all cases of dyspepsia. Duodenal ulcers affect males twice as frequently as females. The peak incidence is between ages 45 and 64 in males and at age 55 in females. Gastric ulcers occur much less frequently than duodenal ulcer and increase in incidence with advancing age. A past history of PUD, *H pylori* infection, NSAID use, male gender, and cigarette smoking all are associated with an increased chance of finding gastric or duodenal ulcers on upper endoscopy.

D. **Gastroesophageal reflux disease (GERD).** GERD is found in 5% to 15% of patients with dyspepsia.

E. **Gastric, esophageal, or pancreatic cancer.** Fewer than 2% of patients with dyspepsia have cancer. The incidence increases with advancing age. Toxins (e.g., nitrosamines or polycyclic hydrocarbons), genetic factors, pernicious anemia, and atrophic gastritis have been associated with gastric cancer.

F. **Cholecystitis or cholelithiasis** (see Chapter 1). For irritable bowel syndrome, see Chapter 1.

G. **Other causes of dyspepsia.** Zollinger–Ellison syndrome, chronic pancreatitis, malabsorption, abdominal angina, and coronary artery disease are uncommon.

III. **Symptoms.** Although symptoms have low specificity in patients with dyspepsia, they may be helpful in guiding the work-up (Figure 19–1).

   A. **Heartburn.** Heartburn, regurgitation, painful swallowing, and chest pain are symptoms suggestive of reflux.

   B. **Alarm symptoms.** The presence of alarm symptoms including age older than 55 years, unexplained significant weight loss ($\geq$10–15 lbs), persistent vomiting, melena, hematemesis, or dysphagia should prompt immediate work-up, usually with endoscopy. (SOR **B**)

   C. **Symptoms that poorly discriminate between specific disease and NUD.** These include relief with antacids or food, nocturnal pain, food intolerance (e.g., fatty food intolerance), duration of pain, pain that occurs within 1 hour of eating, and anorexia.

   D. **Symptoms that may identify patients with complications of PUD.** Symptoms that indicate complications of PUD or other specific causes of dyspepsia are:
      1. Hematemesis, melena, or both indicate GI bleeding.
      2. Dizziness, especially upon sitting or standing, or syncope may indicate significant blood loss.
      3. Persistent vomiting is a symptom of gastric outlet obstruction.
      4. Pain that radiates straight through to the back may indicate a penetrating ulcer, leaking abdominal aneurysm, pancreatitis, or pancreatic cancer.
      5. Pain radiating to the shoulder may result from diaphragmatic irritation caused by pus, blood, or free air in the peritoneum.

IV. **Signs.** In general, the physical examination is not helpful in determining the cause of dyspepsia. In uncomplicated cases, the examination usually reveals only mild to moderate epigastric tenderness. The following signs may be helpful in identifying patients with complications of PUD or serious systemic illness.

   A. **Unexplained tachycardia** (pulse $\geq$ 120) or postural hypotension (orthostatic change in blood pressure $\geq$ 20 mm Hg) may indicate significant blood loss from GI bleeding.

   B. **Abdominal rebound or rigidity** suggests peritoneal irritation. A perforated viscus, blood, or infection in the peritoneal cavity can cause peritoneal irritation.

   C. **Blood in the stool** may indicate upper GI tract bleeding.

   D. **Jaundice** may indicate biliary tract obstruction from pancreatic cancer or cholelithiasis.

   E. **Palpable mass** in the upper abdomen may indicate a hepatic, gastric, or pancreatic malignancy.

V. **Laboratory Tests.** In general, the laboratory evaluation consists of testing for *H pylori* in those individuals without alarm symptoms. This is referred to as the "test and treat" strategy (see Figure 19–1).

   A. **Tests that may be useful** include:
      1. **Tests for *H pylori*.** These can be either noninvasive (serology, urea breath test, urine or stool-based antigen tests) or invasive (rapid urease test or biopsies, obtained at the time of upper endoscopy). Serology is the easiest and least expensive, though the urea breath test is preferred. (SOR **B**)
      2. **Upper GI series.** The upper GI series is noninvasive and relatively inexpensive. It is sensitive in detecting gastric and duodenal ulcers (80%–90%). Its accuracy improves with disease severity. The double-contrast technique including spot views during vigorous compression with the barium-filled bulb improves detection of duodenal ulcers. In patients with GERD, only severe esophagitis may be detected, although reflux and motility disorders of the esophagus can be seen. The presence of a hiatal hernia does not correlate with GERD.
      3. **Upper GI endoscopy.** Upper GI endoscopy is the gold standard for identifying esophagogastroduodenal pathology and is the investigation of choice for patients older than

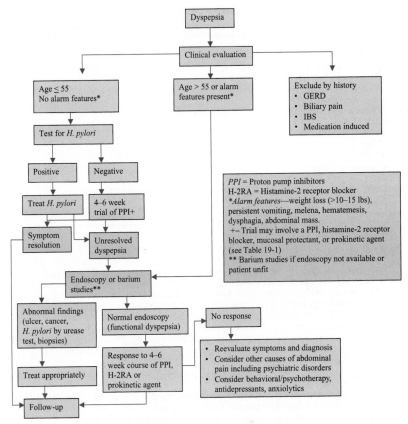

FIGURE 19–1. Management of dyspepsia.

55 with uninvestigated dyspepsia or in the presence of alarm features. (SOR **A**) Upper endoscopy is preferred to upper GI barium study, because lesions can be directly visualized and biopsy can be performed. In addition, testing for *H pylori* can be performed.

4. **Intraesophageal pH monitoring.** Most physicians consider this procedure to be the single best test for diagnosis for GERD. (SOR **A**) Coupled with a symptom diary, 24-hour monitoring has a sensitivity between 87% and 93% and a specificity of 92% to 97% for GERD.

5. **Scintigraphy.** Scintigraphy is best used to detect delayed gastric emptying. GERD and delayed gastric emptying can be detected using [^{99m}Tc] sulfur colloid, although intraesophageal pH monitoring is a better test for reflux.

B. **Indications for further testing.** Diagnostic testing should be started promptly in patients with severe systemic illness, bleeding, perforation, symptoms of upper GI tract obstruction, or evidence of cancer.

1. **Persistence of symptoms** after empiric treatment requires further evaluation with endoscopy or upper GI series.

2. In patients who experience a **recurrence of dyspepsia** following empiric treatment, a specific diagnosis should be made.

TABLE 19-1. MEDICATIONS USED IN THE TREATMENT OF DYSPEPSIA

Medication	Dose/Frequency
H₂blockers	
Cimetidine	400 mg twice daily
Famotidine	20 mg once or twice daily
Nizatidine	150 mg twice daily
Ranitidine	150 mg twice daily
Proton pump inhibitors	
Esomeprazole	20–40 mg once daily
Lansoprazole	15–30 mg once daily
Omeprazole	20 mg twice daily
Pantoprazole	40 mg once daily
Rabeprazole	20 mg once daily
Cytoprotective agents	
Sucralfate	1 g 4 times daily
Misoprostol	100–200 μg 2–4 times a day
Prokinetic agent	
Metoclopramide	10–15 mg 30 min before each meal and at bedtime

VI. Treatment. Figure 19–1 presents the "test and treat" approach to a patient with dyspepsia.

  A. A practical approach for patients with dyspepsia who are younger than 55 years and have no alarm symptoms, complications of PUD, or serious systemic illness is to treat empirically with an H_2 blocker or a PPI (SOR **B**) (see Table 19–1 for medications, dose, and frequency) and test for *H pylori*. If they test positive for *H pylori,* treat (see Chapter 82). Helidac (bismuth subsalicylate–metronidazole–tetracycline) plus a PPI or Prevpac (amoxicillin–clarithromycin–lansoprazole) administered for 14 days are both effective in the treatment of *H pylori* (80%–90% response). (SOR **A**) Patients should also be encouraged to discontinue ulcerogenic medications (e.g., alcohol or NSAIDs) and cigarette smoking. (SOR **C**) If NSAIDs need to be used, a PPI, H-2 blocker, or a cytoprotective agent may be used concomitantly (see Table 19–1) or consider switching to a COX-2 inhibitor (e.g., celecoxib). (SOR **C**)

  B. For **individuals with dyspepsia who are older than 55 years,** empiric treatment should be followed by the establishment of a definitive diagnosis with upper endoscopy. If symptoms worsen or persist despite therapy, the patient should undergo further evaluation (see Section V.B).

  C. **When the cause of the patient's dyspepsia is known,** the following therapeutic measures may be helpful:

   1. **NUD.** At present, the best therapy for NUD is unclear. Fortunately, in most individuals, abdominal discomfort resolves within several weeks. Treatment for *H pylori*, if identified, may resolve dyspeptic symptoms. (SOR **B**) In *H pylori* negative patients with pain, nausea, or bloating as predominant symptoms, a 4 to 6 week course of PPI, H-2 receptor blocker, or a prokinetic agent may be used (see Figure 19–1). (SOR **A**) Patients with prominent somatic complaints, anxiety, or depression are more likely to have a psychologic basis for their symptoms and may benefit from behavior therapy, antidepressants, or anxiolytics. (SOR **B**)

   2. **PUD** (see Chapter 82).

   3. **GERD.** Patients with mild GERD symptoms benefit from adopting antireflux measures, which include losing weight, avoiding lying down or bending over after meals, consuming few large meals and bedtime snacks, elevating the head of the bed on 4- to 8-inch blocks, modifying the diet (avoiding caffeine, chocolate, peppermint, fatty foods), and discontinuing alcohol consumption and cigarette smoking. (SOR **C**) (See sidebar for pediatric GERD.)

     a. In patients with a dominant symptom of heartburn or acid regurgitation, a PPI, H-2 blocker, or a prokinetic agent are options (see Table 19–1). (SOR **A**)

     b. **Antireflux surgery** should be considered in patients with severe esophagitis with inability to tolerate medication (including noncompliance), development of Barrett's esophagus, persistent reflux symptoms despite acid suppression, or severe asthma or aspiration pneumonia in association with GERD. (SOR **C**)

PEDIATRIC GERD

Gastroesophageal reflux is fairly common in infants. It is marked by regurgitation with normal weight gain. The peak incidence is at 1 to 4 months and is usually resolved by age 1. "Happy spitters" can be treated conservatively by reassuring parents and using thickened feedings, hypoallergenic formula, and upright positioning after feedings.

Infants who present with regurgitation and alarm symptoms such as respiratory problems (stridor, wheezing, cough), poor weight gain or growth, or irritability require further evaluation. GERD should be considered in the differential diagnosis of these children. In older children and adolescents, GERD usually presents with heartburn, regurgitation, or lower chest pain. Infants or children with esophageal atresia with repair, neurologic impairment/delay, bronchopulmonary dysplasia, asthma, or cystic fibrosis have an increased risk of GERD. A pediatric gastroenterologist can help guide the work-up of GERD. Medical management includes H_2 blockers and PPIs. Prokinetic agents may have a role.

4. **Gastric or pancreatic cancer.** The primary treatment of gastric or pancreatic cancer is surgery. At present surgery offers the only chance for cure; chemotherapy and radiation therapy are experimental.

REFERENCES

American Gastroenterological Association medical position statement. Evaluation of dyspepsia. *Gastroenterology.* 2005;129:1753-1755.

Institute for Clinical Systems Improvement (ICSI). *Initial Management of Dyspepsia and GERD.* Bloomington, MN: Institute for Clinical Systems Improvement (ICSI); 2006. http://www.guideline.gov/summary/summary.aspx?ss=15&doc_id=9658.

Jung AD. Gastroesophageal reflux in infants and children. *Am Fam Physician.* 2001;64:1853-1860.

Manes G, Menchise A, de Nucci C, Balzano A. Empirical prescribing for dyspepsia: randomized controlled trial of test and treat versus omeprazole treatment. *BMJ.* 2003;326:1118.

Rudolph CD, Mazur LJ, Liptak GS, et al. Guidelines for evaluation and treatment of gastroesophageal reflux in infants and children: Recommendations of the North American Society for Pediatric Gastroenterology and Nutrition. *J Pediatr Gastroenterol Nutr.* 2001;32(suppl 2):S1-S31.

Talley NJ, Vakil MB, Moayyedi P. American Gastroenterological Association technical review on the evaluation of dyspepsia. *Gastroenterology.* 2005;129:1756-1780.

Veldhuyzen van Zanten SJ, Flook N, Chiba N, et al. An evidence-based approach to the management of uninvestigated dyspepsia in the era of *Helicobacter pylori. CMAJ.* 2000;162:S3-S23.

20   Dyspnea

Mark R. Stephan, MD, James C. Chesnutt, MD, Scott A. Fields, MD, & William L. Toffler, MD

KEY POINTS

- Dyspnea is mainly caused by cardiac or pulmonary disorders.
- The history and physical examination will reveal the cause in most cases.
- The ABCs should be used to screen for life-threatening disorders, with further diagnostic testing as indicated.

I. **Definition.** Dyspnea is an unpleasant, subjective sensation of difficult breathing (breathlessness). Respiratory physiology relies on sensory input from peripheral and central chemoreceptors (monitoring P_{O_2}, P_{CO_2}, and pH) and mechanoreceptors (located in the heart, lung, vessels, and chest wall) with central processing and control in the medulla, receiving additional input from higher brain centers, including the cerebral cortex. The sensation of dyspnea is related to a mismatch of sensory input, central respiratory drive, and peripheral ventilatory performance. Dyspnea can vary in quality and intensity and is affected not only by physiologic disturbances but also by psychologic, social, and environmental factors.

II. **Common Diagnoses.** Dyspnea is an extremely common complaint of patients presenting for acute medical care. A chief complaint of shortness of breath accounts for 16% to 25% of nonsurgical admissions from the emergency department. Seventy percent of patients with advanced cancer have dyspnea, of which one-quarter have moderate or severe symptoms. The most common causes of dyspnea relate to either cardiac or respiratory disorders. (See the sidebar for life-threatening causes of dyspnea.)

TEN LIFE-THREATENING CAUSES OF DYSPNEA

1. Myocardial infarction
2. Ventricular tachycardia
3. Status asthmaticus
4. Anaphylactic laryngeal edema
5. Tension pneumothorax
6. Bacterial epiglottitis
7. Pulmonary embolism
8. Carbon monoxide poisoning
9. Guillain-Barré syndrome
10. Diabetic ketoacidosis

A. **Pulmonary disorders**
   1. Those at risk for **obstructive lung disease** include pediatric patients (asthma, bronchiolitis, bronchitis), adults with asthma, and adults with a chronic cigarette smoking history (chronic bronchitis and emphysema).
   2. Dyspnea caused by **restrictive lung disease** is more likely with an occupational exposure (asbestos, coal, beryllium, silica, uranium, cotton dust, grain dust, hay mold), those with severe scoliosis, the morbidly obese, and pregnant patients (caused by uterine growth restricting lung expansion). Chest wall trauma and smoking are associated with pneumothorax.
   3. Severe **pneumonia** also causes dyspnea; those at risk include immunocompromised patients (e.g., *Pneumocystis carinii* pneumonia in HIV disease), the very young, the very old, and those at risk for aspiration (e.g., alcoholics or individuals with stroke or history of swallowing disorders).
B. **Cardiac dyspnea.** Risk factors for cardiac dyspnea include known valvular heart disease, congestive heart failure, known ischemic cardiovascular disease (angina, myocardial infarction, claudication, or stroke), individuals with comorbid conditions (diabetes mellitus, hypercholesterolemia, or tobacco abuse), and those with a strong family history of premature coronary disease (i.e., myocardial infarction in the 40s or 50s in first-degree relatives). Arrhythmias (e.g., sick sinus syndrome, atrial fibrillation, and ventricular tachycardia) can cause dyspnea.
C. **Mixed cardiopulmonary dyspnea.** Risk factors for mixed cardiopulmonary dyspnea include hypercoagulable states, immobilization, major surgery or trauma, malignancy, and pregnancy and oral contraceptives (pulmonary embolism). Morbid obesity and a sedentary lifestyle contribute to deconditioning.
D. **Noncardiopulmonary causes**
   1. Uncommonly, **neuromuscular diseases** (Parkinson's disease, amyotrophic lateral sclerosis, and Guillain-Barré syndrome) can cause dyspnea, owing to respiratory muscle paralysis or dysfunction.
   2. In the presence of clinical findings supporting them, the following **systemic diseases** can cause dyspnea, anemia, thyrotoxicosis, diabetic ketoacidosis, metabolic acidosis, and carbon monoxide poisoning.
   3. A **psychogenic cause** for dyspnea should be considered in patients with a known history of psychiatric disease, multiple life stressors, and poor coping skills or a history of ill-defined somatic complaints. Extreme pain or hyperventilation can cause dyspnea.

TABLE 20-1. FINDINGS IN COMMON CAUSES OF DYSPNEA

Cause	Symptoms	Signs
Pulmonary	–"Chest tightness" (bronchospasm)	–Tachypnea/Tachycardia
–OLD	–"Air hunger" (hypoxemia)	Rales/rhonchi/wheezes
–RLD	–"Increased effort of breathing" (COPD, RLD)	–Nasal flaring, sternal retractions, and accessory muscle use (more severe)
–Pneumonia	–Exercise-induced coughing/wheezing (asthma)	–Cyanosis or clubbing
	–Daily sputum production (COPD)	–Increased A-P chest diameter
	–Cough, purulent sputum (dark or rust)	–Scoliosis, or chest wall deformity
	–"Air hunger" (hypoxemia)	–Fever $\geq$38.5°C (101°F)
	–Pleuritic chest pain	–Tachypnea, cyanosis
	–Chills, rigors	–Coarse rales, dullness to percussion, egophony
Cardiac	–Anginal chest pressure/pain, palpitations	–Tachycardia, arrhythmia
	–Orthopnea, dyspnea on exertion, fatigue	–Abnormal heart sounds (murmur, rub, gallop)
		–Cardiomegaly, JVD
		–Dependent edema
		–Basilar fine rales and decreased breath sounds
Mixed cardiopulmonary	–"Air hunger" (hypoxemia associated with PE)	–Tachypnea/Tachycardia, cyanosis
	–Pleuritic chest pain, syncope, unilateral leg pain, or swelling (PE)	–Calf tenderness, edema, positive Homan's sign (PE)
	–"Heavy breathing" (deconditioning)	–Obesity (deconditioning)
Noncardiopulmonary	–"Increased effort or work of breathing"	–Tachypnea/Tachycardia
–Neuromuscular	Fatigue, weakness, tremor, motor dysfunction (neuromuscular weakness)	–Abnormal muscle tone, strength, gait, or reflexes (neuromuscular disease)
–Systemic disease	–Polyuria, polydipsia, polyphagia (DM)	–Pale (anemia)
–Psychogenic	–Headache, confusion, dizziness (CO)	–Red skin CO poisoning
	–Anxiety, depression, pain (psychogenic)	–Hyperventilation
	–Dysphagia, gagging, drooling, sore throat, hoarseness (epiglottitis)	–Tachypnea distress, inspiratory stridor, high fever (epiglottitis)
–Upper airway obstruction	–Allergic exposure: food, cat, drug, bee sting (anaphylaxis/laryngeal/edema)	–Cyanosis, urticaria (angioedema)
	–Snoring, sleep apnea, daytime fatigue (OSAS)	–Tonsil hypertrophy, nasal obstruction, obesity, large neck (OSAS)

AP, anteroposterior; CO, carbon monoxide; COPD, chronic obstructive pulmonary disease; DM, diabetes mellitus; JVD, jugular venous distention; OLD, obstructive lung disease; OSAS, obstructive sleep apnea syndrome; PE, pulmonary embolism; RLD, restrictive lung disease.

    4. Upper airway causes of dyspnea are more likely in children (tonsillar hypertrophy, croup, epiglottitis, or foreign body aspiration) and in alcoholics or individuals with a history of stroke or of swallowing disorders.

III. Symptoms (Table 20–1). Assessing the patient for dyspnea severity, onset (acute versus chronic), descriptive qualities, and associated symptoms and signs can be extremely helpful in identifying the underlying cause of the dyspnea.

    Various studies show that different descriptive qualities of dyspnea are related to distinct physiologic abnormalities.

IV. Signs (Table 20–1). In order to quickly and accurately identify severe or life-threatening causes of dyspnea, special attention should be given to a rapid assessment of the patient's general level of distress and vital signs. In addition, cardiopulmonary examination is most helpful in identifying underlying causes of dyspnea.

    A. Vital signs. The patient's respiratory rate, temperature, pulse, and blood pressure should be determined. An increased respiratory rate ($\geq$20 respirations per minute) helps quantify dyspnea, but it is a nonspecific sign. Fever ($\geq$38.5°C [101°F]) is associated with respiratory infection. An increased pulse rate (≥ 100 beats per minute) may be associated with pulmonary embolism, dysrhythmia, or metabolic disorder.

B. Focused examination

1. The **pulmonary examination** should consist of auscultation and percussion of the lungs to assess for the presence of rales, rhonchi, wheezing, decreased breath sounds, egophony, or dullness to percussion. Inspection of the oral/nasal cavities, chest wall, and extremities can reveal airway obstruction, an increased thoracic anteroposterior diameter, chest wall deformity, or clubbing. Nasal flaring, sternal retractions, and accessory muscle use indicate more severe respiratory distress.

2. The **cardiac examination** should include an evaluation for rhythm, abnormal heart sounds (S_3 and S_4), murmurs, rubs, increased jugular venous distention, peripheral edema and pulses, and pulmonary rales in the lower lung fields.

3. The extent of additional **noncardiopulmonary examination** should be driven by the symptoms. If a dyspneic patient has weakness, tremor, gait problems, or other muscular or neurologic complaints, a screening neurologic examination should be performed, including testing gait, reflexes, sensation, motor strength, tone, and coordination.

V. Laboratory Tests. The need for testing should be based on the patient's history and physical examination and ordered only if needed to help establish the cause or severity of the illness. A stepwise **"ABC and D"** approach to dyspnea diagnosis and testing may simplify the diagnostic process and decrease both cost and patients discomfort. When dyspnea is severe, a rapid assessment for life-threatening medical problems should focus on the ABCs (**A**irway, **B**reathing, and **C**irculation). Further diagnostic (**D**) testing can focus on evaluating the common causes of dyspnea.

A. Airway. A **peak expiratory flow rate (PEFR)** of ≤ 150 L/min (normal value, 400–600 L/min) predicts a pulmonary cause for dyspnea, indicating significant obstructive airway disease that may require hospitalization. The PEFR is easily measured with a handheld peak flow meter and should be compared to the patient's baseline value and help guide a stepwise asthma/chronic obstructive pulmonary disease (COPD) treatment plan.

B. Breathing

1. **Pulse oximetry** can be used as a rapid and accurate assessment of oxygenation. For hypoxemia of $\leq 90\%$ po_2 on pulse oximetry, an **arterial blood gas analysis (ABG)** profile should be considered, which provides precise levels of oxygenation, carbon dioxide, and pH (normal values: pH, 7.40; Pco_2, 40 mm Hg; Po_2, 90–100 mm Hg). An ABG can aid in the diagnosis of severe dyspnea or dyspnea of unclear origin.

2. **Chest x-ray** is the next step. This can demonstrate an infiltrate, effusion, pneumothorax, sign of congestive heart failure (e.g., pulmonary vascular congestion or cardiomegaly), or lung disease (e.g., fibrosis or tumor).

C. Circulation. An **electrocardiogram (ECG)** is imperative for evaluation of cardiac arrhythmia or ischemia and can aid in the diagnosis of pulmonary embolism, pericarditis, or other cardiac problems. The ECG should be correlated with blood pressure and an assessment of perfusion.

D. Diagnostic testing. Further testing can be based on likely disorders guided by the acuity and severity of symptoms, initial testing, and pertinent examination findings.

1. **Cardiac tests**

   a. **BNP (brain or b-type natriuretic peptide)** is a validated test to evaluate for the presence of congestive heart failure (CHF) in patients with dyspnea. A low value (≤ 100 pg/mL) makes CHF unlikely. Values ≥ 100 and ≤ 500 pg/mL require clinical judgement and further diagnostic testing to confirm CHF. Levels ≥ 500 pg/mL make CHF the most likely diagnosis. (SOR **B**)

   b. **Other useful cardiac studies** may include **echocardiography, cardiac catheterization, cardiac event monitors, and exercise treadmill testing** but likely should be reserved to evaluate abnormal ECG or examination findings or suspicious unexplained symptoms. Exercise testing is helpful in the evaluation of cardiac abnormalities as well as in the diagnosis of exercise-induced asthma.

2. **Pulmonary tests.** These tests can evaluate possible lung disease. **Formal spirometry** is useful in the assessment of patients with lung disease. In **restrictive disease,** forced vital capacity (FVC) is low, and forced expiratory volume in 1 second (FEV_1) and the maximal midexpiratory flow ($FEV_{25\%-75\%}$) may be low. The FEV-FVC ratio may be normal or even high. In **obstructive disease,** FVC, FEV, FEV_1-FVC ratio, or $FEV_{25\%-75\%}$, or all four, may be low. In mixed disease, all these values are low.

3. **Mixed cardiopulmonary.** Pulmonary embolism can cause pleuritic chest pain, dyspnea, tachycardia, and hypoxemia. The following tests can help clarify the diagnosis.
   a. **D-dimer** is useful when negative to exclude deep venous thrombosis (DVT) and pulmonary embolism (PE): a low result has a high-negative predictive value for DVT and PE, especially when combined with a clinical prediction rule that scores a low pretest probability of venous thromboembolism. A high result is nonspecific. SOR Ⓐ (see Chapter 23).
   b. **Multidetector computerized tomography (CT) scan of the chest** is evolving toward standard practice in many hospitals to diagnose or exclude PE.
   c. **Ventilation/perfusion (V/Q) scan** should be used in cases where CT scan is not available or is not conclusive for suspected PE. The result is often inconclusive, which may necessitate the use of **pulmonary angiogram** to clarify the diagnosis.
   d. **Doppler venous flow studies** are a noninvasive, accurate method to identify DVTs, which are correlated with PE (see Chapter 23).
4. **Noncardiopulmonary**
   a. **A complete blood cell count** can establish the presence of anemia or a possible underlying infection. Anemia leads to decreased oxygen-carrying capacity and therefore reduced oxygen delivery.
   b. **Blood glucose, basic metabolic test set, and thyroid-stimulating hormone** may be useful to assess metabolic status in unclear cases. Thyrotoxicosis results in increased oxygen demand. High levels of glucose can cause ketoacidosis. Renal or electrolyte abnormalities can cause dyspnea.
   c. A **carbon monoxide level** (normal value, $\leq 2\%$) may document a toxic exposure to smoke or exhaust from a furnace or other sources. Levels are elevated in active smokers ($\leq 10\%$), thereby decreasing oxygen-carrying capacity. Carbon monoxide binds to hemoglobin with 200 times the affinity of oxygen, severely compromising oxygen delivery to tissue. Lethal levels ($\geq 50\%$) can occur despite relatively normal arterial blood gas levels.
   d. Further neurologic testing or imaging should be guided by abnormal physical examination findings and is unlikely to be cost-effective if a screening neurologic examination is normal.

VI. **Treatment.** Once the underlying diagnosis has been made, treatment strategies should involve increasing oxygen delivery and correcting the underlying disease process, which usually relieves the sensation of dyspnea. For treatment of specific medical problems, please see the following chapters: Asthma (Chapter 68), Chronic obstructive pulmonary disease (Chapter 70), Congestive heart failure (Chapter 72), Cough (Chapter 13), Ischemic heart disease (Chapter 77), and Wheezing (Chapter 65).

Medical therapies aimed at alleviating the symptoms of dyspnea can be used while the disease process is being treated or in cases where the cause of dyspnea is uncertain or related to a terminal condition such as cancer or end-stage COPD.

A. **Oxygen.** Oxygen delivered via nasal cannula at 1 to 4 L/min can provide good relief for mild or severe hypoxemia, at rest or with exercise, regardless of initial oxygen saturation; in COPD patients oxygen therapy can suppress respiratory drive and cause CO_2 retention, which can present as sedation.

B. **Bronchodilators.** Both beta-agonists and anticholinergics alone or in combination provide symptomatic relief in COPD. (SOR Ⓐ)

C. Intravenous **steroids** do not help dyspnea acutely; prolonged use of oral steroids can cause muscle weakness; inhaled steroids do show improved airway reactivity in asthma and COPD and are associated with decreased symptoms and hospitalizations.

D. **Pulmonary rehabilitation programs** relieve dyspnea and fatigue in patients with COPD. (SOR Ⓐ)

E. A Cochrane review found strong evidence that **opioids** relieve dyspnea and improve exercise tolerance in patients with cancer and severe COPD.
   1. Immediate-release forms (e.g., Roxicodone/oxycodone IR) are more effective than sustained-release forms (e.g., OxyContin/oxycodone SR).
   2. Constipation is a problem, but tolerance develops to other side effects.
   3. Studies show opioids do not severely suppress respiration or cause early death in terminally ill patients.

F. Anxiolytics. In end-stage COPD and cancer, oral buspirone (e.g., Buspar, 5–10 mg 3 times daily) or lorazepam (e.g., Ativan, 0.5–2 mg every 4 hours as needed) may relieve anxiety associated with dyspnea rather than dyspnea itself.

G. Nonpharmacologic methods. Use of fans, open windows, cognitive therapy, stress management for patient and caregiver, and nutritional, spiritual, and emotional support have all proved useful in decreasing dyspnea.

REFERENCES

Legrand SB et al. Opioids, respiratory function, and dyspnea. *Am J Hospice Palliat Care.* 2003;20: 57.

Mueller C, Scholer A, Laule-Kilian K, et al. Use of B-type natriuretic peptide in the evaluation and management of acute dyspnea. *N Engl J Med.* 2004;350:647-654.

Segal JB, Eng J, Tamariz LJ, Bass E. Review of the evidence on diagnosis of deep venous thrombosis and pulmonary embolism. *Ann Fam Med.* 2007;5:63-73.

Lacasse Y, Goldstein R, Lasserson TJ, Martin S. Pulmonary rehabilitation for COPD. *Cochrane Database Syst Rev.* 2006(2) CD003793.

Barr RG, Bourbeau J, Camargo CA, Ram FSF. Tiotroprium for stable COPD. *Cochrane Database Syst Rev.* 2005(2) CD002876.

Sestini P, Renzoni E, Robinson S, Poole P, Ram FSF. Short-acting beta-2 agonists for stable COPD. *Cochrane Database Syst Rev.* 2002(2) CD001495.

---

21   Dysuria in Women

L. Peter Schwiebert, MD

KEY POINTS

- In women with dysuria, consideration of historic risk factors should drive differential diagnosis and evaluation.
- Urinalysis or leukocyte esterase dipstick testing is the most important laboratory study in diagnosing urinary tract infection.
- Findings compatible with an acute uncomplicated urinary tract infection warrant empiric treatment for *Escherichia coli.*

I. **Definition. Dysuria** is a discomfort associated with micturition, commonly caused by **bacterial urinary tract infection** (UTI). Among uncomplicated UTIs, 80%–85% are caused by *E coli,* approximately 5%–10% are caused by *Staphylococcus saprophyticus,* and 5%–10% are caused by *Proteus mirabilis.* The foregoing organisms may also cause recurrent or difficult to eradicate (i.e., complicated) UTIs; such infections may also be caused by *Serratia, Pseudomonas aeruginosa, Klebsiella,* enterococci, and Enterobacteriaceae species. Other causes of dysuria include:

   A. **Bladder or urethral irritation** (e.g., interstitial cystitis [IC]).

   B. **Urethral trauma, bubble baths, or dietary factors.**

   C. **Vaginal atrophy** (postmenopausal or other hypoestrogenic state).

   D. **Urethritis,** often caused by sexually transmitted diseases (STDs), including *Chlamydia trachomatis, Neisseria gonorrhoeae, Trichomonas vaginalis,* or herpes simplex virus (HSV) virus infection.

   E. **Psychogenic dysuria** (often a component of somatization disorder, depression, chronic pain, or sexual abuse).

II. **Common Diagnoses.** Clinical syndromes associated with dysuria account for 5% to 15% of visits to family physicians. Approximately 25% of American women report at least one bout of acute dysuria per year. UTI accounts for more than 7 million visits and affects at least 50% of women once in their lifetime. Twenty-five percent of these women suffer recurrent UTIs.

A. **Acute bacterial cystitis** (25%–35% of cases) is more likely with a past history of cystitis, sexual intercourse, diaphragm/spermicidal contraception, douching, or postponement of micturition. Risk factors for complicated UTIs include pregnancy, indwelling urinary catheter, urinary tract instrumentation within the past 2 weeks, urinary tract anomaly or stones, recent systemic antibiotic use, or immunosuppression (e.g., poorly controlled diabetes mellitus).

B. **Vulvovaginitis** (21%–38% of cases) is a more frequent cause of dysuria in college-aged women than are UTIs.

C. The likelihood of **acute or subclinical pyelonephritis** (up to 30% of cases) is increased in women who are symptomatic for more than 7 days before seeking medical attention, of lower socioeconomic status, presenting to an inner-city emergency room, are pregnant, or having recurrent UTIs (more than three in the past year), or in women with a history of first UTI before age 12, with recurrence of a UTI within 7 days of completion of appropriate antibiotic therapy, or with other risk factors for complicated UTI (see Section II.A). Approximately one-third of women with lower UTI symptoms will have unrecognized or subclinical pyelonephritis.

D. The likelihood of **dysuria without pyuria** (15%–30% of cases) is increased with a history of urethral trauma, in women in a postmenopausal state and not receiving estrogen replacement therapy, or with physical/chemical irritants (e.g., douching or consumption of citrus, ethanol, caffeinated carbonated beverages, sugar, or spicy foods). Ninety percent of patients with IC are women (up to 700,000 US women are affected); patients with this syndrome have a median age of 40 and tend to have a past history of childhood or adult UTIs.

E. **Urethritis** (3%–10% of cases) should be considered in women with a recent new sex partner, multiple partners, or a partner with urethritis. Thirty to fifty percent of nongonococcal urethritis is caused by *C trachomatis;* other organisms implicated include urea plasmids and *T vaginalis.*

III. **Symptoms.** The onset of symptoms is usually abrupt, and the patient may describe "internal" dysuria (i.e., suprapubic pain), as opposed to stinging of the skin (i.e., "external dysuria").

A. **Dysuria**

1. Dysuria is the cardinal symptom of an acute bacterial cystitis. Other symptoms of this condition include urinary frequency, mild anorexia or nausea, nocturia, urgency, the voiding of small amounts, urinary incontinence, and suprapubic pain. A recent meta-analysis found that four factors significantly correlate with a diagnosis of UTI: frequency, hematuria, dysuria, and back pain. This same study found four factors (i.e., absent dysuria or back pain, history of vaginal discharge or vaginal irritation) that decrease the likelihood of UTI; women with one or more symptoms of UTI have approximately a 50% likelihood of this diagnosis and combinations of the eight findings can raise the probability of UTI to $\geq$90%.

2. The dysuria accompanying urethritis often has a stuttering, gradual onset and is "internal." Increased frequency and urgency of urination may indicate dysuria without pyuria.

3. Patients who complain of external dysuria, or a burning sensation as the urine passes the inflamed labia, may have vulvovaginitis.

B. **Vaginal discharge**

1. Dysuria and an associated increase in vaginal discharge from concomitant cervicitis may indicate urethritis.

2. Patients with vulvovaginitis complain of vaginal discharge, odor, or itching.

C. **Pain.** Localized pain in the flank, low back, or abdomen and systemic symptoms, such as fever, rigors, sweats, headaches, nausea, vomiting, malaise, and prostration, can occur with UTI, particularly pyelonephritis.

D. **Interstitial cystitis (IC)** is characterized by persistent pelvic or perineal pain, temporarily relieved by voiding, and consistent urinary urgency and voiding 16 to 40 times daily, in the absence of a history of radiation, tuberculosis, or chemical cystitis.

IV. **Signs**

A. **Acute bacterial cystitis**

1. Fever almost never develops when a UTI is localized to the bladder.

2. Suprapubic tenderness is present in only 10% of patients with cystitis. If this sign is present, however, it has a high-predictive value for cystitis.

B. **Vulvovaginitis.** For signs of this condition, see Chapter 64.

    C. Pyelonephritis. The patient often has a fever (temperature of 38–39°C [101–102°F]), costovertebral angle tenderness, and tachycardia.

    D. Dysuria without pyuria. In this case, the physical findings just described are absent. However, the pelvic examination may show some periurethral or vulvar irritation.

    E. Urethritis. Urethritis is frequently associated with mucopurulent cervicitis.

V. Laboratory Tests (Figure 21–1).

    A. A **clean-catch midstream urinalysis (UA)** is readily available in most offices and essential for evaluating patients with dysuria. Using the definition of significant bacteriuria as $\geq 10^2$ of a single uropathogenic bacterial species per milliliter in a symptomatic patient, pyuria (≥ 5 white blood cells [WBCs] per centrifuged high-power field) is found in up to 95% of patients with an acute cystitis, and $\geq 10^5$ bacteria per milliliter and in more than 70% of patients with acute cystitis and 10^2 to 10^5 bacteria per milliliter. The **leukocyte esterase dipstick** test is 75% to 95% sensitive and specific in detecting pyuria and is a reasonable substitute if urine microscopy is unavailable. Microscopic hematuria is present in up to 60% of women with acute bacterial cystitis, but its absence does not rule out this diagnosis. Twenty percent of women with IC have gross hematuria without bacteriuria or WBCs.

    B. Culture (Figure 21–1).

        1. Urine culture is indicated in the following situations:

            a. If an acute bacterial cystitis is suspected, but clinical findings and UA leave the diagnosis in question.

            b. If the patient has symptoms and signs of upper or complicated UTI (see Section II.C).

            c. Two to four days after a patient completes treatment for a complicated UTI.

            d. After a patient self-administers antibiotics (see Section VI.A.2).

        2. In women in whom **urethritis** is suspected, urethral and cervical cultures for *N gonorrhoeae* and *C trachomatis* should be performed.

    C. IC can be diagnosed with findings verifiable only with **cystoscopy** (i.e., glomerulations or ulcers, absence of bladder tumor). **Urodynamic studies** will also demonstrate small bladder capacity, i.e., ≤ 350 mL and urge to void at 150 mL.

VI. Treatment of women with dysuria is based on the clinical picture, supplemented by appropriate laboratory studies. In patients with findings compatible with an acute, uncomplicated bacterial cystitis, it is reasonable to initiate treatment for *E coli* based on UA findings alone.

    A. Acute, uncomplicated bacterial cystitis (Table 21–1).

        1. Short-course antibiotics

            a. Short course (3 days) treatment is equivalent to treatment for 5 or more days for symptomatic cure. (SOR **Ⓐ**) Trimethoprim-sulfamethoxazaole-double strength (TMP-SMX-DS), one tablet twice daily for 3 days, is the first-line treatment in non-sulfa-allergic women. However, 5% to 15%% of *E coli* are resistant to TMP-SMX, and the likelihood of resistance increases with recent hospitalization, use of TMP-SMX during the previous 6 months, or recurrent UTIs during the past year. If resistance is likely, a 3-day course of a fluoroquinolone is reasonable.

            b. In patients with sulfa allergy, the following alternative regimens are effective: trimethoprim (TMP), 100 mg orally twice daily, nitrofurantoin, 100 mg orally 4 times daily, ciprofloxacin, 250 mg orally twice daily, ofloxacin, 200 mg orally twice daily, or fosfomycin, 3 g orally. All of these medications are taken for 3 days, except fosfomycin, which is taken as a single dose.

        2. Recurrent UTIs. Women with one to two uncomplicated UTIs per year can be given a prescription for an appropriate short-course antibiotic (see Section VI.A.1.b). Women who experience three or more symptomatic UTIs over the preceding 12 months or two or more symptomatic UTIs over 6 months warrant prophylaxis.

            a. Measures shown to decrease the number of UTIs include frequent bladder emptying (especially following sexual intercourse), discontinuation of diaphragm use, and urine acidification using cranberry juice (≥ 300 mL daily) or oral ascorbic acid.

            b. Since symptoms develop in 85% of women with recurring infections within 24 hours following sexual intercourse, postcoital antibiotics (1 dose orally after sexual intercourse) may be helpful. Acceptable regimens include TMP-SMX, one single-strength tablet; nitrofurantoin, 50 to 100 mg; or sulfisoxazole, 500 mg.

            c. If a postcoital regimen is not effective, long-term prophylaxis is indicated. Recommended regimens include one of the following: TMP-SMX, one single-strength tablet taken each evening or thrice weekly; TMP, 100 mg once daily at bedtime.

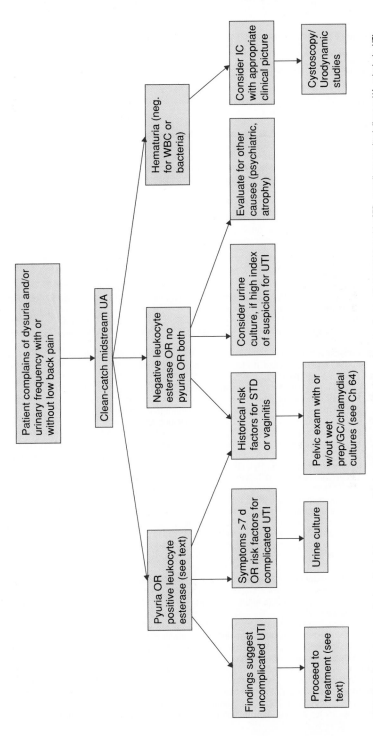

FIGURE 21–1. Approach to evaluation of ambulatory women with urinary tract symptoms. GC, *Neisseria gonorrhoeae*; IC, interstitial cystitis; STD, sexually transmitted disease; UA, urinalysis; UTI, urinary tract infection; WBC, white blood cells.

TABLE 21–1. ANTIBIOTICS RECOMMENDED FOR AMBULATORY MANAGEMENT OF UTIS IN WOMEN

Drug	Dosage (mg)
Trimethoprim-sulfamethoxazole (TMP-SMX)*	160/800 twice daily
Trimethoprim (TMP)[†]	100 twice daily or 200 daily
Nitrofurantoin[†]	100 4 times daily
Ciprofloxacin[†,‡,§]	250 twice daily
Ofloxacin[†,§]	200 twice daily
Fosfomycin[†,§]	3000 (single dose)

*Consult full prescribing information before administering any of these drugs. *Preferred agent in non-sulfa-allergic patients (3-day or 10- to 14-day regimen); in populations with low likelihood of resistance.
[†] Short-course (3-day) alternatives to TMP-SMX in sulfa-allergic patients.
[‡] Preferred oral medication for ambulatory treatment of pyelonephritis (500 mg twice daily orally for 7 days).
[§] Relatively expensive.

or norfloxacin, 200 mg thrice weekly at bedtime. Antibiotics should be discontinued 3 to 6 months after initiating treatment to identify patients who will remain disease-free; women experiencing recurrences should receive extended (1–2 year) prophylaxis.

B. Vulvovaginitis (see Chapter 64).

C. Pyelonephritis

1. Febrile, ill-appearing patients should be hospitalized for treatment with parenteral antibiotics; those with mild symptoms (temperature $\leq$ 38.3°C, no nausea or vomiting, good oral intake) in whom close follow-up is feasible can be treated as outpatients. A recent study found that 7 days of ciprofloxacin, 500 mg orally twice daily, resulted in greater bacterial and clinical cure rates than a standard 2-week course of TMP-SMX-DS.

2. Patients with complicated UTI are at risk for subclinical pyelonephritis and should be treated with a standard 10- to 14-day regimen (Table 21–1).

D. Dysuria without pyuria

1. Offending agents identified through careful history should be eliminated.

2. Postmenopausal women whose symptoms are believed because of estrogen deficiency may benefit from estrogen replacement (see Chapter 78).

3. Other measures that may prove helpful include taking warm baths, avoiding acidic foods (e.g., coffee, citrus fruits, tomato products, chocolate) and alcohol, artificial sweeteners, and carbonated beverages; increasing fluid intake (water is best) to dilute urine; drinking 8 oz water with 1 tbsp baking soda; or taking antispasmodics, such as phenazopyridine (e.g., Pyridium) 100 to 200 mg orally 3 times daily, or hyoscyamine sulfate (e.g., Levsin), 0.125 to 0.250 mg orally every 4 hours.

4. For **IC**, a variety of agents have been used, without convincing evidence of efficacy in large, placebo-controlled trials (though there has been an evidence of success in open-label trials). These agents include tricyclic antidepressants (e.g., amitriptyline or imipramine, 25–100 mg orally at bedtime), antihistamines (e.g., cimetidine, 300 mg orally twice daily, or hydroxyzine, 25–75 mg orally at bedtime).

   a. The only agent approved for IC by the US Food and Drug Administration is pentosan polysulfate (e.g., Elmiron), 100 mg orally 3 times daily. (SOR **B**) Twenty-eight percent of women receiving pentosan (versus 13% receiving placebo) noted improvement in pain/urgency/pressure but no appreciable improvement in frequency, nocturia, or volumes voided. Patients may take 3 to 6 months to respond and may experience side effects, including diarrhea, dyspepsia, headaches, rashes, or abdominal pain.

   b. Patients responding poorly to oral therapies and patients with severe symptoms may benefit from urologic referral for further management, such as intravesical dimethyl sulfoxide (DMSO). Fifty to ninety percent of these women respond to DMSO, with relapse in up to 40% of those discontinuing therapy. (SOR **B**)

E. Urethritis. Empiric therapy for *C trachomatis* or *N gonorrhoeae* can be instituted in high-risk individuals, while one is awaiting culture results. Because of the coprevalence of *N gonorrhoeae* and *C trachomatis* infection, patients should be treated with ceftriaxone (e.g., Rocephin), 250 mg intramuscularly (1 dose), and doxycycline, 100 mg orally twice a day for 7 days. Alternatives to ceftriaxone for *N gonorrhoeae* include cefixime (e.g., Suprax), 400 mg, ciprofloxacin (e.g., Cipro) 250 mg, or ofloxacin (e.g., Floxin), 400 mg orally for 1 dose. Alternatives to doxycycline for *C trachomatis* include azithromycin, 1.0 g orally for 1 dose, or erythromycin base, 500 mg, or erythromycin ethylsuccinate, 800 mg orally 4 times daily for 7 days. **Pregnant or breast-feeding women should receive ceftriaxone plus erythromycin.** (Also see the sidebar on asymptomatic bacteriuria.)

ASYMPTOMATIC BACTERIURIA

Asymptomatic bacteriuria (ASB) is present in between 5% and 10% of pregnant women, with an increased likelihood in women who are sexually active or have diabetes, increased parity, or lower socioeconomic status. In 20% to 35% of women with ASB in pregnancy, overt UTI eventually develops. The American College of Obstetrics and Gynecologists recommends screening all pregnant patents with urine culture at the initial prenatal visit and in the third trimester.

Recommended antibiotics for treating UTI in pregnancy include nitrofurantoin (e.g., Macrobid), 100 mg orally every 12 hours for 7 days, or a cephalosporin (e.g., cephalexin), 250 to 500 mg orally 4 times daily for 7 days, with follow-up culture after treatment and monthly for the duration of the pregnancy, and consideration of prophylactic nitrofurantoin following a bout of pyelonephritis.

The evaluation and management of **elderly women with symptomatic UTI** is as described in the main text. In a healthy, **elderly women with asymptomatic bacteriuria,** there is no evidence that treatment reduces long-term renal problems; treatment increases cost, the likelihood of drug reactions (or drug–drug interactions), and the likelihood of drug-resistant microorganisms.

REFERENCES

Bent S, Saint S. The optimal use of diagnostic testing in women with acute uncomplicated cystitis. *Am J Med.* 2002;113(1 A):20S.

Bent S et al. Does this woman have an acute uncomplicated urinary tract infection? *JAMA.* 2002; 287:2701.

Bremnor JD, Sadovsky R. Evaluation of dysuria in adults. *Am Fam Physician.* 2002;65:1589.

Katchman EA, Milo G, Paul M, et al. Three-day vs longer duration of antibiotic treatment for cystitis in women: systematic review and meta-analysis. *Am J Med.* 2005;118:11.

Nicolle LE. Urinary tract infection: traditional pharmacologic therapies. *Dis Mon.* 2003;49:111.

Rosamilia A. Painful bladder syndrome/interstitial cystitis. *Best Pract Res Clin Obstet Gynecol.* 2005; 19:843.

---

22   Earache

David Berkson, MD, & Carmelo DiSalvo, MD

KEY POINTS

- Most causes of otalgia are benign and are easily diagnosed and managed in the office setting.
- Not all causes of otalgia are intrinsic to the ear itself. Referred pain may be the etiology and can be indicative of a serious problem such as an underlying cancer or other non-ear diseases.
- Unexplained otalgia or otalgia not resolving with appropriate therapy should be evaluated by an otolaryngologist.

I. **Definition.** Earache (otalgia) is pain or discomfort perceived in the ear or surrounding structures. It can be primary, including pain from diseases of the auricle, external canal, middle ear, or inner ear, or referred, occurring secondary to the complex innervations of the head and neck. The ear is innervated by sensory branches of the trigeminal, facial, vagus, and glossopharyngeal cranial nerves and by the lesser occipital and great auricular cervical nerves.

II. **Common Diagnoses.** Earache most commonly originates from middle ear or external auditory canal pathology.

  A. **Acute otitis media (AOM)** occurs most frequently during the winter months, thus coinciding with the peak incidence of viral upper respiratory tract infections. The peak age incidence is 6 months to 7 years. Native Americans and Eskimos experience otitis media more frequently than do people of other races. Otitis media is also more prevalent in children with Down syndrome or cleft palate. The two major risk factors for AOM in children are group daycare involvement and exposure to second-hand smoke. Other risk factors include a family history of AOM, bottle-fed infants, Eustachian tube dysfunction, and enlarged adenoids.

  B. **Otitis externa (OE)** is a generalized inflammation of the external ear canal, which may involve both the pinna and/or tympanic membrane (TM). AOE requires the presence of pathogens and the breakage of skin to cause disease. It is 10 to 20 times more common in the summer than in cooler months, particularly in individuals who swim in lakes or pools. This condition is more likely to affect diabetic patients and other immunocompromised persons, who are also more likely to develop invasive disease. Local trauma with cotton swabs and scratching are among the highest known causes. Other risk factors include, but are not limited to, moisture in the ear canal, canal occlusion, and conditions of abnormal keratin production (i.e. psoriasis, atopic and seborrheic dermatitis).

  C. **Barotrauma** most commonly occurs either after flying in an unpressurized aircraft or after scuba diving. Acute upper respiratory infections and allergies increase susceptibility to this condition.

  D. **Direct trauma** is seen more frequently in young males, resulting from fights or automobile accidents; in military personnel or miners, who may work near explosions; or in hikers, mountain climbers, or outdoor workers in cold climates, who may suffer frostbite.

  E. **Referred otalgia**
   1. **Temporomandibular joint dysfunction** tends to occur in patients with the following conditions: (1) dental malocclusion or poorly fitting dental prostheses, (2) bruxism (nocturnal tooth grinding), (3) trauma to the mandible, or (4) degenerative temporomandibular joint disease, especially in women in the third or fourth decade of life.
   2. **Dental diseases**, such as **abscesses**, are likely to develop in individuals with poor oral hygiene.
   3. **Cancers** of the ear, nose, and throat region have an increased risk in patients with a history of heavy tobacco or alcohol use or serous otitis (in adults), those of Chinese ancestry, and those with dysphagia or hemoptysis.

III. **Symptoms**

  A. **Pain**
   1. Severe deep pain or ear pain that interferes with normal activity or sleep may indicate **AOM.**
   2. Moderate pain, especially with lying on the affected side or movement of the jaw may be present in **OE.**
   3. Pressure progressing to moderate to severe pain over a few hours may be related to **barotrauma**.
   4. Pain in the injured part of the ear is evident with **direct trauma**; frostbite of the auricle usually causes burning pain lasting several hours.
   5. Pain in **referred otalgia** depends on the cause (Table 22–1).

  B. **Tinnitus** can be present with **barotrauma** or may indicate more serious disease.

  C. **Hearing loss**
   1. If unilateral, may be a sign of an effusion or other underlying pathology that may warrant further investigation.

  D. **Otorrhea**
   1. A purulent nonmalodorous discharge in the canal may be seen with TM rupture in **AOM;** perforation often occurs near the annulus, necessitating clear view of the entire TM.
   2. A bloody, serous, or foul smelling discharge may indicate **trauma** with or without accompanying infection.

TABLE 22–1. CAUSES OF REFERRED OTALGIA

Cause	Mechanism	Symptoms	Signs	Laboratory Tests	Treatment	Comments
TMJ dysfunction	Internal derangement of joint, malocclusion, poorly fitting dental prostheses, bruxism	Deep pain that becomes worse with eating	Pain on palpation, crepitus, asymmetry of motion	None	NSAIDs plus jaw-opening exercises; moist heat; mechanical soft diet. Refer if not relieved in 3–4 weeks	
Dental disease	Inflammation or pressure on nerves by abscessed teeth, impacted molars	Dull to lancinating pain worse with eating, tooth sensitive to cold	Carious teeth, tender teeth, red or necrotic gingiva	None	Dental referral; pain control; consider antibiotics	
Head and neck tumors	Traction on or inflammation of nerves	Hoarseness, dysphagia, lump, pain or pressure slowly increasing	Tumor in nasopharynx or larynx	CT, MRI	Refer for excision/biopsy and further treatment	
Infection of sinuses, pharynx	Nerve irritation from infection	Retro-orbital or frontal pain, sore throat	Sinus tenderness, poor transillumination, exudative pharyngitis	Strep screen, consider further sinus evaluation	See Chapters 55 and 57	
Carotodynia	Pain referred along same nerve pathways as ear	Throat pain, dysphagia	Tender bifurcation of carotid artery	Consider radiographic evaluation of carotid anatomy	Consider steroids, moist heat to affected area	
Temporal arteritis	Collagen vascular disease with inflammation	Pain near affected arteries, weight loss, fever, jaw claudication	Tender, indurated temporal artery	Elevated ESR, temporal artery biopsy	Long-term oral steroid taper is mainstay of therapy	Treat to prevent visual loss. Use ESR to monitor therapy. Differential includes arteritis and dissection
Trigeminal, glossopharyngeal, or sphenopalatine neuralgia	Compression of nerves	Lancinating pain triggered by chewing or swallowing cold liquids	Trigger points in nasopharynx	None	Multiple options for oral neuropathic pain tx. Surgical therapy or ablation for nonresponders	Significant potential side effects with medications—monitoring may be necessary
Gastroesophageal reflux disease	Nerve irritation from acid stimulation	Worse at night or with stimulating foods	None	pH study, upper GI study	Diet and behavioral changes. Antacids H_2 blockers, PPIs (see Chapters 19 and 82)	Caution of potential long-term side effects with PPIs (osteopenia)

ESR, erythrocyte sedimentation rate; CT, computerized tomography; GI, gastrointestinal; MRI, magnetic resonance imaging; TMJ, temporomandibular joint.

  E. Itching may be present in **OE** or following minor **trauma**.
  F. Referred pain (see Table 22–1).
  G. Associated symptoms
    1. Fever, dizziness, nausea, and vomiting may occur with **AOM.**
    2. Parents of infants and small children with **AOM** may observe irritability, decreased feeding, or pulling at the ears.
IV. Signs. Examination of patients with otalgia should be directed by the risk factors and symptoms and should include systematic evaluation of the auricle, auditory canals, and TMs, as well as sources of referred otalgia as indicated (Table 22–1).
  A. Auricle
    1. OE may cause erythema or crusting if this portion of the ear is involved.
    2. OE also causes painful movement of the auricle or pressure on the tragus.
    3. In **direct trauma,** injury to the auricle is evident from inspection; frostbite may initially present with auricular pallor, followed by erythema and sometimes, bullae. Examination of the posterior aspect of the auricle is essential to avoid missing signs of **trauma.**
  B. External auditory canal
    1. The canal in **OE** is red and edematous, usually with purulent drainage. The presence of spores or black colored material may signify a fungal infection. A greenish discharge may indicate *Pseudomonas.*
    2. Canal injuries with **direct trauma** include lacerations, abrasions, or hematomas.
  C. Tympanic membrane
    1. A **normal** appearing TM is a pearly colored, partially translucent tissue that vibrates as it transmits sound to the inner ear. The presence of a reddened TM alone, without pneumatic otoscopic evidence of immobility, is not sufficient to diagnose AOM, as an erythematous TM may also be because of increased intravascular pressure (e.g., a crying infant or child). In performing pneumatic otoscopy, it is imperative that a speculum of proper shape and diameter be selected to ensure a proper seal in the external auditory canal.
    2. A diagnosis of AOM requires (1) a history of acute onset of signs and symptoms, (2) the presence of middle-ear effusion, and (3) signs and symptoms of middle-ear inflammation. Pneumatic otoscopy is the primary method for evaluating the presence of effusion with AOM. (SOR **Ⓐ**) Positive predictive values in the 90% range compared to myringotomy have been achieved with the following findings: an opaque TM, a bulging TM, and impaired TM mobility. An air–fluid level seen behind the TM indicates the presence of middle-ear effusion.
    3. A **cholesteatoma** (pearl tumor) can appear as white or yellow flecks and/or as chronic debris behind the TM. Suspicion should arise when there is a perforated or retracted TM with debris that is difficult to clear. Severe complications include central nervous system infection and thrombosis.
    4. In **barotrauma,** the TM initially appears red, later becoming blue or yellow. With continued blockage, bubbles or air–fluid levels may be seen. Other manifestations of barotraumas may include TM rupture, rupture of the inner ear membrane, ova, or round window. It may present with otorrhea, hemotympanum and/or vertigo.
V. Laboratory Tests. The cause of otalgia is usually evident from the history and examination. The following laboratory tests may be helpful in delineating the cause in certain situations:
  A. Tympanometry, a technique that measures immittance of the middle ear at various levels of air pressure, may be helpful for follow-up examination of patients treated for AOM, especially for confirming the resolution of AOM with effusion. See Chapter 35 for more information on tympanometry.
  B. The **white blood cell count** in cases of AOM is frequently elevated and shifted to the left, particularly in children. The complete blood count is not routinely done in non-toxic-appearing children with AOM.
  C. Radiography and **computerized tomography** are useful to determine the presence of other associated injury when occult fractures of the skull or intracerebral injury are suspected. When dealing with otalgia, computerized tomography is most valuable for evaluating the middle ear and the mastoid, when infections of these structures are suspected. MRI with contrast is more appropriate for the evaluation of the soft tissues, lesions around the ear, diseases of CN VII and VIII, and when evaluating the cerebellar pontine angle.
  D. Referred pain (see Table 22–1 for details).

VI. Treatment

A. Otitis media

1. **AOM**: Numerous antibacterial agents are available and clinically effective. Consideration should be used based upon the organisms most likely to be present. In most cases, amoxicillin is used as first-line therapy. In patients with severe illness (moderate to severe otalgia or fever $\geq 39.0°$C) and when additional coverage to treat β-lactamase positive organisms is required (i.e., *Haemophilus influenzae* and *Moraxella catarrhalis*), therapy should be initiated with high dose amoxicillin–clavulanate (90 mg/kg/d of amoxicillin and 6.4 mg/kg of clavulanate per day in 2 divided doses). Based on limited and controversial data, there are currently no recommendations for treatment of AOM with complimentary and alternative medicine.

   a. **Antibiotic selection:** It is important to remember that the bacteria most commonly isolated with middle ear effusions are *Streptococcus pneumoniae* (50%), *H influenzae* (30%), and *M catarrhalis* (25%). Of these, the most important pathogen is *S pneumoniae*, which if left untreated can progress to more invasive disease. Drug-resistant *S pneumoniae* is common and develops resistance by alterations in penicillin-binding proteins, not β-lactamase mechanisms. Therefore, in all but highly resistant organisms, resistance is overcome by higher doses of penicillin, not adding β-lactam stabilizers (e.g., clavulanic acid). Check your local susceptibility patterns for resistance to recommended antibiotics. AOM caused by viruses, nontypeable *H influenzae*, or *M catarrhalis* is likely to resolve spontaneously and is unlikely to progress to more invasive disease. See Table 22–2. (SOR **B**)

   b. **Decongestants/antihistamines:** There is no grade A or grade B evidence that suggests these products shorten the course of the illness, but they are useful for symptomatic care (see Chapter 55 for dosage). In fact, a Cochrane-based review found that in AOM with effusion, not only was no statistical or clinical benefit found, but treated subjects experienced 11% more side effects than untreated subjects. Regardless of whether or not antibiotics are going to be prescribed, the otalgia should be addressed and dealt with appropriately. (SOR **A**) See Table 22–3 for treatments for otalgia.

   c. **Education:** The parents of young patients with AOM should be educated concerning the importance of having the child finish the course of antibiotics as well as keeping follow-up appointments. They should also be made aware of signs of possible invasive disease (i.e., extreme irritability or somnolence, worsening pain, persistent fever). Clinicians should encourage the prevention of AOM through reduction of risk factors. (SOR **C**) Risk factors include tobacco smoke exposure and group daycare (6 or more households represented).

   d. **Follow-up**

      (1) The patient should be **reevaluated in 48 to 72 hours if fever or pain persists** at pretreatment levels. In this case, a 10-day course of a different oral antibiotic, or possibly a short course of IV/IM antibiotics, should be instituted. (See Table 22–2. SOR **C**) If the symptoms fail to improve after this intervention, the patient should be referred to a physician who can perform tympanocentesis for further evaluation, fluid culture, and management. At this point, inpatient care and intravenous antibiotics may be necessary.

      (2) The patient should then **be reevaluated at 4- to 6-week intervals** if an effusion has not resolved. An effusion may require up to 3 months to clear. Antibiotics are not indicated for persistent middle ear effusion in the absence of AOM. Effusions persisting beyond 3 months should be evaluated by an otolaryngologist.

2. **AOM in infants**

   a. Infants younger than age 2 months should be hospitalized for fever even if a source (e.g., AOM) is identified. Children with fever and AOM between ages 2 and 6 months may be treated as outpatients after careful evaluation by a seasoned clinician. Children older than 6 months may be treated with an outpatient course of antibiotics if there is no complicating history or physical finding (TM perforation, craniofacial abnormality, recurrent or chronic infection, or immunocompromise). Controlled trials concluded that a wait and see prescription approach substantially reduced unnecessary use of antibiotics in children with AOM seen in an emergency department and may be an alternative to routine use of antimicrobials for treatment of such children. (Table 22–4. SOR **B**) Providing there are no further complications, follow-up examination should take place in 4 weeks.

TABLE 22–2. RECOMMENDED ANTIBACTERIAL AGENTS FOR AOM AT DIAGNOSIS, AFTER 48 TO 72 HOURS OF OBSERVATION, OR TREATMENT FAILURE AFTER 48 TO 72 HOURS

Temperature ≥39°C and/or Severe Otalgia	At Diagnosis for patients being treated initially with antibacterial agents		Clinically defined treatment failure at 48–72 h after initial management with observation option		Clinically defined treatment failure at 48–72 h after initial management with antibacterial agents	
	Recommended	Alternative for Penicillin Allergy	Recommended	Alternative for Penicillin Allergy	Recommended	Alternative for Penicillin Allergy
No	Amoxicillin, 80–90 mg/kg/d	Non-type I: cefdinir, cefuroxime, cefpodoxime; Type I: azithromycin, clarithromycin	Amoxicillin, 80–90 mg/kg/d	Non-type I: cefdinir, cefuroxime, cefpodoxime; Type I: azithromycin, clarithromycin	Amoxicillin–clavulanate, 90 mg/kg/d of amoxicillin component with 6.4 mg/kg/d of clavulanate	Non-type I: ceftriaxone, 3 d; Type I: clindamycin
Yes	Amoxicillin–clavulanate, 90 mg/kg/d of amoxicillin component with 6.4 mg/kg/d of clavulanate	Ceftriaxone, 1 or 3 d	Amoxicillin–clavulanate, 90 mg/kg/d of amoxicillin component with 6.4 mg/kg/d of clavulanate	Ceftriaxone, 1 or 3 d	Ceftriaxone, 3 d	Tympanocentesis, clindamycin

Reproduced with permission from the AAP/AAFP Clinical Practice Guideline; Subcommittee on Management of Acute Otitis Media: Diagnosis and Management of Acute Otitis Media. *Pediatrics*. May 2004;113:1451-1465.

TABLE 22–3. TREATMENTS FOR OTALGIA IN AOM

Modality	Comments
Acetaminophen, ibuprofen	Effective analgesia for mild to moderate pain, readily available, mainstay of pain management for AOM
Home remedies (no controlled studies that directly address effectiveness)	May have limited effectiveness
Distraction	
External application of heat or cold	
Oil	
Topical agents benzocaine (Auralgan, Americaine Otic)	Additional but brief benefit over acetaminophen in patients ≥ 5 y
Naturopathic agents (Otikon Otic Solution)	Comparable with amethocaine/phenazone drops (anesthetic) in patients ≥ 6 y
Homeopathic agents	No controlled studies that directly address pain
Narcotic analgesia with codeine or analogs	Effective for moderate or severe pain; requires prescription; risk of respiratory depression, altered mental status, gastrointestinal upset, and constipation
Tympanostomy/myringotomy	Requires skill and entails potential risk

Reproduced with permission from the AAP/AAFP Clinical Practice Guideline; Subcommittee on Management of Acute Otitis Media: Diagnosis and management of Acute Otitis Media. *Pediatrics.* May 2004;113:1451-1465.

    b. **A polyvalent pneumococcal vaccine** is available for infants and has been shown to decrease the incidence of AOM and invasive pneumococcal disease.

3. **Recurrent AOM**

    a. **Recurrent disease** is defined as three episodes of AOM in a 6-month period or four or more episodes in a 12-month period. Underlying conditions predisposing to recurrent disease should be treated when associated with recurrence. Such disorders include enlarged adenoids, allergies, immunodeficiencies, nasal septal deviation, and sinusitis.

    b. **Tympanostomy tube** insertion, which results in immediate improvement in hearing, has been advocated for the prevention of recurrent otitis media. However, surgical management has not been proved superior to antibiotic prophylaxis or interval treatment of recurrences for preserving hearing. The interpretation of these data is controversial. Tympanostomy tubes for persistent effusion in children younger than 3 years have not been shown to improve multiple developmental outcomes up to 9 to 11 years. (SOR **B**)

    c. **Prophylactic** antibiotics for recurrent otitis media include **amoxicillin,** 25 mg/kg/d at bedtime; **sulfisoxazole,** 75 mg/kg/d at bedtime; and **trimethoprim-sulfamethoxazole,** 25 mg/kg/d at bedtime, based on the sulfamethoxazole component.

TABLE 22–4. CRITERIA FOR INITIAL ANTIBACTERIAL AGENT TREATMENT OR OBSERVATION IN CHILDREN WITH AOM

Age	Certain Diagnosis	Uncertain Diagnosis
≤ 6 mo	Antibacterial therapy	Antibacterial therapy
6 mo to 2 y	Antibacterial therapy	Antibacterial therapy if severe illness; observation option* if nonsevere illness
≥ 2 y	Antibacterial therapy if severe illness; observation option* if nonsevere illness	Observation option*

*Observation is an appropriate option only when follow-up can be ensured and antibacterial agents started if symptoms persist or worsen. Nonsevere illness is mild otalgia and fever $\leq 39°C$ in the past 24 hours. Severe illness is moderate to severe otalgia or fever $\geq 39°C$. A certain diagnosis of AOM meets all three criteria: (1) rapid onset, (2) signs of MEE, and (3) signs and symptoms of middle-ear inflammation.

Reproduced with permission from the AAP/AAFP Clinical Practice Guideline; Subcommittee on Management of Acute Otitis Media: Diagnosis and Management of Acute Otitis Media. *Pediatrics.* May 2004;113:1451-1465.

B. Otitis externa

1. **AOE** is frequently a polymicrobial infection usually involving *Pseudomonas aeruginosa*, *Staphylococcus aureus*, or both.

2. In 2006, the American Academy of Otolaryngology created the first, explicit, evidence-based clinical practice guidelines for **AOE**:

   a. Assess pain and recommend analgesic treatment based on severity. (SOR **B**)

   b. Distinguish AOE from other causes of otalgia. (SOR **C**)

   c. Evaluate patient for factors that modify management such as nonintact TM, tympanostomy tubes, immunocompromised, and/or prior radiotherapy. (SOR **C**)

   d. Use topical preparations for initial therapy of uncomplicated AOE. (SOR **B**)

   e. Avoid systemic antibiotics unless there is extension of cellulitis outside of the ear canal, DM, immunodeficiency, or other factors prohibiting the delivery of topical therapy. Oral antibiotics may cause adverse reactions and be less effective than eardrops. (SOR **B**)

   f. Topical antibiotic therapy of AOE should be based on efficacy, low incidence of adverse events, likelihood of adherence to therapy, and cost. Patients should be informed with proper instruction of use. (SOR **B**)

   g. When the ear canal is obstructed, enhance delivery of topical preparations with aural toilet, placing a wick, or both. (SOR **C**)

   h. Nonototoxic topical preparations should be prescribed for patients with TM rupture or with tympanostomy tubes. Quinolone antibiotic drops are approved for this purpose and do not contribute to hearing loss. (SOR **C**)

   i. If a patient fails to respond within 48 to 72 hours after initiation of treatment, reassess for confirmation of AOE and to rule out other causes, which includes but is not limited to obstructed ear canal, poor adherence to therapy, misdiagnosis, microbiologic factors, host factors, or contact sensitivity to eardrops. (SOR **C**)

   j. Ear candles are not recommended for treating AOE because efficacy has not been demonstrated. In addition, they may cause adverse effects such as burning and TM rupture.

   k. Patients should abstain from water-related sports for a period of 7 to 10 days after the diagnosis of AOE.

   Meta-analysis of topical treatment for AOE found that 65% to 90% of subjects improved within 7 to 10 days of initiation of treatment, irrespective of the type of topical treatment used. No statistically significant differences in clinical outcomes of AOE existed for antiseptic versus antimicrobial, quinolone antibiotic versus non-quinolone antibiotic(s), or steroid plus antimicrobial versus antimicrobial alone. The combination of antimicrobial and steroid appeared superior to steroid drops alone. Generally, 7 to 10 days of treatment are necessary for the resolution of AOE. Although the use of clinical guidelines is helpful in treating and managing AOE, clinical judgment should take precedence when treating patients.

3. Patients with **necrotizing otitis externa,** formerly malignant otitis externa, a severe infection involving the deeper periauricular tissue, should be hospitalized and treated with parenteral antibiotics providing adequate pseudomonal coverage. Necrotizing otitis externa should be suspected when there is no resolution of either the otalgia or headache despite adequate treatment. In addition, pain out of proportion to clinical findings, and/or the presence of granulation tissue at the bony cartilaginous junction should prompt further investigation. High clinical suspicion for diabetic patients and other immunocompromised patients is warranted.

C. Barotrauma

1. The **acute episode** may be treated with decongestants (e.g., **pseudoephedrine,** 30–60 mg every 4–6 hours) and analgesics (**acetaminophen,** 325–650 mg every 4–6 hours, or **codeine,** 30–60 mg every 4–6 hours).

2. **Patients with multiple episodes** of barotrauma should use a long-acting oral decongestant, such as timed-release **pseudoephedrine,** 120 mg once or twice daily, or a topical nasal decongestant such as **phenylephrine,** two sprays 5 minutes apart in each nostril 30 minutes prior to flying or diving. Individuals who use topical decongestants should be cautioned to limit use to 3 days and/or apply them only intermittently to avoid rhinitis medicamentosum. To prevent future recurrences, the diver or flier should be instructed in the proper methods of equalizing middle ear and ambient pressure, such as swallowing hard or exhaling against closed nostrils.

D. Direct trauma
1. **Abrasions and small lacerations** of the auricle should be treated as are other minor skin injuries (see Chapter 41).
2. **Hematomas** of the auricle should be aspirated, and a pressure dressing should be applied to prevent formation of a cauliflower ear.
3. **Traumatic perforations** of the TM are treated by keeping the canal dry. If the perforations do not heal within several weeks, the patient should be referred to an otolaryngologist.

E. Referred otalgia (see Table 22–1).

REFERENCES

American Academy of Pediatrics, Subcommittee on Management of Acute Otitis Media. Diagnosis and management of acute otitis media. *Pediatrics.* 2004;113(5):1451-1465.
Flynn CA, Griffin GH, Schultz JK. Decongestants and antihistamines for acute otitis media in children. *Cochrane Database Syst Rev.* 2004;(3):CD001727.
Onusko E. Tympanometry. *Am Fam Physician.* 2004;70(9):1713-1720.
Paradise JL, Feldman HM, Campbell TF, et al. Tympanostomy tubes and developmental outcomes at 9 to 11 years of age. *N Engl J Med.* 2007;356(3):248-261.
Rosenfeld RM, Brown L, Cannon CR, et al.; American Academy of Otolaryngology–Head and Neck Surgery Foundation. Clinical practice guideline: acute otitis externa. *Otolaryngol Head Neck Surg.* 2006;134(4 Suppl):S4-S23.
Spiro DM, Tay KY, Arnold DH, Dziura JD, Baker MD, Shapiro ED. Wait-and-see prescription for the treatment of acute otitis media: a randomized controlled trial. *JAMA.* 2006;296(10):1235-1241.

23   Edema

Joshua H. Barash, MD

KEY POINTS

- Edema is a common complaint in primary care and often the manifestation of a serious underlying disease process.
- The underlying etiology causing a patient's edema is best determined based on the distribution of the accumulated fluid, in combination with a targeted history and carefully chosen diagnostic tests.
- Various nonpharmacologic measures are effective in controlling edema.

I. **Definition.** Edema is the excessive accumulation of fluid in the tissues. Responsible factors include (1) **increased capillary pressure,** (e.g., congestive heart failure [CHF], deep vein thrombosis [DVT], venous insufficiency, pregnancy, or drugs); (2) **decreased plasma proteins,** (e.g., nephrotic syndrome, denuded skin areas [wounds], hepatocellular failure, or severe malnutrition); (3) **increased capillary permeability,** (e.g., allergic reactions, bacterial infections, burns, prolonged ischemia, or idiopathic edema); and (4) **lymphatic blockage,** (e.g., local lymphatic blockage from cancer or generalized lymphatic blockage [retroperitoneal]).

II. **Common Diagnoses.** Edema is a common complaint in primary care and often the manifestation of a serious underlying disease process.

A. **Bilateral lower extremity edema**
1. This condition **usually results from systemic conditions** (CHF, hepatocellular disease, or venous insufficiency). **Risk factors for CHF** include coronary artery disease or an acute ischemia, valvular disease, alcohol excess (leading to alcoholic cardiomyopathy), and hypertension. **Risk factors for hepatocellular disease** include a past history of alcoholism or hepatitis B or C infection. **Risk factors for chronic venous insufficiency** include a history of prior DVT, congenital valvular incompetence, or any

TABLE 23–1. MEDICATIONS KNOWN TO CAUSE PERIPHERAL EDEMA

Antidepressants
Monoamine oxidase inhibitors

Antihypertensive medications
Calcium channel blockers
Direct vasodilators
Beta-blockers
Centrally acting agents
Antisympathetics

Diabetic medications
Insulin sensitizers such as rosiglitazone

Other medications
Hormones
Corticosteroids
Estrogens/Progesterones
Testosterone
Nonsteroidal anti-inflammatory drugs (NSAIDs)

---

process that destroys or damages deep venous valves. **Risk factors for pulmonary hypertension** include sleep apnea.

2. Certain **drugs** (Table 23–1), as well as **hyperthyroidism and hypothyroidism,** can also cause bilateral lower extremity edema. **Lipedema** (leg swelling because of abnormal accumulation of fatty substances in the subcutaneous tissues) is commonly mistaken for lymphedema. This condition usually spares the feet and is found almost exclusively in young women.

B. **Unilateral lower extremity edema**

1. The most common causes are DVT (acutely) (see sidebar), or lymphedema (chronically). **DVT risk factors** include immobilization, malignancy, recent leg trauma, surgery, and hypercoagulable states. **Risk factors for lymphedema** include any process that results in obstruction of the lymphatic channels, such as malignancy, infection, surgery, trauma, or radiation exposure.

2. Other common causes of unilateral lower extremity edema include cellulitis, osteomyelitis, burns, and trauma (ruptured gastrocnemius, compartment syndrome, or soft tissue injury).

C. **Upper extremity edema** is rare and most commonly is caused by the superior vena cava syndrome, usually from malignancy.

D. **Idiopathic edema** (hormone-related edema) occurs only in menstruating women and is most common in the 20s and 30s. Symptoms persist throughout the menstrual cycle, and it is felt to be hormonally mediated.

III. **Symptoms** (Figure 23–1).

A. In **bilateral swelling,** CHF is suggested by dyspnea on exertion, orthopnea, and paroxysmal dyspnea, whereas abdominal fullness in the absence of pulmonary symptoms is more common in patients with hepatocellular disease (cirrhosis). Sleep apnea, which can cause pulmonary hypertension, is suggested by loud snoring, apnea noted by the sleep partner, or daytime somnolence.

B. In **unilateral swelling,** historical factors suggesting chronicity include old trauma, surgery, radiation, or old infection. Recent trauma suggests a ruptured gastrocnemius or compartment syndrome. Trauma (e.g., puncture wound) followed by a focal area of erythema and pain suggests cellulitis. Recent inflammation may suggest a burn. Presence of risk factors may suggest an acute DVT.

C. In **idiopathic edema** (also referred to as **hormone-related edema**), the patient may gain several pounds during the day and exhibit significant edema of the hands, breasts, abdomen, and legs by evening. Upon lying down at night, the edema is mobilized, and nocturia often causes overnight loss of the excess weight.

IV. **Signs** (Figure 23–1).

A. **Bilateral pitting edema** with jugular venous distention, bibasilar fine rales, and wheezes points to CHF (see Chapter 72).

B. **Bilateral lower extremity edema** with ascites and absent pulmonary findings suggests hepatocellular disease.

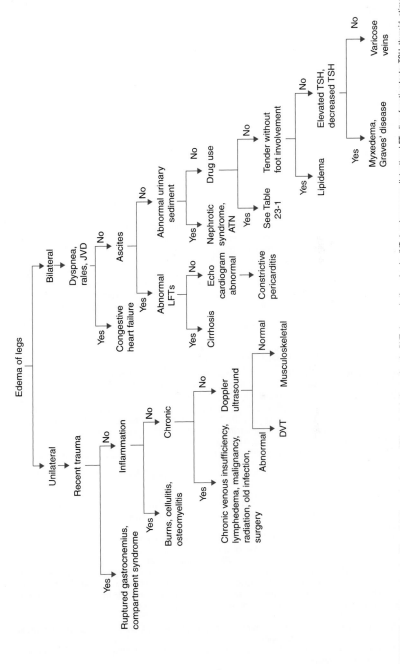

FIGURE 23-1. Approach to the differential diagnosis of edema. ATN, acute tubular nephrosis; DVT, deep vein thrombosis; JVD, jugular venous distention; LFTs, liver function tests; TSH, thyroid-stimulating hormone.

TABLE 23-2. MODEL FOR CLINICAL PREDICTION OF DVT*

Clinical Feature	Score
History	
Active cancer	1
Paralysis, recent plaster cast	1
Recent immobilization or major surgery	1
Physical examination	
Tenderness along deep veins	1
Swelling of entire leg	1
$\geq$3 cm difference in calf circumference	1
Pitting edema	1
Collateral superficial veins	1
Clinical assessment	
Alternative diagnosis likely	-2

*Pretest probability of deep vein thrombosis: high if score of 3 points or greater; intermediate if score of 1–2 points; and low if score of 0 or less.

Reproduced with permission from Wells PS et al: Value of assessment of pretest probability of deep vein thrombosis in clinical management. *Lancet.* 1997;**350**:1795.

   C. Chronic skin changes (stasis dermatitis, brawny induration, ulcers) and absent pulmonary findings suggest chronic venous insufficiency.
   D. Kaposi-Stemmar sign (the inability to pinch a fold of skin on the dorsum of the foot at the base of the second toe) is a sign of lymphedema.
   E. Unilateral edema associated with tenderness, a palpable cord, or a Homan's sign (calf pain with passive dorsiflexion of the foot) suggests an acute DVT.
   F. Erythematous inflamed skin may suggest an underlying cellulitis or osteomyelitis.
   G. The **lack of involvement of the feet** characterizes lipedema and distinguishes it from lymphedema.
   H. Neck circumference $\geq$17 inches suggests sleep apnea.

DEEP VEIN THROMBOSIS

Deep vein thrombosis. DVT can lead to significant morbidity and mortality, if unrecognized and untreated. Although it is not possible to make a definitive diagnosis clinically, reasonable estimates of pretest probability for DVT can be made by ascertaining clinical features found to be independent predictors of DVT (see Table 23–2). Using an estimate of pretest probability in conjunction with results of noninvasive testing allows one to determine the need for anticoagulation, no anticoagulation, or further testing. For example, a person with a low-pretest probability and a normal ultrasound test is effectively ruled out for DVT.

DVT below the knee carries a minimal risk of embolization ($\leq$1% per year), if the clot does not propagate into the thigh.

 V. Laboratory Tests (Figure 23–1 and Table 23–3). After the physician does a targeted history and physical examination, a limited number of laboratory and diagnostic tests may be necessary to arrive at a diagnosis.
   A. In patients with **ascites in the absence of pulmonary signs,** abnormal liver function tests may suggest hepatocellular disease or cirrhosis.
   B. If a cardiac etiology is suspected, an **EKG, echocardiogram, and chest x-ray** should be ordered. If the patient has dyspnea, a **BNP** (brain natriuretic peptide) determination can help detect heart failure. An **echocardiogram** can also detect pulmonary hypertension.
   C. Thyroid-stimulating hormone can point to either hyperthyroidism or hypothyroidism in the absence of findings suggesting a cardiac or liver etiology, or in the absence of a drug side effect as a suspected cause of edema.
   D. A **urinalysis** demonstrating proteinuria may implicate the kidneys, for example, nephrotic syndrome or glomerulonephritis.
   E. Patients with unilateral lower extremity swelling and risk factors suggesting DVT may need the following tests.

TABLE 23-3. TESTS THAT MAY BE USEFUL IN EVALUATING THE CAUSE OF PERIPHERAL EDEMA

Test	Indication
Urinalysis	Glomerulonephritis, acute tubular necrosis, nephrotic syndrome
Thyroid-stimulating hormone	Hyperthyroidism, hypothyroidism
Liver function tests	Cirrhosis
Prealbumin	Malnutrition
D-dimer	Deep vein thrombosis
Chest x-ray	Congestive heart failure, lung cancer
Bone scan	Osteomyelitis
Ultrasound	Deep vein thrombosis, popliteal cyst
CAT scan	Malignancy, cirrhosis
Echocardiogram	Constrictive pericarditis, congestive heart failure

1. **Venous Doppler ultrasound** may be helpful in making a definitive diagnosis. The sensitivity and specificity of this test improve as pretest probability rises; in symptomatic patients sensitivity approaches 93% and specificity approaches 98%. In asymptomatic patients, the sensitivity falls to 59% while specificity remains at 98%.

2. The **plasma D-Dimer test** is highly sensitive but not specific. It is useful in ruling out DVT in low-probability patients in conjunction with a normal Doppler ultrasound. Because of its low specificity, noninvasive testing is needed when a "positive" D-dimer test result is obtained. (SOR **B**)

3. **Impedence plethysomography** detects changes in leg volumes using a thigh blood pressure cuff. In DVT, the normal pattern is altered and detected by plethysmography.

4. **In questionable cases,** a venogram (nearly 100% sensitive and specific) usually provides a definitive diagnosis.

VI. **Treatment.** Specific diseases underlying edema should be treated (Chapter 72 for CHF, Chapter 84 for chronic renal failure, Chapter 71 for cirrhosis). The following measures may be useful in managing other causes of edema discussed in this chapter.

A. In patients with **varicose veins** and **venous insufficiency,** knee-length elastic stockings can aid venous return. In addition, periodic elevation throughout the day can help prevent edema; ideally, the leg should be above the level of the heart for this to be effective. Women should avoid the use of tight girdles, which can restrict superficial venous return at the thigh level. Finally, prolonged standing should be avoided if at all possible. (SOR **C**) Horse chestnut seed extract (300 mg, standardized to 50 mg of escin, twice a day) has been found to be effective and can be obtained in health food stores. (SOR **B**)

B. Patients with **idiopathic edema (hormone-related edema)** should avoid diuretics because they can increase edema. Chronic diuretic use increases aldosterone secretion, exacerbating edema. Angiotensin converting enzyme (ACE) inhibitors have been used with success because of their suppression of aldosterone and salt and water retention. A common ACE inhibitor used for this purpose is captopril (Capoten), 25 to 50 mg by mouth 2 to 3 times each day. Sodium restriction may also benefit idiopathic edema. If diuretics have been discontinued for ≥4 weeks and there is no improvement in the edema, then **spironolactone** can be initiated at a dose of 50 to 100 mg daily, and increased up to a maximum of 100 mg, 4 times daily. (SOR **C**)

C. If an **offending medication** is implicated in edema, then a trial without the medicine should be instituted, substituting an alternative medication, if necessary. (SOR **C**)

D. Patients with **DVT** need initial clot stabilization with heparin followed by oral anticoagulation with Coumadin.

1. Acute DVT is generally treated with **low-molecular-weight heparin,** such as enoxaparin. A typical regimen is enoxaparin, 1 mg/kg twice daily by subcutaneous injection. Therapy is continued until an effective INR (in the range of 2.0-3.0) is achieved with oral Coumadin. Advantages of low-molecular-weight heparin include its efficacy, safety, and twice-daily dosing without the need for partial thromboplastin time (PTT) monitoring. (SOR **A**)

2. **Anticoagulation with oral Coumadin** is usually continued for 3 months for a first-time DVT with known precipitant (e.g., surgery or trauma). Recurrent DVTs or those without a clear etiology require treatment for at least 6 months and sometimes longer (e.g., if serum lupus anticoagulant is identified). (SOR **C**)

REFERENCES

Cho S, Atwood JE. Peripheral edema. *Am J Med.* 2002;113:580.

Ely J, et al. Approach to leg edema of unclear etiology. *J Am Board Fam Med.* 2006;19:148.

O'Brien JG, et al. Treatment of edema. *Am Fam Physician.* 2005;71:2111.

Rose BD. Approach to the adult with edema. In: Rose BD, ed. *UpToDate.* Wellesley, Mass. UpToDate; 2006. Accessed April 2007.

Wells PS, et al. Value of assessment of pretest probability of deep vein thrombosis in clinical management. *Lancet.* 1997;350:1795.

---

24   Enuresis

Kalyanakrishnan Ramakrishnan, MD

KEY POINTS

- Primary monosymptomatic enuresis (enuresis in children without lower urinary tact symptoms (LUTS) other than nocturia and no evidence of bladder dysfunction) is the most common form of enuresis.
- Parents of children in whom primary monosymptomatic enuresis is not distressing should receive reassurance about their child's physical and emotional wellbeing and should be counselled about eliminating guilt, shame, and punishment. Pharmacotherapy and/or alarms should be used only when enuresis poses a significant problem for the child. (SOR **B**)
- Enuresis alarm is an effective treatment for monosymptomatic nocturnal enuresis in older children with motivated families. (SOR **A**)
- Desmopressin is most effective in children with monosymptomatic enuresis with nocturnal polyuria and normal bladder capacity, or when enuresis alarm is impractical or ineffective. (SOR **A**)

I. **Definition. Enuresis** (primary nocturnal urinary incontinence) is repeated spontaneous voiding of urine into the bed or clothes at least twice a week for at least 3 consecutive months in a child who is at least 5 years of age.
   A. **Primary monosymptomatic enuresis** is bed-wetting without a history of nocturnal continence and unassociated with other symptoms.
   B. **Secondary monosymptomatic enuresis** is recurrence of bed-wetting after at least 6 months of nocturnal continence.
   C. **Non-monosymptomatic enuresis** is bed-wetting associated with urinary urgency, frequency, straining, dribbling, pain, chronic constipation, or encopresis.
   D. Children 5 years or older with involuntary or intentional urination into clothing while awake or asleep are said to have daytime incontinence and enuresis. The term diurnal enuresis is considered obsolete.
II. **Common Diagnoses.** An estimated five to seven million children in the United States have primary enuresis; 80% are monosymptomatic, and 5% may have an organic cause.
   A. Risk factors for **primary monosymptomatic enuresis** include the following:
      1. **Family history.** Five to seven times risk if one parent affected; more than 11 times risk if both parents affected.
      2. **Maturational delay.** Affects 6.7% of children between 4 and 6 years, decreasing to 2.8% by 11 to 12 years (15% spontaneous resolution every year). These children may manifest delay in central nervous system maturation, delay in development of language and motor skills.
      3. **Male gender.** Seen 3 times more often in boys.
      4. **Deep sleep.** Abnormally deep sleep patterns in children with enuresis.
      5. **Bladder function.** Smaller functional bladder capacity and inability to hold urine.
      6. **Lower nocturnal levels of antidiuretic hormone (ADH).**
   B. Twenty percent of enuretic children experience some daytime wetting. Risk factors include constipation, urinary tract infection, psychologic stress (dysfunctional home, abuse),

TABLE 24–1. IMPORTANT HISTORY IN CHILDREN WITH ENURESIS

Question	Significance/Suggests
To distinguish primary from secondary enuresis: Has your child ever been consistently dry at night?	"Never dry" suggests primary enuresis
To distinguish uncomplicated from complicated enuresis:	
Does your child wet his or her pants during the day?	Yes, see daytime incontinence and enuresis
Does your child appear to have pain with urination?	Urinary tract infection
How often does your child have bowel movements?	Infrequent stools: constipation
Are bowel movements ever hard to pass?	Constipation
Does your child ever soil his or her pants?	Encopresis
To distinguish possible functional bladder disorder from nocturnal polyuria:	
How many times a day does your child void? (frequency)	More than 7 times a day: functional bladder disorder
Does your child have to run to the bathroom? (urgency)	Positive response: functional bladder disorder
Does your child hold urine until the last minute?	Positive response: functional bladder disorder
How many nights a week does your child wet the bed?	Most nights: functional bladder disorder 1 or 2 nights: nocturnal polyuria
Does your child wet more than once every night?	Positive response: functional bladder disorder
Does your child seem to wet large or small volumes?	Large volumes: nocturnal polyuria Small volumes: functional bladder disorder
To determine how parents have handled bed-wetting: How have you handled the nighttime accident?	Elicits information on interventions that have already been tried; be alert for responses suggesting that the child has been punished or shamed

Adapted with permission, from Thiedke CC. Nocturnal enuresis. *Am Fam Physician.* 2003;67:1499-1506, 1509-1510. Copyright © 2003 American Academy of Family Physicians. All Rights Reserved.

sickle cell disease, obstructive sleep apnea (OSA), chronic renal failure, and diabetes mellitus.

III. **Symptoms.** When evaluating a child with enuresis, responses to several key questions will assist in assessing causes and management for the problem. (See Table 24–1.)

IV. **Signs.** Most children presenting with enuresis in primary care settings, will have a normal physical examination. A focused evaluation is important to detect underlying or contributing causes.

   A. **Blood pressure.**

   B. **Growth chart.** Poor growth, elevated blood pressure, or both suggests renal disease.

   C. **Abdomen/genital examination** to detect renal and bladder enlargement, fecal masses indicating encopresis, genital anomalies (hypospadias, meatal stenosis, ectopic ureter).

   D. **Neurologic examination,** including gait, power, muscle tone, sensation, reflexes, and rectal tone (for underlying neurologic disease).

   E. **Observed voiding** for stream/ability to initiate and interrupt in midstream (for neurologic disease or urethral stricture).

V. **Laboratory Tests.** Most children presenting in ambulatory primary care will have a **normal physical examination;** in these patients, the only testing indicated is **urinalysis (UA)** and **estimation of bladder capacity.** Bladder capacity is estimated by measuring the postvoid residue (PVR). The normal bladder capacity in ounces is age plus 2; the normal PVR in children should be less than 10% of maximal bladder capacity.

   A. **Children with normal physical examination, UA** and a normal PVR require no further evaluation.

   B. **Children with abnormal examination, UA, or both** may require further evaluation.

   1. **Urinalysis. Specific gravity** (SG $\leq$1.005 seen in diabetes insipidus, acute tubular necrosis, pyelonephritis; SG of 1.010 that remains unchanged despite fluid intake is seen in chronic renal disease; high $\geq$1.035 seen in dehydration, congestive heart failure, liver failure, and shock. **Glycosuria** may indicate diabetes mellitus or low renal glycemic threshold (e.g., pregnancy). **Proteinuria** may be benign or indicate underlying disease (see Chapter 53). **Hematuria** can indicate cystitis or urinary calculi and warrants further evaluation (see Chapter 36). **White blood cells** with significant pyuria on a clean-catch specimen suggests urinary tract infection, a cause of polysymptomatic enuresis (see Chapter 21); antibiotic treatment should be instituted.

2. **Blood count, serum chemistry.** Useful in diagnosing chronic renal insufficiency, sickle cell disease.
3. **Imaging studies.** Renal and bladder ultrasound, voiding cystourethrogram. Useful in evaluating vesicoureteral reflux in children with urinary tract infection. Magnetic resonance imaging of the lumbosacral spine if abnormal neurologic examination (detects spinal dysraphism).
4. **Urodynamic studies.** Measurement of residual urine, cystometry. Useful in evaluating voiding dysfunction.

VI. **Treatment.** Treatment should not commence until the child is approximately 7 years old, unless enuresis causes severe emotional distress. The child must comprehend and perceive the condition as a problem and be a willing participant in therapy. Parental involvement is essential to the treatment success. It is important to educate or reassure parents about rates of spontaneous resolution of enuresis (see Section II.A). Secondary causes identified should be treated. (SOR **C**) Encopresis-associated enuresis responds to fecal disimpaction and bowel retraining. Children with OSA respond to surgical correction of the upper airway. Psychotherapy or family therapy is indicated in psychogenic enuresis. Biofeedback is an option for motivated children with dysfunctional voiding. Enuresis associated with infection responds to antibiotics.

A. **Nonpharmacologic measures.** Tried for 3 to 6 months.
1. **Lifestyle modifications** effective in monosymptomatic enuresis include the following:
   a. Goal-setting for **the child to get up at night and use the toilet.** Alarm or parent-awakening approaches can be used.
   b. Improve **access to the toilet**—provide a bedside potty.
   c. Have the child consume 40% of fluids before noon, 40% in early afternoon, and only 20% in the evening. **Avoid giving excessive fluids** and **caffeine-containing products before bedtime.**
   d. **Encourage the child to empty the bladder** at bedtime.
   e. **Discontinue diapers** or pull-ups so that the sensation of wetness is recognized.
   f. **Include the child in morning cleanup** in a nonpunitive manner; criticism and punishment can cause secondary psychologic problems.
   g. Provide a **diary or chart** to monitor progress.
   h. Use **positive reinforcement** (have the child place a favorite sticker on the calendar for dry days).
2. **Behavioral conditioning** may be effective in children with frequent daytime voiding, few or no dry nights, or ≥ 1 enuretic episode per night; these children may have low functional bladder capacity and benefit from an alarm.
   a. **Enuresis alarm** (Table 24–2). Small transistorized mini-alarms are attached to the patient's bed or underwear and are activated (via sound, vibration, or both) with the release of first few drops of urine. Eventually, a conditioned response occurs. Useful in older children with motivated families. (SOR **A**) Cures occur in approximately 50% of children.
   b. **Nighttime alarm** (Table 24–2). An alarm clock is set for 3 hours after going to sleep to awaken the child to get up and void.
3. **Self-hypnosis** with posthypnotic suggestion that the child will wake up and use the bathroom. The cure rate is reported at 77% for children 5 years and older.
B. **Pharmacologic therapy** (Table 24–2)
1. **Desmopressin (DDAVP),** reduces urine volume by reabsorbing water from the distal convoluted and collecting tubules. Sixty to seventy percent of children respond during treatment; most (80%) relapse following treatment cessation. It is available in nasal spray and tablet. It is most effective in children with monosymptomatic enuresis, nocturnal polyuria, and normal bladder capacity, less frequent bed-wetting, positive family history, and family unwilling or unable to cooperate with nonpharmacologic measures. (SOR **A**)
2. Anticholinergics such as the tricyclic antidepressant **imipramine (Tofranil)** and oxybutynin (Ditropan) decrease detrusor tone, improve bladder capacity, and decrease frequency and urgency. They are useful in children with urgency, restricted bladder capacity as a result of detrusor hyperactivity, day-time incontinence and enuresis, and unresponsiveness to desmopressin. (SOR **C**) Side effects include dry mouth, blurred vision, headache, nausea, dizziness, gastrointestinal disturbance, and tachycardia.
C. **Follow-up.** Regular follow-up visits are important to address issues or concerns, answer questions, and encourage the child and parents. In children receiving medications for

TABLE 24-2. INTERVENTIONS FOR ENURESIS

Intervention	Mechanism	Dosage/Instructions	Side Effects/Comments	Efficacy
Dry bed training program	Timed voiding to empty bladder	Parent awakens child 3 hrs after bedtime	Side effects: none Safe. Does not require bed-wetting to initiate alarm	Insufficient evidence if used alone. 75% efficacy when combined with alarm Relapse rate: 20%
Enuresis alarm*	Alarm system activated by wetness that awakens child so child can get up to void	Worn nightly for 2–3 mo	Side effects: sleep disruption to child and family members.	Most effective intervention. Initial cure rate: 75%–84% Relapse rate: 15%–30% with discontinuance
Desmopressin*	Synthetic analogue of vasopressin; reduces urine production by increasing water retention and urine concentration in the distal tubules	1 spray each nostril 20 μg (10 μg) nightly Oral: 0.2–0.6 mg qhs	Common side effects: headache, abdominal discomfort, nausea, nasal congestion, epistaxis, visual disturbances, bad taste. Comments: Contraindicated in patients who have habit polydipsia, hypertension, or heart disease. Caution in cystic fibrosis.	Initial cure rates: 86% Relapse rate with discontinuation: 94%. With Propiverine: 97% efficacy. Desmopressin plus anticholinergic may be appropriate for children bladder instability.
Imipramine	Increases bladder capacity and tightens bladder neck sphincter	Initially 25 mg at night 7–12 y– increase to 50 mg if no response at 25 mg ≥ 12y: increase to 75 mg	Common side effects: drowsiness, lethargy, agitation, depression, sleep disturbance gastrointestinal upsets. Rare adverse effects: seizures, cardiac arrhythmias, accidental overdose. Caution in individuals with epilepsy.	40%–60% efficacy for more than 4–6 mo. Relapse rate with discontinuation: 50% Uused until child has achieved dry (at minimum) 14–28 consecutive dry nights then gradually tapered.
Oxybutynin Oxytrol* Tolterodine Propiverine	Anticholinergic, antispasmodic effects reduce uninhibited detrusor contractions	2.5–5 mg bid–tid 1 patch twice weekly 1–2 mg twice daily 0.4 mg/kg twice daily	Common side effects: dry mouth, blurred vision, headache, nausea, dizziness, gastrointestinal upset and tachycardia Comments: drug of choice for polysymptomatic enuresis.	Relapse rate with discontinuation: Anecdotal reports of benefit; prospective double-blind study showed no benefit versus placebo. See data regarding Propiverine above.
Indomethacin	Inhibits nitric oxide and prostaglandin synthesis, decreases urine volume, and bladder and urethral contractions	50 mg rectally every night for 2–3 wk	Nausea, vomiting, diarrhea, gastric discomfort, renal dysfunction. Risk of side-effects low with short courses.	More effective than placebo. Duration of response still under investigation.

*Associated with greatest efficacy.

161

enuresis, follow-up is recommended 2 weeks after initiation of therapy, then monthly for 3 months.

REFERENCES

Canadian Pediatric Society position statement (CP 2005–2002). Management of primary nocturnal enuresis. *Paediatr Child Health.* 2005;10:611-614.

Evans JHC. Evidence based management of nocturnal enuresis. *BMJ.* 2001;323:1167-1169.

Fritz G, Rockney R, Bernet W, Arnold V, et al. Practice parameter for the assessment and treatment of children and adolescents with enuresis. *J Am Acad Child Adolesc Psychiatry.* 2004;43:1540-1550.

Hjalmas K, Arnold T, Bower W, et al. Nocturnal enuresis: an international evidence based management strategy. *J Urol.* 2004;171:2545-2561.

Makari J, Rushton HG. Nocturnal enuresis. *Am Fam Physician.* 2006;73:1611-1613.

Neveus T, von Gontard A, Hoebeke P, et al. The standardization of terminology of lower urinary tract function in children and adolescents: report from the standardisation committee of the international children's continence society. *J Urol.* 2006;176:314-324.

Thiedke CC. Nocturnal enuresis. *Am Fam Physician.* 2003;67:1499-1506, 1509-1510.

---

25 Failure to Thrive

Cathy Kamens, MD

KEY POINTS

- Growth of children must be measured over time and plotted on a standardized growth chart at every visit.
- A thorough history and physical examination and selective laboratory tests are the foundation for accurate diagnosis and management in failure to thrive (FTT).
- Provision of calories and a multidisciplinary approach are keys to treating children with FTT.

I. **Definition. FTT** is defined as a diagnosis to describe infants and children who lose weight or fail to gain weight in accordance with standardized growth charts. It is a symptom or a sign of an underlying problem, but FTT itself is not a disease or disorder. At each office visit, all infants and children should be accurately measured for weight, length (recumbent, younger than 2 years), or height (standing, 2 years and older), and head circumference. These measurements should be plotted on standardized growth curves (available through the Centers for Disease Control at www. cdc.gov/growthcharts). Growth should be evaluated over time with attention to growth velocity and any change in growth percentiles. Weight should be compared to length (or height), as well as head circumference, to identify children with disproportionate growth. There is no consensus on criteria for FTT, but investigation is appropriate in any child

   A. whose weight or height for age is below the fifth percentile;
   B. whose growth slows to cross two major percentiles;
   C. whose weight for height is less than the fifth percentile.

II. **Common Diagnoses.** FTT occurs in 3% to 10% of children and is usually identified in the infant or young child. It is important for health care providers to consider FTT, because many parents will not recognize the subtle slowing of growth that characterizes most FTT. The differential diagnosis for FTT is long (see Table 25–1), but the etiology can be classified into four categories. There are often multiple contributing factors.

   A. Inadequate caloric intake, as in feeding errors or mechanical feeding difficulties.
   B. Inadequate absorption, as because of gastrointestinal disease.
   C. Defective utilization, as in metabolic or congenital disorders.
   D. Excess metabolic demand, as seen in metabolic, cardiopulmonary, or renal disease.

TABLE 25–1. DIFFERENTIAL DIAGNOSIS, PRESENTATION, AND LABORATORY EVALUATION OF FAILURE TO THRIVE

Cause	History	Signs	Laboratory Tests
Psychosocial			
Breast-feeding problems	Sore nipples, lack of engorgement or milk letdown	Asymmetric FTT (see Section IV.B.1), cracked nipples	None
Feeding errors	Insufficient quantity offered, formula preparation error, excessive juice intake	Asymmetric FTT	None
Infant behavior/ bonding	Refusal of bottle, irritability, ignorance of infant cues	Apathetic, withdrawn behavior, minimal smiling, decreased vocalizations	None
Abuse or neglect	Maternal depression or mental illness, parental drug use, "chaotic" family style, spousal abuse	Poor hygiene, bruises in different stages of healing, characteristic patterns of injury	None
Economic deprivation	Homelessness, public assistance, "rationing" food supplies	Asymmetric FTT, poor hygiene	None
Gastrointestinal			
Gastroesophageal reflux	Very frequent "wet burps"	Emesis, cough, wheezing	Esophageal pH probe
Craniofacial abnormalities Cleft lip/palate Choanal atresia Micrognathia	Nasal regurgitation, choking, unilateral rhinorrhea	Cleft or small jaw seen on examination, unable to pass catheter through nose	None
Malabsorption Celiac disease Lactose intolerance Milk protein intolerance Pancreatic insufficiency	Diarrhea, abdominal pain, foul-smelling stools	Abdominal distention, dehydration, fatty stools	Lactose tolerance test, stool pH, electrolytes, sweat test, fecal fat, jejunal biopsy, anti-endomysial antibodies
Inflammatory bowel disease	Abdominal pain, diarrhea, melena	Heme-positive stool, fever	Stool Hematest, ESR, barium enema
Biliary disease Atresia Cirrhosis	Pale stools	Jaundice, hepatomegaly	LFTs, abdominal ultrasound, liver biopsy
Obstruction Pyloric stenosis Malrotation Hirschsprung disease	Vomiting, may be projectile vomiting after meals	Abdominal distention, palpable mass (olive), dehydration	Electrolytes, KUB, abdominal ultrasound
Renal			
Renal tubular acidosis	Polyuria, vomiting	Tachypnea, muscular weakness	Renal US, electrolytes, blood gas
Chronic renal failure	Listlessness, pruritus	Pallor, edema	Serum, BUN, creatinine, US, UA, electrolytes
Diabetes insipidus	Polyuria, thirst	Dehydration, irritability	
Cardiopulmonary			
Congenital heart defects	Shortness of breath, blue lips	Cyanosis, murmur	CXR, ECG, echocardiogram
Congestive heart failure	Shortness of breath, swelling, blue lips	Cyanosis, rales, edema	CXR, echocardiogram
Asthma	Cough, shortness of breath	Tachypnea, wheezing	Pulmonary function tests
Bronchopulmonary dysplasia	History of prematurity or respiratory disease	Tachypnea, retractions	Pulse oximetry, pulmonary function tests

(Continued)

TABLE 25–1. (*Continued*)

Cause	History	Signs	Laboratory Tests
Cystic fibrosis	Frequent respiratory infections	Tachypnea, wheezing	Sweat test
Anatomic upper airway abnormalities Tracheoesophageal fistula Vascular slings	Slow feeding, coughing and choking, history of pneumonia	Stridor, inability to pass a catheter into the stomach	CXR, barium esophagogram
Obstructive sleep apnea	Snoring, mouth breathing	Adenotonsillar hypertrophy	Sleep study
Endocrine			
Thyroid disease	Dry or moist skin, cold or heat intolerance	Irritability or slow movements, warm or cold skin	Serum thyroxine, TSH
Diabetes mellitus	Polydipsia, polyphagia, polyuria	Lethargy, Kussmaul respirations	UA, serum glucose, pH
Adrenal disorder	Obesity, poor sleeping	Hypertension or hypotension, diabetes mellitus	Urine-free cortisol, plasma, ACTH
Parathyroid disorders	Muscle pain and cramps, abdominal pain	Tetany, cataracts	Calcium, PTH
Pituitary disorders Growth hormone deficiency	May have none	Prominent forehead, large abdomen	"Provocative" growth hormone test
Neurologic			
Developmental disorder	History of developmental delay	May be normal or with dysmorphic features	None
Hydrocephalus	Irritability, lethargy, vomiting	Increased head circumference, wide bulging fontanelle, dilated scalp veins	Head CT or MRI
Neuromuscular disorder Cerebral palsy Hypotonia Myopathy	History of developmental motor delay	Spasticity or hypotonia, microcephaly	Head CT or MRI
Cerebral hemorrhages	Headache, vomiting, history of trauma	Nuchal rigidity, hemiparesis	Head CT or MRI
Infectious			
UTI	Fever, irritability	Fever, suprapubic tenderness	UA and culture
Infectious diarrhea	Diarrhea, melena	Abdominal distention, pain, fever	Stool culture, ova, parasites
Thrush	Refuses bottle	White plaque on oral mucosa	None
Recurrent tonsillitis	Sore throat, bad breath, mouth breathing	Tonsillar hypertrophy, cervical lymphadenopathy	Throat culture
Tuberculosis	Travel in high-risk area or exposure to high-risk persons	Lymphadenopathy	PPD, CXR
Human immunodeficiency virus	Maternal history of high-risk behaviors	Fever, lymphadenopathy	HIV antibody test
Hepatitis	Maternal history or risk factors for hepatitis	Jaundice, hepatomegaly	LFTs, hepatitis serology
Immunologic deficiency	Frequent infections	Lymphadenopathy	CBC, quantitative serum IgG, IgM, IgA
Metabolic			
Inborn errors of metabolism	Lethargy	May be normal	Newborn screen

(*Continued*)

TABLE 25–1. (*Continued*)

Cause	History	Signs	Laboratory Tests
Congenital			
Chromosomal abnormalities Turner syndrome Down syndrome	Advanced maternal age, loose neck skin, and hand puffiness	Dysmorphic features such as short/webbed neck, cubitus valgus, epicanthal folds, simian crease	Chromosomes
Skeletal dysplasias	Positive family history	Short extremities, trident hands	Pelvic, lumbar, extremity x-rays
Congenital syndromes Fetal alcohol syndrome	Maternal history of alcohol ingestion or drug use, delayed development	Symmetric FTT, short palpebral fissures, epicanthal folds, maxillary hypoplasia, micrognathia	None
Miscellaneous			
Malignancy	Fever, fatigue	Lymphadenopathy, tumors	CBC, ESR
Drugs or toxins Lead poisoning Accidental intake	Exposure to lead paint, medication errors	May be normal	Lead levels, toxicology screen
Nutritional deficiencies Iron deficiency Zinc deficiency	Exclusive breast-feeding, unsupplemented formula	Pallor, dermatitis	CBC
Vitamin D deficiency (rickets)	Exclusive breast-feeding, no exposure to sunlight	Large fontanelle, bony deformities	X-rays, calcium, alkaline phosphatase
Connective tissue disease	Fever, arthralgia, myalgia	Arthritis, rash, myositis	ESR, CBC, ANA
Normal variants			
Familial short stature	Short members of family	Symmetric FTT (see Section IV.B.2), normal examination	Bone age x-rays
Constitutional delay of growth	Family history of late puberty	Symmetric FTT, normal examination, delayed puberty	Bone age x-rays
Intrauterine growth retardation	Small for gestational age at birth or prematurity	Hepatosplenomegaly, chorioretinitis	Viral antibody titers, urine for CMV

ACTH, adrenocorticotropic hormone; ANA, antinuclear antibody; BUN, blood urea nitrogen; CBC, complete blood count; CMV, cytomegalovirus; CT, computerized tomography; CXR, chest radiograph; ECG, electrocardiogram; ESR, erythrocyte sedimentation rate; FTT, failure to thrive; HIV, human immunodeficiency virus; KUB, kidney/ureter/bladder (abdominal plain radiograph); LFTs, liver function tests; MRI, magnetic resonance imaging; PTH, parathyroid hormone; PPD, purified protein derivative (TB test); TSH, thyroid-stimulating hormone; UA, urinalysis; US, ultrasound; UTI, urinary tract infection.

FTT must be distinguished from the following normal variants, in which growth failure is usually symmetric (see description below):

1. **Familial short stature,** in which growth deceleration represents a physiologic adjustment for the child's growth potential. Approximately 25% of normal babies have a downward shift in the first 2 years. Calculation of the midparental height (see sidebar) can be helpful in establishing a child's growth potential.

MIDPARENTAL HEIGHT

Girls:

$$\frac{\text{Father's height } + \text{ Mother's height } - 13 \text{ cm [5 inch]}}{2}$$

Boys:

$$\frac{\text{Father's height } + \text{ Mother's height } + 13 \text{ cm [5 inch]}}{2}$$

Familial short stature can be diagnosed when
   a. there is a proportional decrease in weight and length;
   b. bone age is consistent with chronological age;
   c. there is a family history of short stature;
   d. the child maintains a normal annual growth rate without further deceleration.
2. **Constitutional growth delay** occurs when growth decelerates in the first 3 years of life, followed by stabilization on a new growth curve until adolescence, when a growth spurt occurs. Constitutional growth delay is suspected in the following conditions:
   a. Weight and height are proportionally decreased.
   b. Bone age is less than chronological age. There may be a 2- to 3-year delay in skeletal maturation.
   c. There is a family history of a parent or sibling with a similar growth pattern.
   d. A work-up does not reveal inadequate intake, or any other cause of growth delay.
3. **Intrauterine growth retardation** is failure of intrauterine growth because of prenatal factors and not genetic predisposition.
   a. These infants are easily identified by their birth weight below the fifth percentile, or less than 2500 g.
   b. Many of these infants catch up to their peers within the first 6 months, but growth may be slow for the first several years.
   c. Careful monitoring over time should show an improvement in growth. Low-birth-weight infants should double their birth weight by age 4 months and triple it by 1 year.
   d. Very low-birth-weight infants (weighing less than 1500 g), owing to prematurity, should be followed up on a specific very-low-birth-weight graph, with postnatal age adjusted for gestational age.

III. **Symptoms.** A thorough history should be elicited in poorly growing children, including the following specific areas (see Table 25–1):
   A. **Feeding history.** Query method, breast-feeding patterns, engorgement and letdown, frequency, quantity, formula preparation, length and quality of feeding time, feeding techniques, and personal and cultural beliefs about food and feeding.
   B. **Dietary history.** Query 24-hour recall or 72-hour food diary.
   C. **Past medical history.** Query birth weight, prenatal and birth history, illnesses, and hospitalizations.
   D. **Developmental history.** Query gross and fine motor milestones, language milestones, behavior, and temperament.
   E. **Social history.** Query living situation, financial constraints, family stressors, parental employment, parental substance abuse, and domestic violence or abuse.
   F. **Family history.** Query mental illness in the family (especially maternal depression), childhood illnesses, mental retardation, genetic abnormalities, history of growth delays in parents or siblings, and midparental height.
   G. **Review of systems.** Query vomiting, spitting up, choking, diarrhea, dyspnea, and tachypnea.

IV. **Signs** (Table 25–1)
   A. A careful examination may identify physical findings that provide clues to the cause of FTT in children and should include the following:
      1. Accurate measurements and plotting of weight, height, and head circumference. Measurement or plotting errors can give the appearance of FTT, or delay the diagnosis. Therefore, the first step in the diagnosis should be to recheck the child's measurements and re-plot them on the growth curve.
      2. General appearance and vital signs.
      3. Dysmorphic features or structural anomalies.
      4. Signs of abuse or neglect.
      5. Cardiac, respiratory, and gastrointestinal findings and checking of the oropharynx and lymph nodes.
      6. Neurologic examination.
   B. Patterns of growth may provide helpful clues to diagnosis.
      1. **Asymmetric FTT,** in which the head circumference is preserved, is generally because of psychosocial factors or a systemic illness. In severe FTT, the height may also be decreased.

2. **Symmetric FTT,** in which weight, height, and head circumference are proportional, may represent a normal variant or a primary central nervous system disorder.

3. **Isolated short stature,** where the weight is preserved, is likely to represent an endocrine or genetic disorder.

V. **Laboratory Tests** (Table 25–1). No routine laboratory tests are indicated in the child with FTT, (SOR **B**) as only approximately 1% of all laboratory tests ordered in a typical FTT work-up provide useful information. Investigations should be guided by the history and physical examination, as well as response to nutrition intervention.

VI. **Treatment.** FTT must be recognized and treated promptly. Treatment must be individualized for each child according to the medical, family, social, and psychological risk factors identified. A multidisciplinary approach is ideal.

   A. Treatment goals:

      1. Identify and treat any underlying disorder.

      2. Provide a high calorie diet for catch-up growth.

         a. High-calorie concentrated formula, or addition of rice cereal or supplements to usual diet, to provide 150% the recommended daily calories.

CALORIE REQUIREMENTS FOR CATCH-UP GROWTH IN kcal/kg

$$\text{RDA kcal/kg weight} = \frac{\text{Age} \times \text{Ideal (median) weight for age in kg}}{\text{Actual weight}}$$

         b. The child may also benefit from a multivitamin with iron and zinc. (SOR **B**)

      3. Close follow-up based on the child's age and severity of growth failure. Several weeks of refeeding may be necessary to demonstrate weight gain, and it may take several months for the child to return to their baseline growth curve.

      4. A multidisciplinary approach to support and educate the family. The team may include the primary care physician, specialist, dietician, social worker, speech pathologist, occupational therapist, psychologist, and social service agencies. The treatment plan should be realistic and sensitive to ethnocultural differences and the feelings of the family.

      5. Hospitalization is rarely indicated, but may be necessary if:

         a. There is evidence of, or high risk for, physical abuse or severe neglect.

         b. The child is severely malnourished or medically unstable.

         c. Outpatient management has failed to demonstrate any appreciable improvement.

VII. **Prognosis.** There appears to be long-term effects on physical, cognitive, and behavioral development for children diagnosed with FTT. These effects are significantly confounded by other risk factors, and seem to diminish with age. It is unclear whether severity or timing of growth failure affects outcomes, and it is difficult to sort out the causes of FTT from the long-term effects.

REFERENCES

Corbett SS, Drewett RF. To what extent is failure to thrive in infancy associated with poorer cognitive development? A review and meta-analysis. *J Child Psychol Psychiatry.* 2004;45(3):641-654.

Jolley CD. Failure to thrive. *Curr Probl Pediatr Adolesc Health Care.* 2003;33:183-206.

Krugman SD, Dubowitz H. Failure to thrive. *Am Fam Physician.* 2003;68(5):879-884.

Rudolph CD et al. Failure to thrive. In: Rudolph AM, Rudolph CD, eds. *Rudolph's Pediatrics.* 21st ed. New York, NY: McGraw-Hill; 2003:7-12.

Samuels RC, Cohen LE. Understanding growth patterns in short stature. *Contemp Pediatr.* 2001; 18(6):94-112.

26   Fatigue

Anthony F. Valdini, MD, MS

KEY POINTS

- The longer a person is fatigued, the more likely it is that a psychological problem is present.
- History and physical examination are much more likely to reveal the cause of fatigue than blind laboratory testing.
- Fatigue can be caused by physical, psychological, physiologic (appropriate, as in lack of sleep), or mixed etiologies. The mixed category is more common than once thought and may explain the difficulty in resolving the symptom.
- Just because an abnormality is discovered, it does not mean that the problem of fatigue is "solved." First, there is often more that one etiology to the complaint. Second, the abnormality discovered may be treated and resolved without changing the patient's complaint of fatigue.
- The majority of patients complaining of fatigue are depressed.

I. **Definition.** Fatigue is a subjective complaint of tiredness, weariness, or lack of energy.
II. **Common diagnoses.** Fatigue is the seventh most common symptom in primary care and accounts for more than 10 million office visits every year. Various studies have found the prevalence of fatigue in primary care to be between 10% and 20%. One group of investigators found that 6.7% of patients presenting to a family medicine clinic had a primary complaint of fatigue. Patients identified as fatigued visit the physician and are admitted to the hospital more often, incur greater charges for prescription medications, develop more new diagnoses, and have a greater proportion of their diagnoses containing a psychological component than do their non-fatigued counterparts. Fatigue may result from virtually every physical and psychological illness. Four major classes of fatigue that are useful in evaluating the tired patient are listed below.
   A. **Physiologic fatigue** is because of overwork, lack of sleep, or a defined physical stress, such as pregnancy. It can normally be expected in a mentally and physically healthy individual experiencing such stress. Females, as a group, work more hours in a day and more years in their lives than males and this may partially account for women visiting physicians more often for fatigue than men. Individuals with irregular or inadequate sleep patterns (including parents of young children), reducing diets, excessive or minimal exercise, or long hours spent commuting and working are at increased risk for physiologic fatigue.
   B. **Physical fatigue** is caused by infections, endocrine imbalances, cardiovascular disease, anemia, and medications (prescription, over-the-counter—OTC, alcohol, or other drugs of abuse); less commonly, cancer, connective tissue diseases, and other ailments cause physical fatigue.
   C. **Psychological illness,** including depression, anxiety, stress, and adjustment reaction, can cause fatigue. Children of alcoholics have an increased incidence of fatigue and depression.
   D. **"Mixed" fatigue,** which is often overlooked, involves any of the above categories occurring in combination.
III. **Symptoms (Table 26–1).**
   A. Fatigue lasting 1 month or less is commonly a result of physical causes; fatigue lasting 3 months or more is likely to be caused by psychological factors.
   B. **Fever, chills, sweats,** and **significant weight loss** are associated with infection and carcinoma.
   C. **Specific historical features** including endocrine and cardiovascular review of systems may indicate psychological, physical, or mixed origins of fatigue. Review of sleep, work, and travel history, in addition to physical functional capacity can help elucidate the cause of fatigue. Fatigue should be distinguished from weakness and hypersomnolence, which indicate a different origin, such as neuromuscular (e.g., myasthenia) or sleep disorder

TABLE 26-1. CHARACTERISTICS PROPOSED TO DISTINGUISH PSYCHOLOGICAL FATIGUE FROM PHYSICAL FATIGUE

Characteristic	Psychological	Physical
Duration	Chronic	Acute
Primary deficit	Desire	Ability
Onset	Stress related	Unrelated to stress
Diurnal pattern	Worse in morning	Worse in evening
Course	Fluctuates	Progressive
Effect of activity	Relieves	Worsens
Associated symptoms	Multiple and nonspecific	Few and specific
Previous problems	Functional	Organic
Family	Stressful	Supportive
Appearance	Anxious/depressed	Ill
Family history	Psychological/alcoholism	None
Placebo effect	Present	Absent
Effect of sleep	Unaffected/worsened	Relieved
Decreased ability to cope	No	Yes

Adapted with permission from Katerndahl DA. Differentiation of physical and psychological fatigue. *Fam Pract Res J.* 1993;13:82.

(obstructive sleep apnea, narcolepsy). The feature most solidly linked with physical versus psychological causes is the chronicity of fatigue; that is, acute fatigue is likely to be caused by physical or physiologic events, while chronic fatigue is associated with psychological and mixed causes. It has been reported that 69% to 80% of primary care patients with depression present with exclusive complaints related to a physical symptom, and that having five or more physical symptoms is an independent predictor of major depression.

D. **Chronic fatigue syndrome (CFS)** is a distinct diagnostic category. The International Chronic Fatigue Syndrome Study Group revised the 1988 case definition in 1994. It includes a duration of 6 months or longer, absence of an identified cause, and the presence of at least four specific symptoms (see Figure 26–1). Among the symptoms and signs associated with CFS, Komaroff and Buchwald (1991) found the following frequencies: low-grade fever (60%–95%), myalgias (20%–95%), sleep disorder (15%–90%), impaired cognition (50%–85%), depression (70%–85%), headaches (35%–85%), pharyngitis (50%–75%), anxiety (50%–70%), weakness (40%–70%), postexertional malaise (50%–60%), arthralgias (40%–50%), and painful lymph nodes (30%–40%). Despite the findings of "subtle and diffuse" immunologic abnormalities and possibly associated viruses—Epstein–Barr virus, enteroviruses, herpes virus type 6, retroviruses, and others—the syndrome remains enigmatic. Ambiguities in the 1994 case definition were addressed in the 2003 publication wherein the study group recommended use of several standardized instruments to quantify key symptom domains and disability.

   1. **Chronic idiopathic fatigue.** Not all patients with chronic fatigue symptoms meet the criteria for CFS. Persons tired for 6 months or longer for no apparent cause who do not meet CFS criteria for severity or specific symptoms after clinical evaluation are classified as having "chronic idiopathic fatigue."

   2. Most patients who are tired for more than 1 year have significant psychological problems.

      Because depression is the most common psychological cause of fatigue, and not all providers feel comfortable making the diagnosis, an instrument to measure depression (such as Beck's) may be useful (see Chapter 92).

IV. **Signs**

   A. The **physical causes** of acute fatigue (e.g., rales, edema, and gallops of congestive heart failure) may be obvious.

   B. **Subtle signs** of infections (e.g., lymphadenopathy or temperature elevation), connective tissue disease (e.g., extra-articular manifestations), and cancer should not be overlooked.

V. **Laboratory Tests (Figure 26–2).** Laboratory investigation based on signs will be more productive than screening based on the complaint of fatigue alone. (SOR **A**) The patient often needs the reassurance of a laboratory investigation. The clinician should bear in mind, however, that laboratory investigations of persons fatigued for more than 1 year have been remarkably unproductive.

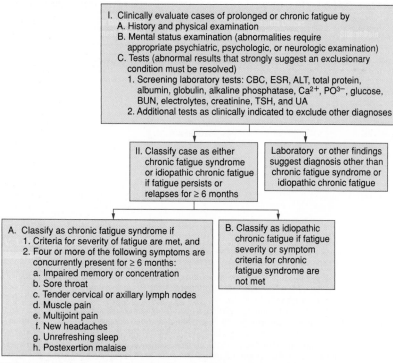

I. Clinically evaluate cases of prolonged or chronic fatigue by
   A. History and physical examination
   B. Mental status examination (abnormalities require appropriate psychiatric, psychologic, or neurologic examination)
   C. Tests (abnormal results that strongly suggest an exclusionary condition must be resolved)
      1. Screening laboratory tests: CBC, ESR, ALT, total protein, albumin, globulin, alkaline phosphatase, Ca^{2+}, PO^{3-}, glucose, BUN, electrolytes, creatinine, TSH, and UA
      2. Additional tests as clinically indicated to exclude other diagnoses

II. Classify case as either chronic fatigue syndrome or idiopathic chronic fatigue if fatigue persists or relapses for ≥ 6 months

Laboratory or other findings suggest diagnosis other than chronic fatigue syndrome or idiopathic chronic fatigue

A. Classify as chronic fatigue syndrome if
   1. Criteria for severity of fatigue are met, and
   2. Four or more of the following symptoms are concurrently present for ≥ 6 months:
      a. Impaired memory or concentration
      b. Sore throat
      c. Tender cervical or axillary lymph nodes
      d. Muscle pain
      e. Multijoint pain
      f. New headaches
      g. Unrefreshing sleep
      h. Postexertion malaise

B. Classify as idiopathic chronic fatigue if fatigue severity or symptom criteria for chronic fatigue syndrome are not met

FIGURE 26–1. International Chronic Fatigue Syndrome Study Group recommendations for evaluation and classification of unexplained chronic fatigue. ALT, alanine aminotransferase; BUN, blood urea nitrogen; CBC, complete blood cell count; ESR, erythrocyte sedimentation rate; po₄, phosphorus; TSH, thyroid-stimulating hormone; UA, urinalysis. (Adapted with permission from Fukada K, Strauss SE, Hickie I, et al.; and the International Chronic Fatigue Syndrome Study Group. The chronic fatigue syndrome: A comprehensive approach to its definition and study. *Ann Intern Med.* 1994;121:953-9.)

  A. Since the most common physical causes of fatigue are infectious (viral infections are the most common), endocrine (thyroid disease and diabetes mellitus predominate), and cardiovascular, (SOR **A**) a level 1 laboratory evaluation would consist of the following tests **(Figure 26–2).**
   1. **Complete blood cell count** with differential, **sedimentation rate, urinalysis,** and **chemistry panel** (e.g., SMA-23).
   2. **Thyroid panel.**
   3. **Pregnancy testing** in females of childbearing age.
   4. **Appropriate cancer screening for age/gender. (USPHS Task Force guidelines). Cancer screening tests will rarely reveal the cause of fatigue, yet they can be reassuring to the patient and physician, and should be a part of a thorough evaluation.**
  B. A **second-level investigation** is rarely useful, but such an evaluation would include the following tests.
   1. **Chest x-ray** for adenopathy, signs of congestive heart failure, pulmonary infections, and tumors.
   2. **Electrocardiogram** to look for silent infarction or ischemia.
   3. **Serologies** (rheumatoid factor, ANA, anti-Ro, and anti-La) to test for connective tissue diseases presenting with fatigue.
   4. A **drug screen** for unreported drug (including alcohol) use can occasionally be productive.

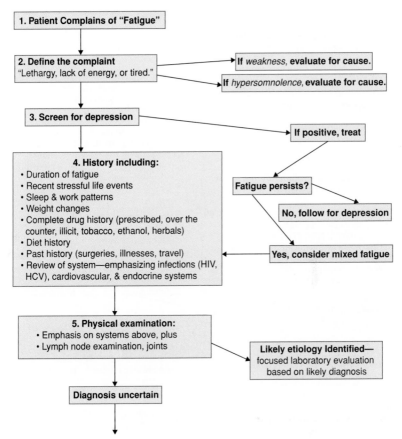

FIGURE 26–2. Evaluation of patient with fatigue. ANA, anti-nuclear antibody; CHF, congestive heart failure; HIV, human immunodeficiency virus; HCV, hepatitis C virus; PPD, purified protein derivative; VDRL, venereal disease research laboratory test. (*Continued*)

5. In appropriate patients and geographic areas, **hepatitis C antibodies, human immunodeficiency virus tests, skin tests for tuberculosis** with controls, **Lyme titers,** and **VDRL tests** should be performed.
C. **Third-level testing** for uncommon causes of fatigue prompted by specific suspicion or sign (e.g., for Addison disease, multiple sclerosis, myasthenia gravis, and poisoning) is best considered last, since these problems represent uncommon causes of fatigue.
D. **Abnormal laboratory findings.** Treatment of the underlying condition until the laboratory abnormality resolves is necessary to determine whether it represented the cause of the fatigue. One should be prepared to resume the search for a cause if a particular laboratory value returns to normal but the patient's condition does not.
VI. **Treatment**
   A. **Etiology identified.** Specific treatments for defined physical and psychological causes should be administered when possible.
   B. **Etiology undetermined**
      1. **Behavioral treatment.** Despite intensive investigation and follow-up, the cause of chronic fatigue often remains undetermined. In such a case, cognitive behavioral

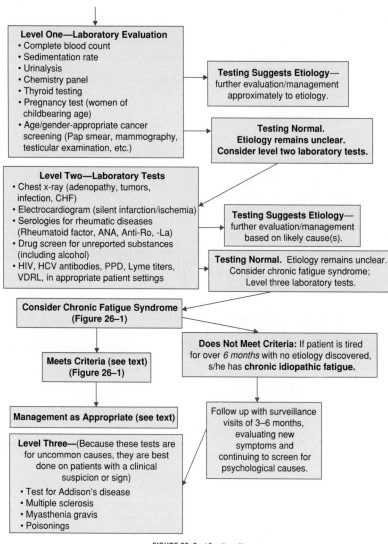

Level One—Laboratory Evaluation
• Complete blood count
• Sedimentation rate
• Urinalysis
• Chemistry panel
• Thyroid testing
• Pregnancy test (women of childbearing age)
• Age/gender-appropriate cancer screening (Pap smear, mammography, testicular examination, etc.)

Testing Suggests Etiology— further evaluation/management approximately to etiology.

Testing Normal.
Etiology remains unclear.
Consider level two laboratory tests.

Level Two—Laboratory Tests
• Chest x-ray (adenopathy, tumors, infection, CHF)
• Electrocardiogram (silent infarction/ischemia)
• Serologies for rheumatic diseases (Rheumatoid factor, ANA, Anti-Ro, -La)
• Drug screen for unreported substances (including alcohol)
• HIV, HCV antibodies, PPD, Lyme titers, VDRL, in appropriate patient settings

Testing Suggests Etiology— further evaluation/management based on likely cause(s).

Testing Normal. Etiology remains unclear. Consider chronic fatigue syndrome; Level three laboratory tests.

Consider Chronic Fatigue Syndrome (Figure 26–1)

Does Not Meet Criteria: If patient is tired for over *6 months* with no etiology discovered, s/he has **chronic idiopathic fatigue.**

Meets Criteria (see text) (Figure 26–1)

Management as Appropriate (see text)

Follow up with surveillance visits of 3–6 months, evaluating new symptoms and continuing to screen for psychological causes.

Level Three—(Because these tests are for uncommon causes, they are best done on patients with a clinical suspicion or sign)
• Test for Addison's disease
• Multiple sclerosis
• Myasthenia gravis
• Poisonings

FIGURE 26–2. (*Continued*)

therapy, and graded exercise programs have often been shown to be effective. (SOR **Ⓐ**) Additionally, group therapy may provide the patient with some solace. These modalities should be offered to all fatigued patients whose problems do not resolve with more specific treatment.

2. **Drug therapy.** A host of medications have been used with limited success to provide relief from fatigue of unknown origin. A partial list includes vitamins, thyroid supplementation (for subclinical hypothyroidism), growth hormone, amphetamines, pemoline, modafinil, and hydrocortisone. The use of any medication for treatment of a symptom without a specific, identified cause is problematic. However, the likelihood of

depression or fibromyalgia causing fatigue in persons with no obvious cause probably warrants a 2-month therapeutic trial of antidepressants.

3. **Diet therapy.** Several unproven diets have been proposed. Although fatigue has been associated with a body mass index of 40 or greater, it is not certain that weight loss will alleviate fatigue in greatly obese persons. Nevertheless, achieving and maintaining ideal body weight through balanced nutrition is recommended for general health and may be helpful in fatigued patients.

4. **Complementary/alternative medical therapy (CAM).** While studies of CAM therapies have not, as yet, provided significant positive benefit, there have been no reports of adverse effects on fatigued patients using CAM. The use of CAM for fatigued patients is empirical.

5. **Patient follow-up.** It is not known exactly how often the fatigued patient should return to the physician. A few bimonthly visits early in the investigation of the complaint will serve to cement the patient–physician relationship and establish good faith. Regularly scheduled visits, even as seldom as twice a year, remind the patient that they are not adrift and that changes in the patient's condition will receive serious consideration. At each visit, a review of physical, environmental, and psychological symptoms and signs should be conducted. Physician support, reassurance, and follow-up are important for the patient whose fatigue appears to have no clear cause.

The natural history of the complaint, "fatigue," was explored in a series in which 73 fatigued and 72 nonfatigued subjects were reevaluated using Rand Index of Vitality scores. After 1 year, 41% of the fatigued patients were no longer fatigued, and 15 of the 72 nonfatigued subjects had become fatigued. The difference in improvement between fatigued patients with physical diagnoses and those with psychological diagnoses was not significant. When patients are classified as CFS they can improve with therapy but their prospects for complete resolution are less than with the general population complaining of fatigue.

REFERENCES

Komaroff AL, Buchwald D. Symptoms and signs of chronic fatigue syndrome. *Rev Infect Dis.* 1991; 13(Suppl 1):S8-11.

Kroenke K, Wood Dr, Mangelsdorff AD, Meier NJ, Powell JB. Chronic fatigue in primary care. Prevalence, patient characteristics and outcome. *JAMA.* 1988;260:929-34.

Fukada K, Strauss SE, Hickie I, Sharpe MC, Dobbins JG, Komaroff A. The chronic fatigue syndrome: A comprehensive approach to its definition and study. *Ann Intern Med.* 1994;121:953-9.

Reeves WC, Lloyd A, Vernon SD, et al.; and the International Chronic Fatigue Syndrome Study Group. Identification of ambiguities in the 1994 chronic fatigue syndrome research case definition and recommendations for resolution. http://www.biomedcentral.com/1472–6963/3/25. Accessed September 15, 2008.

Whiting P, Gagnall AM, Sowden AJ, et al. Interventions for the treatment and management of the Chronic Fatigue Syndrome. *JAMA.* 2001;286:1360-1368.

---

27   Fluid, Electrolyte, & Acid–Base Disturbances

Lara Carson Weinstein, MD, & Marc Altshuler, MD

KEY POINTS

- In the ambulatory care setting, fluid, electrolyte, and acid-base disturbances often present initially as abnormal chemical screening panels in patients with known chronic disease, new medications, previously undiagnosed endocrine disorders, or acute gastrointestinal illnesses.
- Disorders of salt and water balance are exceedingly common in geriatric patients.
- Primary hyperparathyroidism is the most common cause of outpatient hypercalcemia and is often diagnosed through incidental hypercalcemia noted on routine screening.

I. Definition and Common Diagnoses

A. **Decreases in effective circulating volume** commonly occur from **gastrointestinal (GI) losses** (vomiting, diarrhea); **loss through skin** (sweating, fever); **renal losses** (diuretics, interstitial renal disease); and **third-space accumulations** (pharmaceutical excess vasodilatation, pancreatitis). **Expansion of interstitial volume** causes edema. The most common edematous conditions seen in the outpatient setting result from congestive heart failure. Edema is also seen in cirrhosis, renal failure, and the nephrotic syndrome.

  1. **Hyponatremia,** serum sodium ≤135 mmol/L, can be characterized by osmolar and volume status. In most cases, hyponatremia is hypo-osmolar.

  a. Hypo-osmolar hypervolemic hyponatremia occurs in patients with congestive heart failure, liver disease, chronic renal failure, or pregnancy.

  b. Hypo-osmolar euvolemic hyponatremia occurs with hypothyroidism, primary polydipsia, and adrenal insufficiency. However, the most common cause is the syndrome of inappropriate secretion of antidiuretic hormone (SIADH). SIADH can be caused by malignancy (i.e., small cell lung cancer), pulmonary disease (i.e., legionella pneumonia), CNS disease (trauma, infection, tumors), or medications (selective serotonin reuptake inhibitors [SSRIs], tricyclics, carbamazepine, metformin, theophylline)

  c. Hypo-osmolar hypovolemic hyponatremia, from decreased real or effective circulating volume, commonly occurs in the outpatieint setting from diuretic use. It is also seen with other renal losses (osmotic diuresis, diabetes insipidus), GI losses (diarrhea, vomiting), severe burns, or sequestration without actual loss (e.g., intestinal obstruction, pancreatitis, peritonitis).

  d. Hyperosmolar hyponatremia is classically seen with severe hyperglycemia.

  e. Iso-osmolar hyponatremia occurs with severe hypertriglyceridemia or paraproteinemia (pseudohyponatremia), or in the post-transurethral prostatic resection syndrome; when massive volumes of a sodium-free irrigant (such as glycine) are systemically absorbed intraoperatively, causing dilutional hyponatremia

  2. **Hypernatremia** is serum sodium ≥145 mmol/L. Hypernatremia results from a relative water deficit or, less commonly, from a primary sodium gain. Risk factors for hypernatremia include: extremes of age, impaired thirst mechanism, and use of medications that can cause nephrogenic diabetes insipidus (DI) (i.e., lithium)

  3. **Hypokalemia,** plasma potassium ≤3.5 mmol/L, most commonly occurs with diuretic use, and GI losses (i.e., large volume diarrhea, eating disorders with laxative use, and vomiting). Other medications that can cause transcellular potassium shifts include: ß2 sympathomimetic agonists, theophylline, and insulin. Less common causes include: primary and secondary hyperaldosteronism, and type I and II renal tubular acidoisis.

  4. **Hyperkalemia,** plasma potassium ≥5 mmol/L, occurs with impaired renal excretion of potassium, or by a shift of potassium into the extracellular space. Hyperkalemia is commonly seen in chronic renal failure, often with medications (e.g., potassium-sparing diuretics, angiotensin-converting enzyme inhibitors, nonsteroidal anti-inflammatory drugs) that interfere with potassium excretion. It can also occur in adrenal insufficiency, acidosis, uncontrolled diabetes, or ingestion of potassium supplements. Pseudohyperkalemia occurs with blood sample hemolysis.

  5. **Hypocalcemia,** serum calcium of ≤8 mg/dL (ionized calcium ≤4 mg/dL), occurs in chronic renal failure, acute pancreatitis, widespread osteoblastic metastases, hypoparathyroidism, or "hungry bone syndrome" following thyroid or parathyroid surgery, vitamin D deficiency, alcoholism, and premature/low birth weight infants.

  6. **Hypercalcemia** is serum calcium ≥10 mg/dL (ionized calcium ≥5.6 mg/dL). Primary hyperparathyroidism or malignancy cause more than 90% of hypercalcemia. Primary hyperparathyroidism occurs in 1/500 elderly women. Rare causes of hypercalcemia include sarcoidosis, hyperthyroidism, lithium use, and the milk–alkali syndrome.

B. Common causes and mechanisms of **primary acid-base disorders** are outlined in Figure 27–1.

II. Symptoms associated with fluid, electrolyte, and acid-base disorders are subtle, nonspecific, and less sensitive than laboratory testing in detecting these disorders. Symptoms are more likely with large or rapid shifts in fluid, electrolyte, or acid-base status. The most common symptoms include lethargy, fatigue/weakness, or irritability.

A. **Seizures** can occur with severe hyponatemia, hypernatremia, or hypocalcemia.

B. **Severe muscle weakness** can occur with hyperkalemia.

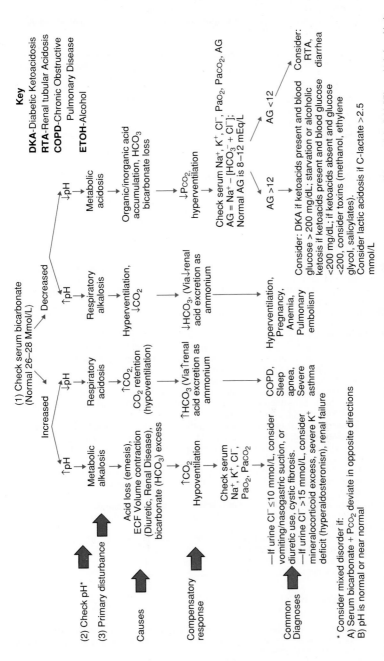

Key
DKA-Diabetic Ketoacidosis
RTA-Renal tubular Acidosis
COPD-Chronic Obstructive
Pulmonary Disease
ETOH-Alcohol

(1) Check serum bicarbonate
(Normal 26–28 Mmol/L)

Increased / Decreased

(2) Check pH*

(3) Primary disturbance

↑pH — Metabolic alkalosis
↓pH — Respiratory acidosis
↓pH — Respiratory alkalosis
↓pH — Metabolic acidosis

Causes

Acid loss (emesis), ECF Volume contraction (Diuretic, Renal Disease), bicarbonate (HCO₃) excess

↑CO_2, CO_2 retention (hypoventilation)

Hyperventilation, ↓CO_2

Organic/inorganic acid accumulation, HCO₃ bicarbonate loss

Compensatory response

↑CO_2 Hypoventilation

↑HCO₃, (Via↑renal acid excretion as ammonium)

↓HCO₃, (Via↓renal acid excretion as ammonium)

↓Pco_2, hyperventilation

Check serum Na⁺, K⁺, Cl⁻, Pao₂, Paco₂

COPD, Sleep apnea, Severe asthma

Hyperventilation, Pregnancy, Anemia, Pulmonary embolism

Check serum Na⁺, K⁺, Cl⁻, Pao₂, Paco₂, AG
$AG = Na^+ - [HCO_3^- + Cl^-]$;
Normal AG is 8–12 mEq/L

AG >12 / AG <12

Consider: RTA, diarrhea

Common Diagnoses

—If urine Cl⁻ ≤10 mmol/L, consider vomiting/nasogastric suction, or diuretic use, cystic fibrosis.
—If urine Cl⁻ >15 mmol/L, consider mineralocorticoid excess, severe K⁺ deficit (hyperaldosteronisn), renal failure

Consider: DKA if ketoacids present and blood glucose > 200 mg/dL; starvation or alcoholic ketosis if ketoacids present and blood glucose <200 mg/dL; if ketoacids absent and glucose <200, consider toxins (methanol, ethylene glycol, salicylates).
Consider lactic acidosis if C-lactate >2.5 mmol/L

* Consider mixed disorder if:
A) Serum bicarbonate + Pco₂ deviate in opposite directions
B) pH is normal or near normal

FIGURE 27–1. Overview of acid-base disorders. AG, anion gap; COPD, chronic obstructive pulmonary disease; DKA, diabetic ketoacidosis; ECF, extracellular fluid; RTA, renal tubular acidosis.

    C. Hypercalcemia is associated with a symptom complex including anorexia/nausea/vomiting, constipation, nephrolithiasis, confusion, and polyuria.

    D. Respiratory alkalosis/hyperventilation is associated with irritability, paresthesias, muscle cramps, and lightheadedness.

    E. Vomiting suggests metabolic alkalosis.

III. **Signs** of common fluid, electrolyte, and acid-base disorders are also less sensitive/specific in diagnosis than laboratory testing; findings associated with particular disorders include the following:

    A. Spasticity, muscle twitching, and hyperreflexia are seen in chronic **hypernatremia.**

    B. Chvostek's sign (facial muscle twitching when the facial nerve is tapped anterior to the ear) occurs with **hypocalcemia.**

    C. Ectopic soft tissue calcifications may be seen with hypercalcemia.

    D. Anxiety and tachypnea may be seen in **respiratory alkalosis** or **acidosis.**

IV. **Laboratory Tests.** Focused **laboratory evaluation** should be based on risk factors/symptoms/signs and will clarify the cause of common fluid/electrolyte and acid-base disorders (Figures 27–1 to 27–4).

    A. In patients with **hyper-** or **hypokalemia,** testing includes: serum electrolytes, creatinine; blood urea nitrogen; glucose; arterial blood gas (ABG); spot urine measurement of sodium, potassium, chloride, creatinine; and electrocardiography (ECG),

        1. In **hypokalemia,** ECG may show flat or inverted T waves, U-wave formation, and ST-segment depression; urine potassium excretion and acid-base status should also be assessed.

        2. In **hyperkalemia,** ECG shows peaked T waves, progressing to QRS widening and eventually ventricular fibrillation.

    B. With **hypocalcemia,** serum ionized (free) calcium, phosphorus, magnesium, chloride, parathyroid hormone, and 25-hydroxyvitamin D levels should be checked.

    C. With **respiratory alkalosis,** flattening or inversion of ECG ST-segments may occur because of hypocapnia.

V. **Treatment** is directed at correcting underlying causes along with identified fluid, electrolyte, and acid-base abnormalities.

    A. Hyponatremia

        1. Fluid replacement in the setting of hyponatremia must be done with caution, the risk of hyponatremia-related cerebral edema must be balanced with the risk of the osmotic demylination syndrome (ODS) from overzealous correction (especially in the setting of chronic, i.e., ≥48 hours, hyponatremia). (SOR **B**) Hypovolemic patients with mild symptoms and chronic hyponatremia may be treated in the hospital setting with 0.9% saline to increase the serum sodium by 0.5 mEq/L/h, with a maximum sodium increase of 10 to 12 mEq/L over 24 hours.

        2. Severe acute hyponatremia with significant neurologic symptoms (i.e., seizures) requires hospitalization with administration of 3% saline intravenously for the first 3 to 4 hours to raise serum sodium concentration at a rate of 1 to 2 mEq/L/h to a goal of 120 mEq/L. (SOR **B**)

        3. Use of an angiotensin-converting enzyme inhibitor, along with fluid and sodium restriction is beneficial in treatment of hyponatremia associated with congestive heart failure.

        4. Syndrome of inappropriate antidiuretic hormone release (SIADH) is treated with water restriction (1000–1500 mL/d) pending correction of the underlying cause.

    B. Hypernatremia

        1. General treatment principles consist of replacing free water; with hypovolemia, volume must be corrected in the hospital setting with initially with isotonic 0.9% saline until the patient is hemodynamically stable.

        a. Water deficit (WD) can be calculated as follows:

$$WD = TBW \times \left(\frac{Plasma\ Na}{140} - 1 \right),$$

        where TBW is total body water. TBW = 0.6 (weight in kg) pediatrics; 0.6 (weight in kg) males; 0.5 (weight in kg) females; 0.5 (weight in kg) elderly males; 0.45 (weight in kg) elderly females.

        b. In general, no more than 50% of the water deficit along with any ongoing losses should be corrected in the first 24 hours, and the remainder over the next 1 to

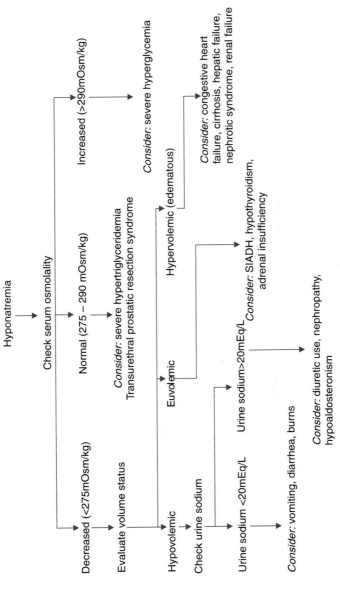

FIGURE 27-2. Evaluation of hyponatremia. SIADH, syndrome of inappropriate antidiuretic hormone release.

177

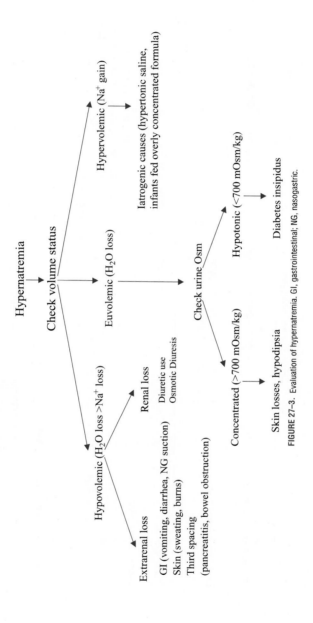

FIGURE 27-3. Evaluation of hypernatremia. GI, gastrointestinal; NG, nasogastric.

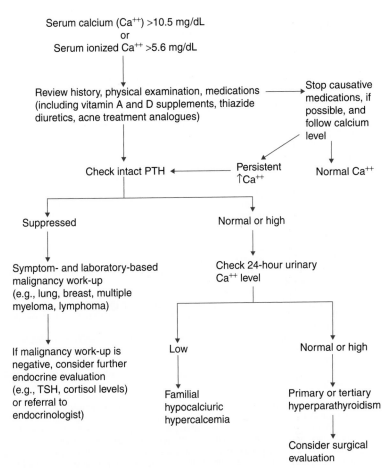

FIGURE 27–4. Evaluation of hypercalcemia. PTH, parathyroid hormone; TSH, thyroid-stimulating hormone. (Adapted with permission from Carroll MF. A practical approach to hypercalcemia. *Am Fam Physician.* 2003;67:1959. Copyright © 2003 American Academy of Family Physicians. All Rights Reserved.)

2 days. To avoid cerebral edema, the serum sodium should be lowered by 0.5 to 1 mEg/L/h, with a maximum decrease of 10 to 12 mEq/L in 24 hours. Initially, free water and volume can be replaced intravenously if necessary. To prevent recurrences, the patient may be given a fluid prescription quantifying recommended daily fluid ingestion.

2. **Central diabetes insipidus** should be treated with desmopressin, starting with 5 μg intranasally per day.
3. **Nephrogenic diabetes insipidus** is managed by treating the underlying disorder.

C. **Hypokalemia**

1. Patients taking **thiazide or loop diuretics** generally require 20 to 60 mEq/d of potassium.

   a. They should be encouraged to increase dietary potassium because this is the safest and least expensive means of supplementation.

   b. If hypokalemia persists, addition of a potassium supplement (e.g., potassium chloride), starting at 20 mEq/d, or potassium-sparing diuretic (e.g., spironolactone) may be considered. Potassium levels require regular monitoring, and this should be initially done weekly, then every 2 to 4 weeks until stable. Patients with chronic renal insufficiency require closer monitoring.

   2. Moderate to **severe hypokalemia ($\leq$3.0 mEq/L)** requires more urgent potassium replacement and management in a hospital setting.

D. Hyperkalemia

   1. Office management of **mild hyperkalemia ($\leq$6 mEq/L)** involves dietary potassium restriction in renal insufficiency and reevaluation of medications.

   2. **Severe hyperkalemia ($\geq$6 mEq/L)** with ECG changes, rapid onset, decreased renal function, or acidosis require urgent inpatient treatment. (SOR **C**) Intravenous calcium gluconate should be used to stabilize the myocardium in patients with ECG changes. (SOR **C**) Insulin and glucose, or a beta$_2$ agonist should be used to lower potassium acutely. (SOR **C**) Sodium polystyrene sulfonate (Kayexalate) can be used to decrease total body potassium. (SOR **C**)

E. Hypocalcemia. Treatment in the office of mild hypocalcemia (ionized calcium of 3.2–3.9 mg/dL) includes oral calcium supplementation (e.g., calcium carbonate, 1–2 g of elemental calcium per day).

   1. **Vitamin D supplementation** with vitamin D2 (ergocalciferol) or vitamin D analogue (e.g., calcitrol) is indicated, with dose depending on the underlying cause. 25-hydroxyvitamin D levels should be maintained above 32 ng/dL to preserve bone health. (SOR **C**)

      a. Severe vitamin D deficiency is treated with 50,000 IU vitamin D daily for 1 to 3 weeks, and then 50,00 IU weekly. (SOR **C**) Once stores have been repleted, maintenance therapy can be started with 800 IU vitamin D daily, or 50,00 IU once or twice a month. (SOR **C**)

      b. Patients with impaired vitamin D metabolism (e.g., chronic renal insufficiency and hypoparathyroidism) may benefit from **calcitrol, (SOR **C**)** 0.25 to 2 μg daily, generally in consultation with an endocrinologist, nephrologist, or both, with close monitoring to avoid hypercalcemia.

   2. **Vitamin D therapy** requires close laboratory monitoring to avoid hypercalciuria, hypercalcemia, and renal toxicity.

   3. **Hospitalization should be considered** for management of ionized calcium levels $\leq$3.2 mg/dL or with signs of neuromuscular irritability (Chvostek's sign or carpopedal spasm).

F. Hypercalcemia

   1. Patients with **serum calcium levels $\geq$13 mg/dL or severe symptoms** require hospitalization for evaluation and treatment. Initial treatment includes aggressive rehydration with normal saline to restore intravascular volume; this may be followed by IV furosemide and other therapies (i.e., calcitonin, bisphosphonates) as indicated.

   2. Patients with mild hypercalcemia ($\leq$13 mg/dL) of known etiology (i.e., known cancer diagnosis) may be treated as outpatients with oral rehydration and possible addition of a loop diuretic.

   3. Asymptomatic patients with primary hyperparathyroidism, who have normal renal and bone status, and only mildly elevated serum calcium, may be candidates for medical management with frequent monitoring. (SOR **C**)

   4. Referral to a neck surgeon for consideration of parathyroidectomy is appropriate in patients with primary hyperparathyroidism with nephrolitiasis, persistently increased serum calcium, hypercalcuria, osteoporosis, decreased creatinine clearance, age $\leq$ 50 years, limited medical surveillance, or patient request.

G. Metabolic acidosis and alkalosis

   1. **Metabolic acidosis** is managed by providing nutrition and rehydration for alcoholic or starvation ketosis (often in a hospital setting), eliminating suspect drugs, or treating underlying diabetes mellitus (Chapter 74), diarrhea (Chapter 16), or causes of lactic acidosis. Renal tubular acidosis should initially be evaluated and managed in consultation with a nephrologist. In addition, the body's compensatory mechanism for metabolic acidosis is to decrease PCO_2 through hyperventilation.

   2. **Metabolic alkalosis** management likewise depends on its cause. Suspected causative medications (e.g., diuretics) should be eliminated if possible, vomiting or nasogastric losses should be replaced (often in the inpatient setting), renal failure should be managed in consultation with nephrology, and mineralocorticoid excess (Cushing's syndrome, primary aldosteronism) should be managed by treating the underlying disease. In metabolic alkalosis, the body's compensatory mechanism is to increase PCO_2 through hypoventilation.

H. Respiratory acidosis is managed by correcting or stabilizing underlying pulmonary or metabolic disorders and improving ventilation. This may include controlling bronchospasm (Chapter 68) and congestive heart failure (Chapter 72). The body tries to reverse the acidosis by increasing HCO_3 through increased renal excretion as ammonium.

I. Respiratory alkalosis treatment also focuses on underlying disorders. For example, patients with symptomatic, anxiety-related hyperventilation may respond to rebreathing (e.g., breathing into a paper bag) when symptoms develop. The compensatory mechanism in respiratory alkalosis involves decreasing HCO_3 through decreased renal excretion as ammonium.

REFERENCES

Carroll MF, Schade DS. A Practical approach to hypocalcaemia. *Am Fam Physician*. 2003;67:1959-1966.

Goh KP. Management of hyponatremia. *Am Fam Physician*. 2004;69;2387-2394.

Higdon ML, Higdon JA. Treatment of oncologic emergencies. *Am Fam Physician*. 2006;74:1873-1880.

Hollander-Rodriguez JC. Hyperkalemia. *Am Fam Physician*. 2006;73:283-290.

Lin M, Liu SJ, Lim IT. Disorders of water imbalance. *Emerg Med Clin N Am*. 2005;23:749-770.

Lynman D. Undiagnosed vitamin D deficiency in the hospital patient. *Am Fam Physician*. 2005;71:299-304.

Sarko J. Bone and mineral metabolism. *Emerg Med Clin N Am*. 2005;23:703-721.

Schaefer TJ, Wolford RW. Disorders of potassium. *Emerg Med Clin N Am*. 2005;23:723-747.

Taniergra ED. Hyperparathyroidism. *Am Fam Physician*. 2004;69:333-339.

Whittier WL, Rutecki, GW. Primer on clinical acid-base problem solving. *Dis Mon*. 2004;50:117-162.

28   Foot Complaints

James R. Barrett, MD, CAQSM, & Kent W. Davidson, MD

KEY POINTS

- One should look for contributing factors, such as improper footwear, when evaluating foot pain since correcting these will decrease the chance of pain recurrence.
- Stress fractures are a common cause of foot pain and may have no initial x-ray findings. A high index of suspicion should be maintained.
- Four types of injuries need to be identified early to reduce morbidity and improve successful treatment: Achilles tendon rupture, Lisfranc injury, and fractures of the fifth metatarsal and navicular bones.

I. **Definition.** The foot, which has 26 bones and 55 articulations, acts as a platform and shock absorber to support the weight of the body as well as a powerful lever to propel the body. Foot complaints are usually related to overuse, trauma, or degenerative changes. Contributing factors include foot type—such as high arch (pes cavus) and flatfoot (pes planus)—foot deformities (i.e., hallux valgus); improper footwear; excessive weight; and underlying systemic diseases (i.e., diabetes or osteoporosis). The foot and ankle can have numerous accessory ossicles that can be confused with a possible fracture.

II. **Common Diagnoses.** Because of the amount of weight that the foot carries every day, it is little wonder that 18% of the population each year will have foot problems, an incidence that increases with age. Diagnosis can be facilitated by considering three distinct regions of the foot: the forefoot, the midfoot, and the hindfoot (Figure 28–1).

A. **Forefoot.** The forefoot, comprising the toes and metatarsals, is the most common site of foot complaints, with a prevalence of 2% to 10%. Most forefoot conditions are caused by poor shoe selection (tight toe boxes, high-heeled shoes); foot deformities (hallux valgus, hammer toes); overuse; or degenerative changes. Common conditions affecting the toes (followed by their prevalence) include calluses/corns (4.5%), plantar warts (2%), onychomycosis (10%), ingrown toenails (3%–5%), phalangeal fractures, and peripheral neuropathy. Common conditions affecting the metatarsals include bunions (hallux valgus) (1.8%), hallux limitus (2%), metatarsalgia, Morton's (interdigital) neuromas, fractures (stress and fifth metatarsal), and sesamoiditis.

B. **Midfoot.** Midfoot complaints, caused by degenerative changes, trauma, or foot deformity, are relatively uncommon but can lead to significant disability. Common conditions affecting the midfoot, which comprises the cuneiforms, cuboid, and navicular bones of the foot, include midfoot sprain, osteoarthritis, tarsal fractures, plantar fibromatosis, posterior tibialis dysfunction, and tarsal coalition. (Also see the sidebars for Lisfranc injury and tarsal navicular bone fractures.)

LISFRANC INJURY

Lisfranc injury is a severe form of midfoot sprain to the tarsometatarsal articulation and is frequently missed. Pain and swelling over the tarsometatarsal articulation and inability to bear weight on tiptoes are clues to the injury. Weight-bearing x-rays of the foot may show avulsed bone between the first and second metatarsals and loss of congruity between the first metatarsal and the first cuneiform, second metatarsal, or both and the second cuneiform. Computerized tomography of the foot may be necessary for diagnosis. Patients with this injury should be placed in a nonweight-bearing cast and referred to orthopedics.

TARSAL NAVICULAR BONE FRACTURES

Tarsal navicular bone fractures are easily missed, because patients may have minimal pain over the midfoot and medial arch; these fractures are important to diagnose early because navicular fractures have a high rate of nonunion. Examination reveals tenderness over the navicular bone and increased pain with hopping on the foot. Plain x-rays of the foot are often inconclusive; therefore, bone scan, computerized tomography, or magnetic resonance imaging may be necessary for diagnosis. Treatment of nondisplaced fractures involves a nonweight-bearing cast for 6 to 8 weeks. Displaced fractures require orthopedic consultation.

C. **Hindfoot.** Hindfoot conditions are the second most common type of foot complaint, with a prevalence of 1%. Common conditions affecting the hindfoot, which comprises the calcaneus and talus, include plantar fasciitis (0.4% prevalence), calcaneal stress fractures, Achilles tendinosis, and bursitis. Most hindfoot conditions are caused by overuse or excessive weight. (Also see the sidebar on Achilles tendon rupture.)

ACHILLES TENDON RUPTURE

Achilles tendon rupture usually causes acute pain in the posterior heel. Examination will often reveal swelling and ecchymosis over the posterior heel, a palpable defect of the Achilles tendon, inability to walk normally, and a positive Thompson test (no plantar flexion when the calf is squeezed). Treatment is usually surgical and warrants an urgent referral to orthopedics.

III. **Symptoms** (see Tables 28–1 to 28–3 and Figure 28–1).
IV. **Signs** (see Tables 28–1 to 28–3 and Figure 28–1).
V. **Laboratory Tests** (see Tables 28–1 to 28–3).
    A. Laboratory tests are generally not necessary in evaluating foot complaints. Atraumatic symmetric foot swelling and pain can be caused by systemic arthritis (such as rheumatoid arthritis and systemic lupus erythematosus) and should be evaluated with tests for sedimentation rate, complete blood count (CBC), rheumatoid factor, antinuclear antibody, and uric acid. Pain caused by peripheral neuropathy is evaluated with a CBC (pernicious anemia, lead poisoning), complete metabolic profile (diabetes, renal disease, liver

TABLE 28–1. EVALUATION AND MANAGEMENT OF COMMON FOREFOOT COMPLAINTS

Diagnosis	Symptoms	Findings	Testing	Treatment
Corn/callus	Pain with pressure on lesion	Skin thickening under bony prominence (calluses) or between toes (corns); tenderness with pressure directly over lesion	None	Paring of calluses* Padding§ Shoes with wide toe box
Plantar wart	Pain with pressure on lesion	Skin thickening or papules that interrupt skin lines and have blood vessels within core; tenderness on squeezing lesion	No routine testing but can do a biopsy for diagnosis	Observation (some spontaneously resolve within 6–12 mo) Wart removal
Onychomycosis (fungal toenail infection)	Thickened nail, occasionally painful	Thickened discolored nail, occasionally crumbles	KOH scraping Fungal culture from scraping	Trimming/thinning of nail Shoes with wide toe box Oral antifungals (SOR **Ⓑ**) Nail removal
Ingrown toenail (Onychocryptosis)	Pain, swelling, and discharge along border of nail	Nail border swollen, erythematous, occasional discharge	None	Ingrown toenail removal† If surrounding cellulitis, use antibiotic
Phalanx fracture	Acute pain and swelling of digit usually after trauma	Bony tenderness, swelling, ecchymosis, pain with toe motion	X-ray	Nondisplaced fracture: Buddy taping to adjacent toe, hard-soled shoe Displaced fracture: Referral to foot specialist
Peripheral neuropathy	Tingling, burning and/or pain initially in toes, then later in a stocking distribution, usually bilateral	May have decreased light touch, vibratory, and temperature sensation over toes. Sensation abnormalities tend to progress to involve entire foot with associated loss of motor strength in foot and loss of Achilles tendon reflex	Electromyography and nerve conduction velocity; laboratory tests to rule out underlying condition	Identify and treat underlying condition if present. Amitriptyline or gabapentin (SOR **Ⓐ**) Pregabalin and duloxetine are alternatives
Bunion or bunionette	Painful bony protuberance of first or fifth metatarsophalangeal joint (MTP)	Tender bony MTP prominence with valgus first MTP deformity (bunion) or varus fifth MTP deformity (bunionette)	X-ray reveals bony angular deformity (angle between first and second metatarsals ≥15 degrees, angle between fourth and fifth metatarsals ≥10 degrees)	Shoes with wide toe box Bunion shield Acetaminophen or NSAID Arch support orthotic Surgical removal if continued pain despite conservative treatment for 6–12 mo
Hallux limitus or hallux rigiditus	Pain and swelling with movement, especially at toe off stage of gait	Loss of motion of first metatarsal, pain with extension of first metatarsal	X-ray may show degenerative spurs and loss of joint space of first MTP	Padding§ Acetaminophen or NSAID Hard-soled shoes Surgery if severe pain despite conservative measures for 6–12 mo
Metatarsalgia	Pain at metatarsal heads	Tenderness on palpation of metatarsal heads	X-ray to rule out fracture, arthritis	Relative rest Padding§ Acetaminophen or NSAID
Morton's neuroma (interdigital)	Pain between metatarsal heads, numbness and tingling into toes, cramping of toes	Tenderness with squeezing metatarsal heads—occasionally accompanied by a click, fullness, or occasional soft tissue mass between metatarsal heads	None	Shoes with wide toe box; Morton's neuroma injection‡ If continued pain referral to foot specialist for excision (SOR **Ⓒ**)

(Continued)

TABLE 28–1. (*Continued*)

Diagnosis	Symptoms	Findings	Testing	Treatment
Metatarsal stress fracture	Pain and swelling over foot with activity, particularly during toe off stage of gait	Exquisite tenderness over metatarsal, occasional swelling and/or ecchymosis	X-ray findings may be absent; periosteal reaction, fracture line, or bony callous formation may be present. Consider bone scan or MRI if negative x-ray result and diagnosis in doubt	Relative rest Padding Short leg removable cast-brace, hard-soled shoe or short leg walking cast for 4–8 wk Orthopedic referral for fifth metatarsal stress fractures as healing is often delayed
Fifth metatarsal fracture	Pain over lateral foot	Tenderness to palpation of fifth metatarsal Swelling over lateral foot	X-ray to evaluate for avulsion fracture versus Jones fracture (Figure 28–2)	Avulsion fracture: Short leg walking cast or air stirrup for 4–6 wk; Jones fracture: Nonweight-bearing short leg cast until callous formation (3–6 wk), then short leg walking cast for 3–6 wk Orthopedic referral if nonunion after 3 mo, displaced fracture, stress fracture, or patient preference
Sesamoiditis	Pain in ball of foot (first MTP) with toe off stage of gait	Tenderness and swelling over plantar first MTP and just proximal to joint	X-ray to rule out sesamoid fracture	Padding§ Relative rest NSAID

*For **paring of calluses,** soak the feet in lukewarm soapy water for 10–15 min. Dry the feet. Using a no. 15 blade scalpel, shave the callus shallowly with the blade parallel to the skin using an up-to-down motion repeatedly. Apply counterpressure with the back of the hand on the patient's foot to prevent slipping and shakiness. Continue until skin lines are apparent or until the callus has been completely removed. Make sure to remove the rim around the callus, not just the center portion. Diabetic patients, in particular, may have an ulcer beneath the callus. If the callus has a boggy feel to it or a bruised appearance underneath, it must be removed to prevent ulcer progression and possible infection.

†For **ingrown toenail removal,** materials needed are a 10-cc syringe with 25-gauge 1½-inch needle; 10 cc lidocaine without epinephrine; alcohol swabs; Betadine; Penrose drain; 2 hemostats; nail lifter; nail separator (can use Beaver blade, sharp scissors, nail nipper, or no. 15 blade scalpel), cotton tip; triple antibiotic cream; 4 × 4 pad; and tape (alternatively, can also use tube gauze, cling, or Coban wrap).

Obtain informed consent from the patient. Perform a digital toe block with 10 cc of lidocaine without epinephrine, evenly distributing anesthetic laterally, medially, inferiorly, and superiorly (Figure 28–3). Sterilely clean the area with Betadine and drape. Apply tourniquet (Penrose drain and hemostat) to the proximal aspect of the toe to reduce the amount of blood in the field; remove as soon as the procedure is finished. Lift section of toenail to be removed (usually 1/4 to 1/3 of nail) with lifter or hemostat blade (blunt end down) all the way to the base of the nail (Figure 28–4). Separate nail to be removed with Beaver blade (no. 61), sharp scissors, nail nipper, or scalpel (no. 15 blade) all the way to the nail bed. Avulse the nail by clamping it with a hemostat, and roll the nail starting at the cut side until the section of the nail is removed, including the ingrown portion. Use a cotton tip to sweep under the fleshy part of the nail–skin border to ensure that the nail has been completely removed. Remove any remaining nail fragments with the hemostat. Dress with antibiotic cream and folded 4 × 4. Hold the dressing in place with tape, tube gauze, cling, or Coban dressing. Advise the patient to change the dressing in 24 h using an adhesive bandage or 4 × 4 until the nail is healed and no longer drains or bleeds. The patient should be advised to limit weight-bearing activity for 2–3 d. The area may be washed after 24 h. Schedule a follow-up examination of the area in 3–5 dto evaluate healing.

‡For **Morton's neuroma injection,** materials needed are a 1-cc syringe; 0.5 cc lidocaine without epinephrine; 0.5 cc triamcinolone acetate (40 mg/mL); topical refrigerant (optional), alcohol swabs, Betadine swabs, or both; and an adhesive bandage.

Obtain informed consent. Place the patient in a seated position. Localize the area to be injected using the metatarsal heads on either side of the neuroma as landmarks. The injection site is 0.5 cm proximal to the space between the metatarsal heads on the dorsal side of the foot. Draw up into a 1-cc syringe a mixture of 0.5 cc lidocaine and 0.5 cc of triamcinolone

(*Continued*)

TABLE 28–1. (*Continued*)

acetate (20 mg). Thoroughly clean the area to be injected with alcohol or Betadine. To provide local anesthesia, apply topical refrigerant (such as ethyl chloride) over the area where the needle will penetrate the skin. Inject using a dorsal approach perpendicular to the skin. Completely inject the mixture within the soft tissue space. Remove the needle. Clean the area and apply the adhesive bandage. Have the patient limit weight-bearing activities for 2 wk.

§For **padding,** materials needed are high-density adhesive foam or felt (or moleskin) and scissors.

Padding takes weight off pressure points or inflamed areas. As a general rule, padding is placed just proximal to the area of irritation to take pressure off that site; the adhesive side is attached to the insole of the shoe. Calluses can be padded by cutting a doughnut-shaped pad and placing the hole of the pad over the callus. Corns need padding cut to a size that separates the two surfaces that are causing friction without being overly bulky.

¶For **wart removal,** this procedure can be performed by two main methods: salicylic acid application (SOR **B**) or liquid nitrogen. (SOR **C**) All methods require debridement of the overlying thickened warty tissue with a no. 15 blade scalpel until there is slight bleeding (at surface of capillary bed) prior to the procedure.

50% salicylic acid paste method: In a 2″ × 2″ piece of 1/8″ adhesive foam, cut a hole slightly larger than the diameter of the wart (alternative—use a nonmedicated corn pad). Place adhesive foam (adhesive side on foot) with the hole centered over the wart. Fill the hole with salicylic acid paste and cover the top with an adhesive bandage. Secure the foam and bandage circumferentially around the foot with tape or Coban dressing, making sure the tape is not restricting circulation. Leave in place for 3–5 d. Remove the bandage and debride the dead skin. The procedure can be repeated in 1–2 wk if the wart is not completely removed.

Liquid nitrogen method: Apply liquid nitrogen with cotton tip applicator or with spray applicator to the wart surface until white coloration of the wart extends past the wart's diameter by approximately 1/8″ and the lesion takes 15 s to return to normal color. Repeat this process 3 times in one session. Warn the patient that the lesion will itch and may form a blister at the base. The skin normally sloughs in 5–7 d. The procedure may be repeated at 1- to 2-wk intervals until the wart is completely removed.

MRI, Magnetic resonance imaging; NSAID, nonsteroidal anti-inflammatory drug.

disease), thyroid-stimulating hormone (TSH), tests for vitamin B_{12}, and, depending on the history, urine heavy metal screen and serum protein electrophoresis (multiple myeloma).

  B. Radiography. X-rays of the foot should be performed on initial presentation in four instances: (1) when bony deformity is present, (2) when fracture is suspected, (3) when trauma to the foot has occurred, or (4) when the diagnosis is in question. Typically, standing anteroposterior, oblique, and lateral views are obtained. **Technetium bone scan** can be used for identifying stress fractures if plain x-ray does not show any abnormality. Bone scan is very sensitive but not very specific in identifying stress fractures. (SOR **A**) **Magnetic resonance imaging (MRI)** is useful in identifying stress fractures and soft tissue abnormalities (e.g., ligament/tendon pathology). It is very sensitive and specific but is frequently more costly than a bone scan. Local expertise and procedure availability may influence the decision between having an MRI or a bone scan. Computerized tomography is useful in evaluating bony pathology such as tarsal fractures if initial x-ray results are negative and there is strong clinical suspicion of fracture.

  C. Electromyography and nerve conduction velocity are frequently ordered to evaluate neurogenic pain when an obvious source is not identifiable or for confirmation of clinical diagnosis. These tests are usually performed by a neurologist or physiatrist and help to anatomically localize the nerve involved or distinguish between mononeuropathies and polyneuropathies.

VI. General Treatment Principles. (Also see Tables 28–1 to 28–3 and Figures 28–1 to 28–4.)

  A. Appropriate footwear can prevent and, in some cases, resolve many problems related to the foot. Characteristics of good footwear include roomy wide toe box, supportive arch, and low heel with a firm cushioned heel counter at the back of the shoe.

  B. Treatment of pain and inflammation involves the use of relative rest, ice, and medications. **Relative rest** means decreasing pain-provoking activity to the point where there is no pain with that activity and substituting alternative minimal weight-bearing activities (i.e., swimming, biking) during healing. Acetaminophen (Tylenol) (500–1000 mg orally 4 times a day) can be used for pain. Nonsteroidal anti-inflammatory medications (e.g., ibuprofen, 400–800 mg orally 3 times daily, or naproxen, 250–500 mg orally twice daily) can be used for pain, inflammation, or both. Chronic neurogenic pain can be treated with amitriptyline, 10 to 100 mg orally at bedtime, or gabapentin (Neurontin), 300 to 800 mg orally 2 to 4 times daily, starting with low doses, slowly titrating the doses higher to obtain pain relief and minimize side effects. (SOR **A**) Pregabalin (lyrica) and duloxetine (cymbalta) are also being used to treat chronic neurogenic pain.

TABLE 28–2. EVALUATION AND MANAGEMENT OF COMMON MIDFOOT COMPLAINTS

Diagnosis	Symptoms	Findings	Testing	Treatment
Midfoot sprain	Swelling and pain diffusely over midfoot with hyperflexion	Tender midfoot diffusely	X-ray to rule out Lisfranc injury	Relative rest Acetaminophen and/or NSAID Shoes with supportive arch cushions Surgical referral if Lisfranc injury
Osteoarthritis	Midfoot pain and stiffness	Diffuse tenderness, occasional diffuse swelling, bony prominence	X-ray may show spurring, loss of joint space; laboratory tests to rule out other types of arthritis	Acetaminophen and/or NSAID (SOR **Ⓐ**) Shoes with supportive arch cushions
Plantar fibromatosis	Painful bumps on bottom of foot	Nodules on plantar aspect of foot	Usually none but can do biopsy for diagnosis	No treatment, as there is high recurrence with excision; scars from excision can cause pain
Posterior tibialis dysfunction	History of twisting injury, sudden loss of arch, pain posterior and inferior to medial malleolus	Medial ankle swelling, asymmetric pes planus, inability to walk on toes, poor internal rotation and inversion, tenderness posterior and inferior to medial malleolus	MRI if rupture suspected (no strength with inversion and internal rotation, tendon not palpable)	Relative rest Arch support (OTC or custom) Surgery if continued pain despite conservative treatment for 6–12 mo
Tarsal coalition	Vague midfoot pain, frequent ankle sprains, lower leg pain with activity	Limited inversion and eversion of foot, tenderness of midfoot and ankle	X-ray may show bony bridge between talus-navicular or talus-calcaneus, CT scan if suspicion but no x-ray findings	Custom arch support Surgery if continued pain despite conservative treatment for 6–12 mo
Tarsal tunnel syndrome	Numbness or burning pain over bottom of foot, worse with walking and sometimes awakens patient from sleep	Positive Tinel's sign (tingling over bottom of foot) on tapping over posterior tibial nerve inferior-lateral to medial malleolus	Laboratory tests for peripheral neuropathy EMG/NCV (SOR **Ⓒ**)	NSAID Arch support (OTC or custom) Physical therapy referral if no improvement in 1–2 mo Referral to foot specialist in cases of severe pain not responsive to conservative management in 2–6 mo

CT, computerized tomography; EMG, electromyography; MRI, magnetic resonance imaging; NCV, nerve conduction velocity; NSAID, nonsteroidal anti-inflammatory drug; OTC, over the counter.

C. **Stretching exercises** are commonly used for foot complaints (especially plantar fasciitis and Achilles tendinosis) and involve stretching the plantar fascia and posterior heel cord muscles (gastrocnemius and soleus). Stretching for the plantar fascia is accomplished in a seated position by grasping the forefoot, dorsiflexing it for 10 seconds, then releasing and repeating this 3 to 5 times a day. The posterior heel cord is stretched by standing facing a wall with one foot placed approximately 24 inches from the wall and the other foot placed 48 to 60 inches from the wall. The patient leans toward the wall with hands on the wall in a "pushing fashion," keeping both heels on the ground. The knee of the leg

TABLE 28–3. **EVALUATION AND MANAGEMENT OF COMMON HINDFOOT COMPLAINTS**

Diagnosis	Symptoms	Findings	Testing	Treatment
Plantar fasciitis	Dull, achy pain in inferior heel, especially upon awakening	Tender calcaneal tubercle and arch	X-ray to rule out stress fracture of calcaneus; calcaneal spurs do not correlate with pain (10%–27% of asymptomatic patients have spurs)	Stretching and strengthening of plantar fascia and Achilles tendon (SOR **B**) NSAID heel cup, arch support (SOR **B**) Night splint (SOR **B**) Physical therapy referral if no improvement after 2–3 mo Plantar fascia injection* Referral to foot specialist if no improvement in 6–12 mo of conservative treatment
Calcaneus stress fracture	Heel pain and swelling with walking, ecchymosis	Squeeze tenderness of calcaneus	X-ray may reveal stress reaction Bone scan or MRI	Relative rest Short leg removable cast-brace or short leg walking cast for 4–8 wk
Achilles tendinosis	Activity-related pain and swelling behind heel	Swelling, tenderness over Achilles tendon (2–6 cm proximal to insertion), weak plantar-flexion	None	Relative rest NSAID Heel lift Glyceryl trinitrate ointment (SOR **B**) Stretching of Achilles tendon Physical therapy if no improvement after 1 mo of above measures
Bursitis (superficial calcaneal or retrocalcaneal)	Pain and swelling localized on posterior ankle near Achilles tendon insertion	Tender posterior ankle, localized swelling/erythema, Haglund's deformity (prominent bony deformity of posterior calcaneus)	None	See Achilles tendinosis treatment

*For **plantar fascia injection**, materials needed are a 3-cc syringe, 1 cc lidocaine without epinephrine; 1 cc bupivacaine (optional); 1 cc triamcinolone acetate (40 mg/mL); topical refrigerant (optional); alcohol swabs, Betadine swabs, or both; and adhesive bandage.

Obtain informed consent from the patient, which should mention the risk of steroid flare and plantar fascial rupture. Ask the patient to lie down. Localize the area to be injected using the calcaneal tubercle as the main landmark. Normally the tubercle is the area of maximal tenderness on examination and can be palpated readily over the plantar aspect of the heel. Draw up into a 3-cc syringe a mixture of 1 cc lidocaine, 1 cc bupivacaine (optional), and 1 cc triamcinolone acetate (40 mg). Thoroughly clean the skin over the medial calcaneus with alcohol or Betadine. To provide local anesthesia, apply topical refrigerant (such as ethyl chloride) over the area where the needle will penetrate the skin. Inject using a medial approach approximately 1 cm up from the plantar aspect of the heel and 3 cm from the rear aspect of the heel using the calcaneal tubercle as a landmark (injection is just distal to the tubercle). Fan the mixture across the area of the fascial insertion. Remove the needle. Clean the area and apply an adhesive bandage. Have the patient limit weight-bearing activities for 2 wk. MRI, magnetic resonance imaging; NSAID, nonsteroidal anti-inflammatory drugs.

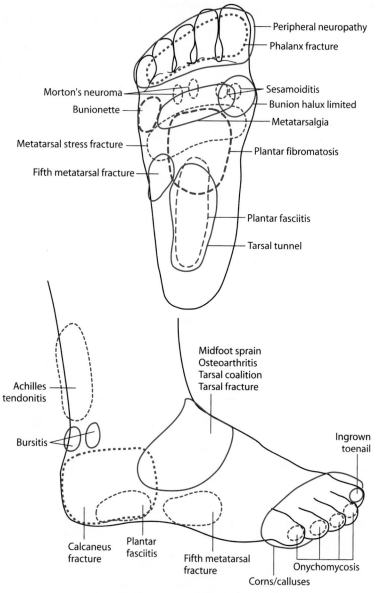

FIGURE 28–1. Foot complaints by location.

in back is extended, while the front knee is slightly flexed. This position is held for 10 to 20 seconds, repeated 3 to 5 times, alternating which foot is forward.

D. Orthotics are used for a wide variety of foot conditions.

    1. Over-the-counter (OTC) **arch cushion insoles** can be used initially for plantar fasciitis, bunions, and posterior tibialis dysfunction. OTC bunion shields, made of felt or silicone, can be used to protect the medial aspect of a bunion.

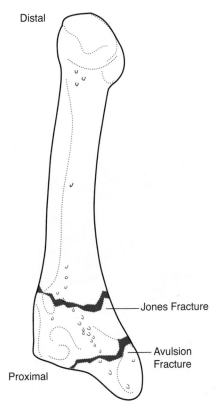

FIGURE 28–2. Fifth metatarsal fractures.

2. **Heel lifts,** made of cork, felt, or visco-elastic material, are commonly used for Achilles tendinosis and bursitis.
3. A **tension night splint for plantar fasciitis** can be commercially obtained or made with fiberglass splinting material, placing the ankle in an 80- to 90-degree angle, with the splint over the plantar aspect of the foot and posterior ankle and calf. ACE bandages secure the posterior splint. (SOR **B**)
4. If these items are not helpful, referral to a foot specialist or orthotist for custom-made arch supports is appropriate.
5. A short leg removable cast brace (cam walker boot) can be used for most stress fractures of the foot.

E. **Systemic antifungal drugs** may be used for onychomycosis. They are expensive, require treatment for 3 months, have a high rate of recurrence of infection (complete cure in ≤50%), and require monitoring of liver function tests (and CBC for terbinafine) at baseline, 6 weeks, and 3 months. Common systemic antifungal drugs given orally include terbinafine (Lamisil), 250 mg daily (for 3 months), and itraconazole (Sporanox), 200 mg twice daily for 1 week, repeated monthly for a total of 3 consecutive months. (SOR **A**) Topical ciclopirox 8% nail lacquer may also be used for onychomycosis. It is applied daily to the nail for 48 weeks but is seldom effective, as only 5% to 8% of patients have a complete cure.

F. **Systemic antibiotics** are used for foot infections such as cellulitis (see Chapter 9).

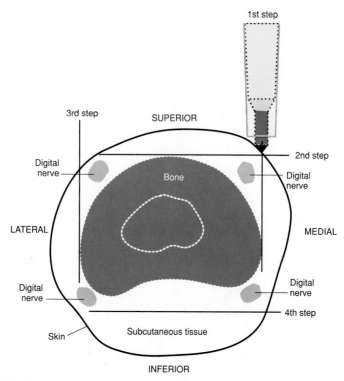

FIGURE 28–3. Digital nerve block. Cross-section through proximal phalanx. **Procedure:** Apply ethyl chloride for topical anesthesia. Insert 25-gauge 1¹/₂-inch needle into the skin at the medial base of the proximal phalanx until bone is touched, aspirating, then injecting a small amount above the bone. Advance the needle along the medial side. While withdrawing the needle, fan 1–2 cc of lidocaine evenly along the side. Repeat this step superiorly, laterally, and inferiorly. Allow at least 5 minutes for the block to become effective.

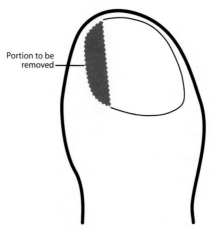

FIGURE 28–4. Toenail avulsion.

REFERENCES

Amundsen G, Ramakrishnan K, Sparks R, Coleman B. *Office Surgery.* FP Essentials, edition no. 290, AAFP Home Study. Leawood, Kansas: American Academy of Family Physicians, July 2003.

Cole C, Seto C, Gazewood J. Plantar fasciitis: evidence-based review of diagnosis and therapy. *Am Fam Physician.* 2005;72:2237-2242.

Corris EE, Lombardo JA. Tarsal navicular stress fractures. *Am Fam Physician.* 2003;67(1):85-90.

Greene WB, Griffin LY, eds. *Essentials of Musculoskeletal Care.* 3rd ed. Rosemont, IL: American Academy of Orthopaedic Surgeons; 2005:574-709.

Pommering T, Kluchurosky L, Hall S. Ankle and foot injuries in pediatric and adult athletes. *Prim Care Office Pract* 2005;32:133-161.

---

29   Fractures

Ted C. Schaffer, MD

KEY POINTS

- After trauma, one should assume a fracture has occurred and immobilize the affected region until x-rays have been obtained.
- The hallmark symptom of a new fracture is pain. Although the amount of pain correlates poorly with fracture severity, the absence of pain with an abnormal x-ray result makes it unlikely that a fracture has occurred.
- When x-ray results are negative but clinical suspicion for fracture is high, a magnetic resonance imaging scan (high cost with high sensitivity/specificity) or bone scan (lower cost but lower specificity) can provide supplemental information.

I. **Definition.** A fracture is a complete or incomplete break in the continuity of a bone. Fractures can be caused by direct trauma to the bone, repetitive forces to a bone (stress fracture), or abnormal bone architecture (osteoporosis or bone tumors).

II. **Common Diagnoses.** Evaluation of musculoskeletal injuries that are potential fractures accounts for 3% to 5% of all office visits. A fracture should be differentiated from a **sprain** (joint injury to ligaments attaching to bone), a **strain** (injury to the musculotendinous unit that attaches to bone) and a **contusion** (injury to the soft tissue surrounding the bone). Conditions associated with fractures include **dislocations** (complete loss of continuity between two articular surfaces) and **subluxations** (partial loss of continuity).

As many as 1% of newborns may sustain a fractured clavicle at the time of delivery. In **childhood,** the incidence of long bone fractures increases, with common areas including buckle fractures of the arm, clavicle fractures, and growth plate injuries. Common **adult** trauma includes finger, metacarpal, and wrist fractures, as well as fractures of the ankle, metatarsals, and toes. The **elderly** are at greater risk for osteoporotic fractures such as vertebral, pelvic, and wrist fractures.

III. **Symptoms**
   A. **Pain** is the hallmark of new fracture occurrence. Often, however, the amount of pain experienced by the patient correlates poorly with the amount of bone damage. In children, pain at an epiphyseal plate is usually a fracture, not a joint sprain, since the growth plate is often the weakest area when a joint is stressed.
   B. **Loss of motion** can occur with fractures, especially when the fracture is located near a joint surface.
   C. **Loss of function** may be noted by the patient, either because of the pain involved or because of soft tissue swelling.

IV. **Signs**
   A. **Tenderness** to palpation should be present over a new fracture site. If there appears to be radiographic evidence of a fracture but the area is not tender on examination, the diagnosis of a fracture is suspected.

B. Swelling and deformity may be apparent when the area of injury is inspected. The deformity may appear either as an obvious angulation at the bone or as an abnormal manner in which the extremity is being held.

C. Abnormal mobility may be observed. Motion of the joint above and the joint below the injured area should always be tested to ensure that these adjacent regions are not also affected by the injury.

V. Laboratory Tests

A. An **x-ray** of any suspected fracture must be performed, since this is the method by which most fractures are confirmed. At least two views directed 90 degrees apart are required, since a nondisplaced fracture may not be visible if only a single view is obtained. Comparison x-rays of the opposite limb should be obtained in children to aid the physician in distinguishing a fracture line from a normal epiphyseal growth plate.

B. A period of immobilization will be necessary for most fractures, especially those of an extremity.

    1. Historically a circumferential cast has been used for most long bone fractures, including those around the wrist and ankle. However, new data suggests that a fitted removable splint may improve function and reduce complications associated with casting. This has been most studied in pediatric buckle fractures of the wrist (SOR **B**).

    2. Time for immobilization will depend on several fractures including the age of the patient and the fracture location. An appropriate guideline is to immobilize children 3 weeks and adults 6 weeks.

C. When clinical suspicion for fracture is great but initial x-ray results are negative, the area can be immobilized and x-rays repeated in 7 to 14 days to look for a new fracture line. If a fracture diagnosis is more urgent, then a **bone scan** or **magnetic resonance imaging (MRI)** scan can be obtained. The MRI is more costly than a bone scan, but its high degree of sensitivity and specificity has made it the diagnostic test of choice for many physicians when initial x-ray results are negative and an early diagnosis is important for management. A bone scan has a high degree of sensitivity but lacks the specificity of an MRI.

VI. Treatment

A. General principles for the management of a potential fracture are as follows.

    1. The physician should assume a fracture has occurred until an x-ray examination has proved otherwise.

    2. A **splint** should be applied to the injured area in order to decrease bone motion and hold the bone in place. This procedure will alleviate pain and prevent further tissue damage.

    3. Ice applied immediately for 20 to 30 minutes will curtail swelling and provide pain relief. The ice should not directly touch the skin. Ice therapy may be repeated at 90-minute intervals.

    4. Most **dislocations** should not be reduced until x-rays have been taken. Reduction before x-ray is advisable when there is evidence of vascular compromise to an extremity that may be relieved by immediate reduction of the dislocation or fracture. Immediate posttraumatic reduction of a dislocation is also permissible when the patient is having substantial pain and the reduction is easily accomplished, such as in an anterior shoulder or finger dislocation.

B. The following **specific fractures** can be managed in an ambulatory setting:

    1. Finger fractures

        a. Distal phalangeal fractures are usually crush injuries, which can be managed by immobilization and protection. If the extensor tendon has been involved, then a mallet finger injury has occurred (see Chapter 33).

        b. Middle and proximal phalangeal fractures can be managed if the injury is nondisplaced, without angulation or rotation. Fracture angulation is evident on x-ray and is caused by the pull of intrinsic hand muscles as they attach to the bone. Rotation is evaluated by having the patient flex their fingers into the palm and observing that the fingers remain parallel and do not overlap. Nondisplaced fractures should be treated with a finger splint on the flexor surface for 2 to 4 weeks, keeping the PIP (proximal interphalangeal) joint at 30- to 50-degree flexion and the DIP (distal interphalangeal) joint at 10- to 20-degree flexion.

        c. PIP joint dislocations often occur with a hyperextension injury, causing a dorsal dislocation of the middle phalanx on the proximal phalanx ("a coach's finger"). These are usually easily reduced by **gentle** traction and **gentle** hyperextension, followed by a flexor surface splint for 2 to 4 weeks.

2. **Metacarpal fractures**
   a. **Fractures of the neck of the fifth metacarpal** ("Boxer's fracture") commonly occur after punching a person or wall. An ulnar gutter splint extending from midforearm to the fingertip is applied for 3 to 6 weeks, keeping the MCP (metacarpal phalangeal) joint in 90 degrees of flexion. (SOR **B**)
   b. **Fracture of the shaft of the fourth and fifth metacarpal** can be treated with an ulnar gutter splint if there is angulation less than 30 degrees and no rotational injury (see Section VI.C.1.b).
   c. **Fractures of the first, second, and third metacarpals** generally require orthopedic referral because of functional problems related to residual angulation.

3. **Wrist and arm fractures**
   a. The **scaphoid** is the most common wrist fracture. Those that involve the distal scaphoid (5% of fractures) or middle scaphoid (80% of fractures) have a good blood supply and can be immobilized for 8 to 12 weeks with a long-arm (extending above the elbow) or a short-arm cast (extending to the proximal forearm); the thumb must be immobilized to the level of the IP (interphalangeal) joint. Fractures of the proximal scaphoid have a poor blood supply and a high risk of nonunion and are therefore referred to an orthopedic surgeon.
   b. **Nondisplaced distal radial fractures** can be treated with short arm cast immobilization for 6 weeks in adults. The cast should extend from the metacarpals to the proximal forearm, with the thumb allowed free mobility.
   c. Children more commonly sustain a nondisplaced fracture of the radius above the growth plate, which is known as a **buckle fracture**. The patient should wear a short arm cast or fitted splint for 3 to 4 weeks. Immobilization should extend from the metacarpal heads to the proximal forearm.
   d. **Proximal radial head** fractures near the elbow can also occur with a fall on an outstretched hand. Unless there is x-ray evidence of a displaced radial head, these fractures can be managed with a long arm splint extending along the ulnar surface from the metacarpals to the proximal humerus, with the elbow at 90 degrees flexion. The splint should be maintained for 3 to 4 weeks with early mobilization to maintain elbow motion, especially in the elderly.
   e. **Humeral head fractures** are common in elderly individuals after falling on an outstretched arm or sustaining a blow to the lateral arm. Eighty percent of proximal humerus fractures are minimally displaced. Treatment, even if the shaft of the humerus is impacted, consists of providing the patient with a shoulder sling for 1 to 2 weeks and, after the sling is removed, providing the patient with range-of-motion exercises. (SOR **A**) The major risk in humeral head fractures of the elderly is loss of shoulder motion after immobilization. Orthopedic referral is needed if there is ≥1 cm fracture displacement between the proximal and distal components.

4. **Clavicle fractures**
   a. **Middle third (midclavicular) fractures** account for 80% of clavicle fractures and are easily managed. A "figure-of-8" or clavicular strap is worn for 3 to 6 weeks by children and for 6 weeks by adults. A residual callus is often left, but the fracture usually heals well.
   b. **Distal fractures,** which are present in 15% of fractures, can be more complicated than midclavicular fractures. If the fracture is nondisplaced, the initial management is the same and can be performed by a family physician. However, a painful acromioclavicular joint arthritis may develop, especially if the fracture is displaced, necessitating orthopedic resection of the distal clavicle.
   c. **Proximal fractures** occur in 5% of cases and should be evaluated carefully. The physician should look for signs of vascular injury owing to the close proximity of the great vessels of the neck. Orthopedic consultation should be strongly considered.

5. **Simple torso fractures**
   a. **Rib fractures** are common in the elderly with only minor trauma. In young adults and children, they are usually the result of greater traumatic force. A chest x-ray should be obtained to exclude pneumothorax or pulmonary contusion. Rib fractures are easily managed if the bones are not displaced.
      (1) **Pain relief** is the main focus of treatment. Oral systemic narcotics (e.g., codeine, 30 mg 4 times daily), and **nonsteroidal agents** (e.g., ibuprofen, 600 mg 3 times daily) are usually adequate, but **intercostal nerve blocks** (usually done by an anesthesiologist) can be considered if a patient is in severe pain. Rib belts

should be avoided, since they cause substantial atelectasis and increase the incidence of pneumonia.

(2) **Hospitalization** should be considered for multiple rib fractures (three or more) because of the increased risk of pulmonary contusion and atelectasis. In the elderly, even a single rib fracture can occasionally lead to pulmonary compromise.

b. **Lumbar compression fractures** are common in elderly patients with osteoporosis and can occur with minimal trauma. They can be seen from the T-4 through L-5 vertebrae, and neurologic compromise is extremely rare. Treatment is aimed at pain relief, with immobilization for a few days followed by ambulation with a support such as a lumbosacral garment.

c. Non**displaced pelvic fractures** are another problem in the elderly, occasionally complicated by blood loss, even with minor fractures. Treatment is aimed at pain relief (see above) and ambulatory support with devices such as a walker or cane until pain resolves.

6. Ankle fractures

a. **Fibular fractures below the tibial dome** are avulsion fractures caused by ligamentous pulling during sudden inversion of the foot. Treatment is a posterior leg splint for 5 to 7 days until the swelling has subsided, followed by a short leg walking cast for 4 to 6 weeks. A pneumatic ankle support (e.g., Aircast) may be considered as an alternative to casting since ankle inversion/eversion will be protected. In children, tenderness over the epiphyseal plate of the distal fibula should be regarded as a Salter I fracture (see Figure 29–1), not an ankle sprain. Treatment consists of a short leg walking cast or walking boot for 3 to 4 weeks.

b. When fibular fractures are **at or above the tibial dome,** greater ligamentous instability occurs, because the syndesmotic ligaments and interosseous membrane are involved. Referral is indicated in these cases, since surgery may be required.

7. Foot and toe fractures

a. **Second, third, and fourth metatarsal** fractures often occur as stress fractures from overuse. Frequently, initial x-ray results are negative, but repeat films in 2 to

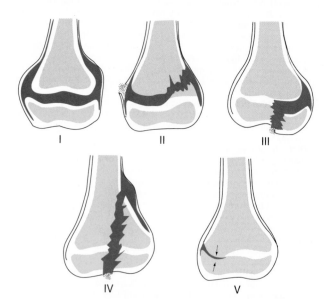

FIGURE 29–1. Salter-Harris classification of epiphyseal injuries in children. (Reproduced with permission from Doherty GM and Way LW, eds. *Current Surgical Diagnosis & Treatment.* 12th ed. Originally published by Appleton & Lange; 2006. Copyright © 2006 by the McGraw-Hill Companies, Inc.)

4 weeks show healing callus. The treatment is relative rest and use of a hard-soled shoe for 2 to 4 weeks until pain subsides. Patient education is important to prevent recurrent injury.

   b. **Fifth metatarsal** fractures can be treated if they are within 1.5 cm of the proximal styloid tip. These are avulsion injuries, which respond to relative rest and a hard-soled shoe. More distal fifth metatarsal fractures have a high incidence of nonunion, often require operative intervention, and are best referred to someone with management experience.

   c. **Toe fractures** are common, and generally require just buddy-taping to an adjacent toe for symptomatic relief of 1 to 2 weeks. A small piece of gauze or tissue should be placed between toes to prevent skin maceration.

C. Special features of **pediatric fractures** are described below.

   1. The time needed for **cast or splint immobilization** for fractures in children is generally one-half to one-third the time needed for immobilization of an adult fracture, since bone healing occurs much faster in children than in adults.

   2. The Salter-Harris classification of pediatric fractures should be understood (see Figure 29–1).

      a. Salter I fractures through the epiphyseal plate are a clinical diagnosis, often with normal x-ray findings. The prognosis is excellent. Salter II fractures through the metaphysis are also stable injuries. Salter I and II fractures are treated like any other fracture with cast or splint immobilization for several weeks.

      b. Salter III and IV fractures, which involve the epiphysis, and Salter V fractures, which are crush injuries to the growth plates, are more serious problems, especially when they involve long bones of the body.

      c. Parents of children with growth plate injuries should be advised of the possibility of growth abnormalities. These abnormalities are quite rare with Salter I and II fractures, except when the fractures are in the distal femur or tibia.

      d. In children, tenderness at the growth plate is assumed to be a bony injury rather than a ligamentous sprain, since the ligaments are stronger than the bone at this age. Immobilization often with casting is indicated, depending on the bone involved. Common growth plate fractures include the ankle and wrist.

D. **Fractures requiring referral.** In an ambulatory setting, the physician must know which injuries should be managed by an orthopedist because of the increased risk of complication. The following list serves as a guideline for situations in which consultation is advisable.

   1. **Open fractures** increase the risk of infection, especially osteomyelitis, and fracture nonunion.

   2. **Neurovascular compromise** is an orthopedic emergency necessitating immediate care by a qualified surgeon.

   3. **Unstable fractures,** where bone alignment cannot be maintained without external forces, usually require open reduction and internal fixation.

   4. **Intra-articular fractures** create a high risk for the development of long-term traumatic arthritis. Open surgical reduction is often required in order to achieve the best possible bone alignment.

   5. **Growth plate injuries** of long bones that involve the epiphysis (Salter III, IV, or V fractures) create a high risk of complications, and therefore the patient may require long-term orthopedic management.

REFERENCES

Eiff MP, Hatch RL, Calmbach WL. *Fractures Management for Primary Care.* 2nd ed. Saunders; 2003.

Griffin LY, ed. *Essentials of Musculoskeletal Care.* 3rd ed. American Academy of Orthopaedic Surgeons; 2005.

Leggit JC, Meko CJ. Acute finger injuries: part III. Fractures, dislocations and thumb injuries. *Am Fam Physician.* 2006;73:827-834.

Plint AC, Perry JJ, Carrell R, Gaboury I, Lanton L. A randomized controlled trial of removable splinting versus casting for wrist buckle fractures in children. *Pediatrics.* 2006;117:691-697.

Simon RR, Sharman SC, Koenigsknecht SJ. *Emergency Orthopedics: The Extremities.* 5th ed. McGraw-Hill; 2007.

30   Gastrointestinal Bleeding

May S. Jennings, MD

KEY POINTS

- Initial assessment of hemodynamic status and appropriate triage of patients with gastrointestinal bleeding are strongly linked to patient outcomes.
- 80% of gastrointestinal bleeding will resolve spontaneously with appropriate supportive care.
- The risk of further upper gastrointestinal bleeding can be minimized by changes in lifestyle and use of medications.

I. **Definition.** Gastrointestinal (GI) bleeding is blood loss from any part of the GI tract, including both symptomatic and occult blood loss.

II. **Common Diagnoses.** The estimated incidence in the United States is 1 per every 1000 people. GI bleeding accounts for 300,000 hospitalizations annually in the United States. The mortality rate for GI bleeding remains around 10% despite modern technological advances.

   A. **Upper GI (UGI) bleeding** is defined as any GI bleeding proximal to the ligament of Treitz.
   1. **Peptic ulcer disease** makes up 50% of significant UGI bleeding. Risk factors include nonsteroidal anti-inflammatory drugs (NSAIDs), alcohol, *Helicobacter pylori* infection, and excess acid production.
   2. **Gastritis** is the presence of subepithelial hemorrhages and erosions in the mucosa. It is associated with NSAIDs, alcohol, and stress.
   3. **Esophagitis** is especially common in geriatric patients and can be associated with drug-induced injury.
   4. **Mallory-Weiss tear** is frequently associated with alcohol ingestion and represents 5% to 15% of UGI bleeding.
   5. **Esophageal and gastric varices** are associated with portal hypertension, generally as a result of cirrhosis. The overall mortality rate from bleeding varices is 30%.

   B. **Lower GI (LGI) bleeding** is defined as any GI bleeding distal to the ligament of Treitz.
   1. **Diverticulosis** is the most common cause of significant LGI bleeding in the older adult population. It is estimated that half of all US adults older than 60 years have diverticuli.
   2. **Vascular ectasias** are the second most common cause of LGI bleeding in the older adult population. Twenty-five percent of geriatric patients have vascular ectasias in the cecum and right colon.
   3. **Colitis** can cause GI bleeding and may be caused by infection, inflammation, radiation, or ischemia.
   4. **Neoplasms and polyps** generally cause occult GI bleeding.
   5. **Hemorrhoids,** both external and internal, can be associated with bleeding after excessive straining and hard stools. They are rarely associated with significant LGI bleeding.
   6. **Anal fissure** is associated with blood around the stool after a painful bowel movement. It is associated with minor LGI bleeding.

   C. **LGI bleeding in children.** UGI bleeding in children is extremely rare in the outpatient setting. Significant LGI bleeding is not common.
   1. **Meckel's diverticulum** is the most common cause of significant GI bleeding in children. It is a congenital abnormality that is generally located in the small intestine. It can present as UGI or LGI bleeding.
   2. **Intussusception** is the second most common cause of significant LGI bleeding. It is caused by the involution of one segment of bowel into another segment of bowel.
   3. **Juvenile polyps** are generally benign, but can be associated with familial polyposis syndromes.
   4. **Colitis** is caused by infection, inflammation, or allergic etiologies. Inflammatory bowel disease often presents in childhood and young adulthood.

    5. Anal fissure or rectal foreign bodies are frequently associated with minor rectal bleeding in children.

III. **Symptoms.** (Also see the sidebar on rare but serious conditions.)

  A. **Bleeding history**

    1. **Hematemesis** is vomiting blood. A careful history must be taken to exclude nasopharyngeal bleeding and hemoptysis.

    2. **Melena** is black, tarry stools. It is generally indicative of UGI bleeding.

    3. **Hematochezia** is passing blood through the rectum. It is indicative of LGI bleeding 85% of the time. If it originates from an UGI source, it denotes a very brisk bleed.

    4. **Currant jelly stool** is blood, mucus, and stool in combination. It is generally seen in intussusception or acute colitis.

  B. **General history.** The history is frequently not helpful in identifying the source of the GI bleeding, especially in UGI bleeding. In fact, the clinical judgment of physicians is only correct 40% of the time. (SOR **B**) Important features of the history are listed below.

    1. **Confusion, dizziness, or syncope.** Any recent history represents a hemodynamically unstable patient who requires urgent attention.

    2. **Abdominal pain.** In UGI bleeding, pain would be more consistent with peptic ulcer disease and gastritis. In LGI bleeding, pain would be most consistent with colitis in adults or Meckel's diverticulum in children. Bowel perforation should always be considered in patients with severe pain.

    3. **Coughing, vomiting, or retching.** These symptoms suggest Mallory-Weiss tear.

    4. **Number of stools.** Knowing the number of stools in the last 24 to 48 hours may be helpful in determining the rate of the bleeding.

    5. **History of prior GI bleeding.** This knowledge may or may not be helpful, since 30% of patients with known varices will bleed from other sites.

    6. **Atherosclerotic disease.** Atherosclerotic disease such as coronary artery disease or peripheral vascular disease raises the possibility for ischemic colitis. Historical features that go along with this diagnosis include abdominal pain after meals and abdominal pain followed by LGI bleeding.

    7. Medications: **NSAIDs, warfarin, and alcohol.** NSAID use increases the risk of UGI bleeding by threefold in adults, fivefold in the elderly. (SOR **A**)

    8. **Weight loss** suggests carcinoma. Colon carcinoma is suggested by weight loss plus a change in bowel habits.

RARE BUT SERIOUS CONDITIONS

  Vomiting, pain and blood in the stool of a young child are suggestive of intussusception.

  History of an aortic aneurysm repair or aortic bypass suggests a potentially life-threatening aortoenteric fistula, usually to the duodenum, as the cause of GI bleeding.

IV. **Signs.** Like the history, the examination may not be very helpful in terms of pinpointing the etiology of the GI bleeding.

  A. **Vital signs.** Orthostasis (rise in pulse by 20 BPM and a fall in systolic blood pressure by 20 mm Hg when standing) indicates hemodynamic instability and rapid bleeding. The presence of orthostasis represents a 20% blood loss and a clinical emergency. Other signs of hypovolemic shock, such as a drop in the patient's usual systolic blood pressure by 40 mm Hg, should be considered an emergency. Beta-blockers may mask the tachycardia normally associated with hemodynamic instability.

  B. **Altered mental status.** Altered mental status is an ominous finding and should be considered a sign of hypovolemic shock until proven otherwise.

  C. **Abdominal examination**

    1. **Peritoneal signs or severe tenderness** raise suspicion for bowel perforation.

    2. **Pain that is disproportional to the abdominal examination** suggests ischemic colitis.

D. Rectal examination. Rectal examination is mandatory in all patients with GI bleeding. This includes the following:

    1. Inspection and digital examination for masses, hemorrhoids, and anal fissures.

    2. Examination of retrieved stool for melena and hematochezia. If no obvious bleeding is noted, stool guaiac testing is indicated.

        a. Stools will appear black (not tarry) after ingestion of iron or bismuth subsalicylate.

        b. Tomatoes, rare meat, and cherries may cause a false-positive stool guaiac study.

        c. Guaiac-positive stools may continue for up to 3 weeks after an acute bleeding episode.

E. Any **sequelae of chronic liver disease** including spider angiomas, ascites, caput medusa, palmar erythema, jaundice, or splenomegaly raises suspicion for variceal bleeding.

F. A **nasogastric (NG) tube** should be placed to try to differentiate UGI from LGI bleeding, regardless of history. (SOR **C**) Bright red blood or "coffee ground" material in the NG tube suggests an UGI source. There is no contraindication to NG tube placement in patients with known or suspected esophageal varices. (SOR **C**) Guaiac testing of the NG aspirate is not recommended. (SOR **C**)

V. Tests

A. Endoscopy (esophagogastroduodenoscopy [EGD], or colonoscopy) is the first step in further evaluation of most patients with GI bleeding. (SOR **A**) In addition to localizing the source of bleeding, endoscopy allows therapeutic interventions including banding of varices, mucosal biopsy to diagnose *H pylori*, sclerotherapy, cauterization, and snaring of polyps.

    1. In patients with hematochezia and hemodynamic instability, EGD should precede colonoscopy.

    2. In patients older than 40 years with occult GI bleeding (guaiac-positive stool with minimal or no symptoms), colonoscopy is indicated. After a negative colonoscopy, further workup may not be productive, unless iron deficiency anemia is present (see Chapter 4).

    3. In patients younger than 40 years with minor rectal bleeding, anoscopy (Chapter 52) or sigmoidoscopy that reveals a likely cause is often a sufficient workup.

    4. Data suggest improved outcomes when EGD is performed within 24 hours of upper GI bleeding onset, likely because this allows early interventions for the 20% of bleeds not resolving spontaneously. (SOR **B**)

B. Hematologic studies

    1. Hemoglobin and hematocrit should be done, though they will be normal early in acute bleeding. A low hematocrit and a low mean corpuscular volume without hemodynamic compromise suggests slow, chronic bleeding.

    2. A **blood urea nitrogen to creatine ratio** ≥ 36 suggests UGI bleeding.

    3. Prothrombin time, partial thromboplastin time, and platelet count assess possible contribution of coagulopathy or thrombocytopenia to the bleed.

C. An electrocardiogram is recommended in adults, especially those with known coronary artery disease. Additionally, ruling out myocardial infarction is recommended for elderly patients and those with a history of coronary artery disease, especially if they are hemodynamically unstable. (SOR **C**)

D. Barium studies and **gastric lavage** (see Section IV.F) are generally not as helpful as endoscopy in diagnosing the etiology of GI bleeding.

E. Technetium red cell scan can locate LGI bleeding sources, but results are not highly reliable. However, the scan is the procedure of choice in confirming Meckel's diverticulum.

F. Angiography is highly sensitive and allows therapeutic intervention during the procedure, but it carries procedure-related risks and cannot locate very slow bleeds.

VI. Treatment. GI bleeding is an emergency until proven otherwise.

A. Hospitalization is always indicated for those with signs or symptoms of hemodynamic instability and those with melena or comorbid disease. (SOR **B**) Hospitalization is also recommended for elderly patients, because of poor functional reserves and frequent comorbidities. (SOR **B**) The inpatient setting allows for aggressive intravenous fluid resuscitation, transfusion (packed red blood cells, fresh frozen plasma, or platelets as indicated), efficient localization of bleeding source (see Section V), and initiation of specific therapy (e.g., octreotide for acute variceal bleeding). **Surgery** is a last resort for bleeding uncontrolled with other interventions.

TABLE 30–1. INITIAL PREDICTORS OF POOR CLINICAL OUTCOME IN GI BLEEDING*

Age ≥60 y

Comorbidities
Presence of 3 or more
Cardiac, pulmonary, renal, or liver disease

Medications
Warfarin
Corticosteroids
Melena
Hemodynamic instability
Bloody nasogastric aspirate

Laboratory tests
Elevated liver function tests
Elevated prothrombin time
Hypoalbuminemia
Thrombocytopenia
Leukocytosis
Elevated creatinine
Hemoglobin ≤10 mg/dL
Electrocardiographic changes

*Poor clinical outcome is defined as risk of rebleeding and risk of death.

    B. Outpatient management is appropriate for patients not meeting criteria for hospital management (e.g., individuals with occult bleeding).

    C. Preventive measures are often effective in minimizing recurrences, once the bleeding source has been identified and controlled (see Chapters **71 and 82**).

    D. Prognosis. In all types of GI bleeding, 80% resolve spontaneously with supportive care. (SOR **B**) Even 60% of variceal bleeds resolve spontaneously without aggressive intervention. Seventy percent of mortality from GI bleeding is attributed to comorbid diseases (Table 30–1, SOR **B**).

REFERENCES

Farrell JJ, Friedman LS. Gastrointestinal bleeding in the elderly. *Gastroenterol Clin.* 2001;30(2):377-407.

Leung AK. Lower gastrointestinal bleeding in children. *Pediatr Emerg Care.* 2002;18(4):319-323.

Manning-Dimmitt LL, Dimmitt SG, Wilson GR. Diagnosis of gastrointestinal bleeding in adults. *Am Fam Physician.* 2005;71:1339-1346.

Pianka JD, Affronti J. Management principles of gastrointestinal bleeding. *Prim Care.* 2001;28(3):557-575.

---

31   Genital Lesions

Tomás P. Owens, Jr., MD

KEY POINTS

- In evaluating patients with genital lesions, a history of sexual preferences/practices is important.
- Most genital lesions can be diagnosed by a careful history and examination, with minimal laboratory testing.
- Human immunodeficiency virus testing should always be considered in patients with genital lesions believed to be sexually transmitted.

I. Definition. Genital lesions are any acquired abnormality of the external genitalia.

II. **Common Diagnoses.** The 2004 National Ambulatory Medical Care Survey describes diseases of the skin and subcutaneous tissue as being the principal diagnosis in 5.2% of all office visits and diseases of the genitourinary system as 4.6% of all office visits.

A. **Ulcerative lesions**

1. **Herpes simplex virus types 1 and 2** (HSV-1 and -2). The presence of antibodies to **HSV-2** varies from 3% in nuns to 70% to 80% in prostitutes and seems to be directly proportional to sexual activity. **HSV-1,** which is present in 90% of the population, can cause genital herpes, although less frequently.

2. **Primary syphilis** (chancre). The United States showed a 90% decline in the number of cases reported from 1991 to 2000, but a 9.5% increase was noted from 2000 to 2005, with the highest incidence among blacks, Hispanics, and in the South. From 2002 to 2005, the incidence has been between 3.1 and 3.2 /100,000. During the last 4 years, there has been an upsurge in cases of men who have sex with men (MSM), and the last year saw for the first time in 10 years an increase in female cases.

B. **Verrucoid/Papillomatous lesions**

1. **Condylomata acuminata** caused by human papillomavirus, most commonly serotypes 6 and 11, are the most common sexually transmitted entity, although this condition can also be transmitted nonsexually. Condylomata are most common during the reproductive years, are commonly associated with other sexually transmitted diseases (STDs), and may grow dramatically with pregnancy, human immunodeficiency virus (HIV), or corticosteroid use.

2. **Secondary syphilis** condyloma latum (see Section II.A.2).

3. Genital lesions of **molluscum contagiosum** are associated with, but not always because of, sexual transmission. HIV infection is associated with an increased number and size of lesions.

4. **Pearly penile papules** are present in up to 30% of men. There are no known predisposing risk factors.

C. **Pruritic lesions**

1. **Balanitis,** irritation of the glans penis, occurs most commonly in uncircumcised diabetic patients, and those with poor hygiene. It can be precipitated by smegma and exogenous contact irritants.

2. **Erythrasma** is a chronic, bacterial infection that occurs more often in obese dark-skinned men.

3. *Phthirus pubis* (pubic lice) occurs only in humans, most commonly in young adults, is very contagious, and is transmitted sexually or by sharing clothing, towels, or bed linens. It prefers moist environments, seldom goes into neighboring skin, and has been described rarely on facial hair.

4. **Vulvar dystrophy/lichen sclerosus et atrophicus (LSA)** is a common process of unknown etiology in postmenopausal women but is seen in all age groups. In men, it is very rare and is called balanitis xerotica obliterans (**BXO**). It is more common in middle-aged diabetic patients but can be seen in all age groups.

D. **Cystic lesions**

1. **Bartholin's gland cysts or inflammation** occurs on either side of the lower vaginal vestibule. They account for 2% of all new patients in a gynecologic practice, are more common after menarche and before menopause, and are unrelated to STDs. Other causes of genital lesions discussed elsewhere include psoriasis, seborrheic dermatitis, scabies, tinea cruris, allergic/contact dermatitis (see Chapter 14); testicular torsion, epididymo-orchitis, spermatocele/epididymal cyst/varicocele (see Chapter 56); folliculitis (see Chapter 9); urethritis (see Chapter 61); and vaginitis, cervicitis, and chlamydia (see Chapters 51 and 64). Causes of genital lesions not discussed here because of their relative rarity include penile cancer, bowenoid papulosis of the penis/vulvar epithelial neoplasia, testicular cancer, lymphogranuloma venereum, granuloma inguinale, lichen planus, fixed drug eruption, erythroplasia of Queyrat, Peyronie's disease, penile/vulvar trauma, penile prostheses, and priapism.

III. Symptoms

A. **Ulcerative lesions**

1. **HSV-1 or -2**

a. The incubation period is 2 to 14 days. Primary infection, which is associated with viremia, may manifest as fever, generalized myalgia, malaise, headaches, and weakness, peaking 3 to 4 days after the onset of lesions. Painful inguinal or deep pelvic lymphadenopathy arises 2 to 3 weeks later. Burning pain and pruritus along with vaginal or urethral discharge and dysuria are common.

    b. There is a prodrome of burning, lancinating pain 1 to 2 days before eruption. Direct local inflammatory changes and cytolysis account for most of the syndrome in recurrences, which rarely cause systemic symptoms.

  2. Chancres are painless, unless secondarily infected. Patients present for evaluation of the lesion or for accompanying lymphadenopathy.

B. Verrucoid/Papillomatous lesions

  1. Condylomata acuminata have an incubation period from weeks to years, are painless, and commonly recur during the first few years. Rarely, a patient may complain of hematuria from a urethral condyloma.

  2. Condyloma lata are painless lesions, although generalized myalgia, fever, chills, and arthralgia may occur in the early phase of eruption, which occurs 6 to 24 weeks after untreated primary syphilis or, rarely, synchronously with the chancre.

  3. The lesions of **molluscum contagiosum** develop slowly over a 2- to 3-month period and rarely are pruritic.

  4. Pearly penile papules are asymptomatic but worrisome to some patients.

C. Pruritic lesions

  1. Balanitis is associated with pruritus and burning pain during or after sexual intercourse or with excessive smegma production. Dysuria and more severe pain occur with more severe disease.

  2. Pruritus and long-standing rash persisting after fungicidal therapy are common presentations for **erythrasma.**

  3. *Phthirus pubis* infestation manifests as pruritus, rarely severe. Some patients describe nits on their pubic hair.

  4. Patients with **vulvar dystrophy/LSA** and **BXO** present with varying degrees of pruritus and concerns about the lesion's appearance.

D. Cystic lesions

  1. Small **Bartholin's gland cysts** are usually asymptomatic. Larger lesions cause discomfort, pruritus, and sometimes dyspareunia. As the lesions become infected, there is at times very severe pain, external dysuria, and vulvar discharge. Systemic symptoms are rare.

IV. Signs

A. Ulcerative lesions

  1. HSV-1 or -2 initially is an erythematous papule, which is followed hours to a few days later by small, grouped vesicles on the glans, on the distal and sometimes proximal shaft of the penis, or on the scrotum in males. The entire vulva can be involved. Pustules, erosions, or ulceration occur, which heal by crusting in 2 to 4 weeks, leaving some hypomelanosis or hypermelanosis. Scarring occurs only with manipulation or secondary infection. **Primary infection** produces larger numbers of lesions than **recurrent infection (see Figure 31–1).**

  2. Primary infection with *Treponema pallidum* produces a **chancre** at the site of inoculation 10 to 90 days after direct contact with secretions of an infected person. The **chancre** is a papule that erodes into a single, round, beefy-red ulcer with hard, raised borders and yellow-green exudative material on its base. Chancres occur in the inside penile foreskin, coronal sulcus, shaft, or base, or on the cervix and vagina (where patients seldom detect it), vulva, or clitoris. Extragenital sites for chancres are the mouth, lips, breast, fingers, and thighs. Multiple chancres can be seen in HIV infection.

B. Verrucoid/Papillomatous lesions

  1. Condylomata acuminata are skin-colored or pink-red tumors, which are localized, fleshy, soft, moist, elongated, and dome-shaped with filiform or conical vegetating projections in grape- to cauliflower-like clusters on moist surfaces (see Figure 31–2.) They can be keratotic and smooth papular warts in dry surfaces or subclinical "flat" warts. Large lesions occur perianally in immunosuppressed persons.

  2. Condylomata lata are soft, flat-topped, moist, skin-colored or pale pink papules, warts, nodules, or plaques, which may become confluent. These lesions occur in any body surface, but have a preference for the anogenital area and intertriginous sites.

  3. Molluscum contagiosum presents as pearly white papules or nodules 2 to 8 mm in diameter, which are mostly round or oval with a classic umbilicated top (see Figure 31–3). The papules are localized in clusters, with preference for the genital area, neck,

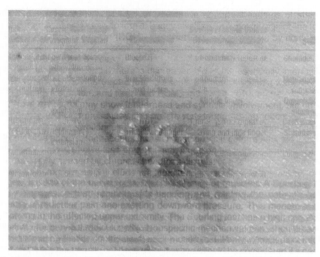

FIGURE 31-1. Tightly grouped vesicles 1 to 3 mm in diameter forming a lobulated irregular plaque over a larger erythematous base represent a herpetic lesion about 2-day-old (see color insert). (Reproduced with permission from Tomás P. Owens, Jr., MD.)

and trunk and may evolve to pustules and small crusts or plaques. Large size or large number of lesions, particularly in the face, suggests HIV.

4. **Pearly penile papules** histologically are angiofibromas that first appear around puberty. They are thin, conical, white, or pale pink uniformly sized groups of papules, forming multiple parallel lines mostly on the corona, but also in the balanopreputial sulcus.

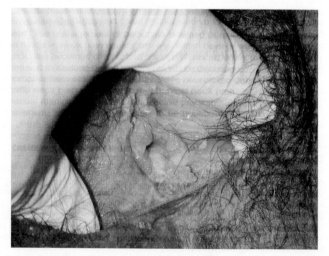

FIGURE 31-2. A peach-colored cauliflower-like lesion is noted on the comisure of the labia majora immediately caudal to the fourchette. Single coniform lighter pink lesions are also present at the R periurethral area, R superior labia majora, and L labia minora (see color insert). (Reproduced with permission from Tomás P. Owens, Jr., MD.)

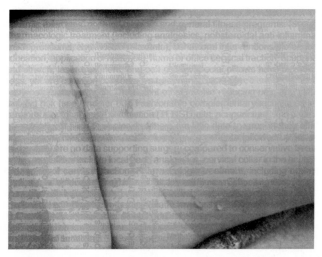

FIGURE 31–3. Umbilicated, tan, volcano-top-like lesions in a very young girl. The inner thigh lesions are coupled, resembling an achrochordon, a more fusiform appearance. Investigation concluded that these were not sexually transmitted (see color insert). (Reproduced with permission from Tomás P. Owens, Jr., MD.)

C. Pruritic lesions

1. Erythema, excess amounts of smegma, and flat white-gray "empty" or erythematous papules suggest **balanitis (see Figure 31–4);** erosions and fine scaling sometimes associated with marked edema of the prepuce suggest **balanoposthitis. Phimosis** (a contraction of the distal foreskin) may be present, revealing only edema and obstructing the view of the glans. In uncircumcised males, phimosis can be a cause or

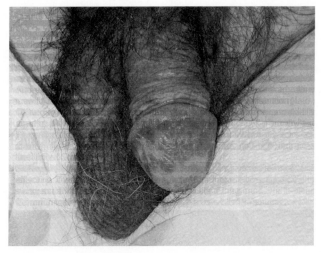

FIGURE 31–4. Irregular erythematous plaques following cleansing of smegma and debris. These lesions completely disappeared after topical antifungals, confirming the absence of Bowenoid disease (see color insert). (Reproduced with permission from Tomás P. Owens, Jr., MD.)

a complication of balanitis (or both). Paraphimosis can occur if the foreskin has been retracted, constricting the glans or the shaft just proximal to the glans, and causing ischemia, which presents as swelling and acute pain. Any papule, plaque, or white discoloration that is not resolved by therapy (see Section VI.C.1.c) is a clue to possible malignancy.

   2. An erythematous to brownish-red plaque with sharp borders and minimal scaling located on the inner thigh extending into the scrotum or vulva suggests **erythrasma.**

   3. Minuscule white-gray nits are seen attached to hair shafts, and brownish-gray lice of similar size (1–2 mm) are seen on the perifollicular skin in *Phthirus pubis* infestation. Papules, lichenification, and excoriations from scratching can be seen.

   4. **Vulvar dystrophy/LSA** varies from nonspecific thinned skin, to multiple flat, irregular pearly/ivory white, or pink/reddish (less common) papules or macules in multiple sites. They may eventually coalesce into white plaques involving the entire perineum. Hyperplastic dystrophy and leukoplakia are less common and considered premalignant; vulvar carcinoma is uncommon. In **BXO,** there is a ring of white sclerotic tissue at the tip of the foreskin (which causes phimosis) or meatus but is not accompanied by inflammatory changes. Kraurosis vulvae (atrophy and shriveling of the skin or mucous membranes) with hypomelanosis, telangiectasias, and a "keyhole" vaginal opening is an old, now abandoned gynecologic term for end-stage atrophy not necessarily caused by sclerosis.

 D. **Cystic lesions**

   1. A rubbery, soft, renitent bulge in the inner aspect of the lower vaginal vestibule (outside of the introitus) suggests **Bartholin's gland cyst;** if infected, the cyst is red and extremely tender.

V. **Laboratory Tests**

 A. **Ulcerative lesions.** Testing for chlamydia, gonorrhea, and HIV (with adequate counseling) should be considered in persons with primary HSV-1 or -2, syphilis, or chancroid (see sidebar), with retesting in 3 to 6 months. In addition, testing for syphilis is recommended in those with primary HSV-1 or -2.

CHANCROID

Chancroid is a highly contagious disease that has declined steadily since 1987 to just 17 cases in 2005. It is caused by *Haemophilus ducreyi,* a gram-negative coccobacillary organism. Occasional discrete outbreaks occur, commonly associated with the influx of Central American, Caribbean, and Southeast Asian immigrants. Underreporting is common because of difficulty in diagnosis. As many as 10% of patients with chancroid may be coinfected with *T pallidum* or HSV. The disease may have an important role in the transmission of HIV, primarily among heterosexuals. Chancroid is a tender, genital papule that erodes into single or multiple round, oval, or serpiginous painful ulcers with sharp, flat, and nonindurated borders. Ulcers can become confluent and large. Regional lymphadenopathy is typical. The diagnosis of **chancroid** is **clinical** and based on excluding other ulcerative processes such as syphilis and herpes. Rapid plasma reagin (RPR) test performed 1 week after identification of the lesion is more reliable than initial RPR in ruling out syphilis. **Gram stain** for coccobacillary clusters is unreliable, and **culture** is difficult and expensive. Commercially available polymerase chain reaction tests can be used but none is approved by the US Food and Drug Administration. Persons with **chancroid** should be treated with azithromycin, 1 g orally in a single dose, *or* ceftriaxone, 250 mg intramuscularly in a single dose, *or* erythromycin base, 500 mg orally 4 times daily for 7 days, *or* ciprofloxacin, 500 mg orally twice daily for 3 days. Ciprofloxacin should not be given to children or pregnant/lactating patients. There has been intermediate resistance to ciprofloxacin and erythromycin worldwide. Uncircumcised males and HIV patients are more resistant to therapy and may require retreatment or longer courses if the condition is not resolved in 7 days.

---

   1. Laboratory studies are rarely necessary in HSV-1 or -2; they are reserved for situations in which the diagnosis is not clear and certainty is imperative, such as a primary infection soon before parturition or when strict confirmation is necessary for medicolegal cases.

      a. In the **Tzanck test,** a vesicle is unroofed and its fluid is smeared on a slide, dried, and stained with Giemsa or Wright's stain. Presence of giant multinucleated acanthocytes is considered a positive test result for **Herpesviridae** (simplex or zoster).

      b. **Viral culture** is expensive and must incubate 7 days before being read. Positive cultures can occur in persons with nonherpetic lesions who shed the herpes virus regularly.

      c. **Microscopic pathology** and **electron microscopy** can be used, although this is rarely necessary.

   2. **Primary syphilis**

      a. **Dark-field microscopic examination** of the lesion's secretions is diagnostic but rarely available to the clinician. It reveals treponemes contracting and kinking, but these may not be seen if the chancre has been treated with topical antibiotics.

      b. **RPR and VDRL tests,** the nontreponemal tests, turn positive 1 week after the appearance of the chancre. These tests become negative up to 1 year after treatment, but may remain positive for life at a low titer in a small percentage of patients.

      c. Confirmatory treponemal tests such as the **fluorescent treponemal antibody-absorption** (FTA-ABS) or *T pallidum* hemagglutination assay (TPHA) may take 2 weeks to become positive. Treponemal tests remain weakly positive for life.

B. **Verrucoid/Papillomatous lesions.** Testing for chlamydia, gonorrhea, and HIV (with adequate counseling, including safe-sex information) should be considered in persons with condylomata acuminata, condyloma lata, or molluscum contagiosum. In addition, testing for syphilis is recommended in those with condylomata acuminata.

   1. The diagnosis of **condylomata acuminata** is clinical.

      a. Occasionally, a **biopsy** confirms the diagnosis.

      b. Subclinical lesions can be soaked with **5% acetic acid** (white vinegar) for 5 minutes, resulting in white epithelium that can be observed with a colposcope or magnifying glass of 4 to 10 × magnification. White papules may be noted, although other changes such as mosaicism and punctation are possible.

   2. RPR and VDRL tests are always positive when **condyloma lata** are present. FTA confirmation is warranted.

   3. Sticking a needle through a lesion releases the semisolid core of **molluscum contagiosum,** which is considered diagnostic. Microscopic observation, rarely necessary, reveals inclusion "molluscum" bodies or Lipschütz cells.

   4. No laboratory is necessary to diagnose **pearly penile papules.** A biopsy reveals an angiofibroma.

C. **Pruritic lesions**

   1. **Balanitis** is a clinical diagnosis; however, biopsy of any associated glanular mass is needed. Biopsy can be done under local anesthesia using a shallow punch at the office.

   2. Wood's lamp examination shows a classic coral-red fluorescence in **erythrasma.** Scraping of the lesions may show gram-positive rods and do not show hyphae.

   3. Lice and nits can be observed microscopically in *Phthirus pubis* infestation. Testing for chlamydia, gonorrhea, syphilis, and HIV (with adequate counseling) should be considered in those who were infested by direct sexual contact.

   4. Biopsy is necessary in **vulvar dystrophy** to distinguish **LSA/BXO** from leukoplakia, vitiligo, lichen planus, or carcinoma. This can be accomplished in the office under local anesthesia using a punch biopsy of the leading edge or a full excision, if the lesion is less than 1 cm in diameter.

D. **Cystic lesions.** Diagnosis of **Bartholin's gland cyst** is clinical. Cultures should be considered only when cellulitis is present.

VI. Treatment

A. **Ulcerative lesions**

   1. Maximal viral shedding in HSV-1 or -2 occurs within 24 hours of the appearance of lesions and diminishes by the fifth day; nevertheless, viral shedding occurs intermittently in the absence of any signs in many persons. Herpes is generally self-limited, with recurrences decreasing over the years. Therapy does not eradicate **HSV-1 or -2,** nor does it affect the severity or rate of recurrences after discontinuation. Significant clinical improvement is seen when therapy is started promptly after onset of symptoms.

      a. **For primary infection,** oral drugs of choice include acyclovir, 400 mg, or famciclovir, 250 mg 3 times per day, *or* valacyclovir 1 g twice a day for 7 to 10 days. (SOR **Ⓐ**)

It is unclear whether higher doses (e.g., acyclovir, 400 mg 5 times per day) are warranted for stomatitis, pharyngitis, or proctitis.

  b. For recurrent infection
- **(1)** At onset, oral acyclovir, 200 mg 5 times per day, or 400 mg 3 times daily, or 800 mg twice daily for 5 days, *or* famciclovir 125 mg or valacyclovir 500 mg twice daily or 1000 mg every day for 5 days, may be prescribed. (SOR **A**)
- **(2)** Oral suppressive therapy options include acyclovir, 400 mg, or famciclovir, 250 mg twice daily, *or* valacyclovir, 500 mg or 1 g once a day for 1 year, (SOR **A**) with consideration of a drug-free period at that point to assess the need for continued therapy.

  c. Counseling regarding potential for recurrence, amelioration of symptoms over the years, transmission through viral shedding in the absence of lesions, and the need for condom use is important.

2. **Primary syphilis** is treated with benzathine penicillin G, 2.4 million U intramuscularly in a single dose. (SOR **A**) Some experts recommend 2 extra doses, a week apart, in patients with HIV. (SOR **B**) Persons who are allergic to penicillin should receive doxycycline, 100 mg orally twice daily for 2 weeks. (SOR **A**) If compliance is an issue, penicillin desensitization should be considered. Dosages and effectiveness of ceftriaxone have not been defined. Azithromycin should not be used and is commonly ineffective.

B. Verrucoid/Papillomatous lesions

1. **Condylomata acuminata** resolve spontaneously in 6 to 15 months, except in immunocompromised persons. Most clinicians treat to avoid persistent growth. Treatment removes only the wart and does not eliminate the virus, which could remain for months to years. Recurrences are common during the first year, even after an adequate removal. An additional Papanicolaou smear is recommended in women at the time of diagnosis with warts. A recombinant vaccine effective against HPV types 6, 11, 16, and 18 (Gardasil, Merck) was approved for females aging 9 to 26 years in June 2006. The vaccine is not intended for treatment.

  a. Most effective therapies include the following:
- **(1)** For **cryotherapy** with liquid nitrogen, the cryotherapy probe, spray "gun," or cotton-tipped applicator is applied until blanching occurs no more than 1 mm around the perimeter of the lesions, which fall off in 24 to 72 hours, leaving a shallow ulcer.
- **(2)** **Trichloroacetic acid** or **bichloroacetic acid** 80% to 90% can be applied, only to warts, and turns them white in seconds. Lesions should be powdered with talc or sodium bicarbonate immediately to remove unreacted acid. Treatment can be repeated weekly as necessary.
- **(3)** **Imiquimod** (Aldara) 5% cream is applied by the patient's finger on each lesion at bedtime and washed off in the morning, 3 times a week for as long as 16 weeks. (SOR **B**)
- **(4)** **Podophyllin,** 10% to 25%, in compound tincture of benzoin, is applied to warts. The total amount applied per session should be limited to 0.5 mL or less than 10 cm^2 to avoid systemic toxicity; medication should be washed off in 4 hours. Treatment may be repeated weekly and is contraindicated in pregnancy.
- **(5)** **Podofilox** (Condylox), 0.5% solution, for self-treatment, is applied twice daily for 3 days followed by 4 days of no therapy. Treatment can be repeated up to 4 cycles and is contraindicated in pregnancy. The health care provider should teach the patient which lesions to treat and how to apply the drug.
- **(6)** **Electrodesiccation** or **electrocautery** is contraindicated in patients with anal lesions or with a pacemaker.
- **(7)** **Surgical tangential shave/scissor excision** or **curettage.**

  b. Alternative therapies include the following:
- **(1)** **Carbon dioxide laser** is necessary only with warts that are very extensive or very resistant to other therapies.
- **(2)** **Interferon alpha-2b** (Intron-A) can be injected on the base of lesions 3 times per week for 3 weeks and repeated as needed. (SOR **C**) This drug is extremely expensive, and its use should be restricted to recalcitrant cases.

2. Treatment for **secondary syphilis,** which is extremely contagious, is the same as for primary syphilis.

   3. Spontaneous remission of **molluscum contagiosum** occurs in weeks to several
   months. **Cryotherapy, curettage,** or **electrocautery** can be done (see Section
   VI.B.1.a).
   4. Reassurance is all that is necessary for **pearly penile papules.**
C. Pruritic lesions
   1. Balanitis
      a. The foreskin should be kept retracted as much as possible.
      b. The glans should be dried thoroughly after showering and micturition.
      c. Candidiasis superinfection should be treated with an **imidazole** cream (ketocona-
         zole, butoconazole, clotrimazole, econazole, miconazole, isoconazole, tioconazole,
         or terconazole), ciclopirox, or **nystatin** cream, topically twice daily, or fluconazole,
         150 mg orally in a single dose. (SOR **A**) Ketoconazole and itraconazole might be
         as effective but have a higher potential for toxicity. Terbinafine should not be used
         as a primary agent for *Candida*.
      d. The glans and prepuce should be washed with soap and water and dried thoroughly
         after sexual intercourse.
      e. Circumcision may be needed if phimosis develops or in resistant cases, since
         chronic balanitis is a potential precursor of premalignant penile glanular changes.
   2. Povidone-iodine soap cleansing can be sufficient for **erythrasma. Econazole** cream
      twice daily for 7 to 10 days or **erythromycin base** 250 mg orally 4 times daily for 14 days
      (SOR **A**) is also effective against the causative agent (*Corynebacterium minutissi-
      mum*).
   3. Lindane 1% shampoo applied for 4 minutes or **permethrin** 1% creme rinse or
      pyrethrins with piperonyl butoxide applied for 10 minutes and then thoroughly
      washed off are effective treatments for **pubic lice.** (SOR **A**) Lindane should be avoided
      in children and during gestation and lactation. **Permethrin** has less potential for toxicity
      than lindane.
   4. Vulvar dystrophy/LSA and BXO
      a. When biopsy reveals intraepithelial neoplasia, either **laser therapy** or conventional
         surgical excision is indicated.
      b. In **LSA/BXO, topical testosterone** is no longer recommended. Highly potent **top-
         ical steroids** (e.g., clobetasol 0.05%) should be carefully rubbed on the lesion
         twice daily for 1 month and then once daily for 2 to 3 weeks followed by lower-
         potency steroids (triamcinolone acetonide 0.1% or betamethasone valerate 0.1%)
         twice daily for a few weeks. (SOR **B**) Tacrolimus ointment 0.1% and pimecrolimus
         cream 1% twice daily are also effective (off-label use). Leukoplakia requires close
         follow-up; 5-fluorouracil topically is often used instead. (SOR **C**)
D. Cystic lesions
   1. Bartholin's gland cysts/inflammation
      a. Hot, wet dressings, or sitz baths may promote spontaneous drainage of cysts.
      b. Incision and drainage are effective in most abscesses.
      c. Marsupialization is recommended for recurrences.
      d. Antibiotic therapy is not necessary unless there is associated cellulitis, generally
         caused by staphylococci, streptococci, coliforms, or anaerobes.

REFERENCES

Wolff K, Fitzpatrick TB, et al. *Fitzpatrick's Color Atlas and Synopsis of Clinical Dermatology.* 5th ed.
   McGraw-Hill; 2005.
Gilbert DN, Moellering RC, Sande MA. *The Sanford Guide to Antimicrobial Therapy.* 37th ed. Antimicrobial Therapy; 2007.
Guidelines for Treatment of Sexually Transmitted Diseases, 2006. *Morb Mortal Wkly Rep.* 2006;55:RR-
   11. http://www. cdc.gov/mmwr/preview/mmwrhtml/rr5511a1.htm.
National Center for Health Statistics. National Ambulatory Medical Care Survey (NAMCS): 2004 Sum-
   mary. Advance Data from Vital and Health Statistics No. 374. National Center for Health Statistics, Centers for Disease Control and Prevention. http://www.cdc.gov/mmwr/preview/mmwrhtml/
   mm5453a1.htm. Accessed June 23, 2006.
Pickering LK, ed. *Red Book: 2006 Report of the Committee on Infectious Diseases.* 27th ed. American
   Academy of Pediatrics; 2006.

32   Hair & Nail Disorders

Amy D. Crawford-Faucher, MD

KEY POINTS

- Ninety-five percent of alopecia cases presenting to primary care physicians are potentially treatable.
- Hirsutism associated with virilization requires hormonal evaluation.
- Only 50% of dystrophic nails are onychomycotic; accurate diagnosis is key to appropriate therapy.
- Melanoma and metastatic cancers sometimes present as nail disorders.

I. **Definition.** Hair follicles produce one of two types of human hair: **vellus hair** is fine, hypopigmented, and barely visible; and **terminal hair,** which is coarse and usually pigmented. Follicles cycle through three stages: anagen (hair growth), catagen (transition), and telogen (rest). Hair shafts mature and are shed after the telogen phase. Scalp hair follicles normally stay in anagen for 2 to 8 years, producing potentially long hairs, then "rest" in telogen for 2 to 3 months. Abnormal hair growth or loss is usually not medically serious, but can indicate systemic disease, and may cause significant emotional distress.

    Alopecia (hair loss) may be localized, patchy, diffuse, or total. It usually occurs when hair follicles are damaged by chemical or physical agents, or by infectious or immunologically mediated inflammation. Metabolic diseases, many medications, and physiologic stresses can also slow or disrupt the normal hair growth cycle and result in alopecia. When hair follicles are retained, there is potential for regrowth, and the alopecia is considered **noncicatricial** (**nonscarring**). If hair follicles are destroyed, the alopecia is **cicatricial** (**scarring**).

    Hirsutism is excess hair growth in a typically male distribution and is because of excess androgen (testosterone and its precursors dehydroepiandrosterone sulfate and 17α-hydroxyprogesterone [17-OHP]) originating in the ovaries, adrenals, or exogenously from medications. These androgens act on a woman's androgen-sensitive follicles (located primarily on the face, chest, upper back, lower abdomen, and inner thighs) to produce terminal instead of vellus-type hair. Hirsutism may be an isolated condition or occur in conjunction with other virilizing symptoms and signs that indicate androgen excess. **Hypertrichosis** refers to excess hair growth that may be diffuse and is not sensitive to androgens.

    Normal nail anatomy includes a vascular and highly innervated nail bed that underlies the nail, which is composed of dead keratin. The proximal end of the nail bed comprises the matrix, from which new nail grows. The perionychium folds around the nail edge proximally and laterally, producing the nail folds. Abnormal nails result from trauma, infection, systemic disease, or congenital conditions or may be variants of normal. Damage to the matrix can cause permanent nail growth abnormalities. Accurate diagnosis of nail disorders is necessary for effective treatment and for prompt evaluation of potentially serious systemic disease.

II. **Common Diagnoses**

    A. **Alopecias** (Table 32–1). Before the era of approved medical therapy for common male pattern baldness, approximately 1 of every 2000 office visits to family physicians was for some form of hair loss; this figure is likely higher today. Nonscarring alopecias account for ≥ 95% of the hair loss seen by primary care physicians. The six causes listed below are the most common and important.

        1. **Androgenetic alopecia,** including male and female pattern baldness, is more common than all other causes of alopecia combined. It affects nearly three-quarters of men to some degree, and probably more than one-third of women. More than half of men show signs of this hair loss by age 50. In genetically susceptible people, androgens gradually transform terminal follicles on the scalp to vellus-like follicles, which eventually atrophy. Androgenetic alopecia is controlled by one dominant, sex-limited, autosomal gene that may be incompletely expressed because of polygenic modifying factors.

        2. **Traumatic alopecia** is relatively common on the occiput of infants who sleep on their backs, and in persons with hairstyles (tight braids, curlers) that put continuous traction

TABLE 32–1. DIAGNOSES AND ETIOLOGIC CLASSIFICATIONS OF ALOPECIA

Cicatricial (scarring) alopecias
Neoplastic: localized or metastatic
Nevoid: nevus sebaceous, epidermal nevus
Physical or chemical: burns, freezing, trauma, radiation, acids, alkalis
Infectious: bacterial, fungal, protozoal, viral, mycobacterial
Congenital or developmental: aplasia cutis, Darier disease, recessive X-linked ichthyosis, keratosis pilaris
  atrophicans
Dermatosis-related: lichen planus, necrobiosis lipoidica diabeticorum, cicatricial pemphigoid, folliculitis
  decalvans
Systemic disease: lupus erythematosus, sarcoidosis, scleroderma, dermatomyositis, amyloidosis

Noncicatricial (nonscarring) alopecias
Drug-induced: antimetabolites, anticoagulants, beta-blockers, antidepressants, lithium, levodopa
Congenital: ectodermal dysplasias, hair shaft disorders
Infectious: secondary syphilis, tinea capitis, human immunodeficiency virus infection
Toxic: arsenic, boric acid, thallium, vitamin A
Nutritional: anorexia nervosa, marasmus, kwashiorkor, "crash" diets, iron or zinc deficiency
Traumatic: trichotillomania, traction, friction, chemical, thermal
Endocrine: hyper- or hypothyroidism, hypopituitarism, hyper- or hypoparathyroidism
Immunologic: alopecia areata
Genetic or developmental: male and female pattern baldness (androgenetic alopecia)
Radiation-induced: x-ray epilation
Physiologic: telogen effluvium (postpartum, postsurgical, febrile illness, severe psychological stress, puberty)

on the follicle. Recurrent, compulsive hair plucking (trichotillomania) can also lead to traumatic alopecia.

3. **Infectious alopecia,** mainly owing to **tinea capitis,** affects up to 4% of all children; it less commonly occurs in adults. Intense inflammation can injure the hair follicles.

4. **Physiologic alopecia,** called **telogen effluvium,** results in diffuse hair loss and most often occurs 2 to 3 months postpartum, following the cessation of oral contraception or corticosteroids, or after serious illness or stress. This hair loss occurs when an unusually large number of follicles (25%–45%) abruptly end anagen and move through catagen and into telogen (rest) phase. Large numbers of telogen hairs then synchronously fall out.

5. **Alopecia areata** has a prevalence of 0.1% of the general population, with lifetime risk approaching 2%. It affects men and women equally. More than half the cases arise by age 40, and there is a familial tendency. Alopecia areata tends to be associated with other autoimmune diseases, such as pernicious anemia, vitiligo, Hashimoto thyroiditis, and atopic dermatitis, and in Down syndrome. While most cases eventually resolve spontaneously, cases that present before puberty, are recurrent, or do not respond to treatment, and carry a poor prognosis for hair regrowth.

6. **Hair loss caused by systemic processes** including thyroid disease, other endocrinopathies, and malnutrition, either slows the rate of hair growth or alters the balance between the anagen and telogen phases in the hair follicles.

B. **Hirsutism** (Table 32–2) affects up to 10% of all women.

1. **Idiopathic hirsutism** is most common in women of Mediterranean ancestry and is thought to represent increased follicle sensitivity to normal levels of circulating androgens. Idiopathic hirsutism is a diagnosis of exclusion.

2. **Polycystic ovarian syndrome (PCOS)** is the most common androgen-excess condition causing hirsutism and affects between 6% and 8% of reproductive-age women.

3. Prevalence of **adult-onset congenital adrenal hyperplasia** is unclear but clearly varies with ethnic background. The disorder is uncommon in women of Northern European ancestry and occurs with greater frequency in Ashkenazi Jews, Hispanics, and Central Europeans.

4. **Cushing syndrome** is a rare cause of hirsutism.

5. **Ovarian or adrenal tumors** are rare causes of hirsutism.

6. **Medications** can cause both hirsutism and hypertrichosis (Table 32–3).

C. **Nail disorders.** The most common nail disorders are listed below.

1. **Onychomycosis,** a fungal infection of the nails, comprises one-half of nail diagnoses, affecting up to 20% of adults, and a much smaller percentage of children. Toenails are

TABLE 32–2. **CAUSES OF HYPERTRICHOSIS AND HIRSUTISM**

Hypertrichosis	Hirsutism
Idiopathic	Polycystic ovarian syndrome (PCOS)
Familial	Congenital adrenal hyperplasia
Puberty	Adrenal or ovarian neoplasm
Pregnancy	Cushing syndrome
Menopause	
Hypothyroidism	
Acromegaly	
Hurler syndrome	
Porphyria cutaneous tarda	
Multiple sclerosis	
Encephalitis	

more commonly involved than fingernails and prolonged or repeated foot dampness and locker room exposure may predispose to infection.

2. **Paronychia,** infection of the proximal or lateral nail folds, is due acutely to local trauma, such as a "hangnail," and chronically to repeated exposure to moisture, as in dishwashers or swimmers.

3. Direct trauma to the nail and fingertip can cause a **subungual hematoma,** with blood from ruptured nail bed vessels collecting in the potential space between the nail bed and plate.

4. **Ingrown nails** are also common, occurring most commonly on the medial edge of the great toenail. Ill-fitting shoes, nail dystrophies, and onychomycosis can all predispose to the condition.

5. **Discolored nails** can be caused by a wide variety of conditions (Table 32–4).

6. **Systemic diseases** can manifest as nail disorders. Alopecia areata, chronic hypoxia, iron deficiency anemia, zinc deficiency, and hypocalcemia can cause nail abnormalities.

III. **Symptoms.** Evaluation of patients with **alopecia** should include duration and location of hair loss, major life changes, physical trauma, drug intake, and hair care habits. For **hirsutism,** the onset, associated signs and symptoms, medication use, ethnic origin, and affected family members are important.

   A. The vast majority of processes leading to alopecia, hirsutism, and hypertrichosis are remarkably symptom-free locally. Trauma or infectious processes such as tinea capitis may cause itching and pain. Women with **hirsutism from androgen excess** commonly report rapid onset of postpubertal virilization and irregular menses. Those with **idiopathic hirsutism** report gradual onset of mild hirsutism, normal menses, and no virilizing signs. Women with hirsutism and *PCOS* often give a history of oligomenorrhea and infertility. Many patients experience psychological distress over their hair loss or excess growth.

   B. **Pain** is a common complaint with ingrown nails from any cause, and from acute or chronic paronychia. Onychomycosis and other nail infections may be painless. Significant throbbing pain at the nail is the hallmark of subungual hematoma, occurring within hours to a day of a crush injury to the fingertip and nail.

TABLE 32–3. **MEDICATIONS CAUSING HYPERTRICHOSIS OR HIRSUTISM**

Hypertrichosis	Hirsutism
Minoxidil (forearms and legs in women)	Anabolic steroids
Cyclosporine	Danazol
Corticosteroids	Reglan
Diazoxide	Aldomet
Streptomycin	Progestins
Interferon	Reserpine
Acetazolamide	Phenothiazines
Phenothiazines	Testosterone
Phenytoin	
Psoralens	

TABLE 32–4. **CAUSES OF DISCOLORED NAILS**

White (leukonychia)
Fungus
Physical stress/mild trauma (transverse lines or spots that grow out with the nail)
Nail bed injury (transverse lines that do not move with the nail)
Heavy metal poisoning (e.g., arsenic) (transverse lines)
Liver disease (all-white nails)
Renal failure and uremia (half white, half pink nails)
Idiopathic (spots and lines)
Congenital

Brown/black
Lines common in dark-skinned persons
Nevus (confined to nail)
Melanoma (may "run over" onto nail fold)
Fungus
Psoriasis or alopecia areata
Chloroquine (bluish)
Quinacrine (bluish)
Several chemotherapeutic agents
Heavy metal poisoning

Yellow
Fungus
Nonpseudomonal bacteria
Psoriasis (usually not uniform)
Alopecia areata (usually not uniform)
Lymphedema
AIDS
Addison disease

Green
Pseudomonal infection

Blue
Minocycline
Doxorubicin (brownish)
Wilson disease
Ochronosis (gray–blue)

Red
Darier disease (longitudinal streaks)

IV. **Signs.** With **hirsutism,** signs of virilization should be sought; including varying degrees of clitoromegaly, cystic acne, decreased breast size, deepened voice, increased libido, increased muscle mass, malodorous perspiration, oligomenorrhea, and temporal hair recession and balding. With **alopecia** a helpful clinical clue is the presence of follicular orifices, which implies a noncicatricial (potentially reversible) process. The following local signs will rapidly narrow the differential diagnosis in alopecia, hirsutism, and nail abnormalities.
   A. **Androgenetic alopecia**
      1. **Male pattern baldness** is most often characterized by frontotemporal hairline recession (in an "M" pattern) with variable hair loss at the scalp vertex.
      2. **Female pattern baldness** predominantly results from diffuse or vertex hair loss. Sometimes the part becomes prominent, but the hair along the frontal hairline is spared.
   B. **Traumatic alopecia** usually shows patchy hair loss but may also be diffuse. Localized breakage with variously shortened hairs suggests mechanical damage.
   C. **Infectious alopecia** caused by tinea capitis exhibits discrete patches of partial hair loss and breakage overlying scaly, inflamed skin. Less commonly, a **kerion** induced by the dermatophyte *Trichophyton tonsurans* causes a deep, purulent folliculitis. With severe fungal infections or marked cellulitis, inflammation and suppuration can cause destruction and scarring. Secondary syphilis, in contrast, leads to a diffuse, moth-eaten appearance of the scalp.

D. Physiologic alopecia is suggested by acute, diffuse, yet reversible hair thinning. When present, transverse nail depressions (Beau lines) imply a subacute physiologic injury.

E. Alopecia areata is characterized by the abrupt onset of patchy but very well-demarcated hair loss. This process leaves discrete areas of smooth, hairless, noninflamed skin that is surrounded by easily plucked hairs. "Exclamation point" hairs are short, heavily pigmented shafts with wide, brush-like distal ends that taper at the skin surface and can sometimes be found at the periphery of areata patches. There can be complete loss of scalp hair (**alopecia totalis**) or of all body hair (**alopecia universalis**), although this is less common than other types of hair loss. Pitted nails are seen in up to one-third of patients.

F. Systemic diseases, such as thyroid disease, exhibit their specific associated signs in addition to diffuse hair loss and thinning.

G. PCOS can be associated with obesity.

H. Adrenal or ovarian neoplasms are associated with rapid onset of significant hair growth many years after puberty and with other virilizing signs. (See sidebar for other neoplasms.)

MELANOMA/CARCINOMA AND NAILS

Malignant melanoma can present as a new hyperpigmented longitudinal line on a nail, especially if it "runs over" onto the proximal nail fold or takes over the entire nail.

Squamous cell carcinoma, melanoma or, rarely, **metastatic cancer** can manifest as a paronychia that does not respond to usual treatments. Biopsy of the nail bed is necessary to diagnose these cancers.

I. Onychomycosis
  1. **Distal onychomycosis** causes nails to become white, yellow, or brownish. The nail thickens and subungual debris collects at the distal tip.
  2. **White superficial onychomycosis** causes soft, rough nails that crumble.
  3. **Proximal onychomycosis** is least common and occurs when *Trichophyton rubrum* invades the proximal nail fold, infects the newly formed nail plate, and moves distally.

J. Acute paronychia presents with significant erythema, tenderness, and fluctuance along the proximal or lateral nail border. **Chronic paronychia** often involves many nails and is less erythematous. Affected nails become tender intermittently, especially after water exposure. The proximal nail folds become edematous but are rarely fluctuant.

K. Subungual hematoma causes an exquisitely tender nail that may appear partially or completely red–blue, purple, or black because of accumulated blood. If significant portions of the bed are affected, the nail may separate partially or completely (onycholysis).

L. Ingrown nails act as a foreign body to cause inflammation and sometimes infection at the site where the corner of the nail grows into the adjacent lateral nail bed. With chronic inflammation, granulation tissue grows over the affected portion of nail. The area is extremely tender to touch and may be fluctuant.

M. Systemic diseases can manifest specific nail abnormalities. **Psoriasis** most commonly causes deep pits in the nails, but can also cause separation (onycholysis), discoloration, and subungual thickening with nail debris accumulation. These findings may be confused with onychomycosis. Usually the nail involvement occurs in conjunction with typical skin symptoms, but it may be the sole sign of the disease. **Alopecia areata** causes shallow pitting with progressive opacification. Clubbing from **chronic hypoxemia** is a chronic and permanent convex nail curvature and swelling of the skin around the proximal nail fold. Occasionally, clubbing occurs as a normal variant. Spoon-shaped (concave) nails in adults can occur with **iron deficiency anemia,** transverse depressions (Beau lines) may indicate **zinc deficiency** or **physiologic stress,** whereas whitish nails may occur in hypocalcemia.

N. Nail curvature, hypertrophy, or splitting may result from repeated nail trauma, such as from constricting shoes, although the etiology is not always clear.

V. Laboratory Tests
  A. Most cases of **alopecia** can be diagnosed by a thorough personal history and a careful physical examination. Ancillary tests may be helpful in certain situations.
    1. The **hair pull or pluck test** involves a moderately firm pull of 10 to 20 closely grouped hairs. Normally, less than 20% of the shafts will be removed, but in telogen

effluvium and active androgenetic alopecia, more than 40% of the shafts will be uprooted.

2. **Potassium hydroxide (KOH) preparation of hair shafts on a gently warmed slide is used primarily to diagnose tinea capitis.** Rarely, **fungal cultures of hair shafts are needed.** Wood's light examination is only helpful in the 5% to 10% of tinea capitis infections that are caused by *Microsporum* species.

3. A **trichogram** involves the microscopic analysis of at least 50 plucked hairs to determine hair structure and the proportion of telogen follicles. These hairs are removed from one area using a hemostat. Telogen hairs have small, unpigmented, ovoid bulbs and no internal root sheath. Anagen hairs have larger, elongated, pigmented bulbs shaped like the end of a broom, with a narrow internal root sheath. In telogen effluvium, between 20% and 60% of the patient's hair will be telogen hairs. Anagen hairs that show atrophied bulbs are typical in patients with androgenetic alopecia.

4. A **hair count** is the actual count of all hairs lost over several days. Up to 100 hairs per day is considered normal. Elevated counts are typical of telogen effluvium.

5. **Scalp biopsy** is usually reserved for cases of uncertain origin but may be helpful in determining the prognosis of patients with alopecia areata and lupus erythematosus based on the degree of perifollicular lymphocytic infiltration and antibody deposition, respectively.

6. **Assessment of endocrine dysfunction** may include thyroid tests (e.g., thyroid-stimulating hormone). Women with androgenetic hair loss should undergo the same evaluation as hirsute women (see Section V.B).

7. **Hematologic, serologic, rheumatologic,** and **blood chemistry tests** should be performed only when systemic disease is suspected, except for balding women, in whom a complete blood cell count, antinuclear antibody test, and ferritin level are routinely indicated.

B. Women with **hirsutism** associated with mild hair growth, normal menses and fertility, and no other virilizing signs may well have idiopathic hirsutism, and may not need extensive laboratory evaluation. However, a PCOS evaluation may still be justified. (SOR **C**) With more significant symptoms/signs, laboratory tests can help detect serious systemic disease; a sequential approach is best (Figure 32–1).

1. With **irregular menses,** thyroid function, prolactin, 17-OHP, and testosterone should be measured; if these are normal, PCOS and anovulation are likely. For suspected PCOS, blood glucose and lipid screening should be done, and measurement of serum insulin levels considered.

2. With **virilization, testosterone, dehydroepiandrosterone sulfate,** and **17-OHP levels** are used in initial screening for ovarian or adrenal tumors. These hormones can be normal or mildly increased in PCOS; marked elevations suggest ovarian or adrenal tumors, respectively. Virilization also requires imaging (computerized tomography or magnetic resonance imaging) of the adrenal glands or ovaries.

C. Many **nail conditions** can be adequately diagnosed by careful history and physical, including search for other signs of systemic illness. Testing primarily confirms the diagnosis of onychomycosis.

1. **KOH stain and fungal cultures** are necessary to diagnose onychomycosis, because only 50% of dystrophic nails are actually mycotic. Although office-based tests exist, the standard remains KOH stain, culture, or both. Affected nail and nail bed should be sampled, using a no. 15 blade or sharp curette to obtain debris from different locations on multiple affected nails. Testing for specific species is generally not warranted, as current treatments are effective against most fungi.

2. **Biopsy** is indicated to diagnose tumors, inflammatory disease, and infections when the diagnosis is unclear. The nail bed, perionychium, or matrix can be biopsied. As nail matrix biopsy can cause permanent nail dystrophy, referral to a dermatologist is usually warranted.

VI. Treatment

A. The goals of **alopecia** treatment are slowing hair loss and maximizing hair regrowth. No "magic pill" exists, and any gains may be subtle. Treatment may be required indefinitely to prevent further hair loss.

1. Androgenetic alopecia

a. **Minoxidil (Rogaine)** solution is a topical agent with unclear mechanism of action that can increase the number of new hairs in thinning scalp. One milliliter is applied to affected areas morning and night.

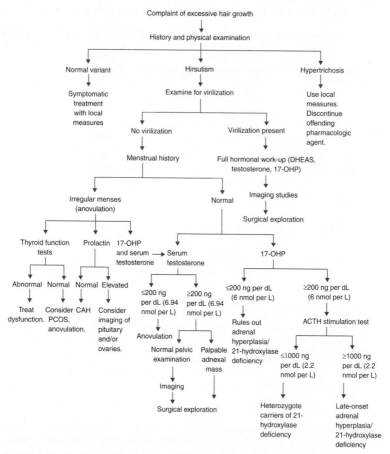

FIGURE 32–1. Algorithm for evaluation of hirsutism. ACTH, adrenocorticotropic hormone; CAH, congenital adrenal hyperplasia; DHEAS, dehydroepiandrosterone sulfate; PCOS, polycystic ovary syndrome; 17-OHP, 17α-hydroxyprogesterone. (Reproduced with permission from Hunter MH, Carek PJ. Evaluation and treatment of women with hirsutism. *Am Fam Physician.* 2003;67:2565-2572.)

    (1) Minoxidil is not effective on receding temporal baldness, and is most successful in those with hair loss of ≤5 years, vertex baldness ≤10 cm, and with the presence of many indeterminate (between vellus and terminal) hairs.

    (2) Approximately 40% of men report acceptable hair regrowth after 1 year of treatment.

    (3) Minoxidil comes as 2% and 5% solutions. Two double-blinded, placebo-controlled, randomized trials compared 5% and 2% minoxidil with placebo. One trial studied only women, the other only men. In both studies, the 5% solution was significantly more effective than either the 2% solution or placebo and was well tolerated, although local irritation did increase with the stronger solution. (SOR **Ⓐ**) The main side effect in women is hypertrichosis of the face and arms that generally resolves over a year of continued use.

  b. **Finasteride (Propecia)** is the only oral medication approved for baldness. Dosed at 1 mg daily, it inhibits 5α-reductase in the follicle to reduce the effects of testosterone.

Results can be slow, but two-thirds of men have increased hair growth after 2 years of treatment. An open label trial comparing finasteride to 5% minoxidil suggests that finasteride may be more effective. Like minoxidil, finasteride must be used indefinitely to maintain hair growth. The most common side effect is sexual dysfunction, affecting 4% of men in one study (compared to 2% on placebo).

(1) Propecia is not effective for alopecia in postmenopausal women, and in fact should be handled cautiously by women of child bearing age, as the drug can theoretically cause genital abnormalities in male fetuses.

c. **Oral contraceptives** do not treat androgenetic baldness in women, but progesterones with low androgen effects (e.g., norgestimate, norethindrone, desogestrel, and ethynodiol diacetate) can help prevent worsening of alopecia.

d. **Other medical therapies** may improve androgenetic alopecia. Oral spironolactone, 50 to 200 mg/d, may be helpful as adjunctive treatment in women, and combination therapy (e.g., minoxidil with finasteride) seems to be somewhat more effective than either drug alone in men. Other 5α-reductase inhibitors are being studied, but safety is a concern as higher doses are required for hair growth than for treatment of BPH.

e. **Surgical methods,** including hair transplantation, remain options for men, but results are generally less satisfactory in women whose hair loss is usually more diffuse.

2. **Traumatic alopecia** is treated by avoidance of the causative action. Trichotillomania can be difficult to treat; a combination of psychological counseling and antidepressant medication may be effective.

3. **Tinea capitis** needs to be treated systemically, as topical antifungals do not penetrate the hair shaft. While only griseofulvin is approved by the US Food and Drug Administration (FDA) in children, terbinafine (Lamisil), itraconazole (Sporanox), and fluconazole (Diflucan) have all been used in children and adults. A meta-analysis comparing terbinafine to griseofulvin found that a 2- to 4-week course of terbinafine is at least as effective as a 6- to 8-week course of griseofulvin for tinea capitis. (SOR **Ⓐ**) The following dosages seem to produce equivalent results after a 3-week course: **terbinafine,** 250 mg daily (125 mg/d if weight 20–40 kg; 62.5 mg/d if ≤20 kg), **fluconazole,** 6 mg/kg/d, or itraconazole, 5 mg/kg/d. (In children, **itraconazole** can be dosed at 100 mg every other day for weight 10–20 kg, 100 mg alternating with 200 mg daily for weight 30–50 kg, and 200 mg/d for children ≥50 kg.)

4. **Telogen effluvium** requires recognition of the inciting event and reassurance that hair growth will normalize.

5. **Alopecia areata** remains challenging to treat.

a. **Intralesional steroid injection** is the treatment of choice for less severe cases (≤50% of the scalp affected). **Triamcinolone (Kenalog)** 5 to 10 mg/mL is used: 0.1 mL is injected intradermally into multiple sites of each patch up to a monthly maximum of 20 to 30 mg. Applying **minoxidil,** a mid-potency topical steroid, or both in between injections may hasten resolution.

b. **Strategies for more severe cases** (affecting ≥ 50% of the scalp) can be complex and include topical immunotherapy, anthralin, and topical or systemic steroids. Therapy for severe alopecia areata is best managed by practitioners experienced with the disorder.

B. **Hirsutism** can be controlled either through hair removal processes, suppression of androgens, or a combination of both.

1. **Hair removal**

a. **Mechanical hair removal** includes shaving, plucking, and waxing. These techniques are relatively inexpensive, but the results are variably short (2–3 days for shaving, 2 weeks for plucking, up to 8 weeks for waxing), can be painful, and often are unacceptable to women.

b. Over-the-counter **chemical depilatories** can provide a 2-week hair-free interval. Local skin irritation is common.

c. **Electrolysis** is performed by specially trained technicians. While considered effective for permanent hair removal, the results are operator- and technique-dependent. Electrolysis is time-consuming, requiring multiple sessions.

d. **Laser therapy** is becoming more popular for hair removal. Lasers direct specific wavelengths of light at the follicles; the absorbed energy damages and sometimes destroys the follicle. Traditionally, lasers worked best on those with dark hair and light skin, because the pigment best absorbs the heat. Advances in laser technology have made laser therapy effective in all hair and skin types; the Nd-YAG laser is a popular type. Often 3 to 6 treatments several weeks apart are needed to produce permanent results.

    e. Eflornithine HCl (Vaniqa) is a topical hair growth modulator that can be effective against unwanted facial hair in women. Eflornithine is applied twice daily to the affected areas of the face; results are usually apparent after 4 to 8 weeks of regular use. Often prescribed by primary care physicians, eflornithine may be used indefinitely, and is most effective when used in conjunction with other modalities of hair removal (such as laser therapy or hormonal treatment).

  2. Several **hormonal therapies** have proved effective in suppressing androgens. These medications are not approved by the FDA for hirsutism, and except for metformin, are labeled pregnancy category D or X; reliable contraception is an important component of therapy.

    a. Oral contraceptives with low androgen effects (see Section VI.A.1.c) can decrease hair growth by 50% to 75%. They confer other benefits to patients with PCOS and are frequently used in conjunction with other medications.

    b. Spironolactone (see Section VI.A.1.d) suppresses testosterone production and inhibits uptake through 5α-reductase in the follicle.

    c. Flutamide (Eulexin) is an antiandrogen dosed at 250 mg orally 2 to 3 times a day. Monthly liver function testing (for 4 months, then periodic monitoring) is necessary.

    d. Finasteride (Proscar) is an antiandrogen; daily dose is 5 mg orally. Results are slow, because effects may be delayed $\geq$1 year.

    e. Metformin (Glucophage) is an insulin-sensitizing agent that results in decreased amounts of free testosterone and minimal hair reduction in women with PCOS. Dosing regimens for metformin include 500 to 1000 mg orally twice daily, or 850 mg 3 times daily. Troglitazone (Rezulin) showed moderate hair reduction, but it is no longer available in the United States.

    f. Gonadotropin-releasing hormone antagonists are potent therapies usually prescribed by endocrinologists or gynecologists experienced with their use. **Leuprolide (Lupron)** is given as an intramuscular injection dosed at 3.75 mg monthly up to 6 months. It may be used for severe or resistant hirsutism, but its side effect profile demands careful risk–benefit analysis. **Cyproterone** is a progestin that acts as a gonadotropin-releasing hormone blocker. It is not available in the United States but is commonly used in other countries as a combination oral contraceptive (**Diane**) for maintenance therapy.

    g. Dexamethasone (0.5 mg nightly) or prednisone (5–10 mg daily) may be helpful in congenital adrenal hyperplasia, but its significant side effect profile may restrict its use by experienced practitioners for resistant or severe hirsutism.

C. Treatment of **nail disorders** is specific to the underlying cause.

  1. Oral antifungal therapy remains the mainstay of treatment for **onychomycosis,** because local agents generally cannot penetrate the nail. Some data suggest that topical amorolfine (Loceryl) can be effective, especially in combination with oral therapy. However, it is not available in the United States. A meta-analysis comparing all oral therapies found terbinafine (Lamisil) to be the most effective agent for dermatophyte infections, followed by itraconazole (Sporanox), either in continuous or pulse therapy. (SOR **A**) Fluconazole (Diflucan) had lower cure rates. The treatment regimens are compared in Table 32–5.

  2. Subungual hematomas respond best to immediate drainage to relieve pressure. Any heated probe, such as an electrocautery probe or even the tip of a paper clip (heated until red hot), is pressed against the nail over the hematoma to make a small puncture. The blood is expressed with gentle pressure, affording almost immediate pain relief.

  3. Ingrown nails with mild inflammation can be treated conservatively with warm soaks, elevating the nail corner with cotton to avoid the inflamed tissue as it grows out, and oral antibiotics if there is a superinfection. Patients should be counseled to trim the nails straight across, which prevents cutting the corners of the nail too short, and to avoid shoes with a narrow toe box. If the ingrown nail does not resolve with these methods, the medial third of the nail should be removed (see Chapter 28).

  4. Acute paronychia usually requires incision and drainage of any fluid collections. The most fluctuant area along the nail fold can be drained by incising with a small blade

TABLE 32–5. ANTIFUNGAL THERAPY FOR ONYCHOMYCOSIS

Continuous Therapy	Dose	Monitoring
Terbinafine (Lamisil)	250 mg/d for 6 wk (fingernails); 12 wk (toenails)	CBC, AST, ALT at baseline, then every 4–6 wk
Itraconazole (Sporanox)	200 mg/d for 6 wk (fingernails); 12 wk (toenails)	AST and ALT at baseline, then every 4–6 wk
Pulse therapy		
Itraconazole (Sporanox)	200 mg twice daily for 7 consecutive days per month; repeat for 2–3 mo (fingernails) and 3–4 mo (toenails)	None recommended
Fluconazole (Diflucan)	150 mg once weekly for 6–9 mo (until nail is improved)	None recommended

CBC, complete blood count; ALT, alanine aminotransferase; AST, aspartate aminotransferase.
Reproduced with permission from Rodgers P, Bassler M. Treating onychomycosis. *Am Fam Physician.* 2001;63:663-672, 677-678.

(either a no. 11 or no. 15 blade), or by gently separating the nail fold from the nail plate to facilitate drainage without cutting the skin. The incision is irrigated and followed up with frequent warm soaks to keep the wound open. Antibiotics are usually not necessary, but are appropriate if local drainage and soaks do not resolve the parony-chia. Sulfamethoxazole–trimethoprim (Bactrim) or clindamycin (Cleocin) are reason-able choices, given the increasing prevalence of methicillin-resistant *Staphylococcus aureus* in some communities.

5. **Chronic paronychia** is more difficult to treat, because several nails are affected and incision and drainage is usually not an option. Treatments include avoiding chronic exposure to moisture (or wearing cotton-lined rubber gloves when unable to prevent exposure) and using 1:1 vinegar–water soaks. A small randomized study reported greater cure rates with the use of topical steroids than with oral antifungals, suggesting that the presence of candidal infection may not contribute significantly to the condition. Areas of inflammation or discharge can be cultured to allow specific treatment as *Staphylococcus* species and *Pseudomonas* have also been implicated and require oral antibiotics. Treatment failures should prompt a search for underlying systemic disease, such as psoriasis.

6. **Nail changes of underlying systemic disorders,** such as psoriasis and alopecia areata, may improve with treatment of the disease, but nail-specific treatment has not been overly successful. Clubbing is usually a permanent change.

REFERENCES

Hordinsky MK. Medical treatment of noncicatricial alopecia. *Semin Cutan Med Surg.* 2006;25(1): 51-55.

Lucky AW, Piacquadio DJ, Ditre CM, et al. Treatment of Alopecia: comparing concentrations of minoxidil. A randomized, placebo-controlled trial of 5% and 2% topical minoxidil solutions in the treatment of female pattern hair loss. *J Am Acad Dermatol.* 2004;50(4):541-553.

Olsen EA, Dunlap FE, Funicella T, et al. A randomized clinical trial of 5% topical minoxidil versus 2% topical minoxidil and placebo in the treatment of androgenetic alopecia in men. *J Am Acad Dermatol.* 2002;47(3):377-385.

Roberts BJ, Friedlander SF. Tinea capitis: a treatment update. *Pediatr Ann.* 2005;34(3):191-200.

Roberts DT, Taylor WD, Boyle J. Guidelines for treatment of onychomycosis. *Br J Dermatol.* 2003; 148(3):402-410.

Tosti A, Piraccini BM, Ghetti E, Colombo MD. Topical steroids versus systemic antifungals in the treat-ment of chronic paronychia: an open, randomized double-blind and double dummy study. *J Am Acad Dermatol.* 2002;47(1):73-76.

33   Hand & Wrist Complaints

Ted Boehm, MD, & Nicole G. Stern, MD

KEY POINTS

- Overuse injuries are common.
- Fractures and tendon injuries should not be missed.
- A normal neurovascular examination should always be documented.
- The contralateral side should be examined for comparison.

I. **Definition.** The hand and wrist consist of 28 bones, numerous articulations, and 19 intrinsic and 20 extrinsic muscles. The surface anatomy can be separated into dorsal, volar (palmar), radial, and ulnar sides. The palm is divided into thenar, midpalm, and hypothenar areas; the **thenar eminence,** containing the small thumb muscles, represents the area just proximal to the thumb, and the opposite side of the palm is the **hypothenar eminence.** Overall, the unique anatomy of the hand and wrist, with closely situated and interrelated structures, allows for extensive variability of movement necessary in functional and recreational activities. Whether occurring acutely or chronically, injuries to the hand or wrist can be debilitating. **Common complaints involving the hand and wrist** include pain, numbness, tingling, instability, weakness, skin discoloration, coldness, swelling, and bony deformity. These are most often owing to overuse, trauma, nerve compression, and underlying systemic diseases such as diabetes mellitus, hypothyroidism, and rheumatoid arthritis. This chapter provides an approach to the differential diagnosis and management of common hand and wrist disorders.

II. **Common Diagnoses.** Hand and wrist injuries are particularly common in certain occupations, hobbies, and sports. Incidence is difficult to assess; however, a study from the University of Rochester Sports Medicine Center reported a 5% incidence of hand injuries in 3431 cases of sports medicine consultations. Knowing which special tests to perform in the clinical setting can assist the examiner in adequately diagnosing the condition of an injured patient. By understanding the functional anatomy of the hand and wrist (Figure 33–1), a careful diagnosis and specific treatment plan can be achieved by the primary care provider.

A. **Tendon injuries,** including tendon ruptures or tendonitis, are common especially in sports and in industrial workers.

1. **Boutonnière deformity** (Figure 33–2) can be seen in athletes, especially those involved in contact or ball sports.

2. **Mallet deformity** (Figure 33–3) occurs in athletes, especially those who hit or catch a ball, and results from an axial blow to the terminal phalanx causing forced flexion of the distal interphalangeal joint, often rupturing the terminal extensor tendon and can cause distal phalangeal avulsion fracture.

3. **Jersey finger** occurs when an athlete attempts to tackle an opponent who is pulling away. In one study, 75% of cases of jersey finger in football and rugby players involved the ring finger. The involved structural injury is avulsion of the flexor digitorum profundus. This can occur with or without a bony avulsion fracture.

4. **Trigger finger** (Figure 33–4) (stenosing tenosynovitis) usually occurs from continuous direct pressure over the distal palm or metacarpophalangeal (MCP) flexion crease in athletes holding a racquet, golf club, or bat.

5. **de Quervain tenosynovitis** occurs in athletes and industrial workers who engage in repetitive wrist motion, which includes radial and ulnar deviation as well as flexion and extension. Sports and activities most commonly associated with de Quervain include racquet sports, golf, and fishing.

B. **Sprains and contusions** represent the most common injuries seen in sporting events (especially basketball, football, and skiing) and likely comprise a majority (incidence unknown) of the hand, finger, and wrist injuries that account for 3% to 9% of all sports-related injuries reported in the literature.

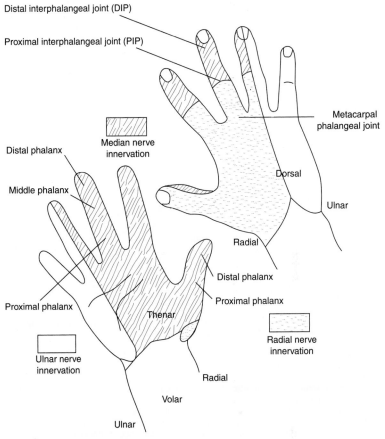

FIGURE 33–1. Sensory distribution of the hand.

1. **Swan-neck deformity** (Figure 33–5) occasionally occurs in athletes playing either contact or noncontact sports. Chronically, swan-neck deformities can also occur in patients with inflammatory arthritis, such as rheumatoid arthritis or gout.
2. **Ulnar collateral ligament injury of the thumb MCP joint** commonly occurs in football players, skiers, and wrestlers when athletes attempt to break their fall with their hand. The mechanism of injury generally involves forced radial deviation of the thumb at the MCP joint.
3. **Triangular fibrocartilage complex (TFCC) tears,** often seen in sports such as baseball and gymnastics, result when the athlete suddenly, or repetitively, loads all their weight on their wrist with or without simultaneous, excessive torque.

C. **Bennett, scaphoid,** and **boxer's fractures** are among the most commonly seen in a primary care provider's office. In addition, **scapholunate dissociation** should not be missed.

1. **Bennett fracture** occurs most often in football players and athletes requiring a strong pinch-grip mechanism in their sport, such as in racquet sports, hockey, or bull riding.
2. **Scaphoid fractures** may represent two-thirds of all carpal fractures. They are usually owing to a fall onto an outstretched hand with the wrist in hyperextension.

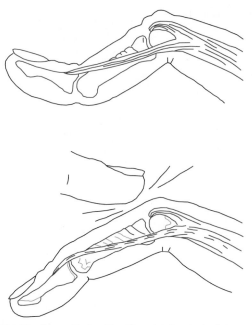

FIGURE 33–2. Boutonnière deformity caused by disruption of the central slip and volar displacement of the lateral bands. The point tenderness test elicits tenderness over the base of the middle phalanx.

    3. Scapholunate dissociation (Figures 33–6 and 33–7) also occurs commonly in those sustaining a fall onto an outstretched hand.

    4. Boxer's fractures involve fracture of the fifth metacarpal after striking an object.

  D. Among **ganglia injuries,** dorsal and volar wrist ganglion cysts are the most common soft tissue masses of the hand and wrist. The incidence is unknown, but there may be a predilection in those with carpal tunnel syndrome, previous wrist impaction injury, or in athletes such as gymnasts.

  E. Arthritis. The hands, notably the base of the thumb, are susceptible to osteoarthritis; carpometacarpal (CMC) arthritis is very common in women, especially those doing repetitive activities (e.g., professional seamstresses). CMC arthritis also occurs idiopathically in women and following trauma in men.

  F. Entrapment neuropathies are commonly seen in the workplace or other situations requiring repetitive hand movement.

    1. Carpal tunnel syndrome is considered the most common entrapment neuropathy and is seen in occupations requiring continuous typing and in athletes, but it may also occur spontaneously in pregnant women or in diabetic, hypothyroid, or acromegalic patients. Approximately 50% of patients have bilateral carpal tunnel syndrome.

    2. Ulnar neuropathy of the hand, also called Guyon canal syndrome, can be seen in cyclists and racquet sport athletes where repetitive power gripping is required. Injury to the ulnar nerve occurs when there is continuous pressure on the nerve, causing inflammation, or from traumatic fractures of the hamate or pisiform.

    3. Radial nerve compression, also known as "handcuff neuropathy," is commonly seen in tennis and other racquet sports in which the athlete performs repetitive ulnar flexion, pronation, and supination.

III. Symptoms (Table 33–1). An accurate history, including occupation, activities, handedness, and mechanism of injury for acute injuries, is critical in diagnosing hand and wrist complaints. An accurate diagnosis may be obtained by a good, detailed history in up to 70% of wrist

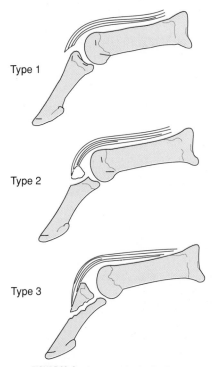

Type 1

Type 2

Type 3

FIGURE 33–3. The three types of mallet finger.

pain cases. In addition, localizing symptoms to specific areas, such as dorsal, volar, radial, or ulnar, can assist in narrowing the differential diagnosis.
IV. **Signs** (Table 33–1). Examination of individuals with hand and wrist complaints is facilitated by knowledge of relevant anatomy and a systematic approach, beginning with inspection (deformity, skin color changes, and edema), followed by palpation (tenderness), range of motion (active, passive, instability check), neurovascular examination (Figures 33–1 to 33–7), and specific provocative testing.
   A. **Special tests**
      1. **Finkelstein test.** This test is used to diagnose de Quervain tenosynovitis, which is inflammation of the extensor pollicis longus, extensor pollicis brevis, and abductor pollicis longus. It is considered positive if the test reproduces a patient's pain when the patient fully flexes the thumb into the palm, followed by passive ulnar deviation of the wrist by the examiner.
      2. **Gamekeeper test.** This test is used to diagnose ulnar collateral ligament (UCL) injury at the thumb MCP joint. Prior to performing this test, an x-ray should be obtained to rule out fracture. If a fracture is seen, the test should not be performed. (SOR **C**) After a fracture has been ruled out, with one hand, the examiner holds the patient's thumb metacarpal, and the other hand holds the patient's thumb proximal phalanx. A gentle radial deviation is applied to the thumb tip MCP joint to stress the UCL. A UCL sprain will show laxity, while a complete rupture (called a **Stener lesion**) can be diagnosed on clinical examination by not feeling an end point during stress testing in either full extension or 30 degrees of MCP flexion. A Stener lesion should not be missed and involves the interposition of the adductor aponeurosis between the torn UCL and its insertion site, preventing ligament healing.
      3. **Grind test.** This test is helpful in diagnosing thumb CMC arthritis. The examiner holds the patient's wrist with one hand and the other hand holds the patient's thumb

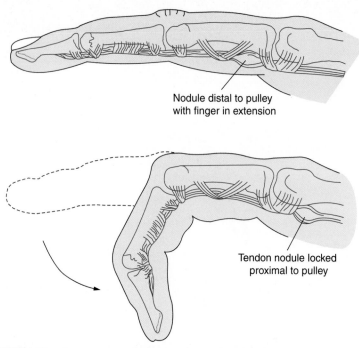

FIGURE 33–4. Trigger finger results from nodular constriction of the flexor tendon by inflammation of the fibrous sheath at the metacarpophalangeal joint. (Reproduced with permission from Greene WB (ed): *Essentials of Musculoskeletal Care, Edition 2*. Rosemont, IL: American Academy of Orthopaedic Surgeons; 2001.)

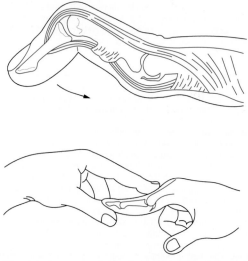

FIGURE 33–5. Volar plate rupture causes swan-neck deformity. A stress test shows an abnormal increase in extension.

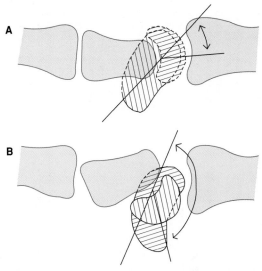

FIGURE 33–6. Scapholunate angle measurements on lateral radiograph. (**A**) Normal scapholunate angle is 30–60 degrees. (**B**) Vertical scaphoid and lunate subluxated palmarward in an abnormal scapholunate angle measured greater than 65 degrees.

metacarpal. The examiner then provides an axial load to the thumb and gently rotates it side-to-side. A positive test reproduces pain and crepitus and sometimes shows instability.

4. **Watson "click" test.** This test is performed to evaluate for scapholunate dissociation. The examiner presses on the scaphoid tuberosity on the palmar side while moving the wrist from ulnar to radial deviation. A "pop" or "click" is present with scapholunate instability or dissociation.

5. **Tinel test.** This test is provocative for carpal tunnel syndrome and is positive if it reproduces the patient's paresthesias (in a median nerve distribution) when the examiner percusses over and just distal to the distal palmar crease midline on the volar wrist. Percussing the distal crease over the radial or ulnar nerve may also assist in diagnosing ulnar or radial neuropathy.

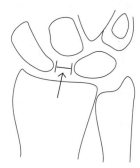

FIGURE 33–7. Distance between the scaphoid and lunate is greater than 3 mm, sometimes called the "Terry Thomas" or "David Letterman" sign.

TABLE 33–1. DIFFERENTIAL DIAGNOSIS AND MANAGEMENT OF COMMON HAND AND WRIST COMPLAINTS

	Diagnosis	Symptoms	Signs	Testing	Treatment
Tendon Injuries	Boutonnière deformity	Pain after sudden forced flexion of PIP	Swelling Flexion of PIP and hyperextension of DIP (Figure 33–2) Tenderness with pressure directly over base of middle phalanx	X-ray anteroposterior and lateral, rule out avulsion fracture	Splint PIP full extension/Leave DIP free Immobilize 6–8 wk and athletes for 4–6 wk more Surgery if fracture
	Mallet deformity	Pain after forceful axial blow causing forced flexion of the DIP	Tenderness on DIP Cannot actively extend distal phalanx (Figure 33–3)	X-ray to rule out fracture	Splint DIP in extension for 6–8 wk, nighttime splint for 3–4 wk, then wean depending on severity of injury
	Jersey finger (flexor digitorum profundus tendon rupture or avulsion)	Pain on flexor side from forced extension of the DIP during maximum contracture	Patient cannot flex at DIP PIP swelling or palm tenderness from FDP retraction in these areas	X-ray to rule out fracture	Early surgical repair of tendon insertion
	Trigger finger (digital flexor tenosynovitis)	Nodule on distal palm, "catching" or "triggering" of finger	Nodular thickening of flexor tendon within distal palm resulting in loss of smooth extension or flexion of the finger (Figure 33–4)	X-ray not necessary unless concern for tumor	Conservative therapy if chronic injury Corticosteroid injection into sheath (Table 33–2) Surgical decompression of the A-1 pulley
	de Quervain tenosynovitis	Pain, swelling near or over radial styloid	Tenderness, swelling over radial styloid (inflammation in first dorsal extensor compartment); positive Finkelstein test (see Section IV.A.1)	X-ray to rule out bony pathology	Thumb/wrist immobilization in thumb spica splint NSAIDs Steroid injection (Table 33–2) and/or surgical decompression if conservative therapy fails
Sprains	Swan-neck deformity	Pain at PIP, deformity often chronic and seen in RA	Tender at PIP, deformity with hyperextension at PIP, and flexion at DIP (Figure 33–5)	X-ray shows deformity	Open repair of volar plate if acute, and if deformity causes disability in chronic cases
	Ulnar collateral ligament (UCL) sprain of thumb MCP (gamekeeper's or skier's thumb)	Pain at MCP of thumb from abduction force across the joint	Tender at MCP of thumb and a positive gamekeeper's test (see Section IV.A.2)	X-ray to rule out avulsion fracture MRI if plain films negative	Grade I/II immobilize in thumb spica cast 2–4 wk, then thumb spica splint 2–4 wk or more Grade III often treated surgically
	Triangular fibro-cartilage complex (TFCC) tears	Dorsal ulnar-sided pain during ulnar deviation with pronation and supination	Pain with forced passive pronation and supination of the wrist; dorsal subluxation of the ulna often with a painful "clunk"	X-ray to rule out radioulnar arthritis or other bony pathology; magnetic resonance arthrogram	Neutral splint NSAIDs, rest; surgical referral for refractory symptoms
Fractures	Bennett fracture	Pain after blow to distal thumb while flexed, swelling base of thumb	Base of thumb metacarpal displaced up and back, while tip of thumb is held into the palm	X-ray to demonstrate oblique fracture of base of thumb metacarpal and dislocation (if present)	Nondisplaced thumb spica (TS) cast 3–4 wk, then splint; dislocation/displaced fracture requires surgery

Category	Condition	History	Examination	Diagnostics	Treatment
	Scaphoid fracture	Radial-sided pain after fall onto outstretched hand	Tender in anatomic snuffbox or volar side of radiocarpal area	X-ray: need longitudinal view of scaphoid. Bone scan/MRI often needed for definitive diagnosis	**Nondisplaced fracture:** Short arm TS cast or splint 4–6 wk. **Middle/proximal fractures:** Long arm TS cast 6 wk, then short arm TS cast 4–14 wk until x-ray union. **Displaced fractures:** Long arm TS cast or splint, refer to hand surgeon
	Scapholunate dissociation	Dorsal radial wrist pain, decreased grip strength, and "clicking"	Tender in anatomic snuffbox or dorsal wrist at the scapholunate joint	X-ray (AP and lateral): scapholunate angle $\geq$ 60 degrees (Figure 33–6) or scapholunate space $\geq$ 3 mm ("Terry Thomas or David Letterman" sign) (Figure 33–7)	Immobilize and refer to hand surgeon
Ganglia	Ganglion cysts	Often originate on tendon sheath; pain or "bump"	Tender or nontender mobile soft tissue mass over radial or dorsal wrist or over flexor/extensor tendon sheath	X-ray to rule out bony pathology; arteriogram as needed to rule out radial artery aneurysm or traumatic pseudo-aneurysm	Observation if asymptomatic; neutral wrist splint, aspiration, injection (Table 33–2) or excision
Arthritis	Carpometacarpal (CMC) of thumb arthritis	Pain at base of thumb with pinching and gripping activities; pain can radiate up arm with "clicking" or "catching" sensation in thumb	Tender over volar or radial sides of CMC joint; positive grind test (see Section IV.A.3)	X-ray shows loss of joint space, subchondral sclerosis, bone spurs, subluxation or dislocation at the CMC joint	Immobilize in TS splint 3–6 wk; injection (Table 33–2); referral to hand surgeon if failed conservative treatment
Neuropathies	Carpal tunnel syndrome	Numbness, tingling, pain in palmar wrist and hand; worse in morning, after repetitive use, and cold sensitivity, color changes	Swelling, weakness, sensation loss in nerve distribution (Figure 33–1); positive Tinel test; negative Spurling test (see Section IV.A.7)	X-ray to rule out bony pathology; nerve conduction studies (NCVs) show delayed terminal sensory latency; c-spine x-ray if indicated to rule out cervical neuroforaminal encroachment	Ergonomic correction, night neutral wrist splints, NSAIDs; injection (Table 33–2) and/or surgery for carpal tunnel release if conservative treatment fails
	Ulnar neuropathy	Numbness and tingling in 4th and 5th digits, pain and weakness (Figure 33–1)	Swelling, weakness, sensation loss; positive ulnar Tinel test (see Section IV.A.4)	X-ray to rule out bony pathology (e.g., hamate fracture); NCVs and Allen test (see Section IV.A.6)	Immobilize, cryotherapy, NSAIDs; surgical decompression for refractory cases
	Radial nerve compression	Pain/numbness/tingling over dorsoradial aspect of wrist and thumb (Figure 33–1)	Swelling, weakness, sensation loss; positive radial Tinel test	X-ray to rule out bony pathology; NCVs, two-point discrimination test (see Section IV.A.8)	Immobilize, NSAIDs, molded orthoses; surgical decompression and nerve transfer for refractory cases

DIP, distal interphalangeal joint; FDP, flexor digitorum profundus; MCP, metacarpophalangeal joint; MRI, magnetic resonance imaging study; NSAIDs, nonsteroidal anti-inflammatory drugs; PIP, tendon proximal interphalangeal joint; RA, rheumatoid arthritis.

6. **Phalen test.** This is another test for carpal tunnel syndrome that is positive if paresthesias occur within 1 to 2 minutes of holding the wrists in maximum flexion.

7. **Allen test.** This test is useful to rule out vascular disorders such as hypothenar hammer syndrome (ulnar artery injury) or Raynaud disease (seen in collagen vascular diseases). The patient rests a hand on the knee or a table while the examiner compresses the radial artery with one thumb and the ulnar artery with the other thumb. Next, the patient clenches and opens the fist 3 times. Then the patient opens the palm and the radial artery is released to see how fast color returns to the palm. The test is then repeated, this time releasing the ulnar artery.

8. **Spurling test.** This test attempts to create neural foraminal narrowing that may or may not reproduce radicular arm pain, numbness, or tingling. With the patient sitting upright on the examination table, the examiner provides gentle axial loading on top of the head while passively extending the neck, then tilting the head to the side. A positive test may represent cervical disk herniation or cervical spondylosis (osteoarthritis).

9. **Two-point discrimination.** To perform this test, use two sterile pins to simultaneously prick the skin on the hand in the area of numbness. The pins are separated at different distances in order to determine when the patient perceives the pins as two points versus one. Fingertip two-point discrimination is normally 2 to 8 mm.

V. **Laboratory Tests** (Table 33–1).

  A. **X-rays.** When diagnosing hand and wrist complaints, initial evaluation often includes obtaining a plain radiograph following physical examination. Finger x-rays should be done with an AP, lateral, and oblique views. (SOR **C**) When reviewing wrist films to evaluate a possible scaphoid or scapholunate injury, a clenched fist view or ulnar deviation view can be obtained. A gap of more than 3 mm in the scapholunate joint should alert the physician to consider scapholunate dissociation until proven otherwise ("Terry Thomas" or "David Letterman" sign). In tendon injuries, it is essential to rule out an avulsion fracture while reviewing a plain x-ray.

  B. **Other radiographic imaging.** MRI can be very beneficial to rule out other injuries to bone, muscle, and tendons. It can also be extremely helpful to evaluate the **TFCC** for a tear. The examiner should make sure to order an MR arthrogram of the wrist to evaluate for a TFCC tear. The dye helps to delineate very small injuries to the TFCC that could otherwise not be visualized. CT scan of the wrist and hand with computerized reconstructions can also be beneficial to evaluate for a small fracture that may be difficult to visualize because of overlapping of the carpal and hand bones on x-ray.

VI. **Treatment** (Table 33–1).

  A. The cornerstone of treatment of most hand and wrist injuries often involves one or more of the following: **nonsteroidal anti-inflammatory drugs (NSAIDs)** (e.g., oral ibuprofen, 600–800 mg with food 3 times daily, or naproxen, 500 mg with food twice daily) for 2 weeks or longer depending on the condition, with precautions for **renal and gastrointestinal toxicity; immobilization; injection** (Table 33–2); or **surgery.**

  B. **Mallet deformity.** All mallet deformity injuries should be placed in a distal interphalangeal joint extension splint of some variety. (See Table 33–1 for duration.) It is important to monitor compliance in patients with these injuries, as it is imperative for successful outcomes. All splints for mallet deformity achieve similar results. (SOR **B**)

  C. **Jersey finger.** All confirmed or suspected jersey finger injuries should be referred to an orthopedic surgeon. (SOR **C**)

  D. **Fifth metacarpal boxer's fracture.** An angulation in the metacarpal neck of 40-50 degrees or less can heal with or without reduction, followed by splinting. An angulation of the metacarpal shaft of 30 degrees or less can also heal without reduction. This, however, should not dissuade the physician from attempting a reduction. (SOR **B**)

  E. **Scaphoid fractures.** Owing to the risk of avascular necrosis, patients with **suspected scaphoid fractures** should be aggressively treated. Patients with a negative x-ray result and scaphoid pain should be placed in a cast until a follow-up x-ray result is obtained in 2 to 3 weeks. Scaphoid fractures, on occasion, may not be visible on x-ray up to 4 weeks after initial injury. Further evaluation with bone scan, CT scan, or magnetic resonance imaging should be considered with continued pain and negative x-rays in this area.

  F. **Carpal tunnel syndrome.** Treatment of **carpal tunnel syndrome** should be conservative if symptoms are mild and of short duration. Patients should first be educated about ergonomic corrections at work or home to prevent further injury. Nighttime neutral wrist splints are usually used to decrease nighttime and morning symptoms. Sometimes NSAIDs help relieve pain, but often patients require local corticosteroid injection if they

TABLE 33–2. HAND AND WRIST INJECTIONS

	Diagnosis	Equipment	Anesthetic	Corticosteroid	Injection Technique
Tendon Injuries	Carpal tunnel syndrome	25–30 gauge, 1.5-inch needle with a 5-mL syringe	2–3 mL 1% lidocaine or 0.25%–0.5% bupivacaine	1 mL betamethasone (Celestone) or 40 mg/mL methylprednisolone	Insert needle at 30-degree angle on volar wrist at proximal wrist crease just ulnar to the palmaris longus tendon aiming at the fourth digit
	1st CMC arthritis	25–30 gauge, 1-inch needle with a 3-mL syringe	0.5 mL 1% lidocaine or 0.25%–0.5% bupivacaine	0.25–0.5 mL Celestone or methylprednisolone	Insert needle on ulnar side of extensor pollicis brevis just proximal to first metacarpal on extensor surface
	de Quervain tenosynovitis	25–27 gauge, 1.5-inch needle with a 5-mL syringe	2 mL 1% lidocaine or 0.25%–0.5% bupivacaine	1 mL Celestone or methylprednisolone	Insert needle into first extensor compartment, direct proximally toward radial styloid (not into tendon)
	Ganglion cysts	18 gauge, 1- to 1.5-inch needle with a 20- to 30-mL syringe	1–2 mL 1% lidocaine or 0.25%–0.5% bupivacaine	1 mL Celestone or methylprednisolone	Insert needle into cyst, aspirate. Use hemostat to stabilize needle, change syringe, then inject
	Trigger finger	25–30 gauge, 1- to 1.5-inch needle with a 3-mL syringe	0.5–1 mL 1% lidocaine or 0.25%–0.5% bupivacaine	0.5 mL Celestone or methylprednisolone	Insert needle at 30-degree angle over palmar aspect distal to the metacarpal head, then direct needle proximally, almost parallel to the skin, toward the nodule

CMC, carpometacarpal joint.

fail conservative treatment. In refractory cases, carpal tunnel release, either arthroscopic or open, is required.

REFERENCES

Daniels J, Zook E, Lynch J. Hand and wrist injuries: part I. Nonemergent evaluation. *Am Fam Physician.* 2004;69(8):1941-1948.

Eiff MP, Hatch RL, Calmbach WL. *Fracture Management for Primary Care.* Philadelphia, PA: Elsevier Science; 2003.

Leggit JC, Meko CJ. Acute finger injuries: part I. Tendons and ligaments. *Am Fam Physician.* 2006;73(5):810-816.

Leggit JC, Meko CJ. Acute finger injuries: part II. Fractures, dislocations, and thumb injuries. *Am Fam Physician.* 2006;73(5):827-834.

Rettig AC. Tests and treatments of hand, wrist, and elbow overuse syndromes: 20 Clinical pearls. *J Musculoskel Med.* 2003;20:136.

Tallia AF, Cardone DA. Diagnostic and therapeutic injection of the wrist and hand region. *Am Fam Physician.* 2003;67:745.

---

34   Headaches

Dan F. Criswell, MD, & Stephen W. Cobb, MD

KEY POINTS

- Most headaches are benign and treatable in the primary care office setting.
- Careful attention to a focused set of symptoms and signs will alert the clinician to more serious causes of headache.
- Neuroimaging is not usually necessary in the evaluation of headaches when the history clearly suggests a primary headache disorder and a careful neurologic examination is normal.

I. **Definition.** Headache, or **cephalgia,** is pain or discomfort perceived in the head, neck, or both. **Primary headache disorders** are recurrent benign headaches whose causes are multifactorial; trigeminal serotonin receptors are felt to play a significant role in the inflammation and vasodilation contributing to pain in migraine headaches. **Secondary headaches** result from an underlying pathology caused by a distinct condition (e.g., aneurysm, infection, inflammation, or neoplasm).

II. **Common Diagnoses.** Most people will experience an episodic headache during their lifetime. The annual prevalence may be as high as 90%, with a minority of those sufferers pursuing medical evaluation. Still, headaches are the second most common pain syndrome in primary care ambulatory practice. There are many headache classification systems. Using the International Headache Society system, **the most common primary headaches in primary care are episodic migraine, tension-type headache, cluster, and analgesic rebound headaches.** Secondary headaches comprise fewer than 10% of headaches in primary care, but include some important treatable and life-threatening entities.

   A. **Episodic migraine.** Migraine affects 18.2% of US women and 6.5% of men each year. Prevalence in the United States was reported for 1999 to be 27.9 million sufferers. The onset of symptoms is usually between adolescence and young adulthood. The peak prevalence is between 30 to 39 years of age, where it affects approximately one in four women and one in 10 men. A strong correlation with family history of migraine has been observed in migraineurs. It is estimated that only 51% of women and 41% of men who experience migraine have actually been diagnosed. More than 60% of migraineurs are treated only by their primary care physicians for headache. Commonly episodic migraine is misdiagnosed as "sinus headache." In one study, 88% of patients who label themselves as having "sinus headaches," actually met criteria for episodic migraine headaches. (SOR **B**)

B. Tension-type headache (TTH), also called muscle contraction headache. Onset varies widely, and can be at any age. Fewer than half of these patients have a positive family history of headache; there is a positive association between chronic TTH and mood disorders. Once felt to be the most common headache diagnosed in the primary care office, a refined definition of migraine has identified migraines that were previously considered tension type. "Mixed headache," another common syndrome consisting of migraine and TTH in the same headache, may actually be a migraine variant or two distinct headache types.

C. Cluster. Although not common in the primary care office, cluster headaches are recognized as one of the more common primary headache disorders in the general population (lifetime prevalence approximately 0.1%). Males are affected more commonly than females, with onset between ages 30 and 50 years. There is a positive association with smoking.

D. Analgesic rebound headaches. The prevalence is 1%, mostly middle-aged women with underlying migraines. Anecdotally, medicines commonly contribute to headache syndromes, particularly in the setting of long-standing **chronic daily headache** and chronic analgesic use. All currently available abortive medications have been associated with overuse or rebound headache. Drugs most commonly associated with rebound headache include acetaminophen, ergot alkaloids, opioids, butalbital, nonsteroidal anti-inflammatory drugs, and Midrin.

E. Secondary headaches. Less than 0.4% of headaches in primary care are from serious intracranial disease. Headaches seen with regularity in primary care include those associated with neoplasm, infections (e.g., meningitis, purulent sinusitis, abscess), temporal arteritis, acute glaucoma, and cerebral aneurysm.

III. **Symptoms.** Differentiation among types of headaches is usually based on the patient's history. Emphasis should be placed on the history of onset, quality and intensity of pain, frequency, provoking influences, and associated symptoms. Patients frequently experience more than one headache type; to avoid misdiagnosis, it is important to define each type carefully. A headache diary can help with ongoing evaluation of episodic headaches. Using standardized inquiries such as the five-item Migraine Disability Assessment Score (MIDAS) questionnaire quantifies the impact of headaches on quality of life and promotes standardization of headache disability (Table 34–1).

A. Migraine. Episodic migraine is classified as migraine with aura (classic) or without (common) (see sidebar). Associated symptoms may include a prodrome (vague symptoms such as smells or emotions), an aura (visual or hemisensory symptoms), or even focal neurologic deficits (complicated migraine). The aura is usually stereotypical, with visual scotomata being the most common. Ninety percent of migraineurs do not exhibit aura or prodrome. Nasal stuffiness, nausea, and vomiting may be prominent symptoms.

DIAGNOSTIC CRITERIA: EPISODIC MIGRAINE WITHOUT AURA

At least five attacks that include the following:
- headache lasting 4 to 72 hours
- at least two of the following:
    - unilateral location
    - pulsating quality (throbbing)
    - moderate to severe intensity (inhibits or prohibits daily activity)
    - aggravated by climbing stairs or similar activity
- at least one of the following:
    - nausea, vomiting, or both
    - photophobia, phonophobia, or both
- mnemonic: POUNDing—**P**ulsatile quality; duration of 4 to 72 h**O**urs; **U**nilateral location; **N**ausea or vomiting, **D**isabling intensity.

B. TTH (see sidebar) originates with pain in the occipital or vertex regions of the skull, evolving into a "band-like" distribution. Though primarily bilateral, unilateral tension headaches also occur. The pain is usually not throbbing, but dull. Nausea is an occasional associated symptom. The duration may be hours to days.

TABLE 34–1. MIDAS QUESTIONNAIRE

INSTRUCTIONS: Please answer the following questions about ALL your headaches you have had over the last three months. Write your answer in the box next to each question. Write zero if you did not do the activity in the last 3 months. Please 'tab' through all five boxes to calculate your MIDAS score.

1	On how many days in the last 3 months did you miss work or school because of your headaches?	0	days
2	How many days in the last 3 months was your productivity at work or school reduced by half or more because of your headaches? *(Do not include days you counted in question 1 where you missed work or school)*	0	days
3	On how many days in the last 3 months did you not do household work because of your headaches?	0	days
4	How many days in the last 3 months was your productivity in household work reduced by half or more because of your headaches? *(Do not include days you counted in question 3 where you did not do household work)*	0	days
5	On how many days in the last 3 months did you miss family, social, or leisure activities because of your headaches?	0	days

Your rating: [   ]   **TOTAL:** [   ] days

A	On how many days in the last 3 months did you have a headache? *(If a headache lasted more than 1 day, count each day)*	0	days
B	On a scale of 0–10, on average how painful were these headaches? *(Where 0 = no pain at all, and 10 = pain as bad as it can be)*	0	days

Grade	Definition	Score
I	Minimal or infrequent disability	0–5
II	Mild or infrequent disability	6–10
III	Moderate disability	11–20
IV	Severe disability	21+

Reproduced with permission from AstraZeneca UK Ltd.
http://www.midas-migraine.net/edu/question/Default.asp.

DIAGNOSTIC CRITERIA: EPISODIC TTH

A. At least 10 previous headache episodes fulfilling B to D below. Fewer than 180 headache days. (If ≥180 days, and B–D are present, then it is chronic TTH.)
B. Headache lasting 30 minutes to 7 days.
C. At least two of the following pain characteristics:
  1. No-pulsating quality—pressing or tightening
  2. Mild or moderate intensity. Not activity prohibiting
  3. Bilateral location
  4. No aggravation by routine physical activity
D. Both of the following
  1. No nausea or vomiting
  2. Either photophobia or phonophobia is absent

C. Cluster headache. These headaches peak very quickly after onset and are "clustered" temporally over weeks to months. Pain-free intervals are variable in length. The pain is sharp, excruciating in intensity, lasting 15 to 180 minutes. The location is usually unilateral and in the orbital, supraorbital, or temporal region. Parasympathetic overactivity (lacrimation and ipsilateral rhinorrhea) is common.
D. Analgesic rebound headache (see sidebar). Since headaches may be caused by medications or medication withdrawal, taking a careful headache and medication history may reveal an association.

DIAGNOSTIC CRITERIA: ANALGESIC REBOUND HEADACHE

1. Headache ≥ 15 days each month

2. Onset after the intake of ergotamines or general analgesics used more than 15 times each month for more than 3 months

3. Disappears after withdrawal therapy

  E. Secondary headaches. Symptoms of a "worrisome" headache that should elicit a search for an underlying cause include the following. (See sidebar on "SNOOP" mnemonic for worrisome headache.)

   1. Headache, new in onset, that is constant, prevents sleep, or progressively worsens over several weeks (indicative of possible intracranial mass lesion or infection). The new headache occurring later in life is less likely to be migraine or tension.

   2. Headache that is abrupt, explosive, and extremely severe (e.g., "the worst headache of my life"), suggestive of intracranial hemorrhage.

   3. Headache beginning with exertion (consider leaking aneurysm, increased intracranial pressure, or arterial dissection). Exertional headache may also be a primary headache type.

   4. Headache in a drowsy or confused patient (consider sepsis, trauma, etc).

   5. New headache in the elderly (consider temporal arteritis, glaucoma, cerebrovascular accident, etc.).

   6. Unremitting moderate or severe headache in obese females (consider pseudotumor cerebri).

"SNOOP" MNEMONIC FOR WORRISOME HEADACHE

  S—Systemic symptoms or signs (fever, weight loss). Systemic disease (cancer, autoimmune).
  N—Neurologic symptoms or signs.
  O—Onset sudden.
  O—Onset late in life.
  P—Pattern change.

IV. Signs. A complete physical examination including careful neurologic, otologic, ophthalmologic, and head and neck evaluation is essential. Vital signs may reveal fever or hypertension. Although there are a few physical examination findings that are common in primary headaches, the examination is most often normal.

  A. Migraine. There may only be evidence of pain behavior (e.g., avoidance of bright light and sound), or there may be focal neurologic deficits, such as hemiparesis or a visual field disturbance.

  B. Tension. A physical examination may reveal muscle tightness, or "trigger points," over the posterior cervical and occipital regions. The neck examination may provide clues to underlying causes of tension headache, such as cervical arthritis (e.g., stiffness, decreased range of motion, or crepitus with movement), inflammatory processes (e.g., trigger points or nodules), or infectious causes (e.g., lymphadenopathy).

  C. Cluster headaches. Photophobia, tearing, nasal stuffiness, or Horner syndrome may be present. The patient may be unable to sit still during the interview.

  D. Secondary headaches. Signs of a "worrisome" headache are listed below.

   1. Fever may indicate meningitis, purulent sinusitis, otitis, dental abscess, etc.

   2. A **stiff neck** may indicate infection or blood in the cerebrospinal fluid.

   3. Focal neurologic deficits or **elevated blood pressure** ($\geq$200 mm Hg systolic or $\geq$120 mm Hg diastolic) may indicate increased intracranial pressure from mass effect, bleed, or accelerated hypertension.

   4. A **palpable, tender temporal artery** suggests temporal arteritis.

   5. Papilledema suggests increased intracranial pressure.

V. Laboratory Tests. Diagnostic testing is unnecessary for most patients with chronic, recurring headaches and for low-risk patients (i.e., young patients who [1] have prior or family history of headache, [2] are improving during their evaluation, [3] have none of the above mentioned "worrisome" symptoms or signs, [4] are alert and oriented, and [5] have no focal neurologic signs). For these individuals, repeated history taking and physical examinations over time, in addition to observations of response to treatment, are the best diagnostic tools. The following tests should be considered in patients not meeting low-risk criteria.

A. **Radiologic evaluation**

   1. **Plain skull films** are rarely useful in the evaluation of headache.

   2. **Computerized tomography (CT)** may assist in evaluating for sinusitis or diagnosing subarachnoid or intraparenchymal hemorrhage in the patient with a severe and acute headache. The acutely ill patient who requires monitoring will be most easily evaluated by CT, although a normal CT scan does not rule out an acute bleed. If the clinical suspicion remains high, a lumbar puncture (LP) should be performed.

   3. **Magnetic resonance imaging (MRI)** is generally more informative than CT in patients with chronic headaches. Characteristic MRI findings have been described in patients with migraine, trigeminal neuralgia, and temporomandibular joint dysfunction. This procedure is also superior to CT in demonstrating subacute subdural hematoma in patients with a history of trauma and is useful in further characterizing lesions detected by CT. MRI has excellent resolution in the posterior fossa. Most patients with primary headache disorders will have an unremarkable study.

B. The purposes of **LP** are (1) to establish the presence or absence of blood or inflammatory cells in the cerebrospinal fluid, (2) to detect hemorrhage or infection in the patient with a stiff neck, and (3) to determine the organism responsible for infection by fluid culture. Although LP is easy to perform and readily available, it is an invasive, uncomfortable procedure that has no role in routine headache evaluation. LP should *not* be performed when increased intracranial pressure is suspected, until mass effect is ruled out. LP opening pressure may also be elevated in pseudotumor cerebri.

C. **Blood analysis.** A complete blood cell count is rarely useful or definitive in the evaluation of headache and has no place except in the febrile patient. The erythrocyte sedimentation rate is indicated in the older patient with a new headache to support a diagnosis of temporal arteritis.

D. **Other studies. Radionucleotide imaging** and **angiography,** which are usually less helpful than CT scans for identifying or ruling out significant intracranial disease, should be reserved for the few patients with normal CT scans and cerebrospinal fluid findings whose evaluations strongly suggest an intracranial lesion. MRI has largely replaced these studies. **Magnetic resonance angiography** is useful to demonstrate small aneurysms. Temporal arteritis should be confirmed by **arterial biopsy;** this procedure should not delay treatment when clinical suspicion is strong. **Electroencephalography** is not routinely helpful for the patient with a new headache, although it may be useful in ruling out seizure disorder in the chronic headache patient responding poorly to therapy.

VI. **Treatment**

A. **Episodic migraine (with or without aura)**

   1. **General measures** include patient education, fatigue avoidance, and life stressor modification. Migraine frequency, duration, and severity are not increased by dietary choices. (SOR **Ⓐ**/d) Regular supplementation with riboflavin (400 mg/d) reduces frequency and intensity of migraines. (SOR **Ⓑ**) Alternative therapies are frequently prescribed for migraine sufferers and include aerobic exercise, biofeedback, progressive self-relaxation, meditation, massage therapy, or acupuncture. The most widely researched botanical for migraine headache is a wildflower called feverfew (*Tanacetum parthenium*), which is modestly efficacious for either acute treatment or prophylaxis (Table 34–2).

   2. **Acute therapy** is appropriate when migraine attacks occur less than 2 to 4 times a month. The most effective approach is individualized and stratified, based on a given drug's ability to preserve normal function and the patient's degree of symptoms. (SOR **Ⓑ**) An abortive medication with receptor-specific therapy (**e.g., a triptan**) should be prescribed initially in patients with moderate to severe symptoms. The triptan should be administered at migraine onset, or in the prodromal/aural phase if possible. Ergot alkaloids are a good alternative to triptans; these drug classes share contraindications. If triptans or ergotamines fail or are contraindicated, **rescue medications,** such as simple analgesics, may be tried. Rescue medications also include combination products, sedatives, antiemetics, and narcotics. These are often effective, but seldom allow the patient to function normally.

   The following specific agents are commonly used (Tables 34–3 and 34–4).

   a. **Triptans** are selective serotonin receptor agonists affecting primarily 5-HT 1B/1D receptors. They have proved to be very effective in the treatment of migraines, with success rates approaching 70%. There are many triptans available, with important

TABLE 34–2. PROPHYLAXIS FOR RECURRENT MIGRAINE HEADACHES

Class	Medication	Tablet Dose (mg)	Oral Dosing/Max	Notes
Beta-blockers	Propranolol (Inderal)	10/20/40/80; 80/120/160—LA	20–40 mg tid–qid	Beta-blockers are first-line preventive drugs; caution with asthma/COPD/bradycardia
	Nadolol (Corgard)	20 mg	20–160 mg	
Tricyclic antidepressants	Amitriptyline (Elavil)	25/50/75/100/125	25–150 mg, HS	Sedating/serotonergic/anticholinergic
	Nortriptyline (Norpramin)	25/50/75/100	25–75 mg, HS	
	Imiprimere (Tofranil)	25/50/75/100	25–150 HS	
Calcium channel blockers	Verapamil (Calan)	120, 180, 240, 360 SR	40–160 mg bid–qid	Agents of choice if beta-blocker intolerant or contraindicated (asthma/CHF/bradycardia)
	Diltiazem (Tiazac)	30, 60, 90, 120 (60, 90, 120 SR)	30–90 mg bid–tid	
Antiepileptic drugs (AEDs)	Divalproex (Depakote)	125, 250, 500	25–500 mg bid	
	Topiramate (Topamax)	25, 100, 200	50–200 mg bid	
	Carbamazepine (Tegretol)	200	200–400 mg bid	
	Tiagabine (Gabitril)	2, 4, 12, 16, 20	4–16 mg qd	
Ergot	Methysergide (Sansert)	2; tid–qid	tid–qid; 16 max	Not commonly used because of reported adverse effects, including retroperitoneal and cardiopulmonary fibrosis
Herbal	Feverfew	125	1 tablet bid	Effective, but concerns with product reliability
Antihistamine	Cyproheptadine (Periactin)	4, 2 mg/5 cc	2–4 mg tid	Useful in childhood migraine
Miscellaneous agents	Fluoxetine (Prozac)	20	20 mg daily	SSRI—modestly effective
	Clonidine (Catapres)	.1, .2 mg	0.1–0.2 mg bid–tid	Central alpha blocker; sedation; possibly effective

Class	Medication	Tablet Dose (mg)	Formulations	Dosing (Tablets Unless Specified Otherwise)	Notes
Combination products	Acetamin/ butalb/ caffeine (Fioricet)	325/50/40	T	T 1–2 po q 4 h. Max 6 tabs/d	Also available with 30 mg codeine
	Acetamin/ dichloralphea/ isometheptine (Midrin)	325/100/65	T	2 at onset, 1 q 30 min. Max 5/d	Effective for mild to moderately intense migraines
Simple analgesics/NSAIDs	Aspirin	325	T	1–2 po q 4 h. Max 4 g/d	Gastrointestinal upset, gastritis, ulcers
	Ibuprofen (Motrin)	200–800	T	1 po q 8 h	Use 50–100 q 6–8 hr
Antiemetics	Chlorpromazine	10, 25	T, RS, IM	25 po q 4–6 hpo	
	Promethazine (Phenergan)	12.5, 25	T, RS, IM, IV	12.5–25 q 4–6 h	25 PR q 12 h, 5–10 mg IV
	Prochlorperazine	5, 10, 25	T, RS, IM, IV	5–10 mg q 6 h	
Narcotic analgesics	Codeine (Tylenol #3)	300/30	T	1–2 q 4 h	
	Oxycodone ± acetaminophen (Lortab)	5 g or 7.5 mg/500 mg	T	1–2 q 6 h	
	Butorphanol tartrate (Stadol NS)	1 mg	IN	1 mg IN, repeated in 1 h, then q 3–4 h	
Sedative hypnotics	Secobarbital (Seconal)	100 mg	T, IM	100 single dose	Sedate—"sleep off" headache
	Triazolam (Halcion)	0.125, 0.25	T	1–2 tablets single dose	Data on efficacy lacking

CHF, congestive heart failure; COPD, chronic obstructive pulmonary disease; HS, hour's sleep (bedtime); SSRI, selective serotonin reuptake inhibitor.
DHE, dihydroergotamine; DT, dissolving tablet; IM, intramuscular; IN, intranasal; NSAIDs, nonsteroidal anti-inflammatory drugs; RS, rectal suppository; SC, subcutaneous; T, tablet.

TABLE 34-3. **MEDICATIONS FOR ACUTE MIGRAINE HEADACHES**

Class	Medication	Tablet Dose (mg)	Formulations	Dosing (Tablets Unless Specified Otherwise)	Notes
Triptans	Zolmitriptan (Zomig)	2.5, 5.0	T/DT	1 po × 1. May repeat in 2 h	
	Sumatriptan (Imitrex)	25, 50, 100	T/SC/IN	1 po × 1. May repeat in 2 h	May repeat SC (6 mg) in 1 h. SC and IN good for early morning migraine
	Rizatriptan (Maxalt)	5, 10	T/DT	1 po × 1. May repeat in 2 h	Caution with propranolol, use 5-mg dose
	Naratriptan (Amerge)	2.5	T	1 po × 1. May repeat in 4 h.	Long half-life
	Almotriptan (Axert)	6.25, 12.5	T	1 po × 1. May repeat in 2 h.	
	Frovatriptan (Frova)	2.5	T	1 po × 1. May repeat in 2 h.	Long half-life, indicated for menstrual migraine 40-mg dose preferred
	Eletriptan (Relpax)	20, 40	T	1 po × 1. May repeat in 2 h	
Ergot alkaloids		D. H.E. 45	1	IV/IM	1 mg IM/IV × 1. May repeat in 1 h × 1.
	Ergotamine/ caffeine	1/100 tab, 2/100 supp	T/RS	1–2 po or PR. May repeat after 30 min	

differences in route of administration (oral tablet, dissolving oral tablet, injectable, intranasal); onset of action; and duration of action. Triptans should be used with caution in patients with suspected coronary artery, cerebrovascular, or peripheral vascular disease, since they have been associated with vasospasm. They should not be used in basilar or complicated migraine. Patients should be limited to two administrations each week, and triptans should not be taken within 24 hours of an ergot alkaloid.

b. **Ergot alkaloids** also target serotonin receptors, but are less selective. These drugs are estimated to be effective within 2 hours in ≥90% of cases when administered parenterally, 80% when given rectally, and up to 50% when given orally. They are

TABLE 34-4. **STRENGTH OF RECOMMENDATION FOR SELF ADMINISTERED ACUTE TREATMENT OPTIONS IN MIGRAINE**

SOR	Treatment (Route of Administration)	Comments
A	Acetaminophen + aspirin + caffeine (po)	NNT 3.9 (3.2–4.9)
A	Aspirin (po)	NNT 3.5–5.5
A	Aspirin + metoclopramide (po)	NNT 3.2 (2.6–4.0)
A	Butorphanol (IN)	Abuse/dependence and rebound risk
A	Dihydroergotamine (IN)	NNT 2.5 (1.9–3.7)
A	Ibuprofen (po)	NNT 7.5 (4.5–22)
A	Triptans (po)	NNT 2.7–5.4
A	Sumatriptan (IN)	NNT 3.4 (2.9–4.1)
A	Sumatriptan (SC)	NNT 2.0 (1.8–2.2)
B	Acetaminophen (po)	NNT 5.2 (3.3–13)
B	Acetaminophen + codeine (po)	Abuse/dependence and rebound risk
B	Isometheptene compounds (po)	Limited clinical trials
D	Butalbital compounds (po)	No clinical trials and rebound risk
D	Ergotamine (po)	Conflicting evidence

po, by mouth; IN, intranasal; SC, subcutaneous.
All numbers needed to treat (NNT) at 95% confidence interval for headache response (reduction in headache severity from "severe" or "moderate" to "mild" or "none" at 2 h.
Reproduced with permission from Polizzotto MJ. Evaluation and treatment of the adult patient with migraine. *J Fam Pract.* 2002;51:2. Table 3, p. 164.

TABLE 34–5. STRENGTH OF RECOMMENDATION FOR PROPHYLACTIC TREATMENT OPTIONS IN MIGRAINE

SOR	Treatment (Route of Administration)	Comments
A	Amitriptyline	NNT 2.3–5.0
A	Divalproex sodium	NNT 2.1–2.9
A	Propranolol	NNT 2.3–5.0
B	Lisinopril	Based on 1 level 1b study
B	Naproxen sodium	Risk of rebound headache
B	Riboflavin	NNT 2.8
D	Verapamil	Limited, poor quality trials

Numbers needed to treat (NNT) are for a 50% reduction in headache frequency compared with baseline.
Reprinted with permission from Polizzotto MJ. Evaluation and treatment of the adult patient with migraine. *J Fam Pract.* 2002;51:2. Table 4, p. 165.

also available in sublingual and intranasal forms. Since ergotamine preparations may result in dependency and rebound headaches, they should not be used more often than 2 d/week.

  c. **Combination products.** A combination of acetaminophen, butalbital, and caffeine (Fioricet) is commonly used for migraine; however, no studies have addressed the efficacy of butalbital.

  d. **Simple analgesics** are effective. The best evidence exists for aspirin, ibuprofen, naproxen sodium, and tolfenamic acid. Acetaminophen is modestly effective when NSAIDs are contraindicated. (SOR **A**)

  e. **Antiemetics** administered either by mouth, intramuscularly (IM), or by rectal suppository may be useful to offset the nausea and gastric stasis associated with migraine. They may be used alone or as adjunctive therapy with narcotics.

  f. Narcotic analgesics such as **codeine** or **oxycodone** are effective during an acute attack, but their use must be carefully balanced with the risks of habituation and rebound headache.

3. **Prophylactic therapy** (Table 34–2 and 34–5) is indicated for more than three or four attacks per month or for headaches occurring on a predictable schedule (e.g., with menses). Effective medications include the following:

  a. **Beta-blockers** are the most important drugs for migraine prevention. Once- or twice-daily dosing improves compliance.

  b. **Tricyclic antidepressants** have also proved useful, probably because of serotonin effects. The full dosages normally used for depression are unnecessary.

  c. **Calcium channel blockers** are not as effective as beta-blockers for prophylaxis. Nifedipine may actually increase headaches.

  d. Reflecting the changing perception of migraine as a neurologic phenomenon perhaps propagated centrally, **antiepileptic drugs (AEDs)** have been used more frequently to suppress migraines. Experience with **divalproex sodium** has been most encouraging. **Topiramate, carbamazepine,** and **tiagabine** may also be effective. Anti-epileptic drugs are generally more expensive than other agents and require monitoring for adverse effects (e.g., abnormalities in liver function).

  e. **Other agents.** ACE inhibitors (Lisinopril) or ARBs are reasonable second-line agents. (SOR **A**) SSRIs are similar to placebo in efficacy for prophylaxis. (SOR **A**) Propranolol, valproic acid, and amitriptyline are effective prophylactic agents in children's migraines. (SOR **B**) Flunarizine is efficacious, (SOR **A**) but not available in the United States.

  f. **Follow-up and education.** Patient education during an acute headache is not very effective. The mutually cooperative, understanding relationship critical to long-term success can be established with frequent visits during medicine trials and titration. Communicating therapeutic goals clearly is essential to success. Follow-up visits to assess response to therapy, patient understanding, and frequency of attacks can be therapeutic.

B. **TTH**

1. **General measures.** A supportive cooperative physician–patient relationship is essential. Education, insight into family and life events, consideration of environmental and emotional triggers, and counseling may help both decrease headache frequency and increase coping skills. Headache diaries, biofeedback, stress management, muscle relaxation techniques, exercise programs, and dietary changes may also help.

Addressing psychiatric comorbidities (see Chapters 89, 92, and 94) contributes to successful treatment of headaches.

Individuals with **chronic tension headaches** may benefit from a multidisciplinary approach using both drug and nondrug treatments, including individual/family therapy and physical therapy.

2. Used sparingly, **muscle relaxants** (e.g., cyclobenzaprine, 10 mg 3 times daily for up to 21 days; chlorzoxazone, 500–750 mg 3 times daily; methocarbamol, 1000–1500 mg 4 times daily; or diazepam, 5 mg 2 to 3 times daily) can be helpful adjunctive therapy. Narcotic analgesics generally should be avoided.

3. **Preventive therapy.** Medications used for migraine prophylaxis (specifically, beta-blockers and tricyclic antidepressants, alone or in combination) have also proved useful in patients with frequent, recurrent, and chronic TTH.

4. **Follow-up**
   a. Most **acute headache patients** will see their primary physician only once for this complaint. Early follow-up is recommended **with new headaches** to gauge response to therapy and reconfirm history and physical findings. Review of headache diaries, precipitating factors, and life stressors may help patients identify/avoid precipitants, thereby reducing the number of headache days.
   b. Clinicians tend to underestimate the therapeutic value of **regularly scheduled follow-up,** often monthly, for **chronic pain complaints like chronic TTH.**

C. **Cluster headaches**
   1. **Acute therapy** during an attack includes (1) **inhalation of 100% oxygen** by mask at a rate of 7 to 10 L/min; (2) **inhaled ergotamine,** one puff every 5 minutes for a maximum of five puffs per day; or (3) **sublingual nifedipine,** 10 to 20 mg, repeated every 6 to 8 hours (not to be used with ergotamine).
   2. **Prevention** is preferable once clusters begin. Effective oral medications, alone or in combination, include (1) **methysergide,** 2 to 8 mg/d; (2) **lithium,** 300 mg 3 times per day (monitoring blood levels weekly to avoid toxicity); (3) **prednisone,** 40 to 60 mg/d for 5 days, followed by tapering over 10 to 14 days; and (4) **calcium channel blockers,** such as nifedipine, 10 to 20 mg 3 times daily. **Indomethacin,** 25 mg orally 3 times a day, is very effective for benign paroxysmal hemicrania, an entity similar to cluster headache.

D. **Analgesic rebound headaches**
   1. Those taking narcotic medication chronically may require inpatient detoxification both to treat the headache and the medication dependence. For non-narcotic agents, treating rebound headaches with ergotamine (DHE 1 mg SQ rescue for excruciating headaches) and stopping the offending agent(s) result in significant improvement within 3 months. (SOR **❻**) Amitriptyline does not affect frequency or severity of rebound headaches, but does improve quality of life. (SOR **❸**) Prednisone (tapering 60–20 mg over 6 days) or naratriptan (Amerge 2.5 mg po bid for 6 days) may reduce need for rescue DHE, but does not affect headache frequency or severity. (SOR **❸**)
   2. **Severe chronic migraine** and **medication-associated headache requiring detoxification** are problems best managed in collaboration with a headache expert.
   3. **Continuity of care** with a single knowledgeable physician remains essential for these patients.

E. **Secondary headaches.** Treatment of the underlying disease, whether medical or neurosurgical, is the best approach.

REFERENCES

Bigal ME, Sheftell FD, Rapoport AM, et al. Chronic daily headache: identification of factors associated with induction and transformation. *Headache.* 2002;42(7):575-81.

Crawford P, Simmons M. What dietary modifications are indicated for migraines? *J Fam Prac.* 2006;55(1):62-66.

Lipton RB, Stewart WF, Diamond S, et al. Prevalence and burden of migraine in the United States: data from the American Migraine Study II. *Headache.* 2001;41:646-657.

McPherson V, Leach L. What is the best treatment for analgesic rebound headaches? *J Fam Prac.* 2005;54(3):265-282.

Polizzotto MJ. Evaluation and treatment of the adult patient with migraine. *J Fam Prac.* 2002;51(2): 161-167.

Tepper SJ, Rapoport A, Sheftell F. The pathophysiology of migraine. *Neurology.* 2001;**7**(5):279-286.

35 Hearing Loss

Robert C. Salinas, MD, & Heather Bartoli, PA-C

KEY POINTS

- Hearing loss is classified as sensorineural, conductive, mixed, or central.
- Sudden deafness is a medical emergency and warrants prompt referral to an otolaryngologist.
- The treatment of hearing loss is dependent on its etiology and involves environmental alteration, assistive listening devices, active medical/surgical intervention, and hearing aids.

I. **Definition.** Hearing loss may be defined as a reduction in an individual's ability to perceive sound. The intensity of sound is measured with the decibel (dB), a logarithmic unit whose reference is 0 on the audiogram. The following classification is frequently used to describe hearing: normal hearing (0 to 20 dB), mild hearing loss (20–40 dB), moderate hearing loss (40–60 dB), severe hearing loss (60–80 dB), and profound hearing loss (above 80 dB). (American Speech-Language-Hearing Association, 2007).

Hearing loss is a common problem encountered in the primary care setting and may be classified as **sensorineural** (caused by deterioration of the cochlea or lesions to the eighth cranial nerve); **conductive** (caused by lesions of the external or middle ear that impede passage of sound waves to the inner ear); **mixed** (sensorineural and conductive); or **central** (caused by lesions of the auditory pathways proximal to the cochlea). Hearing loss may further be described as congenital or acquired. A more complete listing of etiologies of hearing loss may be found in Table 35–1. (Also see the sidebars on acoustic neuroma and sudden deafness.)

ACOUSTIC NEUROMA

Ninety-five percent of acoustic neuromas are idiopathic; 5% occur in patients with neurofibromatosis, in which tumors cases are more aggressive and more likely to undergo malignant transformation. The most common presenting symptoms are tinnitus and progressive hearing loss. Approximately 50% of patients also experience disequilibrium.

Audiometric findings include loss of discrimination that is disproportionate to pure-tone results, and high-frequency sensorineural loss. Approximately 5% have normal audiograms. Thin-section magnetic resonance imaging (MRI) with gadolinium can detect temporal bony acoustic neuromas measuring just a few millimeters. Treatment for acoustic neuroma is surgical excision; however, since acoustic neuromas are usually very slow-growing, the elderly or those with multiple comorbid medical conditions may choose observation as an alternative to surgery.

SUDDEN DEAFNESS

Sudden deafness is a sensorineural deafness that occurs instantly or is noticed over hours or days. The degree of hearing loss may range from mild to complete and is typically unilateral. Potential causes include **localized lesions** of the temporal bone (i.e., acoustic neuroma, aneurysm of the anteroinferior cerebellar artery), **systemic diseases** (i.e., macroglobulinemia, leukemia, polycythemia, sickle cell disease, syphilis, bacterial infection, ototoxic drugs, mumps, multiple sclerosis), **barotrauma**, or **head trauma.** Sudden deafness should be thought of as a medical emergency, requiring prompt referral to an otolaryngologist. Prognosis is dependent on the timeliness of therapy, which may include treatment of identified causes or supportive/empiric therapies (e.g., corticosteroids, vasodilators, anticoagulants, bed rest, sedation, or a low-sodium diet).

TABLE 35–1. COMMON ETIOLOGIES OF HEARING LOSS ENCOUNTERED IN PRIMARY CARE

Conductive	Sensorineural
Cerumen impaction	Genetic*
Cholesteatoma	Alport's syndrome
Cysts	Usher's syndrome
Exostosis	Waardenburg's syndrome
Eustachian tube dysfunction	Meniere's disease
Foreign body	Multiple sclerosis
Hemotympanum	Noise-induced
Ossicular malformations	Ototoxicity
Ossicular discontinuity	Presbycusis
Otitis externa	Sarcoidosis
Otitis media	Sudden idiopathic hearing loss
Otosclerosis	Syphilis
Previous ear surgery	Trauma
Trauma	Vascular
Perforated tympanic membrane	Migraine
Temporal bone fracture	
Tumors	
Tympanic membrane perforation	
Tympanic membrane retraction	
Tympanosclerosis	

*Many genetic syndromes causing hearing loss have been identified; some of the more common examples are listed above.

II. **Common Diagnoses** (Table 35–1). Approximately 15 million people in the United States are hearing impaired, and approximately 2 million Americans are functionally deaf. Hearing loss is also the third most prevalent, chronic condition in older Americans (after hypertension and arthritis) and rises with age to a prevalence of approximately 64% by age 80. It is also estimated that 15% of school-aged children have a 16-dB hearing loss. One of every 2000 individuals is deaf or severely hearing impaired. At least 90% of these hearing problems are secondary to middle ear disorders that are potentially treatable.

A. **Sensorineural loss.** More than 90% of hearing loss is sensorineural. Some common etiologies of sensorineural loss include presbycusis, acoustic damage, ototoxicity, and Meniere's disease.

1. **Presbycusis** is the most common type of hearing loss in the United States, is associated with aging, and may begin in middle age.

2. **Acoustic damage** (noise-induced hearing loss) may be caused by chronic exposure to excessive noise levels or from more acute acoustic trauma (i.e., shotgun blast or firecracker explosion).

a. **As many as 30 million Americans are exposed to excessive noise levels at work.** As many as 17% of these workers have measurable hearing loss, making hearing loss caused by noise exposure one of the most common occupational diseases.

b. **Males are affected more frequently than females** presumably because of occupational noise exposure, military service, and recreational shooting.

c. **Noise exposure is not limited to the workplace.** Noise-induced hearing loss has been demonstrated in children and adolescents.

3. **Ototoxicity** is caused primarily by exposure to drugs and is the most common cause of deafness in children. However, a correlation between ototoxicity and plasma drug levels has not been observed. An increased risk of ototoxicity has been associated with decreased creatinine clearance, advanced age, certain drug classes such as aminoglycosides (especially if administered parenterally), and drug treatment longer than 14 days. Environmental exposure and workplace exposure are less common causal agents. Cigarette smokers are 1.69 times as likely to have hearing loss as nonsmokers.

4. **Meniere's disease** is the most common type of hearing loss that occurs between the fourth and sixth decades but may occur at any age.

5. **Congenital sensorineural hearing loss,** a form of significant hearing loss, is one of the most common major abnormalities present at birth. One in 200 children is born with

some degree of congenital hearing loss, and one-third to three-fourths of these losses have a genetic component. More than 70 syndromes have been identified that involve a genetic basis for hearing loss. Increased risk of congenital hearing loss is associated with a family history of congenital hearing loss; low-birth-weight; craniofacial abnormalities; syndromes known to cause hearing loss (Usher's syndrome, Waardenburg's syndrome, etc); intrauterine infections (i.e., toxoplasmosis, syphilis, cytomegalovirus, rubella); hyperbilirubinemia; prolonged stay in the neonatal intensive care unit; and low Apgar score.

B. Conductive loss. This type usually involves abnormalities of the middle and external ear, and generally has a mechanical cause (e.g., perforated eardrum, fluid in the middle ear, external otitis, cerumen impaction).

   1. Obstruction. Hearing loss often results from obstruction of the external ear canal by cerumen or foreign bodies, such as crayons, food, or toys. Cerumen sometimes accumulates in the auditory canal of individuals with either excessive production of cerumen or ineffective self-cleaning mechanisms. In the third and fourth decades of life, the hairs found in ear canals become coarser and longer, which secondarily reduces natural clearance of cerumen. Edema associated with otitis externa may also obstruct the canal.

   2. Otosclerosis, a progressive sclerotic fixation of the stapes in the round window dampening sound conduction to the cochlea, causes deafness in 50% of affected adults. Otosclerosis is transmitted through autosomal dominant inheritance with variable expression, typically occurs in women during the second or third decades of life, and is 10 times more common among whites than blacks.

   3. Otitis media (suppurative or serous), a collection of fluid behind the tympanic membrane, most commonly causes hearing loss in children younger than 5 years with a history of recurrent ear infections.

C. Central hearing loss. This may be caused by demyelinating disease, ischemia, neoplasm, or hematoma.

III. Symptoms

A. Reduced hearing acuity

   1. Presbycusis may not cause reduced hearing acuity until late in the disease process and may manifest as difficulty in understanding conversation when ambient noise levels are relatively high, as in crowded or large areas or on the telephone. Some patients complain of sensitivity to loud noises or that people mumble.

   2. Patients with **noise-induced hearing loss** first notice some muffling of sound, but they usually consult a physician only when they begin to experience difficulties hearing speech, which is a late finding.

   3. With **conductive hearing loss,** patients tend to hear conversation better in noisy rooms than in quiet rooms. Reduced hearing acuity is common in patients with impacted cerumen.

B. Timing/Onset of symptoms may suggest particular etiologies.

   1. Noise-induced hearing loss may be most pronounced shortly after the patient leaves the workplace, and the patient's hearing may improve while away from work.

   2. A temporal relationship between the **use of a toxic agent** and the symptomatology is generally present in patients with ototoxicity.

   3. Symptoms of hearing loss from **impacted cerumen** frequently begin suddenly following bathing or swimming, when a drop of water closes the passageway.

   4. Hearing loss associated with **presbycusis** is typically of gradual onset and bilateral.

C. Associated symptoms

   1. Vertigo, imbalance, nausea, and disequilibrium may occur in patients with ototoxicity.

   2. High-pitched tinnitus may occur in individuals with presbycusis, noise-induced hearing loss, and otosclerosis.

   3. Pain, discomfort, or itching can occur in patients with hearing loss from impacted cerumen, otitis media, or otitis externa.

   4. Chronic cough may be present in patients with impacted cerumen if the impaction abuts the tympanic membrane. The cough should disappear with removal of the impaction.

   5. In **Meniere's disease** fluctuating, unilateral hearing loss is classically associated with vertigo, tinnitus, and aural fullness.

6. **Behavioral changes** resulting from isolation and depression caused by hearing loss may include fear, anger, depression, frustration, embarrassment, or anxiety. Elderly people with hearing loss suffer depression twice as often as the general population.

IV. **Signs. Physical findings may be limited.**

A. **Otoscopic examination**

1. **Impacted cerumen or a foreign body** may be evident.
2. Findings consistent with **otitis externa or otitis media** (see Chapter 22) may be seen.
3. The medial wall of the middle ear promontory may appear reddish in patients with **otosclerosis.**

B. **Tuning fork tests**

1. **The Weber test** is performed by placing the handle of a vibrating tuning fork (512 cycles/s) against the midline of the patient's forehead. A patient with normal sensorineural function and no conductive hearing loss hears the sound equally in both ears. Lateralization of the Weber test to one side means either a conductive loss on that side or a sensorineural loss on the opposite side.
2. The **Rinne test** assesses air and bone conduction. The handle of a vibrating 512-cycles/s tuning fork is placed against the mastoid until the patient can no longer hear it and then the tines are held near the ear canal to assess whether the patient can still hear it. Air conduction persists longer than bone conduction in a patient with no hearing loss. Equal hearing levels at both positions are consistent with hearing loss of mixed cause. If air conduction is louder, either normal hearing or sensorineural loss may exist. If bone conduction is louder, conductive loss exists.

C. **Developmental milestones.** The primary care practitioner should be familiar with milestones associated with normal speech and hearing. Any deviation from these norms should alert the clinician to consider audiologic testing.

1. From **birth to 3 months,** infants should have a startle reflex to loud sounds. At this age, they are generally comforted by familiar voices.
2. The **ability to localize sound usually develops at around 6 months**, while responding to their name and mimicking environmental sounds usually takes place around 9 months.
3. Infants usually learn to say **their first meaningful word around 12 months,** and by 24 months usually have a vocabulary of approximately 20 words.

V. **Laboratory Tests**

A. **Audiometry** measures the threshold levels (i.e., the intensity at which the patient is able to perceive sound correctly 50% of the time). This level is usually measured by presenting pure tones to the individual at preset frequencies through air conduction and occasionally through bone conduction.

1. **Indications**

a. Screening audiometry for toddlers, preschoolers, and school-aged children should be administered as needed, requested, mandated, or when conditions place them at risk for hearing disability. (American Speech and Language Association)
b. Screening audiometry for hearing loss in adults is voluntary, but is recommended every 10 years until age 50 and then every 3 years thereafter. (SOR **B**) (American Speech and Language Association)
c. **Audiometry is indicated in all patients with hearing loss,** except those patients with a foreign body or an acute infection whose hearing normalizes following treatment.
d. **Baseline audiometry should be performed within 3 days of institution of therapy with ototoxic agents** for patients who are alert enough to cooperate with the examination. Serial audiometry on an individual basis should be considered.
e. **Follow-up should be performed annually** after treatment, if indicated by the patient's condition.

2. **Findings**

a. **Sensorineural loss** causes lower thresholds in low frequencies than in higher frequencies.

(1) Individuals with **presbycusis** display a pattern with a greater high-frequency loss at 8000 than at 4000 cycles, often described as a smooth, ski slope–shaped curve, and the loss is generally bilateral. It is not always possible to distinguish, from an audiogram alone, whether the hearing loss is the effect of presbycusis, noise exposure, or ototoxic agents.

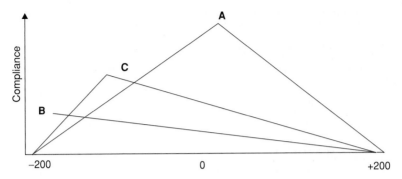

FIGURE 35-1. Tympanogram patterns. (A) Type A tympanogram, with normal compliance of the tympanic membrane. (B) Type B tympanogram, with no impedance peak. (C) Type C tympanogram, with a peak in the negative range.

      (2) The classic **noise-induced pattern** on the audiogram shows high-frequency loss, greatest at 4000 cycle, with improvement at 8000 cycles. The audiogram should be measured at least 14 hours after the last significant noise exposure in order to minimize the confusion of temporary versus permanent threshold shifts.

    b. Conductive loss causes low-frequency (i.e., 125–500 cycles) loss rather than high-frequency loss. Bone conduction testing in patients with conductive hearing loss reveals normal hearing thresholds.

    c. Mixed loss causes audiometric patterns with features of both sensorineural and conductive hearing loss.

B. Tympanometry. Tympanometry is a simple, reliable test that may be rapidly performed in the clinic setting. This test assesses function of the tympanic membrane and Eustachian tube. A small probe is inserted into the external auditory canal and a tone of fixed characteristics is presented via the probe. The compliance of the tympanic membrane is measured electronically while the external canal pressure is artificially varied.

    1. Indications. Tympanogram is useful to confirm an otoscopic diagnosis, aid in diagnosis when otoscopy is equivocal or difficult (especially in children), and as a screening test for ear disease.

    2. Findings (Figure 35–1). In general, tympanograms provide information on presence/absence of fluid in the middle ear, mobility of the middle ear, and ear canal volume. They may be described as type a, type b, or type C. Compliance is greatest when pressures are equal on both sides of the tympanic membrane. A peak will be present when the compliance is normal. **Type A tympanogram** describes normal compliance of the tympanic membrane. **Type B tympanogram** looks flat, because no impedence peak may be identified. There is little or no mobility, often because of fluid in the middle ear. Type B may also be seen with patent pressure equalization tubes and perforations. **Type C tympanogram** shows a peak in the negative range, which is consistent with a retracted tympanic membrane and Eustachian tube dysfunction.

C. Otoacoustic emission (OAE) and/or auditory brainstem response (ABR). Without screening, congenital hearing loss is often not diagnosed until as late as 2.5 years of age, and therefore results in impaired speech, language, and cognitive development. It has been estimated that if exclusively risk-based screening were to be used, up to 42% of profoundly hearing-impaired individuals would be missed. Those that do not pass the screen are often given a second screen to confirm findings along with referrals for follow-up medical and audiologic evaluations. These evaluations should occur no later than 3 months of age. Over 30 states have mandated newborn screening with OAE and/or ABR testing. (SOR **B**)

VI. Treatment

    A. General points/preventive measures. Effective measures to prevent or minimize hearing loss are described below.

1. **The treatment of hearing loss is dependent upon its etiology** and involves environmental alteration, assistive listening devices, active medical/surgical intervention, and hearing aids.
2. **Both conductive and sensorineural hearing loss may benefit from environmental alteration** and usage of assistive listening devices. Perhaps the most important way the listening environment may be altered is by minimizing the amount of background noise.
3. Physicians should **minimize the use of ototoxic drugs** and carefully monitor patients taking these drugs.
4. **Individuals with exposure to noise at home or work** should receive education concerning the use of ear protection during noise exposure and should be fitted for proper ear protective devices such as earmuffs or earplugs.

B. **Sensorineural loss**
  1. **Presbycusis.** Patients with a presumptive diagnosis of presbycusis should be referred to an audiologist for further testing to confirm the diagnosis and for rehabilitation. Patients may increase the effectiveness of communication by cupping the hand behind the ear, reducing distractions and background noise levels, using good lighting to see the speaker and understand gestures, and learning lipreading. Hearing aids or other assistive devices may be beneficial. Psychologic support, particularly for elderly patients, is very helpful. Left untreated, presbycusis can lead to social isolation and depression.
  2. **Noise-induced loss.** Patients with this type of loss should be referred to an otolaryngologist for assessment of asymmetric hearing loss, rapid and progressive hearing loss, permanent threshold shift, or an occasional finding of low-frequency loss. All patients with losses presenting at threshold $\geq$25 dB are candidates for hearing aids.
  3. **Ototoxicity.** For patients with ototoxicity, early removal of the offending agent will reduce the likelihood of permanent hearing loss. Hearing impairment may be either permanent (e.g., when caused by drugs such as mercury, arsenic, lead, or aminoglycosides) or temporary (e.g., when caused by drugs such as aspirin, quinine, or certain diuretics). Actual recovery may be delayed and is often incomplete. Thus, follow-up with an audiologist may be necessary to evaluate for ototoxic sequelae.

C. **Conductive hearing loss**
  1. **Foreign bodies or cerumen** in the external auditory canal can almost always be removed by irrigation with or without the use of ceruminolytics, ceruminolytics alone, or manual removal with forceps, suction, or curette. Patients with objects wedged in place should be referred to an otolaryngologist because of potential risks of damage to the tympanic membrane or bony structures by attempted removal.
      a. **Hard cerumen can be softened** fairly quickly prior to irrigation with a few drops of over-the-counter cerumen softener. The ear can be irrigated with water approximately 20 minutes after the softening agent is applied. The use of water at a temperature of 35 to 37.8°C (95–100°F) will prevent vertigo.
      b. **Water irrigation is contraindicated** with vegetable foreign bodies (i.e., dry beans) because it can cause swelling. Alcohol solutions should be used in such cases. A perforation in the tympanic membrane is an absolute contraindication to irrigation.
      c. **Ear candling is a home remedy that patients should be instructed to avoid because of risks of ear wax occlusion, local burns, and tympanic membrane perforation.**
  2. **Otitis externa** or **otitis media** should be treated with appropriate medication (see Chapter 22); hearing should normalize following treatment of infection and resolution of middle ear effusion, which may take up to 3 months.
  3. Patients with **otosclerosis** can be successfully treated with stapedectomy and should be referred to an otolaryngologist.

REFERENCES

Bogardus ST, Jr., Yueh B, Shekelle PG. Screening and management of adult hearing loss in primary care: clinical applications. *JAMA.* 2003;289(15):1986.

Daniel E. Noise and hearing loss: a review. *J Sch Health.* 2007;77(5):225-231.

El Dib RP, Verbeek J, Atallah AN, Andriolo RB, Soares BGO. Interventions to promote the wearing of hearing protection. Art No.: CD005234. DOI: 10.1002/14651858.CD005234.pub2: 2006.

Isaacson JE, Vora NM. Differential diagnosis and treatment of hearing loss. *Am Fam Physician.* 2003;68:1125.
McCarter DF, Courtney U, Pollart SM. Cerumen impaction. *Am Fam Physician.* 2007;75:1523-1528, 1530.
Onusko E. Tympanometry. *Am Fam Physician.* 2004;70(9):1713-1720.
Robinson TE, White GL, Houchins JC. Improving communication with older patients: tips from the literature. *Fam Pract Manag.* 2006;13(8).
Wrightson AS. Universal newborn hearing screening. *Am Fam Physician.* 2007;75(9):1349-1352.
Yueh B, et al. Screening and management of adult hearing loss in primary care: scientific review. *JAMA.* 2003;289(15):1976.

36   Hematuria

Cynthia M. Waickus, MD, PhD

KEY POINTS

- Hematuria is a common finding on urinalysis in both children and adults and it may be the sign of a benign condition or the symptom of a life-threatening disease.
- Microscopic hematuria should be confirmed by repeat testing and urine microscopy.
- One of the first steps in the evaluation of hematuria is to distinguish between glomerular and extraglomerular bleeding.

I. **Definition.** Hematuria is the presence of an abnormal quantity of red blood cells (RBCs) in the urine, and it may be grossly visible or microscopic (apparent only on urinalysis). It becomes clinically significant when the presence of three or more (adults), or five or more (children) RBCs are visible per high-power field in the sediment of two of three consecutive centrifuged, freshly voided, clean-catch, midstream urine specimens.

II. **Common Diagnoses.** The etiology and pathophysiology of hematuria are varied. Population based studies identify the prevalence of microscopic hematuria to vary from 0.16% to 21% in adults, with some studies reporting an even higher prevalence among women and older persons. Causes of hematuria can be classified as either glomerular or nonglomerular, important prognostically and for subsequent evaluation, as an evidence of glomerular involvement precludes the need for urologic workup.

A. Nonglomerular causes

1. Infections: **Cystitis, urethritis, pyelonephritis,** and **prostatitis**; infectious etiologies are the most common cause of hematuria, accounting for 30% to 35% of both gross and microscopic hematuria. Renal tuberculosis and *Schistosoma haematobium* are rare causes but need to be considered in persons who have traveled to endemic areas.

2. Calculi: **Nephrolithiasis** and **urolithiasis,** (primarily calcium oxalate and calcium phosphate) occur in approximately 5.2% of the overall population, with higher rates in males and whites, and older individuals. Gross hematuria occurs in most patients presenting with kidney stones.

3. Neoplasms:

   a. Renal tumors: **Renal cell carcinoma,** originating in the renal cortex, accounts for 80% to 85% of all primary renal tumors. **Transitional cell carcinomas,** originating in the renal pelvis, are the second most common primary renal tumor (8%). Renal tumors occur primarily after age 60, and are unusual before age 40. Risk factors for renal tumors include: smoking, toxin exposure (cadmium, asbestos, and petroleum by-products), obesity, male gender, acquired cystic disease of the kidney, analgesic abuse nephropathy, and genetic predisposition. The presence of hematuria indicates the tumor has invaded the collecting system. **Wilm's tumor** (nephroblastoma) is the most common renal tumor in children.

   b. **Bladder carcinoma** is the most common malignancy affecting the urinary system, occurring primarily after age 60, and occurs predominantly in males. Exposure to environmental chemicals (aromatic amines) used in the dye, paint, aluminum, textile, and rubber industries and cigarette smoking are the primary risk factors for bladder cancer.

  c. **Prostate cancer** is the most common nonskin cancer, and the third leading cause of death in American men. Age is the most important risk factor; prostate cancer is rare before age 40. It is more common in blacks than whites and has a strong genetic component. Although hematuria is not a common initial presentation, its presence should prompt consideration of prostate cancer.

  d. Benign tumors and polyps: **Benign prostatic hypertrophy** (BPH) and abnormal, benign growths (**polyps**) in the bladder and ureters may cause hematuria. The cellular proliferation in these conditions is associated with the formation of fragile, new blood vessels prone to bleeding.

4. Genetically transmitted diseases: **Polycystic kidney disease** (occurring in 1/400–2000 live births), **medullary cystic kidney disease** (incidence of 0.13/10,000 live births), and **sickle cell disease/trait** often include hematuria as a clinical presentation.

5. Vascular disease: **Arteriovenous malformations or fistulas** of the urologic tract typically present symptomatically as gross hematuria. **Renal infarction**, caused by thrombo or atheroemboli in patients with atrial fibrillation or atherosclerotic disease, presents with the acute onset of nausea, vomiting, flank and abdominal pain, fever, and gross or microscopic hematuria (33%–50% of patients).

6. Mechanical: **Strictures** (ureteral and meatal), solitary renal **cysts, foreign bodies** in the urinary tract may all present with hematuria.

7. Anticoagulation therapy: Routine use of **Coumadin** (warfarin) should not cause either gross or microscopic hematuria unless there is an underlying abnormality, and these patients should be evaluated in the same manner as other patients presenting with hematuria. The incidence of hematuria in patients taking anticoagulant therapy is the same as that of the general population.

8. Hematuria secondary to urinary tract **trauma** is the result of direct cellular and vascular damage. **Exercise-induced hematuria**, is a benign, short-term condition (resolves within 1 week), and is a diagnosis of exclusion. It occurs after noncontact sport activities, and may be the result of brief renal ischemia, and is reported in up to 30% of long-distance runners. It is important to differentiate exercise-induced hematuria from myoglobinuria (caused by rhabdomyolysis), and hemoglobinuria.

B. Glomerular causes: Causes of glomerular hematuria (glomerulonephritis) include:

1. **IgA nephropathy** is the most common cause of primary glomerulonephritis, and it results from an abnormal globular deposition of IgA in the kidney. It has a peak incidence in the second and third decades of life, and is more common in males, Asians and Caucasians. Gross hematuria is a presenting symptom in 40% to 50% of cases, while microscopic hematuria with proteinuria is the presentation in 30% to 40% of cases.

2. **Thin basement membrane nephropathy** (benign familial hematuria) is a common cause of asymptomatic hematuria. It is characterized pathologically by diffused thinning of the glomerular basement membrane, and clinically by persistent microscopic hematuria. It is familial, with an autosomal dominant inheritance, and has a totally benign prognosis as patients maintain normal renal function throughout their lives.

3. **Hereditary nephritis** (Alport syndrome) is an uncommon (1 in 5000 persons), X-linked disorder that causes chronic glomerulonephritis progressing to end-stage renal disease. It presents early in life (before age 10) and is often associated with neural hearing loss and ocular difficulties.

4. **Acute interstitial nephritis** is an important cause of an acute renal failure resulting from immune mediated tubulointerstitial injury.

  a. Drugs (71% of cases): Although any drug can potentially cause a hypersensitivity reaction to the kidney, the most commonly implicated drugs are: antibiotics (penicillins, cephalosporins, sulfas, quinolones, rifampin), diuretics, non-steroidal antiinflammatory drugs (NSAIDs), anticonvulsants, and allopurinol.

  b. Infection (15% of cases): Bacterial (streptococci, legionella, mycoplasma, syphilis), viral (cytomegalovirus [CMV], Epstein-Barr virus [EBV], HIV, Hepatitis B), fungal (histoplasmosis), and parasitic (toxoplasmosis, leptospirosis).

  c. Autoimmune disorders: Most autoimmune disorders eventually cause chronic interstitial nephritis (Sjogren's syndrome, systemic lupus erythematosis [SLE], sarcoidosis, Wegeners' granulomatosis).

III. **Symptoms**
  A. Concurrent symptoms of **dysuria, frequency/urgency**, are classically indicative of an infectious etiology (urinary tract infection [UTI], cystitis, urethritis, prostatitis), but may also be caused by bladder cancer. The presence of **blood clots** in the urine rarely occurs with glomerular bleeding.
  B. **Unilateral flank pain with radiation to the groin** typically suggests an obstructive cause in the kidney or ureter (calculi, clot, stricture, tumor).
  C. **Unilateral flank pain without radiation**, but with **fever, dysuria**, and **frequency/urgency** is suggestive of pyelonephritis. **Pain** is not indicative of glomerular disease.
  D. Prostatic obstruction (benign prostatic hypertrophy [BPH], prostate cancer) in older men may present as **urinary hesitancy** and **dribbling,** with or without **other symptoms of UTI.**
  E. Complaints of **recent weight gain, edema, facial swelling**, and **decreased urine output** or **oliguria** suggests a glomerular cause.
  F. Complaints of **recent upper respiratory symptoms, sore throat** may suggest glomerulonephritis (poststreptococcal glomerulonephritis or IgA nephropathy); also present may be complaints of **fever, rash**, and **joint tenderness**.
  G. **Gross hematuria** can be a presenting symptom with any of the above diagnoses (benign causes to malignancies). A visible color change can be caused by as little as 1 mL/L of blood in the urine, and the color change does not necessarily reflect the amount of blood loss.
  H. The most common presenting symptom for bladder cancer is **intermittent, painless, gross hematuria**, typically present **through micturation**.
IV. **Signs:** Like symptoms and complaints presented by the patient in the history, physical examination findings may be helpful in differentiating between glomerular and nonglomerular etiologies for hematuria, although clinical signs are often absent.
  A. **Vital signs:** Fever typically indicates an infectious or inflammatory cause; elevated blood pressure and weight gain are clues to glomerular injury, whereas weight loss may be sign of a malignancy.
  B. **Costovertebral angle tenderness** may be present with pyelonephritis or renal calculi.
  C. **Digital rectal examination** revealing a firm, enlarged prostate gland will typically provide clues to benign prostatic hypertrophy, and may be present in prostate cancer. A tender, warm, enlarged, "boggy" feeling prostate will add clinical evidence for a diagnosis of prostatitis (Chapter 61).
  D. **Examination of the external genitalia** and urethra/meatus is performed if local trauma is suspected as the cause of the hematuria.
V. **Laboratory Tests** (Figure 36–1): No studies support routine testing for hematuria among the general public for screening, and in general, screening for hematuria (microscopic) in asymptomatic patients (those without signs or symptoms of urinary tract disease) is not recommended. (SOR **Ⓒ**) There are however, certain groups of patients with microscopic hematuria who possess risk factors for significant disease, most specifically malignancy, who should undergo diagnostic workup (see Section II.A.3.c). Diagnostic workup should likewise assist the clinician to sort through glomerular versus nonglomerular etiologies. The identification of glomerular disease or injury as the source of hematuria is important both diagnostically and prognostically. Urologic etiologies can be ruled out, and nephrologic referral is typically warranted.
  A. **Urine dipstick** is a simple, fast, inexpensive, reagent based colorimetric assay tool used in the office setting for screening urinalysis. The test, based on the peroxidase activity of hemoglobin, is at least as sensitive as urinalysis for the detection of microscopic **hematuria**. It can detect trace amounts of hemoglobin, equivalent to 1 to 2 RBCs per high-power field, but it does not distinguish between RBCs, hemoglobin, myoglobin, and therefore has a high-false positive rate; however, false-negatives are unusual. Dipstick reagents may also detect **proteinuria** (although albumin is the only protein detected by dipstick, and does not detect protein excretion below 300 mg/d), **leukocyte esterase**, and **nitrites**. All positive dipstick results should confirmed by microscopic urinalysis of a properly obtained centrifuged urine specimen, or by appropriate quantitative methods.
  B. **Urinalysis:** The initial evaluation of patients with red urine is **microscopic examination** of the **sediment** of the urine specimen. The sample should be a midstream, cleancatch (foreskin retraction or labial separation followed by local disinfection of the meatus and mucosa) specimen, voided into a sterile container. Ideally, especially if infection is

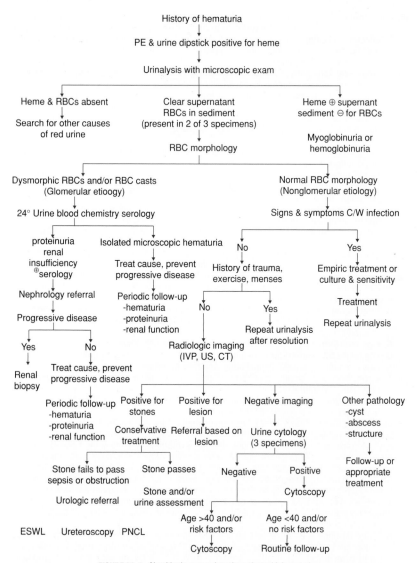

FIGURE 36–1. Algorithmic approach to the patient with hematuria.

suspected, the specimen should be examined within 60 minutes, or refrigerated for less than 24 hours. The specimen is then evaluated for:

1. RBCs: The urine sediment is carefully examined for the presence of erythrocytes (three or more per high-powered field), as hematuria is only present if RBCs are present in the sediment and the supernatant remains clear. If the supernatant remains red (discolored), it must be tested for the presence of hemoglobin; red supernatant that is positive for heme is caused by myoglobinuria (secondary to rhabdomyolysis) or hemoglobinuria; a red supernatant that tests negative for heme may be because of a variety of medications, certain food dyes, beets, or blackberries. **RBC morphology** by phase contrast microscopy may be helpful in distinguishing between glomerular and nonglomerular causes, as the presence of a significant number of dysmorphic RBCs suggests a renal (glomerular) source of the hematuria.

2. White blood cells (**WBCs):** Urinary tract infection without pyuria ($\geq$10,000 WBCs/mL of uncentrifuged urine, or 2–5 WBCs per hpf in sediment) is unusual, and is typically substantiated by a positive urine culture; however, sterile pyuria with hematuria may be indicative of tuberculosis.

3. **Casts:** Urinary casts (tubules of precipitated or aggregated protein) are only formed in the distal convoluted tubules or the collecting ducts, and therefore are indicative of kidney involvement (except for hyaline casts). The presence of **RBC casts** is typically diagnostic of glomerulonephritis. **WBC casts** indicate an inflammatory process in the kidney and are most typical for acute pyelonephritis or glomerulonephritis.

4. **Crystals:** Crystals may be present in the urine sediment of patients with hematuria secondary to calculi, but there is no clear defined association between crystal formation and urolithiasis.

5. **Bacteria:** Bacteria are typically present in the urine of patients with suspected UTI, but contamination is common (normal genital microbes). The diagnosis of bacteruria requires confirmation by urine culture.

C. **Urine culture:** A midstream, clean-catch specimen should be sent for culture, colony count, and antibiotic sensitivity whenever a UTI is suspected.

D. **24-hour urine collection:** The complete collection of all urine excreted in a 24-hour period by a patient with hematuria may provide important clues to the presence of glomerular disease, especially when **proteinuria** (more than 150 mg/d or 10 mg/dL) is present. In addition, the sample may be analyzed for creatinine clearance, and a number of other compounds.

E. **Blood work:** The choice of the hematologic evaluation should be dictated by the signs and symptoms identified clinically, the urinalysis, and the "preliminary" diagnosis in the patient with hemturia. Blood chemistry, including **electrolytes,** renal function (Blood urea nitrogen [**BUN**], creatinine [**Cr**], **albumin/protein levels,** and calculated glomerular filtration rate (**GFR**) are indicated when renal disease is suspected as the cause of the hematuria. Complete blood count (**CBC**) may provide clues to the degree of blood loss, and/or the presence of infection, and **coagulation studies** should be performed in patients with a clear history of a bleeding disorder. In certain populations, a **sickle cell prep** or a **hemoglobin electrophoresis** may help establish the diagnosis of sickle cell disease or trait. Serologic testing including complement levels (Compliment **C3 & C4**), antinuclear antibody titers (**ANA**), erythrocyte sedimentation rate (**ESR**), and antistreptolysin (**ASO) titers** may support a glomerular etiology for the hematuria.

F. **Imaging studies:** Like the hematologic evaluation, radiologic testing should be based on the preliminary diagnosis. If a glomerular etiology is ruled out, it is necessary to examine the upper urinary tract radiographically, to detect any neoplasms, urolithiasis, cystic disease, and obstructive lesions. (SOR **C**)

1. **Intravenous pyelogram (IVP):** The IVP, or excretory urography, was traditionally the first imaging examination of the upper urinary tract in patients with hematuria since it defines the anatomy of the upper tract well. It is limited in its ability to identify small masses ($\leq$3 cm), and it cannot differentiate between cystic and solid lesions. In addition, it necessitates the use of a potentially nephrotoxic contrast dye. Except for the detection of urothelial transitional cell carcinoma, its use is often replaced by high-quality renal ultrasound and/or spiral CT scan.

2. **Renal ultrasound (US):** Ultrasonography, compared with other imaging techniques of the urinary tract, is rapid, noninvasive, readily available, does not require toxic contrast media, and causes no radiation exposure so it may be used in pregnancy. It is therefore thought to be the safest, least expensive imaging choice for the evaluation of hematuria. It is highly sensitive in identifying large masses ($\geq$3 cm), cysts, hydronephrosis, and hydroureter. US is not likely to detect nonobstructing ureteral stones or small urothelial masses (as in transitional cell carcinoma), and is limited in its ability to detect small masses ($\leq$3 cm).

3. **Computerized tomography (CT scan):** Unenhanced (no intravenous [IV] or oral contrast) spiral CT scan of the abdomen and pelvis, is the most sensitive imaging method for detecting urinary tract calculi (96%–100% sensitive). It is also indicated in the patient with hematuria and a history of trauma. Contrast-enhanced CT scan of the

abdomen and pelvis is superior to US or IVP for identifying small (≤3 cm) masses, and is typically used to further evaluate all masses identified by IVP or US.

4. **Abdominal plain films:** Plain films of the abdomen (kidneys, ureters bladder [KUB]) are not typically used in the workup of hematuria, except for a quick detection of radiopaque stones (calcium, struvite, or cystine stones); however, small stones, uric acid stones, or stones behind bony structures are usually not seen. It also fails to detect obstruction. Plain films may be utilized to monitor progression of renal calculi down the urinary tract.

G. **Urine cytology:** Examination of the urine for the presence of malignant cells may be used in patients with hematuria who also have risk factors for urothelial cancers. (SOR **C**) The sensitivity of urine cytology is greatest for high-grade lesions and carcinoma in situ of the bladder (66%–79% sensitivity). This sensitivity is increased by analyzing first-void specimens on three consecutive days, or by obtaining sample during cystoscopy. The utility of urine cytology is very limited for upper tract malignancies (renal cell & transitional cell carcinoma), and for low-grade lesions of the bladder. Positive urine cytology is routinely followed by cystoscopy.

H. **Cystoscopy:** Cystoscopic examination of the bladder, urethra, and ureteral orifices is utilized to exclude the diagnosis of bladder malignancy. It is indicated in all patients older than 40 years with hematuria, in those patients younger than 40 years who present with hematuria and risk factors for bladder cancer, and in those patients who are younger than 40 years with unexplained, persistent hematuria or gross hematuria. Cystoscopy is rarely indicated in children. Cystoscopy typically requires urologic referral.

I. **Renal biopsy:** Renal biopsy, with subsequent microscopic examination of the tissue (light, immunofluorescence, and electron microscopy) is not routinely performed to establish a diagnosis for glomerular hematuria. It is typically considered only if there is an evidence of progressive disease (increasing proteinuria, worsening blood pressure, increased creatinine excretion, worsening renal function).

VI. **Treatment**

A. **Infections: Urinary tract infections** (see Chapter 21) The same principles apply to the treatment of prostatitis (see Chapter 61).

B. **Calculi:** The mainstay treatment for most calculi (80%–85%) is conservative, watchful waiting, involving, hydration, analgesic medication, and often prophylactic antibiotic treatment. Stones larger than 6 mm in diameter are unlikely to pass with conservative treatment and will require intervention. Urologic consultation is indicated for removal of large stones, patients with sepsis, and for obstructive symptoms. Urologic modalities include:

1. **Extracorporeal shockwave lithotripsy (ESWL).**
2. **Percutaneous nephrolithotomy (PCNL).**
3. **Ureteroscopy.**

C. **Neoplasms:** (see Chapter 61).

D. **Glomerular disease:** Treatment of glomerular causes of hematuria are directed primarily toward slowing progression of the disease. In the case of IgA nephropathy or hereditary nephritis, treatment is directed at maintaining normal blood pressures (angiotensin converting enzyme [ACE] inhibitors and angiotensin II receptor blockers [ARBs]), and decreasing cardiovascular risk (statins). Poststreptococcal glomerulonephritis usually resolves gradually after treatment of the infection. Acute interstitial nephritis caused by drugs is treated by removing the causative agent, and autoimmune etiologies are typically treated with immunosuppressants by nephrologists and rheumatologists.

REFERENCES

Choyke PL, Bluth EI, Bush WH, et al. *Expert Panel on Urologic Imaging. Radiologic Investigation of Patients with Hematuria.* Reston, VA: American College of Radiology (ACR); 2005.

Cohen RA, Brown RS. Clinical practice. Microscopic hematuria. *NEJM.* 2003;348:2330.

Grossfield GD, Litwin MS, Wolf JS, et al. Evaluation of Asymptomatic Microscopic Hematurai in Adults: The American Urological Association Best Practice Policy – Part I: Definition, Detection, Prevalence, and Etiology. *Urology.* 2001;57(4):599 & Part II: Patient Evaluation, Cytology, Nephrology Evaluation, and Follow-up. *Urology.* 2001;57(4):604.

Kincaid-Smith P, Fairley K. The investigation of hematuria. *Semin Nephrol.* 2005;25(3):127.

McDonald MM, Swagerty D, Wetzel L. Assessment of microscopic hematuria in adults. *Am Fam Physician.* 2006;73:1748.

37   Insomnia

Jeffrey L. Susman, MD, & Bryan Cairns, MD

KEY POINTS

- Short-term insomnia is a problem for approximately 30% of people, with chronic insomnia affecting approximately 10%.
- When assessing sleep problems, explore the role of underlying medical and psychiatric illnesses, medication use, and current sleep habits.
- Implement good sleep hygiene for all sleep disorders and consider nonpharmacologic approaches to treatment whenever possible.
- The accurate diagnosis of many primary sleep disorders requires full polysomnography in an accredited sleep laboratory; currently, actigraphy and home polysomnography are inadequate substitutes for such an evaluation.

I. **Definition.** Adequate sleep is essential for healthy tissue growth and repair, regulation of immune function, and memory integration. Normal sleep may be divided into five stages. **Non-rapid eye movement (non-REM) sleep** includes the transition period from wakefulness to sleep or light sleep (stages 1 and 2) and deep sleep (stages 3 and 4). Deep sleep is characterized by decreased muscle tone, blood pressure, and respiratory rate. **REM sleep,** or "dream sleep," is associated with skeletal muscle atonia, variability of vital signs, and dreaming. A person normally goes from wakefulness through stages 1 to 4 followed by the first REM period after approximately 90 minutes of sleep. Cycles of REM and non-REM sleep occur at 1- to 3-hour intervals, with decreasing amounts of deep sleep in later cycles. Most adults require 6 to 8 hours of sleep each day. Approximately 2% require less than 5 hours, and another 2% require more than 9 hours each day. **Insomnia** is the inability to fall asleep (long sleep latency) or stay asleep (excessive or prolonged awakenings), and sleep disorders may be associated with disruption of the quality, quantity, or timing of one or more stages of sleep. A 2002 survey by the National Institutes of Health Center for Complementary and Alternative Medicines found that more than 1.6 million Americans use some form of complementary and alternative medicines to treat insomnia (www.nih.gov).

II. **Common Diagnoses.** A National Sleep Foundation poll reported in 2003 that more than two-thirds of Americans older than 55 years reported sleep problems, but only one in eight had their problem diagnosed. More than two-thirds of children experience frequent sleep problems, according to the 2004 survey of the National Sleep Foundation. While the relative incidence of sleep disorders in primary care populations is less clear, almost all individuals suffer from occasional sleep disturbance. The major categories of insomnia include:

A. **Transient conditions** resulting from situational stress or conflict; environmental factors, such as excessive noise, bright light, and improper temperature; travel problems, including jet lag and adjustment to new sleeping environments; hospitalization or institutionalization; and shift work.

B. **Psychiatric diseases** including alcohol and drug abuse (see Table 37–1); depression (Chapter 92); bipolar disorder, mania, or dementia (Chapter 73); delirium (Chapter 11); posttraumatic stress disorder or other anxiety disorders (Chapter 89); ADHD (Chapter 90); and patients with excessive neurotic symptoms or the inability to deal effectively with anger and emotions.

C. **Physiologic, age-, or gender-related insomnia.** More than 50% of elderly people will admit to sleep problems, and females are more likely to complain of insomnia than males.

D. **Medical disorders** such as symptomatic prostatic hypertrophy, congestive heart failure, and gastroesophageal reflux.

E. **Primary sleep disorders**
   1. **Disturbances of the sleep–wake cycle or circadian rhythm sleep disorders** are common in people who are hospitalized, institutionalized, do night or changing shift work, or have jet lag.

TABLE 37–1. MEDICATIONS ASSOCIATED WITH SLEEP DISTURBANCE

Excessive wakefulness
Theophylline
Amphetamines
Caffeine
Anticonvulsants
Antidepressants (e.g., many of the selective serotonin reuptake inhibitors)
Alcohol
Nicotine
Triazolam (rebound phenomena)
Thyroid hormone
Methylphenidate
Sympathomimetics including herbals (e.g., ma huang, ephedra)

Nightmares
Beta-blockers (especially lipophilic agents such as propranolol)
Tricyclics
Antiparkinsonian agents
Quinidine
Buspirone
Selective serotonin reuptake inhibitors (SSRIs)

Excessive somnolence
Benzodiazepines
Antihistamines
Anticonvulsants
Antidepressants
Antipsychotics (both typical and atypical)
Tricyclics (especially amitriptyline, doxepin, and trazodone)
Monoamine oxidase inhibitors
Antihypertensives (especially clonidine)

Other symptoms
Diuretics (nocturia)
Levodopa and tricyclics (sleep-related myoclonus)
Caffeine (nonrepetitive muscle contractions at sleep onset or hypnic jerks)

2. **Sleep-related movement disorders** include restless legs syndrome and nocturnal myoclonus. One-third of patients with **restless legs syndrome** have a family history of this disorder. This problem is sometimes associated with iron deficiency, motor neuron disease, renal disease, or circulatory problems. **Nocturnal myoclonus** is more common in older individuals.

3. **Parasomnias** include nightmares, sleep terrors, sleepwalking, REM sleep behavior, and sleep paralysis. The first three are more common in the pediatric population.
   a. **Nightmares** occur in REM sleep and may be associated with posttraumatic stress disorder.
   b. **Night terrors** are a non-REM phenomenon; in adults, night terrors may be associated with neurologic or psychiatric disorders.
   c. **Sleepwalking** is a non-REM phenomenon, is seen most frequently in children, and new-onset somnambulism in an adult may suggest a central nervous system or psychiatric disorder.

4. **Disorders of excessive somnolence**
   a. **Sleep apnea syndrome.** Central sleep apnea (CSA) usually has a readily apparent cause such as stroke, brain stem infarction, or neoplasia. CSA is often associated with advanced COPD and CHF. Obstructive sleep apnea (OSA) is associated with an upper airway abnormality and with medical conditions such as thyroid dysfunction, hypertension, cor pulmonale, obesity, and severe pulmonary dysfunction. OSA is most common in men and in older individuals.
   b. **Narcolepsy.** Narcolepsy is most likely to occur in young to middle-aged males.

F. **Conditioned or learned insomnia.** These conditions often occurs as patients develop poor sleep habits and come to associate bedtime with a frustrating experience trying to fall asleep or maintain sleep.

G. **Drug-/alcohol-related insomnia** (Table 37–1).

TABLE 37–2. SLEEP DIARY

Date and day of the week
Habits prior to sleep, including food, drink (especially alcohol and caffeine), and medication
Activities prior to bedtime, including reading, television, telephone, sex, work, exercise, and socializing
Bedtime
Time it takes to fall asleep
Quality of sleep, including awakenings and nightmares
Dreams, snoring, or unusual movements
Time awake
Total sleep time
Symptoms and alertness upon awakening
Daytime sleepiness and naps
Other unusual or important factors

III. **Symptoms.** Patients with insomnia may present with unusual or nonspecific symptoms, such as headache and irritability, in addition to complaints of difficulty in initiating or maintaining sleep. A sleep diary for a week (see Table 37–2), a tape recording of the patient's sounds while sleeping, and a history of the patient's sleep patterns provided by the patient's bed partner are useful tools in diagnosing the causes of insomnia.

A. **Snoring** is common in the general population and becomes more common as the patient ages. More than 60% of men and 45% of women older than the age of 60 snore. Unusually loud or disruptive snoring (especially when accompanied by periods of apnea), however, may be a symptom of a more serious problem such as sleep apnea syndrome.

B. **Pain, paresthesias, cramps, cough,** and **breathlessness** may indicate that the insomnia is caused by illness or disease.

C. **Sleep phase disorders**
   1. **Delayed sleep phase.** Patients with this problem have difficulty falling asleep, have no problems once asleep, and awaken later than usual.
   2. **Advanced sleep phase.** Patients cannot stay awake in the evening, have no difficulty once asleep, and awaken early in the morning.
   3. **Irregular sleep phase.** Patients complain of frequent drowsiness and naps and excessive time in bed.

D. **Difficulty maintaining sleep, periodic hypersomnolence, headache, impotence, enuresis, personality changes, unusual movements,** and **loud sounds or snoring** during sleep may indicate sleep apnea syndrome.

E. **Excessive daytime sleepiness** and **"sleep attacks," hypnagogic or bizarre hallucinations,** and **cataplexy** (sudden muscle weakness, especially at times of extreme emotion) are common symptoms of narcolepsy. The symptoms usually begin before age 30.
   1. **Cataplexy** is pathognomonic; however, episodes of cataplexy may be very short, infrequent, and easily overlooked.
   2. **Periodic amnesia** or **accidents** may be the presenting symptoms because of the patient's "sleep attacks" and cataplexy.

F. **Restless legs syndrome** is characterized by a "creepy" or "crawling" sensation and an irresistible urge to move one's legs, particularly when just retiring and frequently during the day when in confined spaces (such as at a movie theatre). A recent medication, pramipexole, is a D3 agonist used in the treatment of RLS, which should be distinguished from akathesia: the constant urge to move as a side effect of antipsychotic medications. **Nocturnal myoclonus** is associated with repetitive stereotypic spasms of the legs in non-REM sleep and with muscle aches and daytime fatigue. These disorders are often coexistent.

G. **Parasomnias** include **nightmares,** which are associated with limited vocalization, vivid recall, and easy arousal; and **night terrors,** which are associated with blood-curdling screams, little recall, and more difficult arousal. There is also minimal recall associated with **somnambulism.**

IV. **Signs** of the psychiatric disorders and medical diseases mentioned previously should be sought, as discussed in detail elsewhere (see Chapters 11, 73, 88, 89, and 92). A large neck, large tongue, or abnormalities in the ear-nose-throat examination may be associated with obstructive sleep apnea.

V. Laboratory Tests. In most cases, a careful history and physical examination will obviate the need for laboratory evaluation and will point to underlying medical conditions. Evaluation of the syndrome should be included in the physical examination, given the relationship between obesity and obstructive sleep apnea. Iron studies (e.g., ferritin) should be ordered in patients with restless legs syndrome; consideration should also be given to renal (blood urea nitrogen, creatinine), folate, and thyroid (TSH) assessment. A TSH level should be ordered in patients with sleep apnea, as well as fasting glucose, lipid studies. A **sleep study** is indicated in the following situations.

A. The diagnosis remains obscure or the problem persists or worsens.

B. There is suspicion of sleep apnea, especially in patients with hypertension, signs of cardiopulmonary difficulties and respiratory symptoms, or daytime somnolence.

C. Periodic hypersomnia is present. A sleep study is particularly important when this is associated with functional impairment.

D. Serious disorders of the sleep–wake cycle, which are not associated with transient changes in work or travel, occur.

E. The patient feels that the problem is becoming more severe and interfering with daily activities.

  The accurate diagnosis of many primary sleep disorders requires full polysomnography in an accredited sleep laboratory; currently, actigraphy and home polysomnography are inadequate substitutes for such an evaluation.

VI. Treatment. Psychiatric and medical disorders associated with sleep disturbance should always be treated optimally, and instituting good sleep hygiene (see Table 37–3) is useful for most sleep disturbances.

A. Transient insomnia

  1. Environmental factors such as proper light, noise levels, and temperature should be optimized. **Drug and alcohol use** should be carefully assessed. **Good sleep hygiene** (Table 37–3) should be instituted.

  2. Adjustments to new sleeping environments, shift work, and **jet lag** should be addressed. Small delays in the sleep–wake cycle (i.e., staying up longer and going to bed later before westbound travel) are more easily accommodated prior to travel than in the opposite situation (i.e., going to bed earlier before eastbound travel). Adjustment to shift work is difficult if the schedule rotates irregularly. If possible, a routine of sleep–wake periods should be established. Melatonin (5 mg of the immediate-release formulation at the desired bedtime) is effective in patients with jet lag, as well is ramelteon, marketed as Rozerem, a melatonin agonist. Exposure to bright light during the day is also helpful.

  3. Pharmacologic agents may be used in select cases of transient sleep disorders unassociated with more serious problems (see Table 37–4). The drug of choice for sleep onset problems is usually zolpidem (Ambien) or eszopiclone (Lunesta). For sleep maintenance difficulty, zaleplon (Sonata) may be used during the middle of the

TABLE 37–3. SLEEP HYGIENE

Awaken at a regular hour
Exercise daily on a regular basis (not close to bedtime)
Control the sleep environment (proper temperature, decreased noise and light)
Eat a light snack before bedtime (if not contraindicated)
Limit or eliminate alcohol, caffeine, and nicotine
Use hypnotics on a short-term basis only
Wind down prior to bedtime
Have a "worry time" early in the evening
Go to bed when sleepy
Avoid excessive sleep on weekends or extremes of sleep
Use relaxation and behavioral modification techniques
Use bed for sleeping only
Eliminate naps unless part of the schedule
Get up if you cannot get to sleep in 15–30 min
Sleep where you sleep best
Recognize the adaptation effect in new environments

TABLE 37–4. PHARMACOLOGIC THERAPY FOR TRANSIENT INSOMNIA

Class and Selected Agents	Initial Dose (mg)	Comments
Nonprescription		
Aspirin or acetaminophen (Tylenol)	325–650	May relieve troublesome aches or pains and thus enhance sleep
Antihistamines		
Diphenhydramine citrate (Excedrin PM)		May be effective transiently but have potential for carry-over, anticholinergic side effects, and can induce paradoxical wakefulness
Diphenhydramine hydrochloride (Benadryl, Nytol)		
Doxylamine succinate (Unisom)		
Hydroxyzine (Atarax, Vistaril)		
Prescription		
Chloral hydrate	500–1000	May cause nausea and displace warfarin and phenytoin from albumin
Trazodone (Desyrel)	50–150	
Gabapentin (Neurontin)	100–400	Sedating; may be associated with priapism, particularly with higher doses
		Particularly useful with neuropathic pain syndromes
Benzodiazepines		
Triazolam (Halcion)	0.125–0.25	Recommended for 1 mo or less of continuous therapy
Alprazolam (Xanax)	0.25	
Lorazepam (Ativan)	1	Decreases sleep latency and nocturnal awakenings. May be associated with withdrawal.
Temazepam (Restoril)	15	
Oxazepam (Serax)	15	Intermediate onset and rapid elimination; may cause rebound insomnia
Estazolam (ProSom)	0.5–2.0	
Flurazepam (Dalmane)	15	Intermediate onset of action and elimination; give at least 1 h prior to bedtime
Chlordiazepoxide (Librium)	5–10	
Diazepam (Valium)	1–5	Slower onset of action; give several hours prior to bedtime
		Intermediate half-life
		Should be used cautiously because of long half-lives and potential for accumulation, especially in elders. Associated with falls and hip fractures.
Non-benzodiazepines		
Zolpidem (Ambien)	5–10	Agent of choice for sleep onset problems; less potential for withdrawal and is more specific for sedative properties alone
Zaleplon (Sonata)	5–10	Best agent for sleep maintenance difficulty; very short elimination half-life
Alternatives		
Melatonin	5 immediate release at time of desired sleep	Effective for jet lag
Valerian		Conflicting data about efficacy but appears to have few substantial side effects; may potentiate other psychoactive drugs
Kava-kava	300–600 of root extract	May be associated with fatal liver failure even after one dose; contraindicated

evening because of its short half-life. Zolpidem controlled-release (Ambien CR) and eszopiclone administered at bedtime may be effective for some individuals. Benzodiazepines should be reserved for nonresponders. Guidelines for hypnotic therapy:

a. Making a presumptive diagnosis and ruling out primary sleep disorders or underlying medical problems that pharmacologic therapy might aggravate.
b. Determining the goals of therapy.
c. Educating the patient on the use of medication.
d. Beginning with a low dose of medication and increasing as needed based on improved sleep and daytime functioning.
e. Following up in 1 week to reassess the patient's condition. Telephone contact is reasonable for reliable patients.

    f. Limiting medication use to no more than 3 to 4 weeks (especially if using a benzodiazepine) or using medications 3 or 4 times per week when longer therapy is warranted. Eszopiclone alone has FDA approval for longer term use based on clinical trial data.

    g. Educating the patient about the possibility of withdrawal symptoms, especially with benzodiazepines.

B. Physiologic or age-related insomnia

    1. The patient should be reassured.

    2. Good sleep hygiene should be recommended.

    3. Medications should be avoided.

    4. In the absence of underlying disease, patients who **snore** should be advised to consider:

        a. Exercise during the day or early evening.

        b. Avoidance of sedatives and alcohol.

        c. Sleeping on the side, not on the back. Sewing a tennis ball in the back of the pajamas may make this position easier to maintain.

        d. Raising the head of the bed 6 inches.

        e. Using a soft collar.

        f. Drinking a cup of coffee before going to bed.

C. Underlying **medical disorders** should be treated whenever possible. Certain problems may be associated with underlying primary sleep disorders (e.g., hypertension and obesity with sleep apnea syndrome). In the absence of contraindications, short-term pharmacologic therapy is often useful for hospitalized patients.

D. Primary sleep disorders

    1. Disturbances of the sleep–wake cycle. Slow advancement or delay of the patient's bedtime, usually in conjunction with a sleep laboratory, is the therapy for this disorder. The irregular sleep phase disturbance will respond to strict structuring of a patient's waking and sleeping hours.

    2. Sleep-related movement disorders. These disorders may respond to the treatment of underlying medical conditions such as iron deficiency or uremia; the avoidance of stimulants, including caffeine; and the judicious use of **benzodiazepines or dopaminergic agents. Oral clonazepam,** 1 to 4 mg, or **carbidopa-levodopa,** 25/100 mg at bedtime; **pergolide,** 0.1 to 0.5 mg 3 times daily; or **pramipexole,** 0.125 to 1 mg 3 times daily, are useful for restless legs syndrome. A trial of iron supplementation is occasionally effective for restless legs syndrome even when iron studies are normal. Opioid analgesics, gabapentin, and a host of other agents are also occasionally used for restless legs syndrome.

    3. Disorders of excessive somnolence

        a. Sleep apnea syndrome. CSA usually requires treatment by a pulmonary or neurologic specialist and is usually directed at the underlying disorder. For patients with **OSA,** consultation with pulmonary and otorhinolaryngology (ORL) specialists is often indicated. Upper airway abnormalities may be amenable to ear, nose, and throat surgery, especially adenotonsillectomy for children, or oral appliances specifically fitted to the patient. (SOR **B**) Obesity and underlying medical conditions should be treated aggressively. Even a small amount of weight loss can translate into a significant reduction in apneas. Patients should sleep on the side and should avoid depressants that affect the central nervous system. Nasal continuous positive airway pressure (CPAP) is the treatment of choice for most patients and positively affects subjective sleepiness, quality of life, and cognition. (SOR **B**) Unfortunately, long-term adherence to CPAP is less than 50%. Many problems can be corrected with refitting of the mask, trial of alternative delivery systems (such as nasal pillows) or the use of BIPAP, and appropriate humidification. Occasionally, uvulopalatopharyngoplasty (UPP) or tracheostomy is necessary if more conservative measures fail. Consultation with a skilled sleep specialist and ORL are important. Intranasal fluticasone has some efficacy in reducing symptoms of OSA, as well as reduction in daytime sleepiness. Similarly nighttime administration of mirtazepine (Remeron) and physostigmine showed reduction in the Apnea Hypopnea Index versus placebo; however, long-term studies are still needed on these agents.

        b. Narcolepsy should be managed by a specialist skilled in the evaluation and control of this disorder. Multiple newer medications (e.g., modafinil) are available to help maintain wakefulness and combat cataplexy.

4. **Conditioned insomnia** will usually respond to strict sleep hygiene, cognitive behavioral measures, and other counseling approaches such as sleep restriction therapy. (SOR **Ⓐ**)
5. **Psychiatric and medical disorders** exacerbating insomnia should be treated (see Chapters 11, 73, 89, and 92).
6. **Alcohol use** should be limited, and alternatives should be sought for drugs felt to be exacerbating insomnia (Table 37–1).

VII. **Follow-up** of sleep disorders and insomnia should be dictated by the severity of the problem. For serious sleep disorders, close supervision and careful follow-up are necessary. On the other hand, when more serious problems have been ruled out, a 2- to 4-week trial of good sleep hygiene is indicated. The identification of hidden medical or psychophysiologic causes of sleep disturbance should be pursued.

REFERENCES

Ambien CR for insomnia. *Med Lett Drugs Ther.* 2005;47:97.

Becker PM. Treatment of sleep dysfunction and psychiatric disorders. *Curr Treat Options Neurol.* 2006;8(5):367-375.

Chiang AA. Obstructive sleep apnea and chronic intermittent hypoxia: a review. *Chin J Physiol.* 2006;49(5):234-243.

Doghramji PP. Trends in the pharmacologic management of insomnia. *J Clin Psychiatry.* 2006;67(Suppl 13):5-8.

Early CJ. Restless legs syndrome. *N Engl J Med.* 2003;384:2103-2109.

Leshner AI, Kvale JN, Baghdoyan HA. National Institutes of Health State-of-the-Science Conference Statement: Manifestations and Management of Chronic Insomnia in adults. http://consensus.nih.gov. Accessed September 3, 2008.

Morin AK, Jarvis CI, Lynch AM. Therapeutic options for sleep-maintenance and sleep-onset insomnia. *Pharmacotherapy.* 2007;27(1):89-110.

Morin CM. Contributions of cognitive-behavioral approaches to the clinical management of insomnia. *Prim Care Comp J Clin Psych* 2002;4(Suppl 1):21.

Schenck CH, Mahowald MW, Sack RL. Assessment and management of insomnia. *JAMA.* 2003;289:2475-2479.

Silber MH. Clinical practice. Chronic insomnia. *N Engl J Med.* 2005;353:803-810.

---

38   Jaundice

Kalyanakrishnan Ramakrishnan, MD, & L. Peter Schwiebert, MD

KEY POINTS

- Most jaundice is produced by one of three underlying mechanisms: excessive hemoglobin degradation/bilirubin overproduction, liver disease, and biliary obstruction.
- Jaundice has many causes but can be effectively evaluated by history (including age of onset), physical examination, and limited laboratory testing.
- Jaundice in newborns can usually be managed conservatively and at home, even if treatment is required.

I. **Definition.** The major source of bilirubin is degradation of hemoglobin from senescent red blood cells. Bilirubin from the periphery is tightly bound to albumin during transport in the blood to the hepatocyte. Inside the hepatocyte, nonpolar bilirubin is enzymatically conjugated by uridine diphosphoglucuronyl transferase (UDPGT) to form water-soluble bilirubin diglucuronide. UDPGT activity is decreased in neonates, resulting in increased levels of unconjugated bilirubin. (In white and African American neonates, bilirubin levels rise steadily, peaking at 5–6 mg/dL between the second and fourth days of life, then slowly declining to adult levels by days 10–12. In Asians and Native Americans, bilirubin levels rise more rapidly, peaking at 8–12 mg/dL by days 4–5, then declining more slowly than in white or African

American neonates.) Conjugated bilirubin is excreted and transported as bile in the biliary system to the gastrointestinal tract, with most being reabsorbed in the ileum and undergoing enterohepatic circulation.

Jaundice is the yellow discoloration of the skin and mucous membranes caused by an elevated serum bilirubin. In adults, clinical jaundice occurs at bilirubin levels of 2 to 3 mg/dL. In newborns, the threshold is higher (5–6 mg/dL). Based on bilirubin physiology, jaundice can be categorized as being owing to (1) **excessive hemoglobin degradation/bilirubin over-production,** as in immune hemolysis (e.g., ABO incompatibility or Rh isoimmunization); non-immune hemolysis (e.g., glucose-6-phosphate-dehydrogenase [G6PD] deficiency or hereditary spherocytosis); extravascular hemolysis (e.g., cephalohematomas in newborns); or intramarrow hemolysis (e.g., "ineffective erythropoiesis" in thalassemia or pernicious anemia); (2) **defective hepatic uptake/conjugation/transport,** as in Gilbert's disease, Crigler-Najjar or Dubin-Johnson syndrome, or hepatitis; or (3) **impaired excretion,** as in hepato-cellular disease, drug effects, primary biliary cirrhosis (PBC), or bile duct obstruction.

II. **Common Diagnoses.** Jaundice is very common in newborns, affecting 60% of full-term and 80% of preterm infants; after the neonatal period, jaundice is less prevalent, accounting for up to 4% of annual acute hospital admissions. Jaundice has myriad causes; while recognizing that more than one pathophysiologic process can be present in a single patient, it is helpful to approach jaundice based on age of onset, risk factors, and fractional elevation of bilirubin, i.e., **unconjugated** (indirect fraction of bilirubin exceeds 80% of total) versus **conjugated** (indirect fraction ranges from 20%–60% of total bilirubin).

A. **Childhood jaundice**
   1. **Unconjugated hyperbilirubinemia**
      a. **Neonatal onset**
         (1) **Physiologic jaundice** is present in as many as 60% of newborns.
         (2) **Jaundice in breast-fed infants. Breastfeeding jaundice** occurs in 5% to 10% of breast-fed infants and is caused by dehydration and decreased caloric intake; dietary supplementation with formula is an additional risk factor. **Breast milk jaundice** occurs in less than 1% of breast-fed infants and is believed to be because of substances in the breast milk inhibiting UDGPT.
         (3) **Hemolytic anemia** is the most common pathologic cause of jaundice, usu-ally resulting from ABO or, less commonly, Rh incompatibility, spherocytosis, enzyme deficiency, or a hemoglobinopathy. African Americans are prone to hemolytic anemias caused by sickle cell disease and G6PD deficiency. Patients of Mediterranean descent and Asians are at increased risk for thalassemias.
         (4) Other causes of unconjugated neonatal hyperbilirubinemia include poly-cythemia, cephalohematoma reabsorption, pyloric stenosis, and congenital hy-pothyroidism.
      b. **Infancy and childhood onset.** Jaundice may result from hemolytic diseases (e.g., G6PD deficiency and spherocytosis), Gilbert's disease, and Crigler-Najjar or Dubin-Johnson syndromes.
   2. **Conjugated hyperbilirubinemia**
      a. **Neonatal onset.** Sepsis, neonatal hepatitis, ToRCHS infections (**t**oxoplasmosis, **r**ubella, **c**ytomegalovirus [CMV], **h**erpes, and **s**yphilis), extrahepatic obstruction in biliary atresia or choledocholithiasis, and metabolic diseases, such as galac-tosemia, α_1-antitrypsin deficiency, or tyrosinemia may result in jaundice.
      b. **Infancy and childhood onset.** Viral hepatitis (see Section II.B.2.a.(1)) is the most common cause of jaundice in a previously healthy child. Less common causes include Wilson's disease and milder forms of galactosemia.
B. **Adult onset**
   1. **Unconjugated hyperbilirubinemia** may occur with **hemolytic anemia, ineffective erythropoiesis** (e.g., thalassemias, sideroblastic anemias, and pernicious anemia), **impaired uptake, and conjugation of bilirubin** (e.g., Gilbert's syndrome, which oc-curs in 3%–7% of the US population, and Crigler-Najjar syndrome type II, an uncom-mon disorder). In addition to risk factors already mentioned, a positive family history may be associated with Gilbert's disease or hemolytic anemia.
   2. **Conjugated hyperbilirubinemia**
      a. **Impaired intrahepatic excretion**
         (1) **Viral hepatitis** accounts for 75% of jaundice in patients younger than 30 years decreasing to 5% in patients older than 60 years. Risk factors for **hepatitis A** include ingestion of raw shellfish, travel to countries with unsanitary water

supplies, household contact with infected persons, and exposure to diapered infants in day care. Risk factors for **hepatitis B** include living in endemic areas (e.g., subSaharan Africa or Asia), fetomaternal transmission, and sexual contact with an infected patient. A history of blood transfusions (especially before 1992), intravenous drug abuse, multiple sexual partners, hemodialysis, and health care occupations are risk factors for both **hepatitis B and C.**

    (2) Cirrhosis causes about one-third of jaundice in 30- to 60-year-old patients. Primary biliary cirrhosis is more common in females; males have a higher risk for alcoholic liver disease.

    (3) Congestive heart failure (CHF) accounts for 10% of jaundice after age 60. Risk factors include a history of hypertension and atherosclerotic cardiovascular disease (see Chapter 72).

    (4) Metastatic disease causes 13% of jaundice after age 60.

    (5) Other causes include drugs (erythromycin, nonsteroidal anti-inflammatory drugs, anabolic steroids, oral contraceptives, phenothiazines, and sulfonylureas), pregnancy, hepatoma, and Dubin-Johnson and Rotor's syndromes.

  b. Extrahepatic obstruction (e.g., gallstones, strictures, and tumors, especially pancreatic cancer) accounts for 60% of jaundice in patients older than 60 years. Gallstones are more common in females.

III. Symptoms

A. Onset of jaundice

    1. A **rapid onset** suggests infection, drug reaction, hemolytic anemia, or acute obstruction caused by common bile duct (CBD) stones.

    2. Intermittent or fluctuating jaundice occurs in Gilbert's disease (typically with fasting or intercurrent illness), Crigler-Najjar syndrome, Dubin-Johnson or Rotor's syndrome, recurrent CBD stones, and CHF.

    3. A **gradual onset** occurs in cirrhosis, liver metastases, pregnancy, or PBC.

B. Pruritus. Severe pruritus and excoriations suggest extrahepatic obstruction.

C. Abdominal pain occurs more often with obstructive jaundice than with hepatocellular disease. Colicky, right upper quadrant pain prior to the onset of jaundice suggests choledocholithiasis, especially in middle-aged and older patients.

D. Fever with chills suggests biliary obstruction and cholangitis. Charcot's triad refers to the triad of pain, jaundice, and fever seen in choledocholithiasis. In Reynold's pentad mental status changes and sepsis are also present. **Flulike symptoms** suggest viral or drug-induced hepatitis.

E. Persisting ($\geq$2-week) history of acholic stools and severe jaundice is also characteristic of **obstructive jaundice.**

F. Sixty to seventy percent of patients with **acute hepatitis C** are asymptomatic, 20% to 30% are jaundiced, and 10% to 20% complain only of fatigue, anorexia, or abdominal pain.

G. In neonates, historical clues include history of premature rupture of membranes (sepsis), delay in clamping the cord (polycythemia), and history of jaundice in a sibling (metabolic disorders or anemias). Both **breast milk** and **breastfeeding jaundice** develop in the first week of life.

IV. Signs

A. Urticaria suggests hepatitis B infection.

B. Cutaneous xanthomas are caused by hypercholesterolemia, and seen in patients with chronic cholestasis (e.g., PBC).

C. Spider angiomata, palmar erythema, clubbing, bilateral parotid enlargement, gynecomastia, testicular atrophy, ascites, and signs of portal hypertension (splenomegaly, enlarged, abdominal wall venous collaterals) are seen in chronic hepatocellular disease or cirrhosis.

D. Kayser-Fleischer rings in the cornea are pathognomonic of Wilson's disease.

E. A **palpable gallbladder** suggests malignant common bile duct obstruction (e.g., cancer of the head of the pancreas). Courvoisier's law states that, in the presence of an enlarged gallbladder, jaundice is unlikely to be caused by gallstones.

F. Large, palpable, nodular liver suggests metastatic cancer.

G. Splenomegaly is found in many patients with cirrhosis, chronic active hepatitis, and alcoholic liver disease. However, it occurs in less than 5% of patients with an acute viral hepatitis, gallstones, or malignant biliary obstruction. Hepatomegaly, especially a tender enlarged liver $\geq$15 cm, suggests alcoholic hepatitis or malignancy.

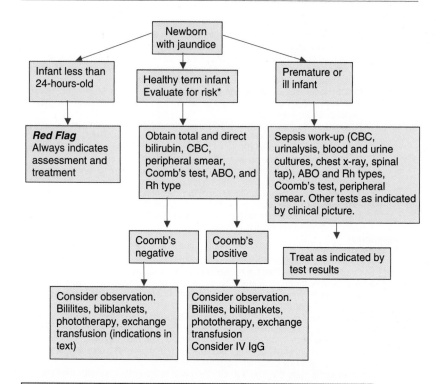

FIGURE 38–1. Evaluation of a newborn with jaundice.

H. **In newborns,** jaundice can be detected by examining the child in a well-lighted room and blanching the skin with digital pressure. Icterus, first seen in the face, progresses craniocaudally to the trunk and the extremities; the degree of progression correlates roughly with bilirubin levels (i.e., the face, approximately 5 mg/dL; midabdomen, approximately 15 mg/dL; and the soles of the feet, approximately 20 mg/dL).

I. **Infants** should be assessed for risk factors for severe hyperbilirubinemia (Figure 38–1), sepsis, polycythemia, metabolic disorders, biliary obstruction.

V. **Laboratory Tests** (Figures 38–1 and 38–2). Most causes of jaundice can be determined by history, physical examination, and simple laboratory evaluation. (SOR **C**)

  A. **Basic tests.** All patients with jaundice should have a complete blood count and total and direct bilirubin levels measured.

   1. In **neonates** (Figure 38–1), Coombs' testing, peripheral smear, and reticulocyte count should also be done; ill or premature infants with jaundice should also have a sepsis workup (chest x-ray, urinalysis, blood/urine cultures).

   2. Liver function tests are recommended in all jaundiced **nonneonates** (Figure 38–2), with further testing based on clinical findings. (SOR **C**)

    a. **Liver profile**

     (1) In classic hepatocellular disease, **alkaline phosphatase** is ≤3 times the upper limit of normal; in obstructive jaundice, values are 3 to 10 times normal.

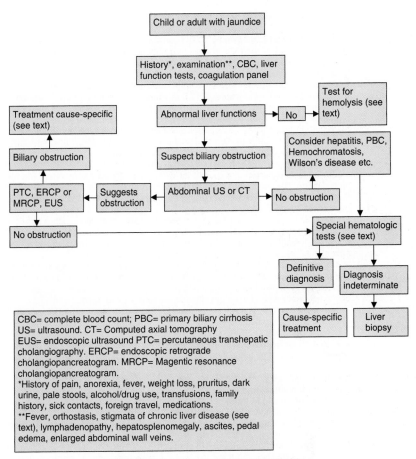

FIGURE 38–2. Evaluation of jaundice in children and adults.

    (2) Transaminase levels (alanine aminotransferase [ALT] and aspartate amino-
transferase [AST]) generally reflect the degree of hepatocellular disease. In
obstructive jaundice, transaminases are typically 2 to 3 times the upper limit
of normal, whereas higher values ($\geq$5 times normal) are seen in hepatocellular
disease.
  b. A peripheral smear, reticulocyte count, and **Coombs' testing** should be performed in all patients with unconjugated hyperbilirubinemia or anemia (checking for
hemolysis). Other features suggesting hemolysis include low serum haptoglobin,
urine hemosiderin, and hemoglobinuria.
  c. A prothrombin time (PT) should be done if obstruction or severe liver dysfunction
is suspected. In **obstructive** jaundice, a prolonged PT may respond dramatically
to 10 mg subcutaneous vitamin K, whereas minimal improvement is seen in hepatocellular disease.
  d. Urinalysis is inexpensive and detects **conjugated bilirubin and urobilinogen.**
B. Additional special testing (Figure 38–2).
  1. Imaging studies.
    a. In patients with extrahepatic obstruction, **ultrasonography (US)** detects dilated
biliary ducts. US is noninvasive and portable, over 90% specific, and, with

jaundice lasting over a week, is close to 90% sensitive in detecting obstruction.

Computerized tomography (CT) scan has greater specificity (93%–100%) and more resolution than US in detecting obstruction, but has similar sensitivity (63%–96%) and is more expensive. CT scan is indicated when US is unsatisfactory because of equivocal findings or technical limitations (e.g., overlying bowel gas).

b. **Endoscopic retrograde cholangiopancreatography (ERCP), percutaneous transhepatic cholangiography (PTC),** or **magnetic resonance cholangiopancreatography (MRCP)** is indicated if extrahepatic obstruction is strongly suspected on clinical grounds (even if US is negative) or if additional anatomic information is required for diagnosis. These tests permit direct imaging of bile ducts and visualization of the periampullary region. The choice of ERCP (sensitivity 89%–98%, specificity 89%–100% in evaluating jaundice) versus PTC (sensitivity 98%–100%, specificity 89%–100%) versus MRCP (sensitivity 84%–100%, specificity 94%–98%) depends mainly on local expertise and availability. ERCP is preferred if sphincterotomy, biliary stenting, pancreatic or CBD stone removal, or biopsy is planned. MRCP is the preferred test for evaluating anatomy because, unlike ERCP, it does not induce postprocedure pancreatitis.

c. Endoscopic ultrasound (EUS) also can detect biliary obstruction, with a sensitivity and specificity comparable with MRCP. EUS also permits biopsy of suspected malignant lesions, and may be combined with ERCP. EUS is most useful when the patient is felt to be at high risk for complications of ERCP or PTC.

d. Nuclear scintigraphy of the biliary tree using radiolabeled derivatives of iminodiacetic acid (e.g., HIDA) is useful in the diagnosis of cholecystitis. It is also useful in evaluating a potential bile leak following biliary surgery (accuracy 87%). Scintigraphy is not useful when the serum bilirubin exceeds 7 to 10 mg/dL.

If biliary obstruction is suspected, US or CT scan is the appropriate initial test. If dilated bile ducts are seen, then ERCP or PTC is followed by therapeutic intervention. If bile ducts are not dilated, and the likelihood of obstruction is low, the patient is evaluated for hepatocellular or cholestatic liver disease. If biliary obstruction is considered likely after a negative US or CT scan, MRCP or EUS is a reasonable next option.

2. **Hematologic testing**
   a. **Viral hepatitis studies**
      (1) **Immunoglobulin M (IgM) hepatitis A antibody** appears at the onset of symptoms of hepatitis A infection and clears within 6 months. The IgM hepatitis A antibody test should be used to confirm the disease in individuals with signs and symptoms suggestive of hepatitis A. (SOR **C**)
      (2) **Hepatitis B surface antigen (HBsAg)** is the first serologic marker to appear in hepatitis B infection, starting 2 to 6 weeks before symptoms. The antigen generally clears within 6 months, but persists in patients with chronic active or persistent infection.
      (3) **Hepatitis B core antibody (antiHBc)** is present in virtually all patients with active hepatitis B infection. AntiHBc appears later than HBsAg, often before symptoms develop, serves to confirm infection, and persists for life.
      (4) **Hepatitis C antibody** becomes detectable by **enzyme immunoassay (EIA)** in 90% of patients by 12 weeks after infection. Because of possible transplacental transmission of maternal antibodies, EIA testing in neonates at risk is not considered reliable until 12 weeks of age. Although EIA is $\geq$97% sensitive in detecting hepatitis C, it cannot differentiate between acute, chronic, or resolved infection and should be confirmed by **recombinant immunoblot assay (RIBA)** testing or a test for Hepatitis C RNA.
         (a) Negative EIA test or positive EIA coupled with negative RIBA rules out hepatitis C; an indeterminate RIBA should be followed with reverse transcriptase-polymerase chain reaction (RT-PCR) for hepatitis C RNA. (SOR **C**)
         (b) Indeterminate RIBA coupled with negative RT-PCR and normal ALT rules out hepatitis C. (SOR **C**)
      (5) **IgM antibody to Epstein-Barr virus and CMV** should also be considered in the appropriate clinical setting, although screening for hepatitis A and B should usually be done first.

    b. Antimitochondrial antibody to screen for PBC should be considered in patients aged 30 to 60 years (especially females) with an evidence of chronic cholestasis. Antibodies are positive in 85% to 90% of patients with PBC.

    c. Antinuclear and smooth muscle antibodies are positive in about one-third of patients with PBC and three-fourths of patients with lupoid hepatitis (autoimmune hepatitis) and should be considered in patients (especially females) who have chronic liver disease without a clearcut cause.

    d. Serum iron, transferrin saturation, and ferritin to screen for hemochromatosis should also be considered in patients with chronic liver disease of unknown cause. In hemochromatosis, the serum iron exceeds 200 U/dL, serum ferritin levels exceed 500 ng/mL, and transferrin saturation exceeds 70%.

    e. Serum protein electrophoresis is useful to screen for α_1-antitrypsin deficiency (decrease in α_1-globulin band).

    f. Serum ceruloplasmin and urine copper levels to screen for Wilson's disease should be considered in patients younger than 30 years of age or in patients with hepatitis and neurologic dysfunction.

    g. An elevated **serum secretory immunoglobulin A** is more reliable than alkaline phosphatase in differentiating mechanical from hepatocellular cholestasis.

    3. Liver biopsy may be useful in the following situations: (1) differentiating chronic active and chronic persistent hepatitis, (2) diagnosing liver malignancy, and (3) documenting or diagnosing hepatocellular disease when the diagnosis is not evident on clinical grounds. (SOR **C**)

VI. Treatment of jaundice is directed at its underlying cause, diagnosed through history, examination and appropriate selective laboratory, and imaging studies.

  A. Therapy for **neonatal jaundice** is directed at underlying causes and preventing kernicterus (unconjugated hyperbilirubinemia-induced neurotoxic basal ganglial/hippocampal damage). At least three factors determine the risk of kernicterus in neonatal hyperbilirubinemia: (1) **gestational age**—in healthy term neonates, risk is low even with markedly elevated total serum bilirubin (TSB), whereas lower levels are tolerated in premature infants; (2) **age at which jaundice is evident**—clinical jaundice at ≤24 hours of life is always nonphysiologic; and (3) **maternal/neonatal features of significant underlying disease.**

    1. With **physiologic jaundice,** which begins between the second and fourth days of life, TSB levels are ≤15 mg/dL, direct bilirubin is ≤1.5 mg/dL. TSB rises by ≤5 mg/dL in 24 hours and resolves by 1 week (in term infants) or by 2 weeks in preterm infants).

    2. Treatment of **breastfeeding jaundice,** which begins on or after the fourth day of life and peaks by day 10 to 15, is more frequent breastfeeding. (SOR **C**)

    3. Breast milk jaundice, beginning on the fourth through seventh day of life and lasting 3 to 10 weeks, can be treated by alternating breast and formula feeding for 2 to 3 days. (SOR **B**, **C**) Breast pumping should be done at formula feedings; full-time breastfeeding can be resumed when jaundice resolves.

    4. Stopping breastfeeding in jaundiced infants does not improve clinical outcomes. Temporarily disrupting or supplementing breastfeeding is associated with premature cessation of breastfeeding. (SOR **B**) There is no significant difference in length of phototherapy, rates of exchange transfusion, or kernicterus between jaundiced breastfed term infants and jaundiced bottle-fed term infants. (SOR **B**)

    5. Phototherapy using blue-range lights and biliblankets, which reflect the light, produce photoisomers of unconjugated bilirubin that are water soluble, and may be excreted in bile or urine without conjugation.

      a. Phototherapy should be considered at TSB ≥15 mg/dL at 25 to 48 hours of age, ≥18 mg/dL at 49 to 72 hours of age, or ≥20 mg/dL in infants over 72 hours of age. A favorable response is a decrease of 1 to 2 mg/dL within 4 to 6 hours, with subsequent continued decrease. Phototherapy may be administered in the hospital or home and discontinued once the TSB is 2 mg/dL below the threshold for initiation of therapy.

      b. The eyes of the neonate must be covered to prevent retinal damage when using bililights. Using biliblankets may allow earlier discharge. Adequate fluid intake also promotes the elimination of bilirubin and counteracts the dehydration associated with phototherapy.

    6. Exchange transfusion is traditionally performed when the TSB exceeds the threshold for phototherapy by 5 mg/dL or if phototherapy fails. (SOR **C**) This threshold should be lowered by 1 to 2 mg/dL when additional risk factors for kernicterus are present; such as perinatal asphyxia, respiratory distress, hypoglycemia, metabolic acidosis (pH $\leq$7.25), hypothermia (temperature, $\leq$ 35°C [95°F]), hypoproteinemia (protein, $\leq$5 g/dL), and signs of clinical or central nervous system deterioration.

7. **Neonates with hemolytic jaundice** (Rh or ABO incompatibilities) may be treated with high-dose intravenous immunoglobulins (IgG) to prevent anemia and hyperbilirubinemia that may develop. (SOR **B**) These infants should have hemoglobin, hematocrit, bilirubin levels, and features of hemolysis monitored serially.

B. **Viral hepatitis.** Most patients can be treated symptomatically as outpatients. Hospital admission is indicated in patients with dehydration, evidence of severe hepatocellular failure, or ascites.

1. If liver enzymes fail to normalize within 6 months, liver biopsy is indicated.

2. Alfa-interferon can induce sustained remissions in some patients with chronic hepatitis B, C, and D. (SOR **A**) Consultation should be sought with a gastroenterologist familiar with its use.

C. **Extrahepatic obstruction**

1. Surgical therapy is generally required.

2. If fever and chills suggestive of cholangitis develop, hospitalization for intravenous antibiotics and surgical consultation is necessary. Nonoperative biliary drainage may be performed in selected patients via ERCP or transhepatically placed stents.

D. **Unconjugated hyperbilirubinemia**

1. **Hemolytic anemia,** particularly if associated with marked hyperbilirubinemia, should be managed with appropriate specialty consultation (e.g., perinatology for neonates, hematology for others).

2. Mild, unconjugated hyperbilirubinemia (e.g., Gilbert's, Dubin-Johnson, Rotor's syndrome) rarely requires treatment to lower bilirubin levels.

E. **Cholestatic jaundice**

1. **Ursodeoxycholate** (usual dose, 13–15 mg/kg/d) significantly reduces ascites, jaundice, and improves liver biochemistry in cholestatic jaundice and is not associated with an increase in adverse events. (SOR **A**) There is marginal therapeutic benefit in PBC—no effect on disease progression, transplantation, or survival.

2. Since **pruritus** may be disabling for some patients, leading to depression and even suicide, early treatment is advisable. Oral agents used to treat pruritus include **cholestyramine** 4 to 6 grams, 30 minutes before meals, antihistamines (e.g., diphenhydramine, 25–50 mg, 3 or 4 times a day, hydroxyzine 25 mg 3 times daily), opioid antagonists such as nalmefene (60–120 mg po daily), and naltrexone (12.5–50 mg po daily), and rifampin (300–600 mg orally daily).

F. **Underlying diseases** contributing to jaundice should be treated (see Chapter 71, "Cirrhosis"; Chapter 72, "Congestive Heart Failure"; Chapter 87, "Thyroid Disease"; Chapter 50, "Pediatric Fever"); drugs contributing to jaundice should be eliminated or substituted.

G. **Other hepatocellular disease.** Periodic monitoring of patients is necessary with clinical examination and liver function tests (see Chapter 43). When the disease is progressive, liver biopsy may be indicated for definitive diagnosis.

REFERENCES

American Academy of Pediatrics Subcommittee on Hyperbilirubinemia. Management of hyperbilirubinemia in the newborn infant 35 or more weeks of gestation. *Pediatrics.* 2004;114:297-316.

Feldman M. *Sleisenger and Fordtran's Gastrointestinal and Liver Disease.* 8th ed. Saunders; 2006.

Goldman L. *Cecil Textbook of Medicine.* 22nd ed. Saunders; 2004.

Chowdhury NR, Chowdhury JR. Diagnostic approach to the patient with jaundice or asymptomatic hyperbilirubinemia. www.uptodate.com. Accessed May 25, 2007.

Roche SP, Kobos R. Jaundice in the adult patient. *Am Fam Physician.* 2004;69:299-304.

Bhutani VK, Johnson LH, Keren R. Diagnosis and management of hyperbilirubinemia in the term neonate: for a safer first week. *Pediatr Clin North Am.* 2004;51:843-861.

39   Joint Pain

L. Peter Schwiebert, MD

KEY POINTS

- In evaluating the complaint of joint pain, it is helpful to differentiate intra-articular from periarticular processes.
- A careful focused history, physical examination, and selective testing allow accurate diagnosis of most common causes of joint pain.
- Physicians should always consider bacterial arthritis in acute monarthritis, because delayed treatment of septic arthritis risks severe joint damage.

I. **Definition.** Joint pain (arthralgia) is discomfort in one or more joints, with or without an evidence of joint effusion, swelling, erythema, or tenderness. Joint pain can be because of **intra-articular** or **periarticular** processes. **Intra-articular** processes include **synovitis** (viral or bacterial infection, transient synovitis, gout/pseudogout, rheumatoid arthritis [RA], rheumatic fever [RF], idiopathic) or **degenerative disease** (osteoarthritis [OA], posttraumatic). **Periarticular processes** include **soft tissue diseases** (fibromyalgia, hypermobility syndromes, viremia, primary Lyme disease) and **idiopathic diseases** (growing pains, psychogenic rheumatism).

II. **Common Diagnoses.** Surveys reveal 11% of patients visiting general and family physicians in the United States have complaints related to the back and the upper or lower extremities. Unspecified arthritis is the 14th most common principal diagnosis seen by these physicians.

A. **Intra-articular processes**

1. **Synovitis**

a. **Bacterial/viral**

(1) **Transient synovitis** occurs in children 3- to 10-year-old, related to recent (within the past week) viral infection. Males are affected more frequently than females.

(2) **Viral synovitis** can occur with a variety of infections, especially hepatitis B, mumps, and rubella.

(3) Over 50% of adult **bacterial arthritis** is caused by *Neisseria gonorrhoeae;* risk factors include past history of gonorrheal infection, multiple sex partners, and nonuse of barrier contraceptives. Other causes of adult **bacterial arthritis** (*Staphylococcus aureus,* group A and B streptococci, gram-negative bacteria) tend to occur with immune compromise (diabetes mellitus, malignancy, human immunodeficiency virus disease); chronic liver disease; periarticular cellulitis or skin ulceration; intravenous drug use; or history of a damaged joint (e.g., with chronic severe RA). Ninety-six percent of bacterial arthritis in children younger than 6-year-old is caused by *Haemophilus influenzae;* children with sickle cell disease are at risk for infection with salmonella species.

b. **Crystal-induced**

(1) **Gouty arthritis,** intra-articular uric acid crystal deposition caused by enzyme deficiency/overproduction/underexcretion, occurs most commonly in men older than 40 years and postmenopausal women, especially with a positive family history of gout. Medications (e.g., thiazide diuretics, aspirin, niacin); myeloproliferative disorders; multiple myeloma; hypothyroidism; chronic renal disease; and alcohol ingestion are also associated with gouty attacks.

(2) **Pseudogout,** calcium pyrophosphate dihydrate deposition disease, most commonly occurs in those who are older than 60 years and can be associated with a variety of metabolic diseases (e.g., hyperparathyroidism, hypothyroidism, diabetes mellitus, Wilson's disease, gout).

c. **Immune-complex**

(1) **Rheumatoid arthritis (RA),** one of a family of autoimmune inflammatory disorders (including systemic lupus erythematosus [SLE], polymyalgia rheumatica, and polymyositis/dermatomyositis) mainly affects synovial membranes. One to

two percent of the US population has RA, with a female: male prevalence of 3:1 and usual age of onset between 20 and 40 years. A positive family history is a risk factor. Eighty-five percent of patients with SLE are women, blacks are affected 4 times as frequently as whites, and positive family history also plays a role. A variety of drugs can cause a lupus-like syndrome; the most common offenders include chlorpromazine, hydralazine, isoniazid, methyldopa, procainamide, and quinidine.

(2) Lyme disease, transmitted by a bite from a tick carrying the spirochete, *Borrelia burgdorferi,* can manifest as autoimmune synovitis in stage 3 (late) disease. Incidence of Lyme disease is highest in summer months, particularly in the Northeastern United States, Wisconsin, Minnesota, and California.

(3) Rheumatic fever (RF), caused by group A β-hemolytic streptococcal (GABHS)–induced immune complex synovitis, is rare ($\leq$1:10,000), and its over-all incidence is progressively declining. RF is most common in 5- to 15-year-old children, with slight male predominance.

2. Degenerative disease

   a. Osteoarthritis (OA) is the most common joint disease, affecting at least 20 million US adults; radiologic evidence of OA is present in weight-bearing joints of 90% of individuals by age 40. Age increases the likelihood of symptomatic disease.

   b. Traumatic arthritis is more likely with a history of recent or remote trauma to affected joint(s) (e.g., falls, motor vehicle accidents, sports injuries, and overuse).

B. Periarticular processes

  1. Soft tissue

    a. Viremia can occur at any age; in winter months in the Northern hemisphere, in-fluenza is commonly implicated.

    b. Joint Hypermobility Syndrome (JHS) is inherited in an autosomally dominant pattern, may be underdiagnosed, may be a common cause of widespread chronic pain and occurs 3 times as commonly in women as in men.

    c. Fibromyalgia is most common in 20- to 50-year-old women, affecting 3% to 10% of the general population; it may be associated with sleep disorders, depression, heightened perception of normal stimuli, and hypothyroidism.

  2. Idiopathic

    a. Growing pains occur in up to 18% of school-aged children, peaking at age 11 years and continuing through adolescence. This problem is more common in females than males and with a family history of similar symptoms.

    b. Psychogenic pain is more common with depression or school phobia (e.g., sepa-ration anxiety or overly dependent parent–child interaction).

III. Symptoms. A systematic history often assists in narrowing the joint pain differential diag-nosis; in addition to evaluating for risk factors, history includes:

A. Location/number of joints involved

  1. Monarticular arthralgia

    a. Septic arthritis typically affects the knee, but may involve the hip, wrist, shoulder, or ankle.

    b. Gout classically presents with first metatarsophalangeal (MTP) arthritis, though it also commonly involves the foot, ankle, or knee.

    c. Transient synovitis typically affects the hip.

    d. Lyme disease is typically monarticular, characteristically targeting the knee.

    e. OA affects large joints (e.g., knee, hip) and the first carpometacarpal (CMC) and distal interphalangeal (DIP) hand joints.

    f. Pseudogout also commonly affects large joints (e.g., knees, wrists) and may also affect metacarpophalangeals (MCPs), hips, shoulders, elbows, or ankles.

  2. Polyarticular arthralgia

    a. Viremia and **growing pains** cause polyarticular arthralgia.

    b. Rheumatologic/autoimmune diseases (e.g., RA) typically present with symmetri-cal multiple joint involvement, often of smaller, non-weight-bearing joints (e.g., hand proximal interphalangeals [PIPs], MCPs, wrists, toes, ankles).

    c. One criterion for **RF** is polyarticular involvement, especially ankles, knees, hips, wrists, elbows, and shoulders.

    d. JHS may be associated with acute or chronic pain, joint clicking, as well as history of dislocation/subluxation.

TABLE 39–1. JONES CRITERIA (MODIFIED) FOR DIAGNOSIS OF RHEUMATIC FEVER

Major Manifestations	Minor Manifestations	Supporting Evidence of Antecedent Group A Streptococcal Infection
Carditis	Clinical findings	Positive throat culture or rapid streptococcal antigen test
Polyarthritis	Arthralgia	Elevated or rising ASO or antiDNAse B titer
Chorea	Fever	
Erythema	Laboratory findings	
marginatum	Elevated acute phase reactants	
Subcutaneous	Erythrocyte sedimentation rate	
nodules	C-reactive protein	
	Prolonged PR interval on ECG	

If supported by evidence of preceding group A streptococcal infection, the presence of two major manifestations or one major and two minor manifestations indicates a high probability of acute rheumatic fever.
ASO, antistreptolysin-O; ECG, electrocardiogram.

B. Chronology
1. The pain of **trauma, gout, pseudogout,** and **septic arthritis** is typically an **acute** onset.
2. Arthralgias associated with growing pains, fibromyalgia, hypermobility, OA, and collagen diseases (e.g., RA) tend to follow an **insidious/chronic/recurrent** pattern.

C. Exacerbating/alleviating factors
1. Osteoarthritis, traumatic arthritis, overuse injuries, and growing pains tend to **worsen with activity.**
2. **Psychogenic pain** associated with school phobia worsens before school and improves on weekends.
3. **Nocturnal worsening** is associated with growing pains; an **acute gout attack** may begin at night.

D. Associated symptoms
1. Complaint of a **red, very tender joint** and feverishness/chills are associated with septic arthritis, gout, and RF.
2. **Stiffness** following immobilization is associated with **osteoarthritis** and **autoimmune arthritis** (e.g., RA); OA stiffness ("gelling") typically abates within 15 minutes of activity, whereas RA stiffness persists at least an hour.
3. Depending on specific underlying disease, **autoimmune arthritis** may be associated with rashes (e.g., butterfly malar rash, sun sensitivity, alopecia, or discoid lesions with SLE).
4. **RF** may be associated with a macular, circinate erythematous truncal rash; Sydenham's chorea (choreoathetoid facial, tongue, or upper extremity movements); and subcutaneous nodules of tendon sheaths (especially in children) (see Table 39–1).
5. **Psychogenic arthralgia** may be associated with symptoms of anxiety, depression, or other psychiatric disease.
6. **Fibromyalgia** frequently is associated with fatigue, sleep disorders, chronic headaches, and irritable bowel symptoms.

IV. Signs. A careful, focused physical examination is crucial in differentiating articular from periarticular processes and, together with symptoms and risk factors, guides testing strategies.
A. Vital signs/general appearance
1. **Fever** is associated with septic arthritis, viral arthralgias, gout, and RF.
2. **Ill or toxic appearance** (or both) raises suspicion of septic arthritis.
3. **Integument/mucous membranes**
   a. **Erythema migrans (EM)** occurs in 90% of patients with early Lyme disease 3 to 30 days following a tick bite. EM begins as a red papule at the site of the bite, enlarging circumferentially over days to a month with central clearing and typical resolution over 3 to 4 weeks.
   b. A generalized evanescent, pinkish maculopapular exanthem makes **viremia** a likely cause of arthralgias.
   c. **SLE** lesions include malar erythema ("butterfly rash,") discoid macular plaquelike lesions, alopecia, or oral ulcers.

B. Joint findings. Intra-articular processes have abnormal findings of affected joints, ranging from heat/erythema, to firm or boggy swelling, to synovial or joint line tenderness, to restricted range of motion (ROM). In **periarticular processes,** by contrast, the joint examination is often normal or minimally abnormal.

1. **Intra-articular processes**
   a. In **transient synovitis,** there is decreased hip ROM, especially internal rotation.
   b. **Bacterial synovitis/septic joint** presents dramatically with a warm/erythematous joint, joint effusion, and restricted ROM.
   c. **Viral synovitis** may show tenderness and synovial involvement, but no deformity.
   d. **Gouty arthritis** presents with swollen, red, tender-to-the touch joint or less dramatically with swollen joint, restricted ROM, and painful weight-bearing. Following multiple attacks, tophaceous invasion may grossly deform affected joints.
   e. **Pseudogout** shows less dramatic inflammation than gout; one may note firm hypertrophy caused by chronic chondrocalcinosis.
   f. **OA** findings typically include crepitus, tender joint line, firm swelling (bony hypertrophy and osteophytes, rather than synovitis), and restricted extremes of ROM.
   g. **Traumatic arthritis** findings are similar to OA; there may be deformity at the site of previous trauma or surgery.
   h. **RA** findings include symmetric, swollen, warm, tender boggy joints; chronic active disease produces deformities, including ulnar deviation of digits, and boutonnière/"swan-neck" digit deformities. The clinical examination is considered the gold standard in diagnosis of synovitis. (SOR **Ⓒ**)
   i. A tender joint, with or without synovitis, occurs with stage 3 **Lyme disease** (late persistent infection).
   j. **RF** may produce tender joints/synovium (large joints); RF may be monarticular in adults.

2. **Periarticular**
   a. Five criteria establish a diagnosis of **JHS;** these include (1) passive opposition of thumb to flexor forearm, (2) passive finger hyperextension parallel to forearm, (3) elbow hyperextension, (4) knee hyperextension, and (5) palms on floor with knees extended. Joint hypermobility may involve only one joint and be associated with stretchability, stretch marks, and paper thin scars.
   b. **Fibromyalgia** is diagnosed by reproducing ≥11 of 18 mainly axial designated tender sites (occiputs, supraspinati, glutei, greater trochanters, upper trapezius borders, anterior cervical 5–7 interspaces, second anterior rib lateral to the costochondral junction, lateral epicondyles, and medial fat pads of knees).
   c. There are no characteristic articular or periarticular findings with **growing pains** or **psychogenic arthralgias.**

V. **Laboratory Tests** (Figure 39–1) can be selective and based on careful history and focused physical examination as described. Because some diagnoses become apparent only over time, serial evaluation and testing may be necessary to arrive at a correct diagnosis. No further testing is necessary if hypermobility syndrome is suspected or for findings consistent with growing pains in absence of articular inflammation. If joint effusion is present and diagnosis is uncertain, or if septic arthritis is suspected, arthrocentesis is indicated (Table 39–2).

A. **Hematologic tests**
   1. In **acute RF,** erythrocyte sedimentation rate (ESR) and antistreptolysin-O (ASO) are elevated, though these are normal in 10% of patients with other findings compatible with RF.
   2. In 75% of patients with **RA, rheumatoid factor** is positive; false-positive results occur with syphilis, sarcoidosis, endocarditis, advanced age, or asymptomatic relatives of patients with autoimmune diseases. Twenty percent of **RA patients** have a positive antinuclear antibody (ANA) test. The minimum laboratory panel in suspected RA includes a complete blood count (CBC), urinalysis (UA), ANA, and transaminases. (SOR **Ⓒ**)
   3. Hematologic abnormalities associated with **SLE** include positive ANA (in 95%–100%), antinative DNA (in 50%), antismooth muscle (in 20%), anemia (in 60%), leukopenia (in 45%), and thrombocytopenia (in 30%).
   4. In acute **gouty** attack, uric level is increased (≥7.5 mg/dL) at some point during the attack, though a single level is normal in up to 25% of acute gouty patients. Commonly, the white blood cell count and ESR are elevated during an acute gouty attack.

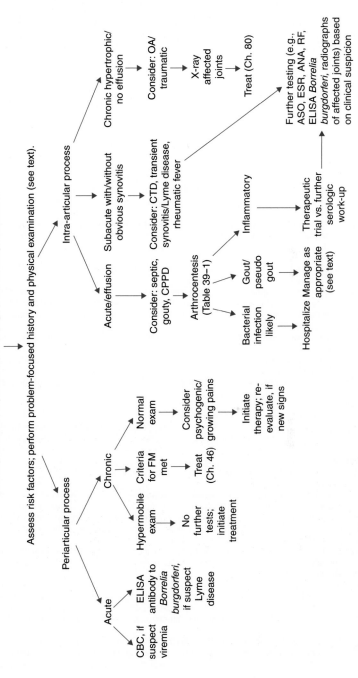

FIGURE 39–1. Approach to evaluating the patient with joint pain. ANA, antinuclear antibody; ASO, antistreptolysin-O; CBC, complete blood count; CPDD, calcium pyrophosphate deposition disease; CTD, connective tissue disease; ELISA, enzyme-linked immunosorbent assay; ESR, erythrocyte sedimentation rate; FM, fibromyalgia; OA, osteoarthritis; RF, rheumatoid factor.

TABLE 39–2. JOINT FLUID FINDINGS

	Normal	Trauma	Infection	Crystalline Disease	Inflammatory
Color	Clear to yellow	Bloody to xanthrochromic	Yellow to cloudy	Yellow to cloudy	Yellow to cloudy
Cell count (cells/μL) WBC/RBC	≤ 200/0	≤ 1000/many	1000–200,000/few	1000–2000/few	1000–20,000/few
Crystals	Negative	Negative	Negative	Yes; pseudogout and gout	Negative
Culture	Negative	Negative	Positive	Negative	Negative

RBC, red blood cell count; WBC, white blood cell count.

5. In **Lyme disease** up to 50% of patients can be enzyme-linked immunosorbent assay (ELISA)-antibody negative during the first several weeks of illness. Repeat titers should be obtained in these cases; a fourfold rise in titer is diagnostic of recent infection. All positive or equivocal ELISA *B burgdorferi* tests should be confirmed with Western immunoblot testing.

B. **Joint fluid examination** (Table 39–2). **Gouty arthritis** is definitively diagnosed by finding urate crystals (needlelike, negatively birefringent); pseudogout crystals are rhomboid-shaped.

C. **Radiology**

1. In **OA,** plain radiographs show joint space narrowing and irregularity, periarticular spurring, and juxta-articular sclerosis.

2. In **RA,** no radiographic abnormalities may be evident during the first 6 months of disease. The earliest changes are evident in the wrists and feet and include soft tissue swelling and juxta-articular demineralization. Later changes include joint space narrowing and periarticular erosions.

3. **Pseudogout** manifests with changes similar to those in OA, along with cartilage calcification.

4. In **transient synovitis,** soft tissue periarticular swelling may be evident, but is a nonspecific finding.

5. In **RF,** one manifestation of carditis may be cardiomegaly and other signs of congestive heart failure on plain chest radiographs.

D. **Other testing**

1. Proteinuria occurs in 30% of **SLE** patients.

2. Electrocardiography (ECG) in RF may reveal increased P-R interval; **echocardiography** may confirm valvular disease or dilated cardiomyopathy with decreased ejection fraction.

VI. **Treatment** is directed at the underlying cause of joint pain, which can accurately be arrived at via appropriate history, focused examination, and selective testing.

A. **Intra-articular diseases**

1. **Transient synovitis** usually resolves on its own over a few days. Bed rest, traction with slight hip flexion, with or without age-appropriate oral nonsteroidal anti-inflammatory drugs (NSAIDs) may increase comfort. Follow-up plain hip radiographs at 1 and 3 months can detect avascular femoral head necrosis, a possible complication of transient synovitis.

2. **Septic arthritis** requires treatment with systemic antibiotics and possible orthopedic consultation, which should occur in a hospital setting.

3. **Gouty arthritis**

a. **Acute attack**

(1) **NSAIDs** (e.g., oral indomethacin, 25–50 mg every 8 hours for 5–10 days or until symptoms are controlled) showed benefit in open label clinical trials but comorbidities (e.g. ethanol use, chronic renal insufficiency, heart disease) may increase their risk.

(2) Alternately, **colchicine** (0.5–0.6 mg orally hourly until symptoms are controlled or diarrhea develops, with maximum of 8 mg) showed significant benefit at 48 hours versus placebo but is limited by gastrointestinal (GI) toxicity. GI symptoms

can be limited using intravenous colchicine, 2 mg in 25 to 50 mL normal saline, with additional 1-mg doses every 6 hours for 2 doses (maximum: 4 mg total). Colchicine should not be used in those with hepatic and renal impairment.

(3) **Intra-articular steroids** (e.g., 10–40 mg of triamcinolone) can be effective for monarticular gout; an oral steroid (e.g., prednisone, 40–60 mg initially and tapered over 7 days) may be effective for polyarticular acute gout.

(4) **Analgesics** (other than aspirin, which may precipitate gout) may be necessary for pain control.

(5) **Bed rest** during the acute attack is also helpful.

b. **Chronic management**

(1) **Patient education**

(a) Patients should be advised to avoid or limit their intake of high-purine foods, including meats, seafood, meat extracts and gravies, yeast and yeast extracts, alcoholic beverages, beans, peas, lentils, oatmeal, spinach, asparagus, cauliflower, and mushrooms.

(b) The following medications can precipitate gouty attacks and should be avoided: thiazide and loop diuretics, low-dose aspirin ($\leq$3 g/d), and niacin.

(2) The decision to initiate **preventive medication** depends on the individual's risk of recurrent gouty arthritis; for example, an individual who had a single attack and is willing to avoid alcohol and lose weight is low risk, while an older individual with multiple attacks, mild chronic renal insufficiency, or requiring a diuretic is considered high risk. One guideline for initiating prophylaxis is to consider it in those with two or more acute gouty flares/year, presence of progressive tophi, or radiographic changes consistent with gout. Once initiated, the target urate level is less than 6 mg/dL. (SOR **A**)

(a) **Oral colchicine,** 0.6 mg twice daily, may be effective prophylaxis in individuals with mild hyperuricemia and few acute attacks; there is a 10% to 100% risk of an acute gouty flare in the first 1 to 3 days of prophylaxis, and colchicine therapy during the first 3 months of prophylaxis decreases this risk.

(b) **The** choice of urate lowering therapy is guided by results of a 24-hour urine collection for uric acid (if $\leq$800 mg/24 h, a uricosuric should be used; if $\geq$800 mg/ 24 h, allopurinol should be used).

(i) **Uricosurics,** which block tubular reabsorption of urate, include oral probenecid, 500 mg initially with gradual increase to 1 to 2 g, or **sulfinpyrazone,** 50 to 100 mg twice daily, increasing as needed to 200 to 400 mg twice daily. Ninety-six percent of those receiving therapeutic doses of uricosurics experienced improvement in pain. Uricosurics should not be used in patients with chronic renal failure (serum creatinine $\geq$2 mg/dL), and patients should consume sufficient fluids to assure at least 2 L urine output daily.

(ii) **Allopurinol,** a xanthine oxidase inhibitor that lowers plasma urate concentrations and can mobilize tophi, is indicated in those with tophi and those who overproduce uric acid, who have failed uricosuric therapy, or who have a history of renal urate stones. Dosing should begin at 100 mg orally daily for the first week, with dose increases depending on serum uric acid response. Most people require 200 to 300 mg/d. Seventy-five percent of those treated with allopurinol for more than 4 months had no further gouty flares. With tophaceous gout, the goal is to maintain uric acid at $\leq$5 mg/dL, and this may require combined allopurinol and uricosuric therapy.

(3) **Prognosis** depends on age at first attack and number of attacks; destructive arthropathy is rare in those having their first attack after age 50.

4. **Pseudogout** treatment is directed at underlying disease. Acute symptoms may be helped with oral NSAIDs, oral colchicine (0.6 mg twice daily may benefit prophylaxis), and joint aspiration followed by intra-articular steroid injection (e.g., triamcinolone, 10–40 mg, depending on joint size), as with monarticular gout.

5. **RA,** like other autoimmune diseases, follows a variable course, with prognosis depending on disease severity; severe disease demands early aggressive treatment with disease-modifying antirheumatic drugs (DMARDs). A recent recommendation is that

RA patients with swelling, pain, or stiffness of more that one joint should be referred to a rheumatologist within 6 weeks of disease onset. (SOR **Ⓑ**)

a. **Supportive therapy**
   (1) Patients should be educated about the disease, its variable course, and their role in self-monitoring and management.
   (2) **Rest** in bed is important for a severe disease flare; 2 hours' rest per day is sufficient for milder inflammation. Activity should be liberalized as tolerated by symptoms.
   (3) **Exercise** depends on disease activity and should start with passive ROM/ hydrotherapy when pain or stiffness is worse, progressing to active then resisted ROM as symptoms abate. Joint stretching may help prevent contractures. Activities producing pain for greater than an hour after activity should be avoided.
   (4) Heat, cold therapy, and assistive devices can also control symptoms and improve quality of life.

b. Response to **medications** can be gauged, based on the patient's stiffness, fatigue, and degree of joint swelling.
   (1) **NSAIDs** (e.g., oral ibuprofen, 600–800 mg, 3–4 times daily, or naproxen, 550 mg twice daily) are first-line anti-inflammatory/analgesic therapy; therapy should be carefully monitored for GI toxicity.
   (2) Poor response to NSAIDs warrants consideration of DMARDs (e.g., methotrexate, gold, tumor necrosis factor inhibitors) and possible rheumatology consultation for drug selection and monitoring.

6. **Lyme disease/EM** (see Chapter 7).
7. **RF**
   a. **Bed rest** is indicated until the patient is afebrile without antipyretics and has a normal pulse rate, ESR, and electrocardiogram.
   b. **Acute medications**
      (1) **Salicylates** (e.g., oral aspirin, 600–900 mg every 4 hours in adults) can markedly improve fever and joint symptoms.
      (2) An **oral steroid** (e.g., prednisone, 40–60 mg, initially and tapered over 7 days) may relieve joint symptoms poorly controlled by salicylates.
      (3) **Benzathine penicillin,** 1.2 million units intramuscularly (IM) in a single dose, or **procaine penicillin,** 600,000 units IM daily for 10 days, will eradicate streptococcal infection in nonallergic patients.
   c. Benzathine penicillin (600,000U IM every 3–4 weeks for those less than 30 kg or 1.2 million U IM every 3–4 weeks for those more than 30 kg) prophylaxis is indicated in those with RF.
      (1) In those without carditis, prophylaxis should be continued until 5 years have elapsed since the last attack or 18 years of age, whichever is longer.
      (2) With a history of carditis, propylaxis should be continued until 10 years after the last attack or age 25 (whichever is longer) for mild mitral regurgitation or lifelong in presence of severe valvular heart disease or following valvular surgery for rheumatic heart disease.

8. **Traumatic arthritis/OA** (see Chapter 80).

B. **Periarticular diseases**
   1. **Viremia-induced arthralgias** should be treated symptomatically and supportively (see Chapter 55).
   2. **JHS** affects quality of life, in that it may be associated with dislocations, osteoarthritis, and osteonecrosis; those with hypermobility may benefit from graded conditioning to provide muscle support of affected joints.
   3. **Fibromyalgia** (see Chapter 46).
   4. Treatment of **growing pains** involves reassurance, symptomatic analgesics, and instructions to follow up, if the symptom pattern worsens.
   5. In **psychogenic arthralgia,** underlying stress or abnormal family dynamics should be identified and treated.

REFERENCES

Bykerk VP, Keystone EC. What are the goals and principles of management in the early treatment of rheumatoid arthritis? *Best Pract Res Clin Rheumatol.* 2005;19:147.

Lane S, Gravel JW. Clinical utility of common serum rheumatologic tests. *Am Fam Physician.* 2002;65:1073.

Mikuls TR, Saag KG. Gout treatment: What is evidence-based and how do we determine and promote optimized clinical care? *Curr Rheum Reports.* 2005;7:242.

Richie AM, Francis ML. Diagnostic approach to polyarticular joint pain. *Am Fam Physician.* 2003;68:1151.

Siva C, et al. Diagnosis of acute monarthritis in adults: a practical approach for the family physician. *Am Fam Physician.* 2003;68:83.

WHO Technical Report Series. Rheumatic Fever and Rheumatic Heart Disease. World Health Organization. 2004.

40   Knee Complaints

Mitchell A. Kaminski, MD, MBA

KEY POINTS

- A working diagnosis is formed using a careful history of the complaint coupled with knowledge of knee anatomy and a focused physical examination.
- Reliable evidence about the accuracy of physical diagnostic tests in diagnosing the cause of acute knee pain is scarce but is being accumulated.
- Evidence-based application of tests (x-ray, magnetic resonance imaging, blood work, and joint aspiration) can cost-effectively enhance diagnosis.
- Knowledge of when to refer to an orthopedist is critical in acute injuries. Medication and an appropriate exercise program benefit the patient with chronic complaints.

I. **Definition.** The knee is a complex, weight-bearing hinge joint comprising ligaments, cartilage, bone, and bursae (Figures 40–1 and 40–2). Knee complaints can be **acute,** most often reflecting medial or lateral external force (collateral ligament tears), excessive anterior or posterior forces with torsion (cruciate ligament injuries), or direct trauma (fractures). Immediate pain and swelling suggest hemarthrosis and more serious injury. **Chronic complaints** reflect overuse, inflammation such as friction between the iliotibial band and the lateral femoral condyle (iliotibial band syndrome) (or both); patellofemoral tracking abnormalities (patellofemoral arthralgia, chondromalacia, and subluxation); or traction trauma (of the calcifying tibial apophysis in Osgood–Schlatter disease, or of the distal pole of the patella in Sinding–Larsen–Johansson syndrome). **Bursitis** results from acute bursal contusion (prepatellar or superficial infrapatellar), overuse (deep infrapatellar or anserine bursa), or intra-articular inflammation (Baker cyst.) The symptoms of **rheumatoid arthritis and osteoarthritis** are chronic, unlike the arthritis of **gout** or **pseudogout,** which flares acutely.

II. **Common Diagnoses.** The knee joint is a frequent source of complaints in primary care practice. Up to 5% of physician visits are related to knee pain. More than one million visits to US emergency departments occur owing to knee trauma, while approximately 11% of patients aged 65 and older have symptomatic osteoarthritis of the knee.

   A. **Acute ligamentous** (collateral, cruciate, or iliotibial band) **and cartilaginous (meniscal) injuries** are more likely in young and active patients. Collateral and cruciate ligament injuries are more common in sports involving contact or torsion of the lower extremity (e.g., football, soccer, and skiing). The medial collateral ligament is more often injured. Cruciate ligament tears are often accompanied by other injuries owing to the severe trauma involved.

   B. **Patellofemoral dysfunction** is an overuse syndrome occurring most often in jumping sports (e.g., basketball). It is most frequent in tall, adolescent females with an abnormal "Q" angle (Figure 40–3). Abnormal patellar tracking in the femoral condylar groove with chronic stresses, recurrent dislocation, or both leads to degeneration of the patellar cartilage (chondromalacia patellae).

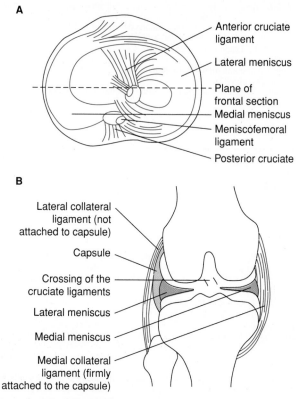

FIGURE 40–1. Relationship between the menisci, the capsule, and the ligaments of the knee. (A) A superior view of the menisci and cruciate ligaments. (B) A posterior view of a frontal section of the knee through the middle third. (Modified with permission from Steinberg GG, Akins CM, Baran DT, et al., eds. *Ramamurti's Orthopaedics in Primary Care.* 3rd ed. Lippincott Williams & Wilkins; 1999.)

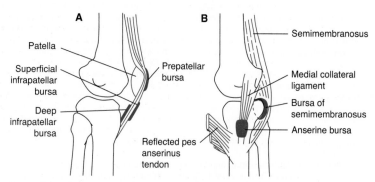

FIGURE 40–2. Bursae about the knee. (A) The lateral view. (B) The medial view. (Modified with permission from Steinberg GG, Akins CM, Baran DT, et al., eds. *Ramamurti's Orthopaedics in Primary Care.* 3rd ed. Lippincott Williams & Wilkins; 1999.)

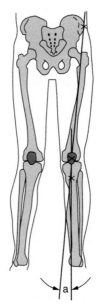

FIGURE 40–3. "Q" angle. A normal "Q" angle is ≤14–15 degrees.

C. The **iliotibial band syndrome** occurs most frequently in runners and can be precipitated by a change in footwear, an increase in a running schedule, or prolonged downhill running.

D. **Bursitis** (prepatellar, infrapatellar, or anserine; Baker cyst) can reflect acute or chronic injury.

E. **Fractures** of the patella or femoral condyles follow acute trauma; compressive, rotational, or lateral stresses can result in tibial plateau fracture. Bone that is pathologically weaker (e.g., osteoporosis) than ligaments will fracture before the ligaments will tear. Distal femoral Salter type I fractures in adolescents may initially mask as a "ligament tear."

F. **Osgood–Schlatter disease** (traumatic apophysitis of the tibial tubercle) and **osteochondritis dissecans** occur in adolescents. Osgood–Schlatter disease is more common in males than females; the additional risk factors for osteochondritis dissecans are unknown.

G. **Arthritis** (rheumatoid or osteoarthritis, gout, or pseudogout) often underlies chronic knee complaints; increasing patient age makes those disorders more likely. Arthritis of the knee is associated with obesity and repetitive trauma, both occupational and recreational. Illnesses such as diabetes mellitus, sickle cell anemia, and recurrent infections often underlie septic arthritis. (See also Chapters 39 and 80.)

H. **Pain referred from the hip** should be considered especially in pediatric patients, and in older patients at risk for metastatic disease and fracture of the hip (Chapter 42).

III. **Symptoms.** In approaching the patient with knee complaints, taking a careful history is a key component to narrow the differential diagnosis. The history should include the mechanism of injury, precipitating factors, or both; chronology; location of symptoms; and exacerbating and alleviating factors. The site of pain and swelling often helps localize the abnormality. Some symptoms are suggestive of specific disorders.

A. **Pain**

1. **Mild pain** over the lateral side of the knee suggests iliotibial band syndrome or collateral ligament strain. **Moderate to severe pain** usually occurs with fractures.

2. **Localized pain** and **effusion** occur with incomplete disruption of ligaments. **Diffuse pain,** especially with climbing stairs or getting up from a squatting position, is a hallmark of chondromalacia patellae.

3. **Pain with weight bearing** often occurs with meniscal tears and with osteochondritis dissecans. Inability to bear weight is common with fractures.

4. **Pain with resisted knee extension** (e.g., from running, climbing, jumping, or kicking) occurs with Osgood–Schlatter disease, Sinding–Larsen–Johansson syndrome, and chondromalacia patellae.

5. **Aching pain** in the knee, even at rest, may indicate osteochondritis dissecans. Knee pain from rheumatoid arthritis is worse after inactivity, while activity tends to precipitate pain in osteoarthritis.

6. **Pain limited to the knee** is common with septic arthritis. Knee pain referred from the hip may be the only symptom of hip disease.

B. Mechanical symptoms

1. A "pop" followed by knee instability may occur with complete ligament disruption, particularly of the cruciate ligaments, and with patellar or quadriceps tendon rupture.

2. **"Locking"** or **"giveway"** suggests a bucket handle meniscal tear.

3. A loose joint body may cause **locking or restricted range of motion** in advanced cases of osteochondritis dissecans.

C. Swelling

1. **Rapid swelling** is usual with hemarthrosis.

2. **Swelling behind the knee** with variable to no pain is seen with Baker cyst.

3. **Swelling with pain over the tibial tubercle** is seen with Osgood–Schlatter disease. **Swelling and pain over the respective bursa** is seen in prepatellar, infrapatellar, and anserine bursitis (Figure 40–2).

4. **Joint swelling** is more common with rheumatoid arthritis than with osteoarthritis (see Chapter 80).

D. Stiffness

1. A patient may feel "**something out of place**" and be unable to flex or extend the knee with patellar dislocation.

2. **Stiffness that is worse after inactivity** is common with rheumatoid arthritis.

E. A **limp** may be noticed in patients who have knee pain referred from the hip.

F. Systemic symptoms

1. Rheumatoid arthritis is accompanied by systemic symptoms more often than is osteoarthritis.

2. **Fever and chills** are common with septic arthritis.

IV. **Signs.** A careful history combined with a systematic knee examination leads to a more accurate diagnosis. (SOR Ⓒ) Examination after a severe, acute injury is often limited by pain and swelling and may require orthopedic referral for examination under anesthesia. Knee examination involves **inspection, palpation, and special maneuvers.**

A. **Inspection. Tense effusion** is seen in patellar fracture, and a tense, hot effusion is common with septic arthritis. Varying amounts of joint effusion are seen with rheumatoid arthritis, osteoarthritis, and the arthritis of gout and pseudogout. **Shortening** and **deformity** may occur with femoral condylar fractures and to varying degrees with rheumatoid arthritis, osteoarthritis, and the arthritis of gout and pseudogout. **Patella alta** (high position) or **patella baja** (low position) are seen with knee flexion in patellar tendon or quadriceps tendon rupture, respectively. **Erythema** may appear in patients with femoral condylar fractures, and it is present to varying degrees in patients with rheumatoid arthritis, osteoarthritis, and the arthritis of gout and pseudogout. **Hemarthrosis** may occur with femoral condylar fractures.

B. **Palpation.** Localization of tenderness by palpation provides diagnostic clues (Figure 40–4). **Localized swelling and tenderness** over the affected bursa will be found in bursitis. Tenderness is also common with femoral condylar fractures. Hip or groin tenderness and pain with rocking of the hip are the primary clues to knee pain referred from the hip. **Crepitance** is palpable with patellar fracture.

C. **Special maneuvers.** Special maneuvers (Table 40–1) may reveal signs of ligamentous or meniscal injury or patellar instability. **Limitation in range of motion** is common with septic arthritis, effusion, and muscle spasm. Irritation with range-of-motion testing and possibly a restriction of range of motion caused by a loose body are seen with osteochondritis dissecans and meniscal tear. **Neural compromise** (altered sensation or loss of motor ability) and **vascular compromise** (loss of peripheral pulse) may occur with femoral condylar fractures. **Increased pain with compression** of the affected side of the joint occurs with tibial plateau fractures.

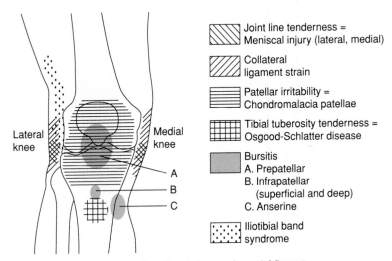

FIGURE 40–4. Sites of knee tenderness and suggested diagnoses.

V. **Laboratory Tests.** In most patients, a careful history and focused examination will allow for accurate diagnosis without additional testing. Additional studies can be ordered if a diagnosis is in doubt, or if findings will affect decisions on additional surgical or medical treatment.
   A. **Imaging studies**
      1. **Plain radiographs** should be ordered whenever the severity of injury or physical signs suggests a fracture. The Ottawa knee rule (Figure 40–5) is a highly validated, sensitive, and specific guideline for accurately determining the need for x-ray in acute knee injury. (SOR **A**)

TABLE 40–1. **SPECIAL MANEUVERS IN THE KNEE EXAMINATION**

Test	Method	Significance	SOR
McMurray	Extend axially compressed knee with internal tibial rotation and then with external tibial rotation	Locking or popping suggests meniscal injury	**C**
Lachman maneuver	With knee flexed 20 degrees and femur supported, pull tibia anteriorly	Step-up from lower patella to tibial tuberosity indicates anterior cruciate ligament instability	**A**
Pivot shift tests	Patient lateral decubitus position: extend knee, internally rotate tibia, apply valgus stress and flex knee	Clunk felt at 30 degrees flexion suggests anterior cruciate ligament rupture	**B**
Collateral ligament stressing	Valgus stress of knee in full knee extension then 30-degree flexion	Laxity with full extension suggests collateral and cruciate ligament injury. Laxity only at 30-degree flexion suggests collateral ligament tear	**C**
Apprehension sign	Valgus varus stress on patella with quadriceps relaxed, knee extended	Extreme guarding suggests patellar subluxation	**C**
Patellar irritability	Compress patella against femoral condyles	Tenderness indicates chondromalacia patellae	**C**
Thigh circumference measurement	Measure thigh circumference at an equal distance above both midpatellae	Decreased circumference of thigh above affected knee suggests subacute or chronic disorder with quadriceps atrophy	**C**

A knee x-ray series is only required for knee injury patients with any of these findings:
1. Age 55 years or older
   or
2. Isolated tenderness of patella*
   or
3. Tenderness at head of fibula
   or
4. Inability to flex to 90 degrees
   or
5. Inability to bear weight both immediately and in the emergency department (4 steps)†

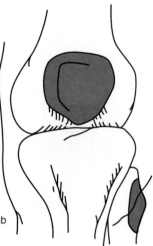

* No bone tenderness of knee other than patella.
†Unable to transfer weight twice onto each lower limb regardless of limping.

FIGURE 40–5. The Ottawa knee rule for the use of radiography in acute knee injuries. (Reproduced with permission from Stiell IG, Wells GA, McKnight, et al. Validity of the "real" Ottawa knee rule. *Ann Emerg Med.* 1999;33(2):241.)

   a. **Anteroposterior, lateral,** and **30-degree sunrise views** are standard.
   b. **A lateral x-ray of the tibial tubercle** will show fragmentation of the apophysis of the tibial tubercle in Osgood–Schlatter disease, but is usually not required.
   c. The **intercondylar notch or tunnel x-ray** view is helpful in searching for loose bodies, such as those that may be found in osteochondritis dissecans.
2. **Magnetic resonance imaging (MRI)** is generally used ahead of diagnostic arthroscopy. It is useful when the diagnosis of acute meniscal care or ACL tear is difficult. MRI may also be useful in assessing bone pathology underlying atypical or chronic knee pain. (SOR **C**)
3. **Arthrography** or MRI definitively diagnose a **Baker cyst.**
B. **Aspiration of effusion** may be done for diagnostic purposes; aspiration of a painful, tense effusion should be performed for pain relief. (SOR **C**) Aspiration of a suspected hemarthrosis is not indicated for diagnosis alone. (SOR **C**)
   1. The anterior knee is prepared with Betadine and covered with a sterile drape. A small area just medial or lateral to the patella is anesthetized with intradermal 1% Xylocaine hydrochloride. A large-bore (16- or 18-gauge) needle is inserted through the anesthetized area, and the syringe plunger is withdrawn until fluid is obtained. Bloody fluid should be sent to the laboratory in a heparinized test tube if cell counts are desired. The aspiration site is then covered with an adhesive bandage or similar dressing.
   2. See Chapter 39 for information on joint fluid analysis.
   C. See Chapter 39 for the laboratory evaluation of arthritis.
VI. **Treatment.** Focused history/examination and testing should differentiate those patients likely to improve with conservative care from those in whom urgent or eventual orthopedic referral is likely. Indications for orthopedic referral are included in Table 40–2. For mild soft-tissue injuries, there is insufficient evidence in the literature to support the traditional use of **RICE** (**R**est, **I**ce, **C**ompression, and **E**levation); however, it is commonly accepted practice for the self-management of a mild soft tissue knee injury in the first 48 to 72 hours. (SOR **C**) There is considerable debate about the efficacy of knee bracing, and insufficient evidence exists at this point to recommend for or against bracing. (SOR **I**)
A. **Ligamentous and cartilaginous injuries**
   1. **Collateral and cruciate injuries** with little or no laxity on testing should be managed as follows.
      a. **Immobilization** is accomplished with a compression dressing (cotton batting wrap with firm Ace wrap application), knee immobilizer (Velcro or strap type with lateral

TABLE 40–2. INDICATIONS FOR ORTHOPEDIC REFERRAL (SOR)

Urgent referral
Red flag signs and symptoms
  Neurovascular damage
  Extensor mechanism rupture
  Infection
  Bleeding disorder
  Possibility of cancer
Severe knee injury
Significant fracture on x-ray

Early referral
Injury to the anterior cruciate ligament or posterior cruciate ligament
A locked knee owing to suspected meniscal entrapment
Equivocal diagnosis

Subsequent referral
Suspected meniscal tear if symptoms persist after a trial of rehabilitation for 6 to 8 wk
At any stage of the rehabilitation process where symptoms persist and clinical milestones are not being achieved

stays), or cylindrical cast. The length of immobilization depends on the extent of injury; protected early range of motion is an option after several days for mild sprains.

    b. Weight bearing is allowed as tolerated. Crutches for aid in ambulation are often initially helpful. **Isometric quadriceps exercises** (tensing of the quadriceps, 10 contractions every few hours while awake) are recommended during immobilization to minimize atrophy.

    c. Cold application with an ice pack through the immobilization apparatus is recommended for 24 to 48 hours after an acute injury. Elevation of the knee above heart level is helpful in decreasing swelling during this period.

    d. Oral nonsteroidal anti-inflammatory drugs (NSAIDs) such as ibuprofen, 400 to 800 mg 3 times a day, with gastrointestinal precautions, are beneficial for treatment of pain and inflammation. (SOR **C**)

    e. After immobilization, **gradual rehabilitation** to full activity is necessary. The rehabilitation interval should be twice as long as the period of immobilization. There is insufficient evidence in the literature to establish the relative effectiveness of the various approaches and methods currently used in physical therapy for the conservative management of soft tissue knee injuries. (SOR **A**) For most knee injuries, strengthening of the quadriceps muscle with straight leg lifting, 10 repetitions 3 times daily, will promote knee stability and decrease the likelihood of repeat injury. The use of ankle weights, with progressive increases in 2- to 4-lb increments, will maximize the benefit of this exercise. Many knee injuries will improve with low-impact activities and exercises to improve muscular strength and flexibility. If the initial examination is limited by pain and swelling, the foregoing regimen can still be followed. An adequate examination will often be possible after 1 week.

  2. Iliotibial band syndrome

    a. Ice should be applied for 24 hours. NSAIDs can also be used (see Section VI.A.1.d).

    b. Rest and avoidance of aggravating activities usually for 1 to 2 weeks until pain and inflammation subside will facilitate the healing process. Resumption of full activity should be gradual. Rehabilitation is recommended (see Section VI.A.1.e).

  3. Meniscal tears are treated acutely the same as ligamentous injuries. After the acute injury, if the knee is persistently locked or if locking or clicking in the knee recurs, orthopedic referral is indicated.

B. Patellofemoral dysfunction

  1. Patellar subluxation is treated like an acute ligamentous injury (see Section VI.A). If the patella is still dislocated, it can be reduced by hyperextending the knee and pushing the patella back into place. Follow-up referral to an orthopedic surgeon within 1 week is necessary.

  2. Acute pain in **chondromalacia patellae** is treated with ice, elevation, and NSAIDs, as for ligamentous injuries (see Section VI.A). The knee should be immobilized for 1 week if pain is severe. Climbing, jumping, running, and squatting should be limited until pain subsides, usually for 2 to 4 weeks. Quadriceps strengthening exercises (see Section VI.A.1.b) are also beneficial.

  3. Patellar or quadriceps tendon rupture. Complete ruptures require surgical repair; partial tears are treated as ligamentous injuries (see Section VI.A.1).

C. Bursitis

  1. For **prepatellar, infrapatellar, and anserine bursitis,** ice should be applied for 24 hours and NSAIDs may be used (see Section VI.A.1.d). Aggravating activities should be avoided until pain and inflammation subside (usually several days to several weeks). A tense, inflamed, noninfected bursa can be aspirated (see Section V.B.1), and corticosteroid solution (e.g., triamcinolone acetonide, 20–40 mg, depending on bursa size) is then injected.

  2. A **Baker cyst** may be aspirated to relieve pressure and pain. The cyst will re-form unless underlying irritation is corrected.

D. Fractures. Most fractures of the patella, femoral condyles, and tibial plateaus require prompt referral to an orthopedic specialist, as noted in Table 40–2.

  1. Patellar fractures without complete disruption of the patella can be immobilized (see Section VI.A.1.a), with orthopedic follow-up in 1 week. Cylindrical casting is usually required for 6 weeks.

  2. Tibial plateau fractures require immobilization and no weight bearing. Surgical reduction is usually required for fracture displacement ≥ 3 mm.

  3. Femoral condylar fractures should be stabilized with a splint until a specialist can attend. If a neurovascular deficit is found, a vascular surgeon should be consulted.

E. Osgood–Schlatter disease and **Sinding–Larsen–Johansson syndrome.** These conditions are treated symptomatically by avoidance of resisted knee extension (running, climbing, jumping, and kicking) until symptoms subside. Immobilization of the affected knee should be considered for 1 to 2 weeks, if walking aggravates pain. **Osteochondritis dissecans** requires limited weight bearing. NSAIDs can be prescribed (see Section VI.A.1.d). Because of the potential for chronic knee pain and the occasional need for removal or fixation of fracture fragments, orthopedic follow-up should be arranged.

F. For the management of **osteoarthritis,** see Chapter 80. Patients with septic arthritis should be hospitalized for parenteral antibiotic therapy to minimize morbidity.

G. Pain referred from the hip (see Chapter 42).

REFERENCES

Bachman LM, Haberzeth S, Steurer J, et al. The accuracy of the Ottawa knee rule to rule out knee fractures: a systematic review. *Ann Int Med.* 2004;140(2):121-124.

Ebell MH. A tool for evaluating patients with knee injury. *Am Fam Physician.* 2005;12(3).

Ellis MR, Griffin KW, Meadows S, et al. For knee pain, how predictive is physical examination for meniscal injury? *J Fam Pract.* 2004;53(11):.

Harris GR, Susman JL. Managing musculoskeletal complaints with rehabilitation therapy: summary of the Philadelphia Panel evidence-based clinical practice guidelines on musculoskeletal rehabilitation interventions. *J Fam Pract.* 2002;51(12).

Holten KB. How should we diagnose and treat osteoarthritis of the knee? *J Fam Pract.* 2004;53(2).

Jackson JL, O'Malley PG, Kroenke K, et al. Evaluation of acute knee pain in primary care. *Ann Int Med.* 2003;139(7):575-588.

New Zealand Guidelines Group (NZGG). *The Diagnosis and Management of Soft Tissue Knee Injuries: Internal Derangements.* Wellington, NZ: New Zealand Guidelines Group (NZGG); 2003:100.

Okazaki KM, Matsuda S, Yasunaga T, et al. Assessment of anterolateral rotatory instability in the anterior cruciate ligament-deficient knee using an open magnetic resonance imaging system [Epub ahead of print March 22, 2007]. *Am J Sports Med.*

Robb G, Reid D, Arroll B, et al. General practitioner diagnosis and management of acute knee injuries: summary of an evidence-based guideline. *N Z Med J.* 2007;120(1249):U2419.

Scholten RJ, Opstelten WI, Van der Plas CG, et al. Accuracy of physical diagnostic tests for assessing ruptures of the anterior cruciate ligament: a meta-analysis. *J Fam Pract.* 2003;52(9).

Solomon DH, Simel DL, Bates DW, et al. Does this patient have a torn meniscus or ligament of the knee?: value of the physical examination. *JAMA.* 2001;286(13):1610-2160.

Zuber TJ. Knee joint aspiration and injection. *Am Fam Physician.* 2002;66:1497-1512.

41   Lacerations & Skin Biopsy

Jason Chao, MD, MS

KEY POINTS

- The goals of laceration repair are to gently appose tissue so that normal healing may take place, and to minimize complications, especially infection and unsightly scars.
- Anesthesia may be accomplished using topical anesthetic or injection.
- Wound closure options include sutures, cyanoacrylate adhesive, staples, adhesive tape, and allowing healing by secondary intention.

I. **Definition.** A laceration is a cut or tear in the skin or mucosa that extends through the epidermis into deeper, underlying tissues. Lacerations may result in two ways: (1) from a **shearing force** that slices through the skin or (2) from **blunt trauma** that compresses or stretches the skin. Blunt trauma requires greater energy and results in more extensive tissue damage. This creates an increased inflammatory response and contributes to additional scarring and greater risk of infection.

Tensile strength of the healing wound increases most rapidly during the first 3 weeks. Unfortunately, sutures must be removed by 2 weeks to minimize suture scars, and dehiscence may occur at this time. Local factors that increase infection rates include poor local blood supply and the presence of any necrotic tissue, foreign bodies, hematoma, or dead space.

II. **Common Diagnoses.** Lacerations and open wound injuries occur in 5 to 10 of every 100 persons each year in the United States. These wounds constitute one-quarter of all injuries in this country, occurring mostly in the home environment. Lacerations are more common among males and happen more frequently during the summer. There is a bimodal age distribution, with one peak of lacerations occurring in persons younger than 5 years and a second peak occurring in persons between 18 and 24 years of age.

A. In **superficial wounds,** the surface epidermis is left intact by contusions or bruises or is abraded, leaving underlying tissue intact.

B. In **puncture wounds,** a small surface opening may hide a deeper, serious injury. An electrical or chemical wound with a break in the skin requires special attention, since the patient may have severe soft tissue injury that is not apparent initially.

C. **Clean lacerations**

D. **Wounds with extensive tissue loss or injury,** including dirty lacerations, compound lacerations, and electrical wounds.

III. **Symptoms.** Lacerations cause **pain, bleeding,** and **swelling.**

IV. **Signs**

A. **Tissue damage**

  1. A partial or complete severing of bones, muscles, tendons, ligaments, major blood vessels, or nerves may occur in **compound lacerations.**

    a. Loss of a pulse or slow capillary refill after the application of pressure distal to wounds may indicate a vascular injury that must be treated.

    b. Sensorineural function distal to wounds should be assessed before anesthesia is administered. Loss of sensation or movement suggests a nerve injury that must be investigated. Poor finger flexion or extension indicative of a tendon injury is common in hand lacerations because the hand lacks subcutaneous fat.

  2. **Dirty lacerations** are contaminated with foreign matter. The depth and degree of contamination of lacerations and the surrounding tissue must be assessed. Full exploration of wounds is best performed after the administration of anesthesia.

  3. Inflammatory reaction with surrounding erythema begins several hours after the patient sustains a laceration. Marked erythema or pus signifies wounds that are not recent and are probably infected.

V. Laboratory Tests

    A. A **deep wound culture** after debridement is usually indicated if the laceration is dirty, more than 24 hours old, or obviously infected. (SOR **C**) The culture results are helpful as a guide in the treatment of the wound if it does not improve with initial therapy.

    B. **X-rays** may be appropriate for patients with compound or deep lacerations to check for a fracture, subcutaneous air, or a foreign body that might be associated with the laceration. Most glass is visible on x-ray.

VI. Treatment. The goals of treatment are to assist the healing process by approximating the wound when possible and to minimize complications, including infection and unsightly scars.

    A. Wound preparation. Most bleeding can be stopped by the application of direct pressure for 10 to 15 minutes. Hemostasis of active bleeders can be obtained using ligation, electrocautery, or Gelfoam.

        1. Thorough cleansing of the wound is performed to ensure that no foreign body is left in the wound.

            a. Gentle rinsing with saline solution is an adequate cleanser for many lacerations. Antiseptic solutions such as hydrogen peroxide, alcohol, Betadine, or Hibiclens should not be used because these disinfectants inhibit the wound repair process. (SOR **B**) Adding antibiotics to the lavage solution does not contribute to wound cleansing. (SOR **A**)

            b. Dirty lacerations should be forcefully irrigated with copious amounts of sterile saline. A 20- to 50-mL syringe and a 19-gauge needle should be used. Sharp debridement with a scalpel or scissors is sometimes necessary to remove the most contaminated tissue. Scrubbing the wound should be avoided if possible in order to prevent additional trauma to the wound.

            c. Areas such as the face or the neck that have a rich blood supply require less debridement than other areas.

        2. If hair removal is required, clipping with scissors is preferable to using a straight razor, to reduce tissue trauma. Eyebrows should not be shaved, since they grow slowly and a defect in the eyebrows is very noticeable.

        3. Wound edges should be perpendicular to the skin surface. If they are beveled, skin should be removed to produce a sharp perpendicular edge that will approximate with the other side. Small skin flaps with inadequate blood supply should be excised to ensure that the skin at the margins of the laceration is vascularized.

        4. If tissue is missing, preventing easy closure of the wound, consider undermining the subcutaneous layers to free the overlying skin, which will allow approximation of the skin margins.

    B. Anesthesia. Anesthesia is used for pain relief and to aid in adequate examination, debridement, and repair. Landmarks that need to be approximated should be identified and marked before local anesthesia is administered in order to prevent distortion.

        1. Local infiltration of the wound with anesthesia is often sufficient. A slow injection (i.e., for more than 10 seconds) of 1% **lidocaine hydrochloride** through a 27-gauge needle is commonly used. Mixing the lidocaine with **sodium bicarbonate** in a ratio of 9:1 will reduce the pain of injection. This procedure provides adequate anesthesia for as long as 2 hours.

        2. Epinephrine, a vasoconstrictor, may be included in an injection with lidocaine except in an area with reduced circulation, such as the fingers, toes, tip of the nose, penis, or earlobes. Contaminated wounds should not be injected with epinephrine because these wounds become easily infected when their blood supply is reduced.

        3. Topical anesthetic avoids painful injection, and does not distort local landmarks. LAT (4% lidocaine, 1:2000 adrenaline, and 0.5% tetracaine) or TAC (0.5% tetracaine, 1:2000 adrenaline, and 11.8% cocaine) can be used, especially in children. However, serious complications including seizures and death have been reported with improper use. Anesthesia using lidocaine and prilocaine (EMLA) cream is more effective but may take up to an hour to become effective, compared with a half hour using LAT or TAC.

        4. A **regional block** may be suitable for wounds that are very large or involve the distal fingers or toes.

    C. Biopsy

        1. For a diffuse skin eruption, a new or fresh lesion should be chosen. In blistering disorders, a rim of normal tissue should be included. Complete removal of a small-to moderate-sized lesion can serve both diagnostic and therapeutic purposes. If malignancy is a concern, adequate margins around the lesion should be obtained.

2. **Shave biopsy** is indicated for benign exophytic lesions such as warts, seborrheic keratoses and skin tags, and superficial nodulo-ulcerative processes. After cleansing the skin and adequate anesthesia, a scalpel blade is positioned almost parallel to the skin surface and the skin specimen is obtained in a single gentle scoop under the lesion, leaving a shallow defect with smooth borders. This wound is left to heal by secondary intention.

3. **Punch biopsy** is indicated for diagnosis in diffuse eruptions, deeper lesions, suspected vasculitis, or other inflammatory lesions requiring direct immunofluorescence. After cleansing the skin and adequate anesthesia, the skin should be stretched perpendicular to skin tension lines. The other hand is used to twist the punch into the skin down to the plastic hub of the punch. The plug of skin is gently removed and cut at the base with scissors or blade. A 4-mm punch is generally adequate. Smaller punches may be useful in cosmetically important areas, but have a lower diagnostic yield. Larger lesions may require up to a 6-mm punch. The wound is closed with sutures as described below.

4. **Excisional or incisional biopsy** is indicated for most pigmented lesions, suspected malignancies, and deep or subcutaneous lesions. After cleansing the skin and adequate anesthesia, a fusiform-shaped cut is made around the lesion. The length of the biopsy should be 3 times its width.

D. **Wound repair**

1. **Wound closure.** When clean lacerations present within 12 to 24 hours, they can be closed primarily. Lacerations closed during this "golden period" are likely to heal without infection. Head wounds with good blood supply may be closed even after 24 hours and still heal well. (SOR **B**)

Lacerations with extensive devitalized tissue or evidence of infection require thorough debriding, but should not be closed primarily. Delayed closure, 3 to 4 days later, may be performed if the wound appears free of infection and is adequately supplied with blood. The following techniques may also be used to close clean surgical wounds.

2. **Equipment.** The equipment required to repair a laceration includes a needle holder, smooth and toothed small forceps, scissors, small hemostats, a scalpel, sterile gauze, suture material, gloves, and drapes. Skin hooks are optional; they allow less traumatic handling of the skin. A disposable skin hook may be created by gently bending a needle with a hemostat. Adequate lighting is essential.

The choice of suture material depends on the location and purpose of the suture (Table 41–1).

a. **Absorbable sutures** should be used for dermal or fascial layer repair or for ligation of vessels. They lose their tensile strength by gradual degradation over days to weeks. Synthetic absorbable polymers (e.g., Dexon, Vicryl, PDS, or Maxon) retain their tensile strength longer than does plain or chromic gut.

b. **Nonabsorbable sutures** should be used for epidermal repair. Nonabsorbable sutures include silk, cotton, synthetic monofilament nylon or polypropylene (e.g., Ethilon, Dermalon, Prolene, Surgilene, or Deklene), and braided polyester. Nonabsorbable sutures remain strong, but induce a cellular reaction and increase the likelihood of infection in dirty wounds. Synthetic monofilament is the most commonly used material for the final epidermal closure.

3. **Placement of sutures.** Tissue should be handled gently to minimize additional trauma to the wound.

TABLE 41–1. WOUND CLOSURE

Site of Wound	Size of Subcutaneous Suture (Absorbable)	Size of Surface Suture (Nonabsorbable)	Time to Removal (d)
Scalp	#4-0 or #5-0	#3-0 or #4-0	5–7
Face	#5-0 or #6-0	#6-0 or #7-0	3–5
Trunk and extremities	#3-0 or #4-0	#4-0 or #5-0	7–10
Hands, feet, and skin over joints	None	#3-0 or #4-0	7–14

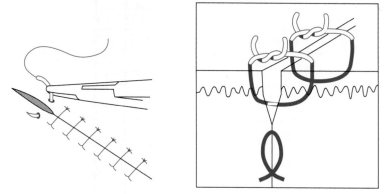

FIGURE 41–1. Simple interrupted suture.

a. **Dermal sutures** are used to approximate larger wounds, close dead space, and provide hemostasis and tensile strength. Sutures in fat lead to infection and should be avoided. An inverted suture will bury the knot deep in the wound.

b. **Skin sutures** should approximate the wound edges and not be tied too tightly. Excessive tightness of sutures restricts blood flow and produces a depressed scar that is more noticeable.

c. **Simple interrupted sutures** (Figure 41–1) are the most commonly used epidermal suture and provide good cosmetic repair. The deep portion of the suture should be wider than the surface to help evert the skin edges and prevent a depressed scar. **Vertical mattress sutures** (Figure 41–2) evert skin edges more than do simple sutures, but they are time-consuming and may lead to increased inflammatory reaction. **Half-buried horizontal mattress sutures** (Figure 41–3) are useful when the patient has skin flaps that appear viable. These sutures are least likely to compromise vascular supply to the flap.

d. **Running simple sutures** (Figure 41–4) provide the fastest repair; however, they are generally not used in cosmetically important areas. **Locked running sutures** (Figure 41–5) are particularly useful when the laceration is in mucosal surfaces, such as the vagina or the rectum. Absorbable suture material should be used. **Subcuticular (buried running) sutures** (Figure 41–6) are time-consuming, but produce good cosmetic results without suture marks when used to close small, clean lacerations. Absorbable sutures may be used. If nonabsorbable sutures are used, the ends should be left on the outside of the skin so the suture can be easily removed.

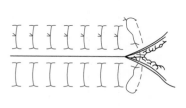

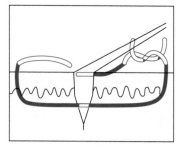

FIGURE 41–2. Vertical mattress suture.

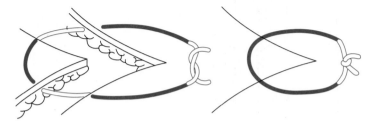

FIGURE 41–3. Half-buried horizontal mattress suture.

e. In patients with facial lacerations, slight misalignments in repair of the eyebrows and the vermilion border of the lips become very noticeable even at a distance. The first sutures that are placed should align the edges of these structures. Lacerations inside the mouth do not need to be closed primarily. For through-and-through wounds, the skin and muscle should be closed, and the oral mucosa should be left alone to heal by secondary intention.

f. For patients with scalp lacerations, choosing a suture of a color different from that of the patient's hair helps the physician in repairing the laceration and during suture removal.

g. Discussion of Z-plasty and other plastic techniques is beyond the scope of this chapter. These techniques may be used on patients with long lacerations that do not follow the natural contours of the body or with lacerations over joints that are likely to involve excessive motion during the healing process.

E. Tissue adhesive for closure

1. **Octylcyanoacrylate** (Dermabond) tissue adhesive has **comparable cosmetic outcome to suturing** in repair of selected traumatic lacerations. (SOR Ⓐ) Tissue adhesive closure is **faster** and **less painful** than suturing. Skin moisture is the catalyst for the adhesive to polymerize, generating heat.

2. Most **facial and selected trunk and extremity lacerations** are suitable for tissue adhesive closure. It should not be used on hands or over joints.

3. When using topical tissue adhesive, care should be taken to **keep adhesive out of the wound,** which would act as a foreign body and inhibit wound healing (Figure 41–7).

4. Wound edges should be apposed when applying the first layer of adhesive, and the adhesive should dry 3 minutes between layers. A minimum of **three layers** of adhesive should be applied.

5. The patient should be instructed to **avoid washing or soaking** the wound, but may get it wet, as in a shower.

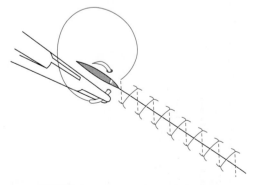

FIGURE 41–4. Running, or continuous, simple suture.

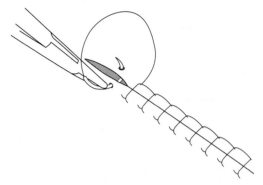

FIGURE 41–5. Locked running suture.

F. Staples. Staples can be applied quickly, but accurate placement may be difficult and they are more painful to remove than sutures. Infection rates are comparable to those of sutures.

G. Prevention of infection

1. The physician should provide **tetanus immunization** if it is indicated (Table 41–2).

2. Prophylactic antibiotics are not necessary except in selected cases, such as in patients with dirty compound lacerations or with lacerations that involve significant tissue ischemia because of blunt trauma. Most patients with bite wounds should receive antibiotics.

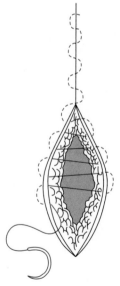

FIGURE 41–6. Subcuticular (buried running) suture. (Adapted with permission from Stillman RM, ed. *Surgery: Diagnosis & Therapy.* Appleton & Lange; 1989.)

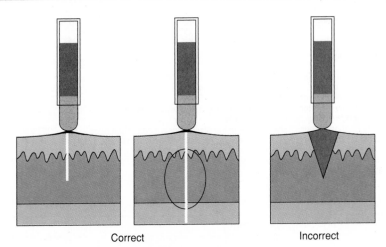

Correct   Incorrect

FIGURE 41–7. Proper tissue adhesive closure (**left, center**); improper use (**right**). (Adapted with permission from Quinn J, Wells G, Sutcliffe T, et al. Randomized trial comparing octylcyanoacrylate tissue adhesive sutures. *JAMA.* 1997;277:1529-1530. Copyright © 1997, American Medical Association. All Rights reserved.)

H. Patient education. Patients should be given the following advice.

    1. Keep the wound clean and dry for the first 24 hours, after which the dressing should be removed, and the wound should be cleaned daily.

    2. Contact a physician if redness, excessive swelling, tenderness, or increased warmth of the skin around the wound occurs; if pus or watery discharge occurs; if there are tender bumps or swelling in an armpit or groin area; if red streaks appear in the skin near the wound; if there is a foul smell from the wound; or if generalized body chills or fever develop.

    3. Elevate an extremity with a laceration to reduce swelling.

    4. Limit activity somewhat for 1 week after the sutures are removed to avoid reopening the wound. Wound healing takes several weeks.

    5. Use sunscreen to protect the scar from sunlight in order to avoid marked pigment changes that occur in lighter-skinned patients. A scar normally appears red and slightly raised or thickened for several months after an injury.

VII. Patient Follow-up. See Table 41–1 concerning the timing of suture removal.

    A. The physician should see patients with contaminated or deep lacerations 48 hours after the sutures are placed in cases in which infection is likely to present.

    B. When lacerations are in areas of tension, every other suture may be removed initially and replaced by adhesive bandages, with tincture of benzoin applied to the normal skin

TABLE 41–2. GUIDE TO TETANUS PROPHYLAXIS

Type of Wound	Immunization Status (Doses of Tetanus Toxoid Received)	
	Uncertain, Less Than 3, or None Within the Last 5 y	3 or More (Booster Within 5 y)
Clean wound	Td*	No prophylaxis necessary
Dirty wound†	Td,*and human tetanus immune globulin, at different site	Consider human tetanus immune globulin

*Adult tetanus and diphtheria toxoids, 0.5 mL intramuscularly. If the patient is younger than 7 years, diphtheria–tetanus or diphtheria–tetanus–pertussis is given intramuscularly.

†A wound that is grossly contaminated, is more than 8 hours old, contains devitalized tissue, or is of a form that prevents adequate irrigation.

(Modified with permission from Chesnutt MS, Dewar TN, Locksley RM. *Office & Bedside Procedures.* Appleton & Lange; 1992.)

to prolong bandage adhesion. The remaining sutures should be removed several days later.

REFERENCES

Attinger CE, Janis JE, Steinberg J, Schwartz J, Al-Attar A, Couch K. Clinical approach to wounds: debridement and wound bed preparation including the use of dressings and wound-healing adjuvants. *Plast Reconstr Surg.* 2006;117(7 S):72S-109S.
Bruns TB, Worthington JM. Using tissue adhesive for wound repair: a practical guide to dermabond. *Am Fam Physician.* 2000;61:1383-1388.
Leach J. Proper handling of soft tissue in the acute phase. *Facial Plast Surg.* 2001;17:227-238.
Wilson JL, Kocurek K, Doty BJ. A systematic approach to laceration repair: tricks to ensure the desired cosmetic result. *Postgrad Med.* 2000;107:77-83, 87-88.
Zuber TJ. The mattress sutures: vertical, horizontal, and corner stitch. *Am Fam Physician.* 2002;66: 2231-2236.

---

42   Leg & Hip Complaints

Geoffrey S. Kuhlman, MD, CAQSM

KEY POINTS

- Leg and hip complaints in children and adolescents often reflect serious conditions and should be treated as such until proved otherwise.
- Leg pain in athletic individuals is usually caused by overuse injuries, including stress fracture or medial tibial stress syndrome.
- The history and physical examination should guide appropriate diagnostic testing in the evaluation of hip and leg complaints.

I. **Definition. Hip complaints** arise from processes in the hip joint (e.g., transient synovitis, bacterial infection, avascular necrosis of the femoral head, slipped capital femoral epiphysis [SCFE], osteoarthritis, rheumatoid arthritis); other soft tissues (e.g., bursitis); or neurovascular structures (e.g., meralgia paresthetica). **Leg complaints** arise in the lower extremity proximal to the ankle from infection (e.g., osteomyelitis of the long bones); joints (e.g., osteoarthritis); muscle (e.g., nocturnal leg cramps); vasculature (e.g., arterial insufficiency, deep vein thrombosis [DVT], or varicose veins); neuropathy; overuse (e.g., stress fracture, medial tibial stress syndrome, or chronic compartment syndrome); or idiopathic etiologies (e.g., growing pains).

II. **Common Diagnoses** (Table 42–1 and Figures 42–1 to 42–4). Hip and leg complaints are common in family medicine. Some causes demand urgent attention, such as osteomyelitis, septic arthritis, and SCFE. Many of the less urgent diagnoses are quite debilitating for patients, causing significant pain, inability to work or exercise, or difficulty sleeping. Likely causes of hip and leg complaints depend on age and activity.

    A. Hip complaints in **children and adolescents** include transient synovitis, septic arthritis, Perthes disease, and SCFE.

        1. Transient synovitis is acute nonspecific inflammation in the hip joint and is the most common atraumatic cause of hip pain in childhood. Risk factors include antecedent upper respiratory infection, recurrent microtrauma, or allergic hypersensitivity.

        2. Septic arthritis of the hip joint can occur at any age but is most common in infants, toddlers, and elderly. Risk factors include wounds, skin infection, hip surgery, diabetes mellitus, HIV, and other immunocompromise.

        3. Perthes disease, avascular necrosis of the femoral head (see sidebar), is bilateral 12% of the time. Low birth weight and family history are risk factors, but the cause is undetermined, and no consistent hereditary pattern exists.

TABLE 42–1. EVALUATION OF COMMON HIP AND LEG COMPLAINTS

Diagnosis	Risk Factors	Symptoms	Signs	Testing
Transient synovitis	3- to 10-y-olds; M:F, 2:1; recent upper respiratory infection	Insidious or acute painful limp	Afebrile, voluntary limited hip range of motion	Hip US
Septic hip arthritis	Infants/toddlers	Rapid-onset, constant hip/thigh/knee pain, worse with movement, failure to thrive	Febrile/ill, thigh edema Flexed/abducted/externally rotated hip	Elevated WBC; plain x-rays show lateral displacement of femoral head; ESR; hip US guides needle aspiration
Perthes disease	4- to 10-y-olds; M:F, 5:1	Insidious pain/stiffness of groin/ lateral hip/medial knee, then limp	Antalgic gait, decreased hip range of motion, occasional flexion contracture	Crescent sign on x-ray (Figure 42–3), followed by progressive changes in femoral epiphysis/femoral head
SCFE	Obese early adolescence; M–F ratio 3:2	Groin/buttock/lateral hip or knee pain, simultaneous pain + limp in 50%	Antalgic gait, hip externally rotated	X-ray (Figures 42–3, 42–4)
OA/RA	90% of adult hip pain	Stiffness after rest, insidious pain referred to groin/thigh/knee	Limp, decreased hip range of motion, especially internal rotation/abduction	X-ray—spurring, narrowed joint space, periarticular sclerosis (OA)
Trochanteric bursitis	40- to 60-y-old females	Thigh, posterolateral hip pain	Tender grt. Trochanter. Increased with resisted abduction (Figure 42–1)	
Ischial bursitis	Prolonged sitting on hard surfaces	Buttock pain, worse with sitting	Tender ischial tuberosity (Figure 42–1), painful SLR	
Iliopsoas bursitis	Sports (e.g., soccer) requiring repetitive hip flexion/adduction	Deep groin pain, worse with hip extension	Tender and cystic mass (30%) over bursa (Figure 42–1), limited hip extension	Hip US detects enlarged bursa; CT confirms
Meralgia paresthetica	Abdominal obesity, middle-aged men, pregnancy	Anterolateral thigh pain, paresthesia	Reproduced by pressing lateral femoral cut. Against anterosuperior iliac spine (Figure 42–2)	None, NCV if diagnosis in question
Growing pains	15% of children 4 to 14 y old	Intermittent bilateral nocturnal thigh and lower leg pain	Normal examination	None

(Continued)

TABLE 42–1. (*Continued*)

Diagnosis	Risk Factors	Symptoms	Signs	Testing
Medial tibial stress syndrome	Adolescent/early adult runners, sudden increased training	Achy posteromedial distal tibia, initially during exercise, progressing to rest pain	Tender medial edge, distal third of tibia	None
Stress fractures	Late teen to early adult athletes, increase in physical activity; oligoamenorrhea/weight loss	Insidious local pain: tibia (34%), fibula (24%), metatarsal (20%), femur (14%), pelvic (6%)	Focal bony tenderness, poorly resolving soft tissue symptoms	X-ray shows periosteal reaction, then fracture (2–4 wk after symptom onset) MRI or radioisotope bone scan more sensitive
Chronic compartment syndromes	Late teen to early 20s, distance runners/sprinters/basketball players/soccer players	Gradual exercise-associated achiness: anterolaterally (anterior tibial compartment) calf pain/plantar paresthesia (posterior compartment), lateral lower leg achiness: lateral compartment	Involved muscle groups tender during/shortly after exercise; normal examination after adequate rest	Compartment pressure measurement (by orthopedist or physiatrist)
DVT	Immobility, leg trauma, hypercoagulable state, major surgery, history of DVT or cancer, estrogen therapy, CHF, pregnancy, atrial arrhythmias	Variable, nonspecific unilateral swelling, pain, erythema	Edema/red/warm (≥50% of DVTs not clinically detectable)	Duplex US (proximal DVT), D-Dimer assay, contrast venography
Nocturnal leg cramps	All ages (especially elderly), occasionally associated with denervation or electrolyte disorders	Abrupt nocturnal calf, plantar cramps	Tender affected muscles	Serum electrolytes if abnormality suspected

CHF, congestive heart failure; CT, computerized tomogram; DVT, deep vein thrombosis; ESR, erythrocyte sedimentation rate; M:F, male:female ratio; MRI, magnetic resonance imaging; NCV, nerve conduction velocity; OA, osteoarthritis; RA, rheumatoid arthritis; SCFE, slipped capital femoral epiphysis; SLR, straight leg raise (seated or supine); US, ultrasound; WBC, white blood cell count.

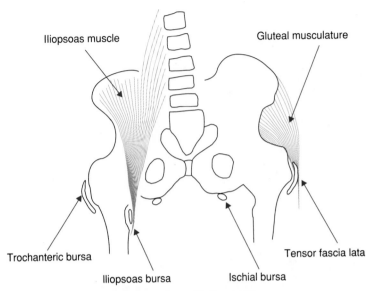

FIGURE 42–1. Bursae of the hip and pelvis.

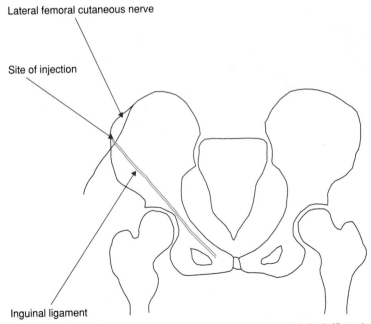

FIGURE 42–2. Meralgia paresthetica. The lateral femoral cutaneous nerve is compressed under the inguinal ligament medial to the anterior superior iliac spine (ASIS). Therapeutic injection is performed 1 cm medial to the ASIS (see text).

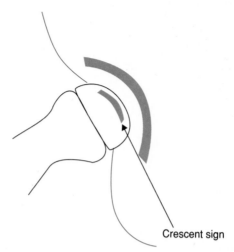

FIGURE 42-3. Crescent sign. In Perthes disease or in avascular necrosis of the hip in an adult, a radiographic finding is the crescent sign, a curvilinear lucency along the articular surface of the head of the femur.

4. **SCFE** is slippage of the proximal femur while the epiphysis remains in its position in the acetabulum. It occurs in early adolescence, and it is bilateral in 25% to 40% of cases. Obesity is a risk factor.

AVASCULAR NECROSIS

Atraumatic **avascular necrosis of the femoral head** begins between ages 25 and 45 years. Predisposing factors in 75% of cases include systemic corticosteroid therapy, alcoholism, sickle cell disease, or dysbaric trauma (underground or undersea work). Avascular necrosis presents with abrupt hip pain followed by progressive, intermittent episodes in 85% of patients, worsened by movement. Rest pain is present in two-thirds of patients and night pain in 40%. Findings on examination include limp and limited abduction/internal rotation.

Plain radiographs have a 19% false-negative rate early in avascular necrosis. Initial plain radiographic findings include a crescent sign (Figure 42–3), with bone collapse and degenerative arthritic changes occurring later.

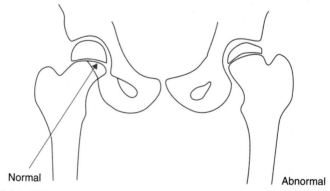

FIGURE 42-4. In SCFE, an early radiographic finding is loss of the triangle of Caper. On the right side of the picture, the entire ischium is seen (normal view). On the left side of the picture, slippage of the femoral epiphysis causes the femur metaphysis to shift medially, obscuring part of the ischium (abnormal view).

Radioisotope bone scans increase sensitivity in detecting avascular necrosis, and magnetic resonance imaging scanning is the most sensitive, specific, and low-risk means of making this diagnosis.

Management of avascular necrosis involves orthopedic consultation for possible core decompression or, for more advanced disease, hip arthroplasty.

B. Hip complaints in **adults** include impingement, osteoarthritis, rheumatoid arthritis, bursitis, meralgia paresthetica, referred pain (lumbar spine or pelvis), avascular necrosis, septic arthritis, and malignancy. Hip bursitis is usually associated with trauma or overuse.

C. **Leg complaints in infants and toddlers** (0–3 years) include septic arthritis of the hip, osteomyelitis (see sidebar), and fracture.

D. **Leg complaints in children** (4–14 years) include transient synovitis of the hip, Perthes disease, SCFE, growing pains, and a variety of injuries. Growing pains are idiopathic.

E. **Common leg complaints in adolescents** (11–16 years) are SCFE, growing pains, and knee disorders such as Osgood-Schlatter disease and Sindig-Larsen-Johansson syndrome (see Chapter 40), risk factors for which include jumping activities, weak hip muscles, and tight quadriceps muscles.

F. **Leg complaints in athletic adolescents and adults**
   1. Medial tibial stress syndrome, periostitis of the origin of the soleus muscle on the distal posteromedial aspect of the tibia, typically develops from repetitive dorsiflexion, as in running.
   2. Stress fractures commonly occur in the tibia or fibula of athletes who run or jump, such as in cross country, track and field, soccer, and basketball. Risk factors include increased activity, abnormal weight loss, inadequate intake of calcium or vitamin D, hyperthyroidism, and hyperparathyroidism.

OSTEOMYELITIS

Risk factors for osteomyelitis in children include male gender (male–female ratio of 2:1), lower socioeconomic status, immunocompromise, and the autumn season. Osteomyelitis presents with rapid-onset leg pain and refusal to walk in children. Findings include fever $\geq$38°C (100.4°F), ill appearance, and redness/warmth/tenderness of the involved region with limited motion of adjacent joints. Early in osteomyelitis, plain radiographs show loss of normal fascial planes and fat shadows because of edema. Bony changes appear 7 to 10 days after symptoms and include (1) destruction, with or without periosteal elevation, (2) fading cortical margins, and (3) absence of adjacent reactive new bone. Radioisotope bone scanning detects osteomyelitis before plain radiographs, and magnetic resonance imaging is the most sensitive, specific, low-risk means of diagnosing osteomyelitis. Suspected osteomyelitis requires hospitalization for blood cultures and prolonged parenteral antibiotics.

   3. Chronic compartment syndrome is ischemic or neuropathic pain resulting from increased muscle mass within an unyielding compartment. **Posterior compartment syndromes** are common in cyclists; **lateral compartment syndromes** are common in football and soccer players.
   4. Other causes include patellofemoral pain, iliotibial band syndrome, muscle strain, and peripheral nerve or artery entrapment.

G. **Leg complaints in adults**
   1. **Deep vein thrombosis (DVT)** occurs in the setting of venous stasis, venous injury, or increased blood coagulability.
   2. **Nocturnal leg cramps** are sudden contraction of the plantar flexor muscles causing painful cramps during sleep.
   3. Other causes include patellofemoral pain (see Chapter 40), iliotibial band syndrome (see Chapter 40), peripheral neuropathy (see sidebar), peripheral arterial disease (see sidebar), acquired spinal stenosis (see sidebar), cancer (see sidebar), osteoarthritis (see Chapter 80), gout and other crystal arthropathies, and rheumatoid arthritis.

PERIPHERAL NEUROPATHIES

Peripheral neuropathies can be classified as **mononeuropathy** (a single nerve affected, usually owing to trauma, compression, or entrapment [e.g., common peroneal neuropathy at the fibular head causing dorsal foot/lateral calf sensory loss and weakened foot dorsiflexion and eversion]) or **polyneuropathy** (affecting multiple nerves simultaneously). Polyneuropathy can be classified as axonal or demyelinating. The **axonal** type involves distal sensory, burning, or tingling progressing proximally in a stocking/glove distribution and initially affecting fine touch and temperature, e.g., diabetes, vitamin B_{12} deficiency, Lyme disease, uremia, drugs, toxins, or human immunodeficiency virus. The **demyelinating** type manifests early with diffuse loss of reflexes and strength, e.g., Guillain-Barré syndrome, multiple myeloma, or chronic inflammatory demyelinating polyneuropathy.

In approaching a patient with peripheral neuropathy, it is important to assess risk factors (e.g., history of recent viral illness, chronic systemic disease, new medications, and occupational or other exposure to toxins, such as alcohol/pesticides/heavy metals); distribution (i.e., likely mono- versus polyneuropathy); and rapidity of onset. (With regard to rapidity of onset, massive intoxications or Guillain-Barré syndrome develop over days to weeks; many toxins will develop over weeks to months; and diabetic, hereditary, or dysproteinemic neuropathies evolve over months to years.) Examination confirms/localizes deficits (i.e., sensation, reflexes, strength, or proprioception). Further testing is based on the foregoing clinical evaluation; helpful basic testing when the cause is not clear includes blood glucose, sedimentation rate, vitamin B_{12} or methylmalonic acid levels, serum blood urea nitrogen and creatinine, and serum protein/immunoelectrophoresis. Electrodiagnostic studies (e.g., nerve conduction velocity) are also helpful in clarifying the type and location of neuropathy. Treatment of neuropathy depends on its causes (e.g., controlling diabetes or renal failure, eliminating inciting drugs or toxins, treating vitamin B_{12} deficiency) and may involve neurologic consultation in puzzling cases.

PERIPHERAL ARTERIAL DISEASE (PAD)

PAD results from endothelial injury, lipid deposits, vasoconstriction, and plaque disruption, which reduce arterial blood flow and oxygen delivery to affected muscles, causing exertional calf or leg angina or nocturnal leg pain improved with walking. (This should be distinguished from neurogenic claudication which is caused by lumbar nerve root compression from spinal stenosis.) Arterial insufficiency pain can also arise from arterial entrapment or malformation, particularly during vigorous exercise. PAD shares risk factors (e.g., hypertension, diabetes mellitus, hypercholesterolemia, tobacco abuse) with coronary artery disease (CAD), and significant CAD coexists in 60% of patients with PAD. The best screen for leg claudication is the ankle-brachial index (ABI), the ratio of systolic blood pressure in the posterior tibial artery/systolic blood pressure in the brachial artery, and is performed supine using a Doppler ultrasound. Since ankle pressure normally is higher, a normal ABI is $\geq$1. Severity of PAD correlates with ABI values, such that $\leq$0.90 diagnoses PAD, 0.70 to 0.89 indicates mild disease, 0.5 to 0.69 indicates moderate disease, and $\leq$0.5, severe disease. Treatment for PAD starts with lifestyle modifications (exercise to develop collateral blood flow, smoking cessation, dietary reduction in cholesterol, glucose control, and blood pressure control) and extends to pharmacologic intervention (lipid-lowering drugs, antiplatelet agents, e.g., aspirin (325 mg daily), cilostazol (50–100 mg twice daily), clopidogrel (75 mg daily), ticlopidine (250 mg twice daily), and red-cell morphology-altering agents, e.g., pentoxifylline 400 mg 3 times daily). (SOR **A**) Revascularization by either angioplasty or bypass grafting is reserved for cases refractory to medical management, for rest pain, tissue loss, persistent ulcers, or gangrene. (SOR **B**)

SPINAL STENOSIS

Spinal stenosis can be congenital or acquired; 75% of cases are acquired, and risk factors include old age (men $\geq$ women) and history of degenerative arthritis, although up to 20%

of adults with spinal stenosis on imaging studies are asymptomatic. Degenerative spinal stenosis can be **central** (circumferential spinal cord compression) or **lateral** (narrowing of neuroforamina).

In differentiating spinal stenosis from disk disease and vasculogenic claudication, it is helpful to know that sciatica caused by spinal stenosis is more commonly bilateral (versus unilateral with lumbar disk disease), that spinal stenosis pain can occur in the hip, thigh, or lower leg, and that the cramping pain in patients with spinal stenosis is relieved with sitting, lying, or leaning forward (versus vascular claudication, which is relieved by decreased muscular activity, without the need to sit or lean forward). In those suspected of having degenerative spinal stenosis, an enhanced magnetic resonance imaging scan is the preferred imaging study; a dural sac with ≤10 mm anteroposterior diameter is consistent with this diagnosis. Initial management of spinal stenosis is symptomatic and using nonsteroidal anti-inflammatory agents (NSAIDs), proper positioning, and physical therapy; surgical decompression is reserved for those patients with significant pain despite medical therapy, those patients whose spinal stenosis significantly impacts daily activities, or those with focal neurologic findings. Surgery is 65% to 80% successful in providing relief, (SOR **Ⓐ**) although approximately 25% of patients develop recurrent spinal stenosis within 5 years.

CANCER

Cancer, most commonly metastatic from breast, prostate, lung, kidney, or thyroid tumors, but also from multiple myeloma in the elderly, causes pain through osteoclastic bone resorption and resulting osteopenia and pathologic fractures. Cancer pain is often nocturnal and described as a deep ache, is exacerbated by movement, and may cause acute disability with pathologic fracture. Typically, physical findings may initially be minimal; later palpable swelling and pain over bony prominences may develop. Pathologic fracture may cause immediate inability to bear weight, though occult fracture may manifest with normal motion, except at extremes of internal or external rotation.

Plain radiographs may show punched-out osteolytic lesions. Cancer patients with osteolytic lesions and increasing pain unresponsive to analgesics (including combination opioids and acetaminophen or NSAIDs) or palliative radiotherapy, in whom radiographs show destruction of ≥50% of bone cortex or lesions ≥3 cm in diameter, should be considered for prophylactic internal fixation, in consultation with an orthopedic surgeon.

III. **Symptoms** (Table 42–1)
  A. **Transient synovitis** pain occasionally will awaken children at night.
  B. In **Perthes disease,** knee pain alone occurs in 15%. The patient usually tolerates symptoms for 1 to 12 months before seeing a physician.
  C. In **SCFE,** approximately 20% of patients present acutely with a history of a sudden twisting or falling injury.
  D. Hip impingement causes anterolateral hip pain worsened by hip flexion, sitting, and leaning forward, such as to tie shoes.
  E. **Osteoarthritis** and **rheumatoid arthritis** (see Chapters 39 and 80).
  F. **Bursitis**
    1. In **trochanteric bursitis,** running or lying on the affected side worsens the pain.
    2. **Iliopsoas bursitis** causes pain with hip extension, as when rising from a chair or lying in bed, and patients often limp with the hip flexed and externally rotated.
  G. In **meralgia paresthetica,** prolonged standing and walking may worsen the pain; sitting may relieve it.
  H. **Chronic compartment syndrome** gradually develops over 1 year or longer, and how far the patient can walk or run before symptoms occur is usually constant, but discomfort may worsen over time.
    1. In **anterior compartment syndrome,** numbness in the web space between the first and second toes and dorsiflexion weakness may occur.
    2. Complaints of ankle instability are common with **lateral compartment syndrome.**
  I. In **stress fractures,** pain initially occurs toward the end of exercise and usually increases over days to weeks; the pain eventually develops early in activity and finally occurs at rest if training is not decreased.

IV. Signs (Table 42–1). Physical examination of hip and leg complaints begins with taking vital signs and observing the patient's general appearance. The hips and legs are inspected for asymmetry, deformity, discoloration, and edema. Gait is observed for symmetry, antalgia (quick soft steps to favor a painful area), hip circumduction (swinging one thigh outward to reduce ipsilateral hip pain), and Trendelenburg sign (dropping one side of the pelvis because of contralateral hip weakness). Palpation of bony landmarks and soft tissue should be done with precision to localize tenderness. Particularly in patients with suspected vascular or neurologic disease, quality of pulses (femoral, popliteal, posterior tibial, and dorsal pedal) and of sensation (light touch, sharp, vibration, temperature) are assessed. Range of motion (ROM) testing should include passive, active, and resisted. Hip (flexion, extension, abduction, adduction, and internal and external rotation) and knee (flexion and extension) ROM are best performed with the patient supine, whereas ankle motion (dorsiflexion, plantar flexion, inversion, and eversion) and Homan's sign (rapid passive dorsiflexion to elicit pain from DVT) are done seated. Tendon reflexes should be tested. If the examination does not clearly localize the problem, then sources of referred symptoms should be examined (e.g., pelvis, lumbar spine).

   A. In **Perthes disease,** thigh and calf circumferences are diminished; late in the process, leg length may decrease.

   B. In **SCFE,** passive hip flexion elicits external rotation and abduction of the hip; half of the patients will have thigh atrophy, and half will have shortening of the extremity up to 1 inch.

   C. In hip impingement, the combination of flexion, adduction, and internal rotation typically causes pain.

   D. Osteoarthritis and **rheumatoid arthritis** (see Chapters 39 and 80).

V. Laboratory Tests (Table 42–1).

   A. In **evaluating hip complaints, plain x-rays** of the involved hip in adults (anterior and lateral views) and both hips in children (often including a frog leg lateral view) are the single-most cost-effective adjunctive test. When combined with age-adjusted history and thoughtful interpretation of physical signs, radiography approaches 90% sensitivity and 90% specificity.

      1. Perthes disease shows the following sequence: crescent sign (Figure 42–3), lateral displacement of the femoral head, widening and increased density of the femoral epiphysis, flattening of the femoral head and widening of the femoral neck, demineralization and fragmentation of the femoral head, and finally, reossification of the femoral head.

      2. The **SCFE** appears widened with irregular margins. The femoral head is displaced posteriorly and medially (Figure 42–4).

      3. Findings in hip impingement can include exostosis of the superior aspect of the femoral head-neck and superior acetabulum osteophytes and fragmentation.

VI. Treatment

   A. The pain of **transient synovitis is relieved with bed rest** at home for 7 to 10 days and **NSAIDs** such as **ibuprofen** (5–10 mg/kg 3 times daily) as needed. Patients may use crutches to resume weight bearing. Most children have only a single attack of transient synovitis, but it may recur. Because 6% to 15% of patients with transient synovitis develop Perthes disease, patients and their parents should be instructed to seek care if hip or leg complaints occur.

   B. Losing weight and avoiding constrictive garments are key to treating **meralgia paresthetica.** Abdominal muscle strengthening is also helpful. Local corticosteroid injection at the site of lateral femoral cutaneous nerve compression may provide relief in refractory cases (e.g., triamcinolone, 10–20 mg with 1 mL lidocaine via a 27-gauge $1^{1}/_{4}$-inch needle, Figure 42–2). Patients should be reassured that this condition is benign and self-limited.

   C. Stretching overlying muscle to reduce friction on a bursa and strengthening weak hip muscles are key to treating **bursitis.** Oral analgesics might be helpful (e.g., ibuprofen, 200–800 mg 3 times daily or naproxen, 375–500 mg twice daily as needed for adults). If pain persists or function is limited, the affected bursa should be injected with 20 to 40 mg of **triamcinolone** or **methylprednisolone** added to 1 to 2 mL of 1% lidocaine. No more than three injections should be given each year.

   D. Hip impingement might respond to physical therapy to improve hip strength, motion, and flexibility, but it often requires arthroscopy.

   E. Osteoarthritis is managed with lifestyle modification (weight reduction, moderate exercise as tolerated), topical and oral analgesia, and assistive devices (see Chapter 80).

F. Surgical intervention

1. A patient with **bacterial infection** of the hip must be hospitalized for **arthrotomy** to drain all purulent material and for intravenous antibiotics. (SOR **C**) Poor prognosis is correlated with delayed action. Results of ultrasound-guided aspiration may allow selection of a smaller high-risk group for operative drainage and may also shorten operative time.

2. Perthes disease requires the orthopedic use of **braces, casts,** or **surgery** in order to retain the normal spherical shape of the femoral head during the natural repair process. (SOR **B**) Under the best of circumstances (e.g., younger age or earlier diagnosis), minimal deformity and normal function will result. Premature osteoarthritis of the hip can develop.

3. **SCFE** is best treated with immediate cessation of weight bearing and **surgical stabilization.** (SOR **A**) Premature osteoarthritis of the hip is common.

4. Under ultrasound or computerized tomography guidance, diagnostic and therapeutic **aspiration and drainage** of an enlarged **iliopsoas bursa** refractory to previously described measures can be accomplished. Prophylactic intravenous antibiotics will lessen the need for repeat aspiration.

G. Because the cause of **growing pains** is unknown, treatment consists of supportive measures including heat, ice, massage, and acetaminophen (10–15 mg/kg every 6 hours as needed) or NSAIDs. If symptoms persist despite a negative work-up, referral to a rheumatologist or pediatric orthopedic surgeon should be considered. (SOR **C**)

H. Chronic compartment syndrome often requires surgical decompression of the affected fascial compartment. Reducing exercise or changing sports is another option. Some cases might respond to a few weeks of stretching the lower extremity musculature 2 to 4 times daily to improve compliance of fascia enclosing compartments. (SOR **C**)

I. Stress fractures

1. Crutches or a leg brace are sometimes required. Weight-bearing exercise should be discontinued until x-ray evidence of healing is seen and there is no tenderness, after which gradual resumption of activity may proceed.

2. Use of analgesics is discouraged because of the possibility of masking pain, which reflects ongoing bone stress.

3. Stress fractures of the pelvis, femur, and anterior tibia have high risk for complications and are best managed by a subspecialist.

J. Medial tibial stress syndrome

1. Initial treatment is rest and ice (15–20 minutes at a time) until pain subsides.

2. Once symptoms resolve, soleus muscle stretching should be initiated, and the patient may gradually return to running. Patients whose feet pronate excessively might benefit from arch support and heel control, such as with off-the-shelf or custom-made orthotics. Physical therapy is sometimes needed. (SOR **C**)

3. In rare instances surgical release of the involved fascia is necessary.

K. DVT (see Chapter 23).

L. Nocturnal leg cramps

1. When cramping occurs, the calf muscles should be stretched by dorsiflexion. Calf stretching at bedtime can prevent symptoms.

2. Quinine sulfate, 200 to 325 mg orally at bedtime, may be helpful. Side effects include nausea, vomiting, headache, tinnitus, hearing loss, vertigo, and vision disturbance.

REFERENCES

Bates SM, Ginsberg JS. Treatment of deep vein thrombosis. *N Engl J Med.* 2004;351:268-277.

Bradshaw C. Hip and groin pain. In: Brukner P, Khan K, eds. *Clinical Sports Medicine.* New York: McGraw-Hill; 2001:375-394.

Dooley PJ. Femoroacetabular impingement syndrome: nonarthritic hip pain in young adults. *Can Fam Physician.* 2008;54(1):42-47.

Edwards PH, et al. A practical approach for the differential diagnosis of chronic leg pain in the athlete. *Am J Sports Med.* 2005;33:1241-1249.

Hart JJ. Transient synovitis of the hip in children. *Am Fam Physician.* 1996;54:1587.

Leet AI, Skaggs DL. Evaluation of the acutely limping child. *Am Fam Physician.* 2000;61:1011.

Loder RT. Slipped capital femoral epiphysis. *Am Fam Physician.* 1998;57:2135.

White C. Intermittent claudication. *N Engl J Med.* 2007;356:1241-1250.

43   Liver Function Test Abnormalities

James P. McKenna, MD

KEY POINTS

- An AST–ALT ratio $\geq$2:1 is highly suggestive of alcoholic hepatitis.
- Persistent elevations of liver function tests for $\geq$6 months suggest chronic liver disease; patients should be evaluated for treatable causes and referred for liver biopsy.
- Alcohol liver disease, hepatitis C, and nonalcoholic fatty liver disease (NAFLD) are the most common causes of persistently abnormal liver function tests.

I. **Definition.** Abnormalities in liver function tests (LFTs) are elevated levels of static biochemical tests, including aspartate aminotransferase (AST) (formerly serum glutamic-oxaloacetic transaminase [SGOT]), alanine aminotransferase (ALT) (formerly serum glutamate pyruvate transaminase [SGPT]), alkaline phosphatase, bilirubin, and albumin. The tests are most frequently obtained as part of LFT panels. Tests other than those mentioned are often included in LFT panels but are less useful in evaluating the spectrum of liver disease, and therefore are not discussed here. Cellular injury in the liver causes release of AST and ALT. ALT is a more specific indication of liver disease, whereas AST elevations may be secondary to damage of other organs (heart, kidney, brain, intestine, placenta). **Alkaline phosphatase** is associated with cellular membranes, and elevated levels may be caused by injury to the liver, bone, kidneys, intestines, placenta, or leukocytes. In the liver, the enzyme is located in the bile canaliculi. Biliary obstruction induces increased synthesis of alkaline phosphatase and spillage into the circulation. **Hyperbilirubinemia** may be caused by increased production (hemolysis, ineffective erythropoiesis); extravasation of blood (hematoma); decreased metabolism (hereditary disease, Gilbert's syndrome, or acquired defects in bilirubin conjugation); or reduced bilirubin excretion caused by bile duct obstruction.

Quantitative LFTs measuring liver metabolism or clearance of caffeine, antipyrine, cholate, or galactose may be used by hepatologists to assess liver function in patients with chronic compensated liver disease.

II. **Common Diagnoses.** In asymptomatic populations, the frequency of abnormal LFTs on routine screening ranges from 1% to 6%. The prevalence of liver disease is approximately 1%.

A. **Elevated aminotransferases** are found to some degree in almost all patients with liver disease and represent hepatocellular dysfunction (Table 43–1).

1. In asymptomatic populations, as many as 6% of patients have abnormal values of AST.

2. Alcohol liver damage, hepatitis C, and nonalcoholic fatty liver disease (NAFLD) are the most common causes of aminotransferase abnormalities in adults.

3. Hepatitis A virus is the most common cause of aminotransferase abnormality in children.

TABLE 43–1. **CAUSES OF ELEVATED AMINOTRANSFERASES**

Alcoholic hepatitis	Drug-induced hepatitis*
Viral hepatitis	Autoimmune hepatitis*
Hepatitis A	Toxic hepatitis
Hepatitis B*	Nonalcoholic fatty liver disease (NAFLD)*
Hepatitis C*	Metabolic hepatitis*
Hepatitis D*	Hemochromatosis
Hepatitis E	α_1-antitrypsin deficiency
Hepatitis G*	Wilson's disease
Cytomegalovirus	
Epstein-Barr virus	

*These conditions may cause chronic active hepatitis.

  B. **Elevated alkaline phosphatase** is secondary to intrahepatic or extrahepatic obstruction, cholestasis from medication, or infiltrative disease (e.g., cancer or granulomas). It has been found in as many as 4% of asymptomatic patients.
  C. **Hyperbilirubinemia** may signify hepatobiliary disease or hemolysis.
    1. Mild degrees of indirect hyperbilirubinemia may be found in as many as 10% of asymptomatic patients with Gilbert's syndrome.
    2. Prior to age 30, hepatitis causes 75% of hyperbilirubinemia.
    3. After age 60, extrahepatic obstruction causes 50% of hyperbilirubinemia (e.g., gallstones or pancreatic cancer).
III. **Symptoms**
  A. Abnormal LFTs in asymptomatic patients may indicate very mild hepatic dysfunction or may represent a more serious illness in its presymptomatic phase. Subsequent testing and follow-up are usually necessary to determine which abnormality exists.
  B. Fatigue, nausea, malaise, pruritus, jaundice, anorexia, or right upper quadrant discomfort are common complaints of patients with compensated liver disease and abnormal LFTs. The severity of the complaints is often related to the acuteness and extent of the illness.

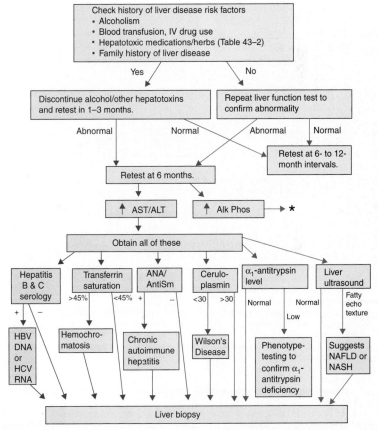

FIGURE 43–1. Evaluation of the asymptomatic patient with abnormal liver function tests. Alk Phos, alkaline phosphatase; ALT, alanine aminotransferase; ANA, antinuclear antibody; antiSm, anti–smooth muscle antibody; AST, aspartate aminotransferase; ERCP, endoscopic retrograde cholangiopancreatography; GGT, γ-glutamyltransferase; HBV DNA, hepatitis B virus deoxyribonucleic acid; HCV RNA, hepatitis C virus ribonucleic acid; IV, intravenous; NAFLD, nonalcoholic fatty liver disease; NASH, nonalcoholic steatohepatitis; ULN, upper limit of normal; US, ultrasound.

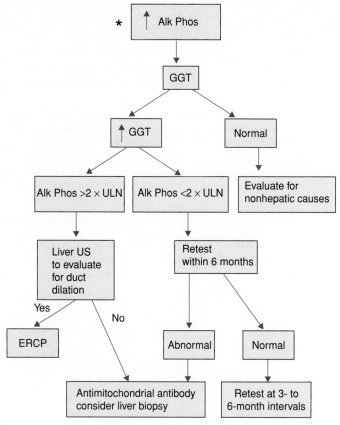

FIGURE 43–1. (*Continued*)

    C. Fatigue, anorexia, weight loss, abdominal distention, hematemesis, hematochezia, con-
fusion, jaundice, and abdominal discomfort are symptoms of hepatic decompensation in
patients with decompensated liver disease and abnormal LFTs.

IV. Signs

    A. Hepatomegaly or an unusually firm liver may be present in asymptomatic patients.

    B. Fever, jaundice, splenomegaly, and a tender, enlarged liver may indicate compensated
liver disease.

    C. Ascites, edema, jaundice, vascular spiders, esophageal varices, splenomegaly, hepatic
encephalopathy, testicular atrophy, gynecomastia, or loss of pubic and axillary hair may
indicate decompensated liver disease.

V. Laboratory Tests

    A. A **stepwise approach to evaluating LFT abnormalities** is recommended (Figure 43–1).
(SOR **C**)

        1. LFTs should be repeated to confirm any abnormalities in asymptomatic patients. Any
offending agents (Table 43–2) should be discontinued, and the test should be repeated
in 1 to 3 months.

           If abnormal LFTs persist for more than 6 months, treatable causes of chronic hep-
atitis should be ruled out. Such causes include hemochromatosis; autoimmune hepatitis; α_1-antitrypsin deficiency; hepatitis B, C, and D; NAFLD; and Wilson's disease
(see Chapters 38 and 71).

TABLE 43-2. **MEDICATIONS THAT MAY ADVERSELY AFFECT LIVER FUNCTION TESTS**

Cholestatic Pattern	Cytotoxic Pattern
Amoxicillin/clavulanic acid	Acarbose
Anabolic steroids	Acetaminophen
Chlorambucil	Allopurinol
Chlorpromazine	Amiodarone
Chlorpropamide	L-asparaginase
Clopridogrel	Aspirin and nonsteroidal anti-inflammatory
Erythromycin estolate	drugs
Estrogen (oral contraceptives)	Carbamazepine
Methimazole	Etretinate
Mirtazapine	HAART drugs
Phenobarbital	Halothane
Terbinafine	Hydralazine
Tolbutamide	Imipramine
Tricyclics	Isoniazid
	Ketoconazole
	Lisinopril
	Lovastatin
	6-Mercaptopurine
	Methotrexate
	Methyldopa
	Nicotinic acid (especially sustained-release)
	Nitrofurantoin
	Omeprazole
	Paroxetine
	Phenytoin
	Propylthiouracil
	Rifampin
	Risperidone
	"Statins"
	Sertraline
	Sulfonamides
	Tetracycline
	Trazodone
	Valproic acid

2. A γ-**glutamyltransferase (GGT) test** should be ordered in patients with abnormal alkaline phosphatase levels to confirm the hepatic origin of the enzyme.
3. Direct and indirect **bilirubin fractions** should be obtained if total bilirubin levels are increased. If the indirect (unconjugated) fraction is elevated ($\geq$80% of the total), a reticulocyte count and a peripheral blood smear should be obtained (see Chapter 4).
4. **Serum albumin** determinations are indicated in any symptomatic patient. Decreased levels reflect decreased synthesis (from poor nutrition or hepatic dysfunction) or increased loss (from the kidneys or the intestines). Serum levels correlate poorly with prognosis in acute liver disease, although patients with decompensated liver disease routinely have low levels.
5. **Prothrombin time (PT)** reflects hepatic synthesis of vitamin K–dependent clotting factors (II, VII, IX, and X) and should be ordered for patients with acute or chronic liver disease or coagulopathy.
   a. Improvement by 30% after a 10-mg subcutaneous injection of vitamin K suggests intact hepatocellular function and makes biliary obstruction the likely cause of the abnormal PT.
   b. If the PT fails to improve after administration of vitamin K, significant loss of hepatocellular function exists and the prognosis is poor.
6. If evidence suggests hepatitis, further serologic testing is indicated to confirm the diagnosis (see Chapter 38).
   Liver biopsy should be considered for any patient with abnormal LFTs for 6 months. (SOR **C**) A biopsy sample should be obtained before the end of the 6-month period if the patient's condition deteriorates. Liver biopsy is the only definitive means of establishing a diagnosis of chronic hepatitis.

B. Interpretation of particular abnormal LFT patterns
  1. Alcoholic liver disease results in modest elevations of the transaminases. An eleva-
      tion of ALT ≥300 IU is not consistent with alcoholic liver damage. The ratio of AST
      to ALT is useful diagnostically, since a ratio of 2:1 or greater suggests a high proba-
      bility of alcoholic liver disease. Elevated mean corpuscular volume and GGT suggest
      alcoholic liver disease.
  2. Viral hepatitis often causes significant elevations of the transaminases, with levels
      exceeding 1000 IU. ALT is typically elevated more than AST; the AST–ALT ratio is
      ≤1.
  3. Medications causing cholestasis (Table 43–2) may result in transaminase and alkaline
      phosphatase elevations that are as much as 10 times the normal levels.
  4. Cytotoxic reactions from medications may cause severe injuries resembling viral
      hepatitis, with transaminase values as high as 500 times the normal levels.
  5. Intrahepatic or extrahepatic obstruction cause values of alkaline phosphatase to
      be 5 or more times higher than normal. The highest values are found in primary biliary
      cirrhosis.
  6. Infiltrative diseases such as neoplasm, granulomas, or amyloidosis may cause mod-
      erate to marked elevations of alkaline phosphatase. Bilirubin is minimally elevated,
      however.
  7. Hemolysis causes an elevated reticulocyte count and an abnormal peripheral smear,
      with the bilirubin level generally ≤5 mg/dL.
  8. Gilbert's syndrome is characterized by indirect bilirubin levels of 2 to 3 mg/dL, normal
      LFTs, and no evidence of hemolysis.
VI. Treatment. For information on the management of the following causes of abnormal LFTs,
      refer to the chapters indicated.
  A. Cholelithiasis (Chapter 1).
  B. Hemolysis (Chapter 4).
  C. Hepatitis (Chapter 38).
  D. Cirrhosis (Chapter 71).
  E. Alcohol and drug abuse (Chapter 88).

REFERENCES

American Gastroenterological Association. Medical position statement: evaluation of liver chemistry
  tests. *Gastroenterology*. 2002;123:1364-66.
Giboney PT. Mildly elevated liver transaminase levels in the asymptomatic patient. *Am Fam Physician*.
  2005;71:1105-10.
Heidelbaugh JJ, Bruderly M. Cirrhosis and chronic liver failure: Part 1. Diagnosis and evaluation. *Am
  Fam Physician*. 2006;74:756-62.
Hoefs JC, Chen PT, Lizotte P. Noninvasive evaluation of liver disease severity. *Clin Liver Dis*.
  2006;10:535-62.
Navarro VJ, Senior JR. Drug-related hepatotoxicity. *N Engl J Med*. 2006;254:731-39.

---

44   Low Back Pain

Dan F. Criswell, MD, & David C. Lanier, MD

KEY POINTS

• Low back pain (LBP) is a broad category of symptomatic low back conditions organized
  into four distinct groups based on duration of symptoms from the initial episode: **acute,**
  ≤6 weeks duration; **subacute,** ≥6 weeks but ≤3 months duration; **chronic,** ≥3 months
  duration; and **acute imposed on chronic,** acute flares with a background of chronic back
  pain.

- Most of the patients seen in primary care settings for acute LBP have no evidence of serious underlying spinal pathology, and diagnostic testing should not be a routine part of their initial evaluation. Seventy percent of patients with LBP clinically improve within 2 weeks and 90% within 4 to 6 weeks. (SOR **A**)
- The clinical history and physical examination are generally effective in identifying the few patients who potentially have serious causes of LBP and need further evaluation immediately. A patient's failure to improve with 6 weeks of conservative treatment is also an indication for further evaluation. (SOR **A**)
- The treatment goal for acute or chronic LBP is for the patient to be active as soon as possible. Bed rest beyond 24 hours should be avoided. (SOR **A**)
- Pain reduction is a primary treatment goal in LBP but attempts at restoration of function is more problematic. Patients with LBP associated with litigation or worker's compensation often have prolonged recovery times. Lack of restored function produces significant disability and costs to industry and the healthcare system.

I. **Definition.** Low back pain (LBP) is pain, muscle tension, or stiffness below the costal margin and above the inferior gluteal folds, with or without pain or neuromotor deficits in the leg (sciatica). Pain may be central (midline) or referred to nonmidline structures including the connective tissues and peripheral nerves innervated by the spinal cord. Most back pain symptoms are **nonspecific** and result from overuse or injury of the ligaments and muscles that hold together the lumbosacral (LS) vertebrae or from degenerative osteoarthritis of the articular processes of the facet joints. All nonmechanical causes of LBP account for less than 2% of all cases. **Specific** mechanisms resulting in LBP include the following:
   A. Herniation of an intervertebral disk, causing inflammation or direct pressure on nerve roots exiting from the LS spinal cord.
   B. Fracture of a vertebra, which may be traumatic or pathologic.
   C. Malignant neoplasm of the spine.
   D. Spinal stenosis, mechanical pressure on neural structures resulting from a degenerative narrowing of the bony spinal canal.
   E. A defect of the vertebral arch (spondylolysis) leading to slippage of all or part of a vertebra on another (spondylolisthesis).
   F. Spinal infection.
   G. Inflammatory diseases.
   H. Referred visceral pain from vascular, genitourinary, or gastrointestinal diseases.

II. **Diagnoses**
   Acute (LBP of ≤6 weeks duration): This is the most common form of LBP and usual causes are mechanical. Nonspecific acute LBP affects both sexes, with men being affected at younger ages (30–50 years) than women (≥50 years). Associated risk factors include repetitive lifting, bending, stooping or pulling, static work positions, sedentary lifestyle especially when coupled with nonaccustomed intense activity, and cigarette smoking. There is only a weak association with obesity. (SOR **A**)
   Specific diagnoses presenting as acute LBP include the following:
   A. Herniated nucleus pulposis (HNP), typically inducing an inflammatory response while compressing the nerve root exiting the LS cord (leg symptoms).
   B. Vertebral fracture—traumatic or pathologic (osteoporosis or tumor).
   C. LBP originating from sources other than the back (e.g., gastrointestinal or genitourinary tract or the abdominal aorta) or associated with systemic symptoms must be ruled out.
   Subacute: or **Chronic (6 weeks to** beyond 3 months): This can be associated with prolonged recovery of acute LBP. but may indicate more serious underlying pathology. Depending upon age and other underlying factors, the following are specific causes of subacute LBP:
   A. Osteoarthritis of the lumbar spine with associated conditions including spinal stenosis, osteoarthritis of the facet joints, osteoarthritis of the sacroiliac joints.
   B. Lumbar disk herniation not spontaneously resolving by 6 weeks. As many as 75% of patients with acute disk rupture do not progress to the subacute category; those with cumulative microdiscal tears are more likely to progress to subacute or chronic LBP.
   C. Those with intrinsic musculoskeletal defects including spondylolysis (pars defects), spondylolisthesis (forward vertebral slippage), scoliosis of greater than 40%, limb length discrepancies of ≥1 cm. are at risk of progression to subacute or chronic LBP. Idiopathic

scoliosis, typically found in young females rarely, causes back pain and the USPSTF has found insufficient evidence for or against routine screening of asymptomatic adolescents. (SOR **Ⓐ**)

D. Patients with bony neoplasms or osteoporosis). Osteoporosis is age related ($\geq$65 years in women and $\geq$70 years in men) and influenced by genetics, but also medication (e.g., corticosteroids). Malignant neoplasms cause less than 1% of subacute or chronic LBP; metastatic lesions from breast, prostate or lung primaries are 25 times more common than primary bone lesions. (SOR **Ⓐ**)

E. Inflammatory diseases (including ankylosing spondylitis, rheumatoid arthritis, and Reiter's syndrome) account for only 0.3% cases of chronic LBP.

F. Infectious diseases (osteomyelitis, diskitis, and abscesses) usually occur in patients with diabetes mellitus, sickle cell disease, immunosuppressive disorders including HIV, IV drug use, history of spinal surgery/instrumentation or previous spinal infections.

G. In the United States, the most common causes of chronic LBP are behavioral or psychological issues leading to secondary gain and prolongation of symptoms. (SOR **Ⓐ**) Patients with chronic LBP are more likely to have poor job satisfaction. Patients with compensation issues have a worse prognosis than patients without compensation issues. In children, psychosocial rather than mechanical factors are associated with LBP. Other associations include emotional problems, conduct problems, headaches, nonspecific abdominal pain, sore throat, and daytime tiredness.

Chronic with acute flares: Any of the aforementioned chronic conditions can be associated with acute flares as well. Typically discogenic lesions maintain a degree of chronic stability until increased activity, devolution of the underlying discal lesion or additional trauma produces an acute flare of the chronic lesion.

III. Symptoms

A. Onset. Back strain typically has an acute, sudden onset, as may the pain from a compression fracture. Pain caused by medical conditions (e.g., inflammation, cancer, or referred visceral pain) generally has a more gradual or insidious onset.

B. Frequency and duration. Most mechanical LBP occurs in intermittent episodes that last from a few days to a few months. A degenerating disk may cause low-grade, persistent discomfort that is exacerbated during acute flare-ups. Patients with osteoarthritis, inflammatory conditions, or cancer usually develop chronic persistent symptoms.

C. Time of day. Inflammatory conditions produce greater back pain and stiffness in the morning; mechanical disorders typically cause pain that increases with the day's activities. Most individuals with spinal cancer complain of back pain that is worse during the night.

D. Location of pain. Most mechanical and medical disorders result in pain localized to the LS spine and surrounding areas. Nerve root irritation (e.g., from a herniated disk, spinal stenosis, or spondylolisthesis) is signaled by pain that radiates from the back to the lower leg or is felt exclusively in the lower leg. Poorly localized pain along nonanatomic routes suggests the presence of social or psychological distress.

E. Aggravating and alleviating factors. Pain caused by mechanical disorders typically improves with recumbency and worsens with activity, whereas patients with back pain caused by inflammatory diseases or tumor often feel worse with bed rest. Relief of pain only with absolute immobility is often a sign of acute infection or a compression fracture.

IV. Signs. The purpose of the physical examination of a patient with LBP is to supplement information obtained in the medical history in searching for serious underlying spinal pathology (e.g., cancer) or possible neurologic compromise. The basic elements of the examination are the following:

A. Vital signs. The presence of fever or weight loss may indicate infection or cancer.

B. Inspection. An **antalgic** gait, resulting from avoidance of weight bearing on the involved leg, may be a sign of nerve root irritation.

C. Spinal range of motion. Very limited range of motion is most common in patients with symptom magnification. However in patients with fever or systemic findings, a significantly reduced range of motion suggests the possibility of a spinal infection.

D. Palpation. Most patients with back strain will exhibit **local tenderness** or **muscle spasm**. These signs, however, are neither highly sensitive nor specific. **Point tenderness** over bony landmarks is a sensitive but nonspecific sign of infection. It is also commonly seen in patients with arthritis or cancer. Pain from percussion of the sacroiliac joints is suggestive but not diagnostic of ankylosing spondylitis.

E. **Neurologic evaluation.** This examination emphasizes ankle and knee reflexes, ankle and great toe dorsiflexion strength, and distribution of sensory complaints.

1. **Diminished or absent ankle reflex, calf weakness or atrophy,** and **sensory loss along the lateral aspect of the foot** are caused by compression of the first sacral nerve root (S1).

2. **Weakness of dorsiflexors of the ankle or great toe** and **sensory loss along the medial foot** are caused by compression of the fifth lumbar root (L5).

3. **Diminished knee jerk** is caused by compression of the fourth lumbar nerve root (L4). This is a relatively uncommon finding.

4. Pain during a **straight leg raising test** indicates nerve root irritation or compression. The examiner raises the affected leg of the supine patient by the heel while keeping the knee fully extended. In a positive test, pain below the knee occurs when the leg is raised 30 to 60 degrees.

F. **Abdominal, rectal, and pelvic examination.** A mass detected on abdominal examination may indicate cancer or aortic aneurysm. A rectal and pelvic examination is especially important if cancer or infection is suspected, or if the patient is new to the practice or has not been examined in the recent past.

G. **Anatomically "inappropriate" signs. These signs** elicited on examination often identify psychological distress as a result, or as an amplifier, of LBP. Such signs include back pain from downward pressure applied to the skull, patient overreaction during the examination, or marked discrepancy between the examination and the patient's ability to dress or move about.

H. **Extremities:** An often neglected but very important physical finding is limb length discrepancy. A greater than 1 cm discrepancy (measured from the anterosuperior iliac spine to the lateral malleolus) can cause LBP. In patients with buttock pain, the Patrick's test (patient supine, thigh and knee flexed, lateral malleolus over the opposite patella, and pain produced by abducting the bent knee) indicates hip pathology instead of neurologic referred pain.

V. **Laboratory Tests.** For most patients with acute LBP, x-rays, imaging studies, and laboratory tests are unnecessary. Table 44–1 lists the signs/symptoms on the initial history and physical examination that suggest a need for immediate testing. Testing is also indicated if significant improvement of LBP is not seen after 2 to 4 weeks of conservative treatment.

A. **Radiologic evaluation** should be used selectively and the results interpreted with care. **Plain films** of the back do not rule out significant LS spine disease and may give false-negative results in as many as 40% of patients with known vertebral cancer. Moreover, conditions such as degenerative arthritis, narrowed disk space, mild scoliosis, facet subluxation, and minor congenital abnormalities (e.g., spina bifida occulta) detected radiographically may be unrelated to back pain, since these conditions are noted with the same frequency in symptomatic and asymptomatic individuals. ACHPR guidelines recommend plain film radiography only with major trauma, age ≤20 or ≥70 years, history of cancer, constitutional symptoms, or back pain worse when supine or resting. (SOR Ⓐ) However adherence to these guidelines still overutilizes plain film radiography. Therefore the clinical recommendation is not to use the age criterion, but to defer x-rays for 2 to 3 weeks unless there is a high risk of other serious disease. (SOR Ⓐ) Lumber x-rays for

TABLE 44–1. SIGNS/SYMPTOMS THAT SUGGEST A NEED FOR EARLY IMAGING IN ADULT PATIENTS WITH ACUTE LOW BACK PAIN

Finding	Rationale for Early Imaging
Major trauma (e.g., fall, MVA)	Possible fracture
Age ≥50 y	Greater risk of cancer, compression fracture
History of cancer	Greater risk of underlying malignancy
Unexplained weight loss	Greater risk of cancer or infection
Fever, immunosuppression, human immunodeficiency virus, IV or injection drug use	Risk for spinal infection
Saddle anesthesia, bladder or bowel incontinence	Possible cauda equina syndrome
Severe or progressive neurologic deficit	Possible cauda equina syndrome or severe nerve root compression

IV, intravenous; MVA, motor vehicle accident.

patients with LBP for $\geq$6 weeks may increase patient satisfaction (at 9 months but not 3 months) but do not improve patient function, severity of pain, or overall health status. (SOR **A**)

Bone scan should be considered for patients with signs or symptoms suggestive of cancer, infection, or occult fractures of the vertebrae—conditions for which bone scans are more sensitive in detecting rather than plain films. However, positive scan results almost always need to be confirmed using other tests.

For patients at risk (Table 44–1), whose symptoms persist despite normal plain films, and those who fail to improve within 6 weeks of conservative treatment, **magnetic resonance imaging (MRI)** is a logical next imaging step. An MRI is inappropriate as a screening test unless neurologic deficits are present or strong suspicions of cancer or cauda equina syndrome are present. Even in the presence of simple radiculopathy, the American Academy of Neurology recommends no MRIs until after 7 weeks of conservative therapy. (SOR **A**) The sensitivity of the MRI may produce false-positive results: bulging disks, focal disk protrusions, and annular tears are common in patients without LBP. Fear may be more disabling for some patients with LBP than any organic condition, and irrelevant radiographic findings probably contribute to this fear.

B. Simple **clinical screening tests** such as the **erythrocyte sedimentation rate** and **serum alkaline phosphatase** can be used to evaluate patients with LBP at risk of having malignancy or an acute infectious or inflammatory process (Table 44–1). Abnormalities of the **urinalysis** may help identify those patients suspected of having referred back pain of urinary origin. However, **serologic tests** (e.g., antinuclear antibodies, rheumatoid factor, and HLA-B27) should not be used for routine screening of patients with LBP since the common spondyloarthropathies affecting the back are seronegative conditions.

C. Electromyography is occasionally useful in assessing a patient with leg symptoms that are possibly back-related and of more than 3 to 4 weeks duration. Test results are not reliable before this time.

VI. Treatment (Table 44–2). When back pain is found to result from medical conditions such as cancer or infection, specific treatment should be directed at the underlying disease. Treatment for almost all other causes of acute LBP (including early treatment of minor neural compression) should be conservative, aimed at relieving pain, maintaining or restoring function, and reassuring the patient that the acute symptoms are self-limited.

A. Activity. Staying active within the limits permitted by the acute pain leads to a more rapid recovery than either bed rest or specific back-mobilizing exercises. Prolonged periods of sitting and activities stressful to the back (e.g., lifting) may need to be limited temporarily. The goal, however, is for the patient to be back to normal activities as soon as possible. Neither prolonged bed rest (i.e., more than a few days) nor spinal traction has any proven efficacy in the treatment of acute LBP. In chronic back pain, most good quality studies indicate that graded activity does not significantly improve pain or long-term function. (SOR **A**)

B. Medication. Nonsteroidal anti-inflammatory drugs (NSAIDs), such as ibuprofen (1600 mg/d), are effective for short-term symptomatic relief in patients with acute symptoms. There is no evidence that any particular NSAID has superior efficacy. **Acetaminophen** (2600 mg/d, every 4–6 hours) is a reasonably safe and effective alternative for patients who are intolerant of NSAIDs. **Muscle relaxants do not exhibit any direct action on skeletal muscle and owe their efficacy to sedation. Such agents,** e.g., cyclobenzaprine (10–20 mg every 24 hours for several days), appear to be as effective as NSAIDs in relieving back symptoms, although drowsiness (which occurs in up to 30% of patients) may limit the patient's ability to ambulate or participate in other activities. There is no added benefit when muscle relaxants are used in combination with NSAIDs. Patients with severe pain not relieved with other conservative treatment may require opioids. Short-acting agents (hydrocodone 5, 7.5, or 10 mg in combinations of acetaminophen from 325–500 mg or ibuprofen 200 mg) are only indicated for treatment of acute LBP and uncontrolled acute flares in chronic LBP. These opioid agents have an effective half-life of only 4 to 6 hours and can be abused if used other than acutely. In those patients with chronic LBP only able to maintain functional capacity with opioids, long-acting opioids (methadone 10–40 mg q 12 h or sustained release morphine or oxycodone 10–160 mg q 12 h) provide steady state analgesia and avoid peaks and valleys of therapeutic effect seen with short-acting opioids. It is important to establish pain contracts in treating patients with potent long-acting opioids and help patients realize the goal of treatment is not pain control but preservation of function. Low-dose **tricyclic**

TABLE 44–2. MAJOR EVIDENCE-BASED RECOMMENDATIONS FOR TREATEMENT OF LOW BACK PAIN

Intervention/Outcome	SOR	Grade of Significance
Acute back pain		
Therapeutic exercise /pain, function/return to work (RTW)	1	C
Continued normal activities vs. forced bedrest/function/pain/RTW	1	A for RTW–C for function
Mechanical traction/pain and global satisfaction	1	C
Therapeutic ultrasound/pain	1	C
TENS/pain	1	C
Subacute low back pain		
Therapeutic exercise/pain, function, global satisfaction	1	A
Mechanical traction/global satisfaction and RTW	1	C
Chronic low back pain		
Therapeutic exercise/pain, function, RTW	1	A for pain/function – C for RTW
Mechanical traction/pain, function, RTW, and global satisfaction	1	C
Therapeutic ultrasound/pain	1	C
TENS/pain and function	1	C
Biofeedback/pain and function	1	C
Massage, electrical stim, thermotherapy	ISD	ISD

Strength of Recommendation Grades
I: Evidence from at least 1 properly randomized controlled trial (RCT)
II-1: Evidence from well-designed controlled trials without randomization
II-2: Evidence from well-designed cohort or case control analytic studies
II-3: Evidence from comparisons between times or places with or without the intervention.
III: Expert opinion, descriptive studies, expert panel
ISD: Insufficient data

	Significance of Recommendations Grades	
Grade	Clinical Significance	Statistical Significance
A	$\geq 15\%$	$p \leq 0.05$ in RCT
B	$\geq 15\%$	$p \leq 0.05$ in non-RCT
C+	$\geq 15\%$	**none,** $p \geq 0.05$
C	$\leq 15\%$	**none,** $p \geq 0.05$
D	$\leq 0\%$	**none,** $p \geq 0.05$

(Data from Philadelphia Panel evidence-based clinical practice guidelines on selected rehabilitation interventions for low back pain. *Phys Ther.* 2001;81(10):1641-1674.)

antidepressants (nortriptyline 25–50 mg at bedtime) in the absence of clinical depression can be useful in the treatment of subacute and chronic LBP by likely improving sleep and serving as adjuvants to other analgesics. Although improving pain, there is no improvement in functional status. (SOR **A**) Selective serotonin reuptake inhibitor (SSRI) antidepressants neither improve pain nor function compared to placebo. (SOR **A**) Alternative medication including **willow bark extract** (standardized to 120–240 mg of salicin) for 4 weeks in treatment of acute LBP is statistically significant for pain relief compared to placebo (p = 0.001, NNT 3–7). (SOR **A**) Systemic **corticosteroids (prednisone 20–30 mg/d for 5–7 days)** significantly improve acute pain associated with acute lumbar disk herniations. **Botulinin toxin A** has been demonstrated to be safe and effective in the treatment of some patients with chronic LBP. (SOR **A**) **Epidural corticosteroid injections** (in consultation with a pain management specialist) may be useful in the treatment of leg pain and sensory deficits early in the course of sciatica secondary to a herniated lumbar disk. Their use should be based on clinical findings rather than imaging results. There is no evidence that injections into facet joints or trigger points improve pain relief or function.

C. **Physical modalities. Spinal manipulation** has been shown in some studies to be effective in reducing acute LBP (and perhaps in speeding recovery) within the first month of symptoms. **Osteopathic manipulation treatment (OMT)** and standard care have similar clinical results but medication use is less in the OMT group. (SOR **A**) Other modalities such as diathermy, ultrasonography, or massage treatments have no proven effect on longer-term outcomes. When compared to control injections alone, prolotherapy, injection of an irritant solution into connective tissue theoretically to strengthen tissue through scarification, demonstrates no clinical superiority in treatment of chronic LBP. (SOR **Ⓐ**) There is limited evidence regarding lumbar supports offer no benefit compared to no treatment for nonspecific LBP and may actually risk worsening pain. (SOR **Ⓑ**)

D. Exercise. The patient should be encouraged to begin low-impact aerobic exercise (e.g., short walks, swimming, or cycling) as soon as possible. More rigorous exercise programs to improve abdominal and paraspinal muscle tone should be delayed for at least 2 weeks following the onset of symptoms. Attainment of aerobic exercise capacity is critical in maintaining functional capacity for patients with subacute and chronic LBP. (SOR **Ⓐ**) *Viniyoga* is more effective than either exercise treatment or self-care in improving functional capacity in patients with LBP. (SOR **Ⓐ**)

E. Patient education. In addition to assuring the patient that in more than 80% of cases the acute LBP will resolve or improve significantly within 4 to 6 weeks, the clinician should focus on the patient's general physical condition. A program of weight loss, exercise, and cessation of smoking can help prevent recurrence of symptoms, which occurs in as many as 75% of patients with occupationally related acute episodes of LBP. For patients with work-related injuries, instruction in body mechanics, (appropriate work stance, lifting, and carrying) with follow-up can reduce incidence of recurrent injury. Job design/redesign to avoid pain-inducing movements may also help prevent recurrences. For patients with subacute or chronic LBP, exploration of psychosocial or behavioral issues can help identify elements that may be contributing to delayed or prolonged recovery.

F. Surgery. The only absolute indication for early lumbar disk surgery is an acute disk herniation associated with either a cauda equina compression or progressive neurologic deficits. Patients with significant pain and unequivocal, disk-related neurologic signs and symptoms may be treated either medically or surgically, depending on individual patient preferences. Surgical diskectomy may substantially improve the short-term symptoms and quality of life for carefully selected patients with painful herniated lumbar disks, although long-term outcomes do not appear to be superior to medical treatment. Surgical consultation is not needed, however, for patients with acute LBP alone who have neither sciatica nor evidence of cancer, infection, or fracture. Surgical treatment of spinal stenosis or spondylolisthesis should be considered only after an adequate trial of conservative therapy as recommended above for treatment of subacute and chronic LBP. There are few randomized controlled trails indicating superiority of surgery to long-term conservative management in terms of pain or function. Operative outcomes for pain but not disability or walking distance are better in patients with spinal stenosis when compared to conservative management. (SOR **Ⓐ**)

VII. Prevention and Screening: The USPSTF concludes insufficient evidence to recommend for or against routine use of interventions as primary prevention of LBP in adults in primary care settings. Specific interventions include: counseling patients to exercise, educational interventions, and use of mechanical supports or risk factor modification. (SOR **Ⓐ**)

REFERENCES

Grover F Jr, Pereira SL. Clinical inquiries. Is MRI useful for evaluation of acute low back pain? *J Fam Pract.* 2003;52(3):229-39.

Harris GR, Susman JL. Managing musculoskeletal complaints with rehabilitation therapy: summary of the Philadelphia Panel evidence-based clinical practice guidelines on musculoskeletal rehabilitation interventions. *J Fam Pract.* 2002;51(2):1042-46.

Kendrick D, Fielding K, Bentley E, Kerslake R, Miller P, Pringle M. Radiography of the lumbar spine in primary care patients with low back pain: randomized controlled trial. *BMJ.* 2001;322:400-405.

Malmivaara A, Slatis P, Heliovaara M, et al. Surgical or nonoperative treatment for lumbar spinal stenosis? A randomized controlled trial. *Spine.* 2007;32:1-8.

Staiger TO, Gaster B, Sullivan MD, Deyo RA. Systematic review of antidepressants in the treatment of chronic low back pain. *Spine.* 2003;28:2540-2545.

U.S. Preventive Services Task Force. Primary care interventions to prevent low back pain in adults: recommendation statement. *Am Fam Physician.* 2005;71(12):2337-38.

45   Lymphadenopathy

Fred Kobylarz, MD, MPH

KEY POINTS

- The majority of patients who present to primary care physicians with lymphadenopathy have benign, easily identifiable causes. The prevalence of malignancy in these patients is as low as 1.1%.
- Risk factors for malignancy include age greater than 40 years, hard texture, fixed lymph nodes, weight loss, and supraclavicular location. Lymph nodes greater than 1 cm in diameter are considered abnormal.
- Localized lympadenopathy involves a single anatomic area and can be observed for up to 1 month. Seventy-five percent of patients with lymphadenopathy will present with localized findings.
- Generalized lymphadenopathy involves two or more noncontiguous anatomic areas, is present in 25% of patients with lymphadenopathy, usually implies a systemic disorder and should always prompt investigation.

I. **Definition.** Lymph nodes are found throughout the body except the central nervous system and serve as filtering sites of lymphatic fluid for microorganisms, malignant cells, particulate debris, or other substances. The normal immune response to acute or chronic infectious or noninfectious substances may lead to lymph node hardening and enlargement. **Lymphadenopathy** is defined as lymph nodes that are abnormal in size, consistency, or number.

II. **Common Diagnoses** (Table 45–1). Lymphadenopathy is common in primary care and occurs because of a vast array of conditions. In the primary care setting, unexplained lymphadenopathy is rare, occurring in only 0.6% of the general population in one study. Of these patients, 3.2% required a lymph node biopsy and only 1.1% were found to have a malignancy. Few additional studies have supported this low prevalence of malignancy. In contrast, in specialized clinics, the prevalence of malignancy on lymph node biopsy is 40% to 60%.

III. **Symptoms.** The patient's history often guides clinical evaluation.

    A. **Age** is an important predictor of diagnosis. The most common causes of lymphadenopathy in children are infectious or benign. The majority of healthy children have palpable

---

TABLE 45–1. **COMMON CAUSES OF LYMPHADENOPATHY IN PRIMARY CARE**

Diagnosis	Etiologies
1. Infectious	Viral infections: infectious mononucleosis, cytomegalovirus (CMV), rubella, herpes simplex, infectious hepatitis, adenovirus, rubeola, and human immunodeficiency virus (HIV)
	Nonviral infections: scarlet fever, cat-scratch disease, brucellosis, tuberculosis, atypical mycobacterial syphilis, histoplasmosis, leptospirosis, tularemia, malaria, toxoplasmosis, typhoid fever, and pyogenic bacterial infections
2. Autoimmune	Connective tissue disorders (e.g., systemic lupus erythematosus and rheumatoid arthritis, dermatomyositis, Sjögren syndrome)
	Benign reactive hyperplasia
3. Iatrogenic	Serum sickness
	Medications (e.g., phenytoin)
4. Metabolic	Gaucher's disease, Niemann-Pick disease, hyperthyroidism
5. Malignant	Leukemia, lymphomas (Hodgkin's and non-Hodgkin's), skin neoplasms, Kaposi's sarcoma, metastatic cancers, malignant histiocytosis, metastases
6. Miscellaneous	Kawasaki disease, sarcoidosis, and chronic pseudolymphomatous lymphadenopathy

(Data from Bazemore AW, Smucker DR. Lymphadenopathy and malignancy. *Am Fam Physician*. 2002;66:2103-2110.)

cervical, axillary, and inguinal lymph nodes. In patients older than 40 years, malignant causes of lymphadenopathy are more likely.

B. Duration. Lymphadenopathy that lasts less than 1 month is usually infectious. Lymphadenopathy persisting for more than 1 month in the absence of an obvious explanation is usually abnormal.

C. Constitutional symptoms (e.g., fatigue, fever, weight loss, unusual rashes, or arthralgias) suggest malignancy, infection, autoimmune diseases, or serum sickness-like syndrome (e.g. medications).

D. Localized symptoms may suggest the cause of lymphadenopathy (e.g., sore throat and cervical lymphadenopathy).

E. Personal/social or family history such as travel, exposure to animals, occupation, dietary habits, hobbies, sexual history and orientation, drug use, infectious contacts, and environmental and family history may help in the diagnosis. For example, travelers to a tropical area have an increased risk of tuberculosis, scrub typhus, and leishmaniasis; patients exposed to cats may have an increased risk of cat-scratch disease or toxoplasmosis; those exposed to lacerations from gardening are at increased risk of sporotrichosis; hunters exposed to wild rodents have an increased risk of tularemia; history of sexual exposure raises the question of gonorrhea, syphilis, genital herpes, or HIV, and patients with a personal history of dysplastic nevus syndrome may have lymphadenopathy from melanoma.

F. A **medication history** may assist diagnosis. Some medications are known to cause lymphadenopathy (e.g. phenytoin) and others (e.g. penicillins or sulfonamides) are more likely to cause a serum sickness-like syndrome with lymphadenopathy.

IV. Signs. When lymphadenopathy is localized, examination should focus on the region drained by the lymph nodes. Since most localized lymphadenopathy is in the head and neck region, physical examination should include ears, nose, throat, and neck examination. If lymph nodes are detected, several characteristics should be noted.

A. Size. Lymph nodes greater than 1 cm in diameter are considered abnormal. Exceptions are epitrochlear nodes, which are abnormal if greater than 0.5 cm, and inguinal nodes, which are abnormal if greater than 1.5 cm. There is little information supporting diagnosis based on size alone.

B. Texture. Softer or fluctuant lymph nodes suggest infectious or inflammatory causes; harder nodes suggest malignancy.

C. Pain. Although nonspecific, tenderness on palpation of lymph nodes suggests an inflammatory cause; absence of pain makes a more serious condition or malignancy more likely.

D. Location of the lymphadenopathy can be helpful in diagnosis (Table 45–2). Seventy-five percent of patients in primary care will present with localized lymphadenopathy: 55% in the head and neck region, 14% in the inguinal region, 5% in the axillary region, and 1% in the supraclavicular region.

E. Lymphadenopathy and splenomegaly suggest infectious mononucleosis, lymphoma, leukemia, or sarcoidosis.

V. Laboratory Tests (Figure 45–1). A careful history and physical examination should allow the physician to determine, if careful observation, treatment, or additional testing is needed. The critical task is to determine which patients with lymphadenopathy have benign, self-limited conditions and which have malignancy or other serious conditions requiring further evaluation and specific treatment. A complete blood cell count with differential often provides useful information and is almost always indicated. Other studies are based on clinical presentation.

A. Lymph node biopsy should be considered when simple measures have failed to provide a diagnosis or if there is a clinical suspicion of serious disorders.

    1. Certain clinical features suggest **the need for an early biopsy.** These features include a diameter of greater than 2 cm, hard and fixed consistency, lack of pain or tenderness on palpation, patient age older than 40 years, an abnormal chest x-ray result (e.g., adenopathy or infiltrate), associated signs and symptoms (e.g., weight loss or hepatosplenomegaly), an absence of upper respiratory tract symptoms, an enlargement of a supraclavicular node, or a cervical node in a smoker. For evaluation of posterior mediastinal lymphadenopathy, endoscopic ultrasound guided fine needle biopsy aspiration (EUS-FNA) is the procedure of choice. (SOR Ⓒ)

    2. Supraclavicular nodes have the highest yield from biopsy and inguinal nodes the lowest.

    3. During follow-up for undiagnosed lymphadenopathy, nodes that remain constant in size for 4 to 8 weeks or fail to resolve in 8 to 12 weeks should be biopsied.

TABLE 45–2. DIFFERENTIAL DIAGNOSIS OF LYMPHADENOPATHY BY LOCATION

Location	Diagnosis
Cervical The most common area of lymphadenopathy and most cases are caused by infections.	*Infections:* Viral upper respiratory infections, bacterial pharyngitis, infectious mononucleosis, cytomegalovirus, toxoplasmosis, mycobacterial diseases, and rubella *Malignancy:* Non-Hodgkin's lymphoma, Hodgkin's disease, head and neck malignancy. *Others:* Kawasaki syndrome, sarcoidosis, Kikuchi's disease, oral injuries, and dental lesions
Supraclavicular This location has the highest risk of malignancy; 90% of patients older than 40 years will have a malignancy when lymphadenopathy is localized here.	*Infections:* Chronic fungal (histoplasmosis) and mycobacterial infections *Malignancy:* Left supraclavicular node (Virchow's node) drains the abdomen or thorax and is associated with breast cancer, lymphoma, and other malignancies. Right supraclavicular node drains the mediastinum, lungs, and esophagus and is associated with pathology in these areas
Axillary Usually secondary to infection or malignancy.	*Infections:* Staphylococcus and strep infections of the arm, tularemia, cat-scratch disease, and toxoplasmosis *Malignancy:* Breast cancer, lymphoma, and melanoma
Epitrochlear Rare in healthy patients.	*Infections:* Infectious mononucleosis, HIV, secondary syphilis, leprosy, rubella, tularemia, and leishmaniasis *Malignancy:* Lymphoma and leukemia
Inguinal Most adults will normally have some degree of inguinal enlargement, and there is a low suspicion of malignancy.	*Infections:* Sexually transmitted diseases, bubonic plague *Malignancies:* Squamous cell carcinoma of the penis/vulva, lymphoma, or melanoma
Generalized Lymphadenopathy found in two or more distinct anatomic regions and needs prompt investigation.	It is more likely to result from serious infections (e.g., HIV), autoimmune disease (e.g., systemic lupus erythematosus), hematologic malignancies (e.g., leukemia), and metastatic cancers

(Data from Ferrer R. Lymphadenopathy: differential diagnosis and evaluation. *Am Fam Physician.* 1998;58:1313-1320.)

4. As many as 25% of patients with nondiagnostic initial biopsy and persistent lymphadenopathy who undergo a second biopsy have cancer.

B. Imaging studies such as ultrasonography, computerized tomography (CT scan), or magnetic resonance imaging (MRI) of the involved area may differentiate lymphadenopathy from nonlymphatic causes. (SOR **C**) CT scan and MRI are useful to demonstrate the presence of mediastinal, mesenteric, or retroperitoneal lymph nodes.

C. A **bone marrow examination** is indicated for patients with severe anemia, neutropenia, thrombocytopenia, or a peripheral smear with malignant blast cells.

VI. Treatment for select conditions.

A. Viral infections. Treatment of viral infections is primarily limited to symptomatic treatment such as warm compresses, analgesics, and the avoidance of trauma to the swollen node.

B. Cat-scratch disease. This disease is usually self-limited, requiring only symptomatic treatment. Aspiration of suppurative glands may reduce swelling and discomfort. Incision and drainage should be avoided to prevent sinus tract formation. For typical cat-scratch disease, there is no proven response to antibiotics. In one study, treatment with oral azithromycin for 5 days afforded significant clinical benefit by decreasing total lymph node size. (SOR **A**)

C. Neoplasm. Neoplastic disease should be referred to an oncologist for treatment.

D. Mycobacterial disease. Nodes affected with atypical mycobacteria are treated by surgical excision. (SOR **A**) A positive culture result or the demonstration of acid-fast bacilli is the most direct method of diagnosis, although treatment of *Mycobacterium tuberculosis* can be initiated on the basis of the clinical presentation and a positive skin test.

E. Acute lymphadenitis. Initial therapy should be directed toward staphylococcal and streptococcal infections. Oral cephalexin (25–50 mg/kg in divided doses up to 500 mg 4 times a day), erythromycin (30–50 mg/kg up to 500 mg 4 times a day), or a semisynthetic

Peripheral lymphadenopathy

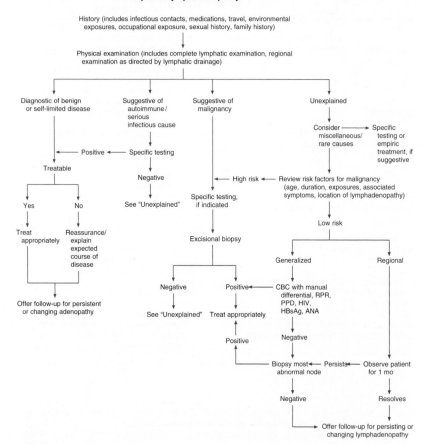

FIGURE 45–1. Algorithm for the evaluation of peripheral lymphadenopathy. CBC, complete blood count; RPR, rapid plasma reagin; PPD, purified protein derivative; HIV, human immunodeficiency virus; HbsAg, hepatitis B surface antigen; ANA, antinuclear antibody. (Adapted with permission from Ferrer R. Lymphadenopathy: differential diagnosis and evaluation. *Am Fam Physician*. 1998;58:1315.)

penicillinase-resistant penicillin such as dicloxacillin (25–50 mg/kg up to 500 mg 4 times a day for 7–10 days) is useful.

REFERENCES

Bazemore AW, Smucker DR. Lymphadenopathy and malignancy. *Am Fam Physician*. 2002;66:2103-2110.

Ferrer R. Lymphadenopathy: differential diagnosis and evaluation. *Am Fam Physician*. 1998;58:1313-1320.

Habermann TM, Steensma DP. Lymphadenopathy. *Mayo Clin Proc*. 2000;75:723-732.

Mcgee SR. ed. Peripheral lymphadenopathy. *Evidence-based Physical Diagnosis*. 2nd ed. Philadelphia, PA: Saunders Elsevier; 2007:chap 24.

Pangalis GA, Vassilakopoulos TP, Boussiotis VA, et al. Clinical approach to lymphadenopathy. *Semin Oncol*. 1993;20:570-582.

Vassilakopoulos TP, Pangalis GA. Application of a prediction rule to select which patients should undergo a lymph node biopsy. *Medicine*. 2000;79:338-347.

46   Myalgia

Tomás P. Owens, Jr., MD

KEY POINTS

- Most common causes of myalgia can be diagnosed through careful history and examination, without laboratory testing.
- Ischemia should be considered in localized myalgia, especially with suggestive risk factors and normal muscle examination.
- Drug-induced rhabdomyolysis should be considered as a potential cause of myalgia.

I. **Definition.** Myalgia is defined as generalized or localized pain perceived as originating in skeletal muscle tissue, usually characterized as a deep, aching sensation but sometimes as a burning or electric sensation. Myalgia can be classified as acute (lasting less than 1 month) or chronic (lasting more than 3–6 months); localized (one or a few muscle groups), or generalized (involving more than 4 areas), or symmetric or asymmetric.

II. **Common Diagnoses.** As many as one-third of patients presenting in an ambulatory primary care setting complain of muscle pain in an extremity or the back. In the general population, as many as 60% of adults have musculoskeletal pain lasting more than 1 month or caused by identified trauma. In one study, 9% of primary care visits were for myofascial pain syndrome.

A. **Viral syndromes** (and other infectious causes). Most **viral syndromes** have seasonal variations, with a winter peak in temperate climates. Arbovirus myalgic syndromes such as West Nile virus predominate between June and October, paralleling the mosquito vectors. Children are particularly at risk for viral syndromes, but myalgia in children is less common than in adults. A rare form of localized myalgia is staphylococcal myositis, which can accompany cellulitis.

B. **Major or minor trauma.** Accumulated metabolic waste products cause myalgia with strenuous exercise in a deconditioned patient. Direct blunt or minor repetitive trauma occurs with occupational hazards (faulty ergonomics, repetitive acts of a monotonous nature), recreational pursuits ("weekend warrior syndrome," with poor conditioning or inappropriate training), or substance abuse (repetitive accidental or self-inflicted trauma), and results in hemorrhage within the muscle tissue and muscle fiber or fascial tears. Trauma also causes muscle spasm or cramping.

C. **Fibromyalgia and myofascial pain** (8%–10% of all visits to a primary care outpatient practice).

1. **Fibromyalgia syndrome** (FMS—former name: fibrositis) affects 5% to 10% of the US population at some point in their lives. It is more common in women than in men (10:1), particularly in women aged 20 to 50 years (with a peak incidence at age 35). **FMS** is the second most common disorder in American rheumatology practices. It has been associated with a history of sexual abuse during childhood, drug use, and eating disorders, but no causal relationship has been established. Depression, personality disorders, and anxiety are also strongly associated. In FMS, there is a clear evidence of regional blood flow abnormalities in the thalamus and caudate nucleus associated with low pain-threshold levels (hyperalgesia) and allodynia, occurring spontaneously or as a neuroimmune response to viral, physical, or psychologic trauma. Biochemical abnormalities are inconsistent and muscle biopsies are unrevealing.

2. Less generalized **myofascial pain syndromes** (not fulfilling **FMS** diagnostic criteria) are seen in up to 50% of the population, are equally common in men and women, and have a much better prognosis with appropriate therapy.

D. **Collagen vascular diseases** (approximately 15% in the general population and more than 1 million newly afflicted patients each year). **Inflammatory articular diseases** such as rheumatoid arthritis and lupus occur primarily in women between ages 20 and 50 years. **Inflammatory nonarticular diseases** such as **polymyositis** and **dermatomyositis** are more common in children and occur equally in men and women, but a particular form occurs in men older than 40 years in association with malignancy of other organ systems. **Polymyositis** may be postviral; it is especially common following enteroviral infections (particularly Coxsackie) or parasitic infection such as trichinosis. Polymyalgia rheumatica **(PMR)** occurs equally in men and women, usually older than 65 years. Myalgia from these conditions is caused by immune-mediated inflammation of periarticular structures or muscle.

   E. Vascular insufficiency ($\leq$1% of patients with myalgia) has a strong association with older age, smoking, hypertension, hyperlipidemia, and diabetes mellitus, and is because of insufficient arterial perfusion.

   F. Primary muscle malignancy is an extremely rare cause of myalgia in primary care, has no specific risk factors, and causes pain from rapid tumor growth with compression of surrounding structures.

   G. Substance-induced (an emerging cause of myalgia).

      1. The "statins" class of lipid-lowering agents have been associated with generalized myalgia by direct toxicity to the muscle (rhabdomyolysis), the so-called **statin-induced myalgia (SIM).** The synchronous use of gemfibrozil or cyclosporine potentiates the effect significantly, as does preexisting renal insufficiency. It is believed that lipid-soluble statins are more likely to produce the syndrome and one has been withdrawn from the market for that reason (cerivastatin).

      2. Excipients in some batches of L-tryptophan (e.g., "peak X") produce a complex immunologic response called **eosinophilia-myalgia syndrome (EMS).**

      3. Other drugs causing myopathy or myalgia but not discussed further here include amphotericin B, chloroquine, cimetidine, clofibrate, glucocorticoids, oral contraceptives, and zidovudine.

III. Symptoms and Signs

   A. Myalgia from **viral syndromes** is relatively mild; the time course parallels the course of the illness and is often accompanied by other systemic viral infection symptoms (malaise, weakness, and any combination of the following: headache, nausea, vomiting, diarrhea, and upper respiratory symptoms, including fever). Viral myalgia is usually generalized, but many patients complain of pain in larger, proximal muscle groups and in the back (particularly the upper back, trapezius, neck, and shoulders). Many experts believe that acute viral infection can precipitate progression to chronic fibromyalgia, in which case patients report a deep, aching discomfort, an inability to be comfortable in any position, and localized, palpable pain. **Well-localized inflammation in relation to cellulitis** is the hallmark of staphylococcal myositis.

   B. Myalgia caused by **trauma** is localized and specific to the trauma history.

      1. Patients sometimes report the **relatively acute onset of localized pain** without associated illness or obvious trauma, but further probing usually reveals some new activity or minor repetitive act (e.g., lifting furniture, gardening, painting, or new work responsibility).

      2. The **pain of major trauma** (e.g., a motor vehicle accident) or overuse usually starts several hours after the event and reaches a peak at 48 hours. The pain may persist for days or weeks, particularly if the offending activity is not identified and stopped. The patient may report some loss of function or pain with a specific movement or position, which sometimes reminds the patient of the precipitating event.

      3. Tenderness on palpation of the specific muscle, sometimes with crepitus, decreased active range of motion, and erythema, is a common finding. Blunt trauma may cause ecchymosis, hematoma, superficial abrasions, pain on palpation, or decreased active and passive range of motion of the involved muscle.

   C. FMS and myofascial pain syndrome

      1. With **FMS,** pain is worse after even minimal activity and may include generalized symptoms such as diffused myalgia, fatigue, a low-grade fever, muscle tension, headache, and skin sensitivity. Sleep disturbance is a particularly prominent and nearly universal complaint. The American College of Rheumatology (1990) diagnostic criteria require the patient to have at least 11 of 18 possible tender points on digital examination and a history of widespread pain (Figure 46–1).

      2. Myofascial pain syndrome includes localized muscle pain in such common areas as the paraspinous regions of the upper and middle back, trapezius, levator scapulae, neck, shoulders, arms, glutei, and legs, often manifesting as **trigger points** (excruciatingly painful foci of muscle from which diffused pain and spasm emanate).

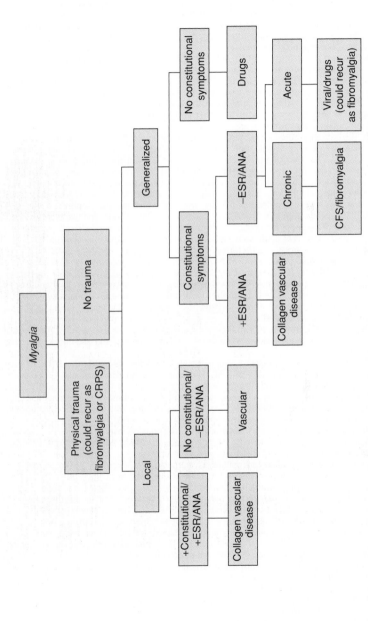

FIGURE 46-1. Evaluation of patients presenting with myalgia. ANA, antinuclear antibody; CFS, chronic fatigue syndrome; CRPS, complex regional pain syndrome; ESR, erythrocyte sedimentation rate. (Adapted from Klippel JH, ed. *Primer on the Rheumatic Diseases.* 13th ed. Arthritis Foundation; 2001.)

D. The myalgia associated with a **collagen vascular disease** parallels the course of the primary disease and is increased with muscle palpation.

1. Signs of the primary rheumatic disease dominate, including joint erythema and swelling or effusion, Raynaud's phenomenon, vasculitis, conjunctivitis, urethritis, or uveitis.
2. The onset of **polymyositis** may be acute, particularly in children, and may include fever. In polymyositis of any cause, the patient reports loss of muscle function either from pain or loss of functioning neuromuscular units. Primary idiopathic **dermatomyositis** can present with multiple abdominal complaints (e.g., pain or dysphagia) and a classic lilac-colored (heliotrope) rash.
3. The pain and stiffness of inflammatory articular disorders such as **rheumatoid arthritis** or lupus are more severe in the morning upon arising.
4. Patients with **PMR** complain of stiffness, weakness, and pain, particularly in the hip and shoulder girdle, along with systemic symptoms such as malaise, fatigue, and headache caused by temporal (giant cell) arteritis.

E. **Vascular insufficiency** causes the most severe myalgia, is intermittent, and physical examination of the muscle is often normal.

1. The pain associated with **arterial insufficiency** (intermittent claudication) occurs with exercise of a predictable type and intensity, is almost always in the lower extremity, and can be described precisely by the patient. It resolves shortly after cessation of the activity. With severe ischemia, rest pain may be present. Peripheral pulses are delayed, decreased, or absent, and extremity blood pressures are asymmetric, with a decreased leg: arm ratio (see Chapter 42). Marked hair loss, dry skin, decreased capillary refill, and pronounced pachyonychia are commonly present.
2. In **thoracic outlet syndrome,** pain, weakness, paresthesias, and claudication occur in one of the upper extremities. Abducting the affected arm and externally rotating the shoulder may precipitate pain with or without cyanosis and pulselessness.
3. The pain of **venous insufficiency** is more vague in onset, nature, and cessation, but is often related to a dependent position of the affected extremity (almost always the leg). Signs may include increased circumference, edema, erythema, brawny hyperpigmentation, and ulceration of dependent areas, particularly the lower legs and ankles ("venous stasis"). Rarely, a **superior vena cava syndrome** will produce symptoms in the upper extremities. These findings are accompanied by facial swelling, cyanosis, and neck vein distention.

F. The pain of **primary muscle malignancy** is gradual in onset and vague in nature, but patients usually report associated weakness and an enlarging, localized mass in the body of the muscle.

G. Generalized, slowly progressive pain, asthenia, and weakness/tenderness of major muscle groups are characteristic of **SIM.** The onset of **EMS** can be abrupt or insidious. Early manifestations include low-grade fever, fatigue, cough, dyspnea, arthralgias, muscle cramping, and myalgia. Arthritis and evanescent erythematous rashes ensue thereafter. Months later, scleroderma-like skin changes, an ascending polyneuropathy with cognitive impairment and, rarely, pulmonary hypertension can develop.

IV. **Laboratory Tests** (Figure 46–1). Laboratory evaluation is not usually indicated in cases of viral syndrome, trauma, or clear-cut myofascial pain or **FMS,** but tests may be indicated in patients with rheumatic symptoms or who have impressive systemic symptoms; whose symptoms have persisted despite conservative, nonspecific therapy for several weeks; who have joint effusions; or whose disease has caused significant disability.

A. **Complete blood cell count.** The white blood cell count may show a neutropenic or inflammatory (leukocytosis) reaction with a viral syndrome, although the **erythrocyte sedimentation rate (ESR)** is usually normal. The ESR helps differentiate fibromyalgia (normal) from collagen vascular diseases (ESR ≥ 50 mm/h). A high ESR may prompt further testing (e.g., antinuclear antibody, rheumatoid factor, and more comprehensive rheumatologic panels) (Chapter 39.) Parasitic infection may cause eosinophilia. Mild anemia and thrombocytosis are common in rheumatic diseases.

B. **Culture of specific infectious lesions** (e.g., primary herpes simplex) should be performed only in appropriate clinical situations. Routine throat swabs and blood cultures are usually unrevealing with viral syndromes.

C. **X-rays** may be required to rule out bony pathology as a result of known or unknown trauma (particularly relating to the hip or pelvis in older persons), or they may be helpful in patients with localized muscle or tendon pain that is difficult to differentiate from bone pain (e.g., lateral epicondylitis).

D. **An empiric trial of a low-daily dose (10–20 mg orally) of prednisone** usually has a dramatic positive effect on almost all collagen vascular diseases and thus has some diagnostic value pending more definitive studies. Unfortunately, corticosteroid use can produce a sense of well-being in patients with almost any pathology. Therefore, empiric corticosteroid use must be adapted to each clinical situation.

E. **Impedance Doppler studies** are required in patients with an evidence of vascular insufficiency (see Chapter 42). These may be followed or, in some instances, supplanted by **arteriography** or **venography.**

F. **Muscle biopsy** should be arranged for any enlarging painful muscle mass not explainable by specific trauma. Abnormal histology on muscle biopsy is the only specific laboratory abnormality in patients with primary muscle tumors.

G. In **SIM,** marked elevations of creatine phosphokinase (CPK) are noted. In **EMS,** the eosinophil count is higher than 1000/mm^3 and biopsy results show eosinophilic fasciitis.

V. **Treatment**

A. Myalgia caused by **viral syndromes** is relieved by treatment with nonsteroidal anti-inflammatory drugs (NSAIDs). **Aspirin,** 650 to 1000 mg orally every 4 hours, is as effective as a prescription NSAID. **Ibuprofen,** 600 mg orally every 6 hours, or **naproxen,** 375 to 500 mg orally every 8 to 12 hours, is an excellent substitute for the anti-inflammatory effects of aspirin, but each is less effective as an antipyretic agent. **Acetaminophen,** 650 to 1000 mg orally every 4 hours (maximum 4 g/d in adults, 3 g/d in the elderly, with strict alcohol avoidance), can be used in addition to the NSAID and, for severe myalgia (particularly associated with severe headache), can be combined with **codeine,** 15 to 30 mg (e.g., Tylenol no. 2 or no. 3), 1 to 2 tablets orally every 4 hours. So-called muscle *relaxants* exert their effects primarily as sedatives and have no true direct muscle action, yet they can be used with caution in selected patients where the risk/benefit ratio is favorable.

B. Myalgia caused by **blunt trauma** or repetitive minor trauma is best treated with rest of the affected muscle, ice and cold therapy (particularly after use of the muscle injured by overactivity or inappropriate athletic training), heat therapy (particularly for generalized myalgia or for localized myalgia with muscle weakness or dysfunction), and immobilization (for localized myalgia caused by trauma with significant dysfunction). Immobilization can be accomplished with either soft (e.g., felt) or rigid (e.g., commercial plastic or metal) splints for only a few days to prevent atrophy and weakness. A more specific diagnosis of the cause of repetitive overuse injuries (recreational or occupational) may lead to specific exercises, strengthening, or avoidance/modification of certain activities in the workplace (ergonomics evaluation) or during leisure time.

C. For myalgia caused by **fibromyalgia,** prescribed reading may give the patient hope by naming the problem and informing the patient that the problem is manageable, and it may help in controlling health care-seeking behavior for the multitude of associated symptoms. Support groups may have similar benefit. Multidisciplinary outpatient treatment programs, even as brief as 1.5 days, can have a significant effect on the impact of illness.

1. An **exercise and stretching program** should be similar to that for rehabilitation of a postmyocardial infarction patient, with specific submaximal heart rate targets (70%–80% of maximum heart rate), frequency (3–5 times weekly), and duration (30–40 minutes with appropriate warm-up and cool down). (SOR **Ⓐ**)

2. **Antidepressant therapy** (e.g., imipramine or amitriptyline, 75–100 mg orally 1–2 hours before bedtime, selective serotonin reuptake inhibitors, heterocyclics, or bupropion) is used in a moderate dosage, primarily for regulation of sleep rather than in the full dosage used for major depressive disorder (SOR **Ⓐ**) (see Chapter 92).

3. **Trigger point injection** can be performed as often as necessary with local anesthetic, (SOR **Ⓑ**) but preferably no more than four or five injections per year should be given if corticosteroids are used. The trigger point should be carefully palpated to determine the point of most exquisite pain. This point is injected intramuscularly using a long 25- or 27-gauge needle that contains 0.5 to 1.0 mL of a long-acting local anesthetic such as bupivacaine 0.25%. There is some evidence of benefit from moving the needle around and pulling back into different parts of the trigger point ("needling"). A corticosteroid, such as 0.5 mL of **triamcinolone,** 40 mg/mL, can be added to the injection, but no evidence exists that the injection will be more effective than any of the local anesthetics or even normal saline.

4. **Cognitive behavioral therapy** is very useful in many patients. Minimal intervention (paradoxical approach) has also been effective, particularly in the outpatient setting.

(SOR **Ⓐ**) Disability claims, with legal and financial repercussions and tremendous secondary gain, make the management of this syndrome complicated in some patients.

5. **Alternative, integrative, complementary,** or **balanced medicine** approaches, including biofeedback, yoga, meditation, tai chi, qi gong, spray-and-stretch techniques, acupuncture, and acupressure, may be helpful, but strong research supporting their efficacy is scarce. (SOR **Ⓑ**)

D. Myalgia caused by **collagen vascular diseases** is managed according to the underlying disease, usually with rheumatologic consultation (see Chapter 39).

1. **PMR,** though self-limited, is treated with low-dose (10–20 mg) oral prednisone daily for symptomatic relief. (SOR **Ⓐ**) If the patient is not nearly asymptomatic in a few days, the diagnosis should be reconsidered. Treatment should continue for 1 year and the disease can be followed clinically, without regard to ESR, tapering off the prednisone over a few weeks and restarting if the pain recurs. Most people are asymptomatic in 24 months, rarely 36 months. Some patients have recurrences early or in a few years, and they respond well to retreatment.

2. If the patient has symptoms of **giant cell arteritis,** treatment with 60 mg of prednisone daily should start immediately to prevent ischemic events, which occur in 20% of all nontreated patients. If the diagnosis is uncertain, a biopsy of the affected arterial segment should be done within a few days. Response to prednisone is rapid and complete in approximately 3 to 4 days. In 4 to 6 weeks the ESR should be normal. Prednisone dose is decreased by 10% per month while continuing a monthly check of the ESR, until a dose of 10 mg/d is reached. That dose is continued for at least 2 years. Approximately 10% of patients may require 3 or more years of therapy. Some patients have recurrences or may require very long or permanent low-dose therapy. Side effects of prednisone include weight gain, worsening of glucose intolerance, and cushingoid features.

E. Myalgia caused by **vascular insufficiency** (see Chapters 23 and 42).

F. Myalgia resulting from **primary muscle malignancy** is relieved by excision of the malignant tumor, in consultation with a surgeon and oncologist.

G. In **SIM,** full resolution of symptoms and normalization of laboratories can be expected within days of drug withdrawal. Intense hydration and loop diuretics are recommended with CPKs higher than 2000. Chronic renal insufficiency can occur secondary to the myoglobinuria. **EMS** has been successfully treated during the acute phase with oral prednisone, 1 to 2 mg/kg/d, for days to weeks. (SOR **Ⓒ**) In the late phase of the illness, no treatment has been helpful. Most symptoms and signs of the illness are resolved in 2 to 3 years, except for cognitive impairment and peripheral neuropathy.

REFERENCES

Goldenberg DL, Burckhardt C, Crofford L. Management of fibromyalgia syndrome. *JAMA.* 2004;292: 2388-2395.

Klippel JH, ed. *Primer on the Rheumatic Diseases.* 13th ed. Arthritis Foundation; 2008.

Rooks DS. Fibromyalgia treatment update. *Curr Opin Rheumatol.* 2007;19(2):111-117.

Sim J, Adams N. Systematic review of randomized controlled trials of nonpharmacological interventions for fibromyalgia. *Clin J Pain.* 2002;18(5):324.

Sprott H. What can rehabilitation interventions achieve in patients with primary fibromyalgia? *Curr Opin Rheumatol.* 2003;15(2):145.

Taylor RR, Friedberg F, Jason LA. *A Clinician's Guide to Controversial Illnesses: Chronic Fatigue Syndrome, Fibromyalgia, and Multiple Chemical Sensitivities.* Sarasota, FL: Professional Resource Press; 2001.

47   Nausea & Vomiting

George R. Wilson, MD, Gabriel D. Paulian, MD, & Frances Emily Biagioli, MD

KEY POINTS

- Nausea and vomiting are common complaints that are usually self-limited.
- Serious etiologies can be ruled out with a thorough history and a directed examination.
- Once any necessary tests show negative results, treatment can be directed toward symptom control and dehydration precautions.
- Complimentary and alternative medical (CAM) therapies provides additional, nonpharmacologic treatment of nausea and vomiting.

I. **Definition. Nausea** is an unpleasant sensation of impending vomiting. **Retching** is a strong, involuntary effort to vomit without bringing up emesis. **Vomiting** is the forceful expulsion of stomach contents in a series of involuntary, spastic movements. **Regurgitation** is the return of gas or small amounts of food from the stomach. It is often, but not always, caused by an incompetent lower esophageal sphincter. **Eructation** is the voiding of gas or, on occasion, small quantities of acidic fluid from the stomach through the mouth. It involves a process similar to regurgitation and is roughly equivalent to belching. Vomiting occurs when the neuroreceptors in the emetic center are stimulated. The emetic center is located in the reticular formation of the medulla oblongata and is rich in histamine (H_1) receptors, muscarinic (M) cholinergic receptors, and serotonin (5-HT_3) receptors. (Figure 47–1) The emetic center can be stimulated through:

    Stomach or **biliary duct distention** via vagal afferents.

    Vestibular dysfunction via H_1 and M receptors.

    Metabolic derangements, toxins, and some medications (cardiac glycosides, chemotherapy, and opiates) via the chemoreceptor trigger zone, which is rich in 5-HT_3 and dopamine (D_2) receptors.

    Inflammation or ischemia of the heart, pericardium, liver, pancreas, gallbladder, or peritoneum.

II. **Common Diagnoses.** Nausea and vomiting are common presenting symptoms in a variety of ailments found in most age and gender groups. Because of lost function, nausea and vomiting inflict significant costs on the patient, their employers, and society. Common etiologies of nausea and vomiting generally fall into one (or more) of a number of groups, irrespective of age or gender (Table 47–1), but there are a few unique patient groups requiring special mention.

    A. **Vomiting in infants** may be associated with acute gastroenteritis or any acute illness (e.g., urinary tract infections, otitis media, or asthma), feeding disorders, hypertrophic pyloric stenosis, or intussusception.

       1. **Hypertrophic pyloric stenosis** is the most common surgical condition encountered in the first 2 to 8 weeks of life. Risk factors include first born, male sex (1:150 males, 1:750 females), and a positive family history.

       2. **Intussusception** usually occurs later, between 6 and 18 months of life, but a small percentage occurs after age 3 years.

       3. **Regurgitation** (spitting up) often is a normal variant and should be distinguished from vomiting. Simple regurgitation usually resolves by 6 months of age. Faulty feeding technique can lead to excessive regurgitation and vomiting, and this should be considered when confronted with an infant with failure to thrive.

    B. **Vomiting in children,** in addition to the above diagnoses, may be from abdominal migraines (cyclic vomiting syndrome). They occur in as much as 1% of all children, at the mean age of 5 years; male incidence is higher in younger children, but male–female incidence equalizes as children grow older. Cyclic vomiting has a familial component and may be associated with migraine headaches.

    C. **Vomiting in women** is common during the first trimester of normal pregnancy and, while discomforting, rarely is of much clinical significance. However, when the vomiting

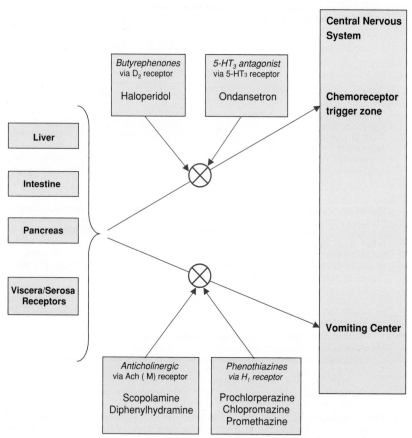

FIGURE 47–1. Schematic representation of interface between vomiting stimuli, therapeutic pathways and site of vomiting impulse.

is excessive and leads to poor weight gain, weight loss or dehydration, other etiologies must be considered. These would include **hyperemesis gravidarum, hydatidiform molar pregnancy,** and **extrauterine pregnancy** (with and without abdominal pain).
   D. **Vomiting in adolescents and adults** is usually caused by common, and benign, disorders. Listed in the approximate order of frequency:
      1. **Acute gastroenteritis,** usually viral (rotavirus, reovirus, adenovirus, Norwalk) and self-limited. Most common between ages 20 and 29 years and occurs most often in autumn and winter. Bacterial etiologies include *Staphylococcus aureus, Salmonella, Bacillus cereus,* and *Clostridium perfringens.*
      2. **Reaction to drugs** (Table 47–2), **toxins** (environmental exposures, alcohol, illicit drugs), or **tumor-produced peptides.**
      3. **Gastrointestinal tract inflammation or infection.** Gastroesophageal reflux disease **(GERD)** and **peptic ulcer disease** are more common with excessive caffeine, alcohol, or nicotine use.
      4. **Pancreatitis** occurs with alcohol, hypertriglyceridemia, or cholelithiasis, and can be idiopathic. Risk factors for **cholelithiasis** include obesity, rapid weight loss, pregnancy, female gender, and older than age 40. It may also be seen in women taking oral contraceptive medication.

TABLE 47–1. DIFFERENTIAL DIAGNOSIS OF NAUSEA AND VOMITING

Medications and Toxic Etiologies	Infectious Causes	Disorders of the Gut and Peritoneum	CNS Causes	Endocrinologic and Metabolic Causes
Cancer chemotherapy	Gastroenteritis	Mechanical obstruction	Migraine	Pregnancy
Severe-cisplatinum, dacarbazine, nitrogen mustard	Viral	Gastric outlet obstruction	Increased intracranial pressure	Other endocrine and metabolic
Moderate-etoposide, methotrexate, cytarabine	Bacterial	Small-bowel obstruction	Malignancy	Uremia
Mild-fluorouracil, vinblastine, tamoxifen	Nongastrointestinal infections	Functional gastrointestinal disorders	Hemorrhage	Diabetic ketoacidosis
Analgesics	Otitis media	Gastroparesis	Infarction	Hyperparathyroidism
Aspirin		Chronic intestinal pseudo-obstruction	Abscess	Hypoparathyroidism
Nonsteroidal anti-inflammatory drugs		Nonulcer dyspepsia	Meningitis	Hyperthyroidism
Auranofin		Irritable bowel syndrome	Congenital malformation	Addison's disease
Antigout drugs		Organic gastrointestinal disorders	Hydrocephalus	Acute intermittent porphyria
Cardiovascular medications		Pancreatic adenocarcinoma	Pseudotumor cerebri	Postoperative nausea and vomiting
Digoxin		Inflammatory intraperitoneal disease	Seizure disorders	Cyclic vomiting syndrome
Antiarrhythmics		Peptic ulcer disease	Demyelinating disorders	Miscellaneous causes
Antihypertensives		Cholecystitis	Emotional responses	Cardiac disease
β-blockers		Pancreatitis	Psychiatric disease	Myocardial infarction
Calcium channel antagonists		Hepatitis	Psychogenic vomiting	Congestive heart failure
Diuretics		Crohn's disease	Anxiety disorders	Radiofrequency ablation
Hormonal prepara-tions/therapies		Mesenteric ischemia	Depression	Starvation
Oral antidiabetics		Retroperitoneal fibrosis	Pain	
Oral contraceptives		Mucosal metastases	Anorexia nervosa	
Antibiotics/antivirals			Bulimia nervosa	
Erythromycin			Labyrinthine disorders	
Tetracycline			Motion sickness	
Sulfonamides			Labyrinthitis	
Antituberculous drugs			Tumors	
Acyclovir			Meniere's disease	
Gastrointestinal medications			Iatrogenic	
Sulfasalazine			Fluorescein angiography	
Azathioprine				
Nicotine				

(Continued)

TABLE 47–1. (*Continued*)

Medications and Toxic Etiologies	Infectious Causes	Disorders of the Gut and Peritoneum	CNS Causes	Endocrinologic and Metabolic Causes
CNS active				
Narcotics				
Antiparkinsonian drugs				
Anticonvulsants				
Antiasthmatics				
Theophylline				
Radiation therapy				
Ethanol abuse				
Jamaican vomiting sickness				
Hypervitaminosis				

(Quigley EM, Hasler WL, Parkman HP. AGA technical review on nausea and vomiting. *Gastroenterology*. 2001;120(1):263-286.)

5. **Hepatitis, appendicitis, pyelonephritis, Reye's syndrome** (a complication of aspirin use in children with viral illnesses, especially with influenza or varicella), and **postgastrectomy states** (often associated with bile reflux or the inability to digest and clear foods normally).
6. **Motility disorders** include diabetic gastroparesis and postvagotomy states, as well as intestinal pseudo-obstruction (gastroduodenal motor dysfunction occurring in patients with neuromuscular disorders).
7. **Gastrointestinal obstruction,** such as gastric outlet obstruction, small-bowel obstruction, incarcerated hernia (femoral or inguinal), volvulus, and achalasia. Risk factors and related diagnoses include having prior abdominal surgeries, being elderly, or having hernias or cancer. Bariatric surgery is a new surgical cause for nausea and vomiting.
8. **Vestibular disorders,** to include motion sickness, Meniere's disease, perilymphatic fistula, or labyrinthitis (either viral or toxic).

TABLE 47–2. MEDICATIONS ASSOCIATED WITH NAUSEA AND VOMITING

Pain medications	Aspirin
	Nonsteroidal anti-inflammatory drugs
	Opiate analgesics (codeine, morphine, etc.)
	Antigout drugs
Infectious disease treatments	Erythromycin or tetracycline
	Nitrofurantoin
	Sulfa drugs
	Acyclovir
	Tuberculosis medications
Cardiac medications	Digoxin
	Antiarrhythmics
	Antihypertensive medications (diuretics, beta-blockers, calcium channel blockers)
Gastrointestinal medications	Sulfasalazine
	Azathioprine
Other medications	Theophylline
	Anticonvulsants
	Nicotine
	Chemotherapy agents
	Lithium
	Quinidine
	Oral contraceptives
	Oral diabetes medications

TABLE 47–3. DIAGNOSIS USING SYMPTOMS OF NAUSEA AND VOMITING IN ADULTS

Timing	Characteristics of Vomitus	± Associated Symptoms	± Associated Past Medical History	Possible Diagnoses
Before breakfast	Projectile	Breast tenderness, fatigue Headache, dizziness		Pregnancy Increased intracranial pressure
		Headache, shakiness	Kidney disease	Alcohol Uremia
Delayed (≥1 h after meal)	Digested food Nonbilious, undigested	Early satiety, nonpainful Painless or colicky pain	Diabetes	Gastroparesis Achalasia, Zenker's diverticula, or gastric outlet obstruction
	Bilious, feculent	Colicky pain		Small-bowel obstruction
After meals		Abdominal pain Abdominal or back pain RUQ abdominal pain		Ulcerative disease Pancreatitis Cholecystitis
Immediately after meals (but can make it to the toilet)		No dysphagia	Psychiatric disorders	Bulimia, anorexia, nervosa, or psychoneurotic vomiting
Intermittent attacks			Migraine headache	Cyclic vomiting syndrome (usually initially diagnosed in childhood)

9. **Increased intracranial pressure,** associated with meningitis or space-occupying lesions (e.g., tumor or subdural hematoma).
10. **Metabolic disorders,** including severe electrolyte derangements, uremia, diabetic ketoacidosis, hypercalcemia, adrenal insufficiency, and thyrotoxicosis.
11. **Psychogenic vomiting** associated with syndromes of physical or sexual abuse, posttraumatic stress, and eating disorders.

III. **Symptoms** (Table 47–3). Because there are many diagnoses associated with nausea and vomiting, an accurate history is essential to determining the underlying cause. Details about the **timing** of symptoms (time of day and any association with eating), **characteristics of the vomitus** (digested chyme, bilious, etc.), any **associated symptoms** (abdominal pain or other symptoms), **associated past history,** and **duration of symptoms** are important. As outlined in Table 47–3, there are some consistencies in symptoms that help in diagnosis; following are some examples:
   A. **Timing and relationship to eating.** Before the first meal of the day, immediately after eating, or delayed for several hours.
   B. **Duration of symptoms.** Acute nausea and vomiting usually lasts for days. Acute symptoms are most often caused by toxins, infections (gastroenteritis, systemic, etc.), inflammation (cardiac, gastrointestinal, etc.), or obstruction. Chronic nausea and vomiting, defined as persistence of symptoms for longer than 1 month, poses a more challenging diagnostic dilemma.
   C. **Past medical history.** Abdominal surgery, previous CNS tumor, or eating disorder (bulimia, anorexia nervosa), regardless of whenever in past, must be explored.
   D. **Specific symptoms.**
      1. **Diffuse abdominal pain** and distention are common findings in mechanical bowel obstruction. Distention without pain, consistent with ileus. Periumbilical pain moving toward the right lower quadrant is associated with acute appendicitis. Right upper quadrant pain is consistent with acute cholelithiasis, acute alcoholic hepatitis, and gastritis. Epigastric pain can be consistent with acute pancreatitis or peptic ulcer disease. Severe flank pain, radiating to the groin, common complaint in renal colic.
      2. **Diaphoresis** related to syncope, vagal stimulation, vestibular dysfunction, dysrhythmia, CNS events.
      3. **Sialorrhea** related to toxins, drugs, and acute gastritis. Associated diarrhea, usual in acute food poisoning (staphylococcus).
      4. **Chills,** fever, cough, rhinorrhea, i.e., viral infections.

IV. **Signs.** The physical examination is unremarkable in many cases of nausea and vomiting, especially when associated with motility disorders, metabolic disorders, drugs, and toxins.
   A. **Vomiting in infants and children.**
      1. No fever, no weight loss, no abdominal distention, child does not appear ill; cause may be a **feeding disorder** or **normal regurgitation.**
      2. **Hypertrophic pyloric stenosis:** weight loss, dehydration, occasionally a palpable "olive" mass in the epigastric area in male infants younger than 8 weeks. Careful observation can identify peristaltic wave progressing across the abdominal wall. Precedes a vomiting episode.
      3. Children with **intussusception:** significant abdominal pain, possible palpable sausage-shaped mass located anywhere in the abdomen, but most common in left side, and hemoccult positive loose stools described as "currant jelly."
   B. **Gastrointestinal tract obstruction**
      1. **Small-bowel obstruction:** high-pitched bowel sounds with occasional visible peristalsis.
      2. **Incarcerated hernia:** painful and represents a medical emergency. Two most common hernias are inguinal and umbilical. Hernias can occasionally be diagnosed by auscultating bowel sounds in the hernia sac. Transillumination in a darkened room can be helpful.
      3. **Volvulus:** associated with acute abdominal distention, periumbilical tenderness.
      4. **Gastric outlet obstruction:** may have distention. Epigastric succussion splash can be demonstrated more than 4 hours postprandial.
   C. **Increased intracranial pressure**
      1. Focal neurologic signs are usually present with **space-occupying central nervous system lesions.** Neurologic signs, changes in mental status are associated with embolic or hemorrhagic stroke (cerebral or cerebellar)
      2. A change in mental status, fever, and neck stiffness; signs of **meningitis,** other CNS infections. Same findings with blood in cerebrospinal fluid. Positive Brudzinski's sign, when present and not appreciated, can lead to a false assumption of no neck stiffness.
   D. For a discussion of signs associated with the following causes of nausea and vomiting, see the chapters indicated below.
      1. Vestibular disorders (Chapter 17).
      2. Pregnancy (Chapter 97).
      3. Gastroenteritis (Chapter 16).
      4. Gastritis (Chapter 19).
      5. Appendicitis (Chapter 1).
      6. Hepatitis (Chapter 43).
      7. GERD (Chapter 19).
V. **Diagnostic Testing:** This is directed by the history and physical examination. Tests and studies that aid in the evaluation of nausea and vomiting are listed in Table 47–4, along with usual costs. The history will guide the examiner toward one or more broad classes of diagnoses. Specific testing can then be directed toward likely etiologies. Pregnancy must be considered and excluded in all female patients capable of childbearing, regardless of age. When symptoms are severe, diagnostic tests should be done to determine the patient's renal function, electrolyte and hydration status before definitive studies to determine etiology. When infection is likely, a complete blood count with differential and urinalysis is required. Further urgent diagnostics may be needed if symptoms, risk profiling, and examination suggest severe etiologies such as increased intracranial pressure, obstruction, meningitis, or drug overdosing. If symptoms become chronic (4 weeks), history and physical examination should be reviewed for elusive diagnoses. When the cause remains cryptic or symptoms persist or worsen, more complex diagnostic testing or gastroenterology referral may be necessary. Following are the additional points to remember:
   A. **Supine and upright abdominal x-ray series** (KUB) are appropriate when pain is present. These are inexpensive, easy to obtain, and helpful when obstruction, incarcerated hernia, perforation, or ileus are considered.
   B. **Upper gastrointestinal series** and **small-bowel follow-through** will help detect obstruction, masses, and large ulcers. But low-grade obstruction and smaller mucosal lesions may not be seen. **Enteroclysis** (small-bowel enema) may also be necessary.
   C. Air-contrast barium enema still has a place in evaluation of the gut, but it has largely been replaced in many situations by contrasted abdominal **computerized tomographic (CT) scan.**

TABLE 47–4. RELATIVE COSTS, BENEFITS, AND RISKS OF DIAGNOSTIC TESTS FOR NAUSEA AND VOMITING

Test	Cost*	Benefit	Risk
Abdominal x-ray	$100	May suggest obstruction, CIIP; may be performed on day of clinical evaluation	Radiation exposure (minimal)
Upper GI barium study	$400	May reveal obstructive or mucosal lesions of upper GI tract	Radiation exposure (modest)
Upper GI and SBFT	$500	Examines small bowel, including terminal ileum	Radiation exposure (modest); may involve prolonged examination
Enteroclysis	$550	Optimal evaluation of small-bowel mucosa	Radiation exposure (modest); oroduodenal intubation
Abdominal CT with oral and IV contrast	$900	Arguably the optimal technique to detect and diagnose cause of obstruction; also examines other intra-abdominal organs	Radiation exposure (modest); possible reaction to IV contrast
Gastric emptying scintigraphy	$600	Quantifies emptying rate of solids and/or liquids	Radiation exposure (minimal)
Esophagogastroduodenoscopy	$950	Optimal examination of esophageal, gastric and duodenal mucosa; biopsies possible	Minimal risk of bleeding, perforation, and sepsis; risks of sedation, if used
EGG	$150	May detect gastric dysrhythmias; indirect measure of gastric motility	None
Antroduodenal manometry	$900	Direct measure of intraluminal pressure changes; detects abnormal motor patterns	Radiation exposure (mild) if fluoroscopy used; nasal intubation

GI, gastrointestinal; IV, intravenous; CIIP, chronic idiopathic intestinal pseudo-obstruction; EGG, electrogastrography.
*Estimated total cost.
(Quigley EM, Hasler WL, Parkman HP. AGA technical review on nausea and vomiting. *Gastroenterology*. 2001;120(1):263–286.)

D. Endoscopy is not first line, but useful for evaluating anatomic lesions, especially if biopsy is required. Included are **sigmoidoscopy, colonoscopy,** or **esophagogastroduodenoscopy** (EGD). Endoscopy is not reliable in diagnosing physiologic gastrointestinal motility disorders, although it can be helpful in diagnoses such as GERD, hiatal hernia, gastric outlet obstruction, and gastroparesis or delayed gastric emptying. Endoscopy of the biliary tract, endoscopic retrograde cholangiopancreatography (ERCP), can assist in diagnosing biliary tract obstruction.

E. Nasogastric tube aspiration that returns significant residual gastric content following overnight fast suggests gastric outlet obstruction or gastroparesis and should be followed by endoscopic evaluation.

F. Formal **psychiatric assessment** should be considered in unexplained chronic nausea and vomiting, especially when there is no associated weight loss, dehydration or electrolyte abnormalities. Psychogenic vomiting (bulimia) can result in severe weight loss and metabolic derangement. This etiology must be considered when a reasonable clinical evaluation has not determined a physiologic cause.

G. Specialized testing is required when a definitive diagnosis is not found and there is clinical evidence to support presence of physiologic dysfunction. These studies are generally entertained on referral to a gastroenterologist.

  1. Radionuclide testing measures gastric emptying rate.

  2. Antroduodenal manometry and **electrogastrography** measure gastric motility and rhythmic functions.

VI. Treatment. Given the various causative etiologies responsible for nausea and vomiting choosing the right therapeutic approach is of utmost importance. When choosing, one has to take into consideration the following basic steps: (1) Identifying the underlying cause for nausea and vomiting. (2) Ability of the patient to follow recommendations. (3) Route of drug administration. (4) Potential side effects of therapy. (5) Patient's ability to afford medication or alternative therapeutic intervention. During diagnostic testing, management is usually symptomatic and must include electrolyte and fluid replacement if needed. If gastrointestinal obstruction is evident, hospitalization for skilled nursing, close monitoring, and surgical consultation are required. If appropriate testing has been done and a definitive diagnosis is still uncertain, symptoms, in a stable patient, may be controlled with a combination of nonpharmacologic measures and antiemetics.

A. **Nonpharmacologic treatment** is appropriate for acute illness when history and physical examination are consistent with a benign process. This can be initiated prior to or in conjunction with pharmaceutical management. In clinically stable adults and older children, limiting oral intake for a period of several hours can be beneficial. This approach can also be used in small children and infants but, because of their small size, careful monitoring is necessary to prevent dehydration and electrolyte problems. Once the patient has been free of symptoms for several hours, reintroducing clear liquids in small quantities and bland foods served cool are helpful.

B. **Complimentary and alternative therapy (CAM)** is an evolving field in medicine but use of alternative therapies is already widespread in the lay population. It is important to inquire about use of these types of therapies since patients are often reluctant to share this information.

   1. **Acupuncture.** Acupuncture has some effect in preventing nausea and vomiting. Stimulation of the P6 acupuncture point has been shown to prevent postoperative nausea and vomiting (PONV) at levels similar to medications. (SOR **Ⓐ**) Acupressure is effective in reducing chemotherapy-related nausea and vomiting, but acupuncture combined with antiemetics and electroacupuncture have been shown to be more beneficial. (SOR **Ⓐ**)

   2. **Ginger extract.** One gram of ginger is more effective than placebo in preventing postoperative nausea and vomiting. (SOR **Ⓑ**)

   3. **Psychological techniques.** Progressive muscle relaxation and guided mental imagery can be used with good effect during chemotherapy treatment. (SOR **Ⓒ**)

   4. **Wrist banding.** Acupressure bands improve nausea on day of chemotherapy treatment, but generally not beyond. Emesis is not reduced. Benefit is due, in part, to placebo effect. (SOR **Ⓐ**)

   5. **Cannabinoids.** Cannabinoids (nabilone, dronabinol, and levonantradol) are slightly superior to conventional antiemetics (prochlorperazine, metoclopramide, chlorpromazine, haloperidol, domperidone, thiethylperazine, or alizpride) and patients prefer them. (SOR **Ⓐ**) Significant side effects such as dizziness, hallucinations, and dysphoria may diminish their widespread use.

C. **Contemporary therapies** are the mainstay of primary care treatment of nausea and vomiting (Table 47–5). Multiple classes of drugs have been found useful and their efficacy has been demonstrated over time. The limiting factors to use of these drugs tend to be route of administration and side-effect profiles. There is a tendency to use these drugs in a linear fashion; however, like other therapies (i.e., antihypertensives and oral hypoglycemics), use of these drugs in a concurrent fashion can often improve efficacy and provide faster relief of symptoms. Drugs useful in treating nausea and vomiting are classified by drug type (e.g., antipsychotics, antihistamines, prokinetic agents) or clinical situation (e.g., bowel obstruction, chemotherapy-induced nausea and vomiting (CINV), and postanesthesia).

   1. **Drug type.**
      a. **Antipsychotics.** The phenothiazines and butyrophenones are useful treatments of acute nausea and vomiting although their side effect profile generally limits long-term therapy. Table 47–5 lists the drugs in this category. Haloperidol and resperidol are butyrophenones. Their site of action is different than the phenothiazines, acting centrally by binding to the dopamine receptors DA_2 and, to a lesser degree, DA_1.

      b. **Antihistamines** are useful in treatment of acute and chronic nausea and vomiting. They are efficacious in treating motion sickness. Examples include dimenhydrinate and meclizine.

      c. **Prokinetic agents** are useful in treating motility disorder, such as diabetic gastroparesis and postvagotomy states. They act centrally, blocking dopaminergic receptors, specifically the D_2 subtype, in the chemoreceptor trigger zone. They improve gastric motility through direct stimulation of gastrointestinal smooth muscle. The only prokinetic agent currently available in the United States is metoclopramide. In addition to its central activity, it augments cholinergic activity peripherally by

TABLE 47–5. PHARMACOLOGIC TREATMENT FOR NAUSEA AND VOMITING

Agents—Receptor Antagonist*—Usual Dose Range	Main Use Situations for This Class	Common Side Effects of This Class
Phenothiazines—D_2 Prochlorperazine (Compazine) 5–10 mg PO/IM q4–6h, 25 mg PR q6h Promethazine (Phenergan) 12.5–25 mg PO/IM q4–6h, 12.5–25 mg PR q6h Chlorpromazine (Thorazine) 10–50 mg po q4–6h, 25–50 IM q3–4, 100 mg PR q6–8h Thiethylperazine (Torecan) 10 mg PO/IM q4–6h, 10 mg PR q6h Perphenazine (Trilafon) 4–8 mg po q6h, 5 mg IM q6h	Chemotherapy, cardiac glycoside, or opiate reactions Radiation therapy effects Postoperative effects Compazine is also used in migraines	Drowsiness Dry mouth Dizziness, hypotension Extrapyramidal reactions (more in children)
Butyrophenones—D_2 Haloperidol (Haldol) 0.5–2 mg q6–12h, 2–3 mg IM q4–6h	Chemotherapy reactions	Less commonly, hypotension Extrapyramidal reactions at higher doses
Serotonin receptor antagonists—5-HT_3 Dolasetron (Anzemet)—100 mg po once, 100 mg IV once Ondansetron (Zofran)—8 mg po twice, 32 mg IV once Granisetron (Kytril)—2 mg po once or 1 mg po bid, 10 μg/kg IV	Chemotherapy reactions Postoperative effects Radiation therapy effects Adjunctively used with steroids	Dizziness, headache Less commonly: prolonged ECG intervals
Prokinetic agents—D_2 Metoclopramide (Reglan)—5–10 mg before meals and qhs, 10 mg IV over 2 min q6h Cisapride (Propulsid)†—No longer on the market	Gastroparesis Gastroesophageal reflux disease	Diarrhea Extrapyramidal reactions
Ethanolamine-antiemetics— H_1Anticholinergic (trimethobenzamide—unknown receptor) Trimethobenzamide‡ (Tigan)—250 mg po qid, 200 IV/PR qid Promethazine (Phenergan)—12.5–25 mg PO/PR q4–6h	Chronic nausea patients Gastroenteritis Less effective, but, fewer side effects than phenothiazines	Drowsiness, dizziness, hypotension May potentiate opiates or other sedatives
Antihistamines—H_1 Dimenhydrinate (Dramamine)—50–100 mg q6–8h, 50–100 mg q12 Meclizine (Antivert, Bonine) 12.5–25 mg q8	Best with vestibular disturbances Motion sickness (best when used in prevention) Meniere's disease	Drowsiness Elders: Confusion Children: Paradoxical CNS stimulation
Anticholinergics—M Scopalamine§ (Transderm Scop)—1 patch 4 h before travel, replace q3 days; for postoperative nausea apply patch the night prior to surgery Hyoscine—150–300 μg q8	Prevention of motion sickness Less effective: postoperative and chemotherapy effects	Dry mouth Fewer side effects when used transdermally
Others Diphenidol hydrochloride¶ (Vontrol)—not on market—Inhibits conduction in vestibular pathways Dronabinol (Marinol)—Cannabinoid—5 mg/m² q1–3	Diphenidol—Use in closely monitored patients, for postoperative, chemotherapy or radiation therapy effects, or labyrinth disturbances	Diphenidol—Auditory and visual hallucinations, disorientation, hypotension Dronabinol—Euphoria, dizziness, paranoia

(Continued)

TABLE 47–5. (*Continued*)

Agents—Receptor Antagonist*— Usual Dose Range	Main Use Situations for This Class	Common Side Effects of This Class
Aprepitant (Emend)—Substance P/neurokinin 1—dose and time vary for pre-anesthesia or chemotherapy. Beware of potential drug interactions	Dronabinol—When other treatments fail Aprepitant—Use with other antiemetics	Aprepitant—Asthenia/fatigue, dizziness

*Serotonin receptor, 5-HT$_3$; dopamine receptor, D$_2$; histamine receptor, H$_1$; muscarinic cholinergic receptor, M.
†Cisapride was removed from the market because of serious cardiac arrhythmias and death. It is available by protocol for patients not responsive to other medications.
‡Trimethobenzamide's receptor is unknown. It is believed to inhibit the chemoreceptor trigger zone.
§Transdermal patch behind the ear every 72 h (removed and reapplied, if necessary).
¶Diphenidol hydrochloride is only available by calling the manufacturer.
CNS, central nervous system; ECG, electrocardiogram.

causing release of acetylcholine from postganglionic nerve endings or by sensitizing muscarinic receptors on smooth muscle. Care must be taken to avoid idiopathic antipyramidal side effects.

    d. Serotonin receptor antagonists are relative newcomers to the treatment of nausea and vomiting. They include the anti-CINV medications such as ondansetron, dolasetron, and granisetron.

    e. Anticholinergic agents include scopolamine, hyoscine, and trimethobenzamide. Trimethobenzamide (Tigan®) should not be used in children when the diagnosis is not clearly defined, since it may worsen Reye's syndrome.

2. Clinical situation.

    a. Bowel obstruction. Treatment of bowel obstruction-induced nausea and vomiting should start with conservative management. Restoring and maintaining adequate hydration, restricting oral intake, and management of pain should be initiated immediately when this diagnosis is considered. In nonsurgical candidates, octreotide is effective. Intravenous haloperidol, at 1 to 2 mgm, is effective in treating nausea and vomiting associated with obstruction.

    b. Vestibular dysfunction. Agents to prevent motion sickness and vertigo (Table 47–5) affect the vestibular system, and probably the emetic center, through antagonism of H$_1$ and M (muscarinic cholinergic) receptors. These agents are most effective if administered prior to the onset of nausea and vomiting. Since acetylcholine mediates impulses from the inner ear, **scopolamine** is an effective motion sickness antiemetic. Side effects include dry mouth and blurred vision. Meclizine is a widely used OTC medication for prevention of nausea and vomiting caused by motion sickness. It exerts its antiemetic effect via depression of labyrinthine excitability and vestibular stimulation.

    c. Infection, toxin, and drug-induced. Treatment of the underlying etiology is paramount. Removal of causative factors (e.g., toxins) and discontinuing or decreasing dose of drugs suspected of inducing nausea and vomiting, should be considered. Infections causing nausea and vomiting are usually viral, and only require maintenance of adequate hydration and electrolytes until resolved. If bacterial infection is suspected, use of appropriate antibiotics is indicated.

    d. Pregnancy-induced nausea and vomiting. Based on the American College of Obstetricians and Gynecologists guidelines, prevention and treatment of pregnancy-related nausea and vomiting should include the following: (1) Taking a **multivitamin** at the time of conception. (2) Taking **vitamin B6** alone or with doxylamine. (SOR **C**) **Ginger extract** will reduce nausea and, to a lesser degree, retching. (SOR **A**) Trials using combination therapy (pyridoxine and metoclopramide) have been shown to be superior to monotherapy with either drug, in the treatment of pregnancy-induced nausea and vomiting. (SOR **B**) Trials of nerve stimulation have been effective in treating pregnancy-induced emesis. (SOR **A**) Corticosteroids used to treat hyperemesis gravidarum are not harmful to the pregnancy or fetus but have not been shown to be beneficial. (SOR **A**)

D. Chemotherapy-induced nausea and vomiting (CINV) is an area where new antiemetics are evolving. **Ondansetron** (Zofran®) and **dolasetron** (Anzemet®) are 5-HT$_3$ receptor serotonin antagonist antiemetics used primarily for prevention of nausea and vomiting associated with chemotherapy. They are generally superior in antiemetic relief compared to prochlorperazine and metoclopramide. (SOR **B**) This may also be true with the combination of a 5-HT$_3$ receptor serotonin antagonist (e.g., ondansetron) plus dexamethasone compared to metoclopramide plus dexamethasone. (SOR **B**) The use of steroids in treating nausea and vomiting should be considered more often for CINV, radiation-induced nausea and vomiting (RINV), and postoperative nausea and vomiting. The 2006 American Society of Clinical Oncology's guidelines for treating CINV in high emetic-risk patients are the three-drug combination: aprepitant, dexamethasone, and a 5-HT$_3$ serotonin receptor antagonist. This treatment is recommended to be given before chemotherapy. (SOR **B**) Dexamethasone alone, or in combination with aprepitant and/or a 5-HT$_3$ serotonin receptor antagonist, is recommended for treatment of delayed emesis following CINV.

E. Radiation therapy-induced nausea and vomiting (RINV) is quite similar to CINV in etiology and treatment. Dopamine receptor antagonists, including metoclopramide, prochlorperazine, and haloperidol have proven to be effective in treating RINV. 5-HT$_3$ serotonin receptor antagonists are also effective RINV antiemetics. Dexamethasone has been the most widely used corticosteroid used in preventing and treating radiation-induced nausea and vomiting. The American Society of Clinical Oncologists recommends antiemetic therapy be instituted before each fraction and continued for at least 24 hours posttherapy.

F. Postoperative nausea and vomiting (PONV) therapy is another area where new treatments are being developed. The following are recommendations for managing PONV:

1. **Serotonin receptor (5-HT$_3$) antagonists** are more effective when given at the end of surgery. They have a favorable side effect (headache, constipation, increased liver enzymes) profile and are considered equally safe to conventional therapies. Ondansetron is one most researched of this group, and there does appear to be some difference in efficacy, but overall their efficacy appears to be equivalent. Refer to Table 47–5 for dosing.

2. **Corticosteroids** are most effective when given prior to anesthesia induction.

3. **Droperidol**, dosed below 1 mg, administered at the end of surgery, is effective in controlling PONV. (SOR **C**) It is effective when used in concert with patient-controlled analgesia (PCA) devices delivering morphine. Droperidol has an FDA warning for induced torsades de pointes, as well as QT prolongation and death, but there are no documented cases of dysrhythmia or cardiac death reported at the doses used in managing PONV. (SOR **C**)

REFERENCES

American Gastroenterological Association. American Gastroenterological Association medical position statement: nausea and vomiting. *Gastroenterology.* 2001;120(1):261-262.

Bsat FA, Hoffman DE, Seubert DE. Comparison of three outpatient regimens in the management of nausea and vomiting in pregnancy. *J Perinatol.* 2003;23(7):531-535.

Kris MG, Hesketh PJ, Somerfield MR, et al. American society of clinical oncology guideline for antiemetics in oncology: update 2006. *J Clin Onc.* 2006;24(18):2932-2947, 5341-5342.

Longstreth GF. Approach to the patient with nausea and vomiting. UpToDate online, version 15.1, current through December 2006. www.uptodate.com.

Longstreth GF, Hesketh PJ. Characteristics of antiemetic drugs. UpToDate online, version 15.1, current through December 2006. www.uptodate.com.

Quigley EM, Hasler WL, Parkman HP. AGA Technical review on nausea and vomiting. *Gastroenterology.* 2001;120(1):263-286.

Yost NP, McIntire DD, Wians FH, Ramin SM, Balko JA, Leveno KJ. A randomized, placebo-controlled trial of corticosteroids for hyperemesis due to pregnancy. *Obstet Gynecol.* 2003;102(6):1250-1254.

48   Neck Pain

Michael P. Rowane, DO, MS, FAAFP, FAAO

KEY POINTS

- Nearly two-thirds of individuals experience uncomplicated neck pain primarily occurring during middle age.
- A careful history and physical examination are usually sufficient to establish a diagnosis, yet in most cases, no definable pathology is found.
- Laboratory investigations play a minor role in most cases of neck pain, but they may help confirm a diagnosis.
- Treatment of problems arising primarily from neck joints and associated ligaments and muscles successfully alleviates symptoms, whereas treatment of problems involving the cervical nerve roots or spinal cord often does not achieve complete pain relief.
- A full recovery occurs in 40% of patients with an acute neck pain, while 80% completely recover within 1 year of a whiplash injury.

I. **Definition.** Neck pain is perceived as posterior cervical discomfort, from the superior nuchal line to the first thoracic spinal process, not equivalent to cervical radicular pain and may present as referred pain to the region. Neck pain may be classified as:

  Mechanical, including nontraumatic (neck strain/torticollis, spondylosis, and myelopathy) and traumatic (whiplash, disk herniation, cervical fracture, neck sprain, and stinger).

  Nonmechanical (rheumatologic/inflammatory, neoplastic, infectious, neurologic, and referred).

  Miscellaneous (e.g., sarcoidosis and Paget's disease).

II. **Common Diagnoses** (Table 48–1). The lifetime prevalence of at least one episode of significant neck pain is estimated at 40% to 70%, whereas nonspecific neck pain over the last 6 months is reported by 40% of adults. Neck pain is most commonly mechanical or because of age-related changes in the cervical spine.

III. **Symptoms** (Table 48–1).

  A. **Pain. Acute torticollis** is a recent, sudden onset of unilateral, muscular pain, whereas **cervical sprain/whiplash** is a severe generalized discomfort in the neck and upper back after an acute trauma. When pain is aggravated by movement, worse after activities, and there is a dull ache in the base of the neck or interscapular region, **osteoarthritis (cervical spondylosis)** should be considered.

  B. **Loss of motion.** Mechanical pain is typically worse on movement and relieved by rest.

  C. **Headache.** Patients with **whiplash** (cervical flexion-extension injuries) frequently have headaches, along with associated nausea, blurred vision, or vertigo.

  D. **Radiating symptoms. Mechanical pain** frequently radiates to the shoulder blades or the top of the arm without any nerve root or spinal cord involvement. **Cervical root irritation** should be considered with radiation of symptoms down the arms, or weakness, numbness, or paresthesias in the arms. With bilateral, radicular symptoms, a **cervical cord compression syndrome** should be considered.

  E. **Precipitating factors.** Tension and stress, along with frequent bouts of pain and depression, may suggest an underlying behavioral or psychiatric diagnosis.

  F. **Difficulty walking,** which could be the presenting symptom of **cervical myelopathy.**

  G. **Other.** A **whiplash injury** especially may be accompanied by anxiety, loss of sleep, dizziness, paresthesias, or nerve root pain. Table 48–2 lists findings suggesting significant underlying disease.

IV. **Signs** (Table 48–1). A focused examination of the patient presenting with neck pain should include **inspection** (for posture, asymmetry, and deformity); **palpation** (for localized tenderness); passive/active/resisted **range of motion (ROM)** (for restrictions and severity of disease); and **provocative maneuvers/neurologic testing** (for radiculopathy).

TABLE 48–1. DIFFERENTIAL DIAGNOSIS OF COMMON CAUSES OF NECK PAIN

Condition	Risk Factors	Symptoms	Signs	Evidenced-Based Testing
Acute nonspecific neck pain	Young adults under some stress	Typically, unilateral neck pain that radiates to the top of the shoulder and periscapular area	Limited ROM; widespread tender/trigger points suggest fibromyalgia	C-spine radiographs are only indicated with positive Red Flags and by Canadian C-spine rules. CT scan is only used when plain films reveal possible fracture.
Chronic mechanical neck pain	Older individuals	Intermittent acute attacks superimposed on chronic pain; pain often radiates to scapular region and top of arms	Limited ROM, tenderness to palpation	Radiographic and CT scans are not indicated. MRI is indicated for work-up of an occult lesion.
Spondylosis/ osteoarthritis	Individuals ≥50 y, history of OA (osteophytes)	Neck stiffness after rest, possible paresthesias/ numbness	Limited ROM, neurologic changes with progression	Cervical spondylosis is the single most common finding on C-spine radiographs, but poorly correlated with symptoms.
Cervical nerve root irritation	History of spondylosis, osteophytes	Discomfort worsening when turning head toward the side of neck pain; paresthesias, weakness	Abnormal Spurling maneuver	**CT** scan can assess for spinal stenosis (older individual with axial stiffness and paresthesias over several dematones); **MRI** provides the best anatomic assessment of disk herniation and soft tissue/spinal cord abnormalities; **EMG** is helpful in localizing radiculopathy/myelopathy.
Acceleration injury/ whiplash	Rear-end or side-impact motor vehicle accidents	Acute pain and stiffness within hours, headache	Limited ROM	**C-spine radiographs** may be indicated by Canadian C-spine rules (Table 48–4)
Torticollis **(cervical dystonia)**	History of congenital or acquired fixed head or C-spine rotation	Usually painless if congenital; usually painful if acquired	Limited ROM; neck is laterally flexed and rotated	No definitive diagnostic test. Consider laboratory tests and neuroimaging to rule out metabolic or structural causes.

CT, computerized tomography; EMG, electromyogram; MRI, magnetic resonance imagery; OA, osteoarthritis; ROM, range of motion.

A. **Tenderness to palpation. Tender points** are common in nonspecific, acute neck pain. Associated widespread tender points, which are sometimes referred to as trigger points, may be indicative of fibromyalgia (see Chapters 39 and 46). Muscle spasm occurs in acute, nonspecific neck pain, whiplash injury, and torticollis.

B. **ROM.** Normal neck ROM includes rotation 60 to 90 degrees, flexion 60 to 90 degrees, extension 60 to 90 degrees, and lateral flexion (side-bending) 30 to 60 degrees. ROM normally decreases with age. Loss of motion is common in an acute, nonspecific, and chronic mechanical neck pain.

C. **Neurologic testing/provocative maneuvers** (Table 48–3). Evaluation for possible levels of sensory and motor involvement, including weakness of the upper extremities, may

TABLE 48–2. RED FLAGS" IN NECK PAIN (THINK "RIFT": CLUES TO POTENTIAL SERIOUS UNDERLYING DISEASE)

Radiculopathy (lower extremity sensory/motor changes/spasticity, bowel/bladder incontinence)
Infection (fever/chills; Immunocompromised population-alcohol/drug abuse, elderly)
Fracture (significant trauma; osteoporosis history)
Tumor (history of cancer; unexplained weight loss; age ≤20/≥50 y, failure to improve with treatment)

TABLE 48-3. EVALUATION FOR CERVICAL NERVE ROOT LESIONS

Nerve Root	Disk Level	Muscle Weakness/ Movement Affected	Reflex	Paresthesia	Site of Pain
C-5	C-4/5	Shoulder abduction, elbow flexion	Biceps	Shoulder	Shoulder, lateral arm
C-6	C-5/6	Wrist extension/ pronation	Brachioradialis and biceps	Thumb	Deltoid, rhomboid muscle areas
C-7	C-6/7	Elbow/finger extension	Triceps	Middle finger	Dorsolateral upper arm, superomedial angle of scapula
C-8	C-7/T-1	Wrist/finger extension	Triceps and finger	Ring and little finger	Scapula, ulnar side of upper arm

suggest lesions of the nerve roots, brachial plexus, or muscles. A **Spurling test,** or the neck compression test, requires side-bending and rotating the patient's head toward the side of radicular pain and exerting downward pressure. This maneuver reproduces symptoms in the affected upper extremity. The Spurling test has a high specificity but low sensitivity for cervical radiculopathy. Nonspecific mechanical pain should be considered when a Spurling test or contralateral neck motion result only in neck discomfort.

V. **Laboratory Tests** are usually not necessary. Testing should be considered if a careful history and physical examination do not clearly suggest a diagnosis, or to guide management (e.g., surgical consultation).

A. **Plain C-spine radiographs** (Table 48-1). A cervical spine injury is unlikely in the absence of neck pain/tenderness, neurologic signs/symptoms, loss of consciousness, and distracting injury, and with a normal mental status examination. The Canadian Cervical Spine Rules (Table 48-4) are a validated tool to determine which patients with neck pain require radiographic evaluation.

B. In the presence of neurologic abnormalities, **other imaging techniques** should be used to resolve lesion anatomy (Table 48-1).

1. A **bone scan** can appraise osseous pathology, including osteomyelitis and neoplastic lesions in bone.

2. **Bone densitometry** diagnoses suspected osteoporosis.

C. **Blood tests** are rarely indicated. Erythrocyte sedimentation rate and complete blood count with differential may help evaluate for suspected serious disorders, including tumor, infection, or inflammatory arthritis, especially with "Red Flag" history or physical examination (Table 48-2).

VI. **Treatment.** The management of neck pain is aimed at relieving symptoms and maintaining good function. Neck pain usually resolves within days or weeks. Approximately 10% of acute neck pain becomes chronic and 5% of patients experience severe disability. Specific conditions and evidenced-based treatments will be discussed.

A. **Uncomplicated neck pain without severe neurologic deficit, including acute, non-specific neck pain and chronic mechanical neck pain**

1. Manual manipulation/mobilization, active physiotherapy, pulsed electromagnetic field treatment, and exercise are likely to be beneficial. Therapeutic exercises, initiated

TABLE 48-4. CANADIAN CERVICAL SPINE RULES

Is there one high-risk factor that mandates immobilization?
   Age $\geq$ 65-year-old, or dangerous mechanism (fall from 1 m or greater, axial load to head, motorized recreational vehicles, bicycle collision, or motor vehicle collision (MVC) with high speed, rollover, or ejection); or
   Numbness/tingling in extremities

Is there one low-risk factor to allow safe assessment of range of motion?
   Simple rear-end MVC; or
   Ambulatory at any time at scene, or
   No neck pain at scene, or
   Absence of midline C-spine tenderness
Is patient able to voluntarily actively rotate neck 45 degrees to the left and right when requested, regardless of pain?

An answer "yes" to the first question or "no" to the second or third question requires radiography.

either in the office or in consultation with a physical therapist, include ROM, isometrics, dynamic exercises, postural training, and general fitness programs. (SOR **B**)
2. Pharmacologic treatment (including analgesics, nonsteroidal anti-inflammatory drugs, antidepressants, and muscle relaxants), behavioral interventions/biofeedback, patient education, application of heat/cold, home or office cervical traction, acupuncture, spray and stretch, laser treatment, and soft collars/special pillows have unknown effectiveness, yet are common conservative treatments. (SOR **C**)

B. **Spondylosis/osteoarthritis.** Treatment must involve reducing pain and stiffness, while minimizing risk (see Chapter 80). Fashionable complementary techniques include transcutaneous electrical nerve stimulation (TENS) units, acupuncture, and a variety of heat, light, magnetic, or filing therapies, but there are little data to support their efficacy.

C. **Cervical nerve root irritation/radiculopathy.** In patients followed up for over a year, there currently are no data supporting surgery compared to conservative treatment. Conservative modalities include local heat, analgesics, cervical collar in the acute phase, and consideration of cervical traction. Pharmacologic treatment, including oral medications and referral for epidural steroid injections, have unknown effectiveness. (SOR **C**)

D. **Acute whiplash injury.** Likely beneficial interventions include early mobilization and return to normal activity, electrotherapy (diathermy and TENS units), and multimodal treatment. (SOR **B**) Multimodal or combined therapy typically refers to intensive programs incorporating exercise as well as pharmacologic, behavioral, and psychosocial interventions. (SOR **C**)

E. **Chronic whiplash injury.** Outcomes are no different comparing physiotherapy alone and multimodal treatment. One study showed significant numbers of pain-free patients 6 months after undergoing percutaneous radiofrequency neurotomy. Another demonstrated significant pain reduction in those undergoing percutaneous radiofrequency neurotomy combined with other modalities, compared to those treated with single modalities. (SOR **C**)

F. **Torticollis (cervical dystonia)** in adults has been typically managed with physical therapy, stretching techniques, gentle manual manipulation, judicious use of a soft cervical collar, and ice/heat. (SOR **C**) Evidenced-based studies have demonstrated benefit of botulinum A and B toxin. (SOR **A**) Medications have unknown effectiveness. (SOR **C**) Physiotherapy in children is likely to be beneficial. (SOR **B**) There is unknown **effectiveness** with surgical treatments, acupuncture, biofeedback, manipulation, and occupational therapy. (SOR **C**)

REFERENCES

Bogduk N, McGuirk B. *Management of Acute and Chronic Neck Pain an Evidence-based Approach.* Philadelphia, PA: Elsevier; 2006.
Binder A. Neck pain. In *Clinical Evidence Concise.* Harrisonburg, VA: Banta Book Group; 2006;15:423-427.
Snaith A, Wade D. Dystonia. *BMJ Clin Eviden.* Y. Charles ed. 2006 Review. *BMJ Publish Group.* 2007.
Devereaux MW. Neck pain. *Prim Care.* 2004;31:19-31.
Swezey RL, ed. Neck pain. *Phys Med Rehabil Clin N Am.* 2003;14(3):455-692 (issue theme).

---

49   Palpitations

Jose E. Rodríguez, MD, & Mike D. Hardin, Jr., MD

KEY POINTS

- Most causes of palpitations are benign and do not require extensive work-up or treatment.
- Palpitations that are sustained or associated with syncope or presyncope require further work-up, electrophysiologic evaluation, or both.
- In general, palpitations are insensitive indicators of arrhythmias.

TABLE 49–1. ETIOLOGIES OF PALPITATIONS

Cardiac	*Habits*
Arrhythmia	Cocaine
Sinus tachycardia	Amphetamines
Ventricular premature contractions	Caffeine
Atrial premature contractions	Nicotine
Re-entrant atrial tachycardias	*Metabolic disorders*
Atrial fibrillation or flutter	Thyrotoxicosis
Sinus bradycardia	Hypoglycemia
Sick sinus syndrome	Pheochromocytoma
Atrioventricular nodal block	Mastocytosis
Conduction defects	Scombroid food poisoning (e.g., tuna fish)
Ventricular tachycardia	
Ventricular fibrillation	*High-output states*
Cardiac and extracardiac shunts	Anemia
Valvular heart disease	Pregnancy
Pacemaker	Paget's disease
Atrial myxoma	Fever
Cardiomyopathy	*Catecholamine excess*
Psychiatric disease	Stress
Panic attack and disorder	Exercise
Generalized anxiety disorder	
Somatization	
Depression	
Medications	
Sympathomimetic agents	
Vasodilators	
Anticholinergic drugs	
Beta-blocker withdrawal	

(Reproduced with permission from Weber BE and Kapoor WN. Evaluation and outcomes of patients with palpitations. *Am J Med.* 1996;100(2):138-148.)

I. **Definition.** Palpitations are an awareness of the heartbeat, are usually benign, and may be either caused by intrinsic cardiac conditions or noncardiac conditions impacting cardiac rate, rhythm, or force (Table 49–1).

II. **Common Diagnoses.** Palpitations are a common chief complaint, accounting for up to 16% of outpatient visits. Relative incidence and risk factors for common causes of palpitations follow:

A. **Cardiac** (43% of cases). Factors increasing the likelihood for a cardiac etiology of palpitations include (1) male sex; (2) description of an irregular heartbeat; (3) history of heart disease; or (4) event duration ≥ 5 minutes. Patients with three predictors have a 71% chance of a cardiac etiology, those with two predictors, a 48% chance; those with one predictor, a 26% chance; and those with zero predictors, a 0% chance of cardiac etiology. The most common cardiac cause is benign supraventricular or ventricular ectopy.

B. **Psychiatric** (31% of cases). Palpitations may be a feature of panic attacks, generalized anxiety disorder, somatization, and depression. Because these disorders are common, they may coexist with other causes of palpitations.

C. Ten percent of palpitations are because of a **variety of defined causes** such as endocrinologic disorders (e.g., hyperthyroidism), cardiac stimulants (e.g., caffeine, over-the-counter sympathomimetics, illicit drugs), and anemia.

D. In 16% of cases, the cause of palpitations is **unknown.**

III. **Symptoms.** Because palpitations can be difficult to characterize, it may be helpful for the patient to tap out the rhythm or for the physician to tap out examples of different rhythms. Important historical features of the palpitations include the following:

A. **Description**

1. **Rate and rhythm.** A **rapid and regular** rhythm suggests paroxysmal supraventricular tachycardia (PSVT) or ventricular tachycardia (VT); **rapid and irregular** suggests atrial fibrillation or atrial flutter with a variable block.

2. A **"flip-flopping"** sensation suggests **ventricular or atrial premature contractions** (VPCs, APCs) with a pause followed by a forceful contraction (postextrasystolic potentiation of ventricular inotropy).

3. A description of "**rapid fluttering in the chest**" may represent a **sustained, ventricular,** or **supraventricular rhythm,** including sinus tachycardia.

4. A "**pounding in the neck**" sensation is caused by A waves resulting from atrial contractions against a closed tricuspid or mitral valve in **atrioventricular dissociation.** Irregular neck palpitations are seen in VPCs, complete heart block, or VT. **Rapid and regular neck pulsations** are typical of atrioventricular re-entrant tachycardia (AVNRT).

B. Onset and offset

1. **Random, episodic,** and last an instant: Premature beats.

2. **Gradual onset and offset:** Sinus tachycardia.

3. **Abrupt onset/termination:** PSVT or VT.

4. Patient able to **terminate with vagal maneuver:** PSVT (especially AVNRT).

C. Positional

1. Initiated by **standing up straight after bending over,** aborted by lying down: AVNRT.

2. **Augmented by supine or left lateral decubitus position:** VPC or APC, secondary to greater awareness of heart activity while relaxed or because of the proximity of the heart to the chest wall.

D. Syncope or presyncope

1. **VT.**

2. **PSVT,** secondary to vasodilation at the onset of the arrhythmia.

E. Reliability of reported palpitations. Although the classic descriptions noted above can be helpful, a recent review of the literature suggests:

1. The vast majority of arrhythmias are unrecognized by patients as symptoms.

2. Of those reporting palpitations, patients with psychiatric disease (e.g., somatization, hypochondriasis) were less accurate historians.

3. Palpitations are insensitive indicators of arrhythmias.

IV. Signs. The physical examination should search for:

A. Cardiovascular abnormalities that could serve as a substrate for arrhythmias:

1. **Mitral valve prolapse:** Midsystolic click (associated with many arrhythmias).

2. **Hypertrophic obstructive cardiomyopathy:** Harsh, holosystolic murmur along the left sternal border that increases with Valsalva's maneuver (associated with atrial fibrillation, VT).

3. **Dilated cardiomyopathy and heart failure:** Diffused and laterally displaced apical impulse, ventricular (S_3) and atrial (S_4) gallops (associated with VT, atrial fibrillation).

B. Signs of other medical disorders such as hyperthyroidism or pheochromocytoma.

V. Laboratory Tests (Figure 49–1). Most palpitations have a benign etiology and extensive evaluation is usually not necessary. The history, physical examination, electrocardiogram (ECG), and limited laboratory tests will yield a diagnosis in over one-third of patients; only a small portion of the remaining cases will require further testing (see Sections V.C and V.D).

A. Laboratory. Limited laboratory tests to rule out hyperthyroidism (thyroid-stimulating hormone), anemia (hemoglobin/hematocrit), and electrolyte disturbances (potassium, magnesium) are sufficient.

B. ECG. An episode of palpitations is rarely captured on a routine ECG. Certain ECG findings, however, may suggest the etiology of the palpitations (Table 49–2).

C. Ambulatory ECG monitoring (AECG). Further AECG testing is used to rule out a serious condition, identify treatable causes of arrhythmias, or reassure a patient.

1. A **Holter (24-hour) monitor** is useful only if a patient has daily palpitations.

2. The preferred study for investigating palpitations is the **continuous loop event recorder,** which is activated by the patient at time of symptoms. Two weeks of monitoring is usually adequate and more cost-effective than the traditional 4 weeks.

3. An **exercise stress test** is useful only for exertional arrhythmias.

D. Electrophysiologic testing is reserved for patients with a high pretest likelihood of serious arrhythmia (e.g., structural heart disease or sustained or poorly tolerated arrhythmia).

VI. Treatment

A. Patients with **sustained supraventricular tachycardia (SVT) or VT.** These patients should be referred to an electrophysiologist (a cardiologist specializing in the pharmacologic and invasive management of arrhythmias) for consideration of radiofrequency ablation (SVT), medical therapy, or implantable defibrillator.

B. Nonsustained ventricular tachycardia (NSVT). NSVT is defined as three or more consecutive beats at a rate of ≥120 beats per minute with a duration of less than 30 seconds. In patients without underlying heart disease, it is a benign finding and no treatment is

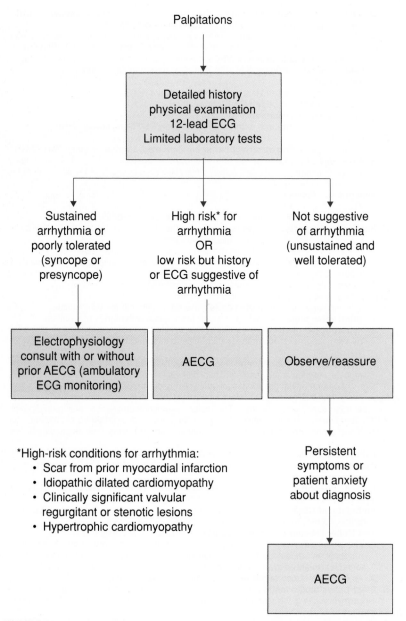

FIGURE 49–1. Decision tree for evaluation of palpitations. AECG, ambulatory electrocardiogram; ECG, electrocardiogram.

TABLE 49–2. ELECTROCARDIOGRAPHIC CLUES TO THE CAUSE OF PALPITATIONS

ECG Findings	Condition	Suggested Etiology
Short PR interval, delta waves	Wolff-Parkinson-White syndrome	Atrioventricular re-entrant tachycardia
P mitrale, left ventricular hypertrophy (LVH), atrial premature depolarizations	Left atrial abnormality	Atrial fibrillation
Marked LVH, deep septal Q waves in I, aVL, and V4–6	Hypertrophic obstructive cardiomyopathy	Atrial fibrillation
Ventricular premature depolarizations, left bundle-branch block with positive axis (in patients without structural heart disease)		Idiopathic VT, right ventricular outflow tract type
Ventricular premature depolarizations, right bundle-branch block with positive axis (in patients without structural heart disease)		Idiopathic VT, left ventricular type
Q waves	Prior myocardial infarction	VPCs, nonsustained or sustained VT
Complete heart block	Complete heart block	VPCs, polymorphic VT (torsade de pointes)
Long QT interval	Long QT syndrome	Polymorphic VT
Inverted T wave in V_2, with or without epsilon wave	Arrhythmogenic right ventricular dysplasia	Arrhythmogenic right ventricular dysplasia

VT, ventricular tachycardia; VPC, ventricular premature contractions.
(Reproduced with permission from Weber BE and Kapoor WN. Evaluation and outcomes of patients with palpitations. *Am J Med.* 1996;100(2):138-148.)

necessary. Patients with heart disease should be referred to electrophysiology for treatment recommendations.

C. **Benign supraventricular or ventricular ectopy.** Reassure the patient and remove precipitating causes (e.g., caffeine, drugs). If symptoms are incapacitating, consider treatment with a beta-blocker to relieve symptoms. (Treatment, however, may not necessarily suppress the arrhythmia, just its symptoms.)

D. **Atrial fibrillation (AF).** There are four principal issues regarding the treatment of AF:

1. **Reversion to normal sinus rhythm (NSR)**
   a. Urgent electrical cardioversion is indicated in **unstable patients** (those with active ischemia, hypotension, or a preexcitation syndrome with an extremely rapid ventricular rate).
   b. In the **stable patient,** rate control is first attained with a calcium channel blocker, beta-blocker, or digoxin (Table 49–3).
   c. Factors that guide drug selection include the patient's medical condition, the presence of concomitant heart failure, the characteristics of the medicine, and the physician's experience with specific drugs. Digoxin is currently recommended as a second-line treatment for rate control, except in heart failure. (SOR **C**)
   d. Recent trials have shown that either rhythm or rate control is acceptable in managing AF. (SOR **A**) Thus, the decision to perform **elective pharmacologic or electrical cardioversion** should be made in consultation with cardiology after consideration of the risks and benefits. Successful reversion to and maintenance of NSR is more likely if:
      (1) The AF has been present less than 1 year.
      (2) The left atrium is not enlarged (diameter ≤4.0 cm).
      (3) A reversible etiologic factor of the AF is present.

2. **Maintenance of NSR**
   a. After successful cardioversion, only 20% to 30% of patients maintain NSR without therapy.
   b. Class IA (quinidine, procainamide, disopyramide), IC (flecainide, propafenone), and III (amiodarone, sotalol, ibutilide, dofetilide) drugs are used to maintain NSR. Although cardiology may initiate this therapy, family physicians are often involved in its maintenance and should be familiar with the numerous drug interactions of antiarrhythmics. (SOR **A**)

3. **Rate control in chronic AF** is achieved using calcium channel blockers, beta-blockers, or digoxin (Table 49–3).

TABLE 49–3. DRUGS USED FOR RATE CONTROL IN PATIENTS WITH ATRIAL FIBRILLATION

Drug	Loading Dose	Usual Maintenance Dose
Digoxin (Lanoxin)	**IV:** 0.25 mg IV every 2 h, up to 1.5 mg **PO:** 0.25 mg every 2 h, up to 1.5 mg	**IV:** 0.125–0.25 mg daily **PO:** 0.125–0.375 mg daily
Calcium channel blockers Diltiazem (Cardizem, Dilacor, Tiazac) Verapamil (Calan, Isoptin, and others)	**IV:** 0.25 mg/kg IV over 2 min **PO:** NA **IV:** 0.075–0.15 mg/kg over 2 min **PO:** NA	**IV:** 5–15 mg/h infusion for ≤24 h **PO:** 120–360 mg/24 h (divided doses or slow-release forms available) **IV:** NA **PO:** 120–480 mg/24 h (divided doses or SR forms available)
Beta-blockers (only two representative members of the class are listed here—others may be used as well) Metoprolol (Lopressor, Toprol) Propranolol (Inderal)	**IV:** 2.5–5 mg IV bolus over 2 min; up to 3 doses **PO:** NA **IV:** 0.15 mg/kg (typically 1–3 mg) **PO:** NA	**IV:** NA **PO:** 25–100 mg/24 h (divided doses or SR forms available) **IV:** NA **PO:** 80–240 mg/24 h (divided doses or SR forms available)

IV, intravenous; NA, not applicable; PO, oral; SR, sustained release.
(Adapted from Fuster V et al: ACC/AHA/ESC guidelines for the management of patients with atrial fibrillation: Executive summary. A report of the American College of Cardiology/American Heart Association Task Force on Practice Guidelines and the European Society of Cardiology Committee for Practice Guidelines (Writing Committee to Revise the 2001 Guidelines for the Management of Patients with Atrial Fibrillation). Developed in collaboration with the European Heart Rhythm Association and the Heart Rhythm Society. *J Am Coll Cardiol.* 2006;48:854-906.)

TABLE 49–4. RISK-BASED APPROACH TO ANTITHROMBOTIC THERAPY IN ATRIAL FIBRILLATION (AF)

Patient Features	Antithrombotic Therapy
Age ≤60 y No heart disease (lone AF)	ASA 325 mg daily or no therapy
Age ≤60 y Heart disease but no risk factors[1]	ASA 325 mg daily
Age ≥60 y No risk factors[1]	ASA 325 mg daily
Age ≥60 y With diabetes or CAD Age ≥75 y, especially women	Warfarin (INR 2.0–3.0) Addition of ASA 81–162 mg/d optional Warfarin (INR ~2.0) Warfarin (INR 2.0–3.0)
Any age patient with: Heart failure LVEF ≤35% Thyrotoxicosis Hypertension Rheumatic heart disease (mitral stenosis) Prosthetic heart valves Prior thromboembolism Persistent atrial thrombus on TEE	Warfarin (INR 2.5–3.5 or higher may be appropriate)

[1]Risk factors for thromboembolism include heart failure, LVEF less than 35%, thyrotoxicosis, or history of hypertension.
AF, atrial fibrillation; ASA, aspirin; CAD, coronary artery disease; INR, international normalized ratio; LVEF, left ventricular ejection fraction; TEE, transesophageal echocardiography.
(Adapted from Fuster V et al: ACC/AHA/ESC guidelines for the management of patients with atrial fibrillation: Executive summary. A report of the American College of Cardiology/American Heart Association Task Force on Practice Guidelines and the European Society of Cardiology Committee for Practice Guidelines (Writing Committee to Revise the 2001 Guidelines for the Management of Patients with Atrial Fibrillation). Developed in collaboration with the European Heart Rhythm Association and the Heart Rhythm Society. *J Am Coll Cardiol.* 2006;48:854-906.)

4. **Anticoagulation** for prevention of systemic embolization:
   a. **While restoring NSR.** If AF is present for more than 48 hours, patients should receive 3 to 4 weeks of warfarin (e.g., Coumadin) therapy (target international normalized ratio 2.5, range 2.0–3.0) prior to cardioversion and continued for 4 weeks after cardioversion. Recent trials have suggested that long-term anticoagulation may be recommended even after cardioversion owing to a 50% risk of recurrent AF. (SOR **A**) Contraindications to warfarin therapy include systemic or intracranial bleeding, noncompliance, or a significant risk of falls.
   b. **Chronic AF.** Determination of a patient's risk for an embolic event guides the selection of anticoagulant therapy (Table 49–4). Risk factors include age, left ventricular dysfunction, hypertension, thyrotoxicosis, and diabetes.

REFERENCES

Arnsdorf MF. Nonsustained VT in the absence of apparent structural heart disease. www.uptodate. com, online version 15.1.

Arnsdorf MF, Podrid PJ. Overview of the presentation and management of atrial fibrillation. www.uptodate. com, online version 15.1.

Barsky AJ. Investigating selected symptoms: palpitations, arrhythmias, and awareness of cardiac activity. *Ann Intern Med.* 2001;134:832.

Fuster V, et al. ACC/AHA/ESC guidelines for the management of patients with atrial fibrillation: Executive summary. *J Am Coll Cardiol.* 2006;48:854-906.

King DE, Dickerson LM, Sack JL. Acute management of atrial fibrillation: part I. Rate and rhythm control. *Am Fam Physician.* 2002;66:249.

Zimetbaum P. Overview of palpitations. www.uptodate. com, online version 15.1.

---

50   Pediatric Fever

Sanford R. Kimmel, MD

KEY POINTS

- Evaluation of the young child with fever is a common but often challenging task for the family physician.
- Most febrile illnesses are viral and self-limited. However, the physician must detect those children with a potentially serious bacterial illness.
- Careful observation and examination along with judicious laboratory testing and close follow-up enable family physicians to evaluate and manage most febrile children.

I. **Definition.** Fever is an elevation of body temperature above the normal range. The normal range for temperature of the body varies according to the age of the children, method of measurement, and time of day. A rectal temperature $\geq 37.8°C$ ($100°F$) in newborns or $\geq 38°C$ ($100.4°F$) in older infants and children denotes fever. Rectal temperature most consistently reflects the body's core temperature and is used in this chapter.

Fever occurs when exogenous pyrogens such as viruses, bacteria, fungi, toxins, drugs, malignancies, metabolic disorders, and antigen-antibody complexes induce release of endogenous pyrogens, such as interleukin (IL) 1β and IL-6. These stimulate the production of hypothalamic prostaglandin E_2 (PGE_2) that raises the "set point" of the body's thermostat. Heat is generated or conserved through shivering or peripheral vasoconstriction. The resulting fever may increase leukocyte migration and antibacterial activity as well as T-cell and interferon production. However, the risk of dehydration also increases, since the body's basal metabolic rate increases 10% for each degree Celsius above normal.

II. **Common Diagnoses.** During the first 2 to 3 years of life, children have an average of four to six acute infections per year. Viral infections cause most febrile episodes, but serious bacterial infections are present in 10% to 15% of febrile infants younger than

3-month-old with a temperature 38°C or higher and in 13% of children aging 3 months to 3-year-old presenting with a fever $\geq$39°C (102.2°F) and a white blood count $\geq$15,000 cells/μL.

A. **Upper respiratory infections (URIs)** (e.g., viral infections, otitis media, pharyngitis, and sinusitis) account for approximately one-third of all visits that children younger than 15 years make to family physicians, while **lower respiratory infections (LRIs)** (e.g., bacterial and viral pneumonias, bronchitis, and bronchiolitis) are less common but significant causes of pediatric fever. Exposure to ill siblings, day care attendance, and parental smoking are some risk factors for respiratory infections.

B. **Gastroenteritis** is a major cause of illness and even death in young children with rotaviruses causing approximately 2 million hospitalizations and 440,000 deaths worldwide per year among children less than 5-year-old. Rotavirus infects 80% of children by 5 years of age, especially during the winter months in countries with temperate climates. The routine administration of rotavirus vaccine to young infants is likely to decrease the future incidence of rotavirus gastroenteritis. The ingestion of contaminated food or water are risk factors for bacterial gastroenteritis caused by *Salmonella* species, *Campylobacter* species, enterotoxigenic *Escherichia coli*, and *Shigella* species.

C. **Bacteremia** occurs in approximately 2% to 3% of febrile children aged 2 to 36 months seen in the emergency department. In addition to young age, risk factors for bacteremia include immunodeficiency or immunosuppression, anatomic or functional asplenia, and household or day care contact with invasive bacterial disease. High immunization rates have made invasive disease because of *Haemophilus influenzae* type b (Hib) rare. Immunization has reduced invasive disease caused by *Streptococcus pneumoniae*. However, pneumococcus causes most cases of occult bacteremia and in some populations, an increase in disease because of nonvaccine serotypes is being seen.

D. **Urinary tract infections (UTIs)** occur in 5% to 7% of girls younger than age 2 presenting with fever and no localizing signs. Uncircumcised male infants have a 10 times greater incidence of UTIs (1%) during the first year of life than do circumcised infants (0.1%). The prevalence of bacteremia is higher in young infants with UTIs.

E. **Bacterial meningitis** can occur throughout the year, but *S pneumoniae* and *Neisseria meningitidis* usually occur during the winter months. If one child has meningococcal meningitis, the rate of a simultaneous case occurring in that family is 1% without chemoprophylaxis. Gram-negative enteric bacteria, group B streptococci, and *Listeria monocytogenes* are important causes of bacterial meningitis in infants younger than 3 months of age. Invasive Hib disease has significantly decreased because of the Hib vaccine. **Viral meningitis** occurs during the summer and fall in temperate climates. Enterovirus is the most common cause and is spread from person-to-person by fecal–oral and respiratory routes and by fomites.

F. Approximately 50% of cases of childhood **osteomyelitis** occur in children younger than 5 years. *Staphylococcus aureus* is the most common cause, but gram-negative bacteria such as *Salmonella* may cause recurrent osteomyelitis in children with hemoglobinopathies such as sickle cell disease, whereas *Pseudomonas aeruginosa* usually causes disease because of puncture wounds of the foot. Approximately 75% of childhood cases of **septic arthritis** occur in children younger than 5 years. Most cases are caused by *S aureus,* but *Neisseria gonorrhoeae* often causes disease in sexually active or abused adolescents. Group B streptococci and enteric gram-negative bacilli are important causes of septic arthritis and osteomyelitis in neonates; Hib may cause bone and joint infections in inadequately immunized children.

G. **Febrile exanthems. Roseola** is caused by human herpesvirus type 6 and usually affects children between ages 6 and 24 months, seldom occurring after 3 years of age. **Measles** is transmitted by direct contact with infectious airborne droplets, predominantly during the winter and spring in temperate climates. Measles cases in the United States have declined as a result of a second measles immunization given prior to school entry. **Scarlet fever** is usually associated with erythrogenic exotoxin-producing group A streptococcal pharyngitis and follows close contact with respiratory secretions of infected individuals. **Varicella** usually occurs by direct contact with persons who have varicella or zoster, and occasionally by airborne spread from respiratory secretions. It is highly contagious among susceptible contacts and is most common during late winter and early spring in temperate climates.

III. **Symptoms.** The febrile child often demonstrates some degree of lethargy, loss of appetite, or irritability.

A. **Respiratory symptoms** include sore throat, nasal congestion, otalgia, cough, and wheezing.

B. **Diarrhea** and **vomiting** usually indicate a gastrointestinal infection, although these symptoms occasionally occur in acute otitis media or UTI.

C. **Fever** may be the only symptom of a UTI in young infants, but older infants and children may **cry with urination or refuse to urinate.**

D. Persistence or worsening of **lethargy** and **irritability** may indicate meningitis.

E. **Refusal to bear weight** or use an extremity may be seen with septic arthritis or osteomyelitis.

F. A transient red maculopapular rash appearing after defervescence of several days of high fever is characteristic of **roseola.** Cough, coryza, and conjunctivitis accompany the confluent red rash of **measles.** A strawberry tongue may be seen with the characteristic sandpaperlike rash of **scarlet fever.** The croplike spread of different stages of macules, papules, and vesicles from the face and trunk to the extremities (but sparing the palms and soles) denotes **varicella. Smallpox** begins on the oral mucosa, face, and upper extremities, then spreads to the trunk and lower extremities, often involving the palms and soles. The initial papules evolve simultaneously into vesicles and then umbilicated pustules.

IV. **Signs**

A. The **degree of temperature reduction in response to antipyretics** is generally not helpful in differentiating viral from bacterial infection.

B. **Observation** of the child's appearance and interaction with the parent or caregiver often determine whether the physician needs to have a high or low index of suspicion of serious underlying disease. Classifying the child aged 3 months and older as toxic or nontoxic in appearance is helpful in determining the extent of investigation necessary to assess the cause of the child's illness.

1. The Acute Illness Observation Scale (AIOS) developed by McCarthy and associates (1982) represented an attempt to predict the presence of serious underlying illness based on the febrile child's clinical appearance and interaction while seated on the caregiver's lap, prior to antipyretic therapy (Table 50–1).

2. A serious underlying disease was found in 92% of children with an AIOS score of 16 or more and in 26% of those with a score of 11 to 15. Only 2.7% of children with a score of 10 or less had a serious illness.

3. No child who smiled normally had a serious illness. In another study, the presence of a social smile did not always exclude the possibility of a serious bacterial illness.

4. In infants 4- to 8-week-old, the AIOS detected ≤50% of those with a serious illness in one study. The sensitivity and positive predictive value of the AIOS also decrease as the prevalence of bacteremia in the population decreases.

C. **Physical findings** associated with specific diseases are presented in Table 50–2.

TABLE 50–1. ACUTE ILLNESS OBSERVATION SCALES

Observation Item	Normal—1	Moderate Impairment—3	Severe Impairment—5
Quality of cry	Strong cry with normal tone, or contented and not crying	Whimpering or sobbing	Weak cry, moaning, or high-pitched cry
Reaction to parental stimulation	Cries briefly and then stops, or is contented and not crying	Cries off and on	Cries continually or hardly responds
State variation	If awake, stays awake, or if asleep and then stimulated, awakens quickly	Closes eyes briefly when awake, or awakens with prolonged stimulation	Falls asleep or will not arouse
Color	Pink	Pale extremities or acrocyanosis	Pale, cyanotic, mottled, or ashen
Hydration	Normal skin and eyes, moist mucous membranes	Normal skin and eyes, slightly dry mouth	Doughy or tented skin, dry mucous membranes or sunken eyes
Response (talk, smile) to social overture	Smiles, or "alert" (≤2 mo)*	Smiles briefly, or "alert" briefly (≤2 mo)*	No smile, anxious face, dull expression, or does not "alert" (≤2 mo)*

*"Alert" applies to children younger than 2 months of age, since these young infants do not have a social smile.
(Adapted with permission from McCarthy PL et al. Observation scales to identify serious illness in febrile children. *Pediatrics.* 1982;70:806. Copyright © American Academy of Pediatrics (AAP).)

TABLE 50–2. PHYSICAL FINDINGS AND CLINICAL CLUES TO ILLNESSES IN FEBRILE CHILDREN

Body Region or System	Physical Findings	Potential Disease(s)
Skin	Petechial rash	Meningococcemia
	Maculopapular rash, followed by petechial rash	Rocky Mountain spotted fever
Head	Bulging fontanelle, nuchal rigidity	Meningitis (later manifestation in children younger than 2 y)
Eyes	Conjunctivitis	Associated otitis media, Kawasaki disease, or measles with cough, coryza
	Redness or swelling around eye	Periorbital cellulitis
Ears	Red, dull, nonmobile tympanic membrane	Otitis media
	Swelling and tenderness behind ear	Mastoiditis
Nose	Purulent rhinorrhea	Sinusitis
	Nasal flaring	Pneumonia or any condition producing respiratory distress
Throat	Stridor	Laryngotracheobronchitis (croup)
	Stridor with drooling, dysphagia, or aphonia	Epiglottitis
	Petechiae on soft palate and uvula	Streptococcal pharyngitis
	Vesicles or ulcers on soft palate and tonsilar pillars	Herpangina
	Vesicles or ulcers on tongue, lips, and buccal mucosa	Herpes stomatitis
	Strawberry tongue	Streptococcal pharyngitis or Kawasaki disease
Chest	Tachypnea, retractions, decreased breath sounds, rales (may not be present)	Pneumonia
	Rhonchi	Bronchitis
	Wheezing	Bronchiolitis, asthma (inhaled foreign body or other causes)
Heart	Murmur	Subacute bacterial endocarditis, rheumatic fever (or normal because of increased cardiac output)
Abdomen	Local tenderness worsening with movement	Appendicitis or condition producing peritoneal irritation
Rectal	Fluctuant mass	Ruptured appendix or perirectal abscess
Musculoskeletal	Refuses to bear weight or use extremity	Septic arthritis or osteomyelitis, especially in the hip

(Reprinted with permission from Kimmel SR, Gemmill DW. The young child with fever. *Am Fam Physician.* 1988;37:202. Copyright © 1988 American Academy of Family Physicians. All Rights Reserved.)

V. Laboratory Tests

   A. **Screening laboratory tests** help determine if further diagnostic studies are needed for moderately ill-appearing children (e.g., an AIOS score of 11–15) who do not have an obvious focus of infection or for well-appearing children with high or persistent fever.

   1. In infants older than 28 days, the following conditions suggest an underlying or occult bacterial illness:

   a. White blood cell count (WBC) of $\geq 15,000$ cells/μL.

   b. Absolute neutrophil count $\geq 10,000$ cells/μL.

   2. The positive predictive value of the above tests for serious bacterial illness (SBI), such as pneumonia, meningitis, or bacteremia is approximately 8% to 10%. Thus, many children with a positive screening test result will not have an underlying SBI.

   3. No test will detect bacteremia or other serious illnesses in all children. Some children with meningitis may have a WBC of $\leq 15,000/\mu$L, and some children with overwhelming sepsis may have a WBC of $\leq 5000/\mu$L.

   4. Careful clinical assessment of the child is necessary in interpreting screening tests. A positive test result is more likely to be significant in an ill-appearing child or one who has underlying risk factors than in one who looks well.

   B. **Further diagnostic tests** (Table 50–3) should be considered in febrile children who appear moderately or severely ill (AIOS score ≥ 10) or who have an abnormal screening test result.

TABLE 50–3. DIAGNOSTIC STUDIES IN FEBRILE CHILDREN WITHOUT AN OBVIOUS FOCUS OF INFECTION

Test	Indications	Comments
Chest x-ray	Fever of sudden onset, tachypnea, decreased breath sounds, or WBC $\geq$20,000/μL	Pneumonia may lack usual auscultatory findings
Urinalysis (UA) with culture and sensitivity (C&S)	Boys $\leq$6 mo or uncircumcised boys $\leq$12 mo . Girls $\leq$2-year-old	Bladder tap newborn; catheterize older children; negative UA does not rule out infection
Lumbar puncture	Child $\leq$3 mo or very irritable or lethargic, feeds poorly, has seizures, bulging fontanelle, or nuchal rigidity	Use needle with stylet; consider hospital admission
Blood culture	Age $\leq$3 y at high risk of bacteremia, acute illness observation score (AIOS) $\geq$11 $\pm$ WBC $\geq$15,000/μL	Draw 0.5–2 mL of blood; one test sufficient for outpatient use
Stool for polymorphonuclear cells (PMNs) with C&S	Abrupt onset or bloody diarrhea, greater than four stools per day, and no vomiting before diarrhea	Positive if $\geq$5 PMNs/hpf

AIOS, acute illness observation scale; hpf, high-power field.

VI. Treatment (Figure 50–1).

A. Hospitalization is indicated in the following circumstances.

1. Infants 0- to 28-day-old with a fever of $\geq$38°C (100.4°F) require a sepsis work-up and parenteral antibiotics pending culture results.

2. Febrile children 29 to 90 days of age not fulfilling the Rochester low-risk criteria (Table 50–4) are at risk for bacteremia or SBI based on their clinical appearance, physical findings, and laboratory studies. These children should be hospitalized for further evaluation and treatment.

3. Hospitalization is also required for any immunosuppressed, toxic appearing, or severely ill febrile child (e.g., AIOS score $\geq$16), or one having an underlying condition placing him or her at high risk of overwhelming infection.

B. Ambulatory management

1. Specific therapy should be initiated for conditions diagnosed and amenable to outpatient treatment (see Chapter 13, for LRIs; Chapter 16, for gastroenteritis; Chapter 22, for otitis media; Chapter 55, for sinusitis; and Chapter 57, for pharyngitis).

2. Infants aged 29 to 90-day-old who fulfil **all** the Rochester low-risk criteria may be managed as outpatients, provided they have reliable caregivers who are able to contact their physician by telephone and obtain medical care within 30 minutes. Parents must be instructed to call or seek immediate medical attention if the child demonstrates worrisome signs such as poor feeding, vomiting, excessive fussiness or sleepiness, skin rash, or color changes. The child must be reevaluated within 24 hours after blood and catheterized urine cultures are obtained (Figure 50–1). A lumbar puncture should be considered prior to empiric antibiotic treatment (see Section VI.B.4). A documented viral infection lowers the likelihood of serious bacterial infection (usually UTI) in this age group by one-half to one-third but does not eliminate it.

3. Febrile children without localizing signs who are 3 months of age or older may be followed up as outpatients if their caretakers are reliable and the children can be reevaluated within 24 to 48 hours.

4. Intramuscular ceftriaxone (Rocephin) at a dose of 50 mg/kg intramuscularly once daily up to 1 g maximum is preferred if the child is given empiric treatment. Amoxicillin–potassium clavulanate (Augmentin) may also decrease the risk of focal infection in bacteremic children, but there is less experience using this antibiotic for this purpose.

   a. Presumptive antibiotic therapy may be begun after obtaining a blood culture and other appropriate diagnostic studies if the child is between 3 months and 3 years of age, the fever is 39°C (102.2°F) or more, the AIOS score is 11 to 15, or the WBC is $\geq$15,000/μL. Antibiotic therapy might be withheld if the child appears nontoxic and has completed a primary series of conjugate pneumococcal vaccine or if prompt reporting of positive blood cultures and callback of the child is feasible.

   b. Therapy should be directed against *S pneumoniae*, which is the most common cause of occult bacteremia, as well as *H influenzae* and *Neisseria meningitidis*.

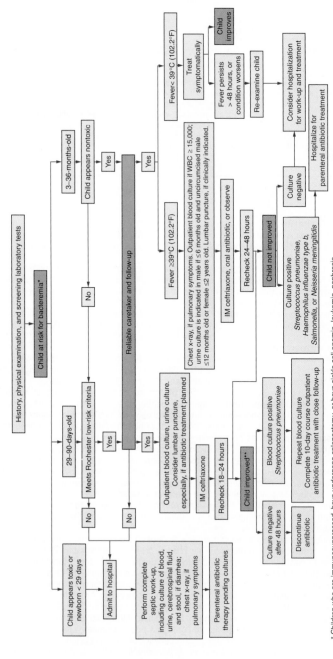

FIGURE 50–1. Guidelines for the management of children with fever without localizing signs. IM, intramuscular; WBC, white blood cell count.

* Children who are immunosuppressed, have undergone splenectomy, or have sickle cell anemia, leukemia, nephrosis, and other conditions placing them at high risk for overwhelming bacterial infection should be managed like toxic children.
**Nontoxic, nonbacteremic, afebrile children with otitis media or urinary tract infection may be treated with outpatient antibiotics.

342

TABLE 50–4. ROCHESTER CRITERIA FOR LOW-RISK INFANTS

1. Infant appears generally well
2. Infant has been previously healthy
Born at term ($\geq$37-wk gestation)
Did not receive perinatal antimicrobial therapy
Was not treated for unexplained hyperbilirubinemia
Had not received and was not receiving antimicrobial agents
Had not been previously hospitalized
Had no chronic or underlying illness
Was not hospitalized longer than mother
3. No evidence of skin, soft tissue, bone, joint, or ear infection
4. Laboratory values
Peripheral blood WBC count 5.0–15.0 $\times$ 10^9 cells/L (5000–15,000/mm^3)
Absolute band form count $\leq$1.5 $\times$ 10^9 cells/L ($\leq$1500/mm^3)
$\leq$ 10WBCs per high-power field ($\times$40) on microscopic examination of a spun urine sediment
$\leq$ 5WBC per high-power field ($\times$40) on microscopic examination of a stool smear (only for infants with diarrhea)

WBC, white blood cell.
(Reproduced with permission from Jaskiewicz JA, McCarthy CA, Richardson AC, et al, and the Febrile Infant Collaborative Study Group. Febrile infants at low risk for serious bacterial infection—an appraisal of the Rochester criteria and implications for management. *Pediatrics.* 1994;94:391.)

5. Follow-up of the older child who has fever and no obvious focus must occur by re-examination or telephone in 24 to 48 hours.
   a. If the child is better and cultures are negative after 48 hours, antibiotic therapy should be discontinued.
   b. If the child's condition is improved and blood culture grows *S pneumoniae,* outpatient antibiotic therapy should be continued for 10 days under close observation. A follow-up blood culture should be obtained to confirm clinical cure.
   c. If the child is improved and afebrile but the urine culture is positive, outpatient antibiotic therapy based on culture results should be continued for 7 to 14 days. Clinical pyelonephritis should be treated for 14 days. A repeat urine culture should be obtained after 48 hours of treatment if the child is not improving, sensitivity testing is not performed, or bacteria are intermediate or resistant to the chosen antibiotic. A structural evaluation of the urinary tract by renal ultrasound followed by voiding cystourethrography (VCUG) should be done in all children 2 months to 2-year-old. The child should continue to receive therapeutic or prophylactic antimicrobial therapy pending the VCUG.
   d. If the blood culture grows Hib, *N meningitidis, Salmonella,* or other pathogenic organisms, the child should be hospitalized for parenteral antibiotic therapy and evaluated for focal sites of infection.
   e. If the child is worse or not improved at follow-up, repeat history, physical examination, and diagnostic laboratory studies should be performed. Hospital admission is often indicated at this time.
6. The primary reason to treat fever symptomatically is to make the child more comfortable. Parents should be instructed as follows.
   a. Fever of 38.9°C (102°F) or greater should be treated with **acetaminophen,** 10 to 15 mg/kg every 4 hours up to a maximum of 5 doses per day. **Ibuprofen,** 5 to 10 mg/kg every 6 to 8 hours, may also be used for fever reduction in children aged 6 months or older.
   b. Children with a temperature $\geq$40°C (104°F) and no response to acetaminophen or ibuprofen should be sponged with lukewarm water. Alcohol or cold water should not be used.
   c. Children should be covered with light blankets and encouraged to drink liquids.
   d. Fever itself is seldom dangerous. It is a symptom of an underlying illness. Observation of children's behavior is even more important than a record of their temperature.

REFERENCES

American Academy of Pediatrics. In: Pickering LK, Baker CJ, Long SS, McMillan JA, eds. *2006 Red Book: 2006 Report of the Committee on Infectious Diseases.* 27th ed. Elk Grove Village, IL: American Academy of Pediatrics; 2006:375-377, 441-452, 591-595, 610-620, 711-725.

American Academy of Pediatrics Committee on Quality Improvement, Subcommittee on Urinary Tract Infection. Practice parameter: the diagnosis, treatment, and evaluation of the initial urinary tract infection in febrile infants and young children. *Pediatrics.* 1999;103:843.

Baraff LJ. Management of fever without source in infants and children. *Ann Emerg Med.* 2000;36:602-614.

Ishimine P. Fever without source in children 0 to 36 months of age. *Pediatr Clin N Am.* 2006;53:167-194.

Peck AJ, Bresee JS. Viral gastroenterititts. In: McMillan JA, Feigin RD, DeAngelis C, Jones MD, eds. *Oski's Pediatrics Principles and Practice.* 4th ed. Philadelphia, PA: Lippincott Williams & Wilkins; 2006:1288-1294.

Ward MA, Lorin MI, Kline MW. Fever without source. In: McMillan JA, Feigin RD, DeAngelis C, Jones MD, eds *Oski's Pediatrics Principles and Practice.* 4th ed. Philadelphia, PA: Lippincott Williams & Wilkins; 2006:908-911.

51   Pelvic Pain

Meredith A. Goodwin, MD

KEY POINTS

- Pelvic pain originates below the umbilicus of the adult female and may be acute (≤ 6 months' duration) or chronic (≥ 6 months' duration).
- Pelvic inflammatory disease, ectopic pregnancy, appendicitis, urinary tract infection, and adnexal mass rupture/torsion/hemorrhage are the most common causes of acute pelvic pain.
- Treatment of chronic pelvic pain is empiric, unless the causative agent is found.

I. **Definition.** Pelvic pain (PP) occurs below the adult female umbilicus. **Acute pelvic pain** (APP) refers to pain for ≤ 6 months. **Chronic pelvic pain** (CPP) lasts ≥ 6 months. **Gynecologic** sources of pain include ectopic pregnancy, acute and chronic pelvic inflammatory disease (PID), adnexal mass and/or torsion, endometriosis, dysmenorrhea, uterine leiomyoma, and chronic pelvic congestion. **Gastrointestinal** pain sources include gastroenteritis, irritable bowel syndrome, appendicitis, intestinal obstruction, hernia, diverticulitis, perirectal abscess, mesenteric ischemia, mesenteric adenitis, and inflammatory bowel disease. **Urologic pain** sources include interstitial cystitis, urolithiasis, and pyelonephritis. Pain from **musculoskeletal disorders** includes hematoma of the abdominal wall, spontaneous rectus sheath hematoma, ilioinguinal and iliohypogastric nerve entrapment, myofascial pain syndrome, and incarcerated hernia. Pain may also be referred from other organs or be psychogenic. This chapter will focus on gynecologic causes of PP in adult women; for other causes see Chapters 1 (Abdominal Pain), 16 (Diarrhea), 21 (Dysuria in Women), 36 (Hematuria), 46 (Myalgia), and 52 (Perianal Complaints).

II. **Common Diagnoses.** PP is a major health problem. It is responsible for 10% for all outpatient visits, 10% of gynecologic referrals, 12% of hysterectomies, and more than 40% of laparoscopies. The annual prevalence of PP in the primary care setting (38 of 1000 patients) is comparable to that of asthma and back pain. Women with PP have a high incidence of concomitant depression, somatization, and substance abuse potentiating their symptoms. The relative frequency of PP is influenced both by patient age and population risk factors. For example, in young women with a high prevalence of sexually transmitted diseases, acute and chronic PID are the most common causes. Reproductive-age patients have a higher prevalence of endometriosis, urinary tract infections, and ovarian cysts. Postmenopausal women have a higher frequency of gastrointestinal and genitourinary disorders. In addition, adnexal masses in this age group are more likely to be malignant.

A. **APP** accounts for 5% of all ambulatory primary care visits. Ten percent of these patients require urgent surgery.

1. **PID.** The exact incidence and prevalence of PID in the United States is unknown, given the frequency of asymptomatic or subclinical infections. The incidence of PID is said

to be 0.10–0.13/100,000 women/year, affecting approximately one million American women aged between 15 and 39 years annually. Risk factors for PID include age 15 to 24 years, a new sexual partner or multiple sexual partners in the preceding 3 months, current Chlamydial or gonococcal cervicitis, history of previous PID, and being within the first few months after placement of an intrauterine medical device (IUD).

2. **Adnexal mass torsion or rupture (16%).** Risk factors for adnexal torsion include reproductive age, prior pelvic surgery, history of ovarian cyst or PID, a pedunculated uterine leiomyoma, and prior tubal ligation. Two-thirds of ovarian tumors happen in the reproductive years, 80% to 85% of which are benign. Functional cysts occur more often in patient who smoke, but less often in patients using oral contraceptives. Most functional cyst ruptures occur on days 20 to 26 of the menstrual cycle, and unruptured corpus luteal cysts can produce symptoms difficult to differentiate from adnexal torsion. The risk of torsion with dermoid cysts is approximately 15%.

3. **Ectopic pregnancy (1%–2%)** occurs in approximately 2% of pregnancies in the United States. Forty percent occur in women aged 20 to 29 years. Predisposing factors include a history of tubal surgery, tubal pathology that alters tubal anatomy or interferes with tubal transport, PID (especially owing to *Chlamydia*), infertility treatment (ovulation induction or in vitro fertilization), endometriosis, uterine leiomyomas (if they obstruct the fallopian tubes), and rarely with in-utero diethylstilbestrol exposure. Contraceptive types influence the risk of ectopic pregnancy, ranging from 0.005/1000 with oral contraceptive pills (OCPs) to 0.020/1000 for IUDs and 0.318/1000 for tubal ligation.

4. **Uterine leiomyomas** are most often asymptomatic, and are clinically apparent in 20% to 25% of women of reproductive age, making this the most common premenopausal solid pelvic tumor in this age group. Leiomyomas are clinically apparent in 20% of women older than 35 years, and 40% of women older than 50 years. Fifty to seventy percent of African American women are affected. Other risk factors include family history (exact genetics are unknown), nulliparity, nonsmokers, and higher BMI owing to increased estrogen production in body fat. Acute degeneration or torsion of pedunculated leiomyoma may cause APP.

B. **CPP** is present in 14% to 16% of women seeking medical care. The incidence is 38.3/1000 women aged 15 to 73 years. In 61% of cases, the cause is not identified. Screening for trauma and posttraumatic stress disorder in these patients is important. (SOR **B**)

1. **Endometriosis** is found in 45% to 50% of women with CPP. Prevalence ranges from 20 to 100/1000 women of reproductive age, and 250–350/1000 of infertile women. Risk factors for endometriosis include family history (sevenfold increased risk in first-degree relatives), genetic abnormalities, immune disorders, Asian ancestry, cigarette smoking, alcohol consumption, lack of exercise, vaginal or cervical stenosis, and uterine anomalies (noncommunicating uterine horn, coelomic metaplasia). The incidence of endometriosis is inversely related to body mass index.

2. **Mittelschmerz** is midcyle pain caused by the release of an egg from the surface of an ovary, accompanied by a small amount of bleeding. It is experienced by **25%** of ovulating females.

3. **Dysmenorrhea (15%).** Approximately **30% to 50%** of all women experience dysmenorrhea, and 15% are incapacitated for 1 to 3 days of each month because of severe symptoms (see Chapter 18).

4. The prevalence of chronic **dyspareunia (35%)** ranges from 8% to 22% (SOR **A**) with more than 60% of women experiencing it at some time in their life. Risk factors for dyspareunia include a history of diabetes, alcohol or marijuana use, PID, medroxyprogesterone use, fatigue, anxiety, stress, depression, sexual abuse, vulvar and perineal surgeries, scarring with immobility or stricture of the vaginal walls, vaginal dryness with friction from inadequate genital sexual arousal, and vaginismus. (SOR **B**) Levator spasm and neuralgia associated with sutures or dissection may also contribute to CPP.

5. **Adhesions** are diagnosed in **25%** of women with CPP, but their causative role remains controversial. Pain caused by adhesions is experienced by 2.9 women per 100 operations, with risk influenced by surgical site—the colon and rectum have the highest incidence, followed by the ovaries. The postoperative adhesion rate does not appear to be different between laparotomy and laparoscopy.

6. **Uterine leiomyomas** are most often asymptomatic, but can be a source of CPP (see Section II.A.4).

7. **Psychogenic pain.** Women with a history of somatization disorder, sexual abuse, posttraumatic stress disorder, and depression frequently experience CPP. The

prevalence of sexual abuse history in CPP is 50%. Depression coexists with CPP in 50% and anxiety in 31% of women.

III. Symptoms (Tables 51–1 to 51–3).

A. Location and quality

1. APP

a. Unilateral sharp moderate/severe pain can occur with ovarian torsion, ruptured ectopic pregnancy, PID, ureteral colic, and diverticulitis.

b. Bilateral or midline diffuse sharp pain can occur with PID, submucosal fibroid rupture, pedunculated fibroid torsion, intra-abdominal hemorrhage, and intestinal obstruction.

c. Dull, pressure pain commonly occurs with mesenteric lymphadenitis, mesenteric ischemia, and diverticulitis.

2. CPP

a. Dull and deep pain characterizes interstitial cystitis and irritable bowel syndrome.

b. Reproducible trigger points confined to one anatomical region on the abdomen and back are found in patients with myofascial syndrome.

c. Pelvic fullness pain can be due to leiomyomas exerting pressure on adjacent structures. They can obstruct a ureter, compress the rectosigmoid with resulting constipation or intestinal obstruction, or compress pelvic veins leading to venous stasis of the lower extremities and possible thrombophlebitis.

B. Onset/chronology

1. APP Sudden onset of pain suggests acute perforation of hollow viscus or intraperitoneal hemorrhage; more gradual onset characterizes inflammation or obstruction.

2. CPP Pain may be dull or sharp, intermittent or constant. Onset is often very gradual, and may be cyclical.

C. Associated symptoms

1. Sexual dysfunction is a prominent feature in 28% of women with endometriosis, dyspareunia, and irritable bowel syndrome.

TABLE 51–1. FINDINGS WITH COMMON CAUSES OF ACUTE PELVIC PAIN

Diagnosis	Location/Quality/ Chronology of Pain	Other Symptoms	Signs
Ovarian cyst	Unilateral dull, pressure-like; severe/diffuse low abdominal (post rupture). Within 7 d of menses, worse with strenuous physical activity	Delayed/scanty menses if lutein cyst	Smooth mobile adnexal mass/fullness; peritoneal signs if ruptured
Pelvic inflammatory disease	Lower abdominal with gradual onset, usually bilateral, worse perimenstrually	Fever, vaginal discharge, dysuria, abnormal vaginal bleeding, backache, rectal pressure, adnexal tenderness/thickening, cervical motion tenderness	See Table 51–3
Adnexal torsion	Unilateral moderate/severe pain; sudden onset, within 24–48 h of presentation	Nausea/vomiting	Adnexal mass and tenderness on the affected side, rebound, guarding may be present
Ectopic pregnancy	Diffuse or localized, colicky or dull lower abdominal, radiating to the shoulder if hemoperitoneum	Amenorrhea or abnormal vaginal bleeding (metrorrhagia/menorrhagia) nausea/breast tenderness	Adnexal tenderness/mass, uterus slightly enlarged, peritoneal signs, abdominal distention and shock if significant hemorrhage
Uterine leiomyoma	Low midline pressure, back pain; moderate to severe pain with torsion/degeneration	Menorrhagia, metrorrhagia, nausea/vomiting with torsion, dysuria (if large), dyspareunia, infertility	Enlarged, nodular uterus, tender if degeneration/torsion; possible anemia

TABLE 51–2. CLINICAL FINDINGS WITH COMMON CAUSES OF CHRONIC PELVIC PAIN

Diagnosis	Location/Quality/ Chronology of Pain	Other Symptoms	Signs
Endometriosis	Variable midline suprapubic, cyclic premenstrual/ menstrual	Dyspareunia, painful defecation, infertility, hematuria	Often none; palpable cysts and nodules on uterosacral ligament
Mittelschmerz	Suprapubic, dull to sharp Midcycle; lasts hours to 3 d	None	None
Psychogenic	Variable	Depression, anxiety, back pain, fatigue, nausea	Signs of depression or anxiety, normal pelvic examination, occasional pelvic tenderness
Dysmenorrhea	Low abdominal starting prior/with menses, dyspareunia, radiates to the rectum	Painful defecation, nausea/vomiting, anorexia, headache, occasional diarrhea	None
Uterine Leiomyoma	Constant mild or no ongoing pain	Menorrhagia, metrorrhagia, pelvic fullness	Enlarged or irregular uterus on examination or TVU
Dyspareunia	Dull pain on vaginal entry or deep pelvic pain during sexual intercourse	Anxiety, depression, sexual dysfunction, vaginal dryness or infection	Anxiety, depression, posttraumatic stress disorder
Adhesions	Colicky, typically unilateral and focal	Bloating, nausea	Diffuse abdominal tenderness without masses; may have decreased mobility of pelvic organs

2. Substance abuse, somatization, depression, and posttraumatic stress disorder are present in 60% to 70% of women with CPP. Up to 25% of these patients have a history of physical abuse.

IV. **Signs** (see Tables 51–1 to 51–3). Also see the sidebars on chronic endometritis, adnexal mass, pelvic congestion syndrome, and ovarian remnant syndrome.

CHRONIC ENDOMETRITIS

Chronic endometritis in nonpregnant women is usually because of infections (PID, tuberculosis), IUD, submucosal leiomyoma, or radiation therapy. CPP, menorrhagia or metrorrhagia, mucopurulent vaginal discharge, and tender enlarged uterus are characteristic findings. Recommended treatment includes removal of an IUD and use of azithromycin or doxycycline (SOR **A**) for *Chlamydia trachomatis* or unknown etiology; *Mycobacterium tuberculosis* should be treated with combination drug therapy for 9 to 12 months. An endometrial biopsy may be needed for diagnosis.

ADNEXAL MASS

A family history of reproductive malignancy (uterine, breast, ovarian), presence of the BRCA gene, nulliparity, early menarche, and late menopause are risk factors for ovarian tumors.

TABLE 51–3. DIAGNOSTIC CRITERIA FOR PELVIC INFLAMMATORY DISEASE

Minimum diagnostic criteria: Uterine or adnexal or cervical motion tenderness.

Additional diagnostic criteria: Oral temperature $\geq 38.3°C$, cervical sampling positive for *Chlamydia trachomatis* or *Neisseria gonorrhoeae,* saline microscopy of vaginal secretions showing WBCs, elevated erythrocyte sedimentation rate, elevated C-reactive protein (CRP), and abnormal cervical or vaginal mucopurulent discharge.

Definitive diagnostic criteria: Endometrial biopsy with histopathologic evidence of endometritis, transvaginal ultrasonography or MRI scan showing thick fluid-filled fallopian tubes, laparoscopic abnormalities consistent with pelvic inflammatory disease.

(From the Centers for Disease Control and Prevention Recommendations, 2006.)

Eighty percent of ovarian masses in girls younger than 15 years are malignant. Thirty to sixty percent of adnexal masses in postmenopausal women are malignant as well. Adnexal masses can cause APP through adnexal mass torsion or ovarian cyst rupture or hemorrhage, and rupture of small (≤4 cm) cysts is usually asymptomatic. The approach to a discovered adnexal mass depends on the patient's age and cyst size. Because of high oncogenic potential (germ cell tumors) in premenarchial patients, all adnexal masses in these individuals should be evaluated by transvaginal ultrasound (TVU) and referred for surgical removal. In reproductive-age women, adnexal masses are commonly follicular or lutein cysts or complications of PID (hydrosalpinx and tubo-ovarian abscess). If pain is not acute or recurrent, palpable cysts ≤6 cm in women of childbearing age may be monitored with repeat pelvic examination in 6 weeks. Any persistent or increasing mass on serial observation or a mass initially ≥6 cm should be evaluated by TVU. Adnexal masses in postmenopausal women have a high risk of malignancy (surface epithelial or stromal tumors) and should be evaluated with TVU, tumor markers (CA-125), and possibly computerized tomography (CT) scanning.

Management of adnexal masses is referral to gynecology for further evaluation and removal, unless a mass in a reproductive-age woman is cystic, small (≤6 cm), and does not persist or increase in size.

PELVIC CONGESTION SYNDROME

Pelvic congestion syndrome is caused by autonomic nervous system dysfunction manifesting as smooth muscle spasm and pelvic vasculature congestion. It is commonly associated with pelvic, vulvar, and thigh varicosities, and psychogenic disorders (depression, anxiety, and posttraumatic stress disorder). Typical symptoms include lower abdominal and back pain, dysmenorrhea, dyspareunia, abnormal uterine bleeding, chronic fatigue, and irritable bowel symptoms. Pain usually begins with ovulation and lasts through menses. Examination reveals an enlarged, tender uterus and ovaries with multiple ovarian cysts and tender uterosacral ligaments. Evaluation for suspected pelvic congestion includes TVU with Doppler flow study and pelvic venography (the gold standard for evaluation of pelvic congestion) looking for delayed disappearance of contrast medium from the uterine and ovarian veins. Because of the cost and possible side effects of treatment, further management should be based on related symptoms rather than the presence of varicosities alone. First-line treatment includes hormonal suppression with continuous progestins (e.g., medroxyprogesterone acetate, 30 mg orally daily for 6 months). Transcatheter embolization of the pelvic veins or hysterectomy with possible oophorectomy are reasonable options in women who have completed their childbearing.

OVARIAN REMNANT SYNDROME

Ovarian remnant syndrome is a rare condition, which develops when functional ovarian tissue is left after intended bilateral oophorectomy. Symptoms usually arise 2 to 5 years after intended oophorectomy, and include cyclic (often with the luteal phase) or constant lateralizing CPP and dyspareunia, with or without adnexal mass. Patients deny menopausal symptoms. Follicle-stimulating hormone and luteinizing hormone typically are in premenopausal range, although occasionally the remaining ovarian tissue may not be active enough to suppress follicle-stimulating hormone levels. TVU or CT scanning helps to identify an adnexal mass. Gonadotropin-releasing hormone (GnRH) agonists often provide relief, but are impractical for long-term use. Patients who achieve relief with GnRH agonists will likely respond to surgical removal of the remnant tissue.

V. **Laboratory Tests** (Tables 51–4 and 51–5).
   A. **Pregnancy test** (urine or serum) must be performed in all patients with PP who are of reproductive age with an intact uterus.
      1. Most currently available **urine pregnancy tests** can detect human chorionic gonadotropin (hCG) levels of 15 to 100 U/mL 3 to 4 days after conception. Dilute urine

TABLE 51–4. TESTS HELPFUL IN DIAGNOSING COMMON CAUSES OF ACUTE PELVIC PAIN

Suspected Diagnosis	Tests
PID	β-hCG, CBC, cervical sampling for *Neisseria gonorrhoeae* and *Chlamydia trachomatis*, ESR, vaginal wet prep, endometrial biopsy, TVU, laparoscopy, LFT if perihepatitis
Ectopic pregnancy	Serum β-hCG, CBC, TVU, laparoscopy
Adnexal mass torsion	TVU with Doppler flow study, CT
Uterine Leiomyomas	TVU, MRI

CBC, complete blood count; CT, computerized tomography; ESR, erythrocyte sedimentation rate; hCG, human chorionic gonadotropin; LFT, liver function tests; PID, pelvic inflammatory disease; TVU, transvaginal ultrasound.

may decrease sensitivity. Most current urine pregnancy tests are 84% to 94% sensitive by the first day of the expected period. By 1 week after the first day of the missed period, sensitivity for urinary hCG is 97%.

2. **Quantitative serum β-hCG** is detected at the level of 2 to 25 mIU at 7 days after conception and doubles every 2 days during the first 4 weeks after implantation. With ectopic pregnancy, quantitative serum β-hCG levels off (plateau) or decrease.

B. **Complete blood cell count.** Fifty-six percent of patients with PID and 36% of patients with acute appendicitis have a normal white blood cell count.

C. **The cervical DNA probe** has a specificity of 99% and a sensitivity of 86% for *Neisseria gonorrhoeae* and a specificity of 98% and a sensitivity of 93% for *C trachomatis*.

D. The sensitivity for adnexal mass detection by **TVU** is 60% to 84%, and specificity is 90% to 98%. TVU with Doppler flow study adds diagnostic efficiency for endometrioma, pelvic congestion syndrome, ovarian and adnexal mass torsion, and ovarian neoplasm.

E. **Magnetic resonance imaging (MRI)** improves visualization of small cystic lesions that are undetectable on TVU (e.g., endometriomas). The sensitivity and specificity of MRI are 71% and 82%, respectively. The fat suppression technique increases sensitivity and specificity to 90% and 98%, respectively. In women desiring future pregnancy, MRI can differentiate between a single leiomyoma (candidate for uterus-preserving interventions) and adenomyosis (necessitating hysterectomy).

F. The sensitivity of **CT** is 92% for diagnosis of peritoneal lesions (e.g., endometriosis or ovarian metastasis). MRI and CT are equally accurate, but more sensitive than TVU for staging of ovarian cancer and localization of endometriosis.

G. **Laparoscopy** is the gold standard for evaluation of CPP. More than 40% of gynecologic laparoscopies are done for this reason. It is reserved for patients with an equivocal diagnosis (e.g., surgical emergency, tubal pregnancy), those unresponsive to treatment (e.g., with PID), or when tissue diagnosis is necessary (e.g., in endometriosis).

H. **Erythrocyte sedimentation rate** is elevated in 75% of patients with PID.

VI. Treatment

A. APP

1. **Treatment of PID** should provide coverage for likely etiologic agents (*N gonorrhoeae, C trachomatis,* anaerobes, enteric gram-negative rods, *Mycoplasma hominis,* and *Ureaplasma urealyticum*), treatment of underlying disease (acute endometritis, salpingitis, or peritonitis), as well as prevention of complications (tubo-ovarian abscess [15% of cases], Fitz–Hugh–Curtis syndrome/perihepatitis [30% of cases], and septicemia).

TABLE 51–5. USEFUL TESTS FOR EVALUATING COMMON CAUSES OF CHRONIC PELVIC PAIN

Suspected Diagnosis	Tests
Adhesions	None
Chronic endometritis	Endometrial biopsy
Dyspareunia	*Neisseria gonorrhoeae* and *Chlamydia trachomatis* study, vaginal wet preparation, vaginal pH, UA, urine culture
Endometriosis	TVU, MRI, laparoscopy
Mittelschmerz	None

CT, computerized tomography; MRI, magnetic resonance imaging; TVU, transvaginal ultrasound; UA, urinalysis.

TABLE 51–6. OUTPATIENT THERAPY FOR PELVIC INFLAMMATORY DISEASE

CDC Recommended Outpatient Regimen
Ceftriaxone 250 mg IM in a single dose

PLUS
Doxycycline 100 mg orally twice a day for 14 d

WITH OR WITHOUT
Metronidazole 500 mg orally twice a day for 14 d

OR
Cefoxitin 2 g IM in a single dose and Probenecid, 1 g orally administered concurrently in a single dose

PLUS
Doxycycline 100 mg orally twice a day for 14 d

WITH OR WITHOUT
Metronidazole 500 mg orally twice a day for 14 d

OR
Other parenteral third-generation cephalosporin (e.g., ceftizoxime or cefotaxime)

PLUS
Doxycycline 100 mg orally twice a day for 14 d

WITH OR WITHOUT
Metronidazole 500 mg orally twice a day for 14 d

(From the Centers for Disease Control and Prevention Recommendations, 2007 Update.)

    a. Inpatient treatment of PID with parenteral antibiotics is recommended for pregnant women, patients with severe illness with fever and vomiting, cases where surgical emergencies (appendicitis, tubo-ovarian abscess) cannot be excluded, or when there is intolerance or poor response to outpatient antimicrobial regimens. Parenteral therapy such as cefotetan 2 g intravenously every 12 hours, OR cefoxitin 2 g intravenously every 6 hours PLUS doxycycline 100 mg orally or intravenously every 12 hours may be discontinued 24 hours after clinical improvement. Oral therapy should continue for 14 days.

    b. Outpatient treatment (Table 51–6) may start presumptively while awaiting culture results.

  2. Ectopic pregnancy

    a. Gynecologic consultation and surgery (laparotomy or laparoscopy) are indicated for ruptured ectopic pregnancy, especially in hemodynamically unstable patients, women unable to comply with monitoring after medical treatment, failure of medical treatment (tubal size $\geq$ 3 cm, serum β-hCG greater than 5000 mIU, or fetal cardiac activity on TVU).

    b. Otherwise, women with ectopic pregnancy are managed either with **methotrexate** or expectantly. Methotrexate is effective in 86% to 94% of patients without indications for surgery (see Table 51–7).

      (1) Complete blood cell count with differential, aspartate aminotransferase, creatinine, blood type, Rhesus (Rh), and weekly monitoring of serum hCG is required. A second IM dose of methotrexate (50 mg/m^2) is recommended if the hCG titer decreases to less than 15% by 4 days after the first injection.

      (2) Methotrexate side effects include stomatitis, diarrhea, leukopenia, thrombocytopenia, anemia, nephrotoxicity, hepatic dysfunction, alopecia, and dermatitis; these are mild, and are reported in 34% of patients.

  3. Urgent gynecologic referral is indicated for **adnexal torsion** and **necrosis of pedunculated leiomyoma.** A torsed ovary may be salvaged by detorsion if pedunculated. Myomectomy and hysterectomy are optional treatments for pedunculated leiomyoma.

  4. Uterine leiomyomas. Stable leiomyomas can be managed medically with nonsteroidal anti-inflammatory drugs (NSAIDs) such as oral ibuprofen 400 mg every 6 hours. Women unresponsive to medical therapy may require gynecologic referral for surgery (myomectomy or hysterectomy). Preoperative GnRH agonists, such as leuprolide 3.75 mg IM monthly, may be given to increase hemoglobin, reduce uterine size, and decrease intraoperative blood loss. Long-term ($\geq$6 month) treatment with

TABLE 51–7. METHOTREXATE PROTOCOLS FOR ECTOPIC PREGNANCY

Day	Single Dose Therapy	Multidose Therapy
0	Labs: hCG, CBC, AST, Cr, type, and Rh	Labs: hCG, CBC, AST, Cr, type, and Rh
1	MTX: 50 mg/m^2 IM	MTX: 1 mg/kg IM
2	—	Leucovorin: 0.1 mg/kg IM
3	—	Labs: hCG; if ≤15% decline then repeat dose cycle on day 3; if ≥15% decline, follow weekly until undetected; max: 4 MTX/Leucovorin cycles total
4	Labs: hCG	—
5	—	—
6	—	—
7	Labs: hCG; if ≤15% decline at days 4–7 then repeat dose; if ≥15% decline, measure weekly until undetected	—

MTX, methotrexate; hCG, human chorionic gonadotropin; CBC, complete blood count; AST, aspartate aminotransferase; Cr, serum creatinine.
(Reprinted with permission from ACP PIER 2007. Ectopic Pregnancy. Drug Therapy: Consider drug therapy with methotrexate to treat ectopic pregnancy. Retrieved from http://pier.acponline.org/physicians/diseases/d050/tables/d050-t3.html)

GnRH agonists is not recommended because of risk of significant bone loss. Another option for leiomyoma treatment is interventional radiology referral for uterine artery embolization.

- **B.** Specific causes of **CPP** should be identified and treated; otherwise, empiric therapy is indicated.
  - **1. Dysmenorrhea** (see Chapter 18).
  - **2. Uterine leiomyomas** are a rare cause of CPP, and should be treated only if symptomatic. See above for specific recommendations.
  - **3. Endometriosis**-associated PP may be treated medically or surgically (via laparoscopy). (SOR **B**) Medications include oral contraceptives (SOR **C**) as first-line therapy if the patient is not trying to conceive, with consideration of a GnRH agonist (SOR **A**) or danazol (SOR **B**) as second-line therapy. (SOR **A**) Add oral norethindrone, with or without conjugated estrogens, to GnRH therapy to prevent hot flushes and bone loss. (SOR **A**) Laparoscopy is often used for a diagnosis of endometriosis, but is not required before a treatment trial with a GnRH agonist. The androgenic side effects of danazol limit its acceptability. Third-line or maintenance therapy with levonorgestrel intrauterine systems has also been effective in reducing both bleeding and pain although this is not an FDA-approved use. (SOR **C**)
  - **4. Dyspareunia** treatment is driven by the suspected etiology. Estrogen deficiency with inadequate lubrication, progressing to loss of elasticity and thinning of the epithelium from vaginal atrophy, is easily treated with local estrogen therapy. Other causes of dyspareunia are managed as indicated by the identified underlying medical or psychological condition.
  - **5. Mittelschmerz** usually requires only patient education and reassurance. Oral NSAIDs may be prescribed for symptoms. OCPs also may be helpful (see Chapter 95).
  - **6.** Gynecologic referral for surgery may be required. Surgical approaches include **laparoscopy** (discussed above), **lysis of adhesions**, and **hysterectomy**. Hysterectomy is effective in some cases; however, 40% of women continue to experience CPP after hysterectomy. The success rate for adhesiolysis ranges from 0% to 65%. Adhesiolysis can significantly improve pain when the adhesions are dense and involve the bowel. Patients with endometriosis may require therapeutic laparoscopy for electrocoagulation or laser ablation of lesions. These patients have a 66% to 80% response rate in clinical trials. (SOR **A**) Approximately 12% of hysterectomies are performed for PP; however, 30% of patients who present to pain clinics have already had a hysterectomy without experiencing pain relief.
  - **7. Symptomatic therapy**
    - **a.** Pharmacologic methods
      - **(1)** Oral NSAIDs (e.g., ibuprofen) act peripherally to create analgesia. Individuals vary widely in their response to different NSAIDs, therefore, at least three unique medications should be tried. COX-2 specific inhibitors may also be used and are

reported to have fewer side effects, although this claim and their safety profile have recently come into question.

(2) Oral opioids that block pain perception centrally (e.g., hydrocodone with acetaminophen 5/500 mg, 1–2 tablets po every 4–6 hours) have a well-recognized role in acute pain management. Their use in the treatment of chronic pain is controversial; however, they may allow the return of normal function without significant side effects in those who have failed other treatments.

(3) Antidepressants such as oral paroxetine, 20 mg po once daily, or amitriptyline, 25 to 50 mg po at bedtime, or both have been used to treat a number of chronic pain syndromes. They are thought to improve pain tolerance, restore sleep patterns, and reduce depressive symptoms.

(4) Continuous oral or intramuscular progestins such as medroxyprogesterone acetate, 5 mg po daily, have been reported to improve symptoms in 73% of patients (see Chapter 95).

(5) OCPs.

(6) Failure to improve symptoms within 3 months suggests the need for laparoscopic confirmation of clinical diagnosis, especially if the results of the psychological evaluation are negative.

b. **Nonpharmacologic approaches** include counseling, acupuncture, behavioral and relaxation feedback therapies, and social interventions, as well as neuroablative treatments. Neuroablative therapies employed in consultation with a pain management specialist or surgeon include presacral neurectomy, uterosacral neurectomy, paracervical denervation, uterovaginal ganglion excision, injection of neurotoxic chemicals, laser treatment, cryotherapy, or thermocoagulation.

REFERENCES

Bordman R, Jackson B. Below the belt—approach to chronic pelvic pain. *Can Fam Physician*. 2006; 52:1556-1562.

Latthe P, Latthe M, Say L, Gulmezoglu M, Khan KS. WHO systematic review of prevalence of chronic pelvic pain: a neglected reproductive health morbidity. *BMC Public Health*. 2006;6:177-183.

Novak E. *Berek and Novak's Gynecology*.14th ed. Philadelphia Lippincott Williams & Wilkins; 2007.

Sexually Transmitted Diseases Treatment Guideline 2006. *MMWR Morbid Mortal Wkly Rep*. 2006; 55(RR11):1-94.

Stones W, Cheong YC, Howard FM. Interventions for treating chronic pelvic pain in women. *Cochrane Database Sys Rev*. 2007;1(2):1-40.

Update to CDC's Sexually Transmitted Diseases Treatment Guidelines 2006. Fluoroquinolones No Longer Recommended for Treatment of Gonococcal Infections. *MMWR Morbid Mortal Wkly Rep*. 2007;56(MM14):332-336.

---

52   Perianal Complaints

Kalyanakrishnan Ramakrishnan, MD

KEY POINTS

- Although benign anorectal diseases such as hemorrhoids, fissures, pruritus ani, and perianal infections are common, in elderly patients a high index of suspicion for colorectal cancer should be maintained in the presence of perianal complaints.
- In young individuals with bleeding-associated defecation and no family history, anoscopy and flexible sigmoidoscopy are sufficient testing. In people older than 50 years, and especially in the presence of fatigue, weight loss, or anemia, colon pathology should be ruled out by a double-contrast barium enema or colonoscopy.
- Most treatment measures for perianal pathology (banding of hemorrhoids, sphincterotomy for fissures, drainage of perianal and pilonidal infections) can be performed as office procedures under local or no anesthesia.

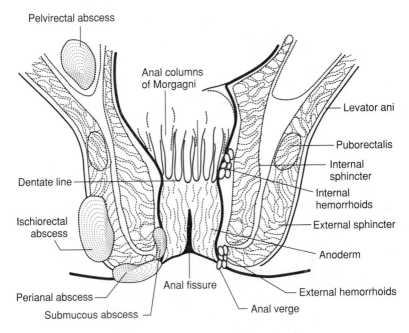

FIGURE 52–1. Anatomy and pathology of the anal canal.

I. **Definition** (Figure 52–1). The **musculature of the anal canal** consists of the **internal sphincter,** the downward continuation of the involuntary circular smooth muscle of the rectum, and the **external sphincter,** an elliptical cylinder of voluntary skeletal muscle that surrounds the anal canal and is continuous with the **levator ani,** which forms the greater part of the pelvic floor. Sympathetic and parasympathetic nerves, both of which are inhibitory, supply the internal sphincter.

The anal mucosa is lined by columnar epithelium above the undulating **dentate line** and supplied by sympathetic nerves (L-1–L-3); the squamous epithelium below the dentate line is supplied by somatic nerves. Above the dentate line are longitudinal folds, 6 to 14 in number, the **columns of Morgagni.** The anal glands, 3 to 10 in number, open directly into an anal crypt at the dentate line.

Perianal complaints include irritation, soreness, or discomfort in the region surrounding the anal canal. Hemorrhoids, fissures, anorectal and pilonidal infections, and pruritus ani are all common causes.

Hemorrhoids are fibrovascular cushions with arteriovenous connections that bulge into the lumen of the anal canal. Their anchoring and supporting connective tissue system deteriorates with aging. Chronic straining secondary to constipation leads to prolapse, thinning, and friability of the overlying mucosa, and results in bright-red rectal bleeding. **Perianal hematoma** is a painful swelling, secondary to thrombosis within a saccule of the hemorrhoidal venous plexus.

Anal fissure is a laceration in the vertical axis of the anal canal caused by repeated trauma by hard stool. Internal sphincter spasm impairs healing.

Anorectal abscesses arise from blockage of the anal glands followed by superimposed polymicrobial aerobic and anaerobic infection.

Fistula-in-ano is a tract lined with granulation tissue connecting a primary opening inside the anal canal to a secondary opening in the perianal skin and is most often caused by rupture or drainage of an anorectal abscess.

Pilonidal cysts develop through in-growth of hair or through trauma to the sacrococcygeal region.

The pain of **proctalgia fugax** results from puborectalis muscle spasm. Suggested causes include laxity of the anal sphincter, levator muscle tension resulting in spasm, and increased contractile activity of the sigmoid colon.

Proctitis, which arises from rectal inflammation (within 15 cm of the dentate line), is because of inflammatory bowel disease (IBD), sexually transmitted diseases—i.e., *Neisseria gonorrhoeae,* syphilis, *Chlamydia trachomatis, Herpes simplex* virus or cytomegalovirus, or from bacterial infections. It may also be because of prior antibiotic use (*Clostridium difficile* proctitis), radiotherapy, or diversion colostomy or ileostomy in patients with an intact rectum. **Pruritus ani** can be caused by benign anorectal diseases producing a discharge, premalignant lesions (Paget and Bowen disease), and nonprimary anal diseases (contact dermatitis, fungal infections, diabetes, pinworm infestations, psoriasis, and seborrhea).

II. Common Diagnoses

A. **The incidence of hemorrhoids** is high (approximately 40%), with equal sexual prevalence, and peak incidence between 45 and 65 years of age. Symptomatic hemorrhoids are associated with aging, pregnancy, pelvic tumors, prolonged sitting and straining, and chronic diarrhea or constipation.

B. **Anal fissures** affect both genders equally; risk factors include the passage of hard stool, chronic diarrhea, habitual use of laxatives, and anal trauma during intercourse or examination.

C. **Anorectal infections**
1. **Anorectal abscess.** The peak incidence is in the third to fourth decades. Male-to-female predominance is 2:1 to 3:1. One-third of patients report similar past episodes. Risk factors include immunosuppression, diabetes mellitus, IBD (predisposes to recurrent/multiple abscesses), and pregnancy.
2. The incidence of **fistula-in-ano** is 8.6 cases per 100,000, and the mean age of occurrence is 38.3 years. Risk factors include trauma, Crohn's disease, fissures, carcinoma, radiation, actinomycoses, tuberculosis, and chlamydial infections.
3. Incidence of **pilonidal disease** is approximately 0.7%, and it is twice as common in men as in women. Precipitants include hyperhidrosis associated with sitting and buttock friction, poor personal hygiene, obesity, and local trauma, and buttock hair characteristics such as kinking, coarseness, and rapid growth rate.

D. **Levator ani syndrome** occurs in 6% to 7% of the general population, slightly more often in women than in men.

E. **Proctalgia fugax** occurs in approximately 13% of adults and is 2 to 3 times more common among women. Stress and anxiety are precipitants. Many patients have other functional bowel symptoms.

F. **Proctitis** occurs predominantly in adults, more in men. Risk factors include high-risk sexual behavior (anal sex, homosexuality, multiple partners), autoimmune disorders, radiation therapy, immunocompromised state, and fecal diversion. Following radiation, 5% to 20% of patients develop proctitis within 3 to 24 months.

G. Idiopathic **pruritus ani** (most common type) is seen more often in men and is typically worse at night. Less common causes include benign anorectal diseases, premalignant lesions, and nonprimary anal diseases.

III. Symptoms. The common symptoms of perianal pathology include pain, bleeding, perianal mass, prolapse, pruritus, and discharge.

A. The most common lesions causing **anorectal pain** are **fissure, abscess, and thrombosed external hemorrhoid.** Anal pain of any etiology may be aggravated by bowel movements.
1. In **anal fissure,** pain occurs during and after defecation and is most acute over the first 2 to 3 days, resolving over a 7- to 10-day period.
2. A dull ache, or throbbing pain in the perianal area worsened by coughing, sneezing, sitting, and relieved by defecation, suggests an **anorectal abscess.** Pain intensifies as the abscess increases in size and becomes superficial.
3. **Perianal hematoma** (external hemorrhoid) appears as a painful swelling soon after straining. **Strangulation** of internal hemorrhoids also causes severe pain, bleeding, and occasionally signs of systemic illness.
4. **Proctalgia fugax** is characterized by the sudden onset of severe pain in the anus lasting several seconds or minutes, which then disappears completely. Approximately one-third of patients suffer attacks following defecation, and some following sexual activity.

   5. Tenesmus, an uncomfortable desire to defecate, is associated with inflammatory conditions. Tenesmus with urgency of evacuation suggests **proctitis.**
   6. The **levator ani syndrome** is associated with chronic or recurrent episodes of rectal pain or aching lasting 20 minutes or longer occurring for at least 3 months, precipitated by prolonged sitting, or by defecation. Some patients have dyschezia or a sense of incomplete evacuation.
B. Bleeding
   1. Hemorrhoids and **fissures** cause bright red blood on stool, toilet paper, or the toilet bowl with, or following, bowel movements. Dark or clotted blood mixed with the stool suggests sources proximal to the anus. Hemorrhoids cause painless bleeding; bleeding with painful defecation suggests a fissure.
   2. Drainage of blood or pus with associated pruritus and pain suggests a **fistula.**
   3. Bleeding with a painful lump not exclusively related to defecation suggests a thrombosed external hemorrhoid; bleeding with tenesmus suggests **proctitis.**
C. Prolapse. Prolapse occurs in second- and third-degree hemorrhoids, usually with a bowel movement, or during walking or heavy lifting, and is associated with an uncomfortable fullness, which resolves on spontaneous or manual reduction.
D. Perianal mass. A painful perianal lump may be an abscess, a thrombosed external hemorrhoid, or a strangulated prolapsed internal hemorrhoid. **Pilonidal abscess** presents with a painful swelling overlying the coccyx, purulent drainage, fever, and constitutional symptoms.
E. Discharge. Blood-stained discharge mixed with mucus, pus, or both is a feature of proctitis, thrombosed or prolapsed hemorrhoids, perianal or pilonidal abscess, fistula, or neoplasm.
F. Miscellaneous. Fever and other constitutional symptoms (anorexia, nausea, vomiting, or diarrhea) may accompany strangulated hemorrhoids, perirectal and pilonidal abscesses, IBD, and proctitis.

IV. Signs
A. Inspection. Skin changes suggestive of psoriasis, seborrhea, ulcerations, or lichenification may indicate the existence of **pruritus ani.** In **pilonidal infections,** a sinus, swelling, and redness overlying the coccyx or purulent drainage may be seen. **Perianal hematoma** presents as a bluish mass at the anal verge and **anorectal abscess,** with localized erythema, purulent drainage, or perianal edema. In **anal fistulas,** external (secondary) openings are seen. Findings in **proctitis** can range from a mild mucoid exudate to marked infection with spontaneous bleeding, purulent discharge, and erosions (in patients with human immunodeficiency virus). Papules, vesicles, shallow ulcerations, and crusts around the anal and genital areas may be seen in **herpetic infections.**
B. Palpation (including digital rectal examination)
   1. A tender fluctuant mass may be palpated at the anal verge (perianal abscess), sacrum (pilonidal abscess), or through the rectal wall (ischiorectal abscess) (Figure 52–1).
   2. Most **fissures** are posterior (Figure 52–1), and can be observed with gentle lateral retraction around the anus or on anoscopy. Anterior fissures have an incidence of 1% in men and 10% in women. **Acute fissures** appear as a fresh laceration, whereas **chronic fissures** have raised edges, exposing the white horizontally oriented fibers of the internal sphincter. The sphincter tone is markedly increased and digital examination or anoscopy reproduces the extreme pain associated with defecation. When fissures are lateral, infections such as syphilis, tuberculosis, occult abscesses, herpes, acquired immunodeficiency syndrome, carcinoma, and IBD should be considered. Secondary changes such as a sentinel pile, induration of the fissure edge, and anal stenosis, because of spasm or a fibrotic internal sphincter, may be seen.
   3. Palpable tenderness of overly contracted levator ani muscles may be noticed in the **levator ani syndrome,** as the examining finger moves from the coccyx posteriorly to the pubis anteriorly.
   4. Uncomplicated internal hemorrhoids are not palpable.
C. Anoscopy. This procedure is performed with the patient in the left lateral position. The instrument is well lubricated to ease insertion. A side-viewing anoscope is inserted with the open portion in the right anterior, then right posterior, and finally the left lateral position to look for hemorrhoidal masses, which will bulge into the anoscope.
   1. Hemorrhoids are classified as internal, external, or combined intero-external. **External hemorrhoids** originate below the dentate line; **internal hemorrhoids** originate above it (Figure 52–1). Internal hemorrhoids are found in the right anterior, right

posterior, and left lateral positions within the anal canal, and graded as first degree (bleeding without prolapse); second degree (prolapse on straining, reducing spontaneously); third degree (prolapse requiring manual reduction); and fourth degree (strangulated, irreducible, prolapsed hemorrhoid).

2. **Fissures** may also be seen, with the characteristics as stated above.
3. Internal openings may be identified in **fistulas.** The **Goodsall rule** states that fistulas with an external opening anterior to a plane passing transversely through the center of the anus will follow a straight radial course to the dentate line. Fistulas with their openings posterior to this line will follow a curved course to the posterior midline.
4. Proctitis owing to *C trachomatis* and *N gonorrhoeae* cause erythema, discharge, and swelling in the anal canal.

V. Laboratory Tests
A. Tests for pruritus ani and proctitis
1. In pruritus ani, skin scrapings (potassium hydroxide preparation) are useful in detecting tinea cruris and yeast infections.
2. In proctitis, diagnosis is confirmed in 92% of patients by anoscopic smears and culture for bacterial, fungal, and viral pathogens, Tzanck testing for multinucleate giant cells, and stool testing for *C difficile* toxin. Syphilis can be confirmed by finding spirochetes on dark-field examination of rectal discharge, and *N gonorrhoeae* through appearance of gram-negative diplococci on Gram staining. If warranted, cultures for *C difficile, N gonorrhoeae, C trachomatis,* and *H simplex,* and serologic testing for syphilis (RPR), should be obtained.

B. Skin biopsy.
Visible abnormalities in the perianal skin may necessitate a skin biopsy (excision or punch biopsy) to rule out Paget or Bowen disease.

C. Endoscopy
1. Rectal bleeding in people older than 50 years warrants a **colonoscopy** to rule out colorectal neoplasm. (SOR **A**)
2. Younger individuals with bleeding-associated defecation, and no family history of colon cancer, require only **flexible sigmoidoscopy.**
3. **Flexible sigmoidoscopy or colonoscopy** may be performed to exclude more proximally located inflammatory disorders with which **anal fistulas** or **perianal pruritus** may be associated. Endoscopic biopsy may show crypt abscesses or other features of IBD.

D. Miscellaneous
1. **Endoanal ultrasound** or **magnetic resonance imaging** is useful before surgery to determine the existence, extent, and location of **anorectal abscesses.**
2. **Ultrasound, fistulography, computerized tomography, and magnetic resonance imaging** may be helpful in identifying an occult cause of **recurrent fistula.**
3. **Electromyography** studies may be used to differentiate the **levator ani syndrome** from pelvic floor dyssynergia, a relaxation abnormality associated with dyschezia and straining.

VI. Treatment
A. Hemorrhoids
causing minor bleeding can be managed with dietary and lifestyle modifications to minimize constipation and straining (see Chapter 12). (SOR **B**) More symptomatic hemorrhoids (e.g., third- or fourth-degree) are likely to require operative intervention. (SOR **B**)

1. **Office procedures**
   a. **Rubber band ligation** is indicated in first-, second-, and third-degree hemorrhoids. (SOR **A**) After rectal examination, the anoscope is inserted and the hemorrhoid to be banded is identified (the largest hemorrhoid is banded first) and grasped with a modified Allis forceps placed through the ligator. In the absence of discomfort, the band is applied by depressing the trigger on the hemorrhoid ligator. Multiple hemorrhoids can be banded at one sitting, or sequentially. A dull persistent ache is common following banding. Significant anal pain owing to band placement below or close to the dentate line requires removal and reapplication. An **anoscope/ligator,** attached to wall suction, is an alternative to traditional banding methods. Complications with both methods are rare (5%) and include urinary retention, bleeding, band slippage, pain, ulceration, thrombosis, and perineal sepsis. Bleeds are self-limited and occur immediately after banding, or 7 to 10 days later. Up to 25% of patients require repeat banding over 5 years.

b. **Infrared coagulation** is most beneficial in first- and second-degree hemorrhoids. (SOR **B**) The coagulator is applied through the anoscope for 1.5 seconds, thrice to the apex of each hemorrhoid.

c. **Sclerotherapy** involves the injection of a sclerosant (sodium morrhuate, 5% phenol, and hypertonic saline) through the anoscope into the submucosa at the apex of the hemorrhoid. (SOR **B**) This causes ischemia, induces fibrosis, and fixes the hemorrhoid to the rectal wall, decreasing bleeding and prolapse. It is performed as an office procedure and requires no special training or equipment. Misplacement may result in perianal infection, anal ulceration, and fibrosis.

d. Most patients with **perianal hematoma** respond to conservative measures (sitz baths twice a day, stool softeners, and analgesics). Surgical excision under local anesthesia is an office procedure. It is considered for patients presenting during the first 2 to 3 days, if ulceration or rupture occurs, or if conservative treatment fails. (SOR **B**) The anoderm overlying the swelling is infiltrated with plain lidocaine and incised with a no. 15 blade, evacuating the clot. Bleeding is controlled with sutures or packing, and conservative measures are continued.

2. **Hemorrhoidectomy** is reserved for large third- and fourth-degree hemorrhoids. (SOR **B**) This is usually performed by a surgeon as a day-case under local anesthesia; patients are generally able to return to work within 2 weeks.

B. **Anal fissures**

1. Acute (superficial) fissures can be managed with fiber supplementation, bulk laxatives, sitz baths, and topical corticosteroid or local anesthetic creams (e.g., Anusol H, Proctosedyl, or 5% lidocaine ointment applied twice daily). (SOR **B**)

2. Other successful topical therapies are nifedipine 0.3% with lidocaine ointment 1.5%, every 12 hours for 6 weeks, topical nitroglycerin ointment 0.2% twice daily for 8 weeks, and diltiazem gel 2% 3 times a day for 8 weeks.

3. Botulinum toxin A, a potent inhibitor of acetylcholine release from nerve endings, injected into the anal sphincter as an outpatient procedure, improves healing in chronic fissures. (SOR **B**)

4. If medical measures fail, a lateral sphincterotomy, performed as an office procedure by a surgeon or a family physician with requisite training, is successful. (SOR **A**)

C. **Anorectal abscess**

1. Outpatient incision and drainage under local anesthesia is reasonable in a healthy patient with a localized abscess. (SOR **B**) The skin over the abscess is cleaned with Betadine and infiltrated with anesthetic, and a no. 11 blade is used to enter the cavity. The skin edges are debrided and the cavity is syringed with saline or hydrogen peroxide, then packed with iodoform gauze. Conscious sedation is useful in the presence of excessive pain or anxiety. Analgesics, sitz baths, and stool softeners are continued. Frequent dressing changes may be necessary, until granulation is well advanced. Complications of drainage include perianal fistula (most common), sepsis, Fournier gangrene, and rarely death owing to sepsis.

2. Drainage in the operating room is advisable in poorly localized infection, septic patients, and in immunocompromised states such as diabetes.

3. The need for routine use of antibiotics has not been established; intravenous antibiotics may be needed in patients who are immunocompromised, septic, have heart valve abnormalities, or following valve replacements or prostheses.

D. Initial management of **perianal fistulas** should be directed at resolving acute infection (including proctitis in IBD). Both outpatient fistulotomy for simple fistulas and more extensive excision in complicated fistulas (postradiation, complicated anatomy) may require a surgical referral. (SOR **C**)

E. **Pilonidal sinus disease**

1. **Conservative, nonexcisional therapy** (shaving the gluteal cleft, improving perineal hygiene, incision and drainage of localized abscesses) effectively controls pilonidal sinus disease in most patients. (SOR **B**) This requires minimal equipment and leads to early recovery. Abscesses are drained under lidocaine infiltration anesthesia after skin preparation with Betadine, with a no. 15 blade. The wound is then syringed and packed as described earlier.

2. **Excisional therapy** should be considered for more extensive or recurrent disease and requires a surgical referral.

F. Treatment options for the **levator ani syndrome** include digital massage of the levator ani muscles 3 to 4 times a week, sitz baths at 40°C, use of muscle relaxants (such as diazepam and methocarbamol), and biofeedback. Recalcitrant cases may benefit from a referral to a gastroenterologist for electrogalvanic stimulation through a rectal probe. (SOR **C**) Surgical division of the puborectalis muscle is associated with a high rate of fecal incontinence and hence is not recommended.

G. Reassurance of the benign nature of **proctalgia fugax,** warm baths, and massage are often all that is necessary. In severe cases, inhaled albuterol, one or two puffs every 3 hours, or oral diltiazem, 2.5 to 5 mg every 6 hours as necessary, may help. (SOR **C**)

H. Proctitis

1. In suspected sexually transmitted disease, oral doxycycline (100 mg twice daily) or trimethoprim–sulfamethoxazole double strength (160/800 mg twice daily) or ciprofloxacin (500 mg twice daily) for 7 days is therapeutic.
2. *Clostridium difficile* proctitis is treated with oral metronidazole (250 mg orally 4 times a day) or vancomycin (250 mg 4 times a day) for 7 to 10 days.
3. In radiation proctitis, rectal corticosteroids as foam (hydrocortisone 90 mg) or enema (hydrocortisone 100 mg or methylprednisolone 40 mg) twice daily for 3 weeks, or mesalamine 4 g enema at bedtime or as suppositories 500 mg once or twice a day for 3 to 6 weeks, are useful. Oral mesalamine (800 mg 3 times a day) and sulfasalazine (500–1000 mg 4 times a day) for ~3 weeks alone or in combination with topical therapy may also be effective. Systemic steroids are reserved for patients unresponsive to these forms of therapy.

I. Treatment of **pruritus ani** depends on recognizing the cause, ruling out other potential diagnoses, addressing precipitating or exacerbating conditions, and relieving the itch/scratch cycle. (SOR **C**)

1. Excessive cleaning, and particularly the use of brushes and caustic soaps, should be avoided.
2. The perianal region should be washed liberally with water to remove any soap after bathing. Following defecation, water-moistened cloths or toilet paper should be used. In between defecation, cotton balls placed next to the anal orifice may help to absorb sweat. Moisture barriers, such as zinc oxide, may ameliorate symptoms.
3. Dietary modifications (restriction of caffeinated or carbonated beverages, dairy products, alcohol, tomato-based food products, cheese, and chocolate) may be useful.
4. A short course of topical steroids (hydrocortisone 1%) may also provide symptom relief, though long-term use should be avoided because of skin atrophy. Anesthetic ointments should also be avoided.
5. *Tinea* and *Candida* respond well to 1% clotrimazole cream applied twice daily for up to 4 weeks.
6. **Pinworms** are treated with one 100-mg dose of mebendazole or a 1-g dose of pyrantel pamoate.
7. **Condyloma acuminata** can be treated effectively with liquid nitrogen or 10% podophyllin. Podofilox applied by the patient every 12 hours for 3 consecutive days is an alternative. Application may be repeated after 4 days.
8. Improvement in symptoms has been noted with the subcutaneous injection of 30 cc of 0.5% methylene blue.

REFERENCES

Cataldo P, Neal Ellis C, Gregorcyk S, et al. Practice parameters for the management of hemorrhoids (revised). The Standards Practice Task Force, The American Society of Colon and Rectal Surgeons, 2005. *Dis Colon Rectum*. 2005;48:189-194.

Kaiser AM, Ortega AE. Anorectal anatomy. *Surg Clin North Am*. 2002;82:1125-1138.

Orsay C, Rakinic J, Brian Perry W, et al. Practice parameters for the management of anal fissures (revised). The Standards Practice Task Force, The American Society of Colon and Rectal Surgeons. *Dis Colon Rectum*. 2004;47:2003-2007.

Pfenninger JL, Zainea GG. Common anorectal conditions: Part I. Symptoms and complaints. *Am Fam Physician*. 2001;63:2391-2398.

Pfenninger JL, Zainea GG. Common anorectal conditions: Part II. Lesions. *Am Fam Physician*. 2001;64:77-88.

The diagnosis and management of common anorectal disorders. gidiv.ucsf.edu/course/things/anorectal.pdf. Accessed January 13, 2007.

Vincent C. Office management of common anorectal problems. *Prim Care*. 1999;26:52-68.

53   Proteinuria

Aamir Siddiqi, MD

KEY POINTS

- Asymptomatic persistent proteinuria on dipstick test needs further evaluation and possible referral to nephrology.
- Urine dipsticks are usually sensitive only to albuminuria and give false-negative results with other urinary proteins.
- Transient proteinuria is a nonpathologic condition.
- Taking a good medication history is an important step in the work-up of proteinuria.

I. **Definition.** Proteinuria is the presence of urinary protein in concentrations ≥ 0.150 g/d in adults and ≥ 0.1 mg/m^2/24 h in children. Nephrotic syndrome is defined as protein excretion of ≥ 3.5 gm/d in adults and 1 gm/m^2/d in children along with hypoalbuminemia, edema, and hypercholesterolemia. **Microalbuminuria** is defined as excretion of 30 to 150 mg of protein per day.

II. **Common Diagnoses**

A. **Transient proteinuria** defined as isolated, self-limited proteinuria is by far the most common, occurring in 4% of males and 7% of females on a single examination. Stressors such as fever and exercise have been considered as potential causes.

B. **Orthostatic proteinuria** appears when a person is upright and accounts for up to 60% of all proteinuria seen in children and adolescents.

C. **Persistent proteinuria** occurs in 5% to 10% of patients with isolated proteinuria. This is commonly associated with underlying extrarenal causes, such as diabetes or hypertension. After the development of proteinuria, as many as 50% of these patients may develop hypertension during the next 5 years, and as many as 20% may develop renal insufficiency during the next 10 years.

D. **Primary renal diseases,** including acute glomerulonephritis, acute renal failure, acute tubular necrosis, and anomalies such as polycystic kidneys, may cause proteinuria.

E. **Drugs** and **toxins,** including antibiotics, analgesics, anticonvulsants, antihypertensives, and heavy metals, may lead to proteinuria (Table 53–1).

F. **Systemic illnesses** (Table 53–2). Approximately 33% of type 1 and 25% of type 2 diabetic patients develop persistent proteinuria. **Overload proteinuria** occurs in systemic diseases, which cause production of abnormal and excessive low molecular weight proteins, as in multiple myeloma.

G. **Nephrotic syndrome** is primarily caused by minimal change disease, focal segmental glomerulosclerosis, membranous glomerulonephritis, membranoproliferative glomerulonephritis, and mesangial proliferative glomerulonephritis. The most common cause in children is minimal change disease accounting for approximately 75% of cases; membranous glomerulonephritis is the most common cause in adults. In children, it is most common from age 2 to 6. The ratio of males to females is 2:1 in childhood and becomes 1:1 in adolescents and adults.

III. **Symptoms.** It is rare to find any symptoms of proteinuria except in patients with the nephrotic syndrome, in whom swelling may be prominent. Characteristic symptoms of primary renal disease or systemic illness may appear in a patient with proteinuria that is caused by the pathologic process of an underlying disease.

A. **Red or cola-colored urine** can be a presenting symptom of acute glomerulonephritis.

B. **Polydipsia or polyuria** can indicate uncontrolled diabetes.

C. **Joint stiffness or pain** may be the presenting complaint of lupus erythematosus.

D. **Fatigue, weakness, anorexia, and malaise** may be associated with chronic renal insufficiency.

E. **Bone pain, especially in the back or chest,** may be associated with multiple myeloma.

TABLE 53–1. DRUGS AND TOXINS CAUSING PROTEINURIA

Acute interstitial nephritis	**Cyclosporine toxicity**
Cephalosporins	**Heavy metals**
Penicillins	Gold
Sulfonamides	Lead
Aminoglycoside toxicity	Mercury
Analgesic nephropathy	**Heroin**
Nonsteroidal anti-inflammatory drugs	**Lithium**
Anticonvulsants	**Penicillamine**
Phenytoin	**Probenecid**
Trimethadione	**Sulfonylureas**
Antihypertensive agents	Tolbutamide
Angiotensin-converting enzyme inhibitors	

IV. **Signs.** If the patient excretes ≤ 2 g of protein daily, signs will usually be absent.
   A. **Periorbital edema, peripheral edema, ascites,** or **pleural effusions** may result from a decrease in serum albumin because of decrease in plasma oncotic pressure.
   B. **Elevated blood pressure** may occur in patients with primary renal disease.
   C. A **toxic neuropathy** may indicate heavy metal poisoning.
   D. **Fever** may be present with infection.
   E. A **heart murmur** may accompany bacterial endocarditis.
   F. **Characteristic signs of systemic illness** may appear in patients whose proteinuria is caused by such illness.
      1. **Adenopathy, organomegaly,** and **masses** can occur with cancer.
      2. **Malar rash** and **joint inflammation** are usually present with lupus erythematosus.
      3. **Diabetic retinopathy** is strongly associated with proteinuria in diabetic patients.
V. **Laboratory Tests** (Figure 53–1)
   A. The **initial screen** for proteinuria is a **dipstick** performed on a random clean-catch urine sample. This is a colorimetric test (quantitative chemical analysis using color) detecting urine protein concentration of ≥ 10 to 30 mg/dL, giving positive results if used in relatively concentrated samples.
      1. **False-positive** dipstick test results can occur with highly concentrated urine, gross hematuria, contamination with antiseptics, or highly alkaline urine (pH ≥ 8.0). Radiographic contrast media, analogues of cephalosporin or penicillin, or metabolites of tolbutamide or sulfonamide can also result in false-positive tests.
      2. **False-negative** qualitative test results may occur with dilute urine. Dipstick qualitative urine tests are relatively insensitive to proteins other than albumin and may give a false-negative result for nonalbumin proteins such as Bence Jones proteins.
      3. **Sulfosalicylic acid test** is a turbidometric test in which one part of supernatant urine is mixed with sulfosalicylic acid. The turbidity is then graded according to a scale. The advantage of this test is detection of proteins besides albumin. This is especially helpful if myeloma kidney is suspected.

TABLE 53–2. **SYSTEMIC ILLNESSES CAUSING PROTEINURIA**

Infections	Cancers	Multisystem Diseases
Acute poststreptococcal glomerulonephritis	Carcinoma	Amyloidosis
Bacterial	Leukemia	Cryoglobulinemia
Endocarditis	Lymphoma—Hodgkin disease	Diabetes mellitus
Syphilis	Multiple myeloma	Goodpasture syndrome
Tuberculosis		Henoch–Schönlein syndrome
Parasitic		Polyarteritis
Malaria		Preeclampsia
Toxoplasmosis		Sarcoidosis
Viral		Systemic lupus erythematosus
Cytomegalovirus		Transplant rejection
Epstein–Barr virus		
Hepatitis B		
Human immunodeficiency virus		

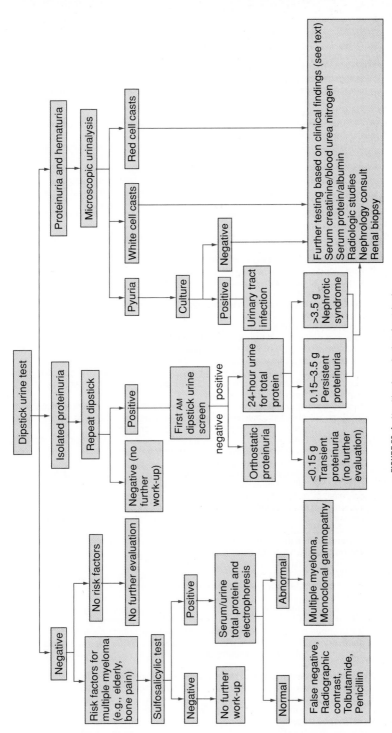

FIGURE 53–1. Algorithm for evaluation of proteinuria.

361

4. A negative qualitative test result on a first, morning specimen (recumbent) followed 2 hours later by a positive test on second sample (upright) indicates orthostatic proteinuria. This can be confirmed by a split urine test in which a 16-hour upright collection is obtained between 7 AM and 11 PM, with the patient performing normal activities and finishing the collection by voiding just before 11 PM. A separate overnight 8-hour collection is obtained between 11 PM and 7 AM. The diagnosis of orthostatic proteinuria is made if urinary protein excretion is normal in the supine collection ($\leq$50 mg/8 h).

B. A **24-hour urine test** for protein and creatinine levels will verify a repeated positive qualitative test result.

1. Urinary creatinine validates an adequate urinary collection; normal creatinine range is 16 to 26 mg/kg body weight per day for males and 12 to 24 mg/kg body weight per day for females. A 24-hour urine creatinine allows calculation of creatinine clearance, which is a good measure of renal function. An alternative to measuring 24-hour urine protein is to measure spot urinary protein to creatinine ratio. In a healthy person, the ratio seldom exceeds 0.1 (100 mg protein per gram creatinine).

2. A normal 24-hour **urinary protein** level indicates a false-positive qualitative test result or transient proteinuria.

C. Urinalysis of a clean-catch midstream specimen is needed to diagnose primary renal disease.

1. Positive urine culture indicates infection.

2. Red blood cell casts indicate glomerulonephritis.

3. White blood cell casts indicate an inflammatory process such as pyelonephritis or interstitial nephritis.

4. Epithelial cell casts may be seen secondary to acute tubular necrosis or toxin ingestion.

D. Blood tests should be performed when systemic disease is suspected.

1. Serum creatinine and **blood urea nitrogen** levels should be determined in order to evaluate renal function. Creatinine clearance is more accurate, especially in elderly patients with decreased muscle mass.

2. Blood glucose or a **glycosylated hemoglobin test** is helpful in the detection of diabetes mellitus. Risk factors for these patients include symptoms of polydipsia, polyuria, and a strong family history of diabetes.

3. Protein electrophoresis or **immunoelectrophoresis** of urine and serum may assist in the diagnosis of multiple myeloma or other monoclonal gammopathies. These patients are usually elderly and may complain of bone pain and fatigue.

4. Complement studies may be helpful in the diagnosis of immune complex diseases. These include autoimmune diseases such as rheumatoid arthritis, systemic lupus erythematosus, and dermatomyositis.

5. Antistreptococcal enzyme titers can help the physician diagnose poststreptococcal glomerulonephritis. This is most common in children younger than age 7 and may be preceded by a skin infection or pharyngitis.

6. Fluorescent antinuclear antibody tests may indicate the presence of systemic lupus erythematosus. Patients usually have arthritis and fatigue and may present with the classic malar rash.

7. Serum albumin levels will be decreased in patients with nephrotic syndrome. These patients usually have significant facial and pedal edema and may have hypertension.

8. Complete blood cell count will help in determining infection or the anemia of renal insufficiency. Systemic infections will cause an elevation of the white cell count. Anemia, if present, is usually characterized by normocytic and normochromic red blood cells.

E. Radiographic evaluation may detect congenital, obstructive, or malignant disease. This should be considered in patients complaining of abdominal pain and hematuria.

1. Intravenous pyelography or **computerized tomographic scans** of the kidney can show structural or obstructive pathology. Caution should be observed using contrast media in patients with diabetes, renal insufficiency, or multiple myeloma because of the risk of renal failure.

2. Renal ultrasonography can be of value in determining renal size, obstruction, and congenital cysts. This should be considered if abdominal examination reveals a mass.

3. Voiding cystourethrogram is useful in documenting reflux. This is usually performed in children who may present with recurrent urinary tract infections.

F. Renal biopsy is reserved for diagnosing and differentiating the glomerulonephropathies and is also performed on most patients with nephrotic-range proteinuria.

VI. Treatment of proteinuria is directed at the underlying cause.
  A. Annual Screening for proteinuria in asymptomatic adults is **not** cost effective.
  (SOR **Ⓐ**)
  B. Transient proteinuria requires no further evaluation or follow-up, as no harmful sequelae
  have been documented.
  C. Orthostatic proteinuria is mostly a benign condition. Patients with this problem have a
  50% chance of remission over 10 years. Follow-up of this problem should occur every 1
  to 2 years, if proteinuria persists, and should involve a blood pressure check as well as
  urinalysis.
  D. Removal of toxins or medications (Table 53–1) can reverse or at least prevent progression of proteinuria.
  E. Appropriate antibiotics can resolve proteinuria associated with urinary tract infections
  (see Chapter 21).
  F. Primary renal disease
    1. **Supportive therapy,** including **sodium** and **fluid restriction** (2 g/d, 1 L/d, respectively)
    may help relieve fluid retention.
    2. **Loop diuretics** such as **furosemide,** 20 to 400 mg/d, can be used to treat circulatory
    congestion, edema, and hypertension. These agents have not been shown to alter the
    course of acute renal failure or to improve the patient's chance of survival.
    3. **Dietary protein restriction** may prevent progression of renal disease and usually
    comprises 20 to 40 g (0.6 g/kg) of protein per day, with 100 g of carbohydrate per day
    if azotemia is present. (SOR **Ⓐ**)
    4. **Corticosteroids** such as **prednisone,** 1 to 1.5 mg/kg/d, and cytotoxic drugs such as
    cyclophosphamide, 1 to 2 mg/kg/d, may be of benefit to patients with certain types
    of nephrotic syndrome and primary glomerulonephritis. These should be prescribed
    in consultation with nephrology. (SOR **Ⓒ**)
    5. **Renal dialysis** is indicated for patients with progressive renal failure and should be
    initiated when any of the following conditions exist: volume overload refractory to
    diuretics, pericarditis, or uremia (blood urea nitrogen $\geq$80–100 mg/dL or creatinine
    $\geq$8–10 mg/dL).
    6. **Renal transplantation** should be considered when a poor quality of life or health exists
    despite dialysis with end-stage renal disease.
  G. Specific treatment of underlying systemic illness (see Table 53–2 and Chapters 74,
  76, and 84) may resolve or improve proteinuria.
    1. **Persistent proteinuria** is associated with a high mortality and risk of death from renal
    disease. Patients with persistent proteinuria from any cause should be referred to
    nephrology. This should be followed up every 6 months to 1 year with urinalysis, blood
    pressure, and renal function studies.
    2. **Antihypertensive therapy** in a patient with nephropathy characterized by proteinuria
    can delay progression of renal failure.
    3. **Corticosteroids** and cytotoxic drugs may improve proteinuria from lupus nephritis.
    4. **Diabetic patients with proteinuria** should all be started on an angiotensin-converting
    enzyme inhibitor or angiotensin receptor blocker to prevent progressive decline in renal
    function. (SOR **Ⓐ**)

REFERENCES

Hogg RJ, Furth S, Lemley KV, et al. National kidney foundation's kidney disease outcomes quality initiative clinical practice guidelines for chronic kidney disease in children and adolescents: evaluation,
  classification, and stratification. *Pediatrics.* 2003;111:1416-1421.
House AA, Cattran DC. Nephrology: 2. Evaluation of asymptomatic hematuria and proteinuria in adult
  primary care. *CMAJ Can Med Ass J.* 2002;166:348-353.
Roth KS, Amaker BH, Chan JC. Nephrotic syndrome: pathogenesis and management. *Pediatr Rev.*
  2002;23:237-248.
Schieppati A, Perna A, Zamora J, Giuliano GA, Braun N, Remuzzi G. Immunosuppressive treatment
  for idiopathic membranous nephropathy in adults with nephrotic syndrome. *Cochrane Database Syst
  Rev.* 2004;(4): CD004293. doi:10.1002/14651858.CD004293.pub2.
Strippoli GF, Craig M, Deeks JJ, Schena FP, Craig JC. Effects of angiotensin converting enzyme inhibitors and angiotensin receptor antagonists on mortality and renal outcomes in diabetic nephropathy: systematic review. *BMJ.* 2004;329:828-839.

54   The Red Eye

Victor A. Diaz, Jr., MD, & Deborah K. Witt, MD

KEY POINTS

- Red eye is the most common ocular problem encountered in ambulatory primary care settings.
- Symptoms suggestive of a medical emergency include eye pain, persistent blurred vision, photophobia, symptoms greater than 1 week in duration, and proptosis.
- Topical corticosteroids or corticosteroid-antibiotic combinations are contraindicated when treating the red eye.
- By paying attention to which ocular structures are involved, the clinician can accurately diagnose and appropriately treat most disorders, as well as determine which cases require referral to an ophthalmologist.
- The differential diagnosis can be clarified by probing the patient's history and physical examination for the following: association with pain, history of preceding trauma, seasonal or recurrent occurrences, changes of the eyelid, and the use of eye drops.

I. **Definition**. An appreciation of normal eye anatomy is the foundation for understanding the differential diagnosis of red eye (see Figure 54–1). The arterial blood supply of orbital structures originates from the ophthalmic artery, which supplies the glands, upper eyelids, ciliary structures, and musculature. The eyelids contain eyelashes and meibomian glands, which secrete a sebaceous substance that prevents the upper and lower lids from adhering to one another.

   "*Red eye*" describes a group of distinct inflammatory or infectious diseases involving one or more ocular structures, i.e., conjunctivae (viral/bacterial/chlamydial/allergic conjunctivitis, pterygium, pingueculum), cornea (abrasion, keratitis), sclera/episclera (scleritis, episcleritis), lids (blepharitis), uveal tract (iritis, uvieits), anterior chamber (acute angle-closure glaucoma).

II. **Common Diagnoses**. The most likely source of red eye is the anterior segment, which consists of conjunctiva, cornea, anterior chamber, and iris (Figure 54-1). Conjunctivitis is the most common eye disease worldwide.

   A. **Conjunctivitis,** inflammation of the mucous membranes lining the eyelid or eyeball, can be because of the following causes:

      1. **Infectious**

         a. **Viral**

            (1) **Adenovirus.** Approximately 85% of viral conjunctivitis is caused by *Adenovirus*, which is highly contagious. It often occurs in epidemics, via respiratory secretions and ocular discharge. Transmission is person-to-person via contaminated fingers, medical instruments, and swimming pool water.

            (2) **Herpes** is the least common cause of viral conjunctivitis and can be caused by *Herpes simplex* virus type 1 or type 2. Herpes zoster virus (HZV) may also affect children and include the eyelid skin up to the midline, as part of the typical dermatomal distribution.

         b. **Bacterial**. Only 15% of conjunctivitis is caused by a bacterial etiology. (Exposures to microbial organisms result in a *papillary* response by the conjunctiva). Adults are primarily infected with *S aureus* and children with *S pneumonia* or *H influenzae*. *N gonorrheae* is the most common cause of conjunctival bacterial infection in neonates and sexually active patients.

         c. **Chlamydia** trachomatis is the leading cause of preventable blindness worldwide and is a major public health concern in developing countries. Inclusion conjunctivitis is usually bilateral and spreads by direct contact with other family members. Spread is often associated with epidemics of bacterial conjunctivitis. Chronic conjunctivitis that resists multiple eye-drop regimens and/or the presence of associated urethritis or salpingitis should raise suspicion for chlamydial infection in sexually active teens

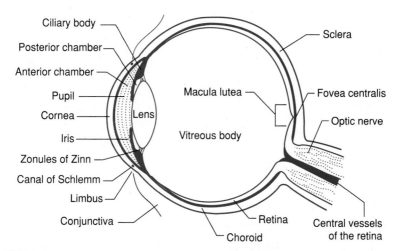

FIGURE 54–1. The eye—cross section. The zonules of Zinn keep the lens suspended, while the muscles of the ciliary body focus the lens. The ciliary body also secretes aqueous humor, which fills the posterior chamber, passes through the pupil into the anterior chamber, and drains primarily via the canal of Schlemm. The iris regulates the light entering the eye by adjusting the size of its central opening, the pupil. The visual image is focused on the retina, the fovea centralis being the area of sharpest visual acuity. The conjunctiva ends abruptly at the limbus. The cornea is covered with an epithelium that differs in many respects from the conjunctival epithelium. (Reproduced with permission from Beers MH, Berkow R, eds. *The Merck Manual of Diagnosis and Therapy.* 17th ed. Merck & Co.; 1999:701. Copyright 1999 by Merck & Co., Inc., Whitehouse Station, NJ.)

and adults. *Inclusion conjunctivitis of the newborn* is the most common cause of conjunctivitis in neonates. Exposure to the organism occurs in the birth canal during delivery and infection may also result in pneumonia.

  d. Noninfectious or allergic conjunctivitis occurs, in individuals with seasonal, environmental, (e.g., dust pollen, animal dander), or chemical (e.g., drugs, chemicals, and/or cosmetics) sensitivities.
B. Corneal abrasion, loss of a portion of the superficial epithelium, likely the most common corneal cause of red eye, typically occurs in individuals who frequently participate in outdoor activities or certain occupations (e.g., tree trimmers, metal shop workers).
C. Blepharitis, is a common inflammatory lesion affecting eyelid margins.
D. Subconjunctival hemorrhage, spontaneous rupture of small conjunctival vessels, usually results from a sudden increase in intrathoracic pressure (e.g., sneezing, coughing, defecating) especially in the elderly, but also occurs with minor trauma, hypertension, and blood dyscrasias and is common in neonates following vaginal delivery.

SCLERITIS AND EPISCLERITIS

Scleritis and **episcleritis** are uncommon conditions, which may occur in association with autoimmune or inflammatory conditions (e.g., rheumatoid arthritis, Wegener's granulomatosis, lupus, polyarteritis noddosa, or herpes zoster). Episcleritis more commonly affects young adults, while sclerities tends to affect women in the fourth to sixth decades. Both **scleritis** and **episcleritis** present with eye pain, more severe in scleritis. In addition, patients with simple episcleritis have photophobia and present with a focal redness of the bulbar conjunctiva in a wedgelike or sector pattern, while nodular episcleritis presents as a hyperemic papule. Scleritis pain is deep, boring, and often interrupts sleep; erythema and decreased visual acuity may be sudden or gradual, unilateral, or bilateral. A bluish hue indicates scleral thinning.

E. Inflamed pingueculum. Extremely common in adults, pingueculae are conjunctival areas of epithelial hyperplasia that become irritated by excessive sun and wind exposure and occasionally become inflamed for periods of weeks. At-risk individuals include farmers, lifeguards, fishermen, and welders.

F. **Pterygium,** a fibrovascular proliferation of the conjunctiva, typically affects individuals in hot, dusty, and windy environments who are exposed to prolonged periods of outdoor ultraviolet light such as farmers, fishermen, and people living near the equator. Rarely seen in children.

KERATITIS

Keratitis is superficial or interstitial (deeper layers) corneal inflammation caused by infection, trauma, decreased tearing, topical medications, ultraviolet exposure, contact lens use, eyelid disorders, or immunosuppression. Intertitial keratitis may also be associated with congenital syphilis or Cogan syndrome (interstitial keratitis, tinnitus, vertigo, and deafness). Keratitis presents with blurred vision, photophobia periocular pain, gritty foreign body sensation, and ciliary flush (circumcorneal conjuctival injection), sometimes associated with corneal opacification or fragmented corneal light reflection.

Fluorescein dye staining often reveals multiple punctuate corneal lesions; however, a dendritic or branching appearance suggests infection with herpes simples virus (HSV). Definitive diagnosis requires ophthalmologic referral for slit-lamp examination and appropriate corneal testing (culture, scraping, or biopsy). Other testing (e.g., serologic testing for syphilis, PPD, ESR, rheumatoid factor, antinuclear antibodies, chest radiographs) may also be indicated.

Cultures should be obtained prior to starting topical antibiotic or antiviral therapy and patients should be referred to an ophthalmologist. Steroids are absolutely contraindicated in the scenario of a possible herpetic infection.

G. **Acute angle-closure glaucoma,** a rare ophthalmic emergency associated with suddenly elevated intraocular pressure (IOP), is most common in middle-aged or older patients with anatomically small anterior chambers or altered iris structure, especially in Asians, Eskimos, and *hyperopic* (farsighted) persons. Comprises 10% to 15% of cases in Caucasians and approximately 5% to 10% of all glaucoma cases. Patients may reveal a recent history of topical or oral mydriatic use or eye surgery and may have a positive family history for glaucoma.

ACUTE ANTERIOR UVEITIS (IRITIS, IRIDOCYCLITIS)

Acute anterior uveitis is an uncommon condition affecting young or middle-aged persons either idiopathically or via autoimmune reaction in conjuction with ankylosing spondylitis (AS), up to 50% of patients, juvenile rheumatoied arthritis (JRA), up to 20% of patients, Reiter's syndrome, sarcoid, herpres simplex or zoster, or Bechet's disease. Anterior uveitis presents with constant periocular achy pain radiating to the brow or temple developing over hours, photophobia, normal or blurred vision, tearing, violaceous ciliary flush, and possibly a constricted, irregular pupil which reacts more slowly to light than the unaffected eye. Occasionally, a layer of white blood cells at the bottom of the anterior chamber (**hypopion**) can be noted on slit lamp examination. **Hyphema** refers to the inferior layer of frank red blood in the anterior chamber that results from trauma to the eye.

III. **Symptoms/Signs (Table 54-1)**
   A. **Viral conjunctivitis** has an incubation period of 7 to 10 days and can last up to 4 to 6 weeks on fomites. Viral conjunctivitis is usually subclinical in nature and resolves in 10 to 14 days. Different manifestations include the following:
      1. Mild follicular involvement. Injected sclera, watery discharge, and burning/itching or foreign body sensation.
      2. Pharyngoconjunctival involvement. Upper respiratory tract symptoms, sore throat, preauricular lymphadenopathy, and fever.
      3. Epidemic keratoconjunctivitis (EKC). Inflammation of the cornea, which produces significant pain, photophobia, and blurred vision. EKC may be difficult to differentiate from other viral forms because it is also associated with preauricular lymphadenopathy, subconjunctival hemorrhage, and purulent discharge.

TABLE 54–1. DIFFERENTIAL DIAGNOSIS OF COMMON CAUSES OF RED EYE

Condition	Risk Factors	Symptoms	Signs	Testing
Viral conjunctivitis	Highly contagious, epidemic person-to-person (e.g., day care, school, swimming pool) HZV—previous history of chicken pox (varicella)	URI/sore throat/itching or FB sensation; HSV—photophobia HZV—pain and tingling precede the rash; high fever and prostration × 1 wk	Injected, watery discharge Palp. Preauricular lymph node; dendrites with HSV HZV—vesicular rash over the distribution of the ophthalmic division of the trigeminal nerve; reddened, edematous conjunctiva with eyelid swelling	HZV—none usually indicated
Bacterial conjunctivitis	N. gonorrhea—sexually active, neonates	Pain/photophobia, pus discharge	Beefy, red conjunctivae; Matted lids; Purulent discharge	Gram stain/culture, if severe persistent
Chlamydial conjunctivitis	Teens and adults—unprotected sexual activity Newborn—via infected birth canal	Tearing/photophobia/pain, pus discharge, redness Failure to respond to traditional antibiotics; possible associated genital symptoms Neonate—onset first 10 d of life	Chronic, bilateral mucopurulent discharge, beefy redness discharge	
Noninfectious conjunctivitis	Seasonal allergies Exposure to chemicals, cosmetics, dust	Itchy/burning/watery discharge; associated allergic rhinitis symptoms	Conjunctival injection/swelling	
Corneal abrasion		Acute discomfort/tearing/blurred vision/FB sensation		Ulcerations with fluorescein staining
Blepharitis	Patients with rosacea and seborrheic dermatitis	Bilateral lid Itching/scaling/burning Associated scalp eyebrow/ear seborrhea Chronic, relapsing nature	Ulcerative eyelash folliculitis; scaling lids Meibomian	Culture, if ulcerative lesion (commonly S aureus)
Subconjunctival hemorrhage	Elderly Trauma, HTN, blood dyscrasia Neonate—vaginal delivery	Painless/unilateral	Localized, sharply circumscribed hemorrhage	Coag profile, CBC and plts, protein C and S levels
Inflamed pingueculum	Sun/wind exposure (farmers, lifeguards, fishermen, welders)	Mild ocular discomfort	Hyperemic yellowsh conju. Nodules at 3 and 9 o'clock positions	No testing
Pterygium	Heat/dust/wind exposure (farmers, fishermen, equatorial environment)	Usually painless, normal or blurred vision	Triangular, yellowish, fleshy injected conjunctival lesion, extension from canthus with possible corneal encroachment	No testing
Acute angle closure glaucoma	Middle age/older, esp. Asians Eskimos, Hyperopia; + FHx	Acute photophobia, periocular pain; "Haloes" around light, N?V, headache; Often onse in dark environment (e.g. theater)	Decreased VA Ciliary flush, hazy cornea Dilated pupil, poor light reaction On gentle palpation, the orbits feel indurated	Schiotz tonometry (applanation tonometry, slit lamp and gonioscopy preferred and more accurate) normal IOP: 10–20 mm Hg

Key:
HSV = herpes simple virus; HZV = herpes zoster virus; DNA= deoxyribonucleic acid; HTN = hypertension; FB = foreign body; CBC = complete blood count; VA = visual activity; IOP = intraocular pressure; N/V = nausea/vomiting.

4. Herpes simplex conjunctivitis is usually monocular; however it can spread to the other eye within the week. There is also photophobia with mild irritation but no discharge. It is possible to see dendrites on the cornea or vesicles on the eyelid.

An important sign that can differentiate viral conjunctivitis from bacterial conjunctivitis is a palpable preauricular lymph node.

B. Bacterial conjunctivitis presents with a beefy red appearance and matted eyelids. Copious and continuous purulent discharge is its distinguishing feature. Patients complain of a gritty sensation.

C. Chlamydial conjunctivitis

1. Trachoma. Symptoms are similar to bacterial conjunctivitis (e.g., tearing, photophobia, pain, and exudates). *Herbert's pits*, small pathognomonic depressions in the connective tissue covered by epithelium, develop over time.

  a. Infant/child infection is insidious and may resolve without complications.

  b. Adult infection may be clinically subacute or acute. Complications develop early in disease.

2. Inclusion conjunctivitis

  a. Adults present with burning, general irritation, redness, and mucopurulent discharge primarily.

  b. Neonates develop tearing, discharge, and swollen eyelids during the first 10 days of life.

D. Allergic conjunctivitis

Symptoms include itching, burning, and watery discharge with some conjunctival swelling.

A clearly delineated injection from the sclera toward the cornea suggests a conjunctival origin.

E. Corneal abrasion is associated with immediate discomfort, photophobia, blurred vision, tearing, and foreign body sensation as a result of exposed nerve endings. Fluorescein dye, which accumulates in areas where the corneal epithelium has been abraded and fluoresces bright green under magnified blue light (Wood's lamp), is the diagnostic tool of choice in the office setting.

F. Blepharitis. Chronic, bilateral itching and burning with foreign body sensation. There is inflammation and crusting of lid margins, usually without discharge.

G. Subconjunctival hemorrhage is usually unilateral, painless, localized, and sharply circumscribed. Extravascular blood is seen underneath the conjunctiva obstructing the view of the sclera; the adjacent sclera is unaffected. Blood pressure should be measured for possible elevation.

H. Episcleritis.

1. *Simple* episclerits presents with eye pain, photophobia, and focal, bright-red injection of the bulbar conjunctiva.

2. *Nodular* episcleritis appears as a painful, hyperemic raised nodule that can be moved slightly over the underlying sclera.

In episcleritis and scleritis, the palpebral conjunctiva is spared, thus distinguishing it from conjunctivits.

I. Scleritis may manifest as *diffused, nodular, or necrotizing*. Severe pain is common to all presentations and is characteristically described as a deep, boring, radiating ache, which interrupts sleep. Onset of redness and decrease in vision may be sudden or gradual and recurring episodes are common. It may be unilateral or bilateral with tenderness to palpation of the globe, photophobia, and lacrimation. Thinning of the cornea or sclera may allow the dark purple/blue color of the underlying uvea to show through. Keratitis and uveitis may occur concomitantly.

The patient with suspected scleritis should be examined in all directions of gaze in daylight or with an adequate room illumination without a slit lamp to best detect the characteristic bluish hue.
Patients with scleritis have tenderness on palpation of the globe, while those with episcleritis do not.

J. **Inflamed pingueculum.** Lesions present as raised, hyperemic, yellowish nodules on the bulbar conjunctiva at the 3- and/or 9-o'clock position. Nasal lesions are more common than temporal ones. Patients report mild ocular discomfort.
K. **Pterygium** is usually painless, with normal or blurred vision. However, changes in vision may occur if the cornea becomes distorted. The conjunctival tissue is triangular, yellowish, fleshy, and injected. It may extend from either canthus and encroach upon or partially cover the cornea.
L. **Keratitis** is characterized by blurred vision, photophobia, periocular pain, foreign body sensation (grittiness), and ciliary flush. Fragmented, corneal, light reflection and corneal opacification may sometimes also be noted on inspection.

Ciliary flush is a term used to describe the concentrated injection of the circumcorneal (limbal) conjunctiva that is characteristic of several red eye conditions such as keratitis, acute angle-closure glaucoma, and acute anterior uveitis.

M. **Acute angle-closure glaucoma** occurs spontaneously, generally in the evening or in darkened settings when reduced light induces mydriasis, causing the iris to block the narrow anterior-chamber angle in these individuals. It is typically unilateral and presents with an acute, periocular pain and congestion, acute photophobia, rapidly progressive loss of vision, ciliary flush, and corneal haziness. Patients often describe the classic symptom of seeing colored haloes around lights. Nausea, vomiting, and frontal headache occur in severe cases. These severe cases have been known to prompt abdominal exploration in an attempt to make the diagnosis.
    The involved pupil is often moderately dilated and unreactive to light, whereas the other pupil is normal. Elevated IOP of the affected eye can be crudely tested by digitally palpating for a hardened globe.
N. **Anterior uveitis.** Patients report periocular "aching" pain, photophobia, normal or blurred vision, and tearing. On examination, there is ciliary flush with a characteristic violaceous hue. As the iris adheres to the anterior lens or the posterior corneal surface, it will cause an irregular pupil which is usually constricted, smaller, and less reactive to light than the fellow eye.

III. **Laboratory tests/Diagnostics**
    A. **Conjunctivitis** overall is a common, self-limiting condition and usually does not require special testing.
        1. **Viral conjunctivitis.** Virus can be grown and identified; however clinical diagnosis is more practical.
        2. **Bacterial conjunctivitis.** Most cases are self-limited; however severe infections can include the following tests:
            a. **Culture** of eye discharge for identification of bacteria and sensitivity to antibiotics.
            b. **Conjunctival scrapings** require local anesthesia to obtain a sample for cytologic evaluation.
                (1) **Gram stain** may also aid in quick identification of the bacterial organism.
                (2) **Giemsa stain** identifies the cell type and morphology of the microbe.
                    (a) **Polymorphonuclear leukocytes** imply bacterial etiology.
                    (b) **Lymphocytes** suggest viral etiology.
        3. **Chlamydial conjunctivitis.** Nonculture tests are now available using DNA amplification testing.

B. Corneal abrasion. Corneal reflection can be observed with a penlight. Fluorescein dye illuminated by a Wood's lamp is used to detect corneal denudment or ulcerations. A short-acting topical anesthetic (e.g., tetracaine 0.5%) is often used to facilitate the examination.

C. Blepharitis. Culturing of the conjunctiva and eyelid margins may yield the bacterial pathogen in patients where ulcerative blepharitis is suspected.

D. Subconjunctival hemorrhage. Coagulation studies, complete blood count with platelets, and protein C and S levels should be considered if hemorrhages are recurrent or there is a history of bleeding problems.

E. Episcleritis. Placement of phenylephrine 2.5% drops in the affected eye followed by re-examination of the vascular pattern 10 to 15 minutes later will reveal blanched episcleral vessels. Appropriate laboratory studies should be done when the history suggests an underlying etiology.

F. Scleritis. Scleral vessels do not blanch on application of topical phenylephrine 2.5%. A complete physical examination with a focus on rheumatologic findings should be performed. Appropriate laboratory tests include a complete blood count (CBC), erythrocyte sedimentation rate (ESR), uric acid, rapid plasma reagent (RPR), fluorescent treponemal antibody-absorption (FTA-ABS), rheumatoid factor (RF), antinuclear antibody (ANA), fasting blood glucose (FBG), angiotensin converting enzyme (ACE), ANCA, CH 50 and C3 and C4 complement levels. Other tests to consider, if suspicious, include purified protein derivative of tuberculin (PPD) with anergy panel and x-rays of the chest and sacroiliac joints.

G. Inflamed pingueculum. No testing is required.

H. Pterygium. No tests are necessary; the diagnosis is clinical.

I. Keratitis. Fluorescein dye staining will often reveal multiple punctuate lesions when the epithelium is disrupted; however, diagnosis requires a slit lamp examination by an ophthalmologist who may also culture, scrape, and/or biopsy the cornea when the cause is uncertain. Appropriate studies (e.g., RPR, FTA-ABS, PPD, ESR, ANA, RF, and chest x-rays) should be ordered to workup the underlying cause.

J. Acute angle-closure glaucoma. Tonometry measures the intraocular fluid pressure using calibrated instruments that can be used in any clinic or emergency department setting; pressures between 10- to 20 mm Hg are considered normal. Slit lamp examination and gonioscopy are the preferred diagnostic methods. Markedly elevated IOP (50–100 mm Hg), a shallow anterior chamber, and corneal edema are hallmark findings.

Applanation tonometry is preferred over Schiotz tonometry in the diagnosis of glaucoma, but requires more training. A Schiotz is portable and easy to learn and use, but requires thorough cleaning between uses. A shallow anterior chamber in a red eye suggests acute angle-closure glaucoma.

K. Anterior uveitis. If there is clinical suspicion, patients should be referred to the ophthalmologist for further work up. The ophthalmologist can visualize a proteinaceous *flare* and cellular debris of the aqueous humor on slit lamp biomicroscopy. Cellular deposits on the corneal endothelium are also a common finding. If pus settles in the anterior chamber, it forms a *hypopion,* a white or yellow-white, flat-surfaced accumulation that is generally visible to the naked eye. IOP may be either markedly elevated or depressed. Adhesions between the iris and the anterior lens surface form *posterior synechiae,* which may lead to decreased vision. Studies may include CBC, ESR, HLA-B27, ACE level, ANA, RPR, FTA-ABS, PPD and anergy panel, chest x-rays, and Lyme titer.

V. Treatment

A. Conjunctivitis

1. **Viral conjunctivitis** is treated with supportive measures including cold compresses and lubricating drops (e.g., artificial tears 1–2 gtts as needed). Preventive measures include frequent handwashing, especially in environments (medical offices, day care centers) where transmission risk is high. (SOR **Ⓐ**) Because of serious ocular side effects (increased duration of viral shedding, risk of corneal ulcerations and perforation), topical corticosteroids are contraindicated in conjunctivitis. (SOR **Ⓑ**)

2. **Herpes conjunctivitis** can be indistinguishable from adenovirus, which is an important reason to avoid topical steroid use. Herpes conjunctivitis can be treated with trifluridine, 1% oph. soln. (1 drop every 2 hours while awake until reepithelialization takes place in

7 to 14 days, then reduce frequency for 7 more days). In cases of HZV, oral acyclovir 800 mg, 5 times daily should be added to the less effective topical regimen in order to decrease pain and minimize the risk of corneal damage and uveitis.

3. **Bacterial conjunctivitis** is usually self-limited, resolving within 7 to 10 days.
   a. Broad spectrum topical antibiotics can be used for severe infections (eye drops are preferred for all patients except infants and young children, for whom ointment is preferable). Examples include bacitracin-polymyxin B (Polysporin oph oint, 0.5 inch q 3–4 hours for 7–10 days), trimethoprim (Polytrim oph soln, 1 gt every 3 hours for 7–10 days), aminoglycosides (gentamicin or tobramycin, 0.3%, 2 gtt or 0.5 inch ointment q 1 hour for 24–72 hours around the clock, then a slow reduction to 3–4 times daily as condition improves) or quinolones (ciprofloxin or ofloxacin, 0.3%, 1–2 gtt q 2–4 hours for 2 days, then qid for 5 more days). (SOR **A**)
   b. Opthalmologic referral is indicated for persistent symptoms beyond 10 days or if there is diminished visual acuity or loss of vision. (SOR **A**)
   c. *N gonorrheal* infection is a medical emergency requiring ophthalmologic referral. If untreated it can lead to corneal ulceration or perforation within 24 hours.
4. **Chlamydial conjunctivitis** is treated with oral erythromycin 250 mg qid or doxycycline 100 mg bid for 14 to 21 days. Sexual partner must be treated. Since coexisting infection with gonorrhea is high in sexually active patient, intramuscular ceftriaxone should be added to the treatment regimen. Neonatal chlamydial infection is best treated with a 2-week course of oral erythromycin.
5. **Allergic conjunctivitis.** Avoidance of offending allergen, application of artificial tears (1–2 gtt as needed) or administration of a topical vasoconstrictor, topical antihistamines, or topical mast cell stabilizer (e.g., naphazoline, 0.025%, 1–2 gtt qid; olopatadine HCl, 0.1%, 1 gt bid at 6–8 hour intervals or cromolyn sodium, 4%, 1–2 gtt 4–6 times daily, respectively) until asymptomatic.

Topical corticosteroid use is contraindicated in treatment of conjunctivitis owing to serious ocular side effects. Documented studies indicate increased duration of viral shedding, prolongation of infectious period, possible corneal ulcerations, and perforations.

B. **Corneal abrasion.** Primary treatment goals are to restore patient comfort, assist in rapid healing, and prevent secondary infections. The corneal epithelium regenerates rapidly, and healing is usually complete within 24 to 48 hours.
   1. Topical cycloplegic drops (atropine oph. sol.) to relieve the pain caused by reflex spasm of the ciliary body muscles
   2. Oral analgesics with codeine (Tylenol #3, 1–2 tabs q 3–4 hours as needed for pain) may occasionally be prescribed.
   3. A topical ophthalmic antibiotic (see topical aminoglycosides or quinolones above) can also be applied. Although soft pressure patches are often used; they are usually not necessary. Contact lens wearers should not receive eye patches at all as this can promote serious corneal/conjunctival infections (e.g., Pseudomonas).

Under no condition should topical anesthetic solutions be prescribed to the patient for pain relief because of their toxic effects on the corneal epithelium.

C. **Blepharitis.** Washing with baby shampoo once daily is an effective way of treating the seborrheic form. An antistaphylococcal antibiotic or topical sulfacetamide, 10% (Bleph-10 ointment, 0.5 inch q 3–4 hours and bedtime for 7–10 days) can be used in the ulcerative form. Most cases are chronic and require long-term therapy.

A cycloplegic (e.g., atropine) is a mydriatic medication that is used in both the diagnosis and treatment of certain ocular conditions by dilating the pupil and paralyzing the muscles of accommodation.

D. Subconjunctival hemorrhage. No treatment is usually required, as hemorrhage sponta-neously clears in 2 to 3 weeks. Treat underlying high blood pressure or bleeding disorder and discontinue any elective aspirin or NSAID use if episodes are recurrent. Artificial tear drops (1–2 gtt as needed) may help for mild irritation. If diagnosis is in doubt or some other abnormality becomes evident on examination, referral to an ophthalmologist is appropriate.

E. Episcleritis is usually self-limited in 1 to 2 weeks. Artificial tears (1–2 gtt as needed) may be used in mild cases. Oral NSAIDs (e.g., indomethacin 25–50 mg 2–3 times daily, naproxen 250–500 mg bid, or ketoprofen 200 mg daily) or mild topical steroids (prednisolone acetate, 0.12%, oph susp, initially 2 gtt q 1 hour for 24–48 hours, then 1–2 gtt 2–4 times daily until resolved) are often successful in more moderate to severe cases. Despite its benign nature, an ophthalmologist best manages these cases, as recurrences may torment the patient for years.

F. Scleritis demands urgent referral to an ophthalmologist. Recurring episodes are common. Patients with RA-associated scleritis seem to have more widespread systemic disease and a higher mortality rate than those without scleritis.

G. Inflamed pingueculum. Topical vasoconstrictors (naphazoline, 0.025%, 1–2 gtt qid) work well. Nonurgent referrals to ophthalmology are appropriate if lesion is unresponsive in 1 week. Surgical removal is not necessary.

Topical vasoconstrictors are to be used with caution especially if redness is not relieved promptly or if other significant problems occur.

H. Pterygia require nonurgent referral to an ophthalmologist for possible surgical excision, if the cornea is involved. No medical treatment is necessary for a long-standing, unchang-ing, asymptomatic growth. Protective glasses are recommended for at-risk individuals to prevent recurrences.

I. Keratitis. Refer emergently to ophthalmology to prevent permanent visual loss.

J. Acute angle-closure glaucoma is an ophthalmic emergency and should be referred. The key to treatment is lowering intraocular pressure. Optic nerve atrophy and irreversible loss of vision can occur within hours after onset of the disorder. The patient should alert relatives about the occurrence of these attacks since it is a highly inheritable condition.

The patient's cardiovascular and electrolyte status needs to be assessed when consider-ing treatment with medications such as beta-blockers, osmotic agents, cholinergics, and carbonic anhydrase inhibitors.

K. Anterior uveitis: Urgent referral to an ophthalmologist is recommended to prevent per-manently impaired vision. Recurrent episodes are not uncommon. Management of the underlying systemic disorder may also require consultation with a rheumatologist.

REFERENCES

Greenberg MF, Pollard ZF. The red eye in childhood. *Pediatr Clin N Am.* 2003;50:105-124.

Leibowitz HM. Primary care: the red eye. *N Engl J Med.* 2000;343(5):345-351.

Patel SJ, Lundy DC. Ocular manifestations of autoimmune disease. *Am Fam Physician.* 2002;66:991-998.

Trobe JD. *Physicians's Guide to Eye Care.* 2nd ed. San Francisco, CA: American Academy of Oph-thalmology; 2000.

Riordan-Eva P, Asbury T, Whitcher JP. *Vaughan & Asbury's General Ophthalmology.* 16th ed. Norwalk, CT: Lange; 2003.

Wirbelauer C. Management of the red eye for the primary care physician. *Am J Med.* 2006;119:302-306.

55 Rhinitis & Sinus Pain

Robert Glen Quattlebaum, MD, Vanessa A. Diaz, MD, MS, & Arch G. Mainous III, PhD

KEY POINTS

- Allergic rhinitis is a common condition that can be managed in the primary care setting with medications and lifestyle interventions.
- Acute sinusitis should be diagnosed using specific criteria in order to decrease overdiagnosis and inappropriate use of antibiotics.
- Most patients with acute sinusitis or rhinitis do not benefit from laboratory tests or imaging studies.
- Initial treatment for acute sinusitis should be analgesics and decongestants. Antibiotics for acute sinusitis should be reserved for patients with persistent symptoms after initial treatment or with severe illness.

I. **Definition. Rhinitis** is an inflammation of the nasal mucous membrane frequently resulting in edema of the mucous membranes, vasodilatation, and rhinorrhea. Common causes include **viruses** and other **infectious agents; type I hypersensitivity reactions** to antigens such as pollens, molds, and animal danders; **autonomic hyperresponsiveness; rebound congestion** from intranasal or certain systemic medications; or **atrophy** of the nasal mucosa.

Five main groups of paranasal sinuses drain through sinus ostia into the nasal cavity: the maxillary, frontal, anterior ethmoid, posterior ethmoid, and sphenoid. The maxillary and ethmoid sinuses are present at birth, whereas the sphenoid sinuses develop by age 3 and the frontal sinuses appear by age 5. Maxillary sinuses are noted radiographically by age 4, sphenoid sinuses by age 6, and frontal sinuses by age 7. However, the sinuses are often asymmetrical and may not be fully developed in as many as 5% of adults.

Sinusitis is an inflammatory process in one or more of the paranasal sinuses, associated with obstruction of the sinus ostia. It is usually caused by **infection.** Viral infections are the most common cause, bacterial infections are usually caused by *Staphylococcus pneumoniae* or *Haemophilus influenzae,* and fungal infections are rarely seen except in poorly controlled diabetic patients or the immunocompromised. Infection of the sphenoid sinus can lead to serious complications because of its proximity to the apex of the orbital cavity, optic nerve, hypophysis, and cavernous sinus.

Other factors predisposing to sinusitis include **allergies; anatomic abnormalities** (e.g., nasal polyps, septal deviation, foreign bodies, or adenoidal hypertrophy); **irritants** (e.g., tobacco, smog, chemicals); **low humidity;** and **systemic diseases** such as cystic fibrosis (abnormally thick mucus), Kartagener's syndrome (immobile cilia within the respiratory tract), and congenital or acquired immunodeficiency syndrome.

II. **Common Diagnoses**

  A. **Common cold or viral upper respiratory infection.** There are nearly 62 million cases annually, resulting in 22 million school days lost. Common colds peak in the winter and occur more commonly in families with children aged 2 to 7 years. The average preschool child has six to ten colds per year; the average adult, two to four. Hand-to-hand contact, as well as contact with wet fomites, are risk factors for spread of the virus.

  B. **Allergic rhinitis** is the most common cause of chronic rhinitis. Twenty to forty million Americans are affected and nine million visits to office-based physicians each year are attributed to allergic rhinitis. The peak incidence occurs in the late teenage years, with another peak between the ages of 30 and 40. It is more common in those with a family history of allergies and is often associated with atopy. It may be seasonal or perennial, depending on the types of allergens involved. The seasonal allergens are mostly encountered outdoors and include pollens and, less commonly, mold spores. The perennial allergens are more likely to be encountered indoors and include dust mites, many mold spores, cockroach feces, and animal dander.

C. **Vasomotor rhinitis** occurs most commonly in the third to fifth decades but is occasionally seen in childhood and adolescence. Vasomotor rhinitis of pregnancy occurs most frequently from the second trimester on and resolves spontaneously by the fifth postpartum day.

D. **Atrophic rhinitis** occurs mainly in elderly adults. Risk factors for its development include chronic granulomatous nasal infections (including sarcoidosis, Wegener's granulomatosis, Churg-Strauss syndrome, and tuberculosis), chronic sinusitis, irradiation, trauma, or radical nasal surgery.

E. **Rhinitis medicamentosum** usually affects young to middle-aged adults, although cases have been reported in children as young as 4 years. Abusers of topical nasal decongestants are at risk (decongestant used more frequently than every 3 hours or for longer than 3 weeks). In some individuals, a form of rhinitis medicamentosum occurs with the use of certain antihypertensive agents (e.g., beta-blockers, guanethidine, methyldopa, or reserpine); aspirin; and oral contraceptives.

F. **Sinusitis** is commonly overdiagnosed, so its overall incidence is unclear. Approximately 32 million adults are diagnosed with sinusitis annually. Chronic sinusitis leads to 11.6 million office-based physician visits annually. The incidence peaks in winter, when viral upper respiratory infections are common.

Based on the time course of symptoms, sinusitis is divided into four categories. **Acute sinusitis** is characterized by symptoms lasting 4 weeks. **Subacute sinusitis** is characterized by symptoms lasting 4 to 12 weeks. **Recurrent acute sinusitis** is more than four episodes of acute sinusitis per year lasting at least 7 days with complete resolution of symptoms between bouts. **Chronic sinusitis** persists for 3 months or more.

G. **Conditions that can mimic sinus pain** include migraine headaches and temporal arteritis (see Chapter 34), periapical dental abscesses of the maxillary teeth, and nasal polyps. **Other causes** of rhinitis not discussed in this chapter include pregnancy (see Chapter 97), endocrine disorders including hypothyroidism (see Chapter 87), nonallergic rhinitis with eosinophilia (NARES), nasal foreign bodies, cocaine snorting, nasal neoplasms, and menstruation-induced rhinitis.

III. **Symptoms (Table 55–1)**

A. For symptoms of common cold or viral upper respiratory infection (URI), allergic rhinitis, vasomotor rhinitis, atrophic rhinitis, and rhinitis medicamentosum, see Table 55–1.

B. **Sinusitis:** Sinusitis typically presents as a syndrome of "double sickening." **Double sickening** refers to patients who start out with symptoms of a viral URI, begin to improve only to have the original symptoms return and also develop sinus pain/pressure, maxillary toothaches (painful mastication), nasal obstruction, high fever, headache, halitosis, hyposmia/anosmia, nausea, and vomiting.

The most common cause of **sinus pain** is sinusitis, with numerous other conditions that can mimic this symptom (see Section II.G). Sinus pain may present as vague, tension-type headaches; or may specifically localize as pain or pressure over the affected sinuses. Pain beneath the eyes suggests **maxillary sinusitis,** pain between the eyes suggests **ethmoid sinusitis,** frontal headache suggests **frontal sinusitis,** and vertex headache suggests **sphenoid sinusitis.** Headache, facial pain, and sinus pressure in sinusitis is often worse in the morning and with head movement.

Orbital swelling or redness, severe swelling over the affected sinus, proptosis, vision changes, and altered mental status may indicate central nervous system complications of sinusitis (e.g., abscesses, meningitis, orbital cellulitis), and warrant immediate surgical consultation.

The symptoms of sinusitis may mimic and overlap those of other diseases, ranging from the common cold to allergic rhinitis. Sinusitis should be suspected when symptoms of these common conditions are prolonged and interfere with daily living or when these symptoms are severe rather than mild or moderate.

IV. **Signs (Table 55–1)**

A. Overview

1. Examination of the nose begins with inspection of the anterior and inferior surfaces, which is aided by a **nasal speculum** and a strong light source. Abnormalities of the nasal mucosa and septum and presence of exudates can help diagnose common causes of rhinitis. A **nasopharyngeal mirror** is required for detection of posterior abnormalities.

2. Examination of the paranasal sinuses begins with **inspection** of the overlying skin for erythema, which can be associated with infection, **followed by palpation for tenderness** of the maxillary and frontal sinuses.

TABLE 55-1. SIGNS AND SYMPTOMS OF RHINOSINUSITIS

Sign/Symptom	Viral URI	Sinusitis	Allergic Rhinitis	Vasomotor Rhinitis	Atrophic Rhinitis	Rhinitis Medicamentosum
Time course	7–10 d	Acute sinusitis: 4 wk; Subacute: 4–12 wk; Chronic: greater than 3 mo	≥2 wk without symptoms without improvement	Occurs with exposure to certain odors, alcohol, spicy foods, intense emotions, pregnancy, and extreme temperatures	Weeks to months	Seen with prolonged use of decongestants, antihypertensive agents (beta-blockers, guanethidine, methyldopa, and reserpine), aspirin, oral contraceptives, and cocaine
Fatigue	Sometimes	Common†	Uncommon	Uncommon	Uncommon	Uncommon
Headache	Sometimes	Sometimes†	Sometimes	Uncommon	Uncommon	Uncommon
Ear pain/pressure	Sometimes	Common†	Uncommon	Uncommon	Uncommon	Uncommon
Sneezing	Common	Sometimes	Common	Uncommon	Uncommon	Uncommon
Rhinorrhea and nasal congestion	Common, usually mucoid but may become mucopurulent after 1–3 d. Usually resolve in 7–10 d.	Common, often purulent and yellow to green, continues for ≥7 d, responds poorly to decongestants. Most often bilateral but may be unilateral. May not have drainage in chronic sinusitis because of occlusion.	Common, usually watery or mucoid	Commonly have unrelenting congestion, rhinorrhea usually very watery	Common	Congestion without rhinorrhea
Nasal obstruction/blockage	Uncommon	Common*	Uncommon	Uncommon	Common	Common
Nasal and conjunctival itching	Uncommon	Uncommon	Common	Uncommon	Uncommon	Uncommon
Hyposmia/anosmia	Uncommon	Common*	Uncommon	Uncommon	Uncommon	Uncommon
Halitosis	Uncommon	Sometimes†	Uncommon	Uncommon	Uncommon	Uncommon
Dental pain	Uncommon	Common†	Uncommon	Uncommon	Uncommon	Uncommon
Pain or pressure over sinuses	Uncommon	Common*	Uncommon	Uncommon	Uncommon	Uncommon
Cough	Common	Common†	Common	Uncommon	Uncommon	Uncommon
Time Course	7–10 d	Acute sinusitis: 4 wk; Subacute: 4–12 wk; Chronic: greater than 3 mo	≥ 2 wk without symptoms without improvement	Occurs with exposure to certain odors, alcohol, spicy foods, intense emotions, pregnancy, and extreme temperatures	Weeks to months	Seen with prolonged use of decongestants, antihypertensive agents (beta-blockers, guanethidine, methyldopa, and reserpine), aspirin, oral contraceptives, and cocaine

(Continued)

TABLE 55-1. (*Continued*)

Sign/Symptom	Viral URI	Sinusitis	Allergic Rhinitis	Vasomotor Rhinitis	Atrophic Rhinitis	Rhinitis Medicamentosum
Fever	Unusual in adults, more common in children	Usually ≤101°F, but may be higher with aggressive sinusitis*	None	None	None	None
Nasal mucosa	Erythematous and swollen	Marked erythema and swelling if acute, varies with chronic.	Pale and boggy or bluish, may have nasal polyp	Bright and red to bluish	Nasal crusting, a shrunken-appearing nasal mucosa, and enlarged nasal cavities Patients may also have epistaxis	Marked erythema or even a hemorrhagic appearance and swelling
Associated Signs/Symptoms	May also have conjunctival erythema and effusions. Frequently with sick contacts	May have nasal or postnasal discharge/purulence.† Second-sickening	Allergic "shiners" (dark rings under the eyes), Dennie-Morgan lines (deep creases below the inferior eyelid), nasal crease (horizontal line across the bridge of the nose)	None	None	None

The presence of two or more major criteria, one major and two or more minor criteria, or nasal purulence on examination constitutes a diagnosis of sinusitis.
*Major criteria (pain/pressure and fever are not major criteria in the absence of another major criterion).
†Minor criteria.

3. **Transillumination** of the sinuses should be performed in a darkened room. A strong, narrow light source is placed snugly under each brow, close to the nose. A dim red glow should be seen as the light is transmitted through the air-filled frontal sinus to the forehead. The maxillary sinuses are transilluminated by shining light downward from just below the inner aspect of each eye while asking the patient to tilt his head back with the mouth wide open. A reddish glow seen at the hard palate indicates a normal air-filled sinus. Asymmetrical or poor transillumination is consistent with sinusitis, although it may also be caused by nonpathologic hypoplastic or aplastic sinuses.

4. Physical examination of children should include evaluation of several key components. The child's **general appearance** should be assessed for lethargy and respiratory distress, which are worrisome signs. The **skin** should be examined for atopic dermatitis, often associated with allergic rhinitis. The **nasal cavity** and **oropharynx** should also be examined for mucosa and anatomy, specifically for nasal obstruction and discharge.

B. **Common cold or viral URI:** On general examination, patients with viral URIs will appear fatigued. The nasal examination will reveal erythematous nasal mucosa and mucoid or mucopurulent discharge. Examination of the throat will reveal erythematous mucosa. Ear examination will occasionally reveal effusions. Cervical lymph nodes may also be present, along with a fever.

C. **Allergic rhinitis:** External examination of the face in patients with allergic rhinitis often reveals a **nasal crease** (a horizontal line across the bridge of the nose caused by repeated upward rubbing of the nose—also known as the **allergic salute**) and allergic **"shiners"** (dark rings under the eyes). The nasal examination will often reveal boggy, pale, bluish-gray mucosa; but erythematous mucosa can also be present. Clear rhinorrhea and nasal polyps may also be present. On the ocular examination, the **conjunctiva** is frequently inflamed, the palpebral conjunctiva may have an edematous and cobblestone appearance, and Dennie-Morgan lines (deep creases below the inferior eyelid) may also be present.

D. **Vasomotor rhinitis:** The physical examination for vasomotor rhinitis is varied, as the nasal examination of this condition can present similarly to infectious, allergic or atrophic rhinitis.

E. **Atrophic rhinitis:** The nasal examination in patients with atrophic rhinitis will reveal **nasal crusting**, a shrunken-appearing nasal mucosa, and enlarged nasal cavities. Patients may also have **epistaxis**. Despite the sensation of nasal congestion, there is no increase in airflow resistance in most of these cases.

F. **Rhinitis medicamentosum:** The nasal examination of patients with this condition reveals **marked erythema** or even a hemorrhagic appearance and swelling of the nasal mucosa.

G. **Sinusitis:** In general, the patient is typically febrile and fatigued. **External signs** of sinusitis include erythema overlying the sinuses. The bony structures overlying the maxillary, frontal, or ethmoid sinuses may be tender to palpation, and eyelid puffiness (chemosis) may be present, especially with maxillary and ethmoid sinusitis. **Sinus transillumination** has very low sensitivity and specificity because of the great variability in sinus anatomy, including asymmetry and underdevelopment. Only normal findings are useful in ruling out maxillary or frontal sinusitis.

In acute sinusitis, infectious rhinitis is also commonly present, and therefore the nasal examination will appear similar to those with viral URIs. When the sinus ostia are visible, purulent discharge may be seen exuding from them. In chronic sinusitis, the appearance of the mucous membranes depends on the underlying cause—pale or bluish and edematous in allergic rhinitis or even relatively normal with anatomic causes, such as choanal atresia or septal deviation.

Signs of complications of sinusitis include periorbital erythema, proptosis, and edema. Cranial nerve deficits, especially an abducens nerve palsy, can indicate invasive infection. Meningitis should be considered in patients with signs of severe acute sinusitis. If these findings are present, prompt surgical consultation is required.

V. **Laboratory Tests** (Table 55–2) may be indicated if medical therapy fails, if there are symptoms and signs of complications, or if there is a serious underlying condition. (SOR **Ⓒ**)

A. **Study of nasal secretions** is not necessary for diagnosis but may help identify the etiology of rhinitis. Nasal secretions are obtained and placed on a glass slide, stained with Hansel, Wright's, or Giemsa stain and examined microscopically. Eosinophils are seen in allergic rhinitis, NARES, and nasal polyposis; large numbers of neutrophils are seen with infection.

B. **Cultures of nasal secretions** from nasal swabs are of limited value because they do not correlate well with bacteria aspirated directly from the sinuses. Endoscopically guided

TABLE 55–2. **INDICATIONS FOR LABORATORY AND IMAGING IN RHINOSINUSITIS**

Laboratory/Imaging Modality	Indications	SOR
Microscopic Nasal Secretion Analysis	Only necessary if unable to distinguish allergic vs. infectious based on history and physical	Ⓒ
Cultures of nasal secretions	Only beneficial in conjunction with fiberoptic rhinoscopy, especially if fungal etiology is suspected	Ⓒ
Fiberoptic rhinoscopy	Patients with recurrent sinusitis or if polyps are suspected	Ⓒ
Allergen skin testing	Patients (not less than 3 y old) who fail medical therapy or have perennial rhinitis that is moderate to severe	Ⓒ
Radioallergosorbent (RAST) testing	Young children ($\leq$ 3 y old), or other patients unable to have skin testing performed	Ⓒ
Sinus films	Patients with uncertain or recurrent sinusitis	Ⓒ
CT scan of sinus	Patients with uncertain, chronic or recurrent sinusitis; or any patient with red flag symptoms	Ⓒ
MRI	Patients suspected of having fungal sinusitis or tumors	Ⓒ

microswab cultures from the middle meatus correlate 80% to 85% with central puncture cultures. Cultures are indicated when acute sinusitis is resistant to one or two courses of antibiotic therapy and in immunocompromised individuals. Cultures are also obtained during most surgical procedures on the sinuses if persistent sinus infection is suspected. Aerobic and anaerobic cultures should be obtained, and fungal cultures should be added if a fungal origin is suspected.

C. **Fiberoptic rhinoscopy** can reveal the presence of nasal polyps, septal deviation, or mucopurulent secretions, and can be used to obtain microswab cultures.

D. **Allergy tests**
   1. **Allergen skin testing** is helpful in diagnosing allergic rhinitis and identifying specific allergens for which avoidance measures, allergen immunotherapy, or both are warranted. It should be considered in patients who fail medical therapy or have perennial rhinitis that is moderate to severe. These tests are relatively inexpensive and fairly reliable. They are not useful in children younger than 3 years because very young children produce inadequate amounts of histamine.
      a. Groups of allergens or single allergens are selected for testing based on the most likely causes of the patient's allergy.
      b. Allergens are introduced into the skin by intradermal injection (which is most accurate but carries a greater risk of anaphylaxis), skin prick test (the easiest, most widely used, and reasonably accurate), or scratch test. (*Note:* Methylxanthines and antihistamines should be discontinued before skin testing.)
   2. **Radioallergosorbent (RAST) testing** is the determination of serum allergen-specific IgE levels by immunoassay. This test is useful in young children, who might not tolerate multiple skin pricks; those with skin conditions such as dermatographia and severe eczema; and those receiving medications that might affect the reliability of skin testing (e.g., antihistamines). However, it is relatively more expensive, is less sensitive, and can test for fewer antigens than skin testing.

E. **Imaging studies (Table 55–2)** may be helpful in uncertain cases, recurrent symptoms despite appropriate treatment, and when symptoms of complications are present. (SOR Ⓒ)
   1. **Sinus films** may be helpful in uncertain or recurrent cases, but not for initial evaluation, since up to 40% of sinus films may be abnormal in viral rhinosinusitis if obtained within 7 days of symptom onset. Four views constitute the sinus series: Waters' view (maxillary sinuses), the Caldwell view (ethmoid and frontal sinuses), the submental vertex view (sphenoid sinuses), and the lateral view. A single Water's view has a high level of agreement with the complete sinus series. A normal series has a negative predictive value of 90% to 100%, particularly for the maxillary and frontal sinuses. A sinus film is read as abnormal if there is mucosal thickening $\geq$6 mm, air–fluid levels, $\geq$33% loss of air space volume, or opacification of one or more sinuses on one or more views. The positive predictive value is 80% to 100%, but sensitivity is only 60%.
   2. The computerized tomography (**CT scan**) has superior sensitivity (95%–98%) and specificity compared to sinus films. The CT scan is particularly valuable in assessing obstruction of the sinus ostia. CT scanning is indicated when medical therapy has

failed to establish the diagnosis of chronic sinusitis in equivocal cases before starting long-term antibiotic therapy or when complications are suspected. A complete series sinus CT scan is required prior to sinus surgery. More than 80% of scan results may be abnormal in viral rhinosinusitis if obtained within 7 days of illness onset.

3. **Magnetic resonance imaging** is used when fungal sinusitis and tumors are suspected. It is not used for routine evaluation of sinusitis.

VI. Treatment

A. Treatment of **common colds** is largely palliative and may include the following strategies.

1. For **fever and headache, acetaminophen** (e.g., Tylenol), 325 mg, one or two tablets orally every 4 to 6 hours for adults (maximum 4 g/24 h) or 10–15 mg/kg every 4 to 6 hours for children younger than 12 years, or **ibuprofen** (e.g., Advil), 200 mg, one or two tablets every 4 to 6 hours for adults (maximum 1200 mg/24 h), or 5–10 mg/kg every 6 to 8 hours for children (maximum 50 mg/kg/d) may be used.

2. For **nasal congestion and rhinorrhea,** oral decongestants such as **pseudoephedrine** (e.g., Sudafed), 30 mg, one or two tablets every 4 to 6 hours for adults and children older than age 12, or 0.5 to 1 tsp every 4 to 6 hours of the liquid for children younger than 12 years, may be used. Short-term use (up to a maximum of 3–4 days) of topical decongestants such as **phenylephrine hydrochloride** (e.g., Neo-Synephrine), 0.125% or 0.25%, two or three sprays in each nostril up to every 4 hours for children and the same dosing schedule of the 0.5% spray for adults, may be helpful. These medications can cause insomnia, nervousness, loss of appetite, and urinary retention in males. They should be used with caution in patients with certain conditions, such as arrhythmias, hypertension, and hyperthyroidism.

3. For **cough,** syrups containing **dextromethorphan** (e.g., Robitussin DM) or **codeine** (e.g., Robitussin AC), 0.5–2 tsp every 4 hours (the exact dose depends on the patient's age), can be prescribed, with **benzonatate** (e.g., Tessalon Perles), 100 mg 3 times daily for adults, a potentially helpful alternative.

4. **Watery rhinorrhea** may be treated with the anticholinergic nasal spray **ipratropium bromide** (e.g., Atrovent 0.06%).

5. **Antihistamines** have not been shown to be beneficial, nor are **antibiotics** indicated or helpful in these patients.

6. **Alternative therapies**

   a. **General supportive measures** in the treatment of **common colds** and **allergies** include adequate sleep, increased fluids, cool vapor steam, and rest. Certainly, adequate fluids (especially water and soups) improve mucous membrane and ciliary function and may also enhance immune function.

   b. The use of other alternative therapies, such as **homeopathic medicines, vitamins, acupuncture,** and **herbs,** is controversial. Although **vitamin C** in high doses (up to 1 g daily) does not seem to prevent illness, it does reduce the duration of symptoms. **Zinc** may also be effective in shortening the duration of symptoms when taken within 24 hours of their onset. Studies indicating **Echinacea** preparations stimulate the immune system, thereby reducing the severity and duration of infection, are debated, although effects appear generally positive.

B. Allergic rhinitis

1. **Environmental control.** Avoidance of inciting factors is fundamental.

   a. For **pollen allergy,** patients should keep doors and windows closed, limit the amount of time spent outdoors, and use air conditioners and a high-efficiency particle air (HEPA) filter.

   b. For **dust mite allergy,** patients should cover bedding (including pillows) with plastic covers, eliminate wall-to-wall carpets (especially in bedrooms), use acaricides such as tannic acid solutions regularly to kill dust mites, avoid or regularly wash stuffed animals in hot water, keep home humidity below 40%, and use HEPA filters.

   c. Patients with **mold allergies** should decrease mold exposure by wiping vulnerable surfaces (e.g., those in the bathroom) with household bleach, keeping indoor humidity below 40%, using air filters, avoiding piles of leaves in the fall, and cutting grass to reduce exposure outside.

   d. **Cat dander** (saliva) is by far the most frequent cause of allergies to animals. If sensitivity develops, contact with the animal should be minimized. The cat should be washed at least once every 2 weeks to remove the antigen-containing cat saliva from its coat.

    e. Elimination of **food allergens** may be beneficial. However, ingested allergens rarely cause isolated rhinitis without involvement of other organ systems. Relatively common food allergens include dairy products, chocolate, wheat, citrus fruits, and food additives such as artificial dyes and preservatives.

2. Pharmacologic therapy includes the following:

    a. Steroid nasal sprays are more effective than antihistamines in the treatment of allergic rhinitis. (SOR Ⓐ) Available preparations include **beclomethasone** (e.g., Beconase or Vancenase), one spray per nostril 2 or 3 times daily; **flunisolide** (e.g., Nasalide), two sprays per nostril twice daily; **triamcinolone acetonide** (e.g., Nasacort), two to four sprays per nostril daily; **budesonide** (e.g., Rhinocort), two to four sprays per nostril daily; and **fluticasone** (e.g., Flonase), one or two sprays daily. Other steroid nasal sprays have good long-term safety records. Local side effects are minimal with proper use, although nasal irritation, bleeding, mucosal erosions, and perforation may occur. Since some nasal corticosteroid preparations have been reported to reduce linear growth (at least temporarily), growth should be monitored when used in children. **Oral steroids** should be avoided, except in severe cases of refractory allergic rhinitis, in rhinitis medicamentosum while topical decongestants are discontinued, and in obstructive nasal polyposis. If used in these situations, short-acting steroids should be used (e.g., in adults, prednisone, 30 mg orally for 3–7 days).

    b. Antihistamines (Table 55–3) reduce sneezing, rhinorrhea, and nasal and ocular pruritus associated with allergic rhinitis, but are less effective for nasal congestion. They are effective when used occasionally for episodic symptoms, but work best when administered on a regular basis. If economic factors are less important, the newer-generation antihistamines are usually preferred, because they have fewer anticholinergic side effects and especially cause less sedation. (SOR Ⓐ) These agents include **desloratadine** (Clarinex), **fexofenadine** (Allegra), **cetirizine** (Zyrtec), and **loratadine** (Claritin), which is currently the only one available over the counter. **First-generation antihistamines** are effective and less expensive than newer agents, but tend to cause more side effects, such as sedation, dry mouth, and fatigue. Even more serious side effects can occur, such as urinary obstruction and slowed reaction times, which can potentially lead to accidents. **Levocabastine** (Livostin 0.05%), one drop into each affected eye 4 times daily, or **Patanol (olopatadine 0.1%), one to two drops in each affected eye twice a day,** can be very helpful in the treatment of allergic conjunctivitis. **Intranasal antihistamines** (e.g., azelastine) offer no therapeutic benefit over conventional treatment.

    c. Antihistamine–decongestant combinations such as **Claritin-D 12 Hour, Claritin-D 24 Hour, Tavist-D,** and **Allegra-D** are also useful, especially if nasal congestion is a prominent symptom. The dose is one tablet twice daily for all except Claritin-D 24 hour, which is taken once daily.

    d. Mast cell–stabilizing agents such as **cromolyn sodium** (e.g., Nasalcrom), one spray per nostril 3 or 4 times per day, can be useful. Ideally, these agents should be started before major symptoms develop because they may take several weeks to be effective.

    e. Anticholinergic agents such as **ipratropium bromide** (e.g., Atrovent 0.03% nasal spray), one or two sprays in each nostril every 6 hours, may reduce rhinorrhea.

3. Immunotherapy is useful especially in severe or refractory cases and in those patients with year-round symptoms (perennial allergic rhinitis). It is the only method demonstrated to favorably modify the long-term course of allergic rhinitis. Criteria for treatment include a history of at least moderate symptoms of allergic rhinitis for ≥2 years or severe symptoms for at least 6 months responding poorly to symptomatic treatment. Other considerations in choosing immunotherapy include comorbidities and failure or unacceptability of alternative treatments. Selection of antigen injection is based on the presence of specific IgE antibodies (see Section V.D) and the patient's history. The patient receives weekly injections of antigen(s), with increasing doses at weekly intervals until a maintenance dose is achieved; injections are then given every 3 to 6 weeks for 3 to 5 years. If therapy does not significantly relieve symptoms within 12 months, immunotherapy should be terminated.

4. Patient education should include information about environmental controls to minimize antigen exposure, management options, and complications.

TABLE 55-3. ANTIHISTAMINES USEFUL IN THE TREATMENT OF ALLERGIC RHINITIS

Class	Generic Name	Sample Trade Name	Dose*	Sedative Effects	Anticholinergic Effects
First-generation Ethanolamines	Diphenhydramine	Benadryl† Allergy tablets Syrup	A: 25–50 mg qid C: 12.5 mg/5 mL 5–10 mL q 4–6 hours	Marked	Mild
	Clemastine	Tavist Tablets Syrup	A: 1.32–2.68 mg bid C: 0.5 mg/5 mL 5–10 mL bid		
Alkylamines	Chorpheniramine	Chlor-Trimeton tablets Triaminic† syrup	A: 4 mg qid C: 1 mg/5 mL 1.5–10 mL q 4 hours	Mild	Mild
Phenothiazines	Promethazine	Phenergan Tablets Syrup	A: 25–50 mg qid C: 6.25 mg/5 mL 5–10 mL tid–qid	Marked	Mild
Piperidines	Cyproheptadine	Periactin tablets	A: 4 mg qid C: 2 mg/5 mL 5–15 mL bid–tid	Moderate	Mild
	Azatadine	Trinalin tablets	A: 1 bid		
Piperazine	Hydroxyzine	Atarax Tablets Syrup	A: 10–50 mg qid C: 10 mg/5 mL 5–15 mL tid–qid	Moderate	Mild
Second generation	Cetirizine	Zyrtec Tablets Syrup	A: 10 mg qd C: 5–10 mL qd (1 mg/mL)	Mild	None
	Fexofenadine	Allegra tablets	A: 60 mg bid	None	None
	Loratadine	Claritin (OTC) Tablets Syrup	A: 10 mg qd C: 10 mL qd (1 mg/mL)	None	None
	Desloratadine	Clarinex Tablets	A: 5 mg qd	None	None

Children's dosages are listed for those medications with available pediatric suspensions. Be aware that a range of dosages are listed. Look up the exact dosages by age before prescribing these medications for children.
*A, adults' dose (mg); C, children's dose (mL).
†A decongestant is added to this formulation.

5. **Alternative therapies**
   a. For more information on **common supportive measures,** see Section VI.A.6.a.
   b. **Other alternative therapies, such as vitamin C, quercetin, homeopathy, acupuncture, and hypnosis, require further study.**
C. Treatment of **vasomotor rhinitis** consists mainly of symptomatic therapy with oral decongestants such as **pseudoephedrine** (e.g., Sudafed), 60 mg 3 or 4 times a day. Anticholinergic agents such as **ipratropium bromide** (e.g., Atrovent nasal spray) (see Section VI.B.2.e) can be very helpful in alleviating profuse watery rhinorrhea. **Intranasal steroids** (see Section VI.B.2.a) may be helpful in treating troublesome exacerbations unresponsive to the therapies listed above. **Intranasal antihistamines** (e.g., azelastine, two sprays per nostril twice daily) are also effective. Severe nonresponsive cases may require surgical resection of the inferior turbinate. Patients should be educated to avoid irritants that may exacerbate this condition; these include tobacco and fireplace smoke,

strong perfumes, chemical and gasoline fumes, and wood dust. Sudden changes in temperature or humidity should also be avoided when possible.

D. In **rhinitis medicamentosum,** topical decongestants should be discontinued. Oral decongestants or a short course of a topical nasal steroid may be helpful (see Section VI.B.2.a). A short course of systemic steroids (e.g., **prednisone,** 40 mg orally initially, tapered over 7–10 days) may be required if other methods are ineffective. The problem usually resolves in 2 to 3 weeks without long-term sequelae. Patients should be educated about the causes of the condition and discouraged from further abuse of topical decongestants.

E. Treatment of **atrophic rhinitis** is directed toward moistening the nasal mucosa. A mucolytic such as **guaifenesin,** 600 to 1200 mg twice daily, can be used in conjunction with nasal preparations such as **Alkalol liquid,** an OTC oral or intranasal mucolytic, **or intranasal saline** (e.g., Afrin saline), two to six sprays in each nostril every 2 hours. **Pulsed irrigators** can also be helpful in helping to cleanse and moisten areas deeper within the nasal cavity. Systemic estrogens in menopausal women may alleviate rhinitis symptoms. Surgical reductions of nasal cavity patency are used only as a last resort. It is important to educate patients that treatment is directed at relieving symptoms and is sometimes only partially successful.

F. **Sinusitis** can usually be managed in the outpatient setting. It can be diagnosed using the major and minor criteria in Table 55–1. Initial treatment should be 10 to 14 days of conservative measures (see Section VI.A) and decongestants. Antibiotics for acute sinusitis should be reserved for patients with persistent rhinorrhea or daytime cough lasting more than 10 to 14 days without improvement after initial treatment or with severe illness (severe facial pain, fever with purulent nasal discharge, periorbital swelling), regardless of duration. (SOR **B**)

Hospital admission is necessary for complicated sinusitis (sinusitis associated with serious complications such as otitis media, asthma, bronchiectasis, fungal infection, multiple antibiotic allergies, or sinusitis that compromises quality of life) or when there is a high risk of complications from a serious underlying disease and close outpatient monitoring is not feasible. (SOR **C**)

1. Humidification with cool steam and increased oral intake of water helps thin nasal secretions.

2. Oral decongestants or short-term use (3–5 days) of **topical nasal decongestants** (see Section VI.A.2) decrease nasal congestion and mucosal edema that can block the sinus ostia.

3. Oral decongestant–antihistamine combinations (Section VI.B.2.c) may be helpful in patients with underlying allergic rhinitis.

4. Guaifenesin in high doses (1200 mg twice daily) may thin tenacious secretions and therefore promote sinus drainage.

5. Nasal irrigation with a normal saline solution is recommended to liquefy secretions. It is especially helpful in infants and young children.

6. Antibiotics (Table 55–4).

   a. The standard has been to treat adults and children with uncomplicated acute sinusitis for a minimum of 7 to 10 days. Data shows as little as 3 days of antibiotic treatment (i.e., with **trimethoprim-sulfamethoxazole [TMP-SMX]**) may be as effective as treatment for 10 days. Thus, the duration of treatment is currently a controversial topic. Antibiotics should be changed if there is no improvement after 3 days of therapy. (SOR **B**)

   b. For initial treatment, the most narrow-spectrum agent active against the likely pathogens, *S pneumoniae* and *H influenzae,* should be used. (SOR **B**) Appropriate first-line therapy in otherwise healthy patients with uncomplicated acute sinusitis who have not received antibiotics in the previous month and are in an area with ≤30% prevalence of drug-resistant pneumococcus includes high-dose **amoxicillin, TMP-SMX, cefuroxime axetil, cefdinir,** and **cefpodoxime.** For patients with penicillin/cephalosporin allergies, other treatment options include **clarithromycin, azithromycin, doxycycline,** or **quinolones.**

   c. If the response to first-line therapy is poor, if there is at least a 30% prevalence of drug-resistant *Pneumococcus,* or if the patient is immunocompromised, reasonable alternative antimicrobials include **amoxicillin-clavulanate** and **quinolones.** Quinolones should only be used in individuals 18 years or older. The American Academy of Pediatrics recommends that for moderate to more severe sinusitis, if

TABLE 55-4. AMBULATORY ANTIBIOTIC REGIMENS IN THE TREATMENT OF UNCOMPLICATED SINUSITIS

Antibiotic	Dose	Relative Cost
Amoxicillin (Amoxil)*	Adult: 500 mg tid Child: (high-dose) 90 mg/kg/d divided bid or tid	$
Trimethoprim-sulfamethoxazole (TMP-SMX)* (Bactrim, 160 mg of TMP and 800 mg of SMX per DS tablet; Septra, 8 mg of TMP and 40 mg of SMX per tsp)	Adult: one DS tablet bid Child: 8–12 mg/kg/d TMP and 40–60 mg/kg/d SMX divided bid	$
Clarithromycin (Biaxin)†	Adult: 500 mg bid or 1 gm qd if extended release Child: 15 mg/kg/d bid	$$$
Amoxicillin-clavulanate (Augmentin)†	Adult: 875/125 mg bid Child: (high-dose) 90 mg/kg/d amoxicillin component divided bid	$$$
Cefuroxime axetil (Ceftin)*	Adult: 250 mg bid Child: 30 mg/kg/d bid	$$$
Cefpodoxime proxetil (Vantin)*	Adult: 200 mg bid Child: 10 mg/kg/d bid	$$$
Azithromycin (Zithromax)†	Adult: 500 mg d 1, 250 mg days 2–5 Child: 10 mg/kg/d 1, 5 mg/kg days 2–5	$$
Levofloxacin (Levaquin)†	Adult: 500 mg qd	$$$

*First-line treatment.
† Second-line treatment.

a child has recently received antibiotics or attends day care, therapy should be initiated with high-dose amoxicillin-clavulanate (80–90 mg/kg/d of amoxicillin component in two divided doses).

d. For chronic sinusitis, antibiotic therapy should continue for at least 3 weeks and until the patient is well for 7 days. Antibiotics with good staphylococcal coverage are often preferred; these include **cloxacillin, dicloxacillin, cephalexin, cefadroxil monohydrate, erythromycin, clarithromycin, amoxicillin-clavulanate,** and **cefuroxime axetil.** With complicated sinusitis, hospital admission for parenteral antibiotics is indicated. If mucormycosis is suspected, parenteral **amphotericin B** should be used.

7. **Other therapies**
   a. **Topical corticosteroids** may be effective adjuncts to antibiotic therapy, but objective data are lacking. The short-term use of **oral corticosteroids** is reasonable in patients with nasal polyps or severe mucosal edema.
   b. **Surgery** should be considered for patients who have frequent recurrences of sinusitis (i.e., three or more attacks in 1 year) despite adequate medical treatment, who have chronic sinusitis responding inadequately to medical therapy alone, or who have an anatomic obstruction amenable to surgery. Functional endoscopic sinus surgery (FESS) has supplanted older surgical techniques. FESS leads to a significant improvement of symptoms in 80% to 90% of patients. It is typically directed at the removal of locally diseased ethmoid tissue to improve ventilation and drainage. When polyps are present and cause marked mechanical obstruction, polypectomy may be indicated. Adenoidectomy may be indicated primarily in younger children with moderate to severe nasal obstruction secondary to adenoidal hyperplasia and may decrease recurrence of sinusitis.

8. **Dental referral** is indicated in patients in whom a tooth abscess is suspected as the underlying cause of maxillary sinusitis.

9. **Patient follow-up**
   a. There are no clear recommendations for follow-up of acute sinusitis; however, it is reasonable to see a patient 10 to 14 days after therapy is initiated to establish whether symptoms and signs of sinusitis have completely resolved.
   b. **Complications** of sinusitis are uncommon. They occur more frequently in children and in patients with immunodeficiency disorders. Patients should be instructed to return to the physician immediately if symptoms worsen or if new symptoms

such as visual disturbance, neck stiffness, or lethargy develop. Complications of sinusitis can be **local, orbital,** or **intracranial.** Prompt surgical consultation should be obtained if any of these complications arise.

(1) Local complications include mucoceles or mucopyoceles. Mucoceles occur most frequently in the frontal sinus, and patients often present complaining of diplopia because the affected eye is displaced.

(2) Orbital complications are the most common, and children with acute ethmoid sinusitis are the most prone to this complication. Preseptal or orbital cellulitis can occur; the latter is more severe because it involves orbital structures. Signs of orbital cellulitis include swelling and inflammation of the eyelids and proptosis of the affected eye. Complete ophthalmoplegia, impairment of vision, and chemosis indicate likely orbital abscess.

(3) Intracranial complications include cavernous sinus thrombosis (signs include bilateral orbital involvement, ophthalmoplegia, progressive and severe chemosis, retinal engorgement, fever, and prostration); meningitis; subdural empyema; and brain abscess.

REFERENCES

CDC. Rhinitis versus Sinusitis in Children: Careful Antibiotic Use. CDC, March 3, 2006. http://www.cdc.gov/drugresistance/community/files/ads/rhini_vs_sinus.htm.

Cummings C, Haughey B, Thomas JR, et al. *Cummings Otolaryngology: Head & Neck Surgery.* 4th ed. Mosby, St Louis, Baltimore, Boston, Chicago; 2004.

Ip S, Fu L, Balk E, Chew P, DeVine D, Lau J. *Update on Acute Bacterial Rhinosinusitis.* Rockville, MD: Agency for Healthcare Research and Quality; 2005. Evidence Report/Technology Assessment 124. AHRQ publication 05-E020-2.

Long A, McFadden C, DeVine D, et al. *Management of Allergic and Nonallergic Rhinitis.* Rockville, MD: Agency for Healthcare Research and Quality; 2002. Evidence Report/Technology Assessment 54. AHRQ publication 02-E024.

McAlister WH, Strain JD, Cohen HL, et al. *Expert Panel on Pediatric Imaging. Sinusitis–child.* Reston, VA: American College of Radiology; 2006. http://www.acr.org/s_acr/bin.asp?CID = 1204& DID = 11846& DOC = FILE.PDF.

Williams JW Jr, Aguilar C, Cornell J, et al. Antibiotics for acute maxillary sinusitis. *Cochrane Database Syst Rev.* 2003;(2):CD000243. doi:10.1002/14651858.CD000243.

---

56   Scrotal Complaints

John A. Heydt, MD, & Ted D. Epperly, MD

KEY POINTS

- A firm grounding in scrotal anatomy is helpful in approaching the patient with scrotal complaints.
- Scrotal complaints affect 0.1% to 0.3% of the male population each year; most causes can be determined by history and limited testing.
- Scrotal pain can have an insidious ($\geq$48 hours) or acute ($\leq$48 hours) onset; a limited history and physical examination, with or without selective testing, will pinpoint the diagnosis.

I. Definition. Scrotal pain refers to discomfort, pain, or an unpleasant sensation originating or referred to the scrotum.

Knowledge of scrotal anatomy (Figure 56–1) is fundamental to diagnosing scrotal complaints.

II. Common Diagnoses

A. Testicular causes

1. Epididymitis most commonly occurs in sexually active males from retrograde spread of prostatitis or urethral secretions through the vas deferens, but may also occur

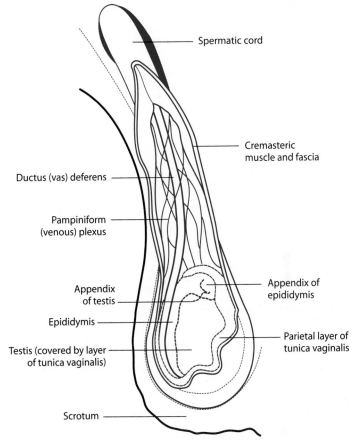

FIGURE 56–1. Testicular anatomy.

in prepubertal boys with urologic abnormalities such as ectopic ureters or congenital/acquired urethral strictures.

    a. In **sexually active men younger than 35 years,** epididymitis is usually associated with urethritis and caused by *Neisseria gonorrhoeae* or *Chlamydia trachomatis* but may be owing to *Ureaplasma* or mycoplasma infections.

    b. In **sexually monogamous men older than 35 years,** epididymitis is usually caused by enteric gram-negative rods (*Enterobacter*) and may occur in association with prostatitis or prostatitis with cystitis.

2. Orchitis is most commonly viral. Approximately 20% to 35% of males who contract mumps develop orchitis, and 35% of those affected have involvement of both testes. Other viral infections known to cause orchitis include influenza, Epstein-Barr, varicella, echo, and Coxsackie. Orchitis can also be associated with a bacterial epididymitis or epididymo-orchitis.

3. Torsion

    a. Testicular torsion occurs most frequently in neonates and pubertal boys. The annual incidence is 1 in 4000 with a peak age of 14. It is rare over age 30. The overall risk of a male having either testicular torsion or torsion of the testicular appendage by age 25 is 1 in 160. Predisposing conditions include the "bell clapper deformity" which occurs in 12% of males, small testicles, excessive exercise, straining, cremasteric spasm, sexual activity, a sudden scare, immersion in cold water, attempted reduction of an inguinal hernia, or trauma.

    b. **Incidence of torsion of the testicular appendage** peaks at age 10, almost always occurs prior to puberty, and shares risk factors with testicular torsion.

4. With **traumatic injuries,** severe scrotal trauma is uncommon and results from either the testicle being compressed against the pubic bone or from straddle injury.

5. **Testicular neoplasms** are the third most common tumors in men between ages 20 and 34 years (incidence of 2–3 per 100,000 men per year). A history of undescended testicle(s), even with correction, increases the risk 2.5 to 20 times over those without such a history.

CRYPTORCHIDISM

Undescended testicle(s) (cryptorchidism) occur in 3% to 5% of term newborns and up to 30% of premature males. Most descend spontaneously, so the prevalence is 1% of boys by age 1 year. Because of the associated risk of testicular neoplasms and decreased fertility, urologic consultation for orchiopexy is indicated between ages 6 months and 1 year.

  B. **Extratesticular causes** can produce scrotal pain and swelling.

    1. **Hernias** can be direct or indirect and are common in all ages. Congenital defects, straining, or both are predisposing factors.

    2. **Prostatitis** (see Section II.A.1.b) can refer pain to the scrotum via the same sensory nerve fibers innervating the testicles.

    3. **Renal colic** from urinary tract lithiases also causes referred scrotal pain. Risk factors include a positive family history, decreased fluid intake, and residency in the southeastern United States.

    4. **Hydrocele,** a fluid-filled mass in the scrotal sac, is usually an idiopathic congenital condition; new-onset hydroceles in young men may be associated with testicular tumor.

    5. **Varicocele,** dilatation, and tortuosity of the pampiniform plexus, rarely occurs before age 10 and is found in up to 15% of adult males.

    6. **Spermatocele** is a small cystic mass just above the testis.

III. **Symptoms** (Table 56–1).

  A. **Testicular causes.** Thirty-three to fifty percent of males with torsion will have experienced similar transient pain in the past. Torsion rarely occurs after trauma, but a history of trauma does not exclude the possibility of torsion.

  B. **Extratesticular causes**

    1. **Renal colic** can produce severe, intermittent flank pain, but the pain can radiate to the abdomen, pubic area, or scrotum. Nausea, vomiting, fevers, chills, and urinary frequency may be present.

    2. **Prostatitis** presents with fever; chills; dysuria; urinary frequency; myalgias; or scrotal, perineal, or back pain. Patients may also experience pain with ejaculation and defecation.

IV. **Signs** (Table 56–1).

  A. **Testicular causes**

    1. **Acute epididymitis** can be difficult to distinguish from testicular torsion.

      a. The **cremasteric reflex** (elicited by stroking or pinching the inner thigh, causing the ipsilateral testicle to retract toward the inguinal canal) is present in epididymitis, but not testicular torsion.

      b. **Prehn's sign** is relief of pain on elevation of the testicle when the patient is supine. This may occur with epididymitis but not with testicular torsion. This maneuver is not specific to epididymitis.

    2. **Torsion**

      a. The **bell clapper deformity,** in which the testicle lacks attachment to the tunica vaginalis and hangs freely, may be noted in older children at risk for testicular torsion. With torsion, the testicle rapidly becomes firm and tender and enlarges with the epididymis into a solitary mass. The scrotum can become erythematous and edematous similar to epididymitis.

TABLE 56–1. DIFFERENTIAL DIAGNOSIS OF COMMON SCROTAL COMPLAINTS

Diagnosis	History	Examination	Tests
Epididymitis	Fevers, chills, rigors, unilateral scrotal swelling, and pain	Swollen/tender upper posterior testicle, presence of cremasteric reflex, Prehn's sign	UA, urethral smear, color Doppler, if diagnosis unclear; VCU and renal/bladder US in prepubertal boys
Orchitis	Unilateral/bilateral testicular pain/swelling; if mumps, occurs 4–10 d after parotitis	Unilateral or bilateral testicular swelling/tenderness	None; color Doppler US, if diagnosis unclear
Torsion	Acute onset, unilateral swelling and pain, nausea and vomiting, ± previous symptoms, no constitutional symptoms (SOR Ⓒ)	Unilateral testicular swelling and retraction transversely—bell clapper deformity; no testicular cremasteric reflex or Prehn's sign	Radionuclide scan/testicular scintigraphy or color Doppler, if diagnosis unclear or symptoms ≥12 h (SOR Ⓒ)
Torsion of the testicular appendage	Moderate pain, acute onset, swelling; no constitutional symptoms	Firm tender nodule upper pole of epididymis; blue dot sign	No tests necessary; color Doppler, if diagnosis unclear
Traumatic epididymitis	Trauma a few days prior, pain and swelling	Possible ecchymosis, unilateral or bilateral edema; cremasteric reflex and Prehn's sign present	No tests necessary; color Doppler, if diagnosis unclear
Testicular hematomas/ hematocele	Trauma, pain, swelling, nausea, or vomiting	Ecchymosis and enlargement of affected testicle	Color Doppler US
Testicular rupture	Trauma history, pain, swelling, nausea, or vomiting	Ecchymosis and enlargement of affected testicle	Color Doppler US
Testicular neoplasms	Enlarging scrotal mass/ testicular nodule; occasional pain, if hemorrhage	Palpable nodule or enlarged testicle; gynecomastia or left supraclavicular node	Scrotal US/tumor markers, biopsy
Inguinal hernia	Variable pain, enlargement in scrotum, or bulge of abdominal wall	Palpable hernia on abdominal wall or through inguinal ring; increases with Valsalva's maneuver	None or CT scan of abdomen and pelvis
Hydrocele	Painless testicular swelling	Minimally tender transilluminating swelling around testicle	Scrotal US
Varicocele	Swelling, dull scrotal heaviness, worse with exercise	"Bag of worms" supratesticular, collapsing with supine position	No tests necessary; color Doppler US, if uncertain
Spermatocele	Asymptomatic	Painless nodule above testicle (spermatic cord)	No tests necessary; US, if diagnosis unclear

CT, computerized tomogram; UA, urinalysis; US, ultrasound; VCU, voiding cystourethrogram.

    b. A small bluish discoloration (the "**blue dot sign**") may be seen through scrotal skin near the upper testicular pole. Coupled with pain, this finding is pathognomonic for appendiceal torsion.
  B. Extrascrotal causes
    1. Renal colic may present with hematuria, there may be tenderness of the flank and hyperparesthesias of the skin of the abdomen, but examination of the scrotum is unremarkable.
    2. In **prostatitis,** a warm, tender, spongy, enlarged prostate can be palpated on rectal examination.
V. Laboratory Tests (Table 56–1). Scrotal complaints can often be diagnosed with a careful history and physical examination, maintaining a high index of suspicion for serious conditions, such as testicular torsion, acute infectious epididymitis, or acute incarcerated inguinal hernia.
  A. Urinalysis detects pyuria or bacteriuria with epididymitis or prostatitis and microscopic or gross hematuria in urinary lithiasis. Urinalysis is normal in testicular torsion or torsion of the testicular appendix.

B. Urethral smear produced by inserting a small, sterile cotton-tipped probe into the urethra for one turn, then layering the secretions on a microscope slide for Gram stain and microscopic examination, is helpful in evaluation of epididymitis in sexually active males younger than 35 years or with suspected sexually transmitted epididymitis. The smear may demonstrate white blood cells (WBCs) and bacteria.

C. An elevated **WBC count** and **erythrocyte sedimentation rate** may occur in febrile patients; an elevated WBC count can occur in torsion, most likely as a stress reaction.

D. Doppler studies measure testicular blood flow.

   1. For most clinicians, **color Doppler ultrasonography** is the preferred diagnostic test, with sensitivity of approximately 90% and specificity of 100% in testicular torsion.(SOR **C**)It is indicated when testicular pain has been present ≥12 hours or the diagnosis of torsion is uncertain. Color ultrasonography can also diagnose incarcerated hernia, varicocele, hematoma, or testicular rupture and can differentiate testicular appendiceal torsion (increased blood flow) from testicular torsion (decreased/ absent blood flow) if the diagnosis is uncertain.

   2. Doppler stethoscope and **conventional gray-scale ultrasonography** are not as accurate as color ultrasonography and should not be used.

E. Radionuclide testicular scan or **testicular scintigraphy** demonstrates decreased blood flow to the affected testicle within a few hours in torsion (sensitivity/specificity ≥90% for an acute torsion when performed by an experienced physician) and increased blood flow with epididymitis. Scintigraphy's main limitation is the delay in results compared to color ultrasonography.

F. Scrotal ultrasound is extremely accurate in distinguishing between solid and fluid-filled masses.

G. In prepubertal boys with epididymitis/urinary tract infection, **renal/bladder ultrasound and voiding cystourethrogram** are indicated to evaluate for urinary tract anomalies.

VI. Treatment

A. Testicular conditions

   1. In **acute epididymitis,** treatment goals include pain relief and addressing underlying infection. In most cases, this is feasible in the outpatient setting.

      a. Pain relief is best accomplished by ice packs for 24 to 48 hours, bed rest, scrotal support, and oral medications, such as ibuprofen, 600 to 800 mg, 3 to 4 times daily (mild/moderate pain); acetaminophen with codeine, 325/30 mg; or hydrocodone, 5 mg 4 times daily (severe pain). A cord block with 5 to 8 mL of a 50/50 mixture or 1% lidocaine and 0.5% bupivacaine can be helpful if administered by an experienced physician.

      b. Antibiotic selection is based on age and sexual history. Generally speaking, in sexually active males older than 35 years, the treatment of choice is either a single intramuscular dose of ceftriaxone (Rocephin), 250 mg, plus doxycycline, 100 mg orally twice daily for 10 days. In males older than 35 years and at low risk for sexually transmitted diseases, treatment options include ciprofloxacin (e.g., Cipro), 500 mg orally twice daily, or ofloxacin, 300 mg orally daily for 10 to 14 days. (SOR **A**)

      c. Hospitalization may be required for males with high fevers, intractable pain, toxic appearance, or suspicion of scrotal abscess.

      d. Surgical drainage, orchiectomy, or both is warranted when severe epididymo-orchitis results in abscess formation.

      e. Urologic consultation and **surgical exploration** are indicated when the diagnosis is unclear or if testicular torsion is suspected (see Section VI.A.3).

   2. The pain of **orchitis** can be managed similarly to that of epididymitis (see Section VI.A.1.a).

   3. Torsion

      a. If **testicular torsion** is confirmed or high clinical suspicion is present, immediate surgical referral should be made. (SOR **C**) If detorsion is accomplished by 10 hours, 70% to 100% of testicles remain viable, after 10 to 12 hours viability drops to 20%, and at 24 to 48 hours 0% of testicles are viable. No testicle is viable after 48 hours. Manual detorsion is successful in 30% to 70% of cases. (SOR **C**) In patients with torsion, bilateral orchiopexy is necessary, because the bell clapper deformity usually exists in both testicles.

      b. Testicular appendage torsion is managed conservatively with analgesics, ice, and scrotal elevation. Activity may worsen symptoms, so it should be restricted. If pain and swelling are severe and the diagnosis is clear, urologic consultation for local nerve block may control pain. If the diagnosis is unclear, prompt diagnostic testing (see Section V.D.1), referral for exploration, or both should be made.

4. Trauma
   a. For **testes rupture** emergent referral should be made for repair; **testicular hematoma** and hematocele also require surgical consultation.
   b. Traumatic epididymitis, which occurs a few days after trauma, is managed conservatively with anti-inflammatory medications, elevation, and ice.

5. Testicular neoplasms should be managed in consultation with a urologic oncologist.

B. Extratesticular causes
   1. Inguinal hernias require urgent surgical consultation if incarcerated or strangulated and elective repair if reducible.
   2. Renal colic (see Chapter 36).
   3. Prostatitis is generally managed with antibiotics (see Chapter 61).
   4. Hydroceles in infants usually spontaneously resolve during the first 1 to 2 years of life. Hydroceles persisting beyond age 1 to 2 years, accompanied by hernia, or occurring in males beyond infancy require surgical consultation for repair.
   5. Because **varicoceles** can affect testicular growth and fertility, consultation with a urologist for elective spermatic vein ligation is prudent. A noncollapsible varicocele raises suspicion for retroperitoneal tumor and requires appropriate imaging study (e.g., abdominal magnetic resonance imaging scan or computerized tomography [CT]) and specialist consultation based on findings.
   6. Only large **spermatoceles** require urologic consultation for excision.

REFERENCES

Gilbert DN, Moellering RC Jr, Sande MA. *The Sanford Guide to Antimicrobial Therapy.* Jeb C. Sanford, FL; 2003:17-18.

Miller KE. Diagnosis and treatment of neisseria gonorrhoeae infections. *Am Fam Physician.* 2006; 73:1779-1784.

Ringdahl E, Teague L. Testicular torsion. *Am Fam Physician.* 2006;74:1739-1743, 1746.

Rupp TJ. Testicular torsion. [emedicine from WebMD]. http://www.emedicine. com/emerg/topic573.htm. Accessed April 27, 2007.

www. cdc.gov/std/treatment/2006/updated

---

57   Sore Throat

L. Peter Schwiebert, MD

KEY POINTS

- Most sore throats encountered in ambulatory family medicine are caused by viruses or irritants.
- Clues to a diagnosis of strep throat include a temperature $\geq 38^{\circ}$C, absence of cough, tender anterior cervical adenopathy, or tonsillar exudate/swelling.
- Antibiotics are not indicated in most patients with sore throat.

I. **Definition.** Sore throat is a pharyngeal sensation of scratchiness or pain because of a wide spectrum of causes, including endogenous/exogenous irritants (e.g., gastroesophageal reflux, allergens, tobacco smoke, low humidity) and infections (viral or bacterial).

II. **Common Diagnoses.** In ambulatory primary care, up to 8% of patient visits per year are for a sore throat, making this complaint second only to cough in ambulatory visits in the United States Common causes:
   A. Irritants. Thirty to sixty-five percent of individuals with sore throat have no specific causative pathogen. Irritants are causative in an undetermined number of these cases. Those at risk include smokers (tobacco is the most common environmental irritant), those

whose clinical picture is compatible with allergies or gastroesophageal reflux disease (GERD) (see below), or who are exposed to irritants (e.g., dust, low humidity, animals, textiles, solvents) in their environment.

B. Viral infections (30%–60% of cases), including common cold viruses (rhinovirus, coronavirus, respiratory syncytial virus, parainfluenza virus); herpesvirus; adenovirus; coxsackievirus; and infectious mononucleosis (IM) viruses (cytomegalovirus and Epstein-Barr virus). Sore throat is more likely because of common cold viruses during community outbreaks in colder months of the year; adenoviral infections are frequent (up to 19%) causes of exudative pharyngitis in children younger than 6 years, and coxsackievirus infections are also most common in young children during the summer and fall. IM is most common in upper-socioeconomic-class adolescents (industrialized societies) living in close contact with one another (e.g., students living in college dormitories).

C. Group A β-hemolytic streptococcal infection (GABHS) (5%–17% of cases in adults and 15%–36% of cases in children). GABHS is most common in 5- to 15-year-olds during the winter/spring months and may, like other infections, occur as epidemics.

III. Symptoms

A. Sore throat
1. Scratchy, dry throat is most common with irritants or common cold viruses.
2. Painful sore throat with dysphagia is typical of streptococcal infection, IM, coxsackievirus, herpesvirus, or adenovirus.

B. Other symptoms
1. Patients with **allergies** classically present with paroxysms of sneezing, watery, itchy eyes, and rhinorrhea associated with exposure to the allergen, although these symptoms may be absent (see Chapters 54 and 55).
2. Individuals with sore throat because of **GERD** often give a history of heartburn/sour eructations, worsening symptoms after a large meal or with recumbency, associated nonproductive cough, and relief with over-the-counter histamine-2 blockers or antacids.
3. The presence of cough, rhinorrhea, conjunctivitis, or diarrhea decreases the likelihood of streptococcal infection and increases the likelihood of irritants, allergies, or viral infection.
4. Individuals with **streptococcal infection** may complain of associated symptoms of chills, malaise, headache, mild neck stiffness, and some gastrointestinal symptoms, though these symptoms are not specific for this diagnosis.

IV. Signs. Since GABHS pharyngitis is the only common cause of sore throat for which antibiotics are indicated and since sore throat and patient requests for antibiotic treatment are common, researchers have investigated clinical scoring systems to predict the likelihood of streptococcal infection. The best-known system is the Centor Strep Score, and McIsaac et al. validated this scoring system in a family medicine population of children and adults (Table 57–1). The Centor criteria can identify those with a low risk of GABHS pharyngitis (one or less positive findings) who do not require antibiotics (SOR **A**). (Also see the sidebars on epiglottitis, retropharyngeal abscess, peritonsillar abscess, and carotidynia.)

TABLE 57–1. MCISAAC MODIFICATION OF THE CENTOR STREP SCORE

1. Add Points for Patient

Symptom or Sign	Points
History of fever or measured temperature ≥38°C (100.4°F)	1
Absence of cough	1
Tender anterior cervical adenopathy	1
Tonsillar swelling or exudates	1
Age ≤15 y	1
Age ≥45 y	−1

2. Find Risk of Strep

Points	LR	% With Strep (Patients with Strep/Total)
−1 or 0	0.05	1 (2/179)
1	0.52	10 (13/134)
2	0.95	17 (18/109)
3	2.5	35 (28/81)
4 or 5	4.9	51 (39/77)

A. The ability of an individual symptom or sign to predict a diagnosis of strep throat is limited. For example:

1. **Exudative pharyngitis** also occurs with viral infections (53% of children younger than 6 years with this sign had adenoviral infection, as do 50% of patients with IM).

2. Fifty-six percent of pediatric patients with adenoviral infection present with fever and temperature $\geq 40^\circ$C (104°F); moderate to high fever is also associated with coxsackievirus and initial outbreaks of herpesvirus infections.

3. More than 90% of patients with IM have **cervical lymphadenopathy** (posterior chain).

B. **Other signs characteristic of common causes of sore throat.** Coxsackievirus infections are associated with erythematous-based small vesicles or ulcers in the pharynx and may be associated with similar papulovesicles on the palms and soles. The shallow, erythematous-based vesicles and ulcers of **herpesvirus** can occur anywhere on the pharynx, gingiva, or vermilion border.

EPIGLOTTITIS

Epiglottitis should be considered when there is a rapidly worsening sore throat, fever, muffled voice, and dysphagia. Epiglottitis is usually caused by *Haemophilus influenzae* (but pediatric incidence of this organism has decreased because of Hib immunization, such that the incidence now peaks between ages 20 and 45 years); *Streptococcus pyogenes, Staphylococcus aureus,* or viruses may also be causative. Lateral neck radiographs are 90% sensitive and show an enlarged epiglottis ("thumb sign") with hypopharyngeal distention. Because of the danger of critical airway obstruction, suspected epiglottitis requires parental antibiotics in an intensive care setting where immediate intubation is available.

RETROPHARYNGEAL ABSCESS

Retropharyngeal abscess is a complication of infected retropharyngeal lymph nodes (usually caused by GABHS) and is more common in pediatric than adult populations. Presenting symptoms of dysphagia and a lateral neck radiograph showing an increased prevertebral space are characteristic.

PERITONSILLAR ABSCESS

Peritonsillar abscess (quinsy), a suppurative complication of superficial tonsillitis, is most common in 20- to 40-year-olds and presents with worsening sore throat, fever, and dysphagia/odynophagia. Likely agents include *S pyogenes, S aureus, H influenzae,* or anaerobes. Examination reveals a muffled "hot potato" voice, trismus (difficulty opening the mouth), and an erythematous, swollen tonsil pushing the uvula to the opposite side. The gold standard for diagnosis is needle aspiration of pus from the abscess (should only be performed with proper training), and the currently recommended treatment is twice-daily clindamycin or a second- or third-generation cephalosporin.

CAROTIDYNIA

Carotidynia is an idiopathic inflammation of the carotid sheath and is a common cause of "sore throat," which, on examination, is actually tenderness over the common carotid sheath. Carotidynia responds rapidly to nonsteroidal drugs (e.g., indomethacin, 25–50 mg, 3 times a day with food, continued 5 to 7 days or until symptoms resolve, whichever occurs first).

V. **Laboratory Tests.** Based on clinical findings alone, one can arrive at a presumptive diagnosis in many patients presenting with sore throat. In those with irritant exposure or a common cold viral infection, no further laboratory work-up of sore throat is indicated, and one can proceed with treatment.

TABLE 57–2. TESTING PATIENTS WITH SORE THROAT BASED ON PRETEST LIKELIHOOD OF STREPTOCOCCAL PHARYNGITIS

Signs	Season Winter/Spring	Summer/Fall
Temperature $\geq 38°$C (101°F), enlarged erythematous tonsils with exudates, enlarged tender anterior cervical nodes	No testing necessary; begin treatment*	Rapid streptococcal screen[†]
Patient with two of the above signs, or all three signs with cough, rhinorrhea, or hoarseness	Rapid streptococcal screen[†]	Blood agar plate culture (BAP)
Patient with one of the three signs or with no signs, but in a high-risk group[‡]	BAP[§]	No testing necessary unless in a high-risk group[‡]

*High pretest likelihood ($\geq 50\%$).
[†] Intermediate pretest likelihood (20%–50%).
[‡] Such patients include those who have diabetes mellitus, have a history of rheumatic fever, or present during a community outbreak of nephritogenic streptococcal infection.
[§] Low pretest likelihood ($\leq 20\%$).

A. **Streptococcal testing.** A decision on which patients with pharyngitis should have a streptococcal screen depends on the physician's goals—minimizing total cost, minimizing risks associated with a missed diagnosis, or minimizing the cost of a missed diagnosis and unnecessary use of antibiotics. The following strategy, which is more cost-effective than mass screening but minimizes chances of missing a case of streptococcal pharyngitis, is recommended. A rapid streptococcal screen should be performed on patients with a sore throat and an intermediate pretest likelihood of streptococcal pharyngitis (Table 57–2).

1. **Rapid streptococcal screen** is a 10-minute test for streptococcal antigens that has a sensitivity of 80% to 95% and a specificity of 70% to 95% for detection of streptococcal pharyngitis. Proper collection requires that the swab contact both tonsils or tonsillar fossae and the posterior pharyngeal wall. Because of its test characteristics and rapid turnaround time, it is the test of choice in confirming suspected streptococcal pharyngitis and should be used in patients with an intermediate pretest likelihood of this diagnosis (Table 57–2). With appropriate test selection, therapeutic decisions can confidently be based on a positive result. However, a negative screen result in the context of clinical suspicion of streptococcal pharyngitis should be followed up with blood agar plate (BAP) culture.

2. **Throat culture.** The BAP culture is 95% sensitive and has a low false-positive rate in diagnosing streptococcal pharyngitis, but it requires 24 hours' incubation. BAP culture should be performed if rapid streptococcal screen result is negative with high suspicion of streptococcal infection or in high-risk, low-prevalence situations (Table 57–2).

3. A **follow-up screen** to test for cure is not recommended or indicated in patients who respond clinically to antibiotic therapy within 5 days. However, in patients with a history of rheumatic fever, posttreatment cultures should be done to ensure eradication of GABHS.

4. The **carrier state** (positive strep screen or BAP with low pretest likelihood or without GABHS antigenemia) usually represents low infectivity. In certain situations, the carrier state warrants treatment; these include a history of rheumatic fever, community outbreak of rheumatic fever or nephritogenic streptococcal infection, or "Ping-Pong" spread of GABHS in a family or other closed community, such as military barracks, prisons, or college dormitories.

B. **Heterophile antibody test.** The Monospot test, which rapidly detects heterophile antibodies, compares favorably with the sensitivity and specificity of older heterophile antibody tests in diagnosing IM. A complete blood cell count (CBC) with differential smear showing at least 50% lymphocytes and at least 10% atypical lymphocytes also confirms this diagnosis.

C. **Other tests**

1. Though not common, *Neisseria gonorrhoeae* should be suspected in patients with pharyngitis and a history of oral-genital sexual relations; in such cases, pharyngeal, endocervical, and urethral cultures for gonorrhea and chlamydia should be done.

2. **Liver function tests,** including serum aspartate aminotransferase (AST) and serum alanine aminotransferase (ALT) as well as serum bilirubin, CBC, platelet count, and Coombs' test, should be performed in patients with IM. These patients are at risk for developing hepatitis, hemolytic anemia, granulocytopenia, and thrombocytopenia (see Chapter 45). Severe hepatitis is indicated by an ALT or AST of $\geq$1000 U/L or a serum bilirubin of $\geq$10 mg/dL.

3. **Abdominal ultrasound, by identifying hepatomegaly or splenomegaly in those with IM, can guide decisions about return to athletic competition.**

VI. **Treatment.** Because 80% to 90% of cases of pharyngitis are caused by viruses or irritants, antibiotics are not indicated for most patients with this complaint. Despite this finding, studies have shown that antibiotics are prescribed for 73% of adults with acute pharyngitis. Dangers of this practice include unnecessary cost, possible allergic reaction, and development of resistant bacterial strains. To avoid these drawbacks, it is important to base antibiotic use on strict criteria and use nonantibiotic treatment in cases not meeting these criteria.

A. **Environmental irritants** should be avoided if possible. In particular, patients should be encouraged to stop smoking, avoid allergens or dusty environments, and humidify low-humidity environments. Treatment of allergies is discussed in Chapter 55, and management of GERD is discussed in Chapter 19.

B. **Viral infections** (e.g., common cold, adenovirus, coxsackievirus, and herpesvirus) are self-limited, lasting from a few days to 2 weeks. Patients may obtain symptomatic relief with the following regimens.

1. **Topical pain relief** may be provided by as-needed lozenges (e.g., Cepastat or Chloraseptic) or saline nasal spray or gargles, made by mixing one-fourth tsp of salt in 4 oz of warm water. Oropharyngeal lesions of coxsackievirus or herpes simplex virus may benefit from viscous Xylocaine 2% or benzocaine 15%, applied to lesions every 3 to 4 hours with a cotton-tipped applicator; soothing rinses (one-fourth tsp of baking soda in 4 oz of warm water or saline, swished orally, then expectorated 3 or 4 times daily); or a variety of coating agents (e.g., diphenhydramine elixir, 12.5 mg/5 mL, mixed with an equal volume of either kaolin and pectin [Kaopectate] or aluminum-magnesium hydroxide antacid [Maalox], 1 tsp swished intraorally for 2 minutes every 2 hours).

2. **Fluid intake** should be increased to up to 2 to 3 quarts of water or juice per day.

3. **Analgesic drugs** include either aspirin, 650 mg every 4 to 6 hours orally in teenagers or adults, or acetaminophen, 5 to 10 mg/kg/d every 4 to 6 hours orally in children. Codeine relieves more severe discomfort; the dosage is 30 to 60 mg orally every 4 to 6 hours in adults or 3 mg/kg/d orally every 4 to 6 hours in children.

4. **Decongestants** (see Chapter 55).

C. **Streptococcal infections.** Antibiotic therapy instituted within 2 to 3 days of onset of symptoms hastens symptomatic improvement in patients with positive culture results or a high likelihood of streptococcal infection, as well as decreasing contagion (especially if the patient lives in close contact with others). The incidence of suppurative complications (e.g., peritonsillar abscess) and immune complications (e.g., glomerulonephritis) is low, regardless of whether antibiotics are used or not. For every 100 patients treated with antibiotics rather than placebo in Cochrane trials, there was one less case of acute rheumatic fever, two less cases of acute otitis media, and three less cases of quinsy (SOR **Ⓐ**).

1. **Indications**
   a. Patients with a positive result on rapid streptococcal screen, throat culture, or both.
   b. Patients with a high probability of having streptococcal infection (Table 57–1).
   c. Some clinicians initiate antibiotic therapy in high-risk patients pending throat culture results (see Section V.A.2), although studies have demonstrated that delaying therapy for 48 hours does not interfere with the antibiotic's reduction in risk of rheumatic fever.

2. **Regimens**
   a. **Penicillin** is the drug of choice (in nonpenicillin-allergic patients); there is no evidence of resistance (e.g., resurgence of rheumatic fever caused by lower rates of GABHS elimination by penicillin) (SOR **Ⓐ**).
      (1) **Oral penicillin V potassium,** 500 mg, 2 to 3 times daily for 10 days, is the treatment for those over 60 lb (27 kg); those weighing less should receive 30 to 50 mg/kg/d in 2 or 3 divided doses, also for 10 days.
      (2) **Penicillin G benzathine** may be preferred for patients in whom compliance with the oral regimen or follow-up is questionable. Adults and children weighing $\geq$27

kg (60 lb) should receive 1.2 million U intramuscularly, and those weighing ≤ 27 kg should receive 600,000 U. A mixture of 900,000 U of benzathine and 300,000 U of procaine penicillin (e.g., **Bicillin C-R**) is also effective and causes less local reaction than penicillin G benzathine alone.

b. **Erythromycin** (e.g., Ery-Tab, Eryc, or E-Mycin) is the drug of choice for penicillin-allergic patients. Adults should receive 500 mg orally twice daily for 10 days. The pediatric dosage is 30 to 50 mg/kg/d, given in 2 or 4 divided doses. Another macrolide, **azithromycin** (e.g., Zithromax), 500 mg orally on day 1 and 250 mg on days 2 to 5, is also effective for adults; the dosage for pediatric patients older than 2 years is 12 mg/kg/d for 5 days.

c. In addition to axithromycin, the following 5-day regimens are FDZ-approved for treatment of GABHS: cefdinir 14 mg/kg (pediatric) or 600 mg (adult) daily, cefpodixime 10 mg/kg/da (pediatric) or 100 mg dosed twice daily. Shorter regimens may improve compliance; disadvantages include higher cost and broader spectrum, which may foster bacterial resistance. Of interest, meta-analysis of 35 studies showed superior bacteriologic and clinical cure with cephalosporins, compared to penicillin (SOR 🅐).

3. **Follow-up**

   a. **Failure to improve.** Antibiotic therapy should improve symptoms within 12 to 24 hours; persistence of symptoms for a week after initiation of antibiotics may be because of noncompliance with the drug regimen, penicillin tolerance, destruction of penicillin by β-lactamase–producing organisms, missed diagnosis, or an undiagnosed second cause of pharyngitis, particularly IM. In addition to evaluating for noncompliance, the following may help:

      (1) Appropriate tests for IM should be performed (see Sections V.B and C).

      (2) **Antibiotic regimens for penicillin tolerance** should be instituted. **Amoxicillin-clavulanate potassium** (e.g., Augmentin), 500 to 875 mg orally twice daily (adults) or 40 mg/kg/d orally in 3 divided doses (children); or a cephalosporin (e.g., **cefadroxil,** 1 g orally in 1 dose for adults or 30 mg/kg/d orally in 2 doses for children) have been shown to be effective in eradicating streptococci in those patients who do not respond to repeated courses of oral penicillin.

   b. **Recurrent episodes** of acute pharyngitis raise the issue of whether **acute streptococcal pharyngitis** or **acute viral pharyngitis with streptococcal carrier state** is occurring. **Viral pharyngitis** is suggested by clinical or epidemiologic findings consistent with viral infection, failure to improve on antistreptococcal antibiotics, no rise in antistreptolysin-O (ASO) titers, or positive throat cultures between episodes of pharyngitis. **Acute, recurrent streptococcal infection** is suggested by appropriate clinical or epidemiologic findings, dramatic response to antibiotic therapy, a rise in ASO titers, or negative throat cultures between episodes of acute pharyngitis.

   c. When eradication of the carrier state is appropriate (see Section V.A.4), the following regimens are effective: clindamycin (e.g., Cleocin), 20 mg/kg/d orally in 3 doses for 10 days, or rifampin (Rifadin), 20 mg/kg/d orally in 2 doses for 4 days, *plus* the standard regimen of phenoxymethyl *or* penicillin G benzathine.

4. **IM**

   a. Ninety-five percent of patients with **IM** recover uneventfully, and supportive treatment will suffice. Such therapy includes avoidance of contact sports or heavy lifting in the first 2 to 3 weeks of illness (especially if the patient has splenomegaly), adequate rest, and analgesics (see Section VI.B.3). Individuals evaluated a month after diagnosis should be afebrile, well hydrated, and asymptomatic without hepatomegaly or splemomegaly before gradual return to competition is allowed (SOR 🅒).

   b. Corticosteroids may be necessary in the following circumstances: impending airway obstruction, severe hepatitis, thrombocytopenia, hemolytic anemia, or granulocytopenia. Treatment should be initiated with prednisone (or any equivalent), 60 to 80 mg/d orally in divided doses, tapered over 1 to 2 weeks.

REFERENCES

Arroll B. Antibiotics for upper respiratory tract infections: an overview of Cochrane reviews. *Resp Med.* 2005;99:255.

Bisno AL. Acute pharyngitis. *N Engl J Med.* 2001;344:205.

Brunton S, Pichichero M. Considerations in the use of antibiotics for streptococcal pharyngitis. *J Fam Prac.* 2006;55:S 9.

Hafener JW. The clinical diagnosis of streptococccal pharyngitis. *Ann Emerg Med.* 2005;46:87.

Vincent MT, Celestin N, Hussain AN. Pharyngitis. *Am Fam Physic.* 2004;69:1465.

Waninger KN. Determination of safe return to play for athletes recovering from infectious mononucleosis. *Clin J Sport Med.* 2005;15:410.

58   Syncope

LeRoy C. White, MD, JD, Dennis P. Lewis, MDH, Brian H. Halstater, MD, & Felix Horng, MD, MBA

KEY POINTS

- A thorough history and physical will reveal a diagnosis in 45% of cases. (SOR **C**)
- An EKG will be diagnostic in only 5% to 10% of cases, but should be done initially because it may reveal clues to underlying cardiac disease. (SOR **C**)
- Most syncope is from neurally mediated reflex mechanisms (e.g., vasovagal or situational) or will be found to be idiopathic and can be effectively managed by the primary care physician.
- Cardiac syncope is associated with a much higher 2-year mortality than all other types and its detection is the primary focus of evaluation. (SOR **C**)

Syncope is a symptom, not a disease, and must be differentiated from conditions that may at first appear as syncope. Nonsyncopal disorders that may present with real or apparent loss of consciousness include seizure disorders, psychogenic "syncope," and metabolic disorders such as hypoglycemia or hyponatremia.

The task of the investigating physician is to determine if the patient has syncope rather than a condition mimicking syncope and then to determine if that condition is life-threatening.

I. **Definition.** Syncope is a transient loss of consciousness followed by prompt recovery without intervention. Syncope is caused by cerebral hypoperfusion. This can be because of decreased cardiac output, cerebrovascular disease, or neurally mediated reflexes. **Decreased cardiac output** can be from hypovolemia, structural heart disease, or arrhythmias. **Neurally mediated syncope (also called neurocardiogenic syncope)** results from reflex decrease in heart rate, blood pressure, or both.

II. **Common Diagnoses** (Table 58–1). At least 10.5% of the population will have a syncopal event within a 17-year period with a 42% prevalence during the life of a 70-year-old person based on the Framingham study. **Thirty-five percent** of patients will have recurrences within 3 years. Eighty-two percent of recurrences occur in the first 2 years. Age older than 45 was associated with a higher recurrence rate. Recurrences are not associated with increased mortality or sudden death rate.

The prevalence of syncope increases with age and is highest in the older institutionalized population. In the United States, syncope accounts for approximately 3% to 10% of emergency department visits and 6% of hospital admissions annually. Approximately 1 million patients are evaluated for syncope each year, at a cost of $750 million.

Syncope can be classified as **neurally mediated, cardiac, cerebrovascular, orthostatic, miscellaneous differentiated causes,** and **idiopathic** (unknown cause). Two-thirds of syncope are either cardiac or neurally mediated, although multiple causes may coexist. A Mayo Clinic study of 987 syncopal patients referred to an electrophysiologic studies series revealed multiple causes in 18.4%, with an increased likelihood of multiple causes in the elderly, those with atrial fibrillation, those taking cardiac medications, or those in New York Heart Association classes II to IV.

TABLE 58–1. DIFFERENTIAL DIAGNOSIS OF SYNCOPE

Category	Risk Factors	Symptoms	Signs
Neurally mediated vasovagal	Young women; exposure to stress, pain, enclosed space	Unpleasant stimulus Prodrome (nausea/lightheadedness/palpitations/tunnel vision/warmth)	Examination is noncontributory
Neurally mediated situational	Elderly	Preceded by micturition/cough/swallow/defecation	Orthostatic hypotension
Neurally mediated carotid sinus	Elderly, atherosclerotic disease	Syncope after head rotation/neck extension, wearing tight collar, shaving	Hypotension or ventricular asystole with carotid sinus massage
Orthostatic	Elderly, autonomic dysfunction, dehydration, prolonged recumbency, certain medications	Prodrome (nausea/lightheadedness/palpitations/tunnel vision/warmth)	Symptoms occur on standing or position change
Cardiac—arrhythmia	Sick sinus, A-V block medications, pacemaker malfunction; recent MI, supra- or ventricular tachycardia, WPW	No prodrome, occurrence while supine	Often normal; may note irregular heart rhythm
Cardiac—structural	VHD, FHx sudden unexplained cardiac death	Occurrence with exertion, change in position, acute shortness of breath	Heart murmur, signs of CHF
Cerebrovascular	HTN, dyslipidemia, diabetes mellitus, old age, cigarette use	Vertigo, dysarthria, diplopia; excessive arm exercise	Carotid bruit, focal neurologic deficit, asymmetric upper extremity BPs
Miscellaneous differentiated	20–40 y old with frequent "fainting," alcohol abuse	Anxiety or depression; multiple somatic complaints	Normal examination or signs of anxiety/depression
Idiopathic		Absence of classic symptoms of other types of syncope	No specific findings

A-V, atrioventricular; BP, blood pressure; CHF, congestive heart failure; FHx, family history; HTN, hypertension; MI, myocardial infarction; VHD, valvular heart disease; WPW, Wolff–Parkinson–White syndrome.

A. **Neurally mediated** reflex syncope accounts for 23% of syncope and refers to a reflex response that when triggered gives rise to vasodilatation and/or bradycardia.
   1. **Classic vasovagal** syncope (18%) is mediated by emotional or orthostatic stress.
   2. **Situational syncope** (5%) is neurally mediated syncope associated with specific inciting factors, e.g., urinating, coughing, defecating.
B. **Cardiac syncope** (18% of cases) has a higher mortality rate than all other etiologies (30% at 2 years, compared to 6% for all other etiologies).
   1. **Arrhythmia** underlies most cardiac syncope.
     a. Risk factors for **bradyarrhythmia** include use of certain medications that delay atrioventricular (A-V) conduction (commonly beta and calcium channel blockers).
     b. Risk factors for **tachyarrhythmia** include use of certain medications that increase A-V conduction (pseudoephedrine and other stimulants, both legal and illicit).
     c. Investigating the family history may reveal familial dysrhythmias such as long Q–T interval.
   2. **Structural heart disease.** Circulatory demands outpace the heart's ability to increase its output. In patients with no known **structural heart disease**, a family history of unexplained sudden cardiac death increases the likelihood of hypertrophic obstructive cardiomyopathy or infiltrative disease such as sarcoid cardiomyopathy.
C. **Cerebrovascular syncope** (10% of syncope) most commonly results from vertebrobasilar artery insufficiency, transient ischemic attack (TIA), stroke (cerebrovascular accident, or CVA), or subclavian steal syndrome. Risk factors for **subclavian steal syndrome** are the same as for CVA and TIA, but also include vigorous use of an upper extremity, and when it occurs in younger populations, a congenital anatomic variant.
D. **Orthostatic syncope** (8%) refers to syncope in which the upright position causes arterial hypotension. The autonomic system is incapacitated and fails to compensate when the upright position is assumed. This is commonly caused by medications. When volume

depletion is present, the autonomic system does not fail, but cannot maintain blood pressure owing to insufficient volume. Note that similar symptoms may occur in vasovagal syncope.

E. Miscellaneous differentiated causes most commonly include psychiatric disorders (roughly 2% of all syncope).

F. Approximately 34% of cases of syncope are considered **idiopathic.** Some **idiopathic** cases are subsequently found to be cardiac syncope in some studies. **Idiopathic syncope** has a slightly higher death rate than the general population.

III. **Symptoms** (Table 58–1). A careful history is essential to accurate assessment of syncope. This should include patient age, details of the syncopal event (timing and onset of the syncope, association with activity or exercise, presence of associated symptoms such as palpitations or chest pain), and previous occurrences and circumstances surrounding these episodes. Risk factor assessment should include chronic diseases, family history, and medication use/substance abuse.

Differentiating between syncopal and nonsyncopal episodes may be difficult. **Prodromal symptoms.** Syncopal episodes typically have some form of premonitory symptoms. Ventricular tachycardia may occur without any prodrome. Syncopal episodes may also have a **precipitating factor.** Tonic/clonic movements followed by a postictal state suggest seizure activity, but pseudoseizures may occur with syncope and many patients are confused after syncopal episodes. Involuntary micturition commonly occurs after neurally mediated syncope.

A. **Neurally mediated reflex syncope**
   1. **Vasovagal syncope** typically occurs after a prodrome of nausea, diaphoresis, or pallor following a sudden unexpected, usually unpleasant sight, smell, or sound, or with pain or fear. Vasovagal syncope also occurs with prolonged standing.
   2. **Situational syncope** may have the same prodromal symptoms as vasovagal syncope with a precipitating factor of coughing, straining at defecation or other events.

B. **Cardiac syncope.** The arrhythmia causing arrhythmogenic syncope may not be present when the patient is evaluated, especially if it is a tachydysrhythmia. The patient may describe a prodrome of palpitations or slow heart beat. In **structural heart disease** of cardiopulmonary origin, the history commonly reveals a prodrome of acute shortness of breath or chest pain (pulmonary embolism, myocardial infarction [MI]). Syncope with obstructive symptomatology may be precipitated with **exertion** (aortic stenosis, pulmonary hypertension, mitral stenosis, hypertrophic obstructive cardiomyopathy, coronary artery disease) or with a **change of position** such as lying down/bending over/turning over in bed (atrial myxoma or thrombus). Pericardial disease may be related to cancer or chest trauma and may be exacerbated by positional changes.

   Young athletes with exertional syncope are at risk for sudden death from hypertrophic cardiomyopathy, an anomalous coronary artery or cocaine-induced coronary vasospasm.

C. **Orthostatic syncope.** Standing up generally precipitates symptoms in this type of syncope. The history may reveal new medications, change in current regimen, polypharmacy, dehydration, alcohol, or diabetes.

D. **Cerebrovascular syncope.** Turning the head or flexing the neck may precipitate symptoms in a patient with vertebrobasilar insufficiency or carotid stenosis. Overhead work or activity may precipitate symptoms in subclavian steal syndrome.

IV. **Signs** (Table 58–1). Physical examination should focus on the **cardiovascular** and **neurologic** systems. **The physical examination is second only to the history in terms of importance in evaluating a patient with syncope.** Vital signs should be recorded, including bilateral supine and standing blood pressures and pulses. Cyanosis or pallor should be noted. Cardiopulmonary auscultation should be performed and carotid/peripheral pulses palpated. Neurologic examination should include orientation and cranial nerves, motor, sensory, and cerebellar testing (gait and Romberg testing).

A. **Neurally mediated syncope**
   1. In **vasovagal syncope,** the patient may manifest hypotension. In patients with **orthostatic hypotension,** standing in place for 3 minutes after 5 minutes of recumbency decreases systolic blood pressure $\geq$20 mm Hg, diastolic blood pressure $\geq$10 mm Hg, or both. Volume-depleted patients may also manifest a postural increase in heart rate of $\geq$30 beats per minute. Patients often are diaphoretic. Classically a patient is hypotensive with bradycardia.
   2. **Situational syncope.** The signs are similar to vasovagal syncope. The history is diagnostic.

3. In **carotid sinus hypersensitivity**, the symptoms may occur after head turning or wearing a tight collar. Symptoms may be reproduced by carotid sinus massage. This maneuver should not be done if carotid bruits or stenosis are present, if the patient has a history of ventricular tachycardia, or with recent TIA, stroke, or MI. Carotid sinus massage is done by vigorously massaging one side only for 5 to 10 seconds. This will produce a ventricular asystole for $\geq$ 3 seconds or fall in systolic pressure of $\geq$50 mm Hg. A false-positive test may occur in the absence of historical risk factors for carotid sinus hypersensitivity.

B. **Cardiac syncope.** With **structural heart disease**, cardiac examination is less likely to be normal than with arrhythmia-induced syncope. Auscultation may reveal murmurs of mitral regurgitation/aortic stenosis/hypertrophic obstructive cardiomyopathy, or murmurs with change in position such as lying down/bending over/turning over in bed (suggestive of atrial myxoma/thrombus/hypertrophy), or findings of pulmonary hypertension (right ventricular lift, loud P2, prominent A-wave in jugular venous pulse).

C. In **cerebrovascular syncope**, carotid bruit may be noted (indicating significant generalized atherosclerosis), **focal neurologic deficit** may be uncovered (after a CVA, but possibly absent after a TIA), or an **asymmetric blood pressure or pulse** between upper extremities may be noted (suggesting subclavian steal syndrome or aortic dissection). In patients at risk, upper extremity activity could reveal pulse discrepancy between extremities (subclavian steal syndrome).

V. **Laboratory Tests.** A systematic history and physical examination alone can elucidate the cause of syncope in up to 45% of cases. Since **cardiac syncope** has a 30% 2-year mortality compared with 6% for all other causes, testing is directed at differentiating cardiac from noncardiac causes.

Initial testing should include a thorough history and physical examination and EKG. **Unless the history and physical and EKG suggest a diagnosis, no further testing should be undertaken** unless patient has recurrent syncope. (SOR 🅒)

The US Preventive Services Task Force states that in screening for coronary heart disease, "the consequences of false-positive tests may potentially outweigh the benefits of screening. (SOR 🅐) False-positive tests are common among asymptomatic adults, especially women, and may lead to unnecessary diagnostic testing, over-treatment, and labeling." However, "for people in certain professions, such as pilots and heavy equipment operators (for whom sudden incapacitation or sudden death may endanger the safety of others), considerations other than the health benefit to the individual may influence the decision to screen for coronary heart disease."

A. All patients with syncope should have an **EKG** even though the diagnostic yield is low (5%). Fifty percent of patients with syncope will have an abnormal EKG even though most will not be diagnostic. In addition to revealing certain structural heart diseases (e.g., previous MI or left ventricular hypertrophy), EKG is primarily helpful in uncovering arrhythmogenic causes of syncope, including **long Q–T interval, conduction delay/block, bundle branch block, fascicle block** (possible bradycardia); atrial and ventricular **ectopy** (nonspecific indicator of arrhythmogenic substrate); **bradycardia** (nonspecific indicator of conduction system disease); and **ventricular preexcitation/delta wave** (Wolff–Parkinson–White syndrome).

B. An **echocardiogram** is recommended in all patients whose evaluation is suggestive of structural cardiac disease. This should include patients with exercise-induced syncope as this may suggest a hypertrophic cardiomyopathy or anomalous coronary artery even in young athletes.

C. **Stress testing** (e.g., exercise treadmill testing or stress echocardiography) is indicated in syncopal patients whose history and risk factors suggest ischemic heart disease.

D. **24-hour Holter monitoring** is recommended in suspected arrhythmogenic syncope (e.g., syncope without prodrome or syncope preceded by palpitations) and with suspected structural heart disease or abnormal EKG.

E. **Long-term ambulatory loop EKG** is a noninvasive method of cardiac monitoring indicated in syncopal patients with a structurally normal heart, but abnormal EKG or 24-hour Holter monitor.

F. Referral to a cardiac electrophysiologist for **intracardiac electrophysiologic studies** is indicated in syncope with structural heart disease (e.g., history of MI, congestive heart failure, cardiomyopathy, coronary artery anomaly), identified arrhythmogenic syncope (e.g., Wolff–Parkinson–White or long Q–T syndrome, ventricular tachycardia, refractory sinus bradycardia/A-V block or supraventricular tachycardia), and also for exertional syncope.

G. Tilt-table testing is recommended in patients with unexplained recurrent syncope in whom cardiac causes of syncope, including arrhythmias, have been excluded. An abnormal result suggests vasovagal syncope, but reproducibility and yield are highly variable.

H. Neurologic testing should be reserved for patients with neurologic signs or symptoms or carotid bruits.

    1. Magnetic resonance angiography of carotid arteries is indicated for bruits or possible vertebrobasilar insufficiency (prolonged loss of consciousness, diplopia, nausea, or hemiparesis).

    2. Focal neurologic signs mandate brain imaging, usually with **computerized tomography** for bleeding or **magnetic resonance imaging** for ischemia.

    3. With evidence of seizure activity, **electroencephalography** may be useful. Cardiac syncope evaluation should be done in patients with seizure activity, normal electroencephalography, and no postictal symptoms, as well as patients with seizures unresponsive to anticonvulsants.

VI. Treatment of syncope is directed at the underlying cause. The prognosis is very good (6% 1-year mortality) even without intervention in those with noncardiac syncope. In cardiac syncope, identification and treatment of underlying causes can reduce the 30% 2-year mortality.

A. Hospitalization is indicated for patients with syncope who have known or suspected cardiac ischemia or arrhythmia, structural heart disease, cardiopulmonary circulatory disease (pulmonary embolus, pulmonary hypertension, atrial myxoma), or stroke. Hospitalization should be considered for diagnostic evaluation of syncope with known or suspected significant heart disease and EKG abnormalities suggesting arrhythmogenic syncope.

B. Cardiology consultation is indicated for syncope with underlying structural, valvular heart disease, or underlying coronary artery disease.

C. Neurologic consultation is indicated for those suspected of a seizure disorder or TIA.

D. Vascular surgery consultation for carotid endarterectomy is clearly beneficial in symptomatic patients with ≥70% carotid artery stenosis and may also benefit those symptomatic with 50% to 65% stenosis. Benefits of endarterectomy versus aspirin therapy are unclear in asymptomatic individuals with significant (≥60%) stenosis; such patients have a 10% to 15% CVA risk over the ensuing 3 to 5 years.

E. Psychiatric evaluation should be considered in young, otherwise healthy patients who faint frequently without any associated injury and in patients presenting with many unassociated nonspecific symptoms such as nausea, lightheadedness, numbness, fear, and dread.

F. Neurally mediated reflex syncope (situational, vasovagal, or carotid sinus hypersensitivity)

    1. Patients should be counseled to:

        a. Avoid situations and stressful events that may trigger fainting, such as hot, crowded rooms or prolonged standing.

        b. Avoid dehydration, ensure adequate fluid and salt intake, (SOR **B**) and proper attire (possibly compression hose or season appropriate).

        c. Minimize situations that trigger syncope, such as coughing excessively or wearing tight collars.

        d. Be aware of warning signs, such as feeling nauseated, sweaty, dizzy, or lightheaded, and sit or lie down to prevent loss of consciousness.

    2. Additional helpful measures include:

        a. Discontinuing or modifying medications (e.g., vasodilating antihypertensives) that increase susceptibility to syncope. (SOR **A**)

        b. Considering pharmacotherapy for resistant syncope, which includes the following:

            (1) Beta-blockers (e.g., metoprolol starting at 50 mg orally twice daily) (SOR ●) increase catecholamine response.

            (2) Alpha adrenergic receptor (midodrine, 2.5–10 mg orally 3 times daily) (SOR **B**) increases peripheral vascular tone.

            (3) Selective serotonin reuptake inhibitors (paroxetine) alter central serotonergic regulation of sympathetic neural transmitters. (SOR **B**)

    3. In **orthostatic hypotension**, treatment is directed at the underlying disorder (e.g., dehydration, medications, endocrine disorders, or neuropathies). In many cases, rising slowly and crossing the legs while standing, combined with use of compression stockings, is helpful.

G. If a thorough history, physical examination, and EKG fail to suggest a cause, the patient should be counseled to return for further evaluation if syncope recurs. (SOR **C**)

REFERENCES

Blatt CM, Graboys TB. Evaluation of the patient with syncope. In: Alpert JS, ed. *Cardiology for the Primary Care Physician.* 4th ed. Philadelphia: Current Medicine LLC; 2005:85-91.
Miller TH, Kruse JE. Evaluation of syncope. *Am Fam Phys.* 2005;72:1492-1500.
Strickberger SA, Benson DW, Biaggioni I, et al. AHA/ACCF Scientific statement on the evaluation of syncope. *J Am Coll Cardiol.* 2006;47(2):473-484.
Brignole M, Alboni P, Benditt D, et al. Task Force on Syncope, European Society of Cardiology. Guidelines on management (diagnosis and treatment) of syncope – Update 2004. *Europace.* 2004;6:467-537.
U.S. Preventive services task force. Screening for coronary heart disease. *Ann Intern Med.* 2004;140: 569-572.

---

59   Tremors & Other Movement Disorders

Aylin Yaman, MD, Hakan Yaman, MD, MS, & Goutham Rao, MD

KEY POINTS

- Tremor is the most common movement disorder in the world. Tremors are basically classified as rest and action tremors.
- Diagnosis is based on history and physical examination.
- Selection of drugs in the treatment of Parkinson disease is based on the age of onset, duration of disease, and existence of complications related to treatment.
- Propanolol and primidone are both effective and first-line treatments for essential tremor. Recent evidence also supports use of topiramate.

I. **Definition.** A **movement disorder** is any condition that disrupts normal voluntary movements of the body or one that consists of one or more abnormal movements. Movement disorders characterized by overall slowness of movement are classified as **hypokinesias**; those characterized by extra or exaggerated movements are classified as **hyperkinesias**. Tremors are the most common hyperkinesias.

   Tremor can be defined as a rhythmical, involuntary oscillatory movement of one or more body parts. A practical classification system divides tremors into rest tremors and action tremors. **Rest tremors** occur in a body part that is not voluntarily activated and is fully supported by gravity. **Action tremors** appear when muscles are voluntarily contracted. Action tremors can be further divided into **postural tremors** (tremor that occurs while maintaining a position against gravity), **isometric tremors** (tremors resulting from muscle contractions against stationary objects), and **kinetic tremors** (tremor occurring during voluntary movement). There are four principal types of kinetic tremors. This typological classification is outlined in Table 59–1.

II. **Common Diagnoses.** Tremor may be associated with many conditions. The list of causes of tremor is very long. A useful starting point is to be able to distinguish among the three most common causes of tremor (Table 59–2). (Also see the sidebars on tic disorders, chorea, myoclonus, dystonia, Wilson disease, and ataxia.)

   A. **Essential tremor, a visible postural tremor of hands and forearms that may have a kinetic component,** is the most common of all movement disorders; prevalence ranges from 4 to 39 cases per 1000 persons. It affects 1.3% to 5% of people older than 60 years. Onset peaks bimodally in the teens and fifth decade of life. A family history of tremor is common, and it may be exacerbated by stress, fatigue, or certain medications. Alcohol may temporarily attenuate symptoms.

TABLE 59–1. **TYPOLOGICAL CLASSIFICATION OF TREMORS**

Rest Tremor	Tremor occurring in a body part that is not voluntarily activated and is supported completely against gravity.		
Action Tremors	Postural tremor		Tremor that occurs while voluntarily maintaining a position against gravity.
	Kinetic tremors (Tremor occurring during any voluntary movement)	(1) Simple kinetic tremor	Tremor occurring during voluntary movements that are not target-directed.
		(2) Intention tremor	Tremor whose amplitude increases during visually guided movements (e.g., finger-to-nose test).
		(3) Task-specific kinetic tremor	Tremor that appears or is exacerbated by specific tasks (e.g., writing).
		(4) Isometric tremor	Tremor that occurs during voluntary muscle contraction against a rigid stationary object (e.g., squeezing examiner's hand).

    B. Parkinson disease is a chronic, progressive, neurodegenerative disorder with several characteristic features; it affects 1% of those older than age 65, and prevalence increases to 4% to 5% in those older than 85 years.

    C. Physiologic tremor, typically a postural tremor with a frequency of 8 to 12 Hz, is present in all subjects to differing degrees. Enhanced physiologic tremor may appear at any age and does not progress in severity. It can be enhanced by stimulants such as caffeine, nicotine, and some illicit drugs as well as medications such as bronchodilators, lithium, neuroleptics, valproate sodium, and tricyclic antidepressants. Other conditions that can augment physiological tremor include thyrotoxicosis, pheochromocytoma, hypoglycemia, withdrawal from opioids and sedatives. The cause is usually reversible.

III. Symptoms (Figure 59–1). The evaluation of a patient with first presentation of tremor begins with a thorough history that includes age at onset, rate of progression, and family history of tremor, medication history, and history of neurologic symptoms other than tremor.

    A. Both essential tremor and the tremor of Parkinson disease usually begin after age 50 and are progressive in severity.

    B. Associated symptoms. In addition to distal resting tremor, patients with Parkinson disease may present with bradykinesia (slowness of movement) and rigidity. Asymmetrical onset is typical for Parkinson disease. Such patients may complain of loss of balance and difficulty with tasks such as turning in bed, rising from a chair, and opening jars.

IV. Signs (Figure 59–1). The focused history should be followed by a physical examination with the goal of (1) identifying the key features of the tremor and (2) identifying features other than tremor that can help establish the diagnosis. A useful first step is to determine if the tremor occurs at rest or during action. A **rest tremor** can be observed by having the patient position his hands on his lap. Postural tremor can be elicited by holding up an arm against gravity. A **kinetic tremor** may be apparent during purposeful movements such as using a spoon, writing, performing a finger-to-nose test, or squeezing an examiner's hand.

    A. Parkinson disease. Obvious tremor at rest should raise suspicion of Parkinson disease. Other common signs of this disease should be elicited.

TABLE 59–2. **THREE COMMON TREMOR SYNDROMES**

Tremor of Parkinson Disease	Slow frequency (4–6/sec) tremor at rest. Tremor inhibited during movement and sleep. Aggravated by emotional and physical stress. "Pill rolling quality."
Classic Essential Tremor	Bilateral, usually symmetric postural or kinetic tremor. Family history of tremor is common. Attenuated by alcohol.
Physiologic Tremor	Present to differing degrees in all normal subjects. Enhanced form is easily visible, mainly postural, and has a high frequency (8–12/sec). No evidence of underlying neurologic disease. Cause is usually reversible (e.g., caffeine).

History:

> Inquire about age at onset, rate of progression, family history of tremor. If age of onset <21 years, consider primary dystonia or Wilson disease. Lack of progression suggests enhanced physiologic tremor. Family history of tremor suggests essential tremor.

↓

> Inquire about use of medications, stimulants, illicit drugs, and alcohol— all secondary causes of tremor.

↓

> Inquire about other symptoms of tremor syndromes and medical illnesses (e.g., bradykinesia in patients with Parkinson disease, symptoms of hyperthyroidism.)

Physical Examination:

> Determine key characteristics of tremor: amplitude, frequency, when it occurs (rest, postural kinetic).

↓

> If rest tremor, assess for other signs of Parkinson disease: bradykinesia detected by slowness of repetitive movements, rigidity of extremities, positive glabella tap test, and festination.

FIGURE 59–1. Systematic approach to the evaluation of tremor.

1. **Rigidity** can be detected by passively flexing and extending the patient's elbow several times. Resistance to movement can be smooth or interrupted (cog wheeling).
2. **Bradykinesia** can be detected by asking the patient to perform any one of a number of repetitive movements such as tapping the fingers or pinching the index finger and thumb repetitively. Obvious slowness in performing such maneuvers increases the likelihood of Parkinson disease.
3. The **glabella tap reflex** is tested by percussing the patient's forehead. The orbicularis oculi muscle reflexively contracts, causing both eyes to blink. The blinking normally stops after 5 to 10 repeated taps. Persistence of blinking is a positive test (Myerson sign) and is more common among patients with Parkinson disease.
4. A sample of writing in a patient with Parkinson disease may reveal **micrographia** (writing that becomes smaller across a page).
5. Late in the course of disease, many patients develop **postural instability.** It becomes difficult for patients to maintain a particular posture. Asking a patient to walk may reveal a tendency to fall or involuntary acceleration forward or backward (festination).
6. During the evaluation of a patient with postural tremor, which suggests essential tremor, the possibility of early Parkinson disease must be excluded since tremors of Parkinson disease may also be of postural and kinetic nature.

B. The possibility of Wilson disease should always be considered in any patient with an action tremor who is younger than 40 years of age.

V. **Treatment.** Therapy for most forms of tremor should target the underlying cause. Specific treatment for Parkinson disease and essential tremor is discussed below.

A. **Parkinson disease** (Table 59–3). Pharmacological therapy has been shown to reduce morbidity and mortality, but requires careful monitoring to determine the optimal dosage.

1. *Neuroprotective* therapy is designed to slow or stop disease progression. The monoamine oxidase B inhibitor (MAO-B) **selegiline** has been shown to delay functional impairment and disease progression. It is unclear whether this is secondary to its neuroprotective effect or its effect on symptoms, which may mask disease progression. There are randomized, controlled trials that found that selegiline delayed the need for levodopa compared with placebo. (SOR Ⓐ) **Rasaligine,** another MAO-B inhibitor, is now being studied as a neuroprotective agent.

TABLE 59–3. **AVAILABLE PHARMACOTHERAPY FOR PARKINSON DISEASE**

Type of Therapy	Class	Agent	Trade Name(s)	Starting Dose	Titration/ Maximum Dose/Special Instructions
Neuroprotective	Monoamine oxidase B inhibitor	Selegiline	Eldepril, Deprenyl	5 mg orally twice daily	5 mg orally twice daily
		Rasagline	Agilect	1 mg once daily	Requires no titration Maximum dose 1 mg/d
Symptomatic	Dopamine precursor	Carbidopa– levodopa	Sinemet, Sinemet CR	Carbidopa 25 mg/levodopa 100 mg 2–4 times daily	Carbidopa 200 mg/levodopa 2000 mg/d
	COMT inhibitors	Tolcapone	Tasmar	100–200 mg 3 times daily	Consider ↓ levodopa dose upon initiation of tolcapone
	Dopamine agonists	Entacapone	Comtan	200 mg orally with each dose of carbidopa– levodopa	1600 mg/d
		Bromocriptine	Parlodel	1.25 mg orally twice daily	Increase by 2.5 mg/d every 2–4 weeks to maximum of 90 mg/d.
		Ropirinole	Requip	0.25 mg orally three time daily	Increase 0.75 or 1.5 mg every week until the optimal therapeutic response is attained. Maximum dose is 24 mg/d.
		Pramipexole	Mirapex	0.125 mg orally 3 times daily	Maximum dosage is 5 mg/d Increase by 0.375 mg/d every 5–7 d until optimal therapeutic response attained. Maximum dosage is 4.5 mg/d

COMT, catechol-*o*-methyltransferase.

2. Most patients with Parkinson disease are treated with *symptomatic* therapy when they begin to experience functional impairment. Factors to consider before instituting symptomatic therapy include whether the patient's symptoms affect the patient's dominant hand, whether symptoms interfere with work or other activities, which features of Parkinson disease are present and whether quality of life is affected. Bradykinesia, for example, is usually more disabling than tremor. Treatment of Parkinson disease with either selegiline, dopamine agonists, or the combination of levodopa and carbidopa or levodopa and carbidopa with entacapone improves symptoms and quality of life, but all these drugs have significant side effects. There is no evidence favoring a medical option, so treatment should be individualized.

There are currently six commonly used types of symptomatic therapy.

a. The dopamine precursor **levodopa** is the most widely used and effective drug. (SOR **B**) To prevent its conversion to dopamine outside the blood–brain barrier, it is combined with the decarboxylase inhibitor, **carbidopa**. Dietary aminoacids may interfere with levodopa absorption; therefore, protein restriction may be necessary for patients with decreased levodopa response. Levodopa is associated with serious adverse effects that increase in severity with prolonged use. These include nausea, vomiting, anorexia, orthostatic hypotension, cardiac arrhythmias, and psychosis. Some serious disadvantages of levodopa treatment are drug-induced dyskinesias and fluctuations in motor response, which are related to long-term treatment. These complications are irreversible. Sustained release preparations of levodopa showed no added benefit for motor complications.

b. Even when combined with carbidopa, only 10% of levodopa reaches the brain. Much of it is converted to an inert metabolite by the enzyme catechol-*O*-methyltransferase (COMT). The COMT inhibitors **tolcapone** and **entacapone** can be administered with levodopa to increase its effectiveness. These drugs are also useful for managing motor fluctuations. (SOR **B**) However, COMT inhibitors are not recommended as initial agents because of their higher cost and lack of proven benefit in patients with early Parkinson disease.

c. The third class of available pharmacotherapy is the dopamine agonists such as **bromocriptine, ropirinole,** and **pramipexole.** They stimulate dopamine receptors. Dopamine agonists are found to reduce dyskinesia and motor fluctuations more effectively compared with levodopa, but were associated with increased treatment withdrawal and poorer motor scores. Also, dopamine agonists are more likely to be associated with hallucinations, somnolence, and edema than levodopa. A dopamine agonist, namely, pergolide should be avoided because of its recent association with restrictive valvular heart disease. A powerful dopamine agonist, apomorphine may be tried in complicated patients who experience sudden, resistant "off" periods, but it must be cautiously used because of severe side effects. Dopamine agonists can be used for initial symptomatic therapy or as adjuncts to therapy with levodopa. (SOR **B**)

d. MAO-B inhibitors selegiline and rasagiline are useful for symptomatic control of disease and as adjuvant therapy for patients with motor fluctuations. Selegiline improves symptoms of Parkinson disease and delays the need for levodopa therapy up to 9 to 12 months. (SOR **A**)

e. Anticholinergics, mainly benztropine and trihexyphenidyl, are useful for symptomatic control, (SOR **C**) but associated with more neuropsychiatric and cognitive adverse effects than other drugs. So, treatment with these agents, especially in the elderly, should be avoided.

f. Amantadine may be effective especially in severe dyskinesias. (SOR **B**) However, effectiveness in the long term is questionable.

g. **Treatment of nonmotor symptoms in Parkinson disease is usually a major challenge for clinicians.**

   (1) In cognitive impairment, doses of antiparkinsonian medications must be adjusted and a cholinesterase inhibitor must be considered. (SOR **C**)

   (2) For depression, selective serotonin reuptake inhibitors are usually used. (SOR **C**)

   (3) With psychosis, hallucinations and delirium, anti-Parkinsonian drugs' doses may be lowered and low-dose clozapine or quetiapine may be considered. (SOR **C**)

   (4) Supportive and symptomatic management for constipation, dysphagia, orthostatic hypotension, sleep disturbances, and urinary urgency may be necessary.

3. Surgical treatment of Parkinson disease is emerging as an effective option for patients in whom pharmacotherapy fails.

   a. **Ablation** of tissue in specific areas of the brain including the ventral intermediate nucleus of the thalamus and globus pallidus pars interna with radio waves, heat, or chemicals is associated with significant improvement. Unilateral pallidotomy improved motor examination and activities of daily living better than medical treatment in one systematic review, but was associated with high incidence of adverse effects. (SOR **B**)

   b. **Deep brain stimulation** of the ventral intermediate nucleus, globus pallidus pars interna, or subthalamic nucleus with an electrode connected to a pulse generator placed subcutaneously over the chest wall is also effective. Controlled trials comparing pallidal deep brain stimulation versus medical treatment are lacking. Adverse effects are probably less frequent with deep brain stimulation than with ablative surgery. (SOR **C**)

   c. **Transplantation of fetal dopaminergic neurons** into the substantia nigra has shown some promise, but remains a controversial and experimental procedure.

4. **Supportive care** is an important component of management. The clinical manifestations of the disease itself are frequently accompanied by a profound psychological and social impact. Stress among caregivers is a significant concern. Health care providers should be sensitive to these problems. Patients with Parkinson disease and their

families should also receive counseling about the clinical features, prognosis, and impact of the disease. A number of support groups are helpful in this regard.

B. Essential tremor

1. Mild essential tremor need not be treated if it causes no functional impairment. Functional impairment as assessed by the severity of symptoms and ability to perform daily tasks (e.g., writing, buttoning) should always be used as a guide to initiate or adjust therapy. Careful monitoring for side effects of medications is essential.

2. **Pharmacological therapy**
   a. The beta blocker **propanolol (Inderal)** and the anticonvulsant **primidone (Mysoline)** are used as first-line treatments for more severe tremor. (SOR **B**) Both are roughly equally effective. Propanolol is initiated at a dose of 20 to 40 mg orally twice daily. Maintenance doses are usually 240 to 320 mg/d. It is usually well tolerated. Patients on propanolol should be carefully monitored for side effects like fatigue, headaches, bradycardia, impotence, and depression. Relative contraindications including asthma, heart failure, atrioventricular block, and diabetes mellitus have limited its use in some patients. In general, 50% to 70% of patients obtain symptomatic relief from propanolol, but dramatic improvement occurs in a much smaller percentage. Primidone should be started at a dose of 25 mg orally once daily and slowly increased as needed to a maximum of 750 mg/d given in 3 divided doses. Long-term treatment with primidone is well tolerated, but some patients will have an acute reaction consisting of nausea, vomiting, or ataxia.
   b. The anticonvulsant **gabapentin (Neurontin)** is also effective, but experience with it as a treatment for essential tremor is limited. (SOR **C**) It can be initiated at a dose of 100 mg orally once daily and increased until tremor is under good control to a maximum of 2400 mg a day (divided into 3 doses).
   c. Topiramate has been shown to be effective as well as gabapentin. It improved tremor scores after 2 weeks' treatment but associated with appetite suppression, weight loss, and paresthesia. Studies addressing the long-term outcomes are lacking. (SOR **C**)
   d. Other classes of medications including benzodiazepines, calcium channel blockers, olanzapine, and theophylline have been used with variable success.

TIC DISORDERS

A tic is a brief, intermittent, repetitive, nonrhythmic, unpredictable, purposeless movement or sound. Tics are preceded by a conscious urge to execute them. Stress results when a tic is suppressed. Stress is relieved upon executing the tic. Voluntary suppression, which is more typical in tics than in other involuntary movements, is a helpful distinguishing feature. Tics are usually intermittent, but may be repetitive and are frequently stereotypical. Motor and phonic tics may persist during all stages of sleep, unlike most other hyperkinesias. Tics have a number of causes. Tourette syndrome, which is the combination of motor and phonic tics occurring before the age of 21, is the most common tic disorder, affecting roughly 5 to 10 of every 10,000 children. Boys are disproportionately affected. Tourette syndrome is frequently accompanied by attention deficit hyperactivity disorder. Dopamine receptor blockers, such as pimozide, fluphenazine and haloperidol, and alpha-receptor agonists such as clonidine provide effective treatment, for the tics. (SOR **C**) Behavioral approaches have also shown some success.

CHOREA

Chorea is an unpredictable, irregular, nonrhythmic, brief, jerky flowing, or writhing movement. Chorea can be consciously incorporated into voluntary movements, such that patients exhibit "semipurposeful" movements known as parakinesias. Chorea has several causes, including Wilson disease, stroke, and as part of an immunologic reaction after streptococcal infection (Sydenham chorea). Chorea may be also drug related, most commonly associated with dopaminergic agents, lithium, phenytoin, and rarely valproate. Huntington disease is a hereditary form inherited in an autosomal dominant pattern. Symptoms typically appear between ages 35 and 50.

Haloperidol (Haldol) and fluphenazine (Prolixin) are effective in treating chorea, but can impair voluntary movements. (SOR **C**) Both are initiated at a dose of 0.5 or 1.0 mg orally once daily and can gradually be increased to a maximum daily dose of 6 to 8 mg/d. The dopamine-depleting drugs reserpine (Serpalan) and tetrabenazine (Nitoman) and the benzodiazepine clonazepam (Klonopin) are also effective. (SOR **C**) Reserpine is initiated at a dose of 0.1 mg orally once daily (maximum dose, 3 mg/d). Tetrabenazine is started at 25 mg orally once daily (maximum dose, 100 mg/d). Klonopin is started at a dose of 0.5 mg orally once daily (maximum dose, 4 mg/d). Wrist weights can improve function by decreasing the amplitude of chorea.

MYOCLONUS

Myoclonus is a brief, sudden movement caused by involuntary muscle contractions or lapse of muscle contraction (*asterixis*). **Generalized myoclonus** refers to synchronous "jerks" in many body parts; **focal myoclonus** affects a single body part. Physiologic myoclonus is benign and includes "sleep jerks" that occur while falling asleep. Rhythmic myoclonus may be confused with tremor and is typically characterized by brief muscle twitches, confined to one limb or to adjacent body region, associated with spike–wave complexes on the electroencephalogram or spinal lesions. Essential myoclonus is disabling and can be treated with clonazepam (starting dose of 0.25 mg orally twice daily, increasing over 3 days to 1 mg/d). (SOR **C**) Most causes of myoclonus are secondary and include drugs such as lithium, toxins, advanced liver disease, infections including human immunodeficiency virus, dementia, and brain lesions. Treatment should target the underlying disorder.

DYSTONIA

Dystonia is a syndrome that includes sustained contractions of opposing muscles that cause twisting, repetitive movements, and abnormal postures. Progressively severe tremor is also common. Primary dystonia is an inherited form that appears before age 21. Dystonic movements are involuntary, but can be diminished by specific maneuvers. In spasmodic torticollis that affects the neck, for example, placing a hand on the chin or side of the face reduces the severity of dystonia. Primary dystonia is generally hereditary and can be treated successfully with high doses of trihexyphenidyl (Artane) alone (starting dose of 1 mg orally per day, increasing gradually to 6–80 mg/d until symptoms are well controlled), or in combination with baclofen (Lioresal) (starting dose of 10 mg orally once daily, maximum dose of 30–120 mg/d). (SOR **C**) The list of secondary causes includes Wilson disease, metachromatic leukodystrophy, Lesch–Nyhan syndrome, stroke, and encephalitis.

WILSON DISEASE

Wilson disease is a rare inherited disorder of copper metabolism that, in addition to hepatic manifestations, often also presents with neuropsychiatric features including progressive tremor, dysarthria, parkinsonism, and dystonia. Very rarely disease presents with isolated action tremor. Symptoms and signs of Wilson disease usually appear at a young age. Tremor in a young patient, therefore, should raise suspicion of primary dystonia or Wilson disease. A low serum ceruloplasmin is a useful screening test although not diagnostic. A slit lamp examination for Kayser–Fleischer rings should also be considered.

ATAXIA

Ataxia is a wide-based, unsteady gait associated with cerebellar dysfunction, proprioceptive defects, or both. Inherited forms include Friedreich ataxia and spirocerebellar ataxia. Ataxia can occur secondary to stroke, trauma, alcoholic degeneration, multiple sclerosis, vitamin

B_{12} deficiency, and hydrocephalus. Treatment, when possible, should target the underlying cause.

REFERENCES

Bhidayasiri R. Differential diagnosis of common tremor syndromes. *Postgrad Med J.* 2005;81(962):756-762.

Clarke C, Moore AP. Parkinson's disease. *Am Fam Physician.* 2007;75(7):1045-1048.

Clarke C, Moore AP. Parkinson's disease. *Clin Evid.* 2005;13:1658-1677.

Ferreri F, Agbokou C, Gauthier S. Recognition and management of neuropsychiatric complications in Parkinson's disease. *CMAJ.* 2006;175(12):1545-1552.

Ferreira J, Sampaio C. Essential tremor. *Clin Evid.* 2005;13:1608-1621.

Jankovic J. An update on the treatment of Parkinson's disease, memorial lecture. *Mt Sinai J Med.* 2006;73(4):682-689.

Rao G, Fisch L, Srinivasan S, et al. Does this patient have Parkinson disease? *JAMA.* 2003;289(3):347-353.

Rao SS, Hofmann LA, Shakil A. Parkinson's disease: diagnosis and treatment. *Am Fam Physician.* 2006;74(12):2046-2054.

Smaga S. Tremor. *Am Fam Physician.* 2003;68(8):1545-1552.

---

60   Urinary Incontinence

Karen D. Novielli, MD, & Barry D. Weiss, MD

KEY POINTS

- Urinary incontinence is extremely common in older patients, particularly older women.
- Middle-aged and older patients should be asked routinely about urinary incontinence, because they are unlikely to spontaneously mention the condition.
- Treatment is based on the cause of urinary incontinence, and behavioral management is a critical management tool.

I. **Definition.** Urinary incontinence is the complaint of any involuntary leakage of urine. Since micturition is controlled through both the central and peripheral nervous systems as well as local anatomic support, incontinence can be caused by numerous conditions affecting the brain, spine, and pelvis.

II. **Common Diagnoses.** Urinary incontinence becomes more frequent with advancing age and is often associated with poor general health and functional status. Among ambulatory, community-dwelling persons older than age 65, urinary incontinence occurs in 17% to 55% of females and 11% to 34% of males. Approximately 14% of older women and 4% of older men are incontinent on a daily basis.

   A. **Transient incontinence** may be present in as many as 20% of incontinent patients and is more likely when incontinence is of recent onset. See Table 60–1 for common causes of transient incontinence.

   B. **Urge incontinence** is the most common cause of persistent incontinence in older individuals. In urge incontinence, involuntary leakage is accompanied by or immediately preceded by urgency and results from uncontrolled contractions of the detrusor muscle. Although most cases are idiopathic, patients with neurologic disorders (including dementia) are particularly at high risk.

   C. **Stress incontinence** is usually present when involuntary leakage occurs from effort or exertion or from sneezing or coughing and is related to increased urethral mobility and/or poor intrinsic sphincter function.

   D. **Overflow incontinence** accounts for ≤5% of incontinence in women but, because of the prevalence of prostate disorders, accounts for 30% to 50% of incontinence in older

TABLE 60–1. CONDITIONS COMMONLY ASSOCIATED WITH TRANSIENT (REVERSIBLE) URINARY INCONTINENCE

Drip mnemonic
  D-delirium
  R-restricted mobility (illness, injury, restraint, gait disorder)
  I-infection, inflammation, impaction
  P-polyuria (diabetes, volume overload), pharmaceuticals (diuretcs, autonomic agents, psychotropics)

men. Overflow incontinence is caused either by obstruction of urinary outflow or impaired detrusor contractility.
  E. **Mixed incontinence** occurs when two or more of the above causes are present si-multaneously, most often urge incontinence in combination with another cause. Mixed incontinence is very common and may occur in as many as 50% of incontinent patients.
  F. **Functional incontinence** is the inability or unwillingness to toilet because of physical, cognitive, psychological, or environmental factors (e.g., a patient with severe depression or who is physically restrained). Functional incontinence is common in the hospital and nursing home settings.
III. **Symptoms.** An assessment of the patient with urinary incontinence should include a general medical history, and specific questioning for symptoms related to the lower urinary tract, bowel and sexual function, and pelvic organ prolapse. Basic elements of the history of the lower urinary tract include duration, frequency, and severity of urine loss; precipitating factors (such as coughing, change in position); and associated symptoms.
  A. **Urgency** is the primary symptom of uncontrolled bladder contractions (i.e., urge incon-tinence). The sensitivity of the symptom of urgency in identifying patients with true urge incontinence, in comparison to formal urodynamic testing, is approximately 60%.
  B. **Loss of urine with coughing,** descending stairs, sneezing, and so on is a classic symp-tom of stress incontinence. The positive predictive value of these symptoms exceeds 85% for identifying patients with true stress incontinence and exceeds 95% when ac-companied by physical examination findings typical of stress incontinence. However, symptoms similar to those of stress incontinence can occur in patients with urge in-continence (pseudo-stress incontinence), because in urge incontinence the bladder is "irritable" and may contract when stimulated by repetitive increases in intra-abdominal pressure, such as from repetitive coughing.
  C. **Dribbling** is a symptom of overflow incontinence, and it may occur with sphincter weak-ness, especially when it is caused by sphincter denervation. It usually increases with postural change or with Valsalva's maneuver.
  D. **Abdominal discomfort** may be present in patients with overflow incontinence because of bladder distention, particularly if urinary retention and overflow are of recent onset.
IV. **Signs.** Physical examination should include an evaluation of the functional and cognitive status of the patient in addition to a thorough neurologic, abdominal, and pelvic evaluation.
  A. **Abnormal mental status** (e.g., dementia) indicates decreased function of cerebral in-hibitory centers associated with urge incontinence.
  B. **Abnormal reflex, motor, or sensory function** suggests the presence of a neurologic disorder leading to neuropathic sphincter, detrusor denervation, or cerebral dysfunction and associated urge incontinence.
  C. **Abdominal distention** or **palpable bladder** is suggestive of urinary retention and asso-ciated overflow incontinence.
  D. **Atrophic vaginitis** indicates the possibility of urge incontinence because of estrogen-responsive irritable bladder.
  E. **Prolapse of pelvic organs** is frequently associated with stress incontinence.
  F. **Prostate enlargement or masses** suggest the possibility of overflow incontinence sec-ondary to bladder outflow obstruction.
  G. **Impacted rectal stool** suggests overflow incontinence from obstruction of urethral out-flow by the fecal impaction.
V. **Laboratory Tests.** Some patients may have preexisting conditions warranting specialized evaluations not discussed in this chapter (Figure 60–1).
  A. **Basic evaluation** (for all incontinent patients)
    1. **Urinalysis.** *Pyuria* or *bacteriuria* suggests infection, and a culture can confirm the di-agnosis. *Hematuria* may indicate neoplasm or calculi, necessitating further evaluation with cystoscopy, renal ultrasound, or radiography.

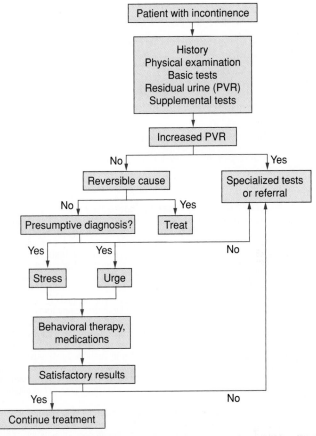

FIGURE 60–1. Urinary incontinence—diagnostic and management strategy for primary care physicians. Note that patients with certain conditions may need specialized evaluation and should not be diagnosed and managed exclusively according to this algorithm. Such patients are those with (1) hematuria or pyuria in the absence of infection, (2) recent (within 2 months) onset of irritative voiding symptoms, (3) previous anti-incontinence surgery or radical pelvic surgery, (4) severe pelvic prolapse, (5) suspicion of prostate cancer, or (6) neurologic abnormalities. PVR, postvoid residual urine.

2. **Postvoid residual urine (PVR)** volume should be measured to exclude overflow incontinence. Normal PVR is ≤50 mL; PVR of 200 mL or more is abnormal and indicates outflow obstruction or diminished detrusor contractility. PVRs between 50 and 200 mL are equivocal, and the test should be repeated on another occasion.
   a. **Postvoid catheterization** is the most common method for determining PVR. A sterile catheter is inserted into the patient's bladder immediately after the patient voids, and the volume of collected urine is recorded. Inability to pass the catheter suggests obstruction from urethral stricture, prostate enlargement, etc.
   b. **Ultrasound** measurement of bladder volume is a noninvasive method for determining the presence of residual urine. Where it is available, ultrasonography may be preferable to catheterization, especially in men with suspected prostate enlargement, because ultrasound involves no risk of infection or urethral trauma, both of which can occur with catheterization.
3. A **cough stress test** should be performed on all females. With the patient in the lithotomy position and with a full bladder, the patient coughs while gauze or a menstrual

TABLE 60–2. PERFORMANCE OF OFFICE CYSTOMETROGRAPHY

1. Have the patient empty his or her bladder by voiding in the toilet, and then have him or her assume the dorsal lithotomy position.
2. Insert a sterile nonballooned no. 12–14 French catheter, and empty the patient's bladder. Measurement of postvoid residual and collection of urinalysis may be performed at this time.
3. Insert the syringe (50 mL, with the plunger removed) into the end of the catheter, and position it 15 cm above the urethra.
4. Fill the bladder by pouring sterile water through the open end of the syringe in 25- to 50-mL aliquots.
5. Record the cumulative total fluid instilled into the bladder, and note the volume at which the patient first reports having the urge to void. Severe urge to void at ≤300–350 mL is suggestive of detrusor overactivity (urge incontinence).
6. Continue adding fluid slowly until the fluid level (meniscus) in the syringe rises, indicating contraction of the detrusor muscle with transmission of intrabladder pressure to the syringe.
   a. The rise in fluid level may be either gradual or explosive.
   b. Detrusor contractions at ≤300–350 mL of bladder volume are generally indicative of urge incontinence.

pad is held over the perineum. Instantaneous leakage onto the pad during coughing suggests stress incontinence. Delayed leakage suggests urge incontinence. If there is no leakage, the test should be repeated with the patient in the standing position.

- B. **Supplemental tests** can be performed if a presumptive diagnosis cannot be reached with a history, physical examination, and the aforementioned tests.
  - 1. **Office cystometrography** (Table 60–2) is a simple office procedure that is useful for detecting the presence of uncontrolled bladder contractions associated with urge incontinence. Cystometrography is safe; urinary infection develops in ≤5% of patients who undergo this test. Compared to formal urodynamic testing, several studies have shown that the sensitivity of simple office cystometrography for diagnosing detrusor instability is between 75% and 100%, the specificity is 69% to 89%, and the positive predictive value is 74% to 91% in patients for whom reversible causes of incontinence have been excluded.
  - 2. **Urinary flow determination** can be useful in male patients suspected of having prostate enlargement causing outflow obstruction. Decreased flow is indicated by either straining or an interrupted stream, or abnormally low flow measurement with a commercially available urine flowmeter. Flow rates in older men are usually ≥20 mL/s; rates ≤10 to 15 mL/s are abnormal.
- C. **Specialized tests** can be performed in selected patients with specific indications or in those for whom a presumptive diagnosis cannot be reached after history, physical examination, and basic and supplemental tests. These tests are usually obtained after referral to a specialist such as a urologist or urogynecologist and include VCUG (video-cystourethrography), videourodynamics, ultrasound, and MRI.
  - 1. **Complete urodynamic testing** (including full cystometrography, perineal electromyelography, urethral pressure profilometry, and other measurements) is commonly performed when a presumptive diagnosis cannot be made, when patients do not respond to treatments for the presumptive diagnosis, when the PVR is increased, and when surgical interventions are being considered.
  - 2. **Endoscopic and imaging studies** of the urinary tract may be indicated in patients with hematuria, sterile pyuria, or recent onset of irritative voiding symptoms (i.e., symptoms of urge incontinence that developed within the previous 2 months). In such patients, these tests may detect neoplasms, stones, diverticula, etc.
- VI. **Treatment.** After the basic and supplemental evaluations described above, in most cases a presumptive diagnosis can be made as to the cause and type of incontinence. Treatment, as outlined below, can be administered based on the presumptive diagnosis. If treatment is unsuccessful, the diagnosis should be reevaluated, and more specialized tests may be indicated to better define the cause of incontinence. The patient can keep a **voiding diary,** in which symptoms and information on the frequency and circumstances of incontinent episodes are recorded. A baseline diary is useful for defining the patient's symptoms and determining the baseline frequency of incontinence to judge subsequent efficacy of therapy.
  - A. **Transient causes** of urinary incontinence are managed by treating the identified cause. If incontinence does not resolve, other causes of transient incontinence should again be considered. If none are found, the patient is then treated for the type of persistent

incontinence (e.g., urge or stress) presumptively diagnosed based on the testing described above. (SOR **C**)

B. Urge incontinence

1. Behavioral therapies are the first-line treatment because they are safe and often effective. In the event that pharmacotherapy is needed, behavioral therapy is an important as adjunctive therapy. Two principles underlie behavioral treatments for urge incontinence: (1) keep the bladder volume low by frequent voiding and (2) inhibit detrusor contractions by retraining cerebral and pelvic continence mechanisms.

    a. Bladder training is the treatment of choice for urge incontinence. It involves progressively lengthening the interval between voiding and encouraging the patient to postpone voiding for increasing lengths of time. Limited data suggest that bladder training is effective and that most patients experience improvement in their incontinence symptoms. At least one study found it superior to drug therapy in cognitively intact women. (SOR **B**)

    b. Pelvic muscle exercises (Kegel exercises) can also improve symptoms of urge incontinence (see Section VI.C.1.a), especially when supplemented with biofeedback. (SOR **C**)

2. Medications are often added as adjunct therapy for the treatment of urge incontinence.

    a. Oral medications for urge incontinence act by diminishing bladder contractions. **Oxybutynin** is an antimuscarinic agent that has a direct antispasmodic effect on the bladder. It is used at doses ranging from 2.5 mg at bedtime to 5 mg 4 times per day. An extended-release preparation is also available that permits once daily dosing and fewer side effects. **Tolterodine** is an anticholinergic drug that has similar efficacy to oxybutynin and may have a lower incidence of dry mouth. The dose of tolterodine ranges from 0.5 mg at bedtime to 2 mg twice a day. Both oxybutynin and tolterodine have significant anticholinergic side effects that may limit their use, particularly in older individuals with comorbid illnesses. Urinary retention, in particular, should be considered in patients with worsening incontinence. There are insufficient data to support the use of other agents including propantheline, tricyclic antidepressants, and calcium channel blockers. (SOR **B**)

3. Other treatments

    a. Electrical stimulation with both implantable and nonimplantable electrodes may improve urge incontinence in some patients. This therapy is used in many centers but is considered investigational. (SOR **C**)

    b. Surgical treatment of urge incontinence with procedures such as augmentation cystoplasty is effective, but is used only in selected patients. Bladder denervation, which reduces detrusor contractility, can be accomplished with subtrigonal phenol injections and a variety of other methods. Cure rates with bladder denervation are low. (SOR **B**)

    c. Intradetrusor injection of botulinum toxin is a new and promising treatment for patients refractory to pharmacotherapy. (SOR **B**)

C. Stress incontinence

1. Behavioral therapies are effective in some patients with stress incontinence.

    a. Pelvic muscle exercises (Kegel exercises) may lessen the severity of sphincter weakness in stress incontinence. Patients are instructed to contract the pelvic muscles for 10 seconds at a time, 30 to 80 times per day, and continue the exercises indefinitely. On average, incontinence is improved in approximately 75% to 85% of patients and eliminated in approximately 10% to 15%. Instruction in proper technique for pelvic muscle exercises is important to improved patient outcomes. (SOR **B**)

    b. Adjuncts to pelvic muscle exercises include **biofeedback** and **vaginal cones.** Each may further improve the effectiveness of treatment, although further research is necessary to quantitate the additional benefit. (SOR **C**)

    c. Bladder training (for urge incontinence as described in Section VI.B.1.a) can result in additional improvement in symptoms of stress incontinence. (SOR **B**)

2. Medications

    a. α-Adrenergic agonists, such as phenylpropanolamine, have significant risk of adverse event such as hemorrhagic stroke. Moreover, since there is limited evidence to support their efficacy for treatment of stress incontinence, they are not recommended at this time. (SOR **B**)

    b. Estrogen, oral, vaginal, or transdermal, can be administered in conjunction with alpha agonists and may result in more improvement than alpha agonists alone. Estrogen alone may improve symptoms of urge or stress incontinence in women with atrophic vaginitis; however, studies to date have not shown a beneficial effect. Concerns about the risk–benefit ratio of estrogen must feature prominently in any decision about its use and if a decision is made to try hormone therapy, the lowest effective dose should be used. (SOR **B**)

    c. Duloxetine is a selective serotonin-noradrenaline receptor inhibitor (SSNRI) that has been shown to be better than placebo at improving quality of life and reducing episodes of stress incontinence by 50%. Duloxetine is not FDA approved for treatment of urinary incontinence. Nausea is common but not serious side effect of treatment. The dose of duloxetine to treat UI is 40 mg twice daily. (SOR **B**)

3. Surgical options including injections of urethral bulking agents, retropubic culposuspension, and suburethral sling are often effective for women with stress incontinence. The appropriate surgical treatment is dictated by whether the patient's symptoms are caused by hypermobility (i.e., descent) of the urethra or by intrinsic weakness of the sphincter muscle (intrinsic sphincter deficiency). Surgery can eliminate incontinence in 70% to 85% of patients with stress incontinence, though older women may have less satisfactory results. For men with stress incontinence, such as occurs after prostatectomy, injections of periurethral bulking agents (e.g., collagen) or surgical implantation of an artificial urethral sphincter can improve or eliminate incontinence. When men are treated with periurethral bulking injections or artificial sphincters, cure (i.e., complete elimination of incontinence) occurs in 20% and 50%, respectively. (SOR **A**)

4. Devices are also available for treating stress incontinence. For women, these include pessaries, suction devices that occlude urethral outflow, and ballooned inserts that lie within the urethral orifice. For men, penile clamps are sometimes used on a temporary basis; clamps sometimes result in injury to the urethra or penile skin. There is little evidence regarding the effectiveness of these treatments. (SOR **C**)

D. Overflow incontinence must be treated by draining the bladder. Failure to drain retained urine may result in hydronephrosis and subsequent renal damage.

1. Intermittent catheterization, performed by patients or their caretakers, is the treatment of choice. The catheter must be clean, but not necessarily sterile, although sterile catheters are recommended for immunocompromised patients. The interval between catheterization varies, depending on how often the individual patient's bladder becomes distended. (SOR **C**)

2. Chronic indwelling catheterization (i.e., Foley catheter) is generally used if intermittent catheterization is not possible. (SOR **C**)

    a. Urinary tract infection. Bacterial colonization is universal among chronically catheterized patients. Antibiotic treatment results in selection of antibiotic-resistant organisms; therefore, only symptomatic urinary tract infections should be treated.

    b. Leakage around the catheter is generally caused by encrustation of the catheter lumen and orifice with calculo-proteinaceous debris, with subsequent drainage of urine around the sides of the catheter. A larger catheter should not be used in an attempt to prevent leakage. Instead, the catheter should be replaced at a frequency dictated by the development of encrustation and leakage. **Acidification of urine** decreases build-up of encrusted material and lengthens the interval between catheter changes. Several medications can acidify urine, for example, **methenamine hippurate** (1 g orally twice a day), **ascorbic acid** (500 mg orally every day), and **acetic acid** (0.25% or less) lavage of catheter and bladder, performed anywhere from once per week to every other day, as needed to prevent encrustation.

    c. Mortality from septic complications is increased among patients who require chronic bladder catheterization.

3. Suprapubic catheterization is useful in selected patients for whom neither intermittent nor chronic urethral catheterization is appropriate. (SOR **C**)

E. Intractable incontinence exists when incontinence from any cause cannot be adequately controlled by the above measures. As noted above, irreversible overflow incontinence always requires catheter drainage. When other forms of incontinence are intractable, the following treatment options are available.

1. Behavioral techniques may be sufficient to decrease incontinence episodes and improve hygiene in some chronically incontinent patients.

    a. **Habit training** involves identification of the patient's natural voiding schedule and development of an individualized toileting schedule designed to preempt involuntary bladder emptying. This technique is used at nursing homes and limited data suggest it may improve outcomes associated with urinary incontinence. (SOR **B**)

    b. **Prompted voiding** involves asking patients whether they need to void and providing them with toilet facilities if they answer affirmatively. It is also used for institutionalized patients and is effective at reducing the frequency of incontinence. (SOR **B**)

    c. **Timed voiding** involves bringing the patient to the toilet on a fixed schedule. Limited data are available to evaluate effectiveness of this treatment. (SOR **B**)

2. **Incontinence underpants** and absorbent pads are useful for collecting and absorbing incontinent urine. The absorbent garment or pad is changed at intervals dictated by the frequency of incontinence. (SOR **C**)

3. **Condom catheters** may sometimes be useful in male patients, especially on a short-term basis. Condom catheters increase the risk of skin problems and urinary tract infections. (SOR **C**)

4. **Intermittent catheterization,** if logistically feasible, can be used to control intractable incontinence from any cause. (SOR **C**)

5. **Chronic bladder catheterization** may be used in patients whose incontinence cannot be managed by other means. (SOR **C**)

6. **Diverting ureteroileostomy** may be appropriate for controlling incontinence in carefully selected patients. (SOR **C**)

REFERENCES

Fantl JA, Newman DK, Colling J, et al. *Urinary Incontinence in Adults: Acute and Chronic Management.* Clinical Practice Guideline No. 2, 1996 Update. US Department of Health and Human Services, Public Health Service, Agency for Health Care Policy and Research; 1996. AHCPR publication 96–0682.

Holroyd-Leduc JM, Straus SE. Management of urinary incontinence in women: scientific review. *JAMA.* 2004;291(8):986-995.

Smith PP, McCrery RJ, Appell RA. Current trends in the evaluation and management of female urinary incontinence. *CMAJ.* 2006;175(10):1233-1240.

Thom D. Variations in estimates of urinary incontinence prevalence in the community: Effects of differences in definition, population characteristics, and study type. *J Am Geriatr Soc.* 1998;46:473-480.

Weiss BD. The diagnostic evaluation of urinary incontinence in geriatric patients. *Am Fam Physician.* 1998;57:2675-2684.

---

61   Urinary Symptoms in Men

Linda L. Walker, MD

KEY POINTS

- Younger men are more likely to present with infectious processes such as **urethritis** and **acute prostatitis**.
- Older men are prone to more insidious conditions such as **benign prostatic hypertrophy**, **chronic prostatitis**, and **cancers of the prostate and bladder**.
  Simple cystitis is not the norm in men; underlying causes of urinary tract symptoms should be sought.

I. **Definition.** Common urinary symptoms in men include voiding pain or discomfort, abnormal urine flow, hematuria, and urethral discharge. Pain is generally caused by infection or inflammation (e.g., urethritis or acute or chronic prostatitis). Flow is influenced by abnormal tone and physical obstruction (e.g., benign prostatic hypertrophy [BPH], prostate cancer, or urethral strictures). Hematuria is pathologic if from bladder or other cancers, but may be because of BPH or infection. Urethral discharge is nearly always infectious.

II. Common Diagnoses

A. Urethritis is pervasive, affecting more than four million males each year, primarily sexually active younger men with multiple partners. There is a resurgence in the number of **gonococcal** cases as a result of male-to-male transmission. However, **nongonococcal urethritis (NGU)** (caused by *Chlamydia trachomatis* in up to 55% of cases, also *Mycoplasma* and *Ureaplasma, Trichomonas* and, infrequently, *Herpes simplex* virus-2) predominates as the **most common sexually transmitted disease** in men. It can be transmitted from asymptomatic partners, and recurrence is widespread. Anal intercourse increases risk for urethritis from enteric pathogens. Chlamydia NGU complications include epididymitis, prostatitis, and Reiter's syndrome.

B. Prostatitis/chronic pelvic pain syndromes (CPPS). Twenty-five percent of adult males presenting with genitourinary symptoms have some form of **prostatitis,** and up to 50% of all men experience the symptoms in their lifetime. This disease spectrum results in more than 100,000 hospitalizations per year. Risk factors for prostatitis include reflux of urine because of bladder, prostate, or urethral abnormalities; anal intercourse; epididymitis; urinary catheters; and urinary tract surgery.

Recently the National Institutes of Health (NIH) classified and redefined prostatitis into the following categories:

1. **Acute bacterial prostatitis**—a fairly uncommon condition primarily affecting men aged 30 to 50 years, consisting of $\leq$5% of all prostatitis cases.
2. **Chronic bacterial prostatitis**—also uncommon, making up 7% of cases, affecting men older than 50 years of age.
3. **Chronic pelvic pain syndrome (CPPS)**—subdivided into two categories, both conditions of men aged 30 to 50 years.
   a. **Inflammatory CPPS**—known also as **nonbacterial prostatitis,** is the largest category of prostatitis syndromes, comprising 40% to 65% of cases overall. The NIH postulates that it is the most prevalent prostate condition, even outnumbering BPH. The cause is unknown.
   b. **Noninflammatory CPPS**—known previously as **prostatodynia,** is also very frequently seen, occurring in 20% to 40% of cases. It also has uncertain etiology, but may be related to internal sphincter failure and pelvic floor relaxation.
4. **Asymptomatic inflammatory prostatitis**—an incidental laboratory finding.

C. BPH is the most common urologic disorder of older men. Twenty-five percent eventually seek care for symptoms, leading to nearly two million patient visits each year. The prevalence is 8% in the fourth decade, 40% to 50% in the fifth decade, and $\geq$80% in the ninth decade of life, reflecting a probable cumulative androgen trophic effect on the prostate. Medications exacerbating BPH obstructive symptoms include antihistamines, anticholinergics, decongestants, and tranquilizers.

D. The most common (nondermal) malignancy in males is **prostate cancer,** affecting 10% of all men. More than 230,000 new cases are diagnosed each year and approximately 30,000 die annually in the United States of this cancer, which is 3% of adult male mortality. However, most men with prostate cancer die of other causes. Aging is the strongest risk factor and long-term androgens may stimulate neoplastic development, as prostate cancer is unknown in eunuchs. Having one, two, or three first-degree relatives with prostate cancer confers a 2-fold, 5-fold, or 11-fold increased risk, respectively. African Americans may have the highest lifetime risk of developing prostate cancer worldwide. At an incidence rate of 200 cases per 100,000, their risk is 1.5 times greater than Caucasians for acquiring the disease and 2 times greater for dying from it. Asian Americans have a lower risk than Caucasians. A diet high in fat or red meat may increase risk. Nutritional practices that may prove protective include intake of antioxidants, lycopenes, soy, garlic, and selenium.

E. Bladder cancer is also age-dependent; 80% of cases occur in individuals older than 50 years of age. It is the fourth most commonly diagnosed cancer in men and the second most prevalent. More than 63,000 people are diagnosed with bladder cancer yearly, and approximately 13,000 die of it; 9000 are men. The greatest risk factor is tobacco use; other risk factors include exposure to dyes and chemicals in metal- and leather-working occupations, long-term urinary catheter use, chronic urinary tract infection, bladder calculi, and pelvic irradiation.

III. Symptoms

A. Urethral discharge is typically copious, purulent, and yellow-green in **gonococcal urethritis,** developing 1 to 14 days after exposure. In **NGU,** the incubation period is 1 to

TABLE 61–1. AMERICAN UROLOGICAL ASSOCIATION SYMPTOM INDEX

Questions—Over the Past Month, How Often Have You	Score
1. had a sensation of not emptying your bladder completely after you finished urinating?	Not at all–0
	≤1 time in 5–1
2. had to urinate again in less than 2 hours after you had finished urinating?	≤half the time–2
	About half the time–3
3. found you stopped and started again several times when you urinated?	≥half the time–4
4. found it difficult to postpone urination?	Almost always–5
5. had a weak urinary stream?	
6. had to push or strain to begin urination?	
7. Over the past month, how many times did you most typically get up to urinate from the time you went to bed at night until the time you got up in the morning?	0–5 points maximum scored here per time reported

Score 7 or less = Mild.
Score 8–19 = Moderate.
Score 19 or more = Severe.

3 weeks, and the discharge is scantier and more mucoid. The marked **dysuria** associated with urethritis is perceived most strongly at the meatus.
   B. Symptoms of **urinary flow abnormalities** in an older man without other complaints most commonly suggest **BPH.** The constellation of lower urinary tract symptoms (LUTS) are divided into two types, and most BPH patients have both.
      1. **Obstructive symptoms** include **hesitant or interrupted stream, decreased stream force/caliber, straining, terminal dribbling, incomplete emptying,** or **frank urinary retention** with possible **overflow incontinence** of small volumes of urine. (*Note:* Obstructive symptoms are so described because of subjective characteristics and cannot be directly correlated with objective findings on urodynamic testing.)
      2. **Irritative symptoms** comprise **frequency, urgency, urge incontinence,** and **nocturia.** These occur in BPH, prostatitis, urinary tract infections (UTIs), and malignancies and with polyuria in systemic diseases (e.g., diabetes mellitus, congestive heart failure, or nephritic syndrome).
         The American Urological Association (AUA) recommends using a symptom index score (Table 61–1) if patients are to be considered for medication for BPH. Since these symptoms are not unique to BPH, the index is a monitoring tool only and should not be the sole basis for diagnosis.
      3. When **pain** is a component of flow abnormalities, then **infectious, inflammatory, and malignant conditions** are higher in the differential diagnosis.
   C. **Pain and discomfort** characterize inflammatory and infectious conditions of the prostate.
      1. **Acute prostatitis** usually has an unambiguous appearance presenting in a younger man who is **febrile, toxic, and acutely ill,** with **moderate to severe pelvic, perineal, and low back pain.**
      2. **Chronic prostatitis and CPPS** present with gradual onset of **vague pelvic pain** or fullness, **ejaculatory or penile pain** (or both), and perhaps **testicular or scrotal aching,** along with irritative voiding and occasionally obstructive symptoms. A key component in the history of patients with chronic prostatitis is **recurrent UTIs** or previous bouts of prostatitis. These individuals often have **anxious or depressive symptoms when CPPS impairs their quality of life.**
   D. **Painless hematuria** can be caused by **BPH** or **bladder cancer.** Urolithiasis and renal cell carcinoma are less common causes. When present in BPH, the blood tends to be seen at the beginning and end of the urine stream. In bladder cancer, the urine is typically uniformly bloody. Patients presenting with more advanced bladder cancer may have irritative voiding symptoms, **flank pain,** or **leg edema.**
IV. **Signs**
   A. **Acute urinary retention** is typically caused by severe **BPH** exacerbated by medications precipitating sudden obstruction, or from **acute prostatitis. Abdominal examination** or ultrasound will reveal **suprapubic tenderness** and a **distended bladder** that may hold ≥1 L of urine, percussable or palpable nearly to the umbilicus.
   B. **Digital rectal examination of the prostate** should be done in all men with urinary symptoms to evaluate for prostate size, consistency, symmetry, and masses.

1. In **acute prostatitis** the gland will be **swollen, boggy, and exquisitely tender.** To decrease the risk of bacteremia and sepsis, the examination should be gently performed in the toxic, ill-appearing patient.

2. **Mild tenderness, sponginess,** or **induration** may be noted in **chronic prostatitis**/CPPS. To collect expressed secretions at the meatus for analysis and culture, the gland is massaged firmly. The examiner uses a rolling motion of the fingerpad from the lateral margins of the prostate to the midline.

3. The gland can be normal or smooth, rubbery, and enlarged in **BPH.** It may compare in consistency to the tip of the nose.

4. **Carcinoma** may be palpable as **lobular asymmetry, induration,** or **mass.**

C. The anus, penis, testes, scrotum, and inguinal region should be evaluated for tenderness, masses, adenopathy, or lesions that could be the source of the patient's genital, urinary, or pelvic complaints (e.g., anal fissure, genital ulcer, inguinal hernia, phimosis).

D. **Neurologic examination** should focus on anal sphincter tone (may correlate with bladder sphincter tone) and on any neurologic deficits (e.g., sudden onset of urinary or fecal incontinence, urinary retention, back pain, extremity weakness, or symmetric extremity or trunk sensory deficits) indicative of spinal cord compression if metastatic prostate cancer is suspected.

V. **Laboratory Tests. Most common nonmalignant urologic conditions in men can be diagnosed using symptoms, physical findings, and laboratory testing available in the primary care setting.** Typical patient presentations with clinical strategies for evaluation follow:

A. **A sexually active young man with a urethral discharge should be treated for Chlamydia and gonorrhea when seen, and have confirmatory testing done.**

1. According to the Centers for Disease Control and Prevention (CDC) guidelines, urethritis in the above setting can be diagnosed by

   a. Observed **urethral discharge.**

   b. **Gram staining a urethral swab. If gram-negative intracellular diplococci are seen, gonococcal infection is present.** This is the most rapid and sensitive method for diagnosing **gonorrhea.**

   At least **5 WBCs per high-power field** indicates the presence of pus, supporting the diagnosis of **NGU** when no gonococci are seen.

   c. A positive **leukocyte esterase dipstick test** of the first voided urine specimen of the day. This test is equivalent to detecting pus in the urethra.

   d. At least **10 WBCs per high-power field** and absence of significant bacteriuria on the first voided urine specimen of the day.

2. In the absence of the above CDC criteria, urethritis cannot be diagnosed, pending further laboratory studies.

   a. The most sensitive test for genitourinary gonorrhea and Chlamydia is **nucleic acid amplification testing (NAAT) on a first-voided urine sample.** However, this is unlikely to be the test selected in a man presenting with acute symptoms of urethritis.

   b. Nucleic acid hybridization technology (**DNA probe**) is 99% sensitive for detection of gonorrhea and Chlamydia on a urethral swab.

   c. An acceptable alternative is **culture of a urethral swab**; however, this is much less sensitive (60%–80%) in detecting Chlamydia.

B. A **toxic-appearing man** in his thirties with the **acute onset of fever and chills, dysuria, severe perineal pain, obstructive symptoms, and a swollen, boggy, very tender prostate** has **acute prostatitis;** prostatic massage is contraindicated, and testing should include a **urinalysis (UA) and culture.** Marked pyuria will be present, and the culture will typically be positive for urethritis organisms in younger men and coliforms in older men.

1. **Blood cultures** should be done in hospitalized, septic-appearing patients.

2. Possible acute urinary retention is evaluated with **abdominal ultrasound;** catheterization for residual urine is very painful and could cause bacteremia, so it should only be done with urologic consultation.

C. A **middle-aged to older aged man** with **insidious complaints of mixed irritative and obstructive voiding symptoms** along with **numerous genitourinary pain complaints and a mildly tender or spongy prostate gland** is presumed to have **chronic prostatitis** or one of the two types of **CPPS.** All such patients should have a **UA and culture** performed. **Expressed prostatic secretions (EPS)** are examined microscopically for white blood cell counts (WBCs) and sent for **culture.**

1. In **chronic bacterial prostatitis**, urinary and EPS cultures are often recurrently positive, with at least 10 WBCs per high-power field in the EPS. Pyuria may also be present.
2. In **inflammatory CPPS,** only WBCs are seen.
3. Culture and WBCs are absent in secretions in **noninflammatory CPP.**

D. An **older man with typical LUTS** and a digital rectal examination consistent with **BPH** is diagnosed on clinical grounds alone. All such patients should have a UA, as a simple screen for other contributing urinary abnormalities (e.g., hematuria, which, if found, demands evaluation—see Section VI.E). (SOR **C**)

1. **Prostate-specific antigen (PSA)** testing should be performed only in men expected to live at least 10 years longer and if the test results would impact clinical management (see Section VI.F).
2. No evidence supports evaluating blood, urea, nitrogen, and creatinine in the absence of clinical suspicion. Elderly men have a high incidence of elevated serum creatinine, not necessarily attributable to their uncomplicated LUTS.
3. **Urinary ultrasound (US)** detects asymptomatic obstructive hydronephrosis in $\leq 2\%$ of otherwise healthy men with BPH and **is not recommended as a screening test** in these individuals.
4. **Postvoid residual (PVR)** urine volume can be measured by "in-and-out" or Foley catheterization, or by US; ≥ 350 mL is a typical threshold for diagnosis of urinary retention. A normal PVR is usually less than 200 mL. However, no correlation exists between PVR volume and symptom severity, urodynamics, or outcomes. (With *acute* urinary retention, a Foley catheter should be left in place because retention recurs in hours to days without a catheter, even if precipitants, such as medications, are corrected.)
5. Referral to urology is necessary for patients with atypical or complex symptoms, when surgical therapy is contemplated, or whenever cancer of the urinary tract is suspected. The urologist decides whether to perform **urodynamic tests (uroflowmetry, cystometrography, and pressure flow studies).** The urologist may also perform **cystoscopy** to visualize the urothelium and obtain tissue biopsy.

E. An **elderly man with a significant smoking history and painless hematuria** should be considered to have **bladder cancer until proven otherwise, as this is the classic presentation.**

1. Evaluation of an otherwise asymptomatic, low-risk patient with hematuria includes UA and culture, urine cytology, and bladder/renal ultrasound.
2. Patients with hematuria and risk factors for bladder cancer, with or without irritative voiding symptoms, require further investigation. This includes cytology on a spontaneously voided urine specimen, and a **CT urogram** for upper tract cancers, stones, or obstruction (or **retrograde pyelography** if there is a contrast dye allergy). Alternative radiologic work-up would consist of **intravenous pyelogram** and **renal ultrasonography.** A urologist performs **cystoscopic biopsy** to definitively diagnose bladder cancer. High-risk patients with a negative initial evaluation need ongoing surveillance for malignancy.

F. When a **patient with BPH requests PSA testing,** he needs thorough counseling on the pros and cons of testing. The AUA and the American Cancer Society (ACS) recommend annual screening for men aged 50 years and older with a life expectancy of at least 10 years. The ACS recommends African American men and those with two affected first-degree relatives begin annual screening at age 35, and the AUA recommends African Americans and those with one affected relative begin annual screening at age 40. The American Academy of Family Physicians (AAFP) recommends counseling about the potential benefits and harms of PSA screening to make individualized patient decisions. The United States Preventive Services Task Force (USPSTF) recommends against PSA screening. The following points should be kept in mind when counseling men about screening PSAs:

1. **Normal PSA levels (≤ 4 ng/mL)** are found in 25% of prostate cancer cases.
2. **Mild elevations (4–10 ng/mL)** are frequently found and 75% of cases are due to benign conditions, usually BPH. Urologic evaluation of these patients with **transrectal ultrasound (TRUS) and biopsy** risks detecting latent microscopic disease, with an unknown natural history and significant treatment-related morbidity (namely, urinary incontinence and erectile dysfunction—see Section VI.E).

3. It is possible that screening results in detection and treatment of indolent cancer that otherwise may never have caused any health problems during the patient's lifetime, but causes considerable anxiety and lifestyle changes from knowledge of test results and decision making relating to treatment.

4. A patient should be referred to a urologist when the PSA is greater than expected for age or ethnicity, as per standardized laboratory norms. Some advocate evaluation for a PSA velocity (rise) more than 0.75 per year.

G. **Advanced prostate cancer.** A minority of men with prostate cancer present with symptoms of advanced disease, including **advanced urinary symptoms, a markedly abnormal prostate examination, gross hematuria, bone pain, elevated alkaline phosphatase (highly suggestive of bony metastases), and generally markedly elevated PSA.** Prostate cancer in most of these men is felt to be so rapidly growing that early laboratory diagnosis would have been impossible, thus patients are only diagnosed clinically relatively late in the course of their illness. When a PSA is ≥ 10, there is at least a 75% chance of prostate cancer, and the risk rises exponentially as PSA values do (in advanced cancer the PSA is ≥ 100). PSA is monitored to look for a response to treatment or rise in refractory cases. All such patients are referred to a urologist for evaluation and management.

H. **If a prostate nodule is detected** in the course of a screening exam or when working up a patient with LUTS, a diagnostic PSA should be ordered. Regardless of the results, urologic referral is indicated for further evaluation. Statistically, there is **at least a 50% chance that the mass is prostate cancer, which often has spread beyond the gland and is incurable**.

VI. Treatment

A. **Urethritis.** Unless results of rapid assays are available, **patients with urethritis (and their sexual partners) should be treated for both NGU and gonococcal urethritis.**

1. For **NGU,** the most common regimen is oral **doxycycline,** 100 mg twice daily for 7 days. **Azithromycin,** 1 g once orally, is more expensive but has the advantage of improved compliance, ideally given when diagnosed in the health care setting. (SOR ●) Alternative oral regimens (for allergy or refractory cases presumed because of resistant mycoplasma or *Ureaplasma*) are metronidazole, 2 g once orally with **erythromycin,** 500 mg 4 times daily for 7 days; or various fluoroquinolones such as **ofloxacin,** 300 mg orally twice daily for 7 days, or **levofloxacin,** 500 mg orally for 7 days. (SOR **B**)

2. **Gonorrhea** is effectively treated with **ceftriaxone,** 125 mg intramuscularly (IM) once; or **cefixime,** 400 mg orally. **Fluoroquinolones are no longer an alternative because of increased resistance.**

3. Testing should be done for other sexually transmitted diseases. Patients should abstain from intercourse for 7 days from the onset of therapy and until all their sex partners from the previous 60 days are treated. Retreatment should be given if symptoms persist or recur and supporting laboratory evidence or objective signs exist per Section V.A.1.

B. **Acute prostatitis**

1. Men younger than 35 years are treated with oral **ofloxacin,** 400 mg initially, then 300 mg twice daily for 10 days; or **ceftriaxone,** 250 mg IM, then oral **doxycycline** 100 mg twice daily for 10 days. (SOR **C**)

2. In older men, coliforms are treated with a fluoroquinalone such as **levofloxacin** 750 mg daily for 10 to 14 days, or **trimethoprim-sulfamethoxazole (TMP-SMX DS)**, twice daily for 10 to 14 days.

3. Oral **nonsteroidal anti-inflammatory drugs (NSAIDs)**, such as **ibuprofen,** 400 to 800 mg thrice daily, are helpful for analgesia. **Opiates,** such as hydrocodone-APAP 5 mg/500 mg (e.g., Vicodin), 1 to 2 tablets orally every 4 to 6 hours as needed, may be used for severe pain. Acute urinary retention may be precipitated by opiate use if the prostate is severely swollen. Opiate side effects of constipation and straining to stool can markedly increase pelvic symptomatology.

4. **Hospitalization** for **intravenous antibiotics** may be necessary for severely ill patients.

C. Optimal treatments for **chronic bacterial prostatitis and CPPS** are being investigated in numerous ongoing clinical trials.

1. **Chronic bacterial prostatitis** is treated with the antibiotics listed for acute bacterial prostatitis, in prolonged courses lasting 4 to 6 weeks for quinolones, and up to 12 weeks for TMP-SMX, repeated as necessary. (SOR **B**)

   a. If recurrences are frequent, data support symptomatic use of oral α-**adrenergic blockers.** These include **doxazosin (e.g., Cardura),** titrated up to 8 mg over several weeks; **tamsulosin (e.g., Flomax),** 0.4 mg once daily, titrated to 0.8 mg after 2 to 4 weeks, can also be used.
   b. Older treatments include repetitive **prostatic massage** and **frequent ejaculation.**
   c. For severe symptoms (Table 61–1) persisting despite medical therapy, urologic consultation for possible surgery (laser or transurethral needle ablation, balloon dilation, or heat therapy) may be beneficial.
2. **CPPS.** Because WBCs are seen in prostatic secretions in **inflammatory CPPS, antibiotics** as above are tried for 4 weeks. **No one therapy has emerged as clearly beneficial for CPPS.** (SOR **B**) In a usual patient several are tried in succession, using individual response as a guide.
   a. For the obstructive symptoms of either type of CPPS, at least a 12-week trial of α-**adrenergic blockers** is recommended.
   b. Pain symptoms are treated with an oral **NSAID** such as **ibuprofen** 400 to 800 mg thrice daily for at least a 6-week trial. If symptoms persist, patients are reevaluated for further therapy.
   c. The most commonly tried **phytotherapy** consists of **quercetin**—a **bioflavenoid** (e.g., **Prosta-Q**), sold as a dietary supplement, taken orally as a 540-mg capsule thrice daily for at least 6 weeks.
   d. Men older than 40 years with inflammatory CPPS can be offered a long-term trial of oral **finasteride (Proscar),** 5 mg daily, or **dutasteride (Avodart),** 0.5 mg daily. These drugs are **5α-reductase** inhibitors, blocking testosterone conversion in the prostate, used primarily in BPH to shrink enlarged tissue, and can be continued long-term if the patient gets symptomatic relief.
   e. **Supportive counseling and psychological treatment** may be necessary for patients severely impacted by lifestyle limitations of their condition. (SOR **C**) It is especially important that any fears patients have about contagion or cancer be addressed and allayed.
   f. Current recommendations for CPPS patients with refractory voiding symptoms include a trial of **Pentosan (Elmiron),** 100 mg orally thrice a day for a limited course of 3 to 6 months, usually under urologic supervision.
   g. As in chronic prostatitis, urologists can offer various surgical interventions as a last resort.
   h. **Biofeedback, acupuncture,** and **neurostimulation** of the pelvic floor muscles are therapeutic adjuncts without proven benefit.
D. **BPH**
1. **Watchful waiting** is the recommendation of choice for patients with mild symptom scores; which should be re-totalled annually (Table 61–1). (SOR **B**) **Lifestyle changes** should include **restriction of caffeine and bedtime fluids, and limitation of any sympathomimetic (e.g., decongestants) and anticholinergic medications. Frequent, regular voiding** may improve quality of life.
2. **Drug therapy.** In patients with moderate or severe symptoms, medications should also be considered.
   a. Patients wishing to begin medication should initially be offered α-**blockers.** These drugs block the reversible component of obstructive symptoms (prostatic smooth muscle contraction), providing fairly prompt relief. (SOR **A**) Traditionally, α_1-**blockers** (e.g., **terazosin** or **doxazosin**) have been used. The α_{1A}-**blockers** (e.g., **tamsulosin [Flomax]**) are a newer class. This drug has effects within days instead of weeks and causes less hypotension than the α_1-blockers, but is more expensive.
   b. Oral **5α-reductase** inhibitors such as **finasteride (Proscar)** or **dutasteride (Avodart)** gradually reduce gland mass up to 50%. (PSA values while taking these medications should be doubled.) Androgen deprivation slowly relieves symptoms over months to years; thus it is reserved for use after, or in addition to, α-blockade trials for larger glands, and for patients with moderate to severe symptom scores. (SOR **A**) 5α-reductase inhibitors cost more than α-blockers but considerably less than surgery and can delay the need for surgery up to several years. Side effects include erectile dysfunction, decreased libido, decreased ejaculatory volume, and testicular pain. Long-term use may be associated with a poorly defined risk of high-grade prostate cancer.

    c. **Saw palmetto** has been a popular choice to help voiding symptoms, although a recent large trial shows no objective benefit. (SOR **A**) It does not affect prostate size, PSA levels, or voiding measurements. A typical dose is 160 mg twice daily.

  3. **Urologic referral** is indicated for BPH patients with marked urinary retention, recurrent UTIs, refractory gross hematuria, bladder calculi, or chronic kidney disease caused by obstruction. Surgical interventions include **transurethral resection of the prostate (TURP)**; **transurethral incision of the prostate (TUIP)**; or **ablation by microwave, laser, or electrode.** The latter procedures are less invasive, with lower complication rates, but provide no surgical specimens to evaluate for occult malignancy. TURP is most effective in relieving symptoms long-term, but retrograde ejaculation ensues in most men. Less frequently seen are impotence, UTIs, and incontinence.

E. Prostate cancer management is based on symptoms; histologic tumor grading (glandular disorganization based on the Gleason system); and clinical staging based on tumor size, local extension, spread to pelvic lymphatics, and metastases to bone, lungs, or liver. The patient's overall expected longevity should be considered based on his age and other medical conditions. The course of prostate cancer is quite variable, from a slow, indolent disease lasting years or decades (most common) to a rapid, invasive illness causing mortality in a few years or less. The 10-year survival rate for localized disease is 85%, and survival for several years is not uncommon in metastatic disease.

  1. In **localized lesions, radical prostatectomy**, several forms of **radiation** therapy, or cryotherapy are offered, in consultation with urology and a radiation oncologist. Risks to be weighed include postoperative urinary incontinence, radiation bowel injury, and erectile dysfunction versus the symptoms of progressive cancer if conservative management is chosen instead.

  2. In more **advanced disease, surgery** can relieve obstruction, while radiation can ameliorate urinary and metastatic symptoms, such as bone pain.

  3. **Widespread disease** is often treated **palliatively,** as no cytotoxic chemotherapy prolongs survival. Various methods are used in succession to cause tumor regression by inducing androgen deprivation. **Orchiectomy** is frequently performed; **leuprolide** injections inhibit pituitary gonadotropins and are often given with oral **flutamide** (an androgen receptor competitor). **Finasteride** may be used, and rarely **DES (diethylstilbestrol),** at risk of thromboembolism. Once the cancer becomes hormone refractory, the median survival is only 1 year.

F. As with prostate cancer, **bladder cancer** management should be coordinated by a urologist knowledgeable in oncology.

  1. **Superficial bladder cancer** can be treated by **local resection.** Bacille Calmette-Guérin (**BCG**) **infusions** into the bladder are given for patients at high risk for recurrence, and **intravesical chemotherapy** infusions are used to prevent and treat recurrence. The 5-year survival varies from 80% to 100% depending on the extent and recurrence of the disease.

  2. For **locally invasive disease, radical cystectomy** offers up to a 50% to 60% 5-year survival rate. **Radiation** is an acceptable alternative.

  3. **Chemotherapy** is the treatment for metastatic bladder cancer; however, there is only a 5% 2-year survival.

REFERENCES

Dale DC, Federman DD, eds. Prostate cancer. *Sci Am Med.* 2004;12:9.

Hua VN, Schaeffer AJ. Acute and chronic prostatitis. *Med Clin North Am.* 2004;88(2):483.

Lyon CJ. Urethritis. *Clin Fam Prac.* 2005;7(1):31.

Meza J, et al. Treatments for chronic prostatitis. *Am Fam Physician.* 2006;74:475.

Rosenberg M, Lakin M, eds. Medical urology for the primary care provider. *Clev Clin J Med.* 2007;74(Suppl 3).

Steinberg GD. Bladder cancer. www.emedicine.com. Accessed November 3, 2005.

62   Urticaria

Robert Ellis, MD, & Montiel Rosenthal, MD

KEY POINTS

- Urticaria or "hives" is a common disorder that causes a raised erythematous intensely pruritic rash or "wheal."
- Natural course is most often self-limited and treatment is aimed at relieving symptoms and avoiding triggers.
- Unless indicated by the history or physical examination, laboratory evaluation and additional tests are usually unnecessary.
- The etiology of urticaria is often not apparent even after careful history, physical exam, and additional tests.

I. **Definition.** Urticaria are **transient,** circumscribed, raised erythematous, sometimes burning, and intensely pruritic skin lesions or wheals of varying size. In the acute form individual lesions can last 24 hours. The evanescent nature of the wheals, or hives with their dermal edema, may lead to diagnostic confusion with other erythematous rashes. These lesions may occur in conjunction with angioedema, a nonpruritic, sometimes painful swelling of subcutaneous, dermal, and often mucosal tissue which can last up to 72 hours. In 30% of cases of urticaria where IgE is implicated, environmental, drug, dietary, and unknown factors serve as triggers to mast cells in the dermis, leading to degranulation of these cells and release of histamine. Other immune modulating substances like prostaglandins, kinins, and leukotrienes also lead to increased vascular permeability, vasodilation, and transudation of fluid from capillaries and small blood vessels into the surrounding tissue, resulting in dermal edema and hyperemia. Chronic urticaria lasts more than 6 weeks and has more complex differential diagnoses.

II. **Common Diagnoses.** Urticaria is one of the most common skin conditions encountered by family physicians. The lifetime incidence is 10% to 20%. Acute urticaria is more common than chronic urticaria and females and young adults have a higher incidence. In 60% to 70% of cases of urticaria there is no identifiable cause. This increases to 80% to 90% in chronic urticaria. The following are specific causes of urticaria.

  A. **Physical factors** (5%–10% of cases).

    1. **Dermographism** ("skin writing") is the most common physical urticaria with a lifetime prevalence of 5% and tends to affect young adults. It presents as the formation of wheals in response to shearing forces on the skin and forms within minutes. Common sites affected include the waist and neck where clothing tends to cause friction.

    2. **Delayed pressure urticaria** is deep and painful swelling that develops over 4 to 8 hours in response to a prolonged static pressure. It lasts 8 to 48 hours, can be associated with fever and malaise, and is typically seen on the soles, palms, buttocks, and posterior thighs. Males are more often affected.

    3. **Cold urticaria** is a reaction to cold stimuli and can also present on rewarming after cold exposure. Women are more likely to be affected. Cold urticaria can be associated with infections, autoimmune disease, and possibly neoplasia.

    4. **Heat urticaria** is a rare form occurring after exposure to temperatures greater than 38°C.

    5. **Solar urticaria** is a rare reaction to either visible or UV wavelengths between 280 and 760 nm.

    6. **Cholinergic urticaria,** induced by heat, emotional stress, or exercise, results in 2- to 3-mm scattered wheals surrounded by large erythematous macules.

  B. **Infections** (10%–15% of cases). Infections are a significant cause of both acute and chronic urticaria. They may account for greater than 80% of pediatric cases. Nonspecific viral infections are considered the most common causative agent. Other infections include Hepatitis A and B, bacterial infections of the nasopharynx, HIV, *Helicobacter pylori*, infectious mononucleosis, TB, syphilis, and parasites. There are no proven associations between urticaria and occult dental abscesses or gastrointestinal candidiasis.

C. Medications (5%–10% of cases). The most common causes include penicillins, cephalosporins, and sulfa drugs. Aspirin and nonsteroidal anti-inflammatory drugs may potentiate urticaria caused by other factors. Codeine and contrast dye may cause direct degranulation of mast cells. Endogenous or exogenous progesterone can also cause urticaria. Preservatives, like methylparaben, used in local anesthetics and medroxyprogesterone can cause urticaria as well.

D. Foods and **food additives** used for color, preservation, and taste may also cause urticaria. Nuts, seafood, eggs, soy, and wheat are among the foods implicated. Food as a true cause of urticaria is much less than that perceived by patients and general physicians and accounts for 1% to 15% of acute and chronic urticaria. Additives are an even rarer cause of urticaria.

E. Other: Insect bites or stings and caterpillar toxins may cause urticaria. Collagen vascular disease, autoimmune disease, antithyroid receptor antibodies, and hereditary conditions predispose to urticaria.

F. Emotional and psychogenic factors are implicated in urticaria, although there is insufficient research to support these in isolation from other factors.

III. Symptoms. Pruritus is most commonly present with urticaria and varies in severity. The intensity of the pruritis, like urticaria itself, is affected by extremes of heat and cold, the consumption of alcohol, and emotional distress. Angioedema manifests as tense swelling of lips and oral or respiratory mucosa and can lead to respiratory arrest if not addressed in sufficient time.

IV. Signs. The characteristic skin lesions of urticaria are evanescent, erythematous, well demarcated, and raised. There may be blanching of edematous central areas. Where the skin has been scratched or exposed to extremes of heat, lesions tend to be more prominent. While examining the patient, the physician should test for dermographism by firmly stroking the patient's skin and should test for other causes of physical urticaria (pressure, cold, heat, contact irritant, aquagenic, solar, and delayed pressure) when the patient's history indicates that further testing would be appropriate.

V. Laboratory Tests (Figure 62–1)

A. Acute urticaria

1. Does not require laboratory evaluation unless suggested by the patient's history and physical examination.
2. Tests usually have little diagnostic value except in urticarial vasculitis.
3. Urticarial vasculitis should be suspected in patients with individual lesions that persist for more than 48 hours, are painful, and are accompanied by ecchymosis or petechiae. Tests include skin biopsy, complete blood count (CBC) with differential, erythrocyte sedimentation rate (ESR), antinuclear antibody (ANA), and serum complement assays.
4. Consider checking for streptococcal infection in pediatric patients.

B. Chronic or persistent urticaria

1. Tests are not required for mild disease that responds to antihistamines.
2. For more severe symptoms and nonresponders, work-up includes CBC with differential, ESR, and thyroid-stimulating hormone (TSH) with antithyroid antibodies.

VI. Treatment (Table 62–1). Removal of the offending agent or management of the underlying cause are the treatments of choice when possible. If the patient has not had life-threatening angioedema as part of their symptom complex, they may benefit from a trial of provocative testing to establish a cause for urticaria if the cause was not apparent at the first visit. Patients with life-threatening angioedema or anaphylaxis should be referred for allergy testing, if no drug was implicated.

A. Patient education. If the cause of urticaria cannot be established during the office visit, the patient should be educated about possible offending agents, ideally with the help of a printed handout. Patients are often their own best detective in sifting through exacerbating factors they encounter between physician visits.

B. General measures

1. The patient should avoid vasodilating influences such as heat, emotional stress, exertion, or alcohol.
2. Cool compresses, oatmeal baths, and antipruritic lotions may provide some relief.
3. Aspirin use probably should be discontinued.
4. Urticaria and angioedema, like other skin conditions, are highly visible to the patient and may contribute to the patient's anxiety which can aggravate the condition. **Reassuring the patient** that the condition is usually self-limited can be beneficial.

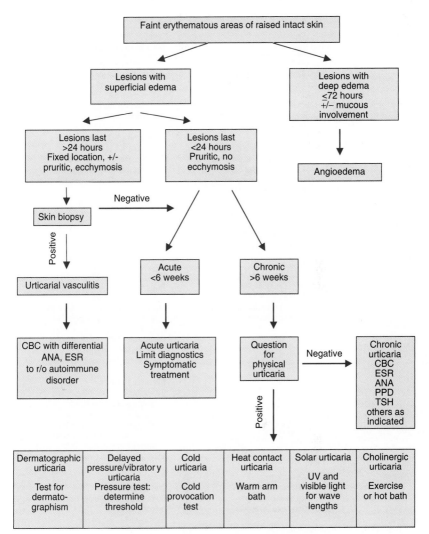

FIGURE 62–1. Diagnostic algorithm for the work-up of a rash suspicious for urticaria.

5. Follow-up care is required when the condition is prolonged ≥ for 6 weeks or more, when the condition worsens, or when new symptoms present.

C. Medications

1. Oral **antihistamines,** including ones likely to cause sedation such as **hydroxyzine, diphenhydramine, chlorpheniramine,** and relatively nonsedating ones such as **loratadine, fexofenadine, and cetirizine,** are commonly used. There is some individual variation in response.

   a. **Hydroxyzine** and **cetirizine** are sometimes more effective than other antihistamines. Cetirizine may cause sedation but less so than hydroxyzine; higher doses of these may be used to control symptoms if tolerated.

TABLE 62–1. TYPES OF URTICARIA WITH TREATMENT OPTIONS

Types of Urticaria	Initial Treatment	SOR	Other Treatment Options	SOR

Acute	H1 antihistamines
	    first generation (sedating)
	    Diphenhydramine 25–50 mg q6 h;
	        for children: 2 mg/kg/d, q 4–6 h
	    Hydroxyzine 25–50 mg q4–6 h
	    Chlorpheniramine 4 mg q4–6 h
	        (used in pregnancy; or
	        4–12 mg bid)
	    second generation (nonsedating)
	    Loratadine 10 mg qd to bid; 5 mg
	        qd for children ages 2–5 y
	    Cetirizine 10 mg qd to bid; for
	        children: 2.5–5 mg qd for
	        6–24 months, 5 mg qd for
	        ages 2–5 y, and 10 mg qd for
	        children ≥6 y
	    Fexofenadine 60–120 mg bid;
	        180 mg qd ≥ 12 y; 30 mg bid
	        6–11 y
	    Desloratadine 5 mg/d
		Ⓐ	H2 antihistamine combined with H1
			    Ranitidine 150 mg qd to bid
			    Famotidine 20–40 mg/d
			    Cimetidine 300–800 mg bid
			        (caution, multiple drug
			        interactions)
			Prednisone 50 mg/d for 3 d
			Prednisolone 1–2 mg/kg/d for
			    children
			Desensitization protocol for aspirin in
			    patients with acute coronary
			    syndrome and cardiovascular
			    disease
			Epinephrine 0.3 ml SQ of 1:1000
				Ⓑ
				
				Ⓒ
				
				Ⓑ
				
				Ⓒ

Chronic	H1 antihistamines (as above)
	Loratadine or Certirizine, and possibly
	    Mizolastine, appear to be
	        treatment of choice for chronic
	        idiopathic urticaria
		Ⓐ	H2 antihistamine combined with H1
			Doxepin 10–25 QHS can increase to
			    10–25 mg tid to qid
			Montelukast 4 mg qd for 1–5 y, 5 mg
			    qd for 6–14 y, and 10 mg qd for
			    ≥14 y
			Prednisone 30–40 mg/d in single or
			    divided dose bid, then taper
			    slowly to lowest dose that controls
			    symptoms
			Nifedipine 10 mg tid
			Cyclosporine 4 mg/kg (effective for
			    severe autoimmune-related
			    urticaria; use limited by side
			    effects and monitoring issues)
			Dapsone 100–200 mg qd (requires
			    intensive monitoring);
			Sulfasalazine 4 g qd (requires
			    intensive monitoring)
				Ⓑ
				Ⓒ
				
				Ⓑ
				
				Ⓒ
				
				Ⓒ
				Ⓐ
				
				Ⓐ
				
				Ⓒ

Physical Dermatographic Delayed pressure Cold Heat contact Solar	Avoidance of triggers H1 antihistamines (as above) High-dose H1 antihistamine H1 antihistamines (as above) Inducing tolerance Inducing tolerance with UV light or PUVA	**Ⓒ** **Ⓐ** **Ⓐ** **Ⓐ** **Ⓒ** **Ⓒ**	PUVA Corticosteroids burst Corticosteroids prolonged treatment Inducing tolerance Montelukast 10 mg qd H1 antihistamines (as above)	**Ⓒ** **Ⓒ** **Ⓒ** **Ⓒ** **Ⓒ** **Ⓐ**
Cholinergic Urticarial vasculitis	H1 antihistamines (as above) Find and treat underlying cause of vasculitis, often autoimmune	**Ⓐ** **Ⓒ**	Danazol 400–600 mg Corticosteroids prolonged treatment	**Ⓒ** **Ⓒ**

   b. Loratadine and **fexofenadine** are especially useful because they are generally nonsedating. In some patients the combination of a nonsedating antihistamine in the morning and a sedating one in the evening will be beneficial.
   c. Diphenhydramine, chlorpheniramine, cetirizine and loratadine are available without a prescription, which may represent an advantage for some patients.
 2. Other medications that are occasionally used include the following.
   a. Systemic corticosteroids are useful in severe and poorly responsive cases of urticaria. **Prednisone** can be used in various doses for adults (see Table 62–1) and

should be added to antihistamine therapy after weighing their benefits and risks. Topical corticosteroids have very little value in the treatment of urticaria.

   b. Leukotriene inhibitors (Montelukast) may be useful in some cases of urticaria. They have been shown to provide benefit in placebo-controlled trials.

   c. The subcutaneous injection of **epinephrine** may be used to confirm the transient nature of the lesions, to provide temporary relief to the acutely symptomatic patient, and in cases of anaphylaxis.

   d. Cimetidine and other H_2 antihistamines sometimes provide benefit when added to H_1 antihistamine treatment but are of little value when used alone. The use of **ephedrine, terbutaline, doxepin, nifedipine, colchicine,** and **dapsone** has been reported to benefit some patients.

REFERENCES

Charlesworth E. Urticaria and angioedema. *Allergy Asthma Proc.* 2002;23(5):341-345.
Grattan C, Powell S, Humphreys F; and British Association of Dermatologists. Management and diagnostic guidelines for urticaria and angioedema. *Br J Dermatol.* 2001;144(4):708-714.
Prodigy Guidance. Urticaria and angio-oedema. http://www.prodigy.nhs.uk, http://www.cks.library.nhs.uk/urticaria/about_this_topic
Ramanuja S, et al. Approach to "Aspirin Allergy" in cardiovascular patients. *Circulation.* 2004;110:e1-e4.
Zuberbier T. Urticaria. *Allergy.* 2003;58:1224-1234.

---

63   Vaginal Bleeding

Judith Kerber Frazier, MD, & Clark B. Smith, MD

KEY POINTS

- Patients of childbearing age with abnormal vaginal bleeding must have a negative pregnancy test result before further work-up is pursued.
- Perimenopausal patients with vaginal bleeding need an endometrial biopsy to rule out a tumor before starting treatment.
- A normal Pap smear (for **cervical** cancer) can never ensure that the patient's uterus (**endometrium**) is normal.
- Identification of the cause of abnormal bleeding determines appropriate treatment.

I. Definition. A **normal menstrual cycle** involves the sequential stimulation and withdrawal of ovarian hormones that affect the uterine endometrium. Immediately after menses, the endometrial layer is thinned and new growth is ready to occur. During the **proliferative phase,** ovarian estradiol 17-β secretion causes spiral arterial elongation and endometrial thickening. Endometrial hyperplasia develops as the epithelium becomes taller. With ovulation, progesterone is secreted by the ovarian corpus luteum (**early secretory phase**). Estradiol levels decrease as progesterone increases, causing coiled arteries to become progressively more tortuous, culminating (**late secretory phase**) in arterial vasoconstriction and ischemia, which in combination with progesterone withdrawal causes the endometrium to slough (**menses**). Normal menstrual cycles are established approximately 2 years after menarche at an average age of 12 to 13 (range: 10–16 years); cycle length averages 28 days (normal range: 21–35 days), with menses lasting 2 to 7 days (average: 4–6 days) and blood loss between 25 and 60 cc/cycle. This translates into approximately 25 pads or 30 tampons (1 box); however, since some women change pads before saturation, pad counts may not provide an accurate assessment of menstrual blood loss.

   Abnormal bleeding is when the cycle length is ≤21 days or ≥35 days, irregular/noncyclic, or involves heavy (≥80 mL per cycle) bleeding. Commonly, this is due to deviations from sequential estrogen/progesterone stimulation and withdrawal just described. Such deviations have many causes as described in the next section.

II. **Common Diagnoses.** The literature suggests that almost 20% of women have abnormal uterine bleeding at some time in their lives.

    A. **Dysfunctional uterine bleeding (DUB)** is abnormal uterine bleeding not caused by other pathology or systemic disease.

        1. **Anovulatory bleeding,** continuous unopposed endometrial estrogen stimulation, accounts for 95% of DUB in women younger than 20 years of age. This incidence falls to less than 20% in women between 20 and 40 years and then rises again to approximately 90% beginning 2 to 3 years prior to menopause.

        2. **Ovulatory bleeding,** caused by fluctuations in estrogen or progesterone levels, occurs in approximately 10% of patients with DUB. More than 50% of women have microscopic mid-cycle spotting caused by mid-cycle decreases in circulating estrogen.

    B. **Pregnancy and its complications** occur most frequently between 18 and 35 years of age. Abnormal vaginal bleeding may complicate up to one in five pregnancies. Common causes include placenta previa, placenta pathology, and spontaneous abortions.

    C. **Medications** cause abnormal vaginal bleeding. Oral contraceptives cause vaginal bleeding in 10% of users. Depot medroxyprogesterone acetate (Depo-Provera), an injectable progestin, frequently causes irregular vaginal bleeding on the first three injections. Other medication culprits include antidepressant, antihypertensive, anticoagulant, and anticholinergic drugs and digitalis, phenothiazines, steroids, tamoxifen, vitamins, herbal supplements, and illegal drugs.

    D. **Sexually transmitted diseases (STDs)** produce vaginal bleeding through cervicitis or endometritis (*Neisseria gonorrhoeae, Chlamydia trachomatis*) or necrosis when blood supply is outstripped (condyloma acuminata). Risk factors include prior history of STDs, multiple sexual partners, and lack of condom use.

    E. **Tumors**

        1. Uterine leiomyomas (fibroids), endometrial polyps, and adenomyomas (adenomyosis) are the most common **benign** tumors of the uterus, are usually seen in the 25- to 45-year age group and cause bleeding by distorting the endometrial cavity or when the tumor outstrips its blood supply.

        2. **Malignant growth,** hyperplasia, or endometrial carcinoma accounts for 10% to 15% of postmenopausal bleeding. Chronically anovulatory women have 3 times the average risk, and women taking tamoxifen have a sevenfold increased risk of endometrial hyperplasia/carcinoma. Other high-risk groups include those who are obese, diabetic, or hypertensive. Vaginal adenosis and adenocarcinoma are uncommon but are often seen in patients who had intrauterine exposure to diethylstilbestrol (DES).

    F. **Trauma and foreign bodies** are not uncommon in children. Sexual abuse of children and young teens frequently presents as abnormal bleeding. Foreign bodies may include objects that can cause abrasions or lacerations.

    G. Blood dyscrasias are very uncommon. Ten percent of women with blood dyscrasia have abnormal uterine bleeding. Twenty-five percent of women with a hereditary coagulation disorder have a negative family history. In adolescents, coagulation disorders cause up to 19% of acute menorrhagia, 25% of severe menorrhagia (hemoglobin $\leq$10 g/dL), 33% of menorrhagia requiring transfusion, and 50% of menorrhagia presenting at menarche.

    H. **Chronic or acute conditions** that can affect vaginal bleeding include weight changes, emotional problems, chronic illness, and endocrine disorders. These include thyroid abnormalities (both hypo- and hyperthyroidism), pituitary adenomas, liver disease, and diabetes

III. **Symptoms.** The history should include the **age of menarche, menstrual pattern**/timing (including last menstrual period and previous menstrual period), **duration** (i.e., number of bleeding days), and estimated **amount of menstrual bleeding.**

    A. **Menstrual pattern**

        1. **Amenorrhea** preceding the abnormal bleeding, without signs or symptoms of pregnancy or recent oral contraceptive use, suggests anovulatory bleeding, particularly in the adolescent or perimenopausal patient. In the perimenopausal or postmenopausal patient, a period of amenorrhea preceding abnormal bleeding suggests endometrial carcinoma.

        2. **Unpredictable bleeding** suggests anovulatory bleeding.

        3. **Mid-cycle predictable spotting** suggests mid-cycle estrogen deficiency.

    4. Predictable **late cycle** spotting or bleeding suggests persistent corpus luteum or luteal phase defect.

    5. Irregular bleeding is common in the **first 3 months of oral contraceptive pill use.**

B. Premenstrual symptoms (e.g., breast tenderness, mood swings, and bloating) tend to be associated with ovulatory cycles.

C. Fever, particularly if associated with pelvic or abdominal pain or dyspareunia, may suggest an STD, pelvic inflammatory disease (PID), or sepsis associated with abortion.

D. A history of **easy bruising** may indicate coagulation defects, drug or medication use, or dietary extremes. **Multiple injuries** may indicate trauma, which can include spouse or child abuse.

E. History of **maternal drug use during pregnancy** (e.g., DES), particularly in adolescents with abnormal bleeding, suggests congenital anomalies of the genitourinary tract, including carcinoma of the upper vagina.

F. Headaches and **visual changes** may suggest a CNS cause, such as a pituitary neoplasm.

IV. Signs. The physical examination should include a pelvic examination, which may require anesthesia in very young girls or those who have not used tampons. Rectal bimanual examination is not a substitute for pelvic examination, since the rectal examination fails to reveal most vaginal or cervical causes or to allow for adequate evaluation of the uterus or adenexal structures.

A. Pallor not associated with tachycardia or signs of hypovolemia suggests **chronic** excessive blood loss such as that found in anovulatory bleeding, adenomyosis, uterine myomas, or blood dyscrasia.

B. If **signs of shock** or impending shock are present, the blood loss is likely related to pregnancy (including ectopic pregnancy).

C. Pelvic masses may represent pregnancy, uterine or ovarian neoplasia, pelvic abscess, or hematoma.

D. Fever, leukocytosis, and **pelvic tenderness** strongly suggest PID.

E. Fine, **thinning hair** and **hypoactive or slow-reactive reflexes** suggest hypothyroidism.

F. Ecchymoses or **multiple bruises** may indicate trauma (including sexual abuse or incest), coagulation defects, drug use, medication effects, or dietary extremes.

V. Laboratory Tests (Figure 63-1) should be directed by history and physical findings. For detailed evaluation of the following causes of vaginal bleeding, see the chapters indicated: PID, Chapter 51; child abuse, Chapter 91; contraceptives, Chapter 95; and pregnancy and complications, Chapter 97. Thyroid-stimulating hormone (TSH) can screen for thyroid abnormalities, prolactin level for pituitary adenoma, and an abnormal blood sugar can lead to the evaluation of possible diabetes or possible polycystic ovarian disease.

A. Endometrial biopsy (EB) is an easy office procedure to sample tissue for pathological evaluation.

    1. Indications

        a. Frequent or exceptionally heavy or prolonged **bleeding refractory to a course of cyclic hormonal therapy.**

        b. Risk factors for endometrial cancer (i.e., unopposed estrogen or patients who are diabetic, hypertensive, or obese).

        c. Women older than 30 years with irregular bleeding or any postmenopausal patient with vaginal bleeding that has become unpredictable and irregular in the last 12 months.

        d. Unexplained vaginal bleeding.

    2. Contraindications to EB include pregnancy, acute infection, PID, or known bleeding disorder (including coumadin use).

    3. Timing and patient preparation. With irregular sporadic menses, EB should be performed on the presumed first or second day of menses; EB can be performed at any time in women with continuous bleeding. Premedication with a nonsteroidal anti-inflammatory drug (NSAID) such as ibuprofen, taken orally about 2 hours before the procedure, is adequate to control postprocedure cramping. Antibiotic prophylaxis is unnecessary for endometrial sampling. A signed consent must be obtained and potential complications (i.e., pain, bleeding, infection, uterine perforation, bowel or bladder injury) explained prior to the procedure. Since this is a blind procedure, a poor sample may be obtained, necessitating repeat of the procedure. There must be documentation in the chart that the risks were explained to the patient.

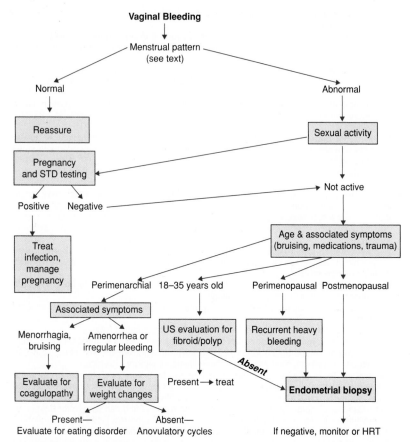

Vaginal Bleeding

FIGURE 63–1. Primary care evaluation of vaginal bleeding. HRT, Hormone replacement therapy; STD, sexually transmitted disease; US, ultrasound.

4. **The procedure** begins with the patient in lithotomy (Pap smear) position. A manual examination will tell the size and orientation of the uterus. A sterile speculum is then placed and the cervix cleaned with povidone iodine. This is easier if ring forceps are used with cotton balls of 4×4 s. A topical anesthetic (e.g., Hurricaine or benzocaine) can be applied to the cervix for patient comfort. A tenaculum is placed on the upper portion of the cervix for counter traction. A sterile sound is gently inserted into the endocervical canal to measure the depth of the uterus; normal is 6 to 8 cm. Pulling the cervix up and outward by placing gentle traction on the tenaculum can facilitate this. If the sound cannot be inserted, a dilator may be necessary to enlarge the cervical canal. The sterile pipette is then inserted through the os and advanced to the depth measured by the sound. At this point the piston on the pipette is pulled back to aspirate a sample. This process is repeated as the pipette is moved to sample multiple areas of the endometrium, in a clockwise fashion. The sample is then evacuated into a specimen cup with formalin preservative. Large volumes of aspirate may necessitate reinserting the pipette and repeating the above procedure, being cautious not to touch the pipette tip to the specimen cup. Blood clots may be seen in the sample; endometrial tissue will be denser. After adequate sample is obtained, the tenaculum and the speculum are

removed. Patients should be cautioned to expect slight bleeding and cramping (like a menstrual period).

5. **Cytologic evaluation** provides information about endometrial cycle stages. (SOR **B**)
   a. **Endometrial hyperplasia with cytologic atypia** progresses to endometrial carcinoma in approximately 25% of cases; without atypia, fewer than 2% progress to carcinoma.
   b. **Adenomatous endometrial hyperplasia** means a superficial carcinoma is present.
   c. **Other cytologic findings** include infection, proliferative versus secretory endometrium, endometrial hyperplasia, or atrophic endometrium and neoplasia.

B. **Hysteroscopy** is a visualization of the endometrium. It is an office procedure but requires special training and equipment. If performed prior to endometrial sampling, hysteroscopy reveals abnormalities missed by endometrial sampling or dilation and curettage (D&C) alone in up to 30% of patients. Hysteroscopy is easier to perform when the patient is not bleeding, but it can be done at any time.

C. **Transabdominal and transvaginal ultrasound** may help delineate **pelvic masses** and can provide information regarding endometrial thickness, uterine size, and the presence of small ovarian cysts such as a persistent corpus luteum cyst that may be significant. In some cases, ultrasound with saline injection will give more detail than ultrasound alone. (SOR **B**)

D. Patients with palpable or ultrasound-proven **pelvic masses** require **computerized tomography** or **magnetic resonance imaging scans**.

VI. **Treatment.** Treatment of abnormal vaginal bleeding should be directed at the underlying cause. Symptomatic treatment depends on the amount of bleeding. A hemoglobin (Hgb) ≤ 7 g/dL requires hospitalization for stabilization, parenteral hormone therapy, and blood transfusion. If Hgb is between 7 and 10 g and the patient is symptomatic (tachycardia, hypoxia, or positive tilt test), hospitalization should also be considered. If Hgb is ≥ 10 g and vital signs are stable, treatment may be with one of the following regimens.

A. **Outpatient therapy** for acute bleeding.
   1. **Progestins** such as medroxyprogesterone acetate (Provera), 20 mg orally initially followed by 10 mg twice daily for 7 days, or aqueous medroxyprogesterone acetate (Depo-Provera), 200 mg intramuscularly.
   2. **Oral contraceptives** such as Lo-Ovral, 4 times daily for 4 days, tapered over 7 to 10 days. (SOR **A**)

B. Once acute bleeding is controlled, **subsequent hormonal therapy** can include:
   1. Provera, 10 mg orally each day for the first 10 days of each calendar month (or from days 16 to 25 of the menstrual cycle) for 3 to 6 months. Alternatively, **oral contraceptives** can be used for a period of 3 to 6 months. However, if bleeding is due to anovulation, oral contraceptives may prolong the problem.
   2. **Estrogen replacement therapy** can be considered in the menopausal patient symptomatic from estrogen deficiency once endometrial or other pelvic malignancy has been excluded (see Chapter 78).
   3. **Gonadotropin-releasing hormone (GnRH) therapy and uterine fibroid embolization** may be used for fibroids (see Chapter 51).
   4. **Hysterectomy** or other surgical treatment may be appropriate in patients with neoplasms, endometriosis, adenomyosis, or chronic PID. (SOR **B**)
   5. With infrequent, asymptomatic bleeding and normal complete blood cell count, reassurance and an accurate explanation of the physiology of the cause are sufficient. Additional oral iron supplementation should be used in anemic patients until iron stores are replenished (see Chapter 4). Forty percent of chronic menorrhagia patients may also respond to a D&C. Oral NSAIDs, such as ibuprofen, 600 to 800 mg thrice daily for 5 days, effectively reduce blood loss in chronic menorrhagia but are ineffective for acute bleeding episodes or in regulating noncyclic bleeding.

REFERENCES

Albers J. Abnormal uterine bleeding. *Am Fam Physician.* 2004;69:195-126.
Evans P. Uterine fibroid tumors: diagnosis and treatment. *Am Fam Physician.* 2007;75:1503-1508.
Schranger S. Abnormal uterine bleeding associated with hormonal contraception. *Am Fam Physician.* 2002;65:2073.
Zuber T. Endometrial biopsy. *Am Fam Physician.* 2001;63:1131, 1137, 1139.

64   Vaginal Discharge

L. Peter Schwiebert, MD

KEY POINTS

- A careful history, physical examination, and office laboratory studies allow arrival at an appropriate diagnosis for common causes of vaginal discharge.
- Sexually transmitted diseases (STDs) often coexist; the presence of risk factors for one should prompt screening for others.
- It is important to base treatment of vaginal discharge on solid clinical documentation to avoid inappropriate treatment and resulting drug resistance, excessive cost, and iatrogenic vaginitis.

I. **Definition.** From menarche to menopause, estrogen stimulates proliferation and glycogen production by vaginal squamous epithelial cells on which lactobacilli depend; these lacto-bacilli produce hydrogen peroxide (toxic to most vaginal pathogens) and lactic acid, resulting in a vaginal pH of 3.5 to 4.5. Normal (physiologic) discharge varies among women and with the stage of a woman's menstrual cycle; normal cervical discharge is clear to slightly opaque.

This chapter focuses on vaginal discharge that is unusual in amount or odor, or causes symptoms, such as itching or burning, and these are often caused by alterations in the physiologic vaginal environment. Such unusual or symptomatic discharge may be related to

A. **Hypoestrogenic states** (in prepubertal or postmenopausal women), which thin the vagi-nal epithelium, decrease glycogen levels, raise pH to ≥ 5.0, and create a mixed vaginal flora.

B. **Sexually transmitted pathogens** (e.g., *Neisseria gonorrhoeae*, *Chlamydia trachomatis*, and *Trichomonas vaginalis*), which stimulate inflammatory response, raise vaginal pH, or both.

C. **Irritants** (e.g., douching, some spermicides), which can alter physiologic vaginal pH and create a favorable environment for pathogens.

D. **Immunocompromise or suppression of normal flora by antibiotics**, which permits overgrowth of opportunistic organisms (e.g., *Candida* species). (*Candida* also grows well in the glycogen-rich vaginas of reproductive-age women, but has no such substrate in premenarchial or postmenopausal females and is therefore rare in these groups.)

II. **Common Diagnoses.** In the ambulatory primary care setting, vaginal discharge is the most common gynecologic complaint and the 10th to 15th most common presenting complaint, resulting in more than 10 million physician office visits annually. These figures underestimate the true prevalence of the problem, however, since many women with discharge or odor do not seek medical attention. Up to 90% of all cases of vaginitis are because of bacterial vaginosis (BV), vulvovaginal candidiasis (VVC), or Trichomonas.

A. **BV** accounts for up to 40% to 50% of cases of vaginitis, with prevalence varying, depend-ing on the population studied (i.e., 15%–19% of ambulatory gynecology patients and 24%–40% of patients attending STD clinics). Risk factors for BV include more than one sexual partner over the previous 3 months, use of intrauterine device (IUD), douching, and pregnancy.

B. **VVC** (approximately 20%–25% of cases) is the second most common cause of vaginitis in the United States and the most common cause in Europe. Up to 75% of women have an episode of VVC at some point and up to 5% have recurrent episodes. Risk factors for VVC include recent antibiotic use (especially penicillins, tetracycline, or cephalosporins); oral contraceptive pills (OCPs) or systemic glucocorticoid use; pregnancy; poorly controlled diabetes mellitus; obesity; immunocompromised state; or diaphragm or spermicide use. *Candida albicans* is the pathogen in 80% to 90% of VVC, with increased likelihood of non*albicans* infection (e.g., *C. glabrata* or *Candida tropicalis*) with immunocompromise, long-term anticandidal treatment, or ≥ 4 documented episodes of VVC more than a year.

C. **Trichomonas vaginitis** (15%–20% of cases), a true STD, is the third most common cause of vaginitis; risk factors include IUD or tobacco use or multiple sex partners. Twenty to

TABLE 64–1. SYMPTOMS AND SIGNS OF VAGINAL DISCHARGE

Condition	Complaint	Appearance of Discharge and Mucosa
Bacterial vaginosis	Odor or vaginal discharge	Thin, watery, grayish discharge; minimal mucosal erythema
Candida vaginitis	Vulvar itching or burning (50% specificity), external dysuria	Curdy white discharge; sometimes erythematous vaginal epithelium
Cervicitis	Mucoid discharge, intermenstrual spotting, dyspareunia	Yellow, mucoid endocervical discharge; inflamed cervix with focal hemorrhage
Trichomonas vaginitis	Discharge, vulvar itching	Typically copious, frothy; green or yellow discharge; punctate cervical hemorrhage sometimes present; vulvar and vaginal erythema
Physiologic discharge	Discharge without itching or odor	Clear to slightly opaque cervical discharge
Atrophic vaginitis	Discharge, burning, or dyspareunia, or all three	Thin and inflamed with loss of rugal folds; discharge, if present, is watery and may be foul-smelling

fifty percent of women with *T. vaginalis* are asymptomatic, and 23% of patients with this infection are also infected with *N. gonorrhoeae*.

D. Cervicitis, caused by *C. trachomatis*, herpes simplex virus, or *N. gonorrhoeae*, accounts for up to 20% to 25% of cases of vaginal discharge. Risk factors include recent new sex partners, lack of contraceptive use (including barrier contraceptives), and age younger than 24 years.

E. Physiologic discharge (10% of cases) is a result of normal variations in cervical or vaginal mucus production.

F. Atrophic vaginitis (10%–40% of postmenopausal women) is because of natural or induced (e.g., radiation/chemotherapy, oophorectomy, and antiestrogenic medications) hypoestrogenic states.

G. Allergic vaginitis (frequency unknown) is caused by topical sensitizers or irritants, such as synthetic tampons, spermicides, hygienic sprays, soaps, perfumes, povidone-iodine solution, latex condoms, or douches.

III. Symptoms and Signs (Table 64–1).

IV. Laboratory Tests (Table 64–2). A careful history and examination, coupled with office laboratory studies, allows confident assessment of common causes of vaginal discharge.

A. A wet preparation is made by adding a drop of normal saline to a drop of vaginal discharge on a glass slide and then examining the slide with a microscope.

TABLE 64–2. OFFICE LABORATORY FINDINGS IN VAGINAL DISCHARGE

Condition	pH (from Vaginal Walls, not Cervix)/ Color of Nitrazine Paper	Wet and Potassium Hydroxide (KOH) Preparations
Bacterial vaginosis	$\geq$4.5/green to purple	Clue cells (bacteria obscuring epithelial cell border in 90% of cases), few WBCs on wet preparation amine "fishy" odor on addition of KOH ($\geq$90% sensitive)
Candida vaginitis	3.5–4.5/yellow to green	Spores and hyphae on KOH preparation (21% sensitive)
Cervicitis	$\geq$4.0/yellow to purple	Mature squames, $\geq$10 WBCs (50%–70% sensitive) on wet preparation
Trichomonas vaginitis	$\geq$4.5/green to purple	Mature squames with many WBCs on wet preparation, motile protozoa can be seen in 60% of cases
Physiologic discharge	$\leq$4.0/yellow	Normal superficial epithelial cells, lactobacilli, no WBCs or spores on wet preparation
Atrophic vaginitis	$\geq$5.0/green to purple	Wet preparation shows many WBCs, small round epithelial cells (parabasal cells) which are immature squames unexposed to sufficient estrogen

WBCs: white blood cells.

B. A potassium hydroxide (KOH) preparation is made similarly using a drop of 10% KOH solution instead of saline.

C. Nitrazine paper changes color in response to changes in the pH of vaginal discharge. A 1- to 2-inch strip of Nitrazine paper is applied to secretions on the vaginal walls or pooled in the posterior fornix.

D. Cultures. Because of the fairly low sensitivity of wet and KOH preparations in diagnosing Candida vaginitis, Trichomonas vaginitis, and cervicitis, cultures for *Candida, Trichomonas, N. gonorrhoeae*, and *C. trachomatis* should be performed in high-risk patients (see Sections II.A–D) if KOH and wet preparations show negative results. In addition, all pregnant women should be screened for *C. trachomatis* and *N. gonorrhoeae*.

> **1.** Culture results for *C. trachomatis* are unavailable for 4 to 7 days. Direct immunofluorescence and enzyme immunoassays are available. The positive predictive value (PPV) depends on the prevalence of *C. trachomatis* studied in the population. So far, studies indicate that direct immunofluorescence has a better PPV than the enzyme immunoassay in populations at intermediate risk. The PPV of neither test has been adequately studied in populations with a low prevalence of *C. trachomatis* infection.
>
> **2.** Culture for cure following treatment of cervicitis with a recommended regimen (see Section V.E.1) is not necessary. However, cultures should be repeated 1 to 2 months after finishing treatment to detect reinfection.

E. Serologic **syphilis test (e.g., VDRL), human immunodeficiency virus (HIV) testing (e.g., enzyme-linked immunosorbent assay [ELISA])**, and counseling should be offered to patients with documented *N. gonorrhoeae* infection.

F. Other tests.

> **1.** The Hansel stain is a modified Wright–Giemsa stain that enhances eosinophils. This test should be considered in women with persistent discharge in whom the usual tests are normal and no other diagnosis is obvious. In one unpublished study of 50 patients with vaginal discharge, 12% had no evidence of infection and also had more than 25% eosinophils in their discharge using the Hansel stain.
>
> **2.** A PCR test (not yet available) offers improved sensitivity/specificity compared to wet mount in diagnosis of trichomonas (84% and 94%, respectively, for PCR versus 52% and 78%, respectively, for wet mount).
>
> **3.** New self-administered tests for BV (e.g., QuickVue Advance pH and Amines test and QuickVue Advance G. vaginalis test) offer rapidity and reasonably high sensitivity/specificity.

V. Treatment

A. General measures. The patient should be instructed to do the following:

> **1.** Discontinue irritating agents (e.g., sprays or bubble baths).
>
> **2.** Wear nonocclusive, absorbent clothing (cotton rather than nylon underclothing).
>
> **3.** Use barrier contraceptives (e.g., condom or diaphragm) to prevent recurrence. (Oil-based intravaginal creams and suppositories may weaken latex condoms and diaphragms and risk unintended pregnancy.)
>
> **4.** Restore a normal vaginal environment (i.e., pH and flora). Some clinicians recommend use of lactobacillus suppositories or oral yogurt.
>
> **5.** Practice good perineal hygiene (i.e., wiping from front to back).

B. BV is diagnosed (90% sensitivity) if three of the following four criteria are met: (1) homogeneous gray discharge adherent to vaginal walls, (2) vaginal pH of ≥4.5, (3) positive "whiff test" (fishy odor on addition of KOH to wet prep), or (4) clue cells are present (Amsel's criteria). Other scoring systems (Nugent, Spiegel) focus on the mix of bacterial morphotypes, with the likelihood of BV increasing with decreasing prevalence of lactobacilli (long gram-positive rods).

> **1.** Metronidazole (e.g., Flagyl or Protostat), 500 mg orally twice a day for 7 days, has been the standard therapy (SOR **A**). Single-dose therapy (2 g) is the least expensive treatment and an effective option when compliance is a problem. Other effective regimens are metronidazole vaginal gel 0.75% (e.g., MetroGel), 5 g vaginally twice daily for 5 days, or clindamycin (e.g., Cleocin), 300 mg twice a day orally or applied vaginally as a 2% cream for 7 days.
>
> **2.** Although BV is associated with sexual activity, there is currently no evidence that treatment of sex partners prevents recurrences.
>
> **3.** BV is associated with adverse pregnancy outcomes (preterm labor, premature ruptured membranes, chorioamnionitis, preterm birth, postpartum endometritis, and postcesarean section wound infection). Although to date there is no evidence of teratogenic or mutagenic effects of metronidazole on newborns, its use is still recommended

TABLE 64–3. TREATMENT OF VULVOVAGINAL CANDIDIASIS

Medication	Proprietary Name	Formulation	Dosage*
Clotrimazole	Gyne-Lotrimin, Mycelex, Mycelex-7[†], Mycelex-G	100-mg vaginal suppository, 1% vaginal cream, 500-mg tablet	Once daily for 7 d or twice daily for 3 d, 1 applicatorful daily for 7–14 d, 1 tablet for 1 d
Miconazole	Monistat 7[†], Monistat 7[†], Monistat 3[†], Monistat 3, Combination[†]	2% vaginal cream, 100-mg vaginal suppository, 200-mg vaginal suppository, 200-mg suppository, 2% cream	1 applicatorful daily for 7 d, 1 tablet for 7 d, 1 daily for 3 d, 1 suppository daily for 3 d; cream prn
Butoconazole	Femstat 3[†], Mycelex-3[†]	2% cream	1 applicatorful daily for 3 d
Tioconazole	Vagistat-1[†]	6.5% ointment	1 applicatorful for 1 d
Terconazole	Terazol 3, Terazol 7, Terazol 3 suppository	0.8% cream, 0.4% cream, 80-mg vaginal suppository	1 applicatorful daily for 3 d, 1 applicatorful daily for 7 d, 1 daily for 3 d
Nystatin	Mycostatin	100,000-U vaginal tablet	1 daily for 14 d
Fluconazole	Diflucan	150-mg tablet	1 orally for 1 d
Ketoconazole	Nizoral	400-mg tablet	1 orally twice a day for 5 d
Itraconazole	Sporanox	200-mg tablet	1 orally either twice a day for 1 d or daily for 3 d

*Unless otherwise indicated, the route of administration is intravaginal; for daily doses, the preferred administration time is at bedtime.
[†] Available over the counter.

only after the first trimester. Dosing with it or clindamycin is as in nonpregnant women. The USPSTF recommends against using intravaginal agents, especially clindamycin, during pregnancy.

4. BV has an overall recurrence rate of 30%; recurrent BV is treated with twice weekly metronidazole gel for 4 to 6 months (70% cure rate during treatment versus 39% for control group) (SOR **B**). There is a high relapse rate if treatment is discontinued.

5. Screening asymptomatic pregnant women for BV is currently not recommended in absence of a prior history of preterm delivery (SOR **A**).

C. **VVC** (Table 64–3). A growing issue in management of VVC is the availability and heavy use of over-the-counter (OTC) medications (VVC preparations are the 10th best-selling OTC products in the United States). In one study, only 28% of women who thought they had VVC actually did and only 11% of women responding to another survey recognized the classic symptoms of VVC. This results in inappropriate treatment, increasing incidence of resistant Candida strains and, in some situations, induction of irritant vaginitis. One guideline (SOR **C**) lists the following criteria for self-medication with OTC antifungals: previous physician diagnosis of VVC, age 16 to 60 years, typical symptoms (vulvar itching, curdy discharge, no odor, two or less acute episodes over prior 6 months).

1. **Uncomplicated infection** (healthy host, infrequent occurrences, mild to moderate symptoms).

   a. Imidazole creams, ointments, or suppositories share similar efficacy ($\geq$80%) in curing uncomplicated VVC.

   b. Tioconazole and terconazole are effective against a broader spectrum of *Candida* species than butoconazole, clotrimazole, or miconazole.

   c. Single-dose fluconazole (e.g., Diflucan) is less expensive, better tolerated, and at least as effective as standard 3- to 7-day intravaginal regimens. Treatment with oral azoles is contraindicated during pregnancy; topical agents should be used.

2. For **complicated VVC** (moderate or severe symptoms or risk factors—see Section II.B), extending standard therapy to 10 to 14 days for acute symptoms may be effective. If using oral therapy, a second 150 mg fluconazole dose 3 days after the initial dose improves response.

3. For **recurrent VVC** ($\geq$4 microscopically or culture-documented episodes in a year), the following may be effective:

    a. Because of the increased likelihood of non*albicans* infection in recurrent VVC, culture is advisable.

    b. Medication should be prescribed for 10 to 14 days, with efficacy confirmed by negative posttreatment fungal culture.

    c. This should be followed by a 6-month maintenance regimen; options include fluconazole, 150 mg/week or clotrimazole, 500 mg vaginally per week. ***Note:*** Chronic daily use of oral medications can interact with other medications (e.g., theophylline, anticonvulsants, anticoagulants, and OCPs), can be hepatotoxic, and may be teratogenic.

    d. Repopulating vaginal lactobacillus using yogurt douches may be effective.

    e. If non*albicans* infection is documented, intravaginal terconazole or oral itraconazole may be more effective than standard regimens.

    f. Studies of complementary and alternative medications in treatment of vaginitis are largely inconclusive and poorly controlled; boric acid suppositories show some promise in women with candida and possibly BV failing traditional topical and oral therapies.

D. Trichomonas vaginitis

    1. Standard regimen. Metronidazole in a single 2-g dose for both the patient and her sex partner(s) shows a $\geq$90% cure rate.

    2. Treatment of pregnant patients. Approximately 30% of symptomatic patients in the first trimester obtain relief with clotrimazole vaginal suppositories (100 mg at bedtime for 7 days). After the first trimester, metronidazole may be given in standard dosing.

    3. Recurrent Trichomonas vaginitis. Metronidazole-resistant *T. vaginalis* has been documented. As of yet, there is no proven effective treatment for it; however, metronidazole, 2 g orally for 3 to 5 days, may be effective (SOR **C**).

E. Cervicitis. Empiric therapy for *C. trachomatis* or *N. gonorrhoeae* can be instituted in high-risk individuals while awaiting culture results.

    1. Because of the coprevalence of *N. gonorrhoeae* and *C. trachomatis* infection, patients should be treated with ceftriaxone (e.g., Rocephin), 250 mg intramuscularly (one dose) and doxycycline, 100 mg orally twice daily for 7 days. Alternatives to ceftriaxone for *N. gonorrhoeae* include cefixime (e.g., Suprax), 400 mg, or ciprofloxacin (e.g., Cipro), 250 mg, or ofloxacin (e.g., Floxin), 400 mg orally for one dose. Alternatives to doxycycline for *C. trachomatis* include azithromycin, 1.0 g orally for one dose, or erythromycin base 500 mg, or erythromycin ethylsuccinate, 800 mg orally 4 times daily for 7 days. **Pregnant or breast-feeding women should receive ceftriaxone plus erythromycin.**

    2. Acyclovir, or a similar nucleoside analogue, should be given in standard doses for herpes simplex virus (see Chapter 31).

F. No treatment other than reassurance is necessary for **physiologic discharge.**

G. Seventy-five to ninty percent of patients with **atrophic vaginitis** obtain relief with standard oral estrogen replacement, with added benefits of relief of vasomotor symptoms and osteoporosis prevention. (However, such benefits must be weighed against potential risks of combined estrogen/progestogen therapy found in the Women's Health Initiative study released in July 2002.) Other therapeutic options include transvaginal estrogen creams, pessaries, or a hormone-releasing ring (e.g., Estring). The latter offers advantages of only needing replacement every 3 months, not being messy, and allowing consistent estrogen release at levels low enough to avoid endometrial stimulation. Topical vaginal lubricants (e.g., Vagisil, Replens) can also provide some relief for symptoms of atrophic vaginitis.

H. Treatment for **allergic vaginitis** is elimination of likely sensitizers.

REFERENCES

Anderson MR, Klink K, Cohrssen A. Evaluation of vaginal complaints. *JAMA.* 2004;291:1368.

Owen MK, Clenney TL. Management of vaginitis. *Am Fam Physic.* 2004;70:2125.

Sobel JD, Ferris D, Schwebke J, et al. Suppressive antibacterial therapy with 0.75% metronidazole vaginal gel to prevent recurrent bacterial vaginosis. *Am J Obstet Gynecol.* 2006;194:1283.

Sobel JD. What's new in bacterial vaginosis and trichomoniasis? *Infect Dis Clin N Am.* 2005;19:387.

US Preventive Services Task Force. Screening for bacterial vaginosis in pregnancy: recommendations and rationale. *Am Fam Physic.* 2002;65:1147.

Van Kessel K, Assefi N, Marrazzo J, Eckert L. Common complementary and alternative therapies for yeast vaginitis and bacterial vaginosis: a systematic review. *Obstet Gynecol Surv.* 2003;58:351.

65   Wheezing

Judith Kerber Frazier, MD

KEY POINTS

- The *cause* of wheezing should be identified based on the patient's age, and diseases other than asthma should be considered.
- **Respiratory distress** (cyanosis, retractions, apnea, or stridor) should be assessed immediately. Oxygen should be applied if needed and evaluation continued in the emergency department.
- **Chest x-ray** should be done in patients who present with new-onset wheezing.

I. **Definition.** Wheezing is a high-pitched musical sound produced by the lungs when airways become narrowed. Wheezing produces a sound similar to deep breathing with a child's party kazoo in the mouth.

II. **Common Diagnoses**

   A. **Infants younger than 2 years**

      1. **Acute viral respiratory tract infections (RTIs)** cause up to 50% of wheezing. Risk factors for RTIs include fall or winter season, child younger than 2 years, history of atopy (allergies or allergic skin conditions), hospitalization, school-aged siblings, day care attendance, passive smoke from parents or caregivers, and bottle-feeding.

      2. **Acute bronchitis and pneumonia** causes 33% to 50% of wheezing in infants. Most cases are caused by viral infection. Risk factors include passive smoke exposure, viral upper respiratory infection (URI), and impaired gag reflex.

      3. **Bronchiolitis** is caused by viral infections, especially respiratory syncytial virus (RSV), and accounts for $\leq$5% of wheezing. RSV is the most important cause of bronchiolitis and pneumonia in children younger than 2 years. It is epidemic in winter and spring in temperate climates. RSV is seen in all age groups, but preterm infants are at greater risk.

      4. **Aspiration** is seen in 1 in 300 infants. Gastroesophageal reflux (GER) is physiologic. It peaks at 1 to 4 months of age and usually resolves by 12 months. True gastroesophageal reflux disease (GERD) is pathologic. It presents with persistent respiratory symptoms, poor weight gain, and esophagitis. Other risk factors include anatomic abnormalities (pyloric stenosis, hiatal hernia, webs, malrotation, etc.). Foreign body aspiration must also be considered.

      5. **Cystic fibrosis (CF)** has an incidence of 1 in 3500 births in whites. It is an inherited autosomal recessive trait that predisposes the patient to respiratory infections. Risk factors include white race and family history.

      6. **Anaphylaxis or hypersensitivity** requires that the patient must have had a prior exposure to the offending agent, often a drug (aspirin), food, bee sting, or exercise.

   B. **Children (age 2 years to teenage)**

      1. **RTIs.**

      2. **Acute bronchitis and pneumonia.**

      3. **Anaphylaxis or hypersensitivity.**

      4. **Asthma** causes 10% to 15% of wheezing in children (see Chapter 68). Risk factors for asthma include viral URI, family history, environmental exposures, passive smoke, age older than 2 years, and allergic rhinitis. Asthma in patients younger than age 2 may be called hyperreactive airway disease (HRAD).

   C. **Adult (young age to middle age)**

      1. **RTIs**

      2. **Acute bronchitis and pneumonia**

      3. **Asthma**

      4. **Anaphylaxis or hypersensitivity**

   D. **Elderly (older than 50 years)**

      1. **RTIs.**

   2. **Acute bronchitis and pneumonia.**
   3. **Chronic obstructive pulmonary disease (COPD)** (see Chapter 70) affects more than 14 million Americans. Risk factors include current or prior smoking history of $\geq$20 pack-years, air pollution, environmental exposures, α_1-antitrypsin deficiency, and family history.
   4. **Congestive heart failure (CHF)** (see Chapter 72) affects more than 5 million people in the United States. Risk factors include hypertension, glucose intolerance, smoking, cardiomegaly, atrial fibrillation, electrocardiogram abnormalities, coronary artery disease, and valvular heart disease.
   5. **Aspiration can be caused by either secretions or a foreign body.**
   6. **Anaphylaxis or hypersensitivity.**
   7. **Pulmonary embolus** is rare and causes wheezing because of clot obstruction of pulmonary vessels. Risk factors include hypercoagulable state, prolonged bed rest, postsurgical changes, and CHF.
III. **Symptoms** (Table 65–1).
   A. Every symptom may not be present in each case.
   B. Additional symptoms may also be present. Must look at the entire picture, not just the patient's lung sounds.
IV. **Signs.** Systematic chest examination is essential and may provide clues to the cause of wheezing.
   A. **Inspection**
      1. **Respiratory rate** should be determined. (Normal is approximately 12–20 breaths per minute in adults; the normal rate in children varies with age.) Patients in trouble can often not speak complete sentences, as they cannot catch their breath.

TABLE 65–1. SYMPTOMS WITH COMMON CAUSES OF WHEEZING

	Wheeze	Fever	Cough	Sore Throat	Rhinorrhea	Lethargy	Onset	Other
Acute viral infection	x	x	x	x	x		Rapid	Coryza
Pneumonia/ bronchitis	x	x	x				Rapid	
Bronchiolitis	x	x	x	x	x	x	Rapid	
GER/GERD	x		x				Gradual	Hoarseness
CF	x					x	Gradual	Irritability Poor feeding Meconium ileus Pancreatic insufficiency
Anaphylaxis	x		x				Rapid	Urticaria Stridor Chest discomfort Lump in throat Flushing N/V/D
Asthma	x		x		x		Gradual	Evening wheezing or coughing
COPD	x		Chronic				Gradual	Recurrent bronchitis Barrel chest
CHF	x		x				Gradual	Lower extremity swelling JVD
PE	x		x				Rapid	Acute shortness of breath Increased respiratory rate

CF, cystic fibrosis; CHF, congestive heart failure; COPD, chronic obstructive pulmonary disease; GER, gastroesophageal reflux; GERD, gastroesophageal reflux disease; JVD, jugular venous distention; N/V/D, nausea/vomiting/diarrhea; PE, pulmonary embolism.

2. **Intercostal retractions,** irregular abdominal breathing motions (or tummy breathing), are clues to respiratory distress.
3. A **barrel chest** is often associated with COPD, asthma, and CF.
B. **Percussion.** Symmetrical resonance is normal, whereas either dullness or hyperresonance may indicate asthma.
C. **Auscultation**
   1. A **prolonged expiratory phase** suggests constricted airways. It is noted by a continued exhale beyond normal duration.
   2. **Localized rhonchi (sounds like velcro coming apart)** may signify pneumonia.
D. **Associated nonpulmonary findings** in wheezing patients.
   1. **Dennie's pleats** (a crease under the eyes from repeated rubbing) and **allergic shiners** (dark circles under the eyes) are often seen in patients with allergic rhinitis or asthma.
   2. **Jugular venous distention** and bilateral dependent edema are associated with CHF (see Chapter 72).

V. **Laboratory Tests**
A. Posteroanterior and lateral views of **chest radiographs (CXR).**
   1. **Patients with a first episode of wheezing** require a CXR.
      a. **Consolidations** suggest pneumonia. A CXR may not show an infiltrate until 3 days into the disease.
      b. **Cardiomegaly** (an enlarged heart) may indicate CHF.
      c. **Hyperexpansion,** noted by ≥ 10 ribs showing and flat diaphragms, may indicate either asthma or COPD.
      d. A **diffuse hazy pattern** is seen in most viral illnesses.
      e. Foreign bodies, such as metallic objects, may be apparent on CXR.
   2. **Known asthmatic patients do not require a CXR** with every episode. If the patient has a fever, rhonchi, or purulent sputum, a CXR is indicated to look for pneumonia.
B. **Lung function tests**
   1. **Peak flow.** This reading can be done in the office or at home. It involves the patient standing upright, placing a peak flowmeter in the mouth, inhaling, then exhaling rapidly and forcefully into the flowmeter. The meter is graduated and will record the FEV_1 (forced expired lung volume in 1 second). It measures how much air patients can rapidly move out of their lungs in 1 second.
      a. Results vary by height, sex, and age.
      b. Peak flow testing **does not** confirm a diagnosis, but is used to monitor the status of lung disease.
      c. Peak flow decreases with obstruction (airway narrowing seen in COPD or asthma) and is a good early indicator of worsening or improving obstruction.
   2. **Pulmonary function tests (PFTs)** can be performed in some clinic settings but are usually done in a pulmonary laboratory. These tests differentiate obstructive from restrictive lung disease, are useful in patients with recurrent lung problems (asthma, COPD), and provide more information than peak flow alone.
C. **Complete blood count (CBC)**
   1. **Elevated white blood cell count (WBC)** can indicate infection.
      a. **Elevated lymphocytes** indicate viral infection.
      b. A CBC with differential will include a band count, but it must be ordered specifically. **Elevated band count** or total polymorphonuclear cells (PMNs) (segs + bands) indicates a bacterial infection (a "left shift").
      c. WBC count can be **falsely elevated** in patients taking intravenous or oral steroids. (Watch for this in asthmatic patients or COPD patients on steroid tapers.)
   2. **Low hemoglobin or hematocrit** is often seen in patients with chronic diseases (anemia of chronic disease).
D. **Nasopharyngeal wash (NP wash)** is also called FA-5 (depending on the institution) and identifies five viruses causing bronchiolitis in infants/children—RSV, adenovirus, influenza A, influenza B, and parainfluenza. The test is performed by placing 2 to 3 cc of normal saline in a syringe; attaching 2 to 3 inches of plastic tubing, such as used for a butterfly venipuncture kit with the needle removed; making sure the patient is upright; and injecting all the saline into one of the patient's nostrils, then quickly pulling back on the plunger so the fluids reenter the syringe. The syringe contents are then emptied into a media test tube, which must be kept on ice and sent to the virology laboratory for evaluation.

Regular RSV NP wash takes approximately 24 hours to process; a rapid RSV test has recently become available, is used in emergency departments, and takes approximately 1 to 1.5 hours for results.

E. Other tests
   1. CF testing
      a. Sweat sodium and chloride testing is usually performed in a hospital setting. It is elevated in 90% of CF patients.
      b. Genetic testing is also indicated to identify CF carriers.
   2. GER/GERD testing
      a. The gold standard in a pediatric patient is a **24-hour pH probe.** (The patient is taken to the endoscopy laboratory for placement, then the device is left in the patient for 24 hours to assess for decreases in pH indicative of reflux.)
      b. Upper gastrointestinal barium swallow study reveals structural defects.
      c. Endoscopy is reserved for patients unresponsive to medical management of GERD symptoms.
   3. CHF testing BNP is a blood test that is now used to help test for a CHF exacerbation in the ED (see Chapter 72).

VI. Treatment
   A. Acute viral respiratory infection (see Chapters 55 and 57).
   B. Acute bronchitis/pneumonia (see Chapter 13 for cough).
   C. Bronchiolitis
      1. Prevention is best. Premature infants may benefit from using either palivizumab (Synagis) or RSV immune globulin, which should be administered just prior to RSV season in November or December. (SOR **C**)
      2. Acute infection necessitates supportive treatment.
         a. Some patients may need to be hospitalized if they cannot maintain acceptable oxygen saturation (above 90% in children). (SOR **D**) They may benefit from a trial of albuterol treatments, 2.5 to 5 mg every 8 hours via nebulizer. If the trial does not lead to clinical improvement it should be stopped. (SOR **B**)
         b. If they are stable enough to be at home, a trial of albuterol by inhaler may be used to relieve bronchial constriction. Outpatient treatment is preferred for otherwise healthy children.
         c. There is no evidence that ribavirin or antibiotics help. (SOR **B**)
   D. Aspiration
      1. Reflux precautions include thickening feeds (1 tbsp rice to 1 oz formula); sitting the infant upright and prone; giving small feeds (feed 1 oz, then burp the baby and repeat after every ounce consumed).
      2. GERD
         a. Patients may need oral medications such as H_2 **blockers** (e.g., ranitidine, 75–150 mg twice daily for adults); children aged 1 month to 16 years use 1 to 2 mg/kg twice daily. A **prokinetic agent** (e.g., metoclopramide, 10–15 mg every 6 hours) may also help control GERD. Proton pump inhibitors are used if the patient has GERD and fails treatment on an H_2 blocker.
         b. In adolescents and adults, caffeine, alcohol, and smoking should be avoided.
   E. Patients with **CF** should be referred to a CF clinic for a team approach to management.
   F. Anaphylaxis. Immediate treatment includes epinephrine injections (such as an Epi-Pen). These patients are then monitored in the hospital or ED. Prevention of recurrences includes behavior modification before another episode occurs.
   G. Asthma (see Chapter 68).
   H. COPD (see Chapter 70).
   I. CHF (see Chapter 72).
   J. Pulmonary embolus requires emergent hospitalization for anticoagulation and supportive care.

REFERENCES

Hosey R, Carek P, Goo A. Exercise-induced anaphylaxis and urticaria. *Am Fam Physic.* 2001;64:1367. Accessed Oct. 28, 2008.

Huntzinger A. AAP publishes recommendations for the diagnosis and management of bronchiolitis. *Am Fam Physic.* 2007;75:2. www.aafp.org/afp/20070115/practice.html. Accessed July 20, 2007.

Jung A. Gastroesophageal reflux in infants and children. *Am Fam Physic.* 2001;64:1853. Accessed Oct. 28, 2008.

Keeley D, Mckean M. Asthma and other wheezing disorders in children. *Am Fam Physic.* 2006;74:11. www.aafp.org/afp/20061201/bmj.html. Accessed Oct. 28, 2008.

66   Acne Vulgaris

Brooke E. Farley, PharmD, BCPS, & Julie A. Murphy, PharmD, BCPS

> **KEY POINTS**
> - Accurate diagnosis of a patient's severity level of acne will ensure optimal medication regimen selection.
> - Education of patients about the disease and the importance of compliance will improve outcomes.
> - Continual assessment of patient progress at regular intervals will enhance success rate of selected medication regimens.

I. Introduction

A. Definitions

1. **Acne vulgaris** is a common, chronic, polymorphic skin disease of pilosebaceous units, consisting of a hair follicle and sebaceous gland, located on the face, chest, and back. It is generally a self-limited condition that begins during adolescence; however, acne can persist into adulthood. In general, acne is not a high mortality disease-state; however, morbidity can be high as the disease can adversely affect self-esteem and can cause scarring and disfigurement.

2. **Noninflammatory (obstructive) lesions**
   a. **Open comedo**, or "**blackhead**", is a wide opening on the skin surface capped with a melanin-containing blackened mass of epithelial debris.
   b. **Closed comedo**, or "**whitehead**", has a narrow or obstructed opening on the skin surface; it may rupture, producing a low-grade dermal inflammatory reaction.

3. **Inflammatory lesions**
   a. **Papule** is a well-defined, elevated, palpable distinct area of skin generally less than 1 cm in diameter.
   b. **Pustule** is a superficial elevation of the skin, filled with purulent fluid, typically surrounding a hair follicle and up to 1 cm in diameter.
   c. **Nodule** is an elevated, firm distinct, palpable, round or oval lesion up to 1 cm in diameter.

4. **Severe acne variants**
   a. **Acne conglobata** is severe cystic acne, characterized by cystic lesions, abscesses, communicating sinuses, and thickened, nodular scars, found on the upper trunk and posterior neck; usually does not affect the face.
   b. **Acne fulminans** is severe scarring acne associated with fever, polyarthralgia, crusted ulcerative lesions, weight loss, and anemia.

B. Epidemiology.
Acne vulgaris is the most common skin disorder in the United States affecting 80% of the population between ages 12 and 25. Prevalence does not appear to differ between gender, race, or ethnicity. Severity of disease may be influenced by race as severity of acne vulgaris appears to be lower in Asians and African Americans than in the Caucasian population.

C. Pathophysiology.
There are four primary pathologic factors, and therefore potential pharmacologic targets, identified as playing a role in the formation of characteristic acne vulgaris lesions.

1. **Excessive sebum production** is caused by androgenic stimulation of the sebaceous glands. Severity of acne may be associated with amount of sebum produced.

2. **Hyperkeratinization of the hair follicle.** The normal process of dead cells being forced out of the follicle by growing hair is interrupted and instead do not leave the follicle as a result of keratin. This results in obstruction of the hair follicle and microcomedone formation. Continued production of sebum and keratin gives rise to visible lesions, which include closed and open comedones, as defined above.

3. **Microbial colonization** of the follicle with *Propionibacterium acnes*. The microcomedone environment is a perfect place for *P. acnes*, an anaerobe, to thrive and ultimately cause inflammatory lesions.

4. **Release of inflammatory mediators** is largely related to the proliferation of *P acnes* and free fatty acid formation within the follicle. Leakage or rupture of the contents of closed comedones into the dermis results in inflammatory acne lesions, including papules, pustules, nodules, and cysts.

II. **Diagnosis.** Diagnosis is based on patient history, clinical signs, and physical examination. Severity is assessed by the number, type, and distribution of lesions.

A. **Mild acne**
   1. **Comedones** (open and closed) are the main lesions (≤20).
   2. **Papules** and **pustules** may be present but are few in number (≤10).

B. **Moderate acne**
   1. **Papules** and **pustules** (10–40) and **comedones** (20–40) are present.
   2. Few **nodules** (≤5) may also be present.

C. **Severe acne**
   1. Numerous **papules** and **pustules** are present (40–100), with many **comedones** (40–100) and occasional larger, deeper **nodules** (up to 5).
   2. **Nodulocystic acne** and **acne conglobata** may be present.
   3. Affected areas usually involve the face, chest, and back.

III. **Treatment.** A summary of treatment recommendations can be found in Table 66–1. The goals of acne management include controlling acne lesions and preventing scarring. Improvement in appearance may not happen for 3 to 6 weeks, with maximum effects not being seen until after approximately 8 to 12 weeks of therapy.

A. **Topical agents** may be available as gels, solutions, creams, or lotions. Gels and solutions are best for patients with oily skin. Creams are better for patients with sensitive or dry skin. Lotions would be appropriate for any skin type. These agents should be applied after the affected area has been washed and patted dry, being sure to avoid the eyes, nose, and mouth.

1. **Benzoyl peroxide (BPO)** (SOR **A**) treats acne through its antibacterial and comedolytic properties. A thin film of BPO is to be used once to twice daily and is available in various concentrations (2.5%–10%) and formulations (lotion, cream, gel, and body washes). Adverse drug reactions that develop in the first few weeks of therapy include contact dermatitis (1%–2%), erythema, peeling, and dryness; this will diminish with continued use. To reduce these reactions, but still maximize the benefits of the medication, the frequency of administration or the concentration of the formulation should be altered. BPO may also cause bleaching of clothing and bed linens. BPO may be used as monotherapy for mild acne or in combination with a topical retinoid for moderate acne.

2. **Retinoids** work as effective comedolytics and have anti-inflammatory effects as well. Common adverse reactions include erythema, scaling, dryness, pruritus, and burning. Patients should be warned of the potential exacerbation of acne within the first few weeks of therapy. Patients should be counseled to avoid prolonged exposure to the sun (this may accentuate the skin irritation), wear effective sunscreen daily (sun protection factor ≥15), and start with no more than a pea-sized amount per application. These agents are indicated for mild to moderate acne.

TABLE 66–1. MANAGEMENT OF ACNE

	First Line	Alternatives	Alternatives for Females	Maintenance
Mild acne	TR +/− TA +/− BPO	Alternate TR or AA +/− BPO	TR	TR
Moderate acne	SA + TR +/− BPO	Alternate SA or OI + alternate TR or AA +/− BPO	OC + TR +/− alternate TA +/− SA	TR +/− BPO
Severe acne	OI	SA + TR + BPO	OC + TR +/− alternative TA	TR +/− BPO

AA = azelaic acid; BPO = benzoyl peroxide; OC = oral contraceptive; OI = oral isotretinoin; SA = systemic antibiotic; TA = topical antibiotic; TR = topical retinoid.

   a. **Tretinoin** (SOR **A**) is to be applied nightly. It is commercially available as Retin-A cream (0.025%, 0.05%, or 0.1%), Retin-A gel (0.01% or 0.025%), and Retin-A Micro gel (0.04% or 0.1%). Although the gel is more potent than the cream, the gel is more likely to be irritating to the patient, particularly at higher concentrations. For patients with sensitive or fair skin, therapy should be initiated with 0.025% cream every other day, and then titrated up as needed. Tretinoin is considered to be a pregnancy category C medication. The newer delivery system (Retin-A Micro) has less irritative effects than the older formulations. This delivery system entraps the drug in microspheres that bring the medication directly to the follicle and serve as reservoirs for the medication.

   b. **Adapalene** (SOR **A**) is to be applied nightly. It is available as Differin gel or cream (0.1%) and although it causes less skin irritation than the other topical retinoids, patients still need to be counseled on these adverse reactions.

   c. **Tazarotene** (SOR **B**) should be considered as a second-line topical retinoid, after tretinoin and adapalene. It is available as a 0.1% gel (Tazorac) or cream (Avage or Tazorac). A thin film should be applied every evening to the affected areas. Tazarotene has been found to be more irritating than the other retinoids and is considered a pregnancy category X medication.

3. **Combined BPO and tretinoin** therapy may be tried in patients who continue to form comedones despite monotherapy with either agent alone. (SOR **C**) BPO is generally applied in the morning and tretinoin in the evening. It is best to initiate therapy by using each medication on alternating days and advancing to day and night applications as the patient tolerates the therapy.

4. **Azelaic acid** (SOR **B**) treats acne through its bacteriostatic and keratolytic properties. It is available as a 20% cream (Azelex) and should be massaged into the skin twice daily. Patients report transient cutaneous irritation and erythema (1%–5%). Azelaic acid is indicated for mild to moderate acne and can be beneficial for postinflammatory hyperpigmentation. Because of the potential for hypopigmentation, it should be used with caution in patients with darker complexions. It is often used when patients are unable to tolerate topical retinoids.

5. **Exfoliating agents**, such as salicylic acid and elemental sulfur, are less effective than BPO or retinoids and should only be used when patients are unable to tolerate the latter agents.

6. **Topical antibiotics** work by inhibiting the growth and activity of *P. acnes* as well as an indirectly effecting comedogenesis. These agents are to be applied once to twice daily. The most common adverse reactions include skin irritation and staining of clothes. When used in combination with BPO there is synergistic antimicrobial action as well as a decreased risk of antibiotic resistance. (SOR **B**) Commonly used preparations include the following:

   a. **Clindamycin** (SOR **A**) is available as a solution, lotion, or gel (Cleocin T 1%). Combination products include the gel formulation Duac, BenzaClin, or Clindoxyl (1% clindamycin & 5% BPO).

   b. **Erythromycin** (SOR **A**) is available as a 2% gel (A/T/S or Emgel), solution (A/T/S or Eryderm), and ointment (Akne-mycin). Combination products include the gel formulation Benzamycin (3% erythromycin & 5% BPO).

B. **Systemic agents**

1. **Systemic antibiotics** are commonly prescribed agents for the treatment of inflammatory acne. Preference should be given for antibiotics that have anaerobic coverage and anti-inflammatory properties. The antibiotics most commonly prescribed for acne are **tetracycline, doxycycline,** and **erythromycin.** Typical duration of treatment is 3 to 4 months. After 4 months of continuous treatment, resistance is more likely to develop. *P. acnes* is developing increasing resistance to erythromycin therefore making it a second-line agent after tetracycline or doxycycline. Side effects for the systemic antibiotics consist primarily of gastrointestinal upset and vaginal candidiasis. Gram-negative folliculitis is a superinfection seen in 1% to 4% of patients on long-term antibiotic therapy.

   a. **Tetracycline** (SOR **A**) is to be administered as 250 to 500 mg twice daily. Tetracycline is contraindicated in pregnant patients and in children younger than 9 years of age because it may stain developing teeth. Tetracycline should be taken on an empty stomach and at least 1 to 2 hours before or 4 hours after antacids or dairy products to avoid chelation of tetracycline.

b. Doxycycline (SOR **B**) is to be administered as 100 mg twice daily. Doxycycline has greater lipid solubility and better penetration into sebaceous follicles than tetracycline. The major limitation of doxycycline is increased photosensitivity.

c. Erythromycin (SOR **B**) is to be administered as 1 to 2 g divided 2 to 4 times daily. This is usually used for those patients who cannot tolerate tetracyclines. Compliance with regimen can be an issue for patients taking this medication.

d. Other antibiotics to consider include minocycline, azithromycin, and trimethoprim-sulfamethoxazole.

2. **Oral contraceptives (OCs)** can effectively block or reduce androgens leading to significant reduction in lesion development. OCs that combine ethinyl estradiol with a progestin agent with low androgenicity (norgestimate or desogestrel) are the best choices. (SOR **A**) OCs containing drospirneone (Yaz or Yasmine), which is structurally similar to sprironolactone, may also be used. (SOR **C**) OCs work best to treat acne when used in combination with other agents, either topically or systemically.

3. **Oral isotretinoin. Isotretinoin** (Accutane) is used for severe acne. (SOR **A**) Mechanistically, it targets all pathophysiological aspects of the disease.

    a. The prescribing of this medication is highly regulated via the FDA managed iPledge Program (see below for program description). Only physicians that are registered with the program may prescribe isotretinoin. The iPledge program also requires that individual pharmacies are registered in order to dispense the medication.

    b. The daily recommended weight-based dose of 0.5 to 1 mg/kg divided twice daily should be administered with food and a full glass of water. Doses of 2 mg/kg may be used in adult patients with severe disease. Side effects often necessitate dose reduction. Initial treatment duration is usually 4 to 5 months. Repeat courses may be necessary and can be initiated after a period of at least 2 months of therapy.

    c. Adverse reactions to isotretinoin are frequent. Mucocutaneous side effects, which include cheilitis, conjunctivitis, dry mucous membranes of the nose and mouth, xerosis, and photosensitivity, are the most common and can generally be managed by the use of topical emollients, artificial tears, or dose reduction. Other side effects include arthralgias and myalgias as well as central nervous system side effects such as headache, nyctalopia, and pseudotumor cerebri. Laboratory changes associated with isotretinoin include hypertriglyceridemia, elevated total cholesterol, and reduced high-density lipoprotein levels, as well as abnormalities in liver function tests and hematologic parameters.

    d. Isotretinoin is a teratogen, resulting in a 25-fold increase in major fetal malformations including hydrocephalus, microcephalus, external ear abnormalities, facial dysmorphia, and cardiovascular abnormalities. All female patients must be educated about risk.

    e. Laboratory tests include a monthly lipid panel and liver function tests (all patients) and a pregnancy test (female patients).

    f. iPledge Program (www.ipledgeprogram.com) was mandated by the FDA in 2006 for the safe prescribing, dispensing, and consumption of the medication, in particular to prevent pregnancies among females taking the medication. All parties involved, including physician, pharmacist, and patient, have monthly responsibilities in an effort to minimize adverse events. Key iPledge points include the following items:

        (1) In order to prescribe the medication, physicians must be registered with the program.

        (2) All patients, female and male, must also be registered and sign an informed consent.

        (3) Isotretinoin cannot be prescribed for greater than a 30-day supply at any one time.

        (4) Two forms of birth control for female patients who can get pregnant is required for at least 1 month before, during, and 1 month after stopping treatment.

        (5) Urine or blood pregnancy tests are required 1 month before, during, and 1 month after treatment.

        (6) Prior to an isotretinoin prescription being dispensed by a pharmacy, patients must log onto the iPledge website monthly to answer comprehension questions and physicians must document, on same website, contraception methods being used and negative pregnancy test. Only when those responsibilities are fulfilled, can a pharmacist dispense the medication.

    (7) The patient has only a 7-day window, from the time of negative pregnancy test, to have prescription filled. If prescription is not filled in that amount of time, another pregnancy test must be done.

  4. Spironolactone is an antiandrogen agent whose role in acne is generally limited to selected females with treatment resistant acne. It is less commonly used in male patients because of potential feminization with long-term therapy. It is administered at a dose of 50 to 100 mg a day in two or three divided doses. Menstrual irregularities are the most common side effects associated with its use. Less common adverse effects include breast tenderness, breast enlargement, reduced libido, and hyperkalemia.

C. Intralesional corticosteroid injection is considered adjunctive therapy in the treatment of nodulocystic acne lesions. Its use will produce a rapid reduction in inflammation and reduces the likelihood of scarring. Diluted **triamcinolone acetonide** (0.63–2.5 mg/mL) is most commonly used and may be repeated in 3 weeks if necessary. The use of a dilute solution reduces the risk of steroid-induced skin changes like atrophy, telangiectasia, and pigmentary changes.

D. Comedo extraction. Both open and closed comedones can be extracted manually by applying gentle pressure with a comedo extractor or with the opening of an eyedropper. Prior to extraction, the pore may be enlarged with a 25-gauge needle.

IV. Management Strategies. The key to successful management of acne is patient education and compliance. Follow-up visits should be routinely scheduled at regular intervals. Important patient education points include the following items:

A. Acne is not a disease of **hygiene**.

B. Patients should **wash** their face twice daily with mild soap and water, **avoiding harsh scrubbing**. Patients should not use alcohol-based astringents that can dry and irritate the skin. Picking at lesions may cause more inflammation.

C. Patients should be instructed to use **oil-free, noncomedogenic cosmetics and lotions**. Oil from hair products and suntan lotions can also exacerbate acne.

D. Acne has no relationship to **diet**.

E. It is thought that acne causes **stress**, not vice versa.

F. Female patients should be told that acne usually worsens during the week before menses.

REFERENCES

Cunliffe WJ, Meynadier J, Alirezai M, et al. Is combined oral and topical therapy better than oral therapy alone in patients with moderate to moderately severe acne vulgaris? A comparison of the efficacy and safety of lymecycline plus adapalene gel 0.1%, versus lymecycline plus gel vehicle. *J Am Acad Dermatol.* 2003;49(Suppl):S218-S226.

Feldman A, Careccia RE, Barham KL, et al. Diagnosis and treatment of acne. *Am Fam Physic.* 2004;69:2123-2130.

James WD. Acne. *N Engl J Med.* 2005;352:1463-1472.

Liao DC. Management of acne. *J Fam Pract.* 2003;52:43-51.

Russell JJ. Topical therapy for acne. *Am Fam Physic.* 2000;61:357-366.

---

67   Acquired Immunodeficiency Syndrome (AIDS)

Jennifer Cocohoba, PharmD, Megan Mahoney, MD, &
Ronald H. Goldschmidt, MD

KEY POINTS

- Assess risk for human immunodeficiency virus (HIV) and sexually transmitted diseases in all patients and perform HIV screening on patients with risk factors. (SOR **A**) Consider one-time HIV screening in all patients between the ages 13 and 64 years, regardless of risk factors. (SOR **C**)

- Consider the diagnosis of acute HIV infection in patients presenting with fever, rash, and myalgias. Assess risk factors for HIV. (SOR **C**)
- Consider HIV infection for patients presenting with thrush, pneumonia, and herpes infections. (SOR **C**) Antiretroviral therapy should be initiated only for patients who are prepared for lifelong multidrug treatment. (SOR **C**) Consultation with experts in HIV treatment is helpful. (SOR **A**)
- Treatment of acute HIV infection is controversial and generally not recommended. (SOR **B**)
- Do not initiate antiretroviral therapy in acutely hospitalized patients except under special circumstances, with expert consultation. (SOR **B**) If the decision is to defer treatment, resistance testing should still be considered. (SOR **C**)
- Do not discontinue antiretroviral therapy in acutely hospitalized patients unless severe toxicity is apparent. (SOR **A**)
- Antiretroviral drug failure can be the result of nonadherence with treatment regimens or virologic resistance. Resistance testing can be helpful in guiding treatment choices. (SOR **A**)

I. Introduction

A. **Definition. HIV disease** is a chronic, progressive disease caused by a retrovirus, the **human immunodeficiency virus. AIDS,** as defined by characteristic opportunistic infections (e.g., *Pneumocystis* pneumonia [PCP], also known as *Pneumocystis jiroveci*, specific cancers [e.g., Kaposi's sarcoma], neurologic conditions [e.g., HIV-related encephalopathy], wasting syndrome, or a CD4$^+$lymphocyte count less than 200 cells per microliter) is the advanced stage of HIV disease.

   1. **Acute syndrome.** This syndrome, which usually occurs approximately 2 to 4 weeks following HIV infection, is difficult to identify because of its nonspecific nature. The symptoms and signs are similar to those of many viral syndromes and can include fever, maculopapular rash, sore throat, lymphadenopathy, oral and genital ulcers, headache, malaise, arthralgias, and myalgias. Oral ulcers in the setting of acute viral symptoms and compatible risk factors for HIV infection are considered pathognomonic pending laboratory confirmation. Abdominal cramps, diarrhea, aseptic meningitis, encephalopathy, and neuropathies can occur rarely. The acute HIV syndrome usually resolves spontaneously within 1 to 2 weeks.

   2. **Asymptomatic HIV infection.** After infection, an asymptomatic phase lasting 5 to 10 years occurs. Although infection persists and the virus continues to proliferate, the immunologic system remains relatively intact.

   3. **Symptomatic HIV infection.** Conditions such as oral candidiasis (thrush), oral hairy leukoplakia, generalized lymphadenopathy, and thrombocytopenia, generally precede the development of clinical AIDS. These conditions can also occur in persons who are not infected with HIV, however, so their presence alone does not define HIV infection.

   4. **AIDS.** Clinical AIDS is characterized by an advanced immunodeficiency with specific opportunistic infections, wasting syndrome, cancers, and encephalopathy. AIDS is also defined by the finding of a CD4$^+$(T-helper) lymphocyte count of $\leq$200 cells per microliter.

   5. **AIDS in children**

      a. Infants and children with AIDS present with recurrent bacterial infections, lymphadenopathy, pneumonia, failure to thrive, loss of developmental milestones, or behavioral problems. Consultation with pediatric AIDS specialists is generally necessary to guide therapy and arrange for clinical trials. (SOR **C**)

      b. Immunization schedules for children with HIV differ from the standard schedules found in Chapter 101. Oral polio vaccine should not be used in children with AIDS or in families with children who are either infected or suspected of being infected with HIV. (SOR **B**)

B. **Epidemiology**

   1. **Prevalence.** At the end of 2005, approximately 470,000 persons in the United States were living with HIV/AIDS; more than 5000 children were living with HIV. Because of extensive testing and treatment, fewer than 200 new vertical transmissions have occurred annually since 2000.

2. **Transmission** of HIV requires the exchange of infectious body fluids, including blood, semen, and vaginal secretions. HIV is not spread by casual contact.
3. The **average period between initial infection and development of clinical AIDS** has been estimated to be approximately 8 to 11 years among homosexual males. AIDS takes less time to develop in children and among intravenous (IV) drug users.
4. Prior to the use of highly active antiretroviral therapy (HAART), the **average length of survival** was $\leq$15 years. In the era of HAART, opportunistic infections and other complications of AIDS have declined and the average length of survival has increased dramatically.
C. **Risk factors.** The seven risk factors, defined by, the Centers for Disease Control and Prevention (CDC) are: male-to-male sexual contact; injection drug use; male-to-male sexual contact and injection drug use; heterosexual (male-female) contact; mother-to-child (perinatal) transmission; occupational exposures; and blood transfusions.

II. **Diagnosis.** Most patients are diagnosed by screening tests rather than by history of opportunistic infections or other manifestations. Early stages of AIDS can be similar to diseases of specific organ systems or nonspecific illnesses such as influenza. Advanced AIDS, with the combination of wasting, infections, and cancers, is rarely confused with other diseases. AIDS complications can be confused with other disorders, so risk assessment, counseling, and HIV testing must be considered.

A. **Symptoms and signs**
1. **Nonspecific symptoms** such as weakness, anorexia, fever, and weight loss are most commonly caused by HIV or opportunistic infections and cancers. Such symptoms can also be caused by bacterial or fungal sepsis, *Mycobacterium avium-intracellulare* complex (MAC) disease or tuberculosis. Cultures can help determine the cause of significant fevers.
2. **Common opportunistic infections and cancers**
   a. **Skin conditions**
      (1) **Kaposi's sarcoma (KS)** of the skin or oral mucosa appears as red to purple lesions, usually $\geq$0.5 cm in diameter.
      (2) **Maculopapular rashes** are exceedingly common and are often associated with drug treatment (either prescription or over-the-counter drugs).
   b. **Eye diseases.** Yellow-white or hemorrhagic patches on the retina can indicate sight-threatening **cytomegalovirus (CMV) retinitis.**
   c. **Oral cavity**
      (1) White plaques or erosive (erythematous) areas suggest **oral candidiasis.** Thrush is common in advanced, symptomatic HIV infection and is seen almost universally in clinical AIDS.
      (2) Painless, white, somewhat hairlike lesions on the lateral borders of the tongue indicate **hairy leukoplakia.** This painless condition, which is caused by the **Epstein-Barr virus,** will disappear and can recur. It requires no treatment.
   d. **Lymph nodes.** Lymph nodes are frequently enlarged, usually reflecting a generalized response to HIV infection. Hard, asymmetrical, or extremely prominent nodes require biopsy to exclude fungal infection or cancer.
   e. **Pulmonary** involvement is the most common condition in patients with AIDS, *Pneumocystis* pneumonia (**PCP**) being the most common pulmonary disease. *Pneumocystis carinii* now refers only to the pneumocystis that infects rodents, and *P jiroveci* refers to the distinct species that infects humans. The abbreviation PCP is still used to indicate *Pneumocystis* pneumonia. Bacterial pneumonias, fungal mycobacterial infections, and KS are also important causes of pulmonary diseases.
      (1) Patients with pulmonary disease can present with symptoms that range from mild shortness of breath or nonproductive cough to severe respiratory distress. Acute PCP is most commonly characterized by shortness of breath, dry cough, and fever. Chest x-rays usually show patchy infiltrates or diffused interstitial disease, although 5% of chest x-rays of patients with pulmonary disease can be normal. Thin-section computerized tomography (CT) scan typically demonstrates patchy ground-glass attenuation in patients with PCP, and might be useful as an adjunctive study in patients with a normal chest x-ray.
      (2) Evaluation of pulmonary disease generally requires examination of induced sputum, bronchial washings, or biopsies. Careful microscopic examination and cultures for *P jiroveci, Mycobacterium tuberculosis,* bacteria, and fungi are essential.

f. Gastrointestinal conditions

   (1) Esophagitis. Dysphagia, odynophagia, and substernal burning pain are symptomatic of **esophagitis.** Esophagitis can be caused by *Candida albicans,* cytomegalovirus CMV, or herpes simplex virus. When an empiric trial of antifungal-medications for patients with concurrent, oral candidiasis fails, endoscopy with biopsies and cultures is essential to establish a diagnosis and direct treatment. (SOR **A**)

   (2) Diarrhea, often copious and frequently associated with malabsorption, can be caused by *Isospora belli, Cryptosporidium, Entamoeba histolytica, Campylobacter,* and other enteric pathogens. Diarrhea from HIV infection alone can occur and requires symptomatic treatment. Diarrhea can also be a complication of HIV medications. Among persons with profuse diarrheal illness, a single-stool specimen is usually adequate for diagnosis. Among persons with less severe disease, repeat stool sampling is recommended. (SOR **B**)

   (3) Liver disease. Increased alkaline phosphatase levels commonly indicate liver infection by *M avium-intracellulare* or *M tuberculosis* or liver involvement by KS or lymphoma. Acute and chronic **viral hepatitis, drug-induced hepatitis, and HIV cholangiopathy** can also occur. Ultrasound examination and CT scan are generally helpful. Biopsy, although rarely helpful, can be considered in some cases in which *M tuberculosis* infections or other treatable conditions might be present. (SOR **C**)

g. Neurologic problems

   (1) Peripheral neuropathies can result in painful dysesthesias of the feet and the legs. Cranial neuropathies can also occur. Presumably, HIV involvement of neural tissue causes this condition.

   (2) AIDS dementia complex is characterized by behavioral changes, deficits in cognitive function, and lack of coordination. Although HIV appears to be the principal cause, other pathogenic conditions (e.g., cryptococcal meningoencephalitis or cerebral toxoplasmosis) can also be involved.

   (3) Meningoencephalitis, most often caused by *Cryptococcus neoformans* infection, is characterized by headache (usually slight, although at times severe), fever, and decreased mental functioning. Neck pain and nuchal rigidity can be present. Examination of cryptococcal antigen determination in serum and cerebrospinal fluid is useful for the diagnosis of *Cryptococcus neoformans* infection. (SOR **A**)

   (4) Mass lesions in the central nervous system can result in encephalopathic symptoms, seizures, or focal neurologic deficits. These lesions can be caused by *Toxoplasma gondii* infection, lymphomas, and, rarely, other opportunistic infections.

B. Laboratory tests

  1. Screening for HIV. A reactive screening test (e.g., enzyme-linked immunosorbent assay [ELISA]) plus a positive specific test (e.g., Western blot or immunofluorescent antibody) confirm HIV infection. Generally, these tests become positive within 1 month of infection; almost all infected persons display positive HIV tests within 3 to 6 months of infection. In most cases, these tests will remain positive indefinitely.

  2. Indicators of progression of HIV disease

   a. A person with advanced HIV disease usually has a CD4$^+$ **count** of $\leq$200 cells per microliter. Normal levels of CD4$^+$ cells usually exceed 800 cells per microliter.

   b. Quantitative plasma **HIV RNA (viral load)** testing is used for staging and monitoring response to therapy. Current tests can now detect viral particles down to 20 to 50 copies/mL.

  3. Initial laboratory evaluation of the newly diagnosed patient includes, in addition to confirmation of the HIV antibody test and baseline CD4$^+$ count and viral load, a complete blood count, chemistry profile, transaminase levels, BUN and creatinine, urinalysis, RPR or VDRL, assessment of latent tuberculosis, *Toxoplasma gondii* IgG, hepatitis A, B, and C serologies, PAP smear in women fasting blood glucose and lipids, and genotype resistance test. (SOR **A**)

  4. Drug resistance testing can be useful in the patient with acute HIV and before initiating therapy for guiding therapy. (SOR **A**) Expert consultation is generally recommended to help interpret the results. (SOR **A**)

III. Treatment. Drug therapy for HIV disease is rapidly changing and is complex. The US Public Health Service guidelines are updated regularly (www.aidsinfo.nih.gov) and serve as the most important single source of comprehensive guidance for HIV care. Starting or changing regimens can have far-reaching implications that affect the availability and efficacy of future therapy. Before one prescribes any medications, consultation with an HIV expert is recommended.

A. HIV antiretroviral (ARV) treatment strategies.

1. **Initiating ARV therapy.** All patients with AIDS and all symptomatic patients with any level of viremia should be offered therapy. (SOR **Ⓐ**) The best time to initiate ARV therapy for asymptomatic patients is not clearly established. Current standards recommend that ARV therapy be initiated in asymptomatic patients if CD4$^+$ cell counts fall below 200 cells/mm^3. (SOR **Ⓐ**) When the viral load is $\geq$100,000 copies per milliliter, ARV therapy should be considered. (SOR **Ⓑ**) Patients whose CD4$^+$ count is $\geq$350 cells/mm^3 have the option to begin or delay therapy. (SOR **Ⓑ**) Note that initiating ARV therapy can induce an **immune reconstitution syndrome** within days or weeks. The manifestations of this syndrome are generally the activation of a quiescent opportunistic infection (such as CMV retinitis, *M tuberculosis* infection, PCP, and many other opportunistic infections).

2. **Constructing an ARV regimen**
   a. First-line therapy consists of a "backbone" of two nucleoside reverse transcriptase inhibitors (nRTIs) combined with either a "boosted" protease inhibitor (PI) or a nonnucleoside reverse transcriptase inhibitor (nNRTI). (SOR **Ⓒ**)
   b. Potent regimens should not be a random selection of agents from different antiretroviral classes. Clinically proven combinations should be considered in conjunction with potential for toxicity, drug–drug interactions, and cross-resistance patterns.
   c. Certain ARV combinations should be avoided because of poor virologic outcomes or overlapping toxicities. (SOR **Ⓒ**) Combinations with poor virologic outcomes include all nRTI and nNRTI monotherapies, nRTI dual therapy, triple nRTI regimens (except for abacavir + zidovudine + lamivudine or tenofovir + zidovudine + lamivudine), delavirdine-based regimens, saquinavir (not boosted with ritonavir)-based regimens, zalcitabine + zidovudine, zalcitabine + lamivudine, lamivudine + emtricitabine, and stavudine + zidovudine. The following ARV combinations should be avoided because of overlapping toxicities, didanosine + stavudine, zalcitabine + didanosine, atazanavir + indinavir.

3. **Classes of antiretroviral agents.** There are several classes of antiretroviral agents that can be used in combination (Table 67–1).
   a. **Nucleoside and nucleotide reverse transcriptase inhibitors (nRTIs)** work by inhibiting HIV viral DNA synthesis. Two nRTIs in combination form the backbone of most HIV regimens. All nucleoside/nucleotide agents can cause nausea, vomiting, liver function test (LFT) elevations, lipoatrophy, and lactic acidosis with hepatic steatosis.
   b. **nNRTIs** inhibit HIV viral DNA synthesis. A single nNRTI can be combined with a nucleoside backbone to form a complete regimen. As a class, nNRTIs commonly cause LFT elevations, hepatitis, rash, and drug interactions.
   c. **Protease inhibitors (PIs)** inhibit formation of HIV viral proteins. PI serum levels are often boosted by the addition of a small amount of ritonavir. A single or boosted protease inhibitor is combined with a nucleoside backbone to form a complete regimen. Protease inhibitors as a class may cause nausea, vomiting, hepatitis, and various metabolic disturbances including lipid, glucose, fat accumulation, and bone disturbances. Medications should be screened for drug interactions with protease inhibitors.
   d. **Fusion inhibitors, entry inhibitors, and integrase inhibitors** are typically reserved for patients who have failed multiple antiretroviral regimens.

4. **Preferred initial regimens**
   a. Therapy should be initiated in consultation with a clinician experienced in managing antiretroviral regimens. Regimen selection should be based on several factors including potency, durability, tolerability, and the patient's ability to adhere. The US Department of Health and Human Services recently published guidelines containing eight preferred initial regimens a clinician can consider starting in an ARV-naïve patient. (SOR **Ⓒ**) Patients initiating abacavir-containing regimens should be screened for HLA-B5701 to assess for hypersensitivity. For information regarding the dose of each ARV agent, please refer to Table 67–1.
      (1) Nonnucleoside reverse transcriptase inhibitor options: Efavirenz (Sustiva) *PLUS EITHER* abacavir/lamivudine (Epzicom) *OR* tenofovir/emtricitabine

TABLE 67–1. HIV ANTIRETROVIRAL AGENTS

Class	Drug	Dosing	Adverse Effects	Administration/Other Notes
Nucleoside/nucleotide RT inhibitors (nRTIs)	Abacavir (ABC, Ziagen)	300 mg po bid	Nausea, vomiting, diarrhea, headache, rash, rare hypersensitivity syndrome (2%–5%)	Hypersensitivity usually occurs during the first 6 wk of therapy. Symptoms include fever, rash, nausea/vomiting, and flulike symptoms. If a patient experiences a hypersensitivity reaction, abacavir should be discontinued. Fatalities have occurred upon rechallenge
	Didanosine (ddI, Videx Videx EC)	200 mg po bid (≥60 kg, buffered) 125 mg po bid (≤60 kg, buffered) 400 mg po qd (≥60 kg, Videx EC) 250 mg po qd (≤60 kg, Videx EC)	Peripheral neuropathy, pancreatitis, diarrhea, GI upset	2 tablets per dose of buffered didanosine must be given to ensure proper absorption. Interactions may occur with drugs impaired by buffered agents.
	Emtricitabine (FTC, Emtriva)	200 mg po qd	Headache, nausea, skin discoloration, diarrhea, rash	Similar to lamivudine, even in resistance patterns
	Lamivudine (3TC, Epivir)	150 mg po bid or 300 mg po qd	Headache, fatigue, insomnia	No known drug interactions. Also used to treat hepatitis B.
	Stavudine (d4 T, Zerit)	40 mg po bid if ≥60 kg 20 mg po bid if ≤60 kg	Peripheral neuropathy, pancreatitis	Stavudine should not be combined with zidovudine because of antagonism
	Tenofovir (TDF, Viread)	300 mg po qd	Nausea, vomiting, diarrhea, flatulence, headaches	Lower dosage of didanosine if given in combination with tenofovir
	Zidovudine (AZT, ZDV, Retrovir)	300 mg po bid	Bone marrow suppression, myositis, GI upset, headache	Beware of drug interactions with probenecid and ribavirin
Fusion inhibitors	Enfuvirtide (T-20, Fuzeon)	90 mg sq bid	Injection-site reactions, fever, asthenia	Reconstituted doses are stable for 24 h. Patients must be taught to self-inject. Availability may be limited.
Nonnucleoside RT inhibitors (nNRTIs)	Efavirenz (EFV, Sustiva)	600 mg po qd	Dizziness, difficulty concentrating, vivid dreams, dysphoria, rash, LFT elevations, hepatitis	Avoid high-fat meals. Monitor for drug interactions.
	Nevirapine (NVP, Viramune)	200 mg po qd × 2 wk, then ↑ to 200 mg po bid	Rash, LFT elevations, nausea, vomiting, diarrhea, fulminant hepatotoxicity, Stevens-Johnson syndrome	Fulminant hepatotoxicity (black box warning) can occur during the first 8 wk of therapy. Dose escalation can reduce incidence of rash. Monitor for drug interactions.
	Delavirdine (DLV, Rescriptor)	400 mg po tid	Rash, nausea, headache, LFT elevations	Monitor for drug interactions. Separate delavirdine from antacids by 1–2 h.
	Etravirine (ETR, Intellence)	200 mg po bid	Rash, nausea, LFT elevations	Monitor for drug interactions. Active against K103N mutants

Class	Drug	Dosage	Side effects	Comments
Protease inhibitors (PIs)	Ritonavir (RIT, Norvir)	100–200 mg qd-bid combined with other protease inhibitors as a "boosting" agent	Nausea, vomiting, diarrhea, anorexia, fatigue, hepatitis, lipid disturbances	Used in small doses to boost the serum levels of other PIs. Monitor for drug interactions.
	Saquinavir (SQV, Invirase)	1000 mg (+100 mg ritonavir) bid	Headache, nausea, GI upset	Must be used (boosted) with low-dose ritonavir to increase absorption. Monitor for interactions.
	Indinavir (IND, Crixivan)	800 mg po tid or 800 mg (+100–200 mg ritonavir) bid	Diarrhea, GI upset, nephrolithiasis, asymptomatic increases in bilirubin	Best on empty stomach unless boosted. Patients should consume at least 6 glasses of water per day to avoid nephrolithiasis. Separate from buffered didanosine and antacids by 1–2 h. Monitor for drug interactions.
	Nelfinavir (NFV, Viracept)	1250 mg po bid or	Diarrhea, nausea, vomiting, GI upset	Monitor for drug interactions. Diarrhea may require symptomatic treatment with loperamide or Lomotil.
	Fosamprenavir (FPV, Lexiva)	1400 mg po bid or 700 mg (+100 mg ritonavir) bid or 1400 mg (+200 mg ritonavir) qd	Rash, nausea/vomiting, diarrhea, perioral paresthesias	Sulfa drug. Monitor for drug interactions.
	Lopinavir/ritonavir (LOP/r, Kaletra)	2 tablets (400/100) po bid or 4 tablets qd in ARV-naive patients	Diarrhea, headache, rash, asthenia	Fixed dose combination tablets. Monitor for drug interactions
	Atazanavir (ATV, Reyataz)	400 mg po qd with food or 300 mg (+100 mg ritonavir) qd	Nausea, vomiting, diarrhea, rash, increased bilirubin, prolonged PR interval	Do not combine with proton pump inhibitors. Monitor for drug interactions.
	Tipranavir (TPV, Aptivus)	500 mg (+200 mg ritonavir) bid	Nausea, vomiting, diarrhea, rash	Reserved for salvage ARV therapy. Must be used (boosted) with low-dose ritonavir. Monitor for drug interactions.
	Darunavir (DRV, Prezista)	600 mg (+100 mg ritonavir) bid	Nausea, vomiting, diarrhea, rash, headache	Must be used (boosted) with low-dose ritonavir. Monitor for drug interactions.
Integrase inhibitors (Int)	Raltegravir (RTG, Isentress)	400 mg po bid	Nausea, vomiting, diarrhea, headache	Can give without regard to food
CCR5 inhibitors	Maraviroc (MVC, Selzentry)	300 mg po bid	Nausea, vomiting, LFT elevations, rash	Monitor for drug interactions. Requires CCR5 tropism test.

GI = gastrointestinal; LFT = liver function tests.

(Truvada). Potential acute side effects include rash, nausea, vomiting, flatulence, anemia, and drug-induced hepatitis. This combination is contraindicated in pregnant patients in their first trimester of pregnancy.

(2) Protease inhibitor options: Lopinavir/ritonavir (Kaletra) *OR* atazanavir/ ritonavir (Reyataz + Norvir) *OR* fosamprenavir/ ritonavir (Lexiva + Norvir) *PLUS EITHER* abacavir/lamivudine (Epzicom) *OR* tenofovir/emtricitabine (Truvada). Potential acute side effects from these regimens include but are not limited to nausea, vomiting, drug-induced hepatitis, and metabolic disturbances in lipids and glucose.

5. **Adherence.** Optimal adherence to antiretroviral therapy is necessary to achieve and maintain durable viral suppression. Patients should be counseled on the risks of developing resistance if adherence is less than excellent. Optimizing ARV regimen characteristics such as reducing overall pill burden with combination pills and aggressively treating ARV side effects can improve adherence. (SOR **C**) Tools such as medication calendars, pill boxes, or watch alarms can be used to help enhance adherence. (SOR **C**)

B. Opportunistic infections and other manifestations

1. **Prophylaxis** to prevent opportunistic infections is indicated when CD4+ levels decrease to specific threshold values, as described in Table 67–2. (SOR **A**)

2. **Kaposi's sarcoma (KS)** of the skin and oral mucosa does not require treatment unless the lesions are uncomfortable or cosmetically disturbing. Widespread disease can be treated with chemotherapeutic agents. Radiation therapy and direct injection with chemotherapeutic agents are effective for some localized disease. Treatment does not appear to prolong life. Antiretroviral treatment may improve KS. (SOR **B**)

3. **CMV retinitis. Ganciclovir, foscarnet, cidofovir,** or oral **valganciclovir** administered for an induction period of 14 to 21 days followed by lifelong maintenance therapy, is effective in retarding the progression of CMV retinitis. (SOR **A**) Selection of drug therapy depends on clinical toxicity variables and availability of supportive care. Valganciclovir is dosed at 900 mg orally twice daily during the induction period, followed by 900 mg orally once daily for maintenance therapy. Ganciclovir is dosed at 5 mg/kg IV every 12 hours during the induction period and 5 mg/kg IV once daily for maintenance therapy. Alternative medications include foscarnet, 90 mg/kg IV every 12 hours (induction), followed by 90 mg/kg IV once daily (maintenance); and cidofovir, 5 mg/kg IV once weekly (induction), followed by 5 mg/kg IV once every 2 weeks. All four medications must be dose-adjusted for renal impairment.

4. **Oral candidiasis** is readily treated with **fluconazole,** 100 mg by mouth daily. (SOR **A**) Standard antifungal troches or solutions such as **clotrimazole** troches, 10 mg 5 times daily, or vaginal suppositories, 100 mg once or twice daily, or **nystatin,** 5 mL swish-and-swallow every 6 hours or 500,000-unit vaginal tablets dissolved in the mouth every 6 hours are suitable alternative therapies.

5. *Pneumocystis* **pneumonia (PCP)**

   a. **Acute PCP.** Three weeks of uninterrupted treatment is successful in treating most episodes of acute PCP, (SOR **A**) Clinical and radiologic evidence of response to therapy usually takes 3 to 7 days. Acute PCP can be treated on an inpatient or outpatient basis. Outpatient therapy is preferred when the disease appears mild and adequate home support is available.

      (1) **Trimethoprim-sulfamethoxazole (TMP-SMZ),** administered intravenously or orally, is the drug of choice in treating acute PCP. (SOR **A**) TMP-SMZ has the advantage of providing additional treatment against most bacterial pulmonary pathogens. The dosage is 15 mg of TMP and 75 mg of SMZ per kilogram daily,

---

TABLE 67–2. PRIMARY PROPHYLAXIS FOR OPPORTUNISTIC INFECTIONS*

CD4+ Count	Provide Prophylaxis Against
≤ 200	*Pneumocystis carinii (Pneumocystis jiroveci)* pneumonia
≤ 100	Toxoplasmosis
≤ 50	*Mycobacterium avium-intracellulare* complex (MAC)

*If antiretroviral therapy results in a CD4+ count increase above prophylaxis thresholds for 6 months, primary prophylaxis can be discontinued.

divided into 4 equal doses or 2 double-strength TMP-SMZ tablets orally every 8 hours. Two- to three-week therapy is recommended. Skin rashes are common; when the rash is mild and does not involve the mucous membranes, TMP-SMZ treatment can usually be continued with the addition of antihistamine therapy. Nephrotoxicity and hepatotoxicity can also occur.

   (2) Other agents can be effective against PCP. Clindamycin, 300 to 450 mg orally every 6 hours, plus 15 mg of **primaquine** base orally every 6 hours; (SOR **B**) **dapsone,** 100 mg orally once daily plus **trimethoprim,** 5 mg/kg orally 3 times daily; (SOR **B**) or **atovaquone,** 750 mg orally twice daily, can be used for mild to moderate PCP. (SOR **B**) **Pentamidine** at 4 mg/kg IV daily is an alternative for severe PCP. (SOR **A**) Adjunctive therapy with corticosteroids such as **prednisone** starting at 40 mg daily and tapered over 21 days, should be considered for patients with moderate-to-severe PCP (pAO2 $\leq$70 mm Hg). (SOR **A**)

  b. PCP prophylaxis. Patients with a CD4^{+} lymphocyte count $\leq$200 cells per microliter should receive **primary PCP prophylaxis.**

   (1) TMP-SMZ is the drug of choice. The dosage is one double-strength tablet daily, (SOR **A**), or 3 times per week. (SOR **B**)

   (2) Dapsone 100 mg orally daily, is a suitable alternative. (SOR **B**)

6. Esophagitis caused by *C albicans* can be treated with oral **fluconazole,** 100 to 200 mg daily, or **itraconazole oral solution,** 200 mg daily. **Caspofungin** 50 mg IV daily and **voriconazole** 200 mg twice daily are effective at treating oral candidiasis but may be more expensive or require intravenous administration. (SOR **B**) Failure to respond necessitates endoscopic evaluation for herpes esophagitis or CMV esophagitis. Intravenous **acyclovir,** 5 mg/kg every 8 hours, followed by oral acyclovir suppression, is effective against herpes simplex esophagitis. **Ganciclovir,** 5 mg/kg IV twice daily for 2 weeks, followed by 5 mg/kg IV daily maintenance; **foscarnet,** 60 mg/kg IV every 8 hours for 2 weeks, followed by 60 mg/kg IV daily maintenance; or **valganciclovir,** 900 mg orally twice daily for 2 weeks followed by 900 mg orally once daily maintenance, may be used to control CMV esophagitis.

7. Diarrhea caused by specific bacterial or parasitic organisms may respond to standard therapy. Symptomatic treatment should be offered when antimicrobial therapy is not effective or when no causative organisms can be identified. Symptoms caused by opportunistic protozoal pathogens such as cryptosporidiosis or microsporidiosis may respond to antiretroviral therapy. (SOR **B**)

8. Cryptococcal meningitis and other cryptococcal infections should be treated acutely with **amphotericin B,** 0.7 to 1 mg/kg daily, in combination with **flucytosine (5-FC)** at 25 mg/kg 4 times daily. (SOR **A**) If the patient is clinically well after receiving 7.5 mg/kg of amphotericin B, **fluconazole** at 400 mg by mouth daily can be given to complete a 10- to 12-week course. (SOR **A**) Long-term suppressive therapy with fluconazole should be given. (SOR **A**)

9. Toxoplasmosis of the central nervous system can be treated with **pyrimethamine,** 50 to 75 mg by mouth daily, plus **sulfadiazine,** 1 g by mouth 4 times daily plus **leucovorin** 25 mg by mouth daily. (SOR **A**) **Clindamycin,** 600 to 900 mg by mouth 4 times daily, can be substituted for sulfadiazine in patients who are allergic to sulfa drugs. (SOR **A**)

10. Mycobacterium avium complex (MAC) can cause a wide range of localized or systemic problems, including hepatic or other gastrointestinal disease, fevers, weight loss, and anemia. Treatment with ethambutol, 15 mg/kg by mouth daily, plus either clarithromycin, 500 mg by mouth twice daily, or azithromycin, 500 mg by mouth daily, can be effective. (SOR **A**) Prophylaxis against MAC disease should be offered to all patients with CD4^{+} counts $\leq$50 cells/mL; azithromycin (1200 mg by mouth once weekly, SOR **B**) or clarithromycin (500 mg orally twice daily, SOR **A**) are the preferred agents.

IV. Management Strategies. Patients with HIV infection require comprehensive primary care. Ideally, one primary care provider who is responsible for health care maintenance, early intervention, and treatment of common opportunistic infections should be identified. Consultation with specialists for specific problems can augment primary care. A team of medical staff, social workers, pharmacists, and family members that is organized around the care of the patient is essential to the treatment of patients with HIV disease.

  A. Patient Education. Special attention to the psychosocial impact of HIV disease is essential to the development of therapeutic strategies. Especially important interventions include discussions about natural history of HIV, infectiousness and transmission, treatment strategies, and consideration of the quality of life. Aftercare for the family of a patient who has died of AIDS is also very helpful.

    1. Primary prevention education. Risk assessment of sexual and drug behaviors and general HIV prevention messages are important for both diagnosis and prevention of HIV and other sexually transmitted diseases, and should be provided to all patients between the ages 13 and 64 years at least annually. (SOR **A**)

    2. Prevention with positives. HIV-positive individuals should be provided with education on ways of preventing transmission and should be screened annually for behaviors associated with HIV transmission. (SOR **A**)

B. Follow-up testing. Generally, the patients should follow-up with their primary care provider every 3 to 6 months for monitoring of disease progression with viral load and $CD4^+$ cell count testing, (SOR **A**).

V. Prognosis. Because of the effectiveness of combination ARV therapy, the prognosis for persons living with HIV infection continues to improve dramatically.

A. The mean survival of HIV-infected persons in the United States before the advent of effective ARV therapy was approximately 11 years from time of infection. The $CD4^+$ count and viral load at the time of diagnosis were closely correlated with the prognosis, with persons with high viral loads and $CD4^+$ counts ≤ 200 cells/μL having an 80% likelihood of developing AIDS within 3 years, whereas persons with high viral loads but $CD4^+$ cell counts ≥ 350 cells/μL having a 40% chance of developing AIDS within 3 years. In contrast, the patient with a $CD4^+$ cell count ≥ 500 cells/μL and viral load $\leq 20,000$ has less than a 20% chance of developing AIDS within 3 years. These data continue to apply to persons with HIV disease who are not receiving effective combination ARV therapy, including the nearly 300,000 persons in the United States infected with HIV disease but unaware of their HIV diagnosis.

B. The life expectancy of most HIV-infected persons who receive effective combination ARV therapy has increased by many years, but the average number of years remains to be determined. Deaths from AIDS have decreased dramatically, and clinical manifestations of HIV infection and AIDS have partially or completely resolved in many patients. The quality of life for persons receiving effective combination ARV therapy can improve dramatically. However, the pill burden and side effects from ARV drugs can be considerable, so quality of life is not invariably improved. The clinician, therefore, needs to help each patient make the best possible decisions about their use of ARV therapy.

REFERENCES

Because advances in HIV/AIDS occur frequently, the principal Federal Guidelines that represent current standards in treatment are continually updated. Following are the essential guidelines in HIV:

Centers for Disease Control and Prevention. Guidelines for the prevention and treatment of opportunistic infections in HIV-1-infected adults and adolescents. June 18, 2008:1-286. http://www.aidsinfo.nih.gov/ContentFiles/.

Centers for Disease Control and Prevention. Incorporating HIV Prevention into the Medical Care of Persons Living with HIV Recommendations of CDC, the Health Resources and Services Administration, the National Institutes of Health, and the HIV Medicine Association of the Infectious Diseases Society of America. *MMWR.* 2003;52(RR-12) 1-24.

Panel on Antiretroviral Guidelines for Adults and Adolescents. Guidelines for the use of antiretroviral agents in HIV-1-infected adults and adolescents. Department of Health and Human Services. January 29, 2008;1-128. http://www.aidsinfo.nih.gov/ContentFiles/AdultandAdolescentGL.pdf. Accessed July 3, 2008.

These and other guidelines can be downloaded from many sites, including the following ones:
    www.aidsinfo.nih.gov
    www. cdc.gov
Additional resources can be found at www.hivinsite.com and www.hopkins-aids.edu.

Jonathan MacClements, MD, FAAFP

KEY POINTS

- Effective control of asthma is necessary to prevent fibrosis of the basement membrane and remodeling of the airways, which can lead to irreversible obstructive lung disease. This control is accomplished by use of anti-inflammatory agents, most commonly inhaled corticosteroids. (SOR **Ⓐ**)
- Successful control of asthma requires high-quality ongoing patient education in which the patients understand their medications and how to avoid factors that aggravate asthma. (SOR **Ⓐ**)
- Common precipitating factors include house dust mites, tobacco smoke, mold, and animal allergens (cat and dog dander and cockroach and rodent products).
- HEPA (high-efficiency particulate air) filtration has become less expensive, more available, and more effective in providing protection from airborne allergens.
- Patients with asthma are at significant risk for high morbidity and death and should be monitored in a systematic and careful manner by their primary care provider. Spirometry and patient-monitored peak flowmeters play an important role in the management. (SOR **Ⓐ**)

I. **Introduction**
   A. **Definition.** Asthma is a disease of the airways, manifested by recurrent or persistent inflammatory and obstructive processes, or both, secondary to multifactorial stimuli, and frequently eventuates in irreversible loss of lung function and major disability. The terms describing the severity of asthma are mild intermittent, mild persistent, moderate persistent, and severe persistent, defined by frequency and severity of symptoms (Table 68–1).
   B. **Epidemiology**
      1. **Onset** is before age 5 in 75% to 90% of cases, with peak prevalence between 10 and 12 years of age.
      2. **Risk factors** include a family history of asthma or atopy, parental smoking, ambient air pollution, and viral respiratory infections, especially bronchiolitis from respiratory syncytial virus. Males and blacks are at greater risk.
      3. The **prevalence** of asthma in the United States has increased during the last two decades, and in 2004, the condition affected approximately 20.5 million persons including 6.2 million children. Five to ten percent of all children experience the disease during childhood with physician visits for the condition doubling over the past decade. Asthma is second only to acute respiratory infection as a cause of pediatric hospital admissions and illness-related school absenteeism.
   C. **Pathophysiology**
      1. **Expiratory airflow obstruction** is initiated by bronchial wall inflammation, resulting in bronchospasm, bronchial gland mucus exudation, airway edema, and airway remodeling.
      2. **Resultant pathophysiologic changes** include increased airway resistance and hyperinflation.
      3. The **etiology** is not completely understood, but encompasses a wide variety of genetic, immunologic, infectious, and environmental factors.
II. **Diagnosis.** The patient's history is most important. Although patients with asthma typically present with recurrent episodes of wheezing, not all asthma are characterized by wheezing, and not all wheezing indicate asthma. Undiagnosed asthma is a common reason for referral to pediatric and adult pulmonary outpatient departments.
   A. **Symptoms and signs**
      1. **Symptoms** usually include wheezing, coughing, dyspnea, chest tightness, and sometimes sputum production. Most patients report symptom-free intervals, but a rapidly changing and variable clinical picture is common.

TABLE 68–1. DESCRIPTION OF ASTHMA SEVERITY

Degree of Severity	Daytime Symptoms	Night-time Symptoms	Pulmonary Function
Mild intermittent	Symptoms ≤ 2/wk	≤ 2/mo	Within 20% of normal; asymptomatic between episodes
Mild persistent	≤ 3 episodes/wk ≤ 1/d	≤ 3 episodes/mo	PEFR within 20% of normal
Moderate persistent	≥ 2/wk to daily episodes	≥ 1 episode/wk	FEV$_1$/PEFR 60%–80%
Severe persistent	Continual symptoms with limited physical activity	Frequent	FEV/PEFR ≤ 60%

FEV$_1$, forced expiratory volume in 1 second; PEFR, peak expiratory flow rate.

   a. **Coughing** may be the initial symptom of asthma and is essentially the only symptom in cough-variant asthma. This form of asthma presents with nonproductive cough occurring both day and night. Pulmonary function studies tend toward normal. Therapy is similar to standard asthma treatment.
   b. **Atelectasis,** often misdiagnosed on chest x-ray as pneumonia, is a common clue to undiagnosed asthma.
   c. A **patient history of atopy** or a family history of atopy or asthma supports the diagnosis.
2. **Signs** may be absent in the asthmatic patient, especially early in the disease and during asymptomatic intervals. Forceful expiration occasionally uncovers otherwise unnoticed end-expiratory wheezing.
   a. **Severe asthma** may be characterized by both expiratory and inspiratory wheezing, prolongation of the expiratory phase, thoracic cage retractions, tachypnea, cyanosis, accessory muscle recruitment, and apprehension.
   b. **Pulsus paradoxus** (a pulse pressure that markedly decreases in size during inspiration), a silent chest, or chest wall crepitus caused by subcutaneous emphysema may signify severe airway obstruction requiring urgent care.
   c. **Chronic changes** may include such chest wall deformities as pectus carinatum or an increased anteroposterior diameter. Clubbing is rarely associated with asthma and should suggest a diagnosis of cystic fibrosis or cancer.
B. **Diagnostic tests**
1. A **peripheral blood smear** and a **sputum examination** showing eosinophilia may suggest allergic asthma.
2. **Allergy skin tests, allergen-specific IgE,** and the **radioallergosorbent test** can be used to test specific allergens. These tests may identify specific allergens that can be avoided or treated with immunotherapy desensitization. Skin tests are the least costly of the three tests. Radioallergosorbent test and IgE blood tests are usually reserved for patients who cannot undergo skin testing because of a history of severe reaction or other intolerance. Positive tests should be correlated with the patient's history of allergies. Total IgE levels are usually elevated in atopic asthma.
3. The **chest x-ray** is useful for selected patients in ruling out other diseases. It may show hyperinflation, atelectasis, pneumonia, or, rarely, pneumomediastinum. Criteria for ordering chest films include tachypnea, tachycardia, localized rales, localized decreased breath sounds, or cyanosis. Portable chest x-rays may be appropriately ordered for the critical patient, but two view posteroanterior and lateral chest films are helpful when the view requires clarification, such as when the physician suspects that a posteroinferior lung infiltrate is concealed behind the cardiac silhouette.
4. **Pulmonary function tests**
   a. **Indications** for pulmonary function tests include confirmation of the diagnosis of asthma, objective measurement of the response to therapy, and measurement of pulmonary dysfunction.
   b. **Forced expiratory volume in 1 second (FEV$_1$)** is very useful in assessing acute asthma, but the **peak expiratory flow rate (PEFR)** parallels the FEV$_1$ and is usually easier to obtain. Devices that measure PEFR are inexpensive and can be prescribed to allow patients with asthma to monitor their progress at home. Patients with a PEFR below 70% of their baseline value should be carefully evaluated. An FEV$_1$ or PEFR below 40% after aggressive therapy indicates severe obstruction, and the

patient should be hospitalized. The accuracy of peak flowmeters varies, however, and can deteriorate over time.

c. The **peak flow–zone system** allows patients to monitor the PEFR and make clinical decisions about their asthma, under the physician's supervision.

    (1) The **green zone** (PEFR = 80%–100% of the patient's best score) indicates that the patient can continue the usual course of medicine.

    (2) The **yellow zone** (PEFR = 50%–80%) is a warning to the patient to take additional medicine or call the physician.

    (3) The **red zone** (PEFR $\leq$ 50%) indicates that the patient should both use the inhaler and call the physician immediately.

5. **Provocative testing** with either methacholine or histamine is indicated for the rare patient for whom a definitive diagnosis is sought when the clinical picture is unclear. These tests carry a minimal risk of producing life-threatening bronchospasm. They must be performed under experienced supervision with resuscitative support immediately available.

6. **Arterial blood gases** are indicated for patients who have poor respiratory status or a poor response to therapy. Impending respiratory failure should be suspected, even when the PCO_2 is normal or slightly elevated ($\geq$40 mm Hg) in the presence of hypoxia ($PO_2 \leq$ 70 mm Hg). Pulse oximetry monitoring is noninvasive and very useful in monitoring the oxygenation of asthmatic patients.

7. **Nitric oxide test system** monitors exhaled nitric oxide levels, which are elevated in the lungs in a variety of inflammatory diseases including asthma. This test has proven beneficial in diagnosing and monitoring the response of lung inflammation with asthma therapy.

C. **Differential diagnosis**

1. **Common diseases** to be excluded are bronchiolitis, cystic fibrosis, foreign bodies, chronic bronchitis, and congestive heart failure.

2. **Less common diseases** to be considered are vocal cord dysfunction, bronchopulmonary dysplasia, allergic bronchopulmonary mycoses, and bronchiolitis obliterans.

III. **Treatment** goals include maintenance of normal activities (including exercise) and optimal pulmonary function values while minimizing symptoms, exacerbations, and adverse drug effects. Long-term therapy directed at suppressing inflammation early in the course of illness is now felt necessary to modify the disease process and prevent irreversible lung dysfunction. (SOR **A**)

A. **Environmental control** can provide significant relief by avoiding triggers identified in the clinical history and known to produce deleterious effects.

1. **Inhaled allergens** cannot be totally avoided, but much of the exposure can be eliminated.

a. **Tobacco smoke** should be banned from the home and automobile. The use of nonsmoking hotel rooms, rental cars, and restaurants is very beneficial.

b. **House dust mites** are difficult to eradicate. Frequent household cleanings can help reduce their numbers.

    (1) **Rooms**, when practical, should be free of carpets, stuffed toys, and other dust-collecting items.

    (2) **Central air-conditioning systems** should have frequently cleaned mechanical or electrostatic air filters. Portable, high-efficiency, particulate air filters can be used in patients' bedrooms.

    (3) **Nonallergenic mattress covers** should be used.

c. **Other irritants** to be avoided include pets, flowering plants, molds, perfumes, hair sprays, paints, and aerosolized chemicals.

2. **Emotional factors** may play a significant role in triggering asthma in some patients and must be minimized.

a. **Parents** should avoid overcompensating behavior that can create opportunities for manipulation by the asthmatic child. They should also avoid the other extreme of ignoring the child's plight.

b. The **home** should offer the child support, consistency, and loving parental guidance.

3. **Exercise** and exposure to cold air frequently aggravate asthma. Acute exacerbations resulting from exercise may be lessened by appropriate premedication and by restricting activities to participation in such sports as water sports, which typically cause less bronchial irritation than do other athletic activities.

B. Drug therapy involves two groups of drugs: long-term-control and quick-relief medications.

    1. Long-term-control medications are usually given daily over the long term to control persistent asthma. They include corticosteroids, cromolyn and nedocromil, long-acting bronchodilators, leukotriene modifiers, and theophylline.

        a. Corticosteroids are very effective anti-inflammatory drugs for treating acute and chronic asthma, (SOR **A**) but can cause many serious adverse effects. In children, suppression of linear growth and adverse effects on the hypothalamic–pituitary–adrenal axis are a major concern of systemic steroids. In adults, bone demineralization, cataract formation, gastrointestinal hemorrhage, and psychiatric problems sometimes occur with systemic usage. Corticosteroids should be initiated early in the course of treatment and in adequate doses for patients with severe asthma. The mode of action of corticosteroids is unclear, but current consensus suggests they improve airflow by decreasing inflammatory activity in the arachidonic acid, leukotriene, prostaglandin, and inflammatory cell systems and by increasing smooth muscle responsiveness to β-agonists.

            (1) Inhaled corticosteroids are first-line drugs and are often prescribed with inhaled β-agonists. (SOR **A**) The FDA has requested that all metered-dose inhaler (MDI) chlorofluorocarbon delivery systems be replaced by hydrofluoroalkane (HFA) to protect the ozone layer. HFA is effective for the delivery of inhaled corticosteroids, β-agonists, and cromolyn. Patients may notice a different taste and lighter canister, but the HFA propellant will not affect the way the medication works. Inhaled corticosteroids available in MDIs include budesonide (Pulmocort), fluticasone (Flovent), beclomethasone (Vanceril or Beclovent), flunisolide (AeroBid), mometasone (Asmanex), and triamcinolone (Azmacort).

                (a) Administration is by MDI with dosages listed in Table 68–2. Budesonide and fluticasone are also available in powder MDI preparations. Budesonide is also available in solution for updraft inhalation.

                (b) Significant adverse effects of inhaled corticosteroids are much less than those of systemic corticosteroids. The safety of long-term treatment with inhaled budesonide with respect to children's growth has been well documented.(SOR **A**) The newer drugs, budesonide and fluticasone, are considered to be more potent and have less gastric absorption and less active metabolites than the older drugs. Minor adverse effects include oropharyngeal candidiasis, cough, and, rarely, dysphonia, but they are seldom severe enough to warrant discontinuation. The use of spacer devices and oral rinses after inhalation can lessen these side effects.

            (2) Systemic steroids are indicated when other modes of therapy fail to control severe asthma.

                (a) Oral tablet-pill preparations—prednisone, methylprednisolone, and prednisolone—are given in doses of 1 to 2 mg/kg/d (usually 20–80 mg/d) and gradually reduced over 1 to 3 weeks, depending on disease severity.

                (b) Liquid preparations of prednisolone include Prelone (15 mg/5 mL) and Pediapred (5 mg/5 mL). Liquid preparations of prednisone include Liquid Pred Syrup (5 mg/5 mL) and Prednisone Intensol (5 mg/1 mL).

        b. Cromolyn sodium and nedocromil

            (1) Cromolyn sodium, an anti-inflammatory medication used prophylactically to control chronic asthma and exercise-induced asthma, (SOR **C**) inhibits both early- and late-response allergic reactions. Although cromolyn's mechanism of action is not fully understood, it probably stabilizes mast cells, preventing their degranulation and release of inflammatory mediators.

                (a) Adverse effects are few, but cromolyn requires dedicated patient compliance, since an adequate therapeutic response may not occur until after 4 to 6 weeks of therapy. Children appear to respond to cromolyn better than adults do.

                (b) Preparations of cromolyn (Intal) include an MDI, an aerosolized solution that can be combined in an aerosol with a β_2 drug, and an inhaled powder capsule. The recommended dosage is 2 inhaled metered sprays (800 μg per spray) 4 times a day at regular intervals. It seems more effective in children with asthma.

TABLE 68–2. COMMONLY PRESCRIBED ASTHMA DRUGS

Drug	Mode of Administration	Adult Dosage	Relative Cost per Month*
β_2-agonists			
Albuterol	MDI	90 μg/puff	++
		1–2 puffs q 4–6 h prn	
	Nebulizer solution	0.63–1.25 mg/3 mL	++
		q 6–8 hours prn	
Levalbuterol	MDI	1–2 puffs q 4–6 h prn	+++
	Nebulizer solution	0.63–1.25 mg/3 mL	++++
		q 6–8 h prn	
Salmeterol	MDI	21 μg/puff	+++++
	Dry powder	1–2 puffs bid	+++++
		50 μg/puff	
Formoterol	Dry powder	1 puff bid	+++++
		12 μg/cap	
		1 puff q 12 h	
Mast cell stabilizers			
Cromolyn sodium	MDI or nebulizer solution	800 μg/puff	++++++
		3–4 puffs tid–qid	
Nedocromil sodium		1.75 mg/puff	+++++
	MDI	2 puffs qid	
Inhaled corticosteroids			
Beclomethasone	MDI	42/84 μg/puff	+++
		6/12–10/20 puffs per day	
Budesonide	MDI	200 μg/puff;	++++++
		1 puff bid to tid	
	Nebulized solution	0.25–0.5 mg/2 mL bid	++++++
Flunisolide	MDI	250 μg/puff	++++
		4–8 puffs per day	
Fluticasone	MDI	44/110/220 μg/puff	++++/+++++/ +++++++
		2–6 puffs per day	++
	Dry-powder inhaler	50/100/250 μg/puff	
		2–6 puffs per day	++++/+++++/ +++++
Mometasone	MDI	220 μg/puff	++
		1–2 puffs per day bid	
Triamcinolone	MDI	100 μg/puff	++++++
		4–20 puffs per day	++++++
Combination medications			
Fluticasone/salmeterol	MDI	45/21; 115/21; 230/21 μg/puff	++++++
		2 puffs bid	++++++
	Dry-powder inhaler	100/50; 250/50; 500/50 μg/dose	
		1 dose inhaled bid	
Methylxanthines			
Theophylline	Extended-release tablets or capsules	300–600 mg/d	+
Leukotriene modifiers			
Montelukast	Tablets	5–10 mg daily	+++++
Zafirlukast	Tablets	20 mg bid	+++++
Zileuton	Tablets	600 mg qid	++++++
Humanized monoclonal antibody			
Omalizumab	Powder for subcutaneous injection after reconstitution	150–375 mg every 2 or 4 wk	++++++

*Cost per month per average dose: +, less than or equal to $25; ++, less than or equal to $40; +++, less than or equal to $60; ++++, less than or equal to $80; +++++, less than or equal to $100; ++++++, more than $100. MDI, metered-dose inhaler.

    (2) Nedocromil (Tilade) is an anti-inflammatory drug available as an MDI. Its action is similar to cromolyn in that it stabilizes mast and other inflammatory cells, but it provides significant clinical improvement within 2 to 4 days. Similar to cromolyn, its adverse side effect profile is very low. It is considered first-line therapy along with β_2-agonist agents in mild and moderate asthma in children 6 years of age and older. (SOR **C**) Up to 20% of patients experience an unpleasant taste with nedocromil.

c. Long-acting β_2-agonists

    (1) Salmeterol (Seravent), available as an MDI and inhaled powder, is a longer-acting (every 12 hours) β-agonist indicated for maintenance therapy and contraindicated for acute treatment. (SOR **A**) It is approved for children 6 years and older. Salmeterol acts as a bronchodilator, relaxing smooth muscle by adenylate cyclase activation and increase in cyclic AMP production. Its onset of action is 15 to 30 minutes and the duration of action is greater than 12 hours. It is especially useful for controlling nocturnal symptoms.

    (2) Formoterol (Foradil Aerolizer) is a dry powder inhaler (DPI), which is similar to salmeterol and is dosed at 12 μg every 12 hours. Both salmeterol and formoterol have an FDA warning that long-acting β_2-adrenergic agonists may increase the risk of asthma-related death. It is recommended to use only as additional treatment if symptoms are not controlled on low-to-medium dose inhaled corticosteroids, or if disease severity warrants initial treatment with two maintenance drugs.

    (3) Albuterol sustained release (Vospire ER) is an oral sustained-release form of albuterol that tends to have more side effects than the inhaled long-acting β_2-agonists.

d. The combination of inhaled fluticasone and salmeterol (Advair Diskus, DPI, and Advair HFA) offers the advantage of improved compliance and may also enhance efficacy through drug synergy. Dosages are listed in Table 68–2.

e. Theophylline is a methylxanthine bronchodilator that is usually well absorbed from the gastrointestinal tract. Theophyllines are considered second-line agents and are used as adjuncts with anti-inflammatory and other bronchodilator drugs. (SOR **A**)

    (1) Dosage requirements of theophylline vary considerably with age and the individual patient. Blood levels should be monitored and maintained between 5 and 15 μg/mL. When possible, therapy should be initiated slowly to minimize side effects. Children tend to clear the drug significantly more rapidly than adults do.

    (2) Adverse effects are similar to those of caffeine and include nervousness, anorexia, irritability, nausea, vomiting, enuresis, insomnia, poor school performance, and behavioral problems. Factors that may increase serum levels of theophylline and give rise to toxicity include impaired liver function, age older than 55 years, chronic heart and lung disease, sustained high fever, viral illnesses, and drug interactions, including those with cimetidine, allopurinol, ciprofloxacin, erythromycin, rifampin, propranolol, oral contraceptives, phenytoin, clarithromycin, and lithium carbonate.

    (3) Overdosage usually manifests as nausea and vomiting but can also cause arrhythmias, seizures, and, very rarely, death. Patients and their family members should be taught to recognize signs of theophylline toxicity.

    (4) Oral preparations of theophylline include liquid, tablets, and capsules. Capsules (Theo-24, TheoCap, and others) can be given to young children by sprinkling the medication on food to facilitate administration and accurate dosing.

f. Leukotriene modifiers are indicated for the treatment of mild-to-moderate nonacute asthma by modifying the inflammatory effects of leukotrienes. (SOR **C**)

    (1) Preparations include orally administered zileuton (Zyflo), a 5-lipoxygenase inhibitor; zafirlukast (Accolate) and montelukast (Singulair), leukotriene receptor antagonists. These drugs offer better compliance because of their oral administration, especially with montelukast's once-a-day dosing. However, they are less effective than inhaled corticosteroids, being indicated for mild intermittent and mild persistent asthma, and are less well supported in their ability to block lung inflammation and sequelae.

    (2) Adverse effects include drug–drug interactions, hepatic toxicity with zileuton, and rare Churg–Strauss vasculitis with zafirlukast and montelukast.

g. Recombinant humanized monoclonal antibody, omalizumab (Xolair), that blocks IgE has shown promise in reducing corticosteroid dosage in patients with persistent and severe allergic asthma who are 12 years of age and older. It is administered subcutaneously every 2 to 4 weeks, but its use may be limited by its cost.

h. Other drugs used to treat asthma

   (1) Antihistamines, which formerly were believed to have adverse effects on asthma, are now considered safe. These agents act as weak bronchodilators.

   (2) Antiviral agents, such as ribavirin for treatment of respiratory syncytial virus, and oseltamivir for influenza not prevented by vaccination, may be helpful.

   (3) Antibacterial drugs are useful for the treatment of patients with pneumonia, bacterial sinusitis, and other specific bacterial infections. Antibiotics are frequently overused in the treatment of patients with asthma, especially when atelectasis is confused with pneumonia.

   (4) Expectorants and **mucolytics** (e.g., guaifenesin and iodides) have not been proven effective. Aerosolized acetylcysteine (Mucomyst) is contraindicated in asthma, since it may cause severe bronchospasm. Sedatives and anxiolytic agents are also contraindicated. (SOR **C**)

   (5) Immunosuppressive drugs such as methotrexate, cyclosporine, and hydroxychloroquine have been considered as therapy, but are not well accepted because of their potential toxicity, low efficacy, or both. **Tumor necrosis factor-α inhibitor** infliximab may be effective in reducing the rate of exacerbations in patients with moderate asthma; (SOR **B**) however, trials are inconclusive.

i. Immunotherapy, also called desensitization, allergy injection therapy, or allergen immunotherapy, remains controversial, inconvenient, and expensive, but may benefit a few selected patients with allergic asthma. (SOR **B**) Immunotherapy also involves a small but significant risk of anaphylaxis and even death.

j. Complementary alternative medicine includes relaxation techniques, herbal medicines, vitamin supplements, dietary changes, acupuncture, homeopathy, and chiropractic spinal manipulation. Although these alternative healing processes are not recommended as substitutes for conventional pharmacologic therapy, they are used in up to 40% asthma patients in the United States and continue to grow in popularity.

   (1) Herbal remedies used to treat asthma have a worldwide origin involving hundreds of plants as well as minerals, animals, and mixtures of all three.

      (a) The **herb ma huang (ephedra)** contains ephedrine (a bronchodilator) and is perhaps the most commonly used agent in alternative medicine. This drug was formerly included in several asthma prescriptions and over-the-counter preparations. However, ephedrine is no longer recommended to treat asthma because of its adverse effects including sudden death, high blood pressure, nephrolithiasis, and hyperglycemia.

      (b) Traditional Chinese medicine is widely used in the United States and involves the use of many unfamiliar herbs, some having been used for hundreds of years. The typical Chinese remedy may contain 10 or more herbs, including ma huang, gingko extracts, Cordyceps, reishi mushroom, flavescent sophora root, licorice, magnolia, and others. While some of these have some efficacy, their clinical value remains unproved. (SOR **B**)

   (2) Hydrotherapy (cold baths) is commonly used in Japan to open constricted airways.

   (3) Acupuncture is very popular, especially in Europe, and has been investigated in a number of controlled studies. It has not been shown to be as effective as conventional therapy. (SOR **B**) Avoidable deaths have been reported in patients with asthma who relied only on acupuncture and avoided conventional therapy. Furthermore, acupuncture carries some risk, including organ puncture or infection from contaminated needles.

   (4) Relaxation techniques are designed to relieve stress, which is believed to aggravate asthma. These include yoga and biofeedback training, especially emphasizing breathing techniques. (SOR **B**)

2. Quick-relief medications

a. Short-acting inhaled β$_2$-agonists are most frequently delivered as aerosols through MDIs and, less commonly, as solutions via compressed-air nebulizers (Pulmo-Aide, among others). The MDI delivery system should be enhanced by the use of reservoir spacer devices (e.g., AeroChamber, Inhal-Aid, InspirEase, or Brethancer). Some spacers have masks that allow for infant and toddler use. Inhaled β_2-agonists are most commonly prescribed as needed, rather than with firm dosage times, because of concerns about tachyphylaxis and adverse side effects.

  (1) **Preparations** include albuterol (AccuNeb, Proair, Proventil, Ventolin), levalbuterol (Xopenex), metaproterenol (Alupent, Metaprel), pirbuterol (Maxair), and terbutaline (Brethine).

   (a) **Albuterol** (Ventolin, Proair HFA, or Proventil) is available in syrup, tablets, MDI, and nebulizer solutions for inhalation. The cost of albuterol inhalers has increased with the recent introduction of the HFA delivery system as generics are presently not readily available.

   (b) **Terbutaline** (Brethaire, Brethine, or Bricanyl) is available in tablets, MDI, nebulizer solution, and an aqueous solution for subcutaneous injection. It is classified as an FDA category B drug in pregnancy.

   (c) **Levalbuterol (Xopenex)**, the *R*-enantiomer of racemic albuterol, is available for nebulization (0.63 mg and 1.25 mg per 3 mL unit-dose vials). Availability as an MDI is anticipated in the near future. Levalbuterol may offer fewer adrenergic effects than albuterol while providing excellent bronchodilatation.

  (2) **Indications** include the rapid relief of acute bronchospasm and prevention of exercise-induced bronchospasm. (SOR **A**) These drugs are generally recommended to be administered on a need basis rather than on a regularly scheduled daily basis. The inhaled route is preferred because of faster onset of action, fewer adverse effects, and greater effectiveness.

  (3) **Adverse effects** include tachycardia, nervousness, irritability, tremor, headache, hypokalemia, and hyperglycemia. The less selective β_2-agonists (epinephrine, metaproterenol, isoproterenol, isoetharine) are no longer recommended for therapy. Patients should be warned against overuse of these drugs (e.g., ≥ 200 puffs of albuterol per month) and encouraged to use more of their anti-inflammatory medications.

 b. Ipratropium bromide (Atrovent), an anticholinergic quaternary derivative of atropine, is indicated for the relief of acute cholinergically mediated bronchospasm. (SOR **A**) This drug is frequently used with a β_2-agonist but has a slightly slower onset of action

 c. Systemic corticosteroids (methylprednisolone, prednisolone, prednisone) are indicated in doses of 1 to 2 mg/kg for patients with acute exacerbations of moderate or severe asthma. (SOR **A**) They are usually given for 3 to 10 days and are continued until the patients' PEFR is 80% of their personal best value. Prolonged therapy, ≥ 1 to 2 weeks, requires tapering of the dosage to prevent pituitary–adrenal–cortical dysfunction, but tapering per se does not prevent relapse of symptoms of asthma.

 C. Bronchial thermoplasty is an experimental outpatient procedure performed through a standard flexible bronchoscope and uses catheter-delivered radiofrequency energy to thermally ablate airway smooth muscle. Ongoing trials show significant decrease in asthma exacerbations in moderate or severe asthma.

IV. Management Strategies

 A. Education is a critical tool in the care of the patient with asthma. Family members, teachers, and athletic coaches must understand the disease process. (SOR **A**) Asthma support groups and camps for asthmatic children can be very helpful also.

  1. Patient compliance is much better when patients are given the opportunity to acquire adequate understanding of both the disease process and the prescribed medications.

  2. Office counseling should be provided to patients and their families, especially to those patients with special educational or behavioral problems.

  3. Referral to an outside counselor may occasionally be necessary to provide parents with additional help in the management of the troubled asthmatic child.

 B. Treatment guidelines. The 2002 (National Asthma Education and Prevention Program) expert committee applied evidence-based methods to review the scientific literature, and the consensus panel's asthma management guidelines include recommendations encouraging the earlier use of inhaled steroids as one of the preferred methods of management for mild persistent and more severe asthma. (SOR **A**)

  1. Patients with **mild intermittent asthma** have acute episodes of illness separated by symptom-free intervals occurring no more than twice weekly. These patients have normal PEFR and no symptoms between exacerbations. They can usually be managed with inhaled β_2-agonists given on an as-needed basis.

2. Patients with **mild persistent asthma** have symptoms more than twice weekly but less than daily. Their exacerbations may affect their daily activities, but their PEFR is at least 80% of predicted. They are usually managed with one inhaled anti-inflammatory drug or oral leukotriene modifier and augmented with an inhaled β_2-agonist for quick relief. Low-dose inhaled corticosteroids are now preferred.

3. Patients with **moderate persistent asthma** have daily symptoms requiring daily use of inhaled short-acting β_2-agonists. They have exacerbations at least twice weekly, which affect their activities and may last for days. Their PEFR values are 60% to 80% of predicted. They are preferably managed with medium-dosed inhaled corticosteroids and long-acting inhaled β_2-agonists (e.g., salmeterol plus low- to medium-dose inhaled corticosteroid) in addition to as-needed short-acting β_2-agonists. Alternative treatment may include medium-dose inhaled corticosteroids with either a leukotriene modifier or theophylline.

4. Patients with **severe persistent asthma** have continual symptoms, limited physical activity, frequent exacerbations, and PEFR less than 60% of predicted. They usually require high-dose inhaled corticosteroids, long-acting bronchodilators, and sometimes augmentation with oral corticosteroids in addition to quick relief with as-needed short-acting β_2-agonists.

5. **Nocturnal asthma** is now easier to manage with the use of longer-acting agents such as inhaled salmeterol, sustained-release preparations of theophylline or albuterol tablets, or the leukotriene modifiers. Nocturnal asthma may be associated with gastrointestinal reflux disease, even with minimal symptoms of the latter. In patients with nocturnal asthma who respond poorly to therapy, diagnosis and therapy for gastrointestinal reflux should be considered.

6. Inactivated flu vaccine is safe in asthmatic patients. Vaccination prevents substantial morbidity from influenza infection and its associated hospitalization costs because of complications. (SOR **A**)

V. **Prognosis**
  A. **Total remission** of symptoms occurs in as few as 16% of patients with asthma by late adolescence or early adulthood. Most patients retain airway hyperreactivity (as demonstrated by provocative testing).
  B. **Onset** of disease is not a reliable factor in predicting either the length or the severity of symptoms.
  C. **Initial severity** of the illness, especially the length of the episode and the need for hospitalization, is a more reliable factor than the time of onset in predicting whether the child's asthma will persist into adulthood.
  D. **Persistence of reduced pulmonary function** and the presence of atopy (eczema, allergic rhinitis, and skin test reactivity to antigens) are associated with continued and more severe disease.
  E. **Control** of the disease process through good pharmacotherapy is not a known predictor of future disease. The relationship of childhood asthma and adult emphysema is unclear.
  F. **Mortality** of patients with asthma in the United States continues to decline, with less than 4100 deaths reported in 2003. Mortality rates are higher in blacks, females, the elderly, and patients with coexistent chronic obstructive pulmonary disease. Historical events of concern for potential fatal outcome include previous history of respiratory acidosis with or without intubation, history of episodes of cyanosis, frequent hospitalizations, multiple emergency department visits during a short period, episodes of loss of consciousness, minimal response to a major therapeutic regimen, and presence of severe anxiety and depression.

REFERENCES

American Lung Association, Epidemiology and Statistic Unit, Research and Program Service, November 2007. Trends in asthma morbidity and mortality. http://www.lungusa.org/atf/cf/{7a8d42c2-fcca-4604-8ade-7f5d5e762256}/ASTHMA_TREND_NOV2007.PDF. Accessed July 16, 2008.

Boushey HA, Sorkness CA, King TS, et al. Daily versus as-needed corticosteroids for mild persistent asthma. *N Engl J Med*. 2005;352:1519-1528.

Bush RK. ed. Asthma. *Med Clin North Am*. 2002;86:925-1164.

Cox G, Thomson NC, Rubin AS, et al. Asthma control during the year after bronchial thermoplasty. *N Engl J Med*. 2007;356:1327-1337.

Lugogo N, Kraft M. Epidemiology of asthma. *Clin Chest Med.* 2006;27:1-15.

National Asthma Education and Prevention Program. Expert Panel Report: Guidelines for the Diagnosis and Management of Asthma Update on Selected Topics–2002. *J Allergy Clin Immunol.* 2002;110: S141-S219.

O'Byrne PM, Pedersen S, Busse WW, et al. Effects of early intervention with inhaled budesonide on lung function in newly diagnosed asthma. *Chest.* 2006;129:1478-1485.

Szefler SJ. Advances in pediatric asthma 2006. *J Allergy Clin Immunol* 2006;119:558-562.

Weinberger M. Clinical patterns and natural history of asthma. *J Pediatr.* 2003;142:S15-S20.

Wen MC, Wei CH, Hu ZQ, et al. Efficacy and tolerability of antiasthma herbal medicine intervention in adult patients with moderate-severe allergic asthma. *J Allergy Clin Immunol.* 2005;116:517.

---

69   Chronic Pain

Michael P. Temporal, MD

KEY POINTS

- The biopsychosocial context is important in the assessment and management of chronic pain conditions to understand both the perception of severity and the effect of treatment.
- Pain scales and pain medication contracts help to decrease the risk of inappropriate pain medication prescription.
- A multidisciplinary approach using multiple modalities is usually needed to manage chronic pain.
- Routine, rather than as-needed, dosing of medications results in better pain control.
- Nonsteroidal anti-inflammatory drugs (NSAIDs) have equivalent efficacy and are used as first-line medications. COX-2 inhibitors may have a role as an alternative in older patients or when first-line NSAIDs fail.
- Narcotic pain medications should be used when patients have failed NSAID therapy alone. They should not be used as a sole agent and should be titrated to the most effective dose and then changed to long-acting preparations when available.
- Adjuvant medications can be particularly helpful for chronic, relapsing pain. Antidepressants are also useful for both the emotional component of pain and analgesia.

I. **Introduction**

    A. Pain is the most common reason because of which people seek medical care. **Pain** is an unpleasant sensory and emotional experience associated with actual or potential tissue damage. **Chronic pain** is defined as recurrent or persistent pain lasting more than 3 months. Chronic pain complaints affect 15% of the population. Annual US monetary loss because of lost productivity from chronic pain is over $60 billion.

    B. Chronic pain may be classified as nociceptive or neuropathic. While acute pain can be protective, a reflexive response to limit further tissue destruction, chronic pain does not have a similar useful purpose.

        1. **Nociceptive pain** stems from ongoing tissue damage such as arthritis or tumor. Pain signals are transmitted through nonmyelinated C-fiber nerves mediated by calcium and sodium. Chronic nociceptive pain is related to *N*-methyl-D-aspartate (NMDA) receptors that are both more easily stimulated and require higher antinociceptive activity to quiet. Released endorphin and enkephalin binding to mu- and gamma-opioid receptors reduce nociceptive pain.

        2. **Neuropathic pain** results from the sustained transmission of pain signals in the absence of ongoing tissue damage. Injury or damage to the sensory nerves or central ganglia has occurred. Common descriptions of this chronic pain include numbness (hypoesthesia), pins-and-needles sensation (paresthesia), or severe pain from usually innocuous stimuli (allodynia). It is more difficult to treat and usually does not respond to treatment with NSAIDs or acetaminophen alone.

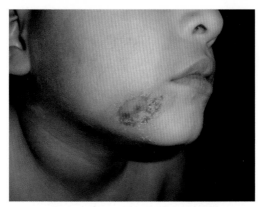

FIGURE 9–1. Erythrasma. (Credit to Dr. Richard Usatine.)

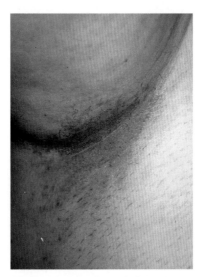

FIGURE 9–2. Impetigo. (Credit to Dr. Richard Usatine.)

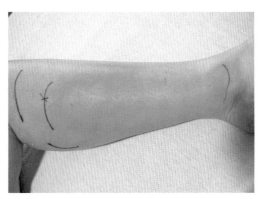

FIGURE 9–3. Cellulitis.

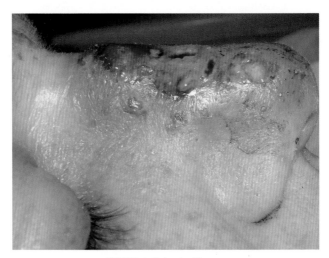

FIGURE 9–4. Carbuncle of the nose.

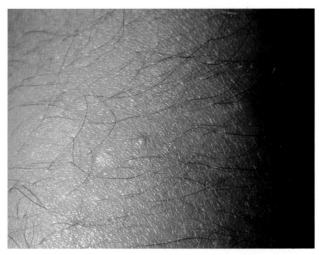

FIGURE 9–5. Folliculitis. (Credit to Dr. Richard Usatine.)

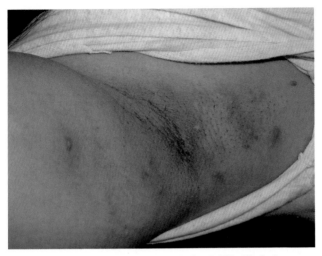

FIGURE 9–6. Hidradenitis suppurativa. (Credit to Dr. Richard Usatine.)

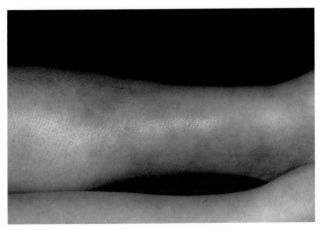

FIGURE 9–7. Erysipelas. (Credit to Dr. Richard Usatine.)

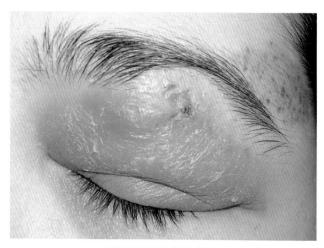

FIGURE 9–8. Periorbital cellulitis.

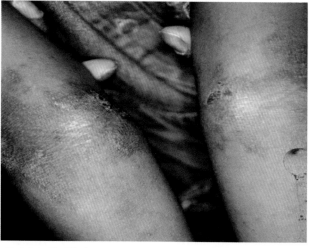

FIGURE 14–1. Atopic dermatitis. (This photograph has been taken by and is the property of Dick Anstett, MD, MPH. Faculty, Family Medicine Residency of Idaho, Boise, Idaho.)

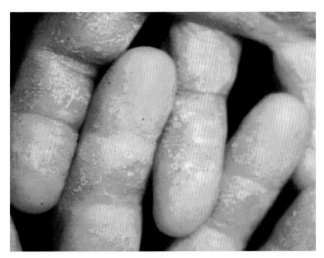

FIGURE 14–2. Contact dermatitis from dishwasher water. (This photograph has been taken by and is the property of Dick Anstett, MD, MPH. Faculty, Family Medicine Residency of Idaho, Boise, Idaho.)

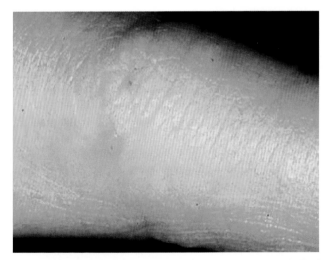

FIGURE 14–3. Scabies. (This photograph has been taken by and is the property of Dick Anstett, MD, MPH. Faculty, Family Medicine Residency of Idaho, Boise, Idaho.)

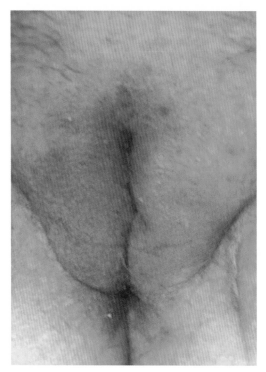

FIGURE 14–4. Lichen simplex chronicus. (This photograph has been taken by and is the property of Dick Anstett, MD, MPH. Faculty, Family Medicine Residency of Idaho, Boise, Idaho.)

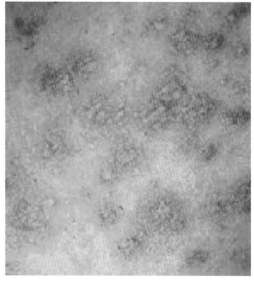

FIGURE 14–5. Lichen planus. (This photograph has been taken by and is the property of Dick Anstett, MD, MPH. Faculty, Family Medicine Residency of Idaho, Boise, Idaho.)

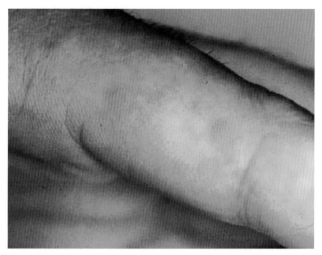

FIGURE 14–6. Dyshidrotic eczema. (This photograph has been taken by and is the property of Dick Anstett, MD, MPH. Faculty, Family Medicine Residency of Idaho, Boise, Idaho.)

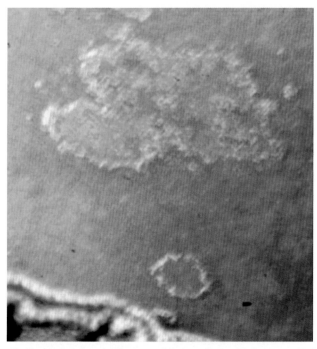

FIGURE 14–7. Herald patch, pityriasis rosea. (This photograph has been taken by and is the property of Dick Anstett, MD, MPH. Faculty, Family Medicine Residency of Idaho, Boise, Idaho.)

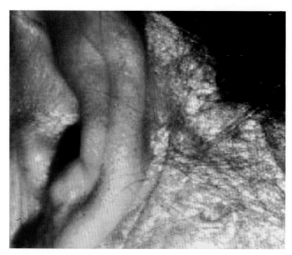

FIGURE 14–8. Psoriasis. (This photograph has been taken by and is the property of Dick Anstett, MD, MPH. Faculty, Family Medicine Residency of Idaho, Boise, Idaho.)

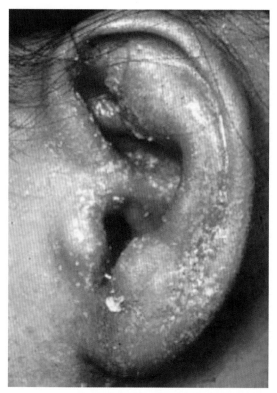

FIGURE 14–9. Seborrhea dermatitis. (This photograph has been taken by and is the property of Dick Anstett, MD, MPH. Faculty, Family Medicine Residency of Idaho, Boise, Idaho.)

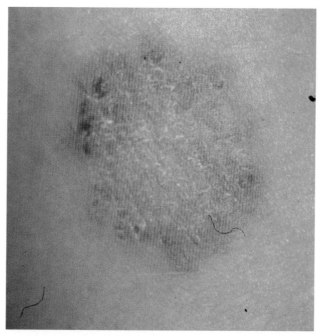

FIGURE 14–10. Nummular eczema. (This photograph has been taken by and is the property of Dick Anstett, MD, MPH. Faculty, Family Medicine Residency of Idaho, Boise, Idaho.)

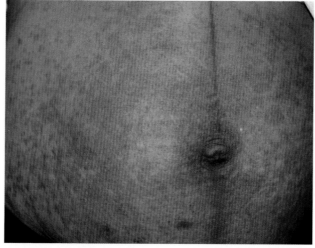

FIGURE 14–11. PUPP. (This photograph has been taken by and is the property of Dick Anstett, MD, MPH. Faculty, Family Medicine Residency of Idaho, Boise, Idaho.)

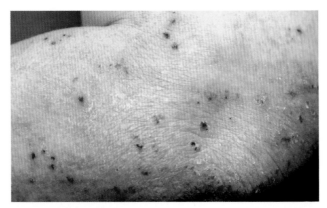

FIGURE 14–12. Delusion of parasitosis. (This photograph has been taken by and is the property of Dick Anstett, MD, MPH. Faculty, Family Medicine Residency of Idaho, Boise, Idaho.)

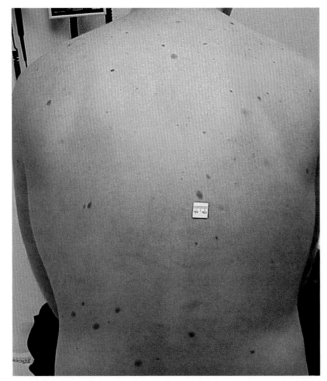

FIGURE 15–1. FAMMS; note multiple macular to papular lesions with variable coloring and size.

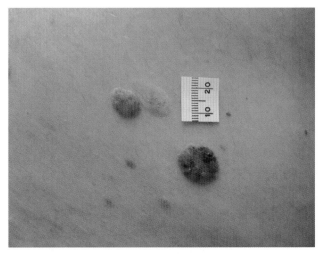

FIGURE 15–2. Multiple macular cherry angiomas. More advanced lesions may be raised or even polypoid. Note several verrucous irregularly pigmented seborrheic keratoses which are also age related.

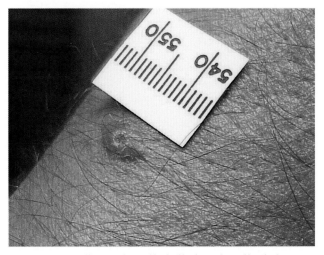

FIGURE 15–3. Keratoacanthoma with raised borders and central keratin plug.

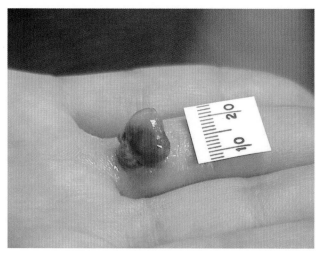

FIGURE 15–4. Pyogenic granuloma with glistening fragile overgrowth of capillaries and epithelium.

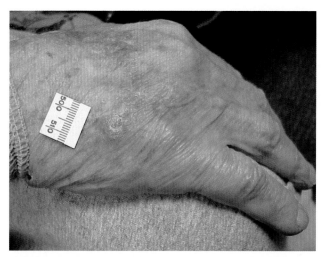

FIGURE 15–5. Actinic keratosis which has reached the raised actinic horn stage and also note the diffuse raised erythematous base of progression to squamous cell cancer.

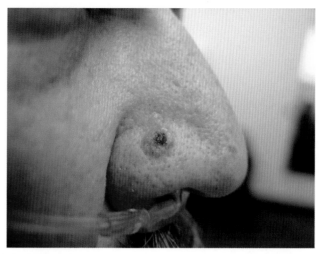

FIGURE 15–6. Basal cell cancer. Note similar appearance to keratoacanthoma with raised borders, but has telangiectasias and central ulceration.

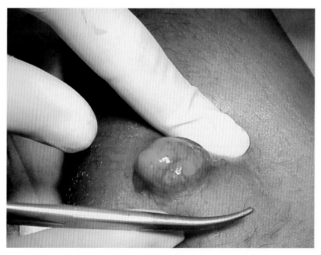

FIGURE 15–7. Lipoma with capsule being expressed after blunt dissection from a relatively small incision.

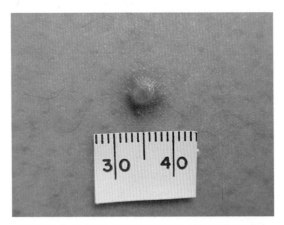

FIGURE 15–8. Dermatofibroma typically pigmented and sometimes raised.

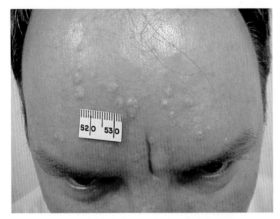

FIGURE 15–9. Sebaceous hyperplasia, common on the forehead and face looks similar to early BCCs, but is often seen as multiple lesions.

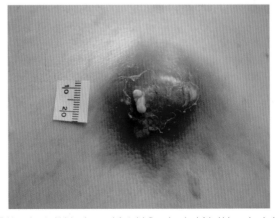

FIGURE 15–10. Epidermal cyst which has become infected, inflamed, and painful which requires incision and drainage.

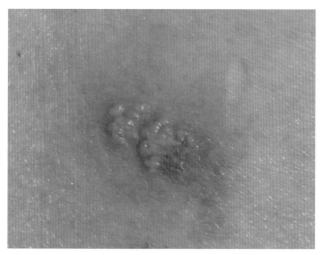

FIGURE 31–1. Thightly grouped vesicles 1 to 3 mm in diameter forming a lobulated irregular plaque over a larger ery-thematous base represent a herpetic lesion about 2-day-old. (Reproduced with permission from Tomás P. Owens, Jr., MD.)

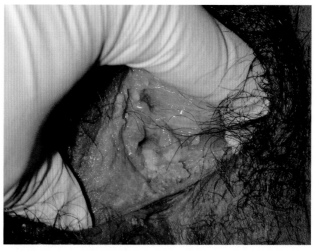

FIGURE 31–2. A peach-colored cauliflower-like lesion is noted on the comisure of the labia majora immediately caudal to the fourchette. Single coniform lighter pink lesions are also present at the R periurethral area, R superior labia majora, and L labia minora. (Reproduced with permission from Tomás P. Owens, Jr., MD.)

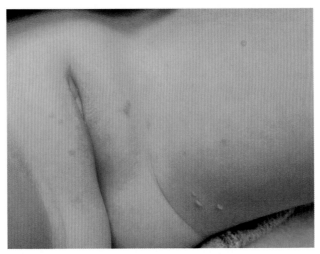

FIGURE 31–3. Umbilicated, tan, volcano-top-like lesions in a very young girl. The inner thigh lesions are coupled, resembling an achrochordon, a more fusiform appearance. Investigation concluded that these were not sexually transmitted. (Reproduced with permission from Tomás P. Owens, Jr., MD.)

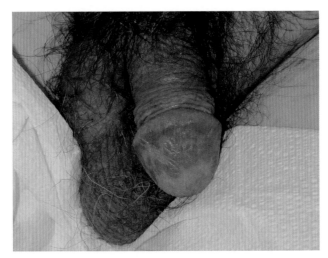

FIGURE 31–4. Irregular erythematous plaques following cleansing of smegma and debris. These lesions completely disappeared after topical antifungals, confirming the absence of Bowenoid disease. (Reproduced with permission from Tomás P. Owens, Jr., MD.)

II. Diagnoses

A. The **assessment of pain** must include the type, severity, onset, location, duration, and previous history. Chronic pain may have variable duration (less than once per week, multiple times per week, daily, or constant). Within a psychosocial context, more intense pain may be associated with certain activities, emotions, or events (work, mood, menstrual cycle).

B. An important **measure of chronic pain** is the associated impairment or loss of function. Associated symptoms such as nausea, dizziness, diaphoresis, and weakness should be sought as well as comorbid conditions such as diabetes mellitus, connective tissue disease, and psychiatric illness (which may affect treatment response) as well as hepatic disease, renal disease, history of gastrointestinal (GI) bleeding, and medication sensitivity (which may limit treatment choices). Previous treatment strategies (including complementary and alternative therapies) and response to those strategies provide important historical information and can guide the current management.

C. **Pain rating scales** allow quantification of baseline and relative response to pain therapies. The simplest range from 0 (no pain) to 10 (worst pain possible). Mild pain ranges from 1 to 3, moderate pain ranges from 4 to 6, severe pain from 7 to 9. While developed for palliative care, the Edmonton Symptom Assessment System scale has the patient rate on a 0 to 10 scale additional domains, including tiredness, nausea, depression, anxiety, drowsiness, appetite, well-being, shortness of breath, and other problems to give a multidimensional perspective.

D. Physical assessment can give more objective data to the necessarily subjective sensation of pain. However, instability of vital signs or alterations of consciousness seen in acute pain situations may be blunted in chronic pain. Important functional information of endurance, range of motion, and palpable inflammation, point tenderness, or spasm should be identified.

III. Treatment

A. **Physical.** Physical therapy has been used in the management of acute pain to help with stretching, strengthening, and improving endurance. The primary impairments, directly caused by the injury, may or may not be responsive to physical therapy. The secondary impairments—lack of exercise, poor body alignment, shortening and weakening of the joint structures, and overguarding of the injured area—which can exacerbate daily functioning and the perception of pain and suffering, often are responsive in the motivated patient. Physical reconditioning in a gradual, directed program will help the patient who has been immobile. With the goal of increasing function, decreasing disability, and establishing effective pain coping and management skills, exercise programs can include the following: aerobic exercise to 65% to 80% of predicted maximal heart rate; stretching exercises for shortened muscles; endurance exercise for major postural muscles; and coordination and stabilization exercises. (SOR **C**)

　1. **Transcutaneous electrical nerve stimulation (TENS)** has been helpful in mild to moderate pain. (SOR **B**) It works through counterstimulation of the pain-transmitting nerves.

　2. Scheduled use of **ice or heat** may provide a similar benefit.

　3. **Occupational therapy** can be used to help moderate total activity and develop compensatory techniques for activities of daily living. The provision of adaptive equipment can enhance the effectiveness of other treatment modalities.

　4. **Biofeedback, self-hypnosis,** and **relaxation** can also be taught to help manage the sensation of pain.

B. **Cognitive.** Understanding the pain cycle and how the individual is affected can be a step toward moving the focus away from the pain and more toward adaptive behaviors. (SOR **C**) Cognitive therapies seek to bring an awareness of the triggers and responses the body has to pain in the context of daily life activities. Educating the patient and the family regarding pain, tension, and the physiologic response is a therapeutic intervention. Reframing the language and associations of pain may bring control for a person who has not had control of pain for a long time. Relaxation techniques, stress management, and pain diary records help to respond productively to pain.

C. **Medical**

　1. **Conventional agents**

　　a. Acetaminophen is an excellent analgesic for mild to moderate nociceptive pain. In the treatment of osteoarthritis, doses to 4 g/d (500 mg, 2 tablets orally 4 times daily) have been associated with long-term efficacy comparable to nonsteroidal agents. (SOR **Ⓑ**) Although it has no anti-inflammatory properties, acetaminophen is thought to work through NMDA receptors and substance P.

b. **NSAIDs** are effective agents for mild to moderate pain with an inflammatory component. They work at the peripheral site of action and are effective in the chronic management of arthritides and myalgias. They also can be effectively combined with centrally acting opioid medications for other chronic pain. Not even one NSAID is superior to others for chronic pain, but periodic substitution between classes may afford an improved response. (SOR **Ⓑ**) The risks of NSAIDs are related to prostaglandin inhibition and include gastric irritation, bleeding, and renal dysfunction. Allergic reactions including angioneurotic edema, asthma, and hypotension have been reported. Because of sodium retention, caution is advised in the setting of congestive heart failure. Choices include:

   (1) Ibuprofen, 200 to 800 mg orally 3 times daily.
   (2) Naproxen, 250 to 500 mg orally twice daily.
   (3) Piroxicam, 20 mg orally every day.

c. **COX-2 inhibitors** are newer medications that inhibit cyclooxygenase-2 and have comparable efficacy to that of NSAIDs. They are reported to have less GI toxicity and bleeding, but ulcers and bleeding have occurred. Another potential risk is cardiovascular complications (i.e., thrombosis). These medications are often used as first-line agents in the elderly or when first-line NSAIDs fail. Celecoxib (Celebrex), 100 to 200 mg orally every day to twice daily is the only COX-2 inhibitor now on the market.

d. **Tramadol (Ultram)** is a centrally acting, synthetic opioid agonist oral analgesic useful in moderate to severe pain. It is discussed here because it is a nonscheduled medication. It binds to mu-opioid receptors and inhibits serotonin and norepinephrine reuptake. Starting doses are 50 mg every 4 to 6 hours and ranges from 300 to 400 mg/d. Like codeine, it can cause nausea, constipation, or drowsiness, but reportedly has less of these effects and it is not associated with the GI and renal effects of NSAIDs. Serious reactions include seizures, angioedema, and Stevens-Johnson syndrome.

2. **Psychopharmacologic agents.** The majority of patients with chronic pain will be prescribed an antidepressant. In chronic pain, antidepressants have a dual role of treating mood disorders and independently addressing pain symptoms. Tricyclic antidepressants work through various degrees of inhibition of norepinephrine and serotonin reuptake. Selective serotonin reuptake inhibitors are effective and have a more favorable side effect profile than older agents. (SOR **Ⓑ**) Atypical antidepressants include norepinephrine and dopamine reuptake inhibitors, serotonin-norepinephrine reuptake inhibitors, and serotonin-2 antagonist reuptake inhibitors. These agents have analgesic qualities and are used for chronic pain but have not been proven in randomized control trials.

a. **Tricyclic antidepressants** have analgesic properties in low doses, but maximal analgesic affect is achieved at increased doses. Dosing then should be titrated over weeks and increased to maximum efficacy as dose-related side effects will allow. Typical agents include tertiary amines imipramine (Tofranil), amitriptyline (Elavil), clomipramine (Anafranil), and doxepin (Sinequan). Each has various degrees of anticholinergic activity, and hypotension and sedation are common side effects. Amitriptyline (0.1 mg/kg/d titrated over a few weeks to maximum 150 mg/d) and imipramine (0.2–3 mg/kg/d up to 100 mg/d maximum in elderly or 300 mg/d) have chronic pain indications. The quaternary amines may be better tolerated in older patients and tend to have less central activity and hypotension. (SOR **Ⓑ**) These include desipramine (Norpramin), nortriptyline (Pamelor), protriptyline (Vivactil), and amoxapine (Asendin). Blood counts should be monitored for agranulocytosis or thrombocytopenia.

b. Selective serotonin reuptake inhibitors were introduced in the late 1980s as a novel antidepressant. They were soon found to be useful in a variety of conditions including panic disorder, generalized anxiety, chronic fatigue, premenstrual syndrome, and chronic pain. (SOR **Ⓑ**) Common side effects include headache; stimulation or sedation; cardiac effects (bradycardia or tachycardia); GI effects (increased or decreased appetite, nausea, vomiting, bloating, diarrhea); sedation; fine tremor; and tinnitus. They variably affect libido. Agents include fluoxetine (Prozac), fluvoxamine

TABLE 69–1. OPIOID THERAPY

Drug	Equianalgesic Dose (mg)	Starting Oral Dose /frequency	Duration of Action (h)
Morphine	10 IM, 30 po	15–30 mg/q 2–4 h	3–4
Codeine	75 IM, 130 po	60 mg/q 4–6 h	3–4
Oxycodone	15 IM, 30 po	15–30 mg /q 4–6 h	2–4
Hydromorphone	1.5 IM, 7.5 po	2–4 mg/q 4–6 h	2–4
Levorphanol	2 IM, 4 po	4–8 mg/q 6–8 h	4–8
Methadone	10 IM, 20 po	5–10 mg/q 8–12 h	4–8
Fentanyl patch	25 μg/h = 1 mg/h	25 μg/q 72 h	72

(Luvox), paroxetine (Paxil), sertraline (Zoloft), citalopram (Celexa), and escitalopram (Lexapro). See Chapter 92 on depression for further dosing information.

   c. Duloxetine (Cymbalta), is a balanced, serotonin-norepinephrine reuptake inhibitor. While also treating depression, it is indicated for the treatment of painful diabetic neuropathy. (SOR **B**) It can be dosed 60 mg daily, and major side effects include nausea. Careful monitoring is indicated if the patient is on multiple serotonin medications or when discontinuing the medication.

  3. Opioid agents (Table 69–1). Whereas opioid medications are readily accepted in the management of cancer pain, their use in chronic, nonmalignant pain is characterized by provider fear of regulatory scrutiny, fostering addiction, and overuse. However, the use of opioids is appropriate when usual modalities have failed to provide adequate analgesia. In cancer pain, opioid dose is titrated to patient response and limited by side effects such as respiratory depression. In chronic nonmalignant pain, there is an evidence that continued escalating doses results in worsened analgesic response. (SOR **B**) This is because NMDA receptors are upregulated and lead to tolerance, while pain receptors become more sensitive to similar stimuli. Low to moderate total dosage of opioid agents may have the best response in chronic pain. (SOR **C**) Short-acting agents can be used initially to titrate quickly to effect, then converted to long-acting agents for chronic use. In situations of tolerance to medication with a desire to change receptor response, it is appropriate to switch from one opioid agent to another, usually starting at half the equivalent dose of the alternate medication. (SOR **C**)

  4. Adjuvant therapies. Randomized, controlled trials have shown the efficacy of tricyclic antidepressants and other agents for management of the pain of diabetic neuropathy, postherpetic neuralgia, trigeminal neuralgia, and peripheral neuropathy. These same agents then have been tried for other chronic pain conditions.

   a. Anticonvulsants. Stabilizing neuronal membranes; alteration of sodium, calcium, and potassium ion channels; and effects on other neurotransmitters (norepinephrine, gamma-aminobutyric acid, serotonin, etc) have been proposed mechanisms for anticonvulsants.

    (1) Gabapentin (Neurontin) has been used for a variety of neuropathic pain conditions. It is indicated in the management of postherpetic neuralgia. (SOR **B**) It has relatively few side effects and its absorption is not affected by food. The starting dose is 300 mg at bedtime, gradually increased to 300 mg 3 times daily, then titrated based on response, to a maximum of 1200 mg 3 times daily. Leukopenia is a serious reaction to monitor. Common side effects include somnolence, dizziness, and fatigue. The dose should be adjusted in renal insufficiency.

    (2) Phenytoin can be started at 100 mg 3 times daily and titrated to patient response. Serum levels can be monitored; ≥ 20 μg/mL are considered toxic. It should be taken after meals to decrease GI irritation. Folate (1 mg/d) supplementation should be given to decrease risk of drug-induced peripheral neuropathy and megaloblastic anemia.

    (3) Carbamazepine (Tegretol) may be started at 200 mg/d and increased by 200 mg every 1 to 3 days to a maximum of 1500 mg/d, with therapeutic response typically at 800 to 1200 mg/d. It should be taken with food. Sedation, nausea, diplopia, and vertigo are common side effects; slower titration may minimize them. Monitoring of the complete blood count and liver function studies are important to monitor for aplastic anemia, agranulocytosis, thrombocytosis, and jaundice.

    (4) Valproic acid can be started at 15 mg/kg/d in divided doses and increased weekly by 5 to 10 mg/kg/d to clinical response or a maximum dose of 60 mg/kg. Baseline and periodic liver function tests should be monitored. GI side effects will often improve over time. An extended release preparation (Depakote ER) can be used for once daily dosing.

    (5) Clonazepam (Klonopin) is a benzodiazepine with anticonvulsant activity. It may be started at 0.5 mg 3 times daily and increased by 0.5 mg every 3 to 4 days until adequate response (typically 1–4 mg/d) or a maximum dosage of 6 mg/d is reached. Typical effects of benzodiazepines can be expected. Abrupt cessation of this medication can result in a withdrawal syndrome.

    (6) Pregabalin (Lyrica) works through calcium channels to mediate neurotransmitter pain response. It can be helpful for diabetic, postherpetic, and other neuropathic pain (B). Dosing begins at 50 mg 3 times daily, titrated to 300 mg total daily dose. Doses of 75 mg twice daily have been efficacious for fibromyalgia. (SOR **B**) It has been associated with thrombocytopenia, though common reactions include dizziness, somnolence, and peripheral edema.

  b. Local anesthetics. Local anesthetics have been used as blocking agents subcutaneously, along nerve roots, and at the spinal cord for acute conditions and procedures. In chronic pain, they may be helpful for continuous and lancinating pain, neuropathic pain of herpes zoster, phantom limb pain, and diabetic neuropathy. The mechanism of action is direct stabilization of nerve membranes and decreased ion flux in sodium channels. A trial with intravenous lidocaine (under appropriate cardiac monitoring) can be infused at 1 to 2 mg/kg over 10 to 15 minutes. During the infusion, the patient may experience tinnitus, perioral numbness, a metallic taste in the mouth, or dizziness. A reported 50% or greater reduction in pain based on pre- and postinfusion questionnaires warrants a trial of mexiletine. Oral mexiletine may be given as 150 mg at bedtime, increased weekly to 150 mg 3 times daily, then up to a maximum dose of 10 mg/kg/d or 1200 mg/d. Side effects may include dizziness, tremor, hypotension, ataxia, dyspepsia, or rash.

  c. Antispasmodics are often used to treat spasticity associated with chronic conditions, but they are also believed to have analgesic properties that may augment opioid-induced analgesia.

    (1) Baclofen has been useful for painful spasticity, trigeminal neuralgia, and lancinating neuropathic pain. Oral dosing begins at 5 mg 3 times daily and increased by 5-mg increments every few days to a maximum 80 mg/d. Side effects include central nervous system depression, fatigue, dizziness, orthostatic hypotension, headaches, insomnia, and headache.

    (2) Cyclobenzaprine (Flexeril) relieves muscle spasm without interfering with muscle function. It should not be used for more than 2 to 3 weeks, so it may not be a good choice for chronic conditions. Typical doses range from 20 to 40 mg/d. It should not be given with monoamine oxidase inhibitors, and side effects include arrhythmia, hyperthyroidism, and urinary obstruction.

    (3) Tizanidine (Zanaflex) is an α_2-agonist that decreases sympathetic transmission at the level of the dorsal horn and is indicated for sympathetic maintained pain as well as pain described as lancinating, electrical, or burning. Dosing begins with 1 to 2 mg orally at bedtime and then is switched to 3 times daily dosing with the usual range from 4 to 12 mg/d; it should not exceed 36 mg/d. Side effects include dry mouth, sedation, dizziness, and weakness.

  d. Clonidine. Through α-adrenergic receptor stimulation in the brain stem, decreased sympathetic outflow results in decreased peripheral resistance, heart rate, and blood pressure. Thus, this drug has been used for sympathetically maintained pain. The transdermal patch is associated with more consistent blood levels and easier administration. Dizziness is a common side effect, as well as dry mouth, drowsiness, fatigue, and headache. Clonidine should be used with caution in the patient with already low blood pressure. The 0.1-mg patch (TTS-1) worn daily for a week is the typical starting dose and can be titrated to a maximum of two TTS-3 patches per week.

D. Topical agents. The use of topically applied gels and ointments can help in painful arthritic conditions and work locally, while other agents have effect at the level of the peripheral nerve. Topical analgesics include methyl salicylate/menthol (Ben-Gay), trolamine salicylate (Aspercream), and camphor/phenol (Campho-Phenique). They are best for

TABLE 69–2. COMPONENTS OF A NARCOTIC MEDICATION PAIN CONTRACT

The risks, side effects, and benefits have been discussed in detail.
Only one physician will be responsible for prescribing narcotic pain medications.
Other providers caring for the patient must be aware of the pain medication plan.
Patient must make regular scheduled visits at least every 2 mo to receive prescriptions.
Narcotic prescriptions will not be mailed.
Patient agrees to random urine or blood tests to assess compliance.
Lost, misplaced, destroyed, or stolen medications will not be replaced. Refills will not be given early for any reason.
If there is no observed improvement in quality of life or function for the
patient, narcotic pain medication will be tapered.

localized pain in muscles and joints. (SOR **⑥**) Capsaicin cream (Capsin 0.025%, Zostrix HP 0.075%) depletes substance P at the local area and can provide relief in postherpetic neuralgia. (SOR **⑧**) Caution should be used in not inadvertently making contact with mucus membranes. Finally, the lidocaine patch (Lidoderm 5%) can be used for postherpetic neuralgia, applied up to 12 h/d. (SOR **⑧**)

- E. **Complementary and alternative therapies.** Patients in chronic pain are usually willing to try anything to help relieve their pain. Complementary approaches including homeopathy, naturopathy, and spiritual healing may have a therapeutic effect on the patient, although randomized, controlled trials have not been conducted. The provider must find the balance between maintaining hope while limiting potential harm to the patient.
- F. **Surgical therapies** include implanted nerve stimulators (TENS), injected anesthetics, nerve blocks, and nerve ablation. Specialized anesthesiologists can assist in these techniques.

IV. **Management Strategies**
- A. Effective care of chronic pain is best delivered using multidisciplines and modalities. The biochemical pain may respond better to usual or adjuvant pharmacotherapies. The physical pain may respond to massage, cold/heat, and medication. The emotional pain response may depend on the effective communication of the provider as much as any other treatment. Caregivers must be included in discussions and may be a critical component to implementing care plans.
- B. The patient and care provider must negotiate and agree on the goals of treatment: the reduction rather than elimination of pain; the improvement or restoration of function; the ability to resume social activities; or the improvement of mood. They must also discuss possible limitations including medication side effects (sedation, confusion) or tolerance and risk of addiction. Both patient and provider must be willing to acknowledge when a particular treatment is not working and should be abandoned. With the use of chronic opioid pain medications, a pain contract should be initiated (Table 69–2).

REFERENCES

American Geriatric Society Panel on Persistant Pain in Older Adults. The management of persistent pain in older persons. *J Am Geriatr Soc.* 2002;50(6 Suppl):S205-S224.

American Pain Society: *Principles of Analgesic Use in the Treatment of Acute Pain and Cancer Pain.* 5th ed. Glenview, IL: American Pain Society; 2003.

Ballantyne J, ed. *The Massachusetts General Hospital Handbook of Pain Management.* 3rd ed. Philadelphia: Lippincott, Williams & Wilkins; 2005.

Ballantyne J, Mao J. Opioid therapy for chronic pain. *N Engl J Med.* 2003;349(20):1943-1953.

Guidelines for using the Edmonton Symptom Assessment System (ESAS). Caritas Health Group. http://www.palliative.org/PC/clinicalinfo/assessmenttools/easa.pdf, accessed August 4, 2008.

H. Bruce Vogt, MD

KEY POINTS

- Chronic obstructive pulmonary disease (COPD) is the fourth leading cause of death in the United States, and the mortality rate continues to rise.
- COPD is divided into two types—emphysema and chronic bronchitis. Although additional risk factors have been identified, cigarette smoking accounts for greater than 80% of cases.
- The primary differential diagnoses for COPD are asthma, bronchiectasis, and congestive heart failure. In acute exacerbations, the physician must consider comorbid disorders causing or contributing to the respiratory deterioration such as infection (pneumonia, purulent bronchitis), congestive heart failure, cardiac dysrhythmias, pneumothorax, pulmonary embolism, and myocardial infarction.
- Spirometry is required to make the diagnosis of COPD, assess disease severity, and monitor response to treatment.
- Bronchodilators via metered-dose inhalers—either anticholinergic (ipratropium bromide [Atrovent], tiotropium [Spiriva]) or β_2-adrenergic agents (e.g., albuterol [Ventolin, Proventil], salmeterol [Serevent Diskus], formoterol [Foradil])—are the initial drugs used in the management of COPD. If symptoms are intermittent, initiate therapy with a short-acting agent (ipratropium or albuterol). If symptoms are persistent, a long-acting agent (tiotropium, salmeterol, or formoterol) should be prescribed with a short-acting agent used in addition as needed. Long-acting drugs are not appropriate for acute bronchospasm. Albuterol is preferred over ipratropium as a "rescue" drug given its quicker onset of action.

I. **Introduction**
  A. **Definition. COPD** is a preventable and treatable disease characterized by airflow limitation that is generally progressive, although it may be partially reversible. It is associated with an inflammatory response of the lung to noxious particles or gases and may be accompanied by airflow hyper-reactivity. It also causes significant extrapulmonary effects. Pathologically, there is a mixture of small airway disease (obstructive bronchiolitis) and parenchymal destruction (emphysema). COPD is manifested clinically as emphysema, chronic bronchitis, or both.

  Chronic bronchitis is defined clinically as the presence of a chronic productive cough for 3 consecutive months in 2 successive years. **Emphysema** is defined morphologically as permanent enlargement of airspaces distal to the terminal bronchioles caused by destruction of alveolar walls.

  B. **Epidemiology. COPD** affects an estimated 16 million persons in the United States. It is the fourth leading cause of death, and mortality rates continue to rise. The prevalence of the disease is significantly higher in those older than 40 years, in men, and in smokers and ex-smokers. Although more common in men, the prevalence of COPD has increased in women as smoking rates in women have increased. The predominant form is chronic bronchitis.

  C. **Pathophysiology/risk factors**
    1. Cigarette smoking, usually at least a 20 pack-year history, is the major cause of COPD, accounting for greater than 80% of cases, although not all smokers develop clinically significant COPD. This suggests that genetic factors modify risk. The age of onset of smoking, total pack-years, and current smoking status are predictive of mortality from COPD. The role of passive smoking (secondhand smoke) is unclear, although it may contribute to COPD.
    2. Occupational exposure to hazardous airborne substances (e.g., dusts, gases, fumes), when intense or prolonged, is an independent risk factor for COPD and, when associated with smoking, increases the risk of disease. Indoor pollution from biomass cooking and heating in poorly ventilated dwellings is a risk factor. Urban air pollution is harmful to persons with lung disease, but its role in the etiology of COPD is uncertain.

3. α_1-Antitrypsin deficiency is a rare genetic abnormality that accounts for less than 1% of COPD. More than 95% of severely deficient individuals are monozygous for the Z allele (PiZZ). Screening for this problem should be considered in patients who present with COPD prior to age 45, a predominance of basilar emphysema in a smoker with dyspnea, unremitting asthma, unexplained hepatic cirrhosis, or a family history of the disorder.

II. Diagnosis

A. Differential diagnosis

1. The primary differential diagnoses for COPD are asthma, bronchiectasis, and congestive heart failure. Asthma and congestive heart failure are discussed in Chapters 68 and 72, respectively. Bronchiectasis is a disease in which destruction of the structural components of the bronchial walls leads to permanent dilation of bronchi. Infection is the primary cause. Clinical features include persistent cough productive of purulent sputum and episodic exacerbations of increased sputum production and fever.

B. Symptoms and signs

1. Dyspnea is the cardinal symptom of patients with emphysema and the reason most patients with COPD seek medical care. Chronic productive cough is the key symptom of patients with chronic bronchitis and is often the first symptom of COPD. Initially, it may be intermittent. Sputum is usually mucoid except during exacerbations, when it may become purulent.

2. Other symptoms of COPD include wheezing, chest tightness, and recurrent respiratory infections. Anorexia and weight loss are common in advanced emphysema. Anxiety and depression are also frequent problems in severe COPD.

3. COPD is characterized by acute exacerbations, with shorter intervals between episodes as the disease progresses.

4. The physical examination may be entirely normal or reveal only prolonged expiration or wheezing on forced expiration with early or mild disease.

5. With later-stage disease, hyperinflation is manifested by a barrel-shaped chest, hyperresonance to percussion, decreased breath sounds, and distant heart sounds. Crackles may be heard, particularly in chronic bronchitis, and wheezing is common. In advanced disease, there is dyspnea at rest and may be cyanosis. The patient often uses pursed lip breathing during expiration and the accessory muscles of respiration are employed. While sitting, the patients may lean forward and rest on their elbows to increase use of the accessory muscles (*tripoding*).

6. Physical findings unrelated to heart failure may include a palpable but normal-sized liver owing to chest hyperexpansion and neck vein distention as a result of increased intrathoracic pressure. When right heart failure is present, increased jugular venous distention, tender hepatomegaly, and peripheral edema are typical.

C. Diagnostic tests

1. **Office spirometry** is necessary to make the diagnosis, assess disease severity, and monitor response to treatment. In addition, it is indicated in COPD patients who will be undergoing an operation. Measurements of airflow include forced vital capacity (FVC), forced expiratory volume in 1 second (FEV_1), forced expiratory flow rate over the interval from 25% to 75% of the total FVC ($FEF_{25\%-75\%}$), and the calculated FEV_1/FVC ratio. Lung volume measurements, important in diagnosing restrictive lung disease, are not routinely used in the office management of COPD. It is logical that an active lung infection, active hemoptysis, unstable angina, and a recent myocardial infarction are among the contraindications to spirometry.

   a. **Spirometry** results should be compared to reference values based on race, gender, age, and height. An FEV_1/FVC ratio less than 70% indicates airflow limitation. If initial testing indicates airflow limitation (particularly Stage II COPD or greater) a short-acting inhaled bronchodilator should be administered and the testing repeated in 10 minutes. A 15% or greater increase in the FEV_1 or a 30% or greater increase in the $FEF_{25\%-75\%}$ indicates a significant component of reversibility. Glucocorticoid reversibility testing may be performed in selective cases (e.g., history of childhood asthma, nocturnal awakening because of coughing or wheezing). For daily monitoring by the patient and during office follow-up visits, the peak expiratory flow rate—which correlates well with FEV_1 in an individual patient—can be easily measured with use of an inexpensive peak flow meter. The spirometric classification of COPD from the Global Initiative for Chronic Obstructive Lung Disease (GOLD) is depicted in Table 70–1.

TABLE 70–1. SPIROMETRIC CLASSIFICATION OF COPD SEVERITY BASED ON POSTBRONCHODILATOR FEV$_1$

Stage I: Mild	$FEV_1/FVC < 0.70$ $FEV_1 \geq 80\%$ predicted
Stage II: Moderate	$FEV_1/FVC < 0.70$ $50\% \leq FEV_1 \leq 80\%$ predicted
Stage III: Severe	$FEV_1/FVC < 0.70$ $30\% \leq FEV_1 \leq 50\%$ predicted
Stage IV: Very Severe	$FEV_1/FVC < 0.70$ $FEV_1 < 30\%$ predicted *or* $FEV_1 < 50\%$ predicted plus chronic respiratory failure

FEV_1, forced expiratory volume in one second; FVC, forced vital capacity; Respiratory failure, arterial partial pressure of oxygen (PaO_2) less than 8.0 kPa (60 mm Hg) with or without arterial partial pressure of CO_2 ($PaCO_2$) greater than 6.7 kPa (50 mm Hg) while breathing air at sea level.
(Reproduced with permission from the Global Initiative for Chronic Obstructive Lung Disease (GOLD). 2006. Global strategy for the diagnosis, management and prevention of COPD. http://www.goldcopd.org. Accessed October 28, 2008.)

2. **Arterial blood gas measurements** are usually normal in early or mild COPD. They should be obtained in patients with an $FEV_1 \leq 50\%$ of predicted, findings suggestive of respiratory or right heart failure, polycythemia, dysrhythmias, or an altered mental state. A $PaO_2 \leq 60$ mm Hg (hypoxemia) with or without a $PaCO_2$ of ≥ 50 mm Hg (hypoventilation, respiratory acidosis) on room air indicates respiratory failure. An O_2 saturation of $\leq 90\%$ also indicates hypoxemia. Arterial blood gases should also be obtained if oxygen therapy is initiated and periodically thereafter. Finger or ear pulse oximetry may be used for follow-up of patients in both the hospital and outpatient settings but is less reliable.

3. **Complete blood counts** are indicated to screen for polycythemia and when the patient is febrile or a superimposed infection is suspected. Eosinophilia suggests atopy and possibly an element of reversible bronchospasm (i.e., allergic asthma).

4. **Chest x-rays** are unremarkable in early disease, but abnormalities are apparent with advanced disease. Findings include hyperexpansion characterized by a low and flat diaphragm, increased anteroposterior diameter of the thorax, hyperlucency, increased retrosternal airspace, and a vertically positioned, narrow heart shadow. Bullae may or may not be seen and, if present, may only indicate focal severe disease, not necessarily diffuse disease. High-resolution computerized tomographic scans of the chest have a much greater sensitivity and specificity, but are not part of routine care unless the diagnosis is in doubt or if a surgical procedure (e.g., bullectomy) is considered.

5. **Electrocardiograms** are not routinely indicated, although in patients with long-standing COPD, may show low voltage, right axis deviation, poor R wave progression, and, when cor pulmonale is present, may demonstrate right atrial enlargement (P pulmonale) and right ventricular hypertrophy with strain.

III. **Treatment.** Treatment goals include prevention of progression, correction of any reversible component, increasing respiratory muscle function, improving exercise tolerance, controlling symptoms (optimum therapy), minimizing and treating exacerbations, treating complications, improving overall health status, and reducing mortality. The various components of treatment are discussed below. A typical drug regimen for treating COPD is outlined in Figure 70–1. No drugs modify the natural history of COPD.

A. **Nutrition**

1. Patients with COPD are prone to nutritional deficiencies and have below-normal muscle mass, including respiratory muscles. Weight loss may be because of reduced caloric intake and hypermetabolism. Low body weight is associated with impaired lung function, exercise capacity, and a higher mortality rate. Unfortunately, a meta-analysis showed nutritional support had no effect on anthropometric measures, lung function, or exercise capacity in patients with stable COPD.

2. Inhaled bronchodilators, as well as chest physiotherapy if part of a patient's treatment plan, should be scheduled 1 hour before or after meals to prevent or reduce nausea.

3. For the patient with advanced disease, frequent small meals may help avoid loss of appetite and the adverse metabolic and ventilatory effects of a high caloric load.

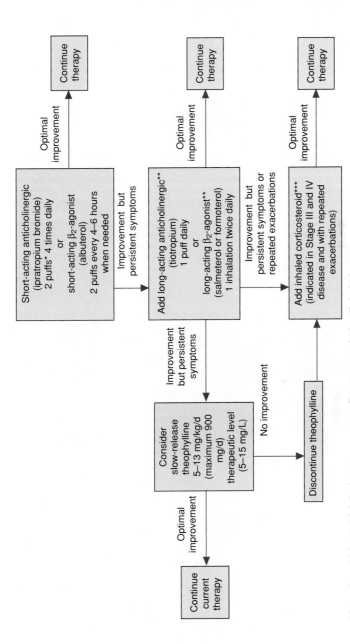

*Sometimes higher total daily dosage necessary. Do not exceed 12 puffs in 24 hours.
**May use both long-acting anticholinergic and β₂-agonist if suboptimal response with single agent.
***If good response, consider combination of a β₂-agonist with a corticosteriod.

FIGURE 70–1. A typical drug regimen for treating chronic obstructive pulmonary disease.

4. Adequate protein intake (approximately 20% of calories or 1.2–1.5 g of protein per kilogram) is important to maintaining muscle mass. Liquid high-calorie protein supplements can enhance caloric intake.

5. Sodium restriction is appropriate in patients with cor pulmonale or congestive heart failure.

6. Fluid intake should be adequate to maintain good hydration and help thin secretions, thereby promoting expectoration.

7. Consultation with a nutritionist may be helpful in developing a plan tailored to the patient.

B. Exercise

1. Exercise has both physiologic and psychologic benefits.

2. A combination of muscle strength and endurance training is beneficial. Programs should relate to daily activities such as walking and use of the arms. Recommendations for frequency, intensity, and duration vary based on baseline functional status, needs, and goals.

3. Regular lower extremity exercise improves exercise tolerance, particularly endurance, enhances performance of daily activities, and reduces dyspnea. Walking, jogging, bicycling, stair climbing, and swimming are examples of aerobic (endurance) exercise. Treadmills, exercycles, and stair steppers are also effective devices, as well as cross-country ski and rowing machines, which provide the added benefit of upper extremity exercise.

4. Upper extremity exercise is associated with a higher ventilatory and metabolic demand than lower extremity exercise. Upper extremity training, endurance and strength, improves arm muscle endurance and sense of well-being.

5. Resistance training (e.g., weightlifting) is the mainstay of strengthening.

6. Breathing retraining and respiratory muscle training are discussed below.

C. Bronchodilators. β_2-agonists, anticholinergics, and methylxanthines are the principal bronchodilators used in COPD. β-Adrenergic agents produce sympathetic-mediated bronchodilation, whereas anticholinergic agents reduce parasympathetic-mediated bronchoconstriction. The methylxanthine, theophylline, is a nonselective phosphodiesterase inhibitor that has a bronchodilatory effect, but primarily decreases dyspnea by enhancing diaphragmatic function. Bronchodilators are either given on a routine basis to prevent or decrease symptoms or as needed for relief of acute or persistent symptoms. Both β_2-agonists and anticholinergic agents improve exercise capacity and reduce symptoms. (SOR **Ⓐ**) Inhaled bronchodilators are preferred. Side effects are less common and resolve more quickly upon cessation than with oral preparations. The potential for theophylline toxicity is also a concern. Regular use of long-acting agents is more convenient and effective (i.e., decreased dyspnea, improved exercise capacity and health-related quality of life) than short-acting bronchodilators, although more expensive. (SOR **Ⓐ**) Combining drugs with different mechanisms of action may improve pulmonary function and health status. Combining a long-acting anticholinergic with a β_2-agonist may improve quality of life more than a β_2-agonist alone. Increasing the number of drugs, however, usually increases cost. Therefore, increasing the dose of one agent is an appropriate strategy as this may offer a similar benefit, assuming side effects are not a problem. Ultimately, the choice of bronchodilator(s) relates to availability, patient response, and cost consideration. Patient education in how to use an inhaler is imperative.

1. **Anticholinergic agents** have an effectiveness at least as good as that of β-adrenergic agents in improving the pulmonary function of patients with COPD. Side effects (dry mouth, metallic taste, urinary retention, and glaucoma secondary to mydriasis) have been reported, though tend to be less troublesome. They have fewer cardiac side effects and tremor. They are supplied as either metered-dose inhalers (MDI), powder dose inhalers (PDI), or aerosols for use with nebulizers. Ipratropium bromide (Atrovent, Atrovent HFA) is the only short-acting agent and tiotropium (Spiriva) is the only long-acting agent currently available in the United States. Given a number of studies demonstrating that anticholinergic agents produce significantly greater bronchodilation than β-adrenergics, and the fact that they reduce mucus hypersecretion, have fewer side effects even at high doses, and do not cause tachyphylaxis, many consider anticholinergics as the initial agents of choice for maintenance therapy. However, a Cochrane database systematic review found any advantage to be small. Ipratropium (Atrovent, Atrovent HFA) has a slower onset of action than short-acting β_2-agonists and is not suited for "rescue" when a rapid response is required. The standard dosage

of an ipratropium (Atrovent, Atrovent HFA) MDI is 2 to 4 puffs 4 times daily, but higher doses may be required and tolerated in selected patients with severe exacerbations. A combined preparation of ipratropium and albuterol is available as an MDI (Combivent) or as a solution for nebulization (Duo Neb), although the same systematic review noted above showed little advantage of the combination drug over a β_2-agonist alone. Tiotropium (Spiriva), a long-acting anticholinergic, is used as one inhalation daily. It has proven to be more effective than ipratropium in improving symptoms, quality of life, decreasing exacerbations and related hospitalizations. (SOR **Ⓐ**) A disadvantage is the markedly higher cost.

2. β-**Adrenergic agents** are available in inhaled (via MDI, PDI, or nebulizer), oral, and subcutaneous preparations. Selective β_2 agents are preferred to minimize the likelihood of β_1 (cardiac) side effects. Inhalation via MDI, PDI, or nebulizer-delivered aerosol is preferential to oral preparations because of their ability to present a high concentration of drug to target receptors with minimal systemic effects. Short-acting (albuterol [Ventolin, Ventolin HFA, Proventil, Proventil HFA], levalbuterol [Xopenex, Xopenex HFA]) and long-acting (salmeterol [Serevent Diskus], formoterol [Foradil]) agents are available. The usual regimen for short-acting agents given via an MDI is 2 puffs 4 times daily. Salmeterol (Serevent Diskus) and formoterol (Foradil) are both inhalation powders, given as one inhalation twice daily. They must not be given more often because of their duration of action. Salmeterol (Serevent Diskus) and formoterol (Foradil) are excellent choices for the patient with nocturnal symptoms. The short-acting agents are required for "rescue" in the scenario of acute bronchospasm with dyspnea. In severe exacerbations, nebulized aerosol can deliver a high concentration of medication; however, the repeated use of an MDI has equivalent effects, particularly when a spacer is employed. Routine use of a spacer is always preferable, but particularly in the setting of an acute exacerbation or for patients who are not facile with use of an MDI. The potential for cardiac dysrhythmias necessitates careful monitoring in patients with known cardiac disease, although complications are rare with usual doses. Levalbuterol (Xopenex, Xopenex HFA) is the *R*-isomer of racemic albuterol and is given as 2 puffs every 4 to 6 hours as needed. Although promoted as safer than albuterol, with less effect on heart rate, there appears to be no significant clinical advantage and is considerably more expensive. See Table 70–2 for inhaled bronchodilator preparations and dosages. Oral β_2 drugs should only be prescribed for patients unable to use inhaled agents, and when employed, should be administered in small doses that are gradually increased. If inhaled dosage is adequate, little additional bronchodilation is gained from an added oral agent and side effects are more common. A subcutaneous preparation of terbutaline (Brethine, Bricanyl) is available with a recommended dose of 0.25 mg every 6 hours.

3. **Theophylline** is effective in COPD through more than one mechanism. Although a bronchodilator, it also improves diaphragmatic function and stimulates the respiratory center. The fact that theophylline can improve cardiac output, decrease pulmonary vascular resistance, and improve the perfusion of ischemic cardiac muscle offers advantages to COPD patients with associated cor pulmonale or cardiac disease. It, however, is not a first-line drug and carries the risk of significant toxicity. It is appropriate to consider adding it in patients who remain symptomatic despite optimum bronchodilator inhalation therapy and in patients who have difficulty with or are noncompliant with MDIs. Potential toxicities include gastrointestinal intolerance (e.g., anorexia, nausea, vomiting, abdominal cramping, diarrhea), headache, tremors, cardiac side effects (e.g., sinus tachycardia, premature ventricular contractions, ventricular tachycardia), and seizures. Ventricular tachycardia and seizures tend to occur at high serum concentrations ($\geq$35 mg/L). Toxicities are more likely in patients who do not metabolize the drug well (e.g., liver disease) and when drug interactions increase the level of theophylline.

a. **Dosage.** The usual starting dose, based on lean body weight, for a nonsmoking patient is 5 to 13 mg/kg/d of a long-acting preparation given every 12 hours. However, the most appropriate dose depends on many factors including age, lean body weight, smoking status (speeds rate of metabolism), liver function, associated congestive heart failure, and concomitant drug use. The therapeutic window is narrow (5–15 mg/L) and serum levels must be checked on a regular basis. Patients with daily fluctuations in symptoms may benefit from peak and trough theophylline levels. A conservative approach is to start with 400 mg/d given as 200 mg twice a day

TABLE 70–2. COMMON INHALANT BRONCHODILATORS

Class	Drug	Formulation*/Adult Dosage	Cost[††]
Anticholinergic	Ipratropium bromide[†,‡] (Atrovent, Atrovent HFA)	MDI/2 puffs qid; maximum 12 puffs daily Nebulized/0.5 mg tid–qid	$$
	Tiotropium[§] (Spiriva)	DPI/1 inhalation once daily	$$$$
β$_2$-agonists[¶]	Albuterol (Proventil, Proventil HFA, Ventolin, Ventolin HFA, Volmax, VoSpire ER, Ventodisk)	MDI/2 puffs q 4–6 h Nebulized/2.5 mg tid–qid	$ $
	Levalbuterol (Xopenex, Xopenex HFA)	MDI/2 puffs q 4–6 h Nebulized/0.63–1.25 mg q 6–8 h	$$$ $$$
	Metaproterenol (Alupent)	MDI/2–3 puffs q 3–4 h Nebulized/0.2–0.3 mL q 4 h	$$ $$
	Pirbuterol (Maxair, Maxair Autohaler)	MDI/1–2 puffs q 4–6 h	$$
	Salmeterol (Servent Diskus)**	DPI/1 inhalation bid	$$$$
	Formoterol (Foradil)**	DPI/1 inhalation bid	$$$
Combination anticholinergic– β$_2$-agonist	Ipratropium[‡]–albuterol (Combivent)	MDI/2 puffs qid; maximum 12 puffs daily	$$$
	(DuoNeb)	Nebulized/2.5 mg (albuterol)/0.5 mg (ipratropium) qid	$$$$$

*MDI, metered-dose inhaler; DPI, dry powder inhaler.
[†] Slower onset of action than short-acting β$_2$-agonists, making the latter preferable for acute bronchospasm.
[‡] Contraindicated in patients with soy & peanut allergy.
[§] Long-acting, given once daily; not used for acute bronchospasm.
[¶] Given there are some β$_1$-receptors in cardiac muscle, a significant cardiovascular effect can occur in some patients, particularly at high dosages.
**Long-acting, given bid; not used for acute bronchospasm.
[††] Range of average monthly cost from $ (low) to $$$$ $ (high).

and increase the dose every 3 to 5 days if tolerated. Starting with a lower dose and gradually increasing it may be of benefit to patients with a history of gastrointestinal intolerance to medication.

- D. **Corticosteroids** given by inhalation are indicated in patients with Stage III and IV COPD. (SOR **A**) Although they do not modify the natural history of the disease, they do reduce the rate of exacerbations. Treatment of exacerbations with oral or parenteral agents improves dyspnea, reduces treatment failure and the need for additional treatment. (SOR **A**) There is no evidence to support long-term use of glucocorticoids in stable patients. (SOR **A**) Parenteral steroids are commonly used during acute exacerbations treated in the hospital setting. A study employing parenteral methylprednisolone (Solu Medrol) reported more rapid improvement of FEV$_1$ over the first 72 hours in patients treated with steroids compared with those who were not. This clinical trial demonstrated that patients treated with systemic steroids had fewer treatment failures, better spirometry, and shorter hospital stays.
  1. **Dosage/route**
     - a. **Oral administration.** For acute exacerbations, **prednisone** can be started in doses of 30 to 40 mg daily for 7 to 10 days. Long-term treatment is not recommended. (SOR **A**)
     - b. **Parenteral administration.** In the Systemic Corticosteroids in COPD Exacerbations clinical trial, methylprednisolone (Solu Medrol) 125 mg was given every 6 hours for 72 hours followed by oral prednisone tapered for up to 57 days.
     - c. **Inhalant administration.** Available inhalant preparations include beclomethasone (QVAR), flunisolide (Aerobid, Aerobid-M, Aerospan), fluticasone (Flovent, Flovent HFA, Flovent Rotadisk), triamcinolone (Azmacort), budesonide (Pulmicort Turbuhaler), and mometasone (Asmanex Twisthaler).
  2. **Side effects.** Oral candidiasis is the most common side effect reported with use of a steroid inhaler and can be prevented by use of a spacer and by rinsing the mouth with water after use.
- E. **Combined bronchodilators/corticosteroids.** Combination therapy with a long-acting β$_2$-agonist and a corticosteroid improves symptoms, spirometric indices, quality of life, and decreases mean rates of exacerbations. (SOR **A**) Fluticasone + salmeterol (Advair

Diskus, dry powder inhaler, 100/50, 250/50, 500/50) is given as one inhalation twice daily. The newer aerosol preparation (Advair HFA 45/21, 115/21, 230/21) is given as 2 puffs twice daily, as is the combination medication budesonide + formoterol (Symbicort).

F. **Antibiotics** are usually indicated for acute exacerbations of COPD. Increased dyspnea is the main symptom of an exacerbation of COPD. Although viral infections may cause an exacerbation, increased sputum volume and purulence suggests a bacterial etiology. Influenza, parainfluenza, coronavirus, and rhinovirus are common viral pathogens. Bacteria may either be the cause of an infection or represent a secondary infection of what originated as a viral syndrome. The GOLD Program recommends antibiotics in patients presenting with the three cardinal symptoms (increased dyspnea, sputum volume, and purulence), in patients with increased sputum purulence and one other cardinal symptom, and in patients requiring mechanical ventilation. Antibiotics reduce short-term mortality and treatment failures for patients with an acute exacerbation. (SOR **A**) The emergence of drug resistance also demands thoughtful consideration in antibiotic selection. The most likely bacterial pathogens include: *Haemophilus influenzae, Streptococcus pneumoniae, Moraxella catarrhalis, and Pseudomonas aeruginosa. Mycoplasma pneumoniae* and *Chlamydia pneumoniae* have also been reported. First-line, less expensive antibiotics include amoxicillin, sulfa-trimethoprim, tetracycline, doxycycline, and erythromycin. Second-line agents offer broader coverage, but are more expensive. Table 70–3 lists first- and second-line oral antibiotics commonly used during exacerbations of COPD. There is no evidence to support prophylactic or continuous use of antibiotics.

G. **Mucolytic agents** are associated with a small reduction in acute exacerbations and total days of disability. (SOR **A**) They may be of the most benefit for patients with exacerbations that are frequent, prolonged, or require repeated admission to the hospital. They may be beneficial during the winter months in patients with moderate or severe COPD who are not on inhaled steroids. Their widespread use cannot be recommended. Hydration (oral, intravenous) and moisture administered by nebulization may be useful.

H. **Chest physiotherapy** (manual or mechanical chest compression, postural drainage) may be of benefit to patients who produce ≥25 mL/d of sputum during acute exacerbations.

TABLE 70–3. **COMMON ORAL ANTIBIOTICS FOR CHRONIC OBSTRUCTIVE PULMONARY DISEASE EXACERBATIONS**

	Drug	Dosage (10-d Course)	Cost*
First-line agents	Amoxicillin (generic, Amoxil, Polymox, Trimox)	500 mg tid	$
	Sulfamethoxazole/trimethoprim† (generic, Bactrim, Septra, Sulfatrim)	160 mg/800 mg bid	$
	Tetracycline (generic, Sumycin)	500 mg qid	$
	Doxycycline (generic, Vibramycin, Doryx, Monodox)	100 mg bid	$
	Erythromycin (generic, Eryc, E-mycin, EES)	1000–2000 mg/d divided dose (bid–qid) depending on agent	$
Second-line agents	Amoxicillin/clavulanate potassium (Augmentin)	500–875 mg/125 mg bid or 250–500 mg/125 mg tid	$$$
	Cerfuroxime (Ceftin)	250–500 mg bid	$$$
	Ceprozil (Cefzil)	250–500 mg bid	$$$$
	Cefixime (Suprax)	400 mg/d (once daily)	$
	Cefpodoxime (Vantin)	100–400 mg bid	$$$$
	Loracarbef (Lorabid)	200–400 mg bid	$$$$
	Cefdinir (Omnicef)	14 mg/kg/d up to 600 mg divided daily or bid	$$$$
	Azithromycin (Zithromax)‡,§	500 mg day 1, then 250 mg days 1–4	$$
	Clarithromycin (Biaxin)§	500 mg bid	$$$
	Levofloxacin (Levaquin)§	500 mg daily	$$$

*Range of daily cost from $ (low) to $$$$ (high).
†Available in single-strength (80 mg/400 mg) or double-strength (160 mg/800 mg) tablets.
‡Five-day course.
§Caution must be taken when using macrolides or levofloxacin (Levaquin) in a patient on theophylline because of drug level increases of the latter.

  I. Antitussives must be used judiciously as cough has a significant protective role. If prescribed, a nonnarcotic agent such as dextromethorphan should be tried. Codeine and other narcotics should be avoided, because they cause respiratory depression and may worsen hypercapnia.

  J. Other treatments

    1. Respiratory stimulants are not currently recommended.

    2. Nebulized opioids have not been sufficiently tested to determine if they are effective.

    3. Antioxidants such as N-acetylcysteine have been shown in small studies to reduce the frequency of exacerbations, but a large randomized controlled trial found no effect except in patients not treated with inhaled steroids.

    4. Phosphodiesterase-4 (PDE$_4$) inhibitors are being studied. The role of these selective agents is yet to be determined.

    5. α_1-Antitrypsin therapy is expensive and not available in most countries. It should only be considered in patients with emphysema related to the deficiency of this protease inhibitor.

    6. Psychoactive agents to treat depression, insomnia, or anxiety can be helpful to improve the quality of life for patients with COPD. Benzodiazepines are best avoided because of the potential for suppressing ventilatory drive. Nortriptyline, sertraline, and buspirone are reported to reduce anxiety in COPD patients and buspirone decreased dyspnea in one small study. The antidepressant bupropion may be of assistance in smoking cessation.

    7. Surgery can be considered in carefully selected patients. Bullectomy, which allows greater lung expansion, is effective in reducing dyspnea and improving pulmonary function. In a large multicenter trial of **lung volume reduction surgery**, patients with upper lobe emphysema and low exercise capacity had a greater survival rate at 4.3 years and improved maximal work capacity and health-related quality of life compared with similar patients who received medical therapy. This palliative operation, however, is expensive and associated with significant morbidity and an early mortality rate of approximately 5%. Other techniques are being studied (e.g., bronchoscopic lung reduction).

IV. Management Strategies. The primary care physician should develop an individualized plan for the patient and coordinate the care given by others.

  A. Smoking cessation. This is often the most difficult challenge faced by the patient with COPD but also the most important, as only smoking cessation modifies the natural history of the disease by decreasing the rate of pulmonary function decline. Smoking cessation decreases cough and sputum production, slows the decline of FEV_1, and reduces the risk of respiratory failure. It can also lower the patient's risk of contracting other smoking-related illnesses. The physician needs to be persistent in educating patients about the benefits of and methods for discontinuing smoking. Since there are various factors that foster smoking, success in cessation often involves combined approaches. Practical counseling, behavior modification, self-help materials, group cessation programs, social support, and pharmacotherapies all have a place in assisting the patient (see Chapter 100).

  B. Hospitalization. The physician should consider hospitalization for the patient with COPD under the following circumstances:

    1. Acute exacerbations failing to respond to outpatient treatment.

    2. Marked increase in the intensity of symptoms.

    3. Onset of new physical findings (e.g., cyanosis, peripheral edema).

    4. Impaired level of consciousness or acute confusion.

    5. Severe COPD or frequent exacerbations.

    6. Significant comorbidities, both pulmonary (e.g., pneumothorax, pleural effusion, pneumonia, pulmonary contusion) and nonpulmonary (e.g., rib or vertebral body fracture, severe steroid myopathy).

    7. New-onset cardiac dysrhythmias.

    8. Lack of sufficient home support either by family or supplementary home care services.

    9. Planned surgical or diagnostic procedure requiring analgesics or sedatives that may adversely affect pulmonary function.

  C. Environmental control

    1. Patients should avoid exposure to secondhand tobacco smoke and remain indoors when air quality is poor.

2. Patients who are sensitive to extremes of humidity and temperature may find that use of a humidifier in the winter and a dehumidifier or air conditioner in the summer improves symptoms.
3. Air cleaners, whether directed against indoor or outdoor generated air contaminants, are ineffective.
4. Commercial aircraft are usually pressurized between 5000 and 10,000 feet. Most patients do not require supplemental oxygen, though hypercapneic patients do. A flow rate of 1 to 3 L per nasal cannula usually suffices. Patients should contact their travel airline a few days prior to flights to learn specifics for making the necessary arrangements. Patients should avoid flying in unpressurized aircraft, and those with large bullae should probably not fly at all because of the significantly increased potential for pneumothoraces.

D. **Home oxygen therapy.** The administration of oxygen for 15 hours or more per day to patients with a PaO_2 less than 60 mm Hg increases survival. (SOR Ⓐ) It positively impacts hemodynamics, hematologic characteristics, exercise capacity, lung mechanics, and mental state. It also improves sleep and cognitive performance. Reversal of hypoxemia supersedes concerns about CO_2 retention, which is rare. Oxygen is the most potent treatment for cor pulmonale and mitigates right heart failure secondary to it.

1. **Guidelines**
   a. $PaO_2 \leq 55$ mm Hg or $SaO_2 \leq 88\%$ (waking values), with or without hypercapnia; OR PaO_2 between 55 mm Hg and 60 mm Hg or SaO_2 of 88% with pulmonary hypertension, peripheral edema suggesting congestive heart failure, or polycythemia (hematocrit $\geq 55\%$).
   b. The goal is to increase baseline PaO_2 to at least 60 to 65 mm Hg or $SaO_2 \geq 90\%$ at rest, with exertion and during sleep using the lowest liter flow rate possible. Start with 1 L/min by nasal cannula. The flow rate should be adjusted upward over baseline for exercise and sleep if required to prevent desaturation.

2. **Sources and delivery systems** include:
   a. Nasal continuous flow, pulse demand, reservoir cannula, and transtracheal catheter.
   b. Liquid gas (in canisters) is the only practical system for active individuals, but is more expensive and may be of limited availability in small communities.
   c. Compressed gas (in high-pressure cylinders) is widely available and lower cost. However, multiple tanks are needed and the tanks are heavy and unsightly.
   d. Concentrators are convenient for home use and lower cost. Disadvantages include the lack of portability, noise, and need for electricity.
   e. Oxygen-conserving devices allow more efficient oxygen delivery. They either collect O_2 flowing during expiration or only permit O_2 flow during inspiration (demand system).

3. **Monitoring.** A patient should initially be assessed via arterial blood gases. Monitoring may then be accomplished by either arterial blood gases or by pulse oximetry done periodically. This is particularly important in the patient with worsening symptoms. Pulse oximetry should also be checked with typical exertion (e.g., walking in the hallway) and sleep, as a patient's resting oxygen saturation may be normal.

E. **Pulmonary rehabilitation** is a multidisciplinary, multidimensional approach to care of patients with chronic respiratory diseases with goals of reducing symptoms, preventing complications, improving quality of life, and achieving the individual's maximum level of independence and functioning in the community. Major components include: education, nutrition counseling, exercise training, breathing re-training, and inspiratory muscle training.

1. **Patients at all stages of disease** appear to benefit from exercise training by demonstrating improved exercise tolerance and less dyspnea and fatigue. (SOR Ⓐ) It is unknown whether repeated rehabilitation courses enable patients to sustain benefits gained in an initial program.
2. **Strength training** has proven benefits, as does **lower extremity strengthening,** the key element of endurance training.
3. **Breathing retraining** should be part of a rehabilitation program with the aim of helping the patient relieve and control dyspnea and of counteracting physiologic abnormalities such as hyperinflation. Pursed-lip and diaphragmatic breathing assist in slowing the respiratory rate and increasing tidal volume, while inhibiting airspace collapse and enhancing gas exchange. Both help alleviate dyspnea. Leaning forward and resting the arms on one's thighs or on a table (*tripoding*) may also help relieve dyspnea.

4. **Inspiratory muscle training** likely increases respiratory muscle strength, but its effect on symptoms and functional limitations is not clearly established.
5. **Baseline assessment** includes:
   a. History and physical examination
   b. Spirometry (pre and postbronchodilator)
   c. Assessment of exercise capacity
   d. Measurement of health status and impact of breathlessness
   e. Assessment of inspiratory and expiratory muscle strength and quadriceps strength in patients with muscle wasting
6. **Outcomes assessment** includes retesting items c, d, and e above.

F. **Personalized patient education** should address the disease process and provide information about medications (e.g., rationale, side effects, inhaler technique, and home oxygen, if prescribed). Patient education and patient–physician agreement on short- and long-term goals improve adherence to the therapeutic regimen. This should include helping identify a way for the patient to monitor progress toward goals. Sensitive issues such as sexual activity should be addressed. Education of family members, particularly those involved in the patient's care, is also important and, given the considerable adaptation they must make in their own lives, caregivers may need supportive therapy themselves.

G. **Immunization** for influenza is recommended on an annual basis for all COPD patients. It can reduce serious illness and death by approximately 50%. (SOR Ⓐ) The value of pneumococcal immunization has also been demonstrated. The vaccine covers more than 80% of pneumococcal strains. The frequency of revaccination is debated. In patients who received the vaccine prior to age 65, a booster should be given after age 65, but at least 5 years after the initial vaccination.

V. **Prognosis**

A. **Death rate.** COPD is the fourth leading cause of death in the United States and is projected to be the third leading cause of death for both men and women by 2020. There has been a dramatic increase in mortality in women over the past 20 years in the United States. It has more than doubled, increasing from 20.1/100,000 in 1980 to 56.7/100,000 in 2000 compared with 73.0/100,000 and 82.6/100,000, respectively, in men. This reflects an increased smoking rate in women. The prevalence of mild and moderate COPD is still greater in men than women and Caucasians than African Americans, but the differences in the age-adjusted death rates have narrowed.

B. FEV_1 declines with normal aging. COPD is characterized by a much greater progressive decline in pulmonary function. Although variable, FEV_1 decreases by an average of 45 mL/y in smokers and by 50 to 75 mL/y in patients with COPD, compared to 25 to 30 mL/y (beginning at around age 35) in nonsmokers without pulmonary disease. Age, lifetime smoking, and the number of cigarettes currently smoked are all risk factors for more rapid decline in pulmonary function. Dyspnea with moderate exertion is usually noticeable when FEV_1 falls to approximately 1.5 L. Dyspnea with any exertion is usually present at an FEV_1 of 1 L. Patients with an FEV_1 of 0.5 L or less are usually invalids. Besides age, FEV_1 is the best predictor of mortality. Other indicators of poor prognosis include resting tachycardia, severe hypoxemia, severe atrial hypoxia, severe hypercapnia, hypoalbuminemia, and cor pulmonale. In severe COPD, death is related to recurrent episodes of hypoxia, leading to the development of pulmonary vascular hypertension and cor pulmonale. Acute respiratory failure, severe pneumonia, pneumothorax, pulmonary embolism, and cardiac dysrhythmias are medical complications often responsible for death. The mortality rate 10 years after diagnosis is ≥ 50%.

C. Regular follow-up is important to the successful management of the patient with COPD. The purpose of such visits includes supporting the patient in smoking cessation, monitoring and modifying as necessary the therapeutic regimen, monitoring changes in pulmonary function, early identification of complications, ongoing education, and emotional support. Attention to the pulmonary illness must not entirely supplant addressing other health promotion/disease prevention issues. Advance directives should also be reviewed periodically.

REFERENCES

American Thoracic Society Standards for the diagnosis and management of patients with COPD. http://www.thoracic.org/sections/copd. Accessed October 28, 2008.

Anzueto A. Clinical course of chronic obstructive pulmonary disease: review of therapeutic interventions. *Am J Med.* 2006;119(10A):S46-S53.

Fabbri LM, Luppi F, Beghe B, Rabe K. Update in chronic obstructive pulmonary disease 2005. *Am J Respir Crit Care Med.* 2005;173:1056-1065.

Global Initiative for Chronic Obstructive Lung Disease (GOLD). December 2006. Global strategy for the diagnosis, management, and prevention of COPD. http://www.goldcopd.org. Accessed December 1, 2006.

Rennard S. Treatment of stable chronic obstructive pulmonary disease. *Lancet.* 2004;364:791-802.

Sutherland E, Cherniack R. Management of chronic obstructive pulmonary disease. *N Engl J Med.* 2004;350(26):2689-2697.

---

71   Cirrhosis

Mark C. Potter, MD, & Mari Egan, MD, MHPE

KEY POINTS

- Cirrhosis is the 12th leading cause of death in the United States. Alcohol abuse is the most common cause of cirrhosis, followed by hepatitis C.
- Treatment for hepatitis C is currently indicated for patients with biopsy-proven active hepatitis and detectable serum levels of hepatitis C RNA, or most patients with viral genotype 2 or 3. (SOR **B**) Regimens for treatment of viral hepatitis have been evolving rapidly. Treating physicians should consider referring to frequently updated sources of treatment recommendations (see References) or consider specialist consultation for treatment initiation. The current regimen of first choice is pegylated interferon alfa 2b (PEG-Intron), 1.5 μg/kg subcutaneously weekly, or pegylated interferon alfa 2 a (Pegasys), 180 μg subcutaneously weekly with ribavirin (Rebetol), 0.8 to 1.2 g/kg/d divided for twice daily for up to 48 weeks' treatment duration. (SOR **A**)
- Other treatments for underlying causes of cirrhosis include treatment of hepatitis B, many current regimens with no clear consensus, (SOR **B**) treatment of primary biliary cirrhosis which consists of ursodeoxycholic acid (UDCA), 13 to 15 mg/ kg/d, (SOR **A**) treatment for Wilson disease with D-penicillamine, 250 to 500 mg orally 3 times daily, OR trientine, 250 to 500 mg orally 4 times daily, (SOR **A**) and treatment for hemochromatosis with phlebotomy (removing 500 mL of blood) weekly for up to 1 year. (SOR **A**)
- The primary care physician should monitor patients with cirrhosis for signs of encephalopathy, fluid retention, infection, gastrointestinal bleeding, and hepatocellular carcinoma. (SOR **C**)

  The physician should use beta-blockers for prophylaxis in patients with a history of variceal bleeding. (SOR **A**) The usual starting dose is propranolol, 10 mg 3 times daily.

  Vaccinations should be administered (influenza and pneumococcus) (SOR **C**) and education should be given on avoiding medical toxicity (e. g., acetaminophen), (SOR **C**) eating a low-salt diet, 1 to 1.5 g protein per kg/d diet, (SOR **B**), and being aware of increased risks for infection. (SOR **C**)
- Patients with cirrhosis are at an increased risk for hepatocellular carcinoma. Patients should be screened for cancer with a serum α-fetoprotein test and liver ultrasound every 6 to 12 months. (SOR **B**)

I. Introduction

   A. Cirrhosis is characterized by diffused liver injury, which progresses with nodular regeneration to eventual irreversible fibrosis. Because of loss of normal hepatocytes and distorted hepatic architecture, the liver is unable to perform its synthetic or metabolic functions normally. As the normal portal architecture is destroyed, the blood flow is diverted around the liver rather than through it (portosystemic shunting). This process has major effects on many other organ systems, which manifest as the important complications of cirrhosis.

   B. Cirrhosis is a frequent cause of death in the United States and is most prevalent in the 36- to 54-year-old age group as chronic liver disease often takes 20 to 40 years to progress from hepatitis to cirrhosis. Once cirrhosis is advanced, liver transplantation is often required to extend life. There are 4 times the number of patients who are candidates for liver transplants in the United States than will eventually get one.

C. When a physician first evaluates a patient with liver disease, it is important to assess risk factors. History should be elicited of prior blood transfusions, hemodialysis, hemophilia, organ transplants, sexual practices, multiple sexual partners, alcohol intake, hepatotoxic drugs (prescription and over-the-counter drugs, vitamins, and herbal remedies), occupational exposures, family history, and other systemic disease.

D. In patients with cirrhosis, the physician must manage complications of liver damage if they occur. However, not all patients with cirrhosis will develop life-threatening complications. In 40% of patients with cirrhosis, the diagnosis will be made at autopsy.

E. Among patients infected with hepatitis C virus (HCV), 20% to 30% will develop cirrhosis in 20 to 40 years.

II. Diagnosis

A. **Symptoms and signs.** The clinical presentation of patients with cirrhosis varies widely. It ranges from asymptomatic patients found incidentally having liver disease to patients presenting with multiple end-stage findings.

The symptoms and signs of cirrhosis can be separated into the three major groups below.

1. **Symptoms and signs of hepatocellular dysfunction.** These include fatigue, weakness, weight loss, jaundice, nausea and vomiting, coagulopathy, palmar erythema, gynecomastia, testicular atrophy, menstrual dysfunction, loss of pubic hair, muscle wasting, spider angiomas, and parotid and lacrimal gland hypertrophy.

2. **Signs and symptoms of portal hypertension.** These are caused by increased intrahepatic vascular resistance, which causes ascites, edema, splenomegaly, esophageal and gastric varices, and dilated abdominal wall veins (caput medusa).

3. **Signs and symptoms caused by the disease underlying the cirrhosis.** These include withdrawal symptoms and signs in chronic alcoholics and cardiomyopathy or arthropathy in patients with hemochromatosis.

B. **Diagnosis of diseases that cause cirrhosis.** A complete diagnostic work-up should be undertaken in all patients with cirrhosis to identify all contributing underlying causes (see Table 71–1). In some types of cirrhosis, treatment can slow the progression of further injury.

1. **Viral hepatitis. Chronic hepatitis C, chronic hepatitis B, and coinfection with hepatitis D** are major causes of cirrhosis. Most patients with chronic viral hepatitis are asymptomatic or have nonspecific symptoms. Some patients will present with complications of cirrhosis as the earliest sign of infection. Patients presenting with cirrhosis should be tested for hepatitis B surface antigen, surface antibody, core antibody, and

TABLE 71–1. COMMON CAUSES OF CIRRHOSIS

Etiology of Cirrhosis	Diagnosis (Biopsy May be Required for Definitive Diagnosis)	Management (Transplant May be Required if Severe, Immunizations and Screenings as in Text)
Alcohol	Alcohol abuse history AST greater than ALT	Abstinence from alcohol (SOR **A**) nutritional support (SOR **B**) Consider PTU or colchicine (SOR **C**)
Hepatitis C	Hepatitis C antibodies, may confirm with quantitative hepatitis C assay	Interferon and ribavirin (SOR **A**) immunization (SOR **C**)
Hepatitis B	HBsAg, HBeAg	Several treatment options (SOR **A**)
Nonalcoholic steatohepatitis (NASH)	No alcohol history hyperlipidemia and diabetes associated	Gradual weight loss (SOR **B**)
Primary biliary cirrhosis	Elevated alkaline phosphatase, antimitochondrial antibodies	UDCA 13–15 mg/kg/d (SOR **A**)
Sclerosing cholangitis	Inflammatory bowel disease, beaded appearance on contrast cholangiography	UDCA 13–15 mg/kg/d (SOR **C**)
Autoimmune hepatitis	Antismooth muscle antibody	Corticosteroids
Wilson's disease	Low ceruloplasmin, high urinary copper excretion	Penicillamine 250–500 mg po tid (SOR **A**)
Hemochromatosis	Elevated transferring saturation and ferritin	Phlebotomy 500 mg weekly for 24–48 wk (SOR **A**)

hepatitis C antibody. Patients with chronic hepatitis C infection will have a positive test for anti-HCV antibody. Patients with a positive anti-HCV antibody test and low or intermediate risk for hepatitis C infection based on risk history should have the presence of HCV RNA confirmed with either a quantitative (preferred if treatment likely) or a qualitative polymerase chain reaction test. (SOR **C**) Patients with positive anti-HCV antibody with a high-risk history for hepatitis C infection (e.g., injection drug users) can be assumed on the basis of the anti-HCV antibody test to have true hepatitis C infection and proceed to quantitative HCV antibody testing, and liver biopsy if they are a candidate for treatment. (SOR **C**) Persistently elevated alanine aminotransferase (ALT) may be seen, though ALT levels often fluctuate, and may have periods in the normal range even with persistent viral infection, and so are not a reliable guide as to the severity of liver injury. A positive test for hepatitis D virus indicates coinfection by hepatitis D.

2. **Alcoholic cirrhosis** usually occurs 10 or more years after a period of excessive alcohol ingestion. Between 8% and 20% of chronic alcoholics develop cirrhosis. Laboratory evidence in patients who are currently drinking can show a ratio of aspartate aminotransferase (AST) to ALT greater than one and usually greater than two. Hypoalbuminemia is commonly seen in malnourished alcoholics as well as hyponatremia, hypomagnesemia, hypophosphatemia, low blood urea nitrogen levels, and elevated mean corpuscular volume. Other toxins (e.g., industrial cleaning solvents) and drugs (e.g., methotrexate, isoniazid, acetaminophen, and estrogen) can cause cirrhosis.

3. **Primary biliary cirrhosis** is a chronic, progressive autoimmune disease of the liver characterized by destruction of the intrahepatic bile ducts. The disease chiefly affects women, with an onset aging from 30 to 50 years. More than half of patients are asymptomatic when diagnosed, although pruritus with fatigue is a common presenting symptom. Hepatomegaly is seen in 50% of patients, and 10% to 50% will have splenomegaly. Laboratory tests may show an isolated elevation of serum alkaline phosphatase often more than twice the upper limit of normal with no other abnormal liver function test findings. Patients will also be positive for antimitochondrial antibodies with high titers.

4. **Hereditary diseases** can be the cause of cirrhosis. **Wilson disease** is a rare, autosomal, recessive disorder of copper metabolism. Cirrhosis occurs, if it is untreated in children and adolescents. Central nervous system damage also occurs. Kayser-Fleischer rings, a deposition of copper in the cornea, are detected by slit-lamp examination when making the diagnosis. Patients are found to have reduced serum levels of ceruloplasmin, increased urine copper excretion, and increased hepatic copper concentrations.

   Hemochromatosis is a more common, autosomal recessive disorder that is associated with increased absorption of iron and deposition of the iron in the liver and other organs. Clinical symptoms of the disease are not seen until after age 40, when the body iron stores reached 4 to 10 times the normal amount. The disease affects men more often than women and at an earlier age. Most patients are asymptomatic when diagnosed, but symptoms of diabetes mellitus, cutaneous hyperpigmentation, fatigue, arthralgias, and impotence are seen. Laboratory tests reveal elevated serum transferrin saturation and an elevated ferritin concentration. Another hereditary disease that can cause cirrhosis is α_1-antitrypsin deficiency.

5. **Nonalcoholic steatohepatitis (NASH):** This entity is diagnosed when a liver biopsy reveals findings indistiunguishable from alcoholic hepatitis or cirrhosis but the patient's history is repeatedly confirmed to exclude significant alcohol consumption. NASH is associated with hyperlipidemia and diabetes. NASH carries a better prognosis than alcoholic liver disease.

6. **Autoimmune hepatitis:** Although uncommon, this entity responds well to corticosteroids and so should be considered and sought in patients for which another diagnosis is not found. Findings suggestive of autoimmune hepatitis include elevated gammaglobulins, which can be further characterized by testing for ANA, antismooth muscle antibody, ANCA 1, and anti-LKM-1 and anti-ALC-1 antibodies.

7. **Other causes of cirrhosis** include chronic biliary obstruction, **primary sclerosing cholangitis,** cardiac cirrhosis, and postnecrotic cirrhosis. In 10% to 15% of patients, there is no identifiable cause of the liver damage, and this is called **cryptogenic cirrhosis.**

C. **Laboratory tests.** Common laboratory findings in cirrhotic patients include mild anemia, normal or slightly decreased white blood cell count, elevated serum globulins, reduced albumin, and moderate thrombocytopenia.

1. **Liver enzymes** (ALT and AST) assess acute liver injury. They are usually moderately increased in cirrhosis, although they may be minimally elevated or normal in as many as 10% of patients. Paradoxically, the enzymes may be virtually normal in severe liver disease, since many of the normal liver cells have been replaced by fibrous tissue. ALT is found predominantly in the liver and is a more specific indicator of liver damage.

2. **Lactate dehydrogenase** is a marker of hepatocyte injury, although less specific than AST or ALT. It is elevated disproportionally after ischemic injury to the liver.

3. **Alkaline phosphatase** originates mostly from liver and bones. Elevated levels are seen when there is a blockage of the bile ducts or impaired bile formation. It is also elevated when there is injury to the bile ducts. It is elevated disproportionately to AST or ALT in primary and secondary biliary cirrhosis as well as primary sclerosing cholangitis.

4. **Serum bilirubin levels, albumin levels, and prothrombin time** represent hepatocyte function rather than acute hepatocellular injury. Hepatocyte injury or destruction inhibits the secretion and conjugation of bilirubin. The conjugated **bilirubin** level will not become elevated until the liver has lost more than 50% of its excretory capacity. **The serum albumin** is often depressed in cirrhosis and can serve as a gauge of the liver's synthetic function. Because the liver manufactures the blood-clotting factors, the **prothrombin time** can be prolonged in cirrhosis. A prolonged prothrombin time that does not correct after parenteral vitamin K (10 mg subcutaneously every day for 3 days) suggests severe liver damage.

5. **Serum ammonia** is often measured in patients with hepatic encephalopathy. Although elevated serum ammonia levels do suggest a hepatic cause for encephalopathy, the ammonium concentration does not correlate tightly with the level of stupor or coma.

6. **Ultrasonogrphy of the biliary tree and liver** is the initial diagnostic imaging modality of choice in evaluating patients with liver dysfunction (SOR **Ⓒ**). Beyond evaluating for obstructive causes of liver dysfunction, the echotexture or nodularity of the liver parenchyma and dimensions of the portal vessels often provides useful information. Ultrasonography is very sensitive for detecting ascites and can detect as little as 100 mL of peritoneal fluid. **Computerized tomography** usually does not add much to ultrasound information. MRI has been used in evaluation of cirrhosis but has not yet gained a clear role. A **radionucleotide scan of the liver and spleen** in cirrhotic patients will show decreased, patchy uptake in the liver and increased uptake in the spleen and bone marrow, but does not often add to information gained by other testing.

7. **Liver biopsy.** A liver biopsy provides information on the grade (inflammatory severity) and stage (degrees of fibrosis) of liver disease. A liver biopsy is usually indicated if a treatable cause of cirrhosis, such as Wilson disease or hepatitis C is suspected. This procedure may also be used to help establish a prognosis and to determine whether a patient with antibody evidence of hepatitis B or C infection would benefit from antiviral therapy.

III. **Treatment.** The treatment of cirrhosis consists of preventing further liver damage, managing the potential complications of cirrhosis, treating the underlying cause of cirrhosis when possible, and considering liver transplantation, see Table 71–1

  A. **Preventing further liver damage:**

   1. **Avoidance of alcohol and drug toxicity.** Safe levels of alcohol consumption in cirrhosis have not been established, so complete abstinence is the most prudent recommendation. Alcohol also acts synergistically with hepatitis C, so abstinence from alcohol should also be recommended to those with chronic hepatitis C even without established cirrhosis. The liver is also vulnerable to injury from medications, vitamins, and herbs. Common hepatotoxic medications include tricyclic antidepressants, muscle relaxants, lipid-lowering drugs, antidiabetic agents, isoniazid, nitrofurantoin, antifungal agents, and anticonvulsant agents. Nonsteroidal anti-inflammatory drugs are especially important to avoid in cirrhosis. Because they inhibit platelet function, they may exacerbate coagulopathy. In addition, as a prostaglandin inhibitor, they may decrease renal blood flow and precipitate renal failure. Acetaminophen should be used with caution if at all, and should be restricted to a dose of 500 mg 4 times a day in well-nourished patients who are not actively consuming alcohol. Patients and physicians should attempt to assess all vitamins and herbal therapies for hepatotoxicity.

   2. **Vaccinations against hepatitis A and B viruses** should be performed in patients with cirrhosis if they are not already immune. (SOR **Ⓒ**) Superinfection with these viruses

can worsen liver disease. In addition, the pneumococcal and influenza vaccines should be given.

3. **Diet.** A nutritious low-salt diet is desirable because cirrhotic patients have increased sodium retention. In early cirrhosis with muscle-wasting malnutrition, a diet containing 1 to 1.5 g of protein per kilogram per day with vitamin supplementation is optimal. (SOR **B**) Dietary treatment in severely malnourished alcoholics has demonstrated short and longer-term survival benefit. (SOR **B**) With worsening cirrhosis and increased risk of encephalopathy, protein should be restricted to no more than 1 g/kg/d. (SOR **B**)

B. **Managing complications of cirrhosis:**

1. **Ascites**: Restriction of sodium intake is the cornerstone of therapy. Sodium intake should be limited to less than 2 g/d. Diuresis can be initiated with **spironolactone,** starting with 25 to 50 mg twice daily if salt restriction alone is ineffective. If there is no effect after 1 week, the daily dose of spironolactone may be increased by 100 mg every 3 to 5 days until a total dose of 400 to 600 mg/d is reached.

   If diuresis remains inadequate, **furosemide** can be added in gradually increasing doses, starting with 20 mg/d. Care must be taken to avoid intravascular depletion. Weight loss should be limited to no greater than 0.5 kg/d for patients with ascites and 1 kg/d for patients with both ascites and edema.

   Repeated therapeutic paracentesis can be useful for patients with diuretic-resistant ascites. If more than 5 L of fluid is withdrawn, giving 25 to 50 g of albumin intravenously is helpful to avoid intravascular depletion.

   Restriction of fluid intake to 1500 mL/d may be necessary for treating ascites in patients with sodium levels less than 125 mEq/L. Evaluation for liver transplant should be undertaken when ascites develops.

2. **Spontaneous bacterial peritonitis (SBP)** is one of the major potential complications of cirrhosis. Paracentesis to exclude SBP should be considered for patients with ascites that is new in onset or who have fever, hypotension, abdominal pain, decreased bowel sounds, and an abrupt onset of hepatic encephalopathy. Ascitic fluid with a total white blood cell count of $\geq$500/mL or a neutrophil count $\geq$250 cells per mm^3 or a positive culture is diagnostic for bacterial peritonitis. Hospitalization and treatment with broad-spectrum antibiotics are required. Several sources have recommended prophylaxis antibiotics to prevent secondary recurrences of SBP.

3. **Hepatic encephalopathy** should be considered when the cirrhotic patient exhibits a change in mental status. Common symptoms are forgetfulness, impaired arousability, and asterixis (flapping tremor). Infection, gastrointestinal bleeding, medications, and increased protein intake are common precipitants of encephalopathy. Use of branched chain amino acids supplements in the setting of hepatic encephalopathy is recommended. (SOR **B**) Dietary protein should be restricted. **Lactulose,** 30 mL orally every 4 to 6 hours, with subsequent adjustment to allow for two or three soft stools a day, is indicated for encephalopathy that is incompletely controlled by diet alone. Antibiotics are added if symptoms worsen. **Amoxicillin, 4 g/d, or neomycin,** 1 to 4 g orally in 4 divided doses, are used. However, chronic usage of neomycin may result in ototoxicity and nephrotoxicity.

4. **Coagulopathy** may be improved by vitamin K, 10 mg subcutaneously every day for 3 days.

5. **Varices** occur secondary to chronic high pressure in the portal veins. Bleeding from varices is the most common cause of death in the cirrhotic patient. Sixty percent of patients with cirrhosis will have varices on endoscopic examination. Patients with cirrhosis should be endoscopically screened for varices. Nonselective beta-blockers are used for primary prophylaxis against bleeding. The usual dose is propranolol, 10 mg 3 times a day, or nadolol, 20 mg once daily. Isosorbide mononitrate is a second-line therapy and is given in a dosage of 20 mg twice daily. Endoscopic sclerotherapy or esophageal banding is effective for variceal bleeding.

C. **Specific treatment for underlying causes of cirrhosis:**

1. **Treatment for alcoholic cirrhosis** includes arranging all necessary support for total alcohol abstinence. Colchicine at 1 mg daily and propylthiouracil at 300 mg daily have demonstrated mortality benefit in some smaller trials but problems with the consistency and strength of these findings and adherence have led to limited use of these treatments. Metadoxin (a combination of pyridoxine and pyrrolidone) has shown some biochemical benefit, and may be approved in the United States in the future.

2. **Treatment for chronic hepatitis C:** Antiviral therapy is indicated when HCV RNA is positive or there is evidence of inflammation, fibrosis, or cirrhosis on liver biopsy and no major contraindications exist (e.g., uncontrolled depression or substance use). Medications consist of pegylated interferon alfa 2b (PEG-Intron), 1.5 μg/kg subcutaneously weekly, or pegylated interferon alfa-2 a (Pegasys), 180 μg subcutaneously weekly with or without ribavirin (Rebetol), 600 mg twice daily for up to 48 weeks' treatment duration. The HCV viral load should be assessed after 24 weeks of therapy. Detection of viremia at 24 weeks predicts viral persistence, and therapy should be discontinued.

3. Treatment for primary biliary cirrhosis is ursodeoxycholic acid (UDCA), 13 to 15 mg/kg/d.[3] The **pruritus of primary biliary cirrhosis** may be improved by cholestyramine, 4 to 16 g/d divided and mixed with food or juice with each meal.[3]

4. **Hemochromatosis** is treated when there is an evidence of iron overload with an elevated serum ferritin concentration. Removing 500 mL of blood weekly by phlebotomy until the hemoglobin is found to be lower than 12 g/dL and the ferritin level is no higher than 50 ng per mL is effective.[3]

5. Treatment for **Wilson's disease** is D-penicillamine, 250 to 500 mg orally 2 to 4 times daily beginning with 250 mg daily and increasing by 250 to 500 mg daily every 4 to 7 days to a maximum of 1000 to 1500 mg daily in 2 to 4 divided doses. After 4 to 6 months of initiation treatment, the dose may be reduced to 750 to 1000 mg daily in 2 divided doses for lifelong maintenance. (SOR **B**) Children should be dosed 20 mg/kg/d divided twice daily. For patients that do not tolerate penicillamine trientine can be used, 750 to 1500 mg orally divided 2 to 3 times daily. Dosing for children can be 20 mg/kg/d divided 2 to 3 times daily. (SOR **C**) Copper excretion, CBC, UA, and serum creatinine should be monitored for patients on treatment.

6. **Treatment for chronic hepatitis B** is indicated when the ALT level is 2 times normal, HBV DNA is positive, and HBe antigen is positive. Hepatitis B treatment consists of interferon alfa 2b, 5 million IU subcutaneously, or IM daily OR 10 million IU subcutaneously/IM 3 times per week for 16 weeks; or lamivudine, 100 mg daily for up to 1 year; or Adefovir dipivoxil, 10 mg daily for up to 48 weeks.

IV. **Management Strategies.** Management of cirrhosis not only consists of treatment but also of monitoring for complications, deciding when hospitalization is required, providing education for the patient, and, if needed, referring the patient for liver transplantation.

   A. **Monitoring**

   1. **Laboratory parameters** to be followed, on an interval based on severity include serum transaminases (AST, ALT), prothrombin times, serum albumin, electrolytes, bilirubin, and complete blood counts. The patient should be checked clinically for ascites, signs of volume depletion, bleeding, and encephalopathy. Surveillance for hepatocellular carcinoma (HCC) should be performed every 6 to 12 months with ultrasound and serum alphafetoproteain (AFP). (SOR **A**)

   2. **Hospitalization** is indicated for gastrointestinal bleeding, worsening encephalopathy, increasing azotemia, or intractable ascites.

   3. **Diagnostic paracentesis** should be considered for new-onset or worsening ascites, or when SBP is suspected.

   4. **Hepatocellular carcinoma** should be suspected in patients with an unexplained clinical deterioration of chronic cirrhosis or watery diarrhea.

   B. **Patient support for adherence to diet is essential.** Abstinence from alcohol is also essential; most patients will require considerable skill and support from the primary care physician, the family, and rehabilitation programs in order to abstain (see Chapter 88).

   C. **Liver transplantation**

   1. A physician should consider referring a patient for a liver transplant when death from cirrhosis is expected in 3 to 6 months, and the patient is without major contraindications to transplanataion (e.g. unstable cardiac disease, metastatic cancer, persistant substance use). Hepatitis C is the most common reason for liver transplantation today. **Absolute contraindications** to liver transplantation include portal vein thrombosis, severe medical illness, malignancy, hepatobiliary sepsis, or lack of patient understanding. Among the **relative contraindications** are active alcoholism, human immunodeficiency virus (HIV) positivity, hepatitis B surface antigen positivity, extensive previous abdominal surgery, and lack of a family or personal support system.

V. **Prognosis.** The prognosis for cirrhosis is determined by the cause and the presence of complications. Complications of cirrhosis include portal hypertension, variceal bleeding, splenomegaly, ascites, edema, and hepatic encephalopathy.

A. Prognosis related to complications of cirrhosis
   1. **Portal hypertension.** Portal hypertension contributes to the development of splenomegaly, varices, and ascites and carries a significant negative prognosis.
   2. **Hepatic encephalopathy** is a complex, neuropsychiatric disorder most likely caused by one or more substances of intestinal origin that are not metabolized because of hepatocellular dysfunction and portal systemic shunting. As a late-stage finding in cirrhosis, unless an acute reversible liver insult is identified and removed, hepatic encephalopathy tends to recur.
B. Patients without gastrointestinal bleeding, encephalopathy, low albumin, and ascites have a better prognosis than those with such complications.
C. The prognosis of alcoholic cirrhosis is dependent on abstinence. The 5-year survival rate is 60% or greater for patients who abstain, compared to 40% for patients who continue to drink alcohol.
D. In a 20-year prospective study of cirrhotic individuals, liver failure, hepatocellular carcinoma, and gastrointestinal hemorrhage accounted for three-quarters of the deaths. The 5-year survival rates were 14% for cryptogenic cirrhosis and 60% for chronic active hepatitis.

REFERENCES

Gilbert D, Moellering RC, Eliopoulos GM, et al., ed. *The Sanford Guide to Antimicrobial Therapy.* 37th ed. Sperryville, VA: Antimicrobial Association, 2008.

Goldberg E, Chopra S. Overview of complications, prognosis and management of cirrhosis. www.uptodate.com. Accessed August 25, 2007.

Goldberg E, Chopra S. Diagnostic approach to patients with cirrhosis. www.uptodate.com. Accessed August 25, 2007.

Pawlotski J. Therapy of hepatitis C: from empiricism to eradication. *Hepatology* 2006;43:S207-S220.

72	Congestive Heart Failure

Philip M. Diller, MD, PhD

KEY POINTS

- Heart failure (HF) is a common progressive terminal condition with a poor prognosis; the prevalence of HF is increasing with the aging of the population.
- Optimal management of the HF patient identifies the stage of HF (A–D), the type of HF (systolic versus diastolic) and uses therapies that prevent HF (BP control, lipid lowering SOR **A**), slow the progression of cardiac remodeling (angiotensin-converting enzymes and beta-blockers SOR **A**), achieve euvolemia (diet and diuretics SOR **B**), and maintain or improve quality of life (exercise SOR **C**, digitalis SOR **A**).
- Angiotensin-converting enzymes, beta-blockers, aldosterone, and angiotensin II receptor blockers have been shown to reduce mortality rates in clinical trials of HF patients with left ventricular systolic dysfunction. (SOR **A**)
- Diastolic HF therapies are directed to the underlying cause—typically ischemia, hypertension, and rate control if a tachycardia is present. (SOR **C**)

I. Introduction
   A. Definition. HF is a clinical syndrome of symptoms and signs that may include fatigue, exercise intolerance, dyspnea, peripheral edema, and pulmonary congestion. HF signs and symptoms result when the heart is unable to fill with or eject blood sufficient to perfuse body tissues and meet metabolic demands. "Heart failure" is preferred over the term "congestive heart failure" because up to one-third of ambulatory patients with HF do not manifest pulmonary or systemic congestion.

B. Classification. In clinical practice, HF is commonly classified in two ways. First, according to left ventricular ejection fraction (LVEF): **systolic** if **LVEF <40%** or **diastolic** if LVEF >45% to 50% and documented diastolic dysfunction. Second, according to the stage of progression, introducing the conceptual framework that recognizes the early, often asymptomatic, onset of HF and its progression to more advanced stages.

1. **Stage A:** At risk for developing HF, but no structural disorders of the heart (in the United States, 50–60 million individuals).
2. **Stage B:** No experience of HF symptoms, but with a structural disorder of the heart (in the United States, 8–10 million individuals).
3. **Stage C:** Structural heart disease and is experiencing or has experienced the HF symptoms (in the United States, 5 million individuals).
4. **Stage D:** Advanced heart disease with severe HF symptoms and specialized treatment approaches (in the United States, 50,000–200,000 individuals).

   This staging system emphasizes the important role of preventing HF for the primary care physician.

C. Epidemiology

1. **Prevalence.** Close to 5 million people in the United States have HF, with nearly 500,000 new cases diagnosed annually. HF is the primary reason for more than 1 million hospital admissions each year and is the most common reason for hospital admission among persons older than 65 years (1 in 5 admissions). Approximately 300,000 HF-related deaths occur each year in the United States, and the number increases despite advances in treatment. Approximately 6% to 10% of people older than 65 years of age have HF.

   In primary care practice, approximately 40% of patients present with signs and symptoms of HF and have normal systolic dysfunction; the other 60% have left ventricular systolic dysfunction. HF causes with a normal LVEF are shown in Table 72–1.

2. **Etiology.** Underlying the signs and symptoms of HF are diverse causes that lead to an inability of the heart to perfuse tissues and meet the metabolic demands of the body. Some of the most important predisposing factors include the following:

   a. **Hypertension.** From the Framingham study, 5143 adults without HF at baseline were followed up for an average of 14 years. Of 392 persons who developed HF, 357 (91%) had hypertension that antedated initial HF diagnosis. Hypertension accounted for 39% of new HF cases in men and 59% of new cases in women. Chronic hypertension that leads to left ventricular hypertrophy (LVH) is a common pathway in the development of HF.

TABLE 72–1. **COMMON CAUSES OF HEART FAILURE WITH NORMAL LVEF**

Inaccurate diagnosis of HF (e.g., COPD)
Inaccurate measurement of LVEF
LV systolic function overestimated by LVEF (e.g., mitral regurgitation)
Episodic LV systolic dysfunction, normal at the time of evaluation (severe
  hypertension, ischemia, tachycardia, infection, volume overload,
  spontaneous variability of EF)
Obstruction of LV inflow (mitral stenosis)
Diastolic dysfunction because of:
  Abnormal LV relaxation
  Ischemia
  Hypertrophy
  Cardiomyopathies
  High-output states
  Volume overload
  Aging
  Diabetes mellitus
  Amyloidosis
  Pericardial disease

COPD, chronic obstructive pulmonary disease; EF, ejection fraction; HF, heart failure; LV, left ventricular; LVEF, left ventricular ejection fraction.

(Adapted from Dauterman KW, Massie BM, Gheorghiade M. Heart failure associated with preserved systolic function: A common and costly clinical oentity. *Am Heart J.* 1998;135:S310-S319.)

   b. **Coronary artery disease.** Coronary artery disease is the cause of HF in two-thirds of patients with left ventricular (LV) systolic dysfunction. Measurable decreases in systolic function may be present for months or years before overt HF symptoms develop. Acute myocardial ischemia and myocardial infarction can result in sudden changes in systolic and diastolic ventricular function and acute HF with systemic congestion.

   c. **Other causes of cardiomyopathy.** Viral infections, diabetes mellitus, and excessive alcohol intake have direct effects on the myocardium and can lead to cardiomyopathy and ventricular dysfunction. Diabetes is emerging as a significant causative factor for the development of HF.

   d. **Valvular disease.** Significant valvular stenosis, regurgitation, or both, particularly in the mitral or aortic valves, are well-documented factors that contribute to ventricular dysfunction, and are commonly seen in the elderly as a contributing factor for HF.

   e. **Cardiovascular changes that occur with normal aging** help explain why HF incidence and prevalence increase with age. Arterial stiffening with increased afterload and peripheral resistance occurs with advancing age even in normotensive individuals. An increase in LV mass that often occurs with aging may lead to impaired ventricular diastolic filling.

3. **Prevention of HF.** The common etiologic factors leading to HF suggest potentially useful strategies to prevent HF. Preventive measures include adequate blood pressure control using medications known to limit or reverse LVH, (SOR **Ⓐ**) smoking cessation, (SOR **Ⓐ**) aggressive lipid lowering, (SOR **Ⓐ**) achieving target blood sugar control in patients with diabetes, (SOR **Ⓐ**) alcohol abstention, (SOR **Ⓒ**) surgical valve replacement when indicated, improvement of coronary blood flow with appropriate revascularization strategies, (SOR **Ⓐ**) and use of angiotensin-converting enzyme inhibitors (ACEIs) for patients with asymptomatic LV systolic dysfunction. (SOR **Ⓐ**)

D. **Pathophysiology**

1. **The HF syndrome is a heterogeneous, progressive condition** caused by various combinations of central and peripheral pathophysiologic mechanisms. These mechanisms are often dynamic, leading to wide fluctuations in measured ventricular function and physical impairment that may be observed over time in individual patients.

2. **Central/cardiac factors.** HF begins with some injury to or stress on the myocardium that leads to impaired ventricular function during systole, diastole, or both. Initially, the effects of inadequate cardiac output may only be experienced with physical exertion, but eventually in advanced HF dyspnea at rest occurs. This progression of symptoms correlates with changes in the geometry of the left ventricle: dilatation, hypertrophy, and assumption of a more spherical shape. Such cardiac remodeling leads to inefficient hemodynamic performance that is sustained and progressive.

3. **Peripheral factors.** Peripheral compensatory responses to diastolic or systolic LV dysfunction or both may initially help maintain cardiac function and organ perfusion, but eventually they lead to worsening HF signs and symptoms.

   a. **Renin–angiotensin–aldosterone system (RAAS).** In response to LV dysfunction, the RAAS is activated, resulting in increased levels of angiotensin II, aldosterone, increased preload and afterload, and sodium and water retention. Initially, RAAS activation may help maintain or even improve LV function, but continued increases in intravascular volume and peripheral resistance become detrimental to LV function and lead to volume overload.

   b. **The sympathetic nervous system.** This system is also activated in response to LV dysfunction in order to maintain blood pressure and organ perfusion through increased catecholamine levels that augment cardiac contractility and increased heart rate. Prolonged sympathetic activation causes chronic elevations in afterload (peripheral vasoconstriction) and eventual worsening of LV function. Elevated resting plasma norepinephrine levels are independent predictors of clinical outcomes and mortality among patients with severe HF.

   c. **Natriuretic peptides and other parahormones.** Atrial natriuretic peptide and brain natriuretic peptide (BNP) are produced from cardiac myocytes in response to increased pressures in the cardiac chambers. These peptides initially promote natriuresis and diuresis, but resistance occurs to these effects over time in chronic HF. Endothelins are endogenous peptides with strong vasoconstrictor and vasopressor activities and are found at high levels in patients with HF. Elevated levels of the natriuretic and endothelin peptides correlate with worsening HF and higher mortality rates among HF patients. N-terminal-proBNP is also available for measurement and this or measurement of BNP is helpful in the diagnosis of HF (see Section II.C.1).

II. **Diagnosis.** HF diagnosis requires first, the recognition of the clinical syndrome based on the characteristic constellation of clinical signs and symptoms, and second, the determination of the underlying structural abnormality of the heart that produced those symptoms. Clinical criteria used to aid in the diagnosis of HF include the Framingham Criteria and the Boston Criteria (Table 72–2). These criteria may not identify individuals with LV dysfunction who have mild or intermittent symptoms. Determination of plasma BNP levels can assist in the differentiation between cardiac and noncardiac causes of dyspnea. (SOR **B**)

   A. Clinical symptoms and signs

   1. Symptoms

   a. Shortness of breath can range from mild to severe. **Exertional dyspnea** may occur with any level of activity, depending on the severity of the HF syndrome. The absence of dyspnea on exertion makes the diagnosis of HF unlikely. (SOR **B**) With **orthopnea,** patients will report feeling short of breath while lying flat, may be using pillows to prop themselves up at night, or may need to sleep sitting up if HF is severe. With **paroxysmal nocturnal dyspnea or night-time cough,** waking from sleep because of dyspnea or experiencing dry cough only while lying down are suggestive of HF. **Dyspnea at rest** occurs in advanced HF or during acute exacerbations and volume overload.

   b. Fatigue and weakness. These symptoms are nonspecific and are in part caused by abnormal autoregulation of blood flow to the extremities and muscle deconditioning.

TABLE 72–2. CRITERIA USED FOR DIAGNOSIS OF CONGESTIVE HEART FAILURE IN CLINICAL STUDIES

The Framingham Heart Study Criteria	The Boston Scale Criteria
Major criteria	*Category I: History*
• Paroxysmal nocturnal dyspnea	• Rest dyspnea (4 points)
• Neck vein distension	• Orthopnea (4 points)
• Rales	• Paroxysmal nocturnal dyspnea (3 points)
• Cardiomegaly	• Dyspnea climbing (1 point)
• Acute pulmonary edema	*Category II: Physical examination*
• S_3 gallop	• Heart rate: 91–110 (1 point): > 110 (2 points)
• Increased venous pressure (>16 cm)	• Jugular venous pressure elevation: > 6 cm H_2O plus hep-
• Circulation time ≥ 25 s	atomegaly or leg edema (3 points)
• Hepatojugular reflux positive	• Lung rales: Basilar (1 point); more than basilar (2 points)
Minor criteria	• Wheezing (3 points)
• Ankle edema	• Third heart sound (3 points)
• Night cough	*Category III: Chest radiography*
• Hepatomegaly	• Alveolar pulmonary edema (4 points)
• Pleural effusion	• Interstitial pulmonary edema (3 points)
• Vital capacity reduced by one-third from predicted	• Bilateral pleural effusion (3 points)
• Tachycardia (≥120)	• Cardiothoracic ratio ≥ 0.50 (3 points)
• Major or minor criterion	• Upper zone flow redistribution (2 points)
• Weight loss of more than 4.5 kg over 5 days in response to treatment	*Determine score*
	• Point value within parentheses and no more than 4 points from each category allowed. The maximum possible is
Definite congestive heart failure	12 points.
• Two major criteria or one major and two minor criteria	*Definite congestive heart failure*
	• 8–12 points
	Possible congestive heart failure
	• 5–7 points

(Data adapted from McKee PA, Castelli WP, McNamarra PM, et al. The natural history of congestive heart failure: the Framingham study. *N Engl J Med.* 1971;285:1441-1446; and Remes J, Miettenen H, Rennanen A, et al. Validity of clinical diagnosis of heart failure in primary health care. *Eur Heart J.* 1991;12:315-321; and Young JB. The heart failure syndrome. In: Mills RM, Young JB, eds. *Practical Approaches to the Treatment of Heart Failure.* Philadelphia: Lippincott Williams & Wilkins; 1998.)

2. **Clinical signs. Physical examination findings for HF (SOR Ⓒ)**
   a. **Tachycardia** is present in many patients with HF and reflects increased adrenergic activity. Other symptoms related to increased adrenergic activity are pallor and coldness of the extremities and cyanosis of the digits (peripheral vasoconstriction).
   b. **Moist crackles,** usually heard in both lung bases, are a consequence of transudation of fluid into the alveoli. Pleural effusion collecting in the bases may lead to dullness on percussion. If the bronchial mucosa is congested, then bronchospasm and associated high-pitched wheezes may also be present.
   c. **Systemic venous hypertension** is suggested by a jugular venous pressure level higher than 4 cm above the sternal angle when the patient is examined sitting at a 45-degree angle. In advanced cases, venous pressure is so high that peripheral veins on the dorsum of the hand are dilated and fail to collapse when elevated above the shoulder.
   d. **Hepatojugular reflux** is helpful in differentiating hepatomegaly resulting from HF from other conditions. The neck veins are observed, and then the right upper quadrant of the abdomen is compressed continuously for 1 minute. The patient is instructed to breathe normally. This maneuver increases venous return to the heart. In HF patients, the jugular veins expand during and immediately after compression, because of the inability of the heart to respond to the increased venous supply.
   e. **Hepatomegaly** is because of congestion of the liver. If this occurs acutely, the liver may be tender to palpation. With advanced HF, the liver is still enlarged, but typically nontender.
   f. **Peripheral edema** is a nonspecific yet very common sign in HF. A corresponding symptom of weight gain may often be elicited from patients. The edema is typically bilateral and symmetrical in the dependent portions of the body. For ambulatory patients, the edema worsens as the day progresses and resolves after a night's rest.
   g. **Cardiomegaly** is also a nonspecific yet very common sign in HF patients. A normal apical impulse is located in the fourth or fifth intercostal space and is a brief tap. It is only palpable in approximately 50% of HF patients. If the apical impulse involves more than one intercostal space, cardiomegaly is present. Precordial percussion is more sensitive than the apical impulse for detecting abnormal LV size. A percussion dullness distance greater than 10.5 cm in the fifth intercostal space has a sensitivity of 91% and a specificity of 30% for increased LV size.
   h. **The presence of an S_3 gallop** occurs from ventricular vibration with rapid diastolic filling. It is a low-pitched sound that is best heard with the bell of the stethoscope over the apical impulse. Having the patient in the 45-degree left lateral decubitus position doubles the yield.
B. **Chest roentgenogram. (SOR Ⓑ)** Findings in HF patients may include the following:
   1. **Cardiomegaly.** A cardiothoracic ratio $\geq$ 50% on an anteroposterior chest x-ray.
   2. **Pulmonary edema** marked by equalization of the caliber of blood vessels in the apex and the lung bases (cephalization), interstitial edema (development of Kerley B lines, sharp linear densities of interlobular interstitial edema), and alveolar edema (central butterfly or cloud-like appearance of fluid around the hila).
C. **Laboratory testing in a patient with a new HF diagnosis should include an** electrocardiogram (for arrhythmia, ischemia, LVH); a complete blood count (anemia); a urinalysis and tests of levels of serum creatinine, potassium (renal function), and albumin; and thyroid studies (T4, thyroid-stimulating hormone; hypothyroidism). Screening evaluation for arrhythmias using Holter monitoring is not routinely warranted.
   1. **Measuring BNP in HF patients.** BNP is elevated in both systolic and diastolic HF. BNP can be helpful when the physician is unclear if the patient has dyspnea caused by HF or to other noncardiac causes. Using a cutoff level of 100 pg/mL, BNP has a sensitivity of 90%, a specificity of 76%, and a positive predictive value of 83% in identifying patients with LV dysfunction compared to the Framingham clinical criteria, which have a sensitivity of 83%, a specificity of 67%, and a positive predictive value of 73%. Elevated pulmonary hypertension and pulmonary embolus can also cause elevations of BNP in the intermediate range between 100 and 400 pg/mL, so if these conditions are suspected based on clinical presentation, then appropriate tests should be obtained to diagnose these disorders.
D. **Diagnosing the heart's structural abnormality (the type of HF)** helps outline the physiologic goals of treatment and individualize pharmaceutical therapy.

1. Two-dimensional echocardiography coupled with Doppler flow (SOR **B**) studies allows the physician to determine whether the structural abnormality is myocardial, valvular, or pericardial, and if myocardial, whether the dysfunction is systolic or diastolic. Measurement of LVEF is determined with this study; patients with LVEF <40% have systolic dysfunction. Physiologic goals and the evidence base for specific therapeutic decisions differ for patients with LV systolic dysfunction and those who have normal LVEF and isolated diastolic dysfunction. Doppler flow measures of diastolic filling need to be interpreted in the context of the individual patient, since they are often abnormal in healthy elderly patients without HF and may be deceivingly normal in patients with progressively restrictive filling patterns or difficult to assess in obese patients.

2. Coronary angiography should be performed in HF patients who have angina or evidence of ischemia and be considered for revascularization if indicated.

E. **Assessing the level of HF severity. The level of functional impairment** from HF is a strong prognostic marker, allows the physician to monitor the effects of treatment, and determines whether patients will benefit from certain therapies (see Section V). **The New York Heart Association (NYHA) Functional Classification** is the simplest and most widely used tool for assessing physical functioning (Table 72–3). Other objective tests of functional capacity include the six-minute walk test (distance covered in 6 minutes), formal exercise testing, and maximal oxygen uptake (VO_{2max}).

III. **Treatment.** The heterogeneous nature of HF mandates an individualized approach to treatment with attention to etiology, type of HF, noncardiac comorbid conditions, and if systolic HF, the stage. Most of the large clinical trials that have influenced the treatment of HF have only included patients with systolic dysfunction. The treatment of diastolic HF continues to be based on the underlying pathophysiologic mechanism(s).

A. **Treatment of specific underlying cardiac factors** may significantly improve ventricular function and HF symptoms. Special attention should be given to surgical correction of significant valvular disease when appropriate and reversal of myocardial ischemia with stent placement or surgical bypass when indicated. Ventricular rate control and conversion to sinus rhythm may improve ventricular function for patients with atrial fibrillation and HF.

B. A number of **noncardiac comorbid conditions** may affect the proper diagnosis and clinical course of HF and should be carefully assessed and treated:

1. **Chronic obstructive pulmonary disease.** Dyspnea, exercise intolerance, night-time cough, and other symptoms of chronic pulmonary disease may be misinterpreted as HF symptoms. Treatment of chronic obstructive pulmonary disease should be optimized.

2. **Diabetes mellitus** may predispose patients to silent myocardial ischemia that worsens LV function, "stiff" ventricles, and diastolic dysfunction. For both types of HF, diabetes control is an important goal. However, the thiazolidinediones class of medications can cause fluid retention and acute volume overload episodes, and therefore, must be used cautiously in HF patients.

3. **Renal insufficiency** will influence fluid and electrolyte problems in HF and may limit usefulness or lead to changes in dosing for HF medications, particularly ACEIs and diuretics.

4. **Significant arthritis** may further limit physical activity and worsen the skeletal muscle changes that occur in HF patients. Nonsteroidal anti-inflammatory drugs and

TABLE 72–3. NEW YORK HEART ASSOCIATION FUNCTIONAL CLASSIFICATION

Class I	No limitation of activity.
	Ordinary activity does not cause undue fatigue, palpitation, dyspnea, or anginal pain.
Class II	Slight limitations of physical activity.
	Patient is comfortable at rest. Ordinary activity results in fatigue, palpitation, dyspnea, or anginal pain.
Class III	Marked limitation of physical activity.
	Patient is comfortable at rest, but less than ordinary activity causes fatigue, palpitation, dyspnea, or anginal pain.
Class IV	Inability to carry out physical activity without symptoms.
	Symptoms of heart failure often present at rest. Increased symptoms or discomfort with even minor physical activity.

(Adapted from Criteria Committee, New York Heart Association. *Nomenclature and Criteria for Diagnosis of Diseases of the Heart and Great Vessels.* 9th ed. Boston, MA: Little, Brown; 1994:253-256.)

COX-II inhibitors can cause sodium retention and peripheral vasoconstriction, leading to reduced efficacy, and can potentially enhance the toxicity of diuretics and ACEIs. Such anti-inflammatory drugs are used cautiously in HF patients.

5. **Depression and poor social support** have been shown to be important predictors of clinical outcomes, hospitalizations, and deaths among patients with ischemic heart disease. Depression is common is HF patients.

6. **Substance abuse.** Smoking cessation should be encouraged. Patients with a component of LV dysfunction resulting from alcohol abuse may show significant functional improvement with abstention from alcohol.

7. **Hypothyroidism or hyperthyroidism** may aggravate HF symptoms.

8. **Nephrotic syndrome, hypoalbuminemia, or both** may worsen volume overload in HF.

C. **Treatment of systolic dysfunction HF.** The treatment of systolic HF is guided by stage. For stage A (asymptomatic, high risk for developing HF), stage B (structural dysfunction without HF symptoms), stage C (LV dysfunction with symptomatic HF), and stage D (refractory HF requiring specialized interventions), the treatment recommendations are shown in Table 72–4.

The centerpiece of these recommendations for the stage congestive heart failure patient is the use of ACEIs and beta-blockers **to reduce mortality in all patients with systolic HF.** (SOR **A**) Additional mortality reductions are possible with the addition of aldosterone antagonists in patients with severe HF. (SOR **A**) In addition to the mortality prevention goal, there are other physiologic goals of treatment for stage C patients. The following discussion reviews the necessary management steps to achieve those goals.

1. **Achieving and maintaining optimal volume status.** Although ACEIs should be considered first-line therapy for chronic HF resulting from systolic dysfunction, the initial presentation of the HF patient with pulmonary and systemic congestion dictates acute treatment with diuretics to lessen fluid overload and rapidly improve symptoms. Intravenous administration of diuretics may be necessary to relieve acute pulmonary

---

TABLE 72–4. TREATMENT RECOMMENDATIONS ACCORDING TO HEART FAILURE STAGE

Stage A. At risk for heart failure but without structural heart disease or symptoms of HF
Treat hypertension
Encourage smoking cessation
Treat lipid disorders
Encourage regular exercise
Discourage alcohol intake, illicit drug use
ACE inhibition in appropriate patients

Stage B. Structural heart disease but without symptoms of HF
All measures under Stage A
ACE inhibitors in appropriate patients
Beta-blockers in appropriate patients

Stage C. Structural heart disease without prior or current symptoms of HF
All measures under Stage A
Drugs for routine use:
  Diuretics
  ACE inhibitors
  Beta-blockers
  Digitalis
Dietary salt restriction

Stage D. Refractory HF requiring specialized interventions
All measures under Stages A, B, and C
Mechanical assist devices
Heart transplantation
Continuous (not intermittent) intravenous inotropic infusions for palliation
Hospice care

ACE, angiotensin-converting enzyme.
(Data from Hunt SA, Abraham WT, Chin MH, et al. ACC/AHA 2005 Guideline Update for the Diagnosis and Management of Chronic Heart Failure in the Adult: a report of the American College of Cardiology/American Heart Association Task Force on Practice Guidelines. *Circulation.* 2005;112:e154-e235.)

congestion. (SOR **Ⓐ**) The discussion that follows is geared more toward management of the patient with chronic HF.

a. **The loop diuretic furosemide (SOR Ⓐ)** is the most frequently prescribed diuretic for treatment of volume overload in HF. Initial oral doses of 10 to 40 mg once a day should be administered to patients with dyspnea on exertion and signs of volume overload who do not have indications for acute hospitalization. Severe overload and pulmonary edema are indications for hospitalization and intravenous furosemide. Other considerations for prescribing diuretics in HF include the following:

   (1) Some patients with mild HF can be treated effectively with thiazide diuretics. Those who have persistent volume overload on 50 mg of hydrochlorothiazide per day should be switched to an oral loop diuretic.

   (2) Oral absorption of furosemide is diminished by physiologic changes in HF, particularly if the oral dose is taken on a full stomach. Torsemide is an alternative loop diuretic that is extremely well absorbed from the gastrointestinal tract in HF patients.

   (3) HF patients with poor oral absorption, renal insufficiency, or both may require much higher doses of a loop diuretic to reach a threshold level for diuresis, up to a maximum of 300 mg twice a day of furosemide.

   (4) Important adverse effects of diuretics that require periodic monitoring include orthostatic hypotension, prerenal azotemia, hyponatremia, hypomagnesemia, and hypokalemia. Most patients taking 40 mg or more of furosemide daily should supplement their oral potassium intake through dietary changes, prescribed potassium supplements, or both.

   (5) Once volume overload is corrected and an ACEI is initiated, the diuretic dose can often be carefully decreased or even eliminated. Some patients may only need intermittent diuretic therapy when symptoms and increases in daily weights signal a return of excess fluid volume.

b. **Adding a second diuretic** is sometimes necessary to maintain optimal fluid balance. (SOR **Ⓒ**) Adding **metolazone**, 2.5 to 10 mg/d, to a daily furosemide dose can significantly increase diuresis for outpatient treatment of moderate volume overload. Prolonged combined therapy with metolazone should be avoided because of the increased risk of electrolyte depletion.

c. **Spironolactone** can also be added to standard regimens (diuretics, ACEI, digoxin, and a beta-blocker) to increase diuresis, but this medication is reserved for NYHA class III or IV patients and those who have a serum potassium level < 5.0 mmol/L, creatinine < 2.5 mL/dL, or creatinine clearance > 30 mL/min. This medication and a more specific aldosterone antagonist, eplerenone (starting dose, 25 mg orally) may improve survival for patients with moderate to severe systolic dysfunction HF. (SOR **Ⓐ**) Serum potassium must be initially monitored frequently and then regularly after the initiation of spironolactone.

d. **Sodium restriction.** (SOR **Ⓒ**) Patients should limit sodium intake to 2 to 3 g/d or less by avoiding salty tasting foods, not adding salt at the table, and reading nutritional labels to choose lower-sodium food options. A sudden increase in dietary sodium intake is a frequent cause of acute fluid overload, pulmonary congestion, and hospitalization.

e. Patients should **weigh themselves daily**, record their weight, and report any gain or loss of more than 3 lbs from their baseline weight. Baseline weight is determined when the patient is at optimal fluid balance on a stable medical regimen. Reliable patients may be instructed to increase daily diuretic dose for 2 to 4 days when they see an increase in daily weights.

2. **Decreasing preload and afterload by blunting the exaggerated peripheral compensatory response** has, as its foundation, treatment with ACEIs, which should be considered first-line therapy for HF resulting from systolic dysfunction.

   a. **ACEIs.** Many clinical trials have provided consistent evidence that ACEIs result in decreased symptoms, improved quality of life, fewer hospitalizations, and reductions in mortality for patients with NYHA class II–IV HF. (SOR **Ⓐ**) In addition, ACEIs slow the progression to HF among patients with asymptomatic LV systolic dysfunction. (SOR **Ⓐ**) **All HF patients with LV systolic dysfunction should be prescribed ACEIs unless they have a contraindication to these drugs.**

   (1) Contraindications to ACEI use include pregnancy, bilateral renal artery stenosis, angioedema or other allergic responses, or documented persistent intolerance to ACEI (symptomatic hypotension, severe renal dysfunction, hyperkalemia, or cough).

(2) The positive effects of ACEI probably apply to all available drugs in this class, but preference should be given to drugs with the most evidence for improved clinical outcomes. Enalapril, captopril, lisinopril, and ramipril have the strongest evidence for mortality reductions. (SOR **A**)

(3) To minimize the risk of symptomatic hypotension, one-half the normal starting dose should be given to patients with hyponatremia (<135 mEq/L), recent increase in diuretic dose, serum creatinine levels > 1.7 mg/dL, and patients older than 75 years. Patients at high risk for symptomatic hypotension should be given a test dose of a short-acting ACEI (captopril, 6.25 mg) and be observed in the physician's office for 2 hours before starting daily ACEI therapy.

(4) Blood urea nitrogen, serum creatinine and potassium concentrations, and blood pressure should be determined before starting ACEI therapy, 1 to 2 weeks after initiating therapy, after changes in dose, and every 3 to 4 months thereafter. The average increase in creatinine is 0.4 mg/dL, with most of the change observed in the first 6 weeks. The reversible renal function caused by ACEIs may resolve with a careful decrease in diuretic dose. As long as creatinine stabilizes at approximately 3.5 or less, and hyperkalemia or symptomatic hypotension is not persistent, ACEIs should be continued and titrated up to target doses (Table 72–5). If target doses are not tolerated, lower doses should be used because they also appear to confer some benefit. (SOR **C**) Systolic blood pressure of 90 to 100 should not deter the physician from titrating to target doses unless hypotension becomes symptomatic.

(5) Nonproductive cough is a common adverse effect of ACEIs, secondary to increased bradykinin levels. Cough may not be attributable to ACEIs in a given HF patient, since it is a common HF symptom. Only 1% to 2.5% of patients in clinical trials discontinued ACEI because of cough. For patients with cough on an initial ACEI trial, switching to an alternative ACEI may diminish cough symptoms.

(6) Concomitant use of aspirin may attenuate the hemodynamic actions of ACEIs and their effects on survival, whereas clopidogrel does not. However, there

TABLE 72–5. TARGET DOSES FOR ACEIs AND HYD-ISDN COMBINATION

	Starting Dose/Maximum Daily Dose (mg)	Target Dose (mg)	Side Effects and Notes	Cost
Preferred ACEIs (see text)			Monitor Renal function with ACEIs	
Captopril*	6.25–12.5 tid/100 qid	50 tid	Rash, angioedema, hyperkalemia, hypotension, loss of taste, cough, neutropenia, increased serum Cr	$
Enalapril	2.5 bid/20 bid	10 bid	For Lisinopril and Ramipril in addition to above, also watch headache and dizziness	$ (trade $$)
Lisinopril	5 qd/40 qd	20 qd		$ (trade $$-$$$)
Ramipril	1 bid/10 bid	5 bid		$$
Other ACEIs indicated for heart failure				
Fosinopril	5 qd/40 qd	20 qd	Same as other ACEIs	$$$
Quinapril	5 bid/20 bid	20 bid	Same as other ACEIs	$$$
Hydralazine-ISDN combination				
Hydralazine (HYD)	25 tid/150 qid	75 qid	Drug induced Lupus like syndrome, fluid & sodium retention; tachycardia, hypotension; caution in renal failure	$
Isosorbide dinitrate (ISDN)	10 tid/80 tid	40 tid	Hypotension, headache, lightheadedness	$

*Give a single dose of captopril 6.25 mg with observation of the patient for 2 hours for patients at high risk for symptomatic hypotension.

ACEIs, angiotensin-converting enzyme inhibitors.

Cost: Average monthly cost to the patient: $, $0 to $10; $$, $10 to $25; $$$, $25 to $75; $$$$, $75 to $150.

is insufficient evidence to not use aspirin and ACEIs together in appropriate patients.

  b. For patients unable to use ACEIs, a trial of **hydralazine and isosorbide dinitrate (HYD-ISDN)** should be initiated to decrease preload and afterload (SOR **Ⓐ**) (Table 72–5). Patients at high risk for symptomatic hypotension should receive lower initial doses and be monitored for adverse effects. The HYD-ISDN combination has shown decreased mortality in HF clinical trials, but compliance with this combination is poor owing to the high number of tablets needed and the high incidence of adverse effects (headache and gastrointestinal complaints).

  c. **Angiotensin II receptor blockers (ARBs)** are an alternative therapy for patients who cannot use ACEIs. (SOR **Ⓐ**) ARBs do not affect bradykinin levels, and thus, do not induce angioedema and cough to the same extent as ACEIs. Evidence is mounting that these medications alone confer mortality reductions equivalent to ACEIs, and that addition of ARBs to standard regimens of ACEIs and beta-blockers reduces hospitalizations for HF. A recent study suggests that addition of ARBs to patients taking ACEIs and a beta-blocker may also lead to further mortality reductions. However, the addition of an ARB to HF patients already on an ACEI and a beta-blocker is not recommended. (SOR **Ⓐ**)

  d. The first- and second-generation **calcium channel blockers** such as nifedipine, diltiazem, and nicardipine may worsen systolic dysfunction symptoms because of their negative inotropic effects. Amlodipine is better tolerated, with evidence of a neutral if not beneficial effect on HF survival. Amlodipine can be considered for patients with continued hypertension who take ACEI and diuretics, or those with symptomatic ischemia not controlled by nitrates, beta-blockers, or both.

  e. **Exercise training** is an effective intervention that reverses some of the exaggerated peripheral compensatory changes in patients with stable mild to moderate (class I–III) systolic dysfunction HF. A series of randomized trials has shown improvements in a number of peripheral hemodynamic parameters, with diminished symptoms and improved physical functioning. Most trials have used supervised aerobic exercise on treadmills or stationary cycles. A single study evaluating the long-term effect of exercise training showed a reduction in hospitalization and deaths. Exercise training should be considered for all stable HF patients, even though there is limited clinical trial evidence using mortality as an endpoint.

3. **Delaying the clinical progression of systolic dysfunction HF** and further improving symptoms may be accomplished with two other pharmaceutical interventions. One has been a part of HF treatment for some 200 years (cardiac glycosides/digoxin), while the other has gained acceptance in recent years (beta-blockers).

  a. **Beta-blockers** inhibit the adverse effects of sympathetic nervous system activation (e.g., cardiac hypertrophy and apoptosis, provoked arrhythmias, increased ventricular volumes) in HF patients. Three drugs have been studied in clinical trials involving >10,000 patients: β_1-adrenergic receptor selective blockers (bisoprolol and metoprolol) and α_1, β_1, and β_2-adrenergic receptor blocker (carvedilol). The collective experience indicates that treatment with beta-blockers in systolic dysfunction HF patients reduces HF symptoms, improves quality of life, reduces the risk of death by 35%, and prevents hospitalizations. (SOR **Ⓐ**) The patients in these trials were also taking ACEIs, diuretics, and digoxin; thus, the benefits of beta-blockers were in addition to those already seen with the ACEIs. **Beta-blockers should be prescribed in all patients with stable HF caused by LV systolic dysfunction unless they have a contraindication** (symptomatic bradycardia, allergy) or are unable to tolerate them (asthmatic patients).

  (1) Starting beta-blockers should be delayed in patients who are not euvolemic. Volume overload should be treated before starting a beta-blocker.

  (2) The starting dose of the medication should be at very low doses, followed by a gradual up-titration once the lower dose is well tolerated (∼ every 2–4 weeks). If fluid retention occurs, then the diuretic can be increased until the weight returns to its pretreatment levels. The goal is to get the patient to the target doses achieved in the clinical trials. Table 72–6 shows the starting and target doses for beta-blockers in HF patients. Some patients may require a longer up-titration period to achieve the target dosing goal.

  (3) Patients should be monitored for the most common complications of beta-blockade: hypotension/poor perfusion, bradycardia or atrioventricular block, and bronchospasm.

TABLE 72-6. STARTING AND TARGET DOSES FOR BETA-BLOCKERS

Drug	Starting Dose/Maximum Daily Dose (mg)	Target Dose (mg)	Side Effects and Notes Should be euvolemic when starting	Cost
Bisoprolol	1.25 mg qd/20 mg qd	10 mg qd	Drowsiness, insomnia, decreased libido, bradycardia, depression, bronchospasm	$$$
Carvedilol	3.125 mg bid/50 mg bid	25 mg bid	Hypotension, dizziness, fatigue/ weakness, hyperglycemia, weight gain, diarrhea, bradycardia, edema, headache	$$$
Metoprolol Immediate release	6.25 mg bid/225 mg bid	75 mg bid	Bradycardia, hypotension, dizziness, fatigue, depression, bronchospasm	$
Extended release	12.5–25 mg qd/400 mg qd	200 qd		$$

Cost: Average monthly cost to the patient: $, $0 to $10; $$, $10 to $25; $$$, $25 to $75; $$$$, $75 to $150.

      (4) Patients should be informed that achieving benefit and desired clinical response might take 2 to 3 months. Fatigue is a common side effect and usually resolves spontaneously after several weeks except in a small percentage of patients.

   b. Digoxin is considered the preferred agent among a number of available cardiac glycoside preparations. Digoxin neither improves nor worsens HF survival, but does decrease symptoms, increase exercise capacity, and decrease the need for hospitalization in systolic dysfunction HF. (SOR **Ⓐ**) Digoxin is particularly appropriate for patients who remain symptomatic on ACEI, beta-blockers, and diuretics, and for patients with atrial fibrillation and rapid ventricular response.

      (1) Loading doses are generally unnecessary. A daily oral dose of 0.125 to 0.25 mg will lead to steady-state serum levels in 1 to 2 weeks.

      (2) Once a steady state is reached, a serum digoxin level, an electrocardiogram, blood urea nitrogen/creatinine levels, and serum electrolytes should be obtained.

      (3) Results of the Digitalis Investigation Group (DIG) trial suggest that a serum concentration in the lower therapeutic range (0.7–1.2 ng/mL) retains the clinical benefit of digoxin while avoiding toxicity. Levels should be checked yearly and at the time of significant changes in HF symptoms or renal function.

D. Isolated diastolic dysfunction. In comparison to the large evidence base for treating systolic dysfunction, there are minimal data available to guide the treatment of HF resulting from diastolic dysfunction. The only evidence for any treatment effects comes from small studies where diastolic HF patients on verapamil increased exercise performance and improved HF symptom score. Treatment is largely empiric and directed toward reversing presumed underlying pathophysiology. (SOR **Ⓒ**) There are a number of ongoing trials of ACEIs, beta-blockers, and ARBs in HF patients with preserved systolic function.

   1. Reduce the congestive state. The methods for achieving and maintaining optimal fluid balance are similar to those described for systolic dysfunction. Rapid or over-diuresis should be avoided since small changes in intravascular volume may cause significant decreases in diastolic filling and cardiac output.

   2. Treatment of cardiac ischemia may improve diastolic function. Nitrates, beta-blockers, and calcium channel blockers may all be useful, but there is little direct evidence for their effectiveness in treating diastolic dysfunction. Coronary revascularization should also be considered for appropriate patients with ischemia.

   3. Effective treatment of hypertension is indicated with drugs that may limit or even reverse LVH (ACEI, ARBs, CCB > beta-blockers) and thus improve the compliance of the ventricle. Beta-blockers are attractive in this regard in addition to their anti-ischemic and rate-limiting properties, all of which may improve diastolic filling. ACEIs are often appropriate, but compared with systolic dysfunction there is no evidence for specific indications for diastolic dysfunction HF. Candesartan has demonstrated decreased hospitalizations in patients with preserved systolic function, but not a mortality benefit (CHARM preserved trial).

4. Conversion of atrial fibrillation to sinus rhythm will restore the atrial component of diastolic filling and may improve cardiac output. If conversion to sinus rhythm is not feasible, then ventricular rate control with a rate-limiting calcium channel blocker or digoxin may allow more complete ventricular filling in diastole.

5. Attention to controlling the heart rate is important in managing HF patients with diastolic dysfunction. Slowing the heart rate will improve cardiac output in HF patients with diastolic dysfunction who have tachycardia. Over-diuresis often leads to tachycardia in these patients, compounding the problem of dyspnea in the acute setting.

6. Theoretically, digoxin would not be indicated for patients with diastolic dysfunction; however, a subgroup analysis of the recent DIG clinical trial showed surprising improvement in clinical outcomes for the small number of patients in the study who had normal LVEF. Until more evidence is available, however, digoxin should be reserved for diastolic dysfunction patients who have a separate indication such as atrial fibrillation.

IV. **Management Strategies**

A. **Patient education and self-care** are important components of maintaining clinical stability. (SOR **B**) Topics include explanation of symptoms, causes, and prognosis; activity recommendations including exercise prescription when appropriate; proper use of medications; sodium restriction; daily weights; and instructions for monitoring symptoms and when to contact the physician (Table 72–7).

B. **Case management strategies** have been shown to improve quality of life and decrease the need for hospitalization. (SOR **B**) Nurse case managers work with patients to improve patient education; promote adherence to medication and dietary regimens; improve home-based self-monitoring; and coordinate medical, community, and social support resources.

C. **Consultation or referral** to a cardiologist or HF specialty clinic should be considered for patients who remain symptomatic on standard HF therapy, have underlying valvular or pericardial infiltrative disease, or have potentially reversible ischemic heart disease. Patients may also benefit from co-management with a cardiologist to ensure reaching target doses of an ACEI or to initiate beta-blocker therapy. Those with symptomatic atrial or ventricular tachyarrhythmias should also be assessed by a cardiologist. Evaluation for possible cardiac transplantation includes exercise evaluation with measurement of VO_{2max}. Patients with VO_{2max} < 14 mL/kg/min and no severe comorbid conditions may be candidates for transplantation.

V. **Prognosis**

A. **Exacerbations and hospitalization** frequently occur in HF. More than 40% of hospitalized HF patients require readmission to the hospital within 6 months of discharge. Patients often experience a fluctuating clinical course marked by periods of fluid overload and diminished exercise tolerance. Common preventable reasons leading to hospitalization include poor adherence to sodium restriction or medication regimens, inadequate social support systems, or failure to seek medical attention when symptoms worsen or daily

---

TABLE 72–7. SPECIFIC INSTRUCTIONS FOR PATIENTS ABOUT WHEN TO CONTACT A PHYSICIAN'S OFFICE

Weight gain $\geq$ 3 lbs, not responding to predesignated diuretic change
Uncertainty about how to increase diuretics
New swelling of the feet or abdomen
Worsening shortness of breath with mild exercise
Onset of inability to sleep flat in bed or awakening from sleep because of shortness of breath
Worsening cough
Persistent nausea/vomiting or inability to eat
Worsening dizziness or new spells of sudden dizziness not related to sudden changes in body position
Prolonged palpitations

If you, the patient, experience any sudden severe symptoms, you may need to call 911 or the equivalent emergency phone number to arrange a trip to the emergency department. (These sudden severe symptoms may include **but are not limited to** chest pain, severe shortness of breath, loss of consciousness not because of sudden standing, new cold or painful arm or foot, sudden new visual changes, or impairment of speech or strength in an extremity.)
Note: This is only a sample list and is not intended to include all potential problems for which a patient with heart failure should seek urgent medical advice.
(Reprinted with permission from Goldman L, Braunwald E. *Primary Cardiology*, 2nd ed. Philadelphia, PA: Saunders; 2003.)

weights increase. Hospitalization rates are similar for patients with systolic and diastolic dysfunction HF.

B. Mortality risk for HF patients is substantial, with annual rates as high as 50% mortality for patients with advanced disease (NYHA class IV). LVEF is one of the most consistent predictors of mortality, with a marked increase in mortality risk for patients with LVEF less than 20%. Hyponatremia, elevated plasma norepinephrine levels, BNP levels, and significant ventricular arrhythmias are also independent markers for increased mortality risk. Mortality rates are lowest for HF patients with normal LVEF.

REFERENCES

Adorisio R, De Luca L, Rossi J, Gheorghiade M. Pharmacological treatment of chronic heart failure. *Heart Fail Rev.* 2006;11:109-123.

Aurigemma GP, Gaasch WH. Clinical practice, diastolic heart failure. *N Engl J Med.* 2004;351:1097-1105.

Fonarow GC, Adams KF, Abraham WT, et al. Risk stratification for in-hospital mortality in acutely decompensated heart failure: classification and regression tree analysis. *JAMA.* 2005;293:572-580.

Heart Failure Society of America. 2006 Comprehensive Heart Failure Practice Guideline. *J Card Fail* 2006;12(1):e1-122. http://www.heartfailureguideline.org/index.cfm?id=131&s=1. Accessed August 4, 2008.

Hunt SA, Abraham WT, Chin MH, et al. ACC/AHA 2005 Guideline Update for the Diagnosis and Management of Chronic Heart Failure in the Adult: a report of the American College of Cardiology/American Heart Association Task Force on Practice Guidelines. *Circulation.* 2005;112:e154-e235.

Jessup M, Brozena S. Heart failure. *N Engl J Med.* 2003;348:2007-2018.

Redfield MM, Jacobsen SJ, Burnett JC, Mahoney DW, Bailey KR, Rodeheffer RJ. Burden of systolic and diastolic ventricular dysfunction in the community: appreciating the scope of the heart failure epidemic. *JAMA.* 2003;289:194-202.

---

73   Dementia

Richard J. Ham, MD

KEY POINTS

- **Dementia** is a syndrome in which memory loss and at least one other cognitive deficit is persistent and severe enough to interfere with daily **function**; it is not a final diagnosis (Table 73–1).
- Most *progressive* dementias are caused by **Alzheimer's disease** (AD), which is extremely slow in its onset, with its early symptoms frequently subtle or only present at times of stress. Consequently, delayed recognition and diagnosis occur frequently.

  Age is the single most potent risk factor for AD; prevalence in individuals aged 85 and older may be as high as 45%.
- **Earlier recognition** by families and professionals of the symptoms and signs of dementia, and thus earlier diagnosis and differential diagnosis of AD than is generally achieved at present is essential. (SOR **C**)
- **Earlier initiation** of comprehensive management—to ensure safety, to relieve and prevent family stress, to provide early education of caregivers especially in behavioral management, to clarify advance directives (including the will) while the person can still participate, and to initiate potentially stabilizing medications while the symptoms are still mild—should be attempted in the primary care practice setting. (SOR **C**)
- **Pharmaceutical treatment,** as soon as the diagnosis of dementia of Alzheimer's type is a strong probability, with a cholinesterase inhibitor (ChEI) is the normal approach at this time for the primary care physician, (SOR **A**) with the addition of memantine when the dementia can be defined as "moderate" recommended for most such patients. (SOR **A**) These are symptomatic treatments, which do not affect the disease process itself (Table 73–2).

  Caregiver stress is considerable and since the qualities of the caregiving arrangements are major determinants of patient outcomes, caregiver support and education is considered vital to management, (SOR **C**) and should include the **Alzheimer's Association** (1–800-272-3900 or www.alz.org or a local chapter) and other caregiver-oriented sources.

TABLE 73–1. WHAT IS DEMENTIA?

Multiple cognitive deficits, i.e., memory impairment and one or more of aphasia, apraxia, agnosia, or disturbed executive
  functioning (i.e., planning, organizing, sequencing, abstracting)
The deficits impair occupational or social function and represent a decline from prior status and do not only occur during
  a delirium

(Data from, American Psychiatric Arlington: American Psychiatric Publishing, Inc, Association, DSM-IV. 1997.)

I. Introduction

   A. **Dementia** is extremely common, particularly in the old. Two careful US studies, sampling
      urban populations older than 85 years, confirmed a prevalence of clinical Alzheimer's
      disease (AD) in approximately 45%. Prevalence in primary care practice is also high,
      with dementia present in 6% of patients older than 65, 2% of those aging 65 to 69, 7%
      of those aging 70 to 79, and 17% of those older than 80 in the practices studied. Even
      allowing for the longevity of women, more women have AD than men (the ratio is 3:2).

   B. The histopathology (still the definitive diagnostic technique, usually at autopsy) was de-
      scribed by Alzheimer in 1907: plaques with a core of beta-amyloid and neurofibrillary
      tangles. These changes do not themselves explain the extent of neuronal degeneration
      that ultimately takes place. Inflammatory changes around the lesions may play a role.
      Estrogen interferes in the processes preceding the formation of both plaques and tan-
      gles. Considerable research continues on the steps in the formation of the beta-amyloid.
      An experimental vaccine to prevent the formation of beta-amyloid was discontinued be-
      cause of the occurrence of encephalopathy in some subjects, but in one patient who
      died of unrelated causes, there appeared to be activity in the plaques. However, stopping
      beta-amyloid formation may not stop the disease process. Extensive research on the de-
      phosphorylation of tau protein, an initial step leading to the neurofibrillary tangles, adds
      to the increasingly precise definition of the pathways to the pathology, and thus to the
      probability of pharmaceutical intervention. Several promising disease-altering medication
      approaches are currently in development in the pharmaceutical field.

   C. Deficits in a number of neurotransmitters, most especially acetylcholine, as well as more
      recently glutamate, are the basis of the approved medical treatments. The "choliner-
      gic hypothesis" (that reducing the known decline in cholinergic neuronal activity would be
      therapeutic) has a literature spanning 20 years. Medications (the ChEIs) that inhibit acetyl-
      cholinesterase, thus preventing the breakdown of naturally occurring acetylcholine, have
      been approved for US prescription since 1997 and offer symptomatic treatment, allowing
      better functioning of the deteriorating nerve cells and are recommended for widespread
      use. (SOR **Ⓐ**) They have been shown to have a robust effect on cognition, function, and
      behaviors in all except the terminal stages of the illness, relative to the changes in control
      groups, and appear effective in some non-Alzheimer dementias. They probably postpone
      nursing home care. They rarely cause any symptomatic change that the patient or family
      will be able to notice and they do not effect the disease process itself.

   D. Genetic "risk factors" are probably crucial. Familial clusters owing to specific, rare genetic
      changes have been defined over the years. Then in 1994, apolipoprotein epsilon 2, 3, and
      4 alleles were shown to be "risk" (apo-E 4) and "protective" (apo-E 2) factors in typical
      late-onset AD. Current efforts continue, seeking the three or more other genetic *partial*
      risk factors which are predicted from the inheritance patterns of typical AD patients.

   E. The presence of plaques and tangles does not correlate fully with the presence of symp-
      toms. All Down syndrome patients apparently develop the plaques and tangles of AD if

TABLE 73–2. ALZHEIMER'S MANAGEMENT PRINCIPLES

Diagnose it Earlier	Care for the Caregivers
Name it, name the proxy	Training, support, respite
Treat it persistently	*Develop community resources*
Cholinesterase inhibitors, vitamin E, memantine	Use them, promote them
Manage it comprehensively	
Cognition, function, behavior	

TABLE 73–3. RISK FACTORS (AND PROTECTIVE FACTORS) FOR ALZHEIMER'S DISEASE

Risk Promoting	Possibly Protective
Age	
Family history	Higher education
Apolipoprotein E4	Apolipoprotein E2
Head trauma	Anti-inflammatory drugs
Female gender	Statins
Cerebrovascular disease	Antioxidants
Cardiovascular disease?	Low glycemic diet
Chromosome changes at 14,19,21	Low cholesterol diet
Down syndrome or FH of it	Continuing intellectual activity
Diabetes mellitus	Continuing regular exercise
Low testosterone?	
Estrogen use?	

they live to be old (55–65 years), but only approximately half have evidence of progressive dementia in late life. A theory which explains the association of other events (e.g., stroke, head injury) with the onset or worsening of speed of decline in persons with dementia is that genetic risk, or even AD pathology, is pushed into clinical symptomatology by such other acute events or by concurrent chronic illnesses, such as diabetes.

F. Cerebrovascular disease (and probably vascular disease elsewhere, such as systolic hypertension) and head injury (especially serious head injury earlier in life) are to be regarded as strongly associated with increasing the risk of the development of clinical AD. (SOR **Ⓐ**) Hypercholesterolemia and diabetes mellitus are also now to be regarded as risk factors (Table 73–3).

G. No environmental factor has yet been convincingly shown to influence the emergence of AD, but chemicals that adversely affect mitochondria (e.g., insecticides, pesticides, and some horticultural and agricultural agents) could be factors.

II. Diagnosis
   A. Symptoms and signs
      1. Early dementia is frequently unreported, not presented for care, denied, or unrecognized. There is lack of recognition not only by the family and the patient, who will often attribute early symptoms to "aging," but also by ourselves, the clinicians. It is fostered by the overriding characteristic of the early symptoms of AD (and other slowly progressive dementias): an extremely *insidious* onset. The symptoms are also commonly present in many older people or are nonspecific (memory loss, functional decline, behavioral changes) and are often initially present only when an individual is stressed (by illness, relocation, anxiety, etc.).The preservation of good social function and speech in many early AD patients (who may look fine in the familiar setting of their own physician's office, but cannot cope with the complexities of life outside) compounds the recognition issue.

      Tables 73–4 and 73–5 summarize some "hints" that early dementia may be present and which may be observed (or sought) in primary care and Table 73–6 lists some medical events which indicate that the patient is at sufficiently increased risk that screening for dementia in the primary care setting should be carried out, both at "baseline" and at intervals (6 months is recommended).

      2. Reasons for making an accurate early diagnosis of an apparent dementia are summarized in Table 73–7. Table 73–8 summarizes the clinical process as it ideally should occur in primary care, from early recognition to a working diagnosis.

      3. Mass screening of asymptomatic people has recently been recommended *against* by the US Preventive Services Task Force, citing a lack of outcome data and the potential creation of unnecessary anxiety. However, asking a simple "review-of-symptoms" type question, such as "How is your memory?" or (this author's recommendation) "Is your memory getting worse?" (or asking a family member—but not in front of the patient and ideally with the patient's implied permission) when the patient is at increased risk (or there have been some potential early symptoms) is recommended in practice. (SOR **Ⓒ**)

TABLE 73–4. EARLY WARNINGS OF ALZHEIMER'S DISEASE: SOME SYMPTOMS

Memory loss that is getting worse
Losing things
Repetitive questions
"Slowing down"
Driving problems
Financial mistakes
Aggressive or inappropriate behavior (e.g., shoplifting, sexuality, explosive outbursts)
"Depressed"
Weight loss
Poor hygiene
Irritability
Suspiciousness

TABLE 73–5. EARLY WARNINGS OF ALZHEIMER'S DISEASE: SOME OBSERVATIONS

Cannot remember recent information
Defers to caregiver
Dresses inappropriately
Poor hygiene or grooming
Trouble expressing thoughts
Persistently a "no show" or comes at wrong day/time
Noncompliant
Procrastinates excessively
Weight loss and/or "failure to thrive"

TABLE 73–6. EARLY WARNINGS OF ALZHEIMER'S DISEASE: MEDICAL CONDITIONS WHERE ALZHEIMER'S DISEASE SCREENING IS RECOMMENDED

Delirium
Depression
Head injury
Stroke
Catastrophic reaction

TABLE 73–7. WHY DIAGNOSE ALZHEIMER'S DISEASE EARLY?

Safety (e.g., driving, compliance, cooking)
Family stress and misunderstanding (e.g., blame, denial)
Caregiver education re early coping skills (e.g., choices, getting started)
Advance planning while patient is competent (will, proxy, power of attorney, advance directives)
Patient's and family's right to know
Stabilizing treatments now available

TABLE 73–8. ESTABLISHING THE ALZHEIMER'S DISEASE DIAGNOSIS EARLIER: THE PROCESS

Be alert to hints, clues, and early warning signs
Question patient and family about memory
When suspicious:
Confirm history: How long? How abrupt? Getting worse? How fast?
Are there other typical early AD symptoms?
Test cognitive status (MMSE, clock drawing test)
Record functional status (FAQ)
In most cases, diagnosis now established
Investigate for contributors, causes, and concurrent conditions

FAQ, Functional Activities Questionnaire; MMSE, Mini-Mental State Examination.

4. **Past medical history** (PMH) may be helpful, especially the cardiovascular history. Specific enquiry should be made about head injury (falls and car crashes may involve head injury which was over shadowed by other aspects of the incident).

5. The **family history** (FH) is significant: having a first-degree relative (especially a sibling) with clinical AD (even with no autopsy—as is usually the case) increases the likelihood of AD. An FH of one or two more distantly related family members should not be allowed to cause extra family anxiety in this very common illness. An FH of Down syndrome has some weight as a risk factor. In two reports all Down syndrome patients autopsied had in late life (late 50s/early 60s) Alzheimer's-type pathology (see above).

6. A thorough **medication history**—current and recent past—is required. Patients with early dementia naturally forget or mix up their medications. Occasionally, medications alone will be the cause of apparent dementia, and often medication adjustment can reduce AD symptoms. The anticholinergic side effects of many over-the-counter allergy, cold, and even pain medications (e.g., diphenhydramine [Benadryl] included in "Tylenol PM") are a frequent cause of abrupt worsening of cognition in old people, and especially in those with dementia of course, in view of the known cholinergic deficit. The anticholinergic effects of different concurrent drugs are additive, so more mildly anticholinergic medications such as furosemide and ranitidine add to this effect. Urinary antispasmodics (oxybutinin [Ditropan] and tolterodine [Detrol]) are sometimes useful in this age group, but this author recommends trying without such medications in all patients with cognitive problems, and avoiding them in general with elders unless the benefits truly outweigh this huge disadvantage.

7. A general **physical examination** is needed; the patient may well have not sought recent medical attention. Throughout these illnesses, **health maintenance** tends to be neglected. Signs of common problems, including abuse or neglect or unreported falls, hearing loss and poor balance or gait should all be sought (Table 73–9). A **review of systems (ROS)** can be done at the same time as the physical examination, improving the likelihood of the patient's recall as each system is examined. (A family member should also be interviewed for the ROS, saving clinical time by using a written format.)

B. **Confirming dementia, staging it, and the differential diagnosis.** Progressive dementias like AD can present for "first-time" diagnosis at any stage of the illness. Sometimes the changes have been so insidious, or the patient's verbal ability and social skills have been so well preserved, that the decline has truly been unnoticed. Sometimes in a patient declining because of one or more chronic and progressive illnesses, and becoming more dependent, the management of the recognized medical problems obscures the cognitive decline or such decline is attributed to the illness itself (e.g., in COPD). As we all know (but can forget when pressed for time!) it is characteristic of older patients to have multiple concurrent conditions; our traditional training of tying all the symptoms together into fewer diagnoses does not apply!

It is clinically useful to describe the manifestations of dementias in three domains: **cognitive, functional, and behavioral** while recognizing that the early symptoms may be in only one or two domains. For both diagnosis and management, it is useful to record characteristic symptoms from these three domains, asking direct questions if necessary.

There are three plus questions (Table 73–10) that help a lot in distinguishing slowly progressive dementias (e.g., AD, dementia of Lewy body type [DLB], and truly vascular dementia) from other dementias (e.g., those that can follow an acute event such as hypoxic brain injury after cardiopulmonary resuscitation) and in differentiating illnesses

---

TABLE 73–9. PHYSICAL EXAMINATION IN DEMENTIA

Nutritional status?
Hearing loss?
Visual loss?
Neglect of mouth, feet, perineum?
Physical abuse or neglect?
Appears safe when standing up or walking?
Localizing or lateralizing motor signs?
Signs of parkinsonism?
Review of systems while examining patient

TABLE 73–10. THREE PLUS QUESTIONS IN ALL MEMORY DISORDERS

How long has this been going on?
How abruptly did it start?
Are the symptoms progressing, and if so, how fast?

that can imitate dementia (e.g., delirium or major depressive episode [MDE, popularly called "clinical depression"]).

1. **Mild cognitive impairment (MCI)** is a term increasingly used, although it is not truly a diagnostic entity and is not in ICD-9 or DSM-IV. It is a syndrome defined in order to research those patients whom we used to reassure as having "benign forgetfulness," who have mild symptoms, not convincingly progressive, and insufficient to cause functional impairment. Research on such patients shows a wide range of "conversion" rates to "clinical AD," i.e., in those patients, the MCI really did represent early AD—before it had progressed to cause the functional impairment of dementia. So it is wrong to reassure patients, particularly the older they are chronologically, that memory loss can be accepted as "normal." Such a patient should be given scheduled follow-up visits (and called if a "no show") in order that cognitive testing (see below), can be carried out at intervals of more than 6 months, thus ensuring early recognition and diagnosis.

2. **Confirmation that a dementia is present** should be as objective as possible. The most widely used instrument (questionnaire) for objective recording of **cognitive symptoms** is the Mini-Mental State Examination (MMSE), a straightforward, easy-to-administer test, which briefly assesses orientation to time and place, registration and short-term recall, visuospatial skills, reading and obeying a written command, naming of objects, and sequencing skills and language skills (writing a sentence and repeating a well-known phrase) (Figure 73–1). The MMSE is not a very sensitive instrument, nor was it designed for the uses to which it has been extended; a well-educated person with early AD may score 100%! However, if there are abnormalities, the test provides quantitative confirmation of the cognitive domains often affected in the dementias, and it is sensitive to change at intervals of 6 months or more in the clinical situations described here.

   a. The physician (or practice nurse) does not need to administer the test personally; a trained interviewer, maybe a medical assistant if available, can accurately record the MMSE. This takes some of the tension out of the examination, making it seem more like the routine acquisition of "vital signs." However, the patient should be informed that his or her memory is to be tested, so that an optimal effort is made; questions of this nature should not be simply inserted into the patient interview. It is important to keep the original written record of the MMSE, as the mere total score does not distinguish the area of difficulty, and some points have considerably more weight than others.

   b. If the results are equivocal, it may help to add tests for **symptoms not assessed by the MMSE.** Abstract thinking can be assessed by the ability to interpret proverbs (e.g., "glass houses" where the typically concrete thinking of even quite early AD, for example, might create a response such as "the glass will break" when asked what the proverb means). A less culturally specific way of testing abstraction is to ask the patient to say what is similar about an arm and a leg, then (getting more complicated), asking the same question about laughing and crying or eating and sleeping. The range of the MMSE may also be enhanced by asking questions to test the retrieval of long-term memories, tested in "category retrieval" questions such as "Name all of the four-legged animals that you can think of in 30 seconds" (should be 10 or more).

   c. The **clock drawing test,** which some have attempted to standardize, can be done quite informally, with a paper and pencil. The patient is asked to "draw a clock." If necessary he or she is prompted to draw the circle, and then prompted/told to place the numbers "like the face of a clock." It is appropriate to state that the hands "should point to 20 past 8" (see Table 73–11). Patients with abstract difficulties may well not be able to find the number that would represent "20 after." The clock does get progressively disorganized as the illness progresses. It is sometimes useful to show the clock to family members if one or several of them (as happens in disputing extended families at times) cannot accept that their parent's mind is failing.

TABLE 73–11. CLOCK DRAWING TEST

"Draw a clock"
"Put the numbers in"
"Put the hands at 20 after 8"

i. Orientation (Maximum score: 10)
"What is today's date" Then ask specifically for parts omitted, such as
and "you also tell me what season it is"

Date (e.g. January 21) ..... 1 ___
Year................................. 2 ___
Month.............................. 3 ___
Day (e.g. Monday) .... 4 ___
Season .... 5 ___

"Can you tell me the name of this hospital"
"What floor are we on?"
"What town (or city) are we in?"
"What country are we in?"
"What state are we in?"

Hospital............................ 6 ___
Floor................................. 7 ___
Town/City......................... 8 ___
Country............................. 9 ___
State................................10 ___

ii. Registration (Maximum score: 3)
Ask the patient if you may test his memory. Then say "ball," "flag," "tree"
clearly and slowly, allowing about one second for each. After you have said
all three words, ask the patient to repeat them. This first repetition determines
the score (0-3), but continue to say them (up to six trials) until the patient
can repeat all three words. If he does not eventually learn all three, recall
cannot be meaningfully tested.

"ball"................................ 11 ___
"flag"................................12 ___
"tree"................................13 ___

Number of trials: _____

iii. Attention and calculation (Maximum score: 5)
Ask the patient to begin at 100 and count backward by 7. Stop after five sub-
tractions (93, 86, 79, 72, 65). Score one point for each correct number.

"93".................................14 ___
"86".................................15 ___
"79".................................16 ___
"72".................................17 ___
"65".................................18 ___
or
Number of correctly
Placed letter.................... 19 ___

If the subject cannot or will not perform this task ask him to spell the word
"world" backward (D, L, R, O, W). Score one point for each correctly placed
letter, e.g. DLROW = 5, DLROW = 3,
Record how the patient spelled "world" backward: _____
D L R O W

iv. Recall (Maximum score: 3)
Ask the patient to recall the three words you previously asked him to
remember (learned in Registration).

"ball"................................20 ___
"flag"................................21 ___
"tree"................................ 22 ___

v. Language (Maximum score: 9)
Naming: Show the patient a wristwatch and ask "What is this?"
Repeat for a pencil. Score one point for each item named correctly.

Watch...............................23 ___
Pencil...............................24 ___

Repetition: Ask the patient to repeat: "No it's, and's or but's." Score one point
for correct repetition.

Repetition.........................25 ___

Three-stage command: Give the patient a piece of blank paper and say
"Take the paper in your right hand, fold it in half and put it on the floor."
Score one point for each action performed correctly.

Takes in right hand ....26 ___
Folds in half ....27 ___
Puts on the floor ....28 ___

Reading: On a blank piece of paper, print the sentence "Close your eyes" in
letters large enough for the patient to see clearly. Ask the patient to read it
and do what it says. Score correct only if he actually closes his eyes.

Closes eyes ....29 ___

Writing: Give the patient a blank piece of paper and ask him to write a sentence.
It's to be written spontaneously. It must contain a subject and verb
and make sense. Correct grammar and punctuation are not necessary.

Writes sentence................30 ___

Copying: On a clean piece of paper, draw intersecting pentagons as illustrated,
each side measuring about 1 inch, and ask the patient to copy it exactly
as it is. All 10 angles must be present and two must intersect to score 1 point.
Tremor and rotation are ignored.

Draws pentagons............. 31 ___

Score: Add number of correct responses, in Section 32: includes items 14 through
18 or item 19, not both, (Maximum total score: 30)
Level of consciousness: — coma — stupor — drowsy — alert.

Total score: _____

FIGURE 73–1. Mini-Mental State Examination. *It has become common practice to substitute "apple, table, penny" to ease registration of the three words. (From Folstein MF, Folstein SE, McHugh PR. Mini-mental state: a Practical method for grading the cognitive State of patients for the clinician. *J Psychiatr Res.* 1975;12:189-198.)

Place a check mark under the column that best describes the patient's
ability to perform the tasks listed below:

	Completely unable to perform task (3 points)	Requires assistance (2 points)	Has difficulty but accomplishes task, or has never done, but the informant feels could do task with difficulty (1 point)	Normal performance, or has never done task, but the informant feels the patient could do the task if necessary (0 points)
1. Writing checks, paying bills, balancing a checkbook	_____	_____	_____	_____
2. Assembling tax records, business affairs, or papers	_____	_____	_____	_____
3. Shopping alone for clothes, household necessities, or groceries	_____	_____	_____	_____
4. Playing a game of skill, working on a hobby	_____	_____	_____	_____
5. Heating water, making a cup of coffee, turning off the stove	_____	_____	_____	_____
6. Preparing a balanced meal	_____	_____	_____	_____
7. Keeping track of current events	_____	_____	_____	_____
8. Paying attention to, understanding, discussing a TV show, book, or magazine	_____	_____	_____	_____
9. Remembering appointments, family occasions, holidays, medications	_____	_____	_____	_____
10. Traveling out of the neighborhood, driving, arranging to take buses	_____	_____	_____	_____
Points per column	_____	_____	_____	_____

Total points _____

FIGURE 73–2. Functional Activities Questionnaire (FAQ). (Adapted and reprinted with permission from Pferrer RI, Kurosaki TT, Harrah CH Jr, Chance JM, Filos S. Measurement of functional activities in older adults in the community. *J Gerontol.* 1982;37:323-329.)

    d. A comparable test of functional impairment is the **Functional Assessment Questionnaire** (FAQ) (Figure 73–2). This is currently the most widely recommended of many instruments that assess "instrumental activities of daily living," that is, the more complex daily activities that one does, not self-care skills, but those which are "instrumental" to daily life: balancing the checkbook, preparing a meal, following a television program, traveling alone, shopping, etc. The FAQ can be completed by family members if necessary, but is best done by having a staff person interview the family and fill in their responses. Each function is scored from three to zero—three meaning that the person cannot perform the task at all (whereas they used to be able to) and zero meaning that they have no difficulty or that it was something they never did. This test gives a measure of the functional impact and can be used to track its progression or stability. Results also give extra insight into the caregiver's role and burden.

    e. Most clinicians working with AD would recommend repeating the MMSE and FAQ at intervals of 6 to 12 months in order to assess progress. Some prescription plans require an MMSE or similar examination in order to justify the continuing expense of ChEIs.

3. Assessing the severity or stage of the dementia. It is helpful to the caregiving family members to assign an approximate stage to the dementing process, and it helps the physician interpret the FDA's medication approvals. Although each patient is truly unique, Galasko's categorization into three stages, defined in terms of the most frequently reported problem areas in multiple reported series of patients, can be useful

TABLE 73-12. MILD, MODERATE, AND SEVERE DEMENTIA: COMMON CLINICAL FEATURES

Mild (MMSE Typically 21–30)	Moderate (MMSE Typically 10–20)	Severe (MMSE Typically <10)
Cognition	*Cognition*	*Cognition*
Recall/learning	Recent memory	Attention
Word finding	Language (names, paraphasias)	Difficulty performing familiar activities
Problem solving	Insight	Language
Judgment	Orientation	*Function*
Calculation	Visuospatial ability	Activities of daily living:
Function	*Function*	Dressing
Work	Instrumental activities of daily living	Grooming
Money/shopping	Misplacing things	Bathing
Cooking	Getting lost	Eating
Housekeeping	Difficulty dressing (sequence and selection)	Continence
Reading	*Behavior*	Walking
Writing	Delusions	Motor slowing
Hobbies	Depression	*Behavior*
Behavior	Wandering	Agitation
Apathy	Insomnia	Verbal
Withdrawal	Agitation	Physical
Depression	Preserved social skills	Insomnia
Irritability		

(Data after Galasko D, Edland SD, Morris JC, et al. The Consortium to Establish a Registry for Alzheimer's Disease (CERAD): XI. Clinical milestones in patients with Alzheimer's disease followed for three years. *Neurology.* 1995;45:1451.)

for this purpose (Table 73–12). The MMSE alone is not the criterion; a more global estimate, based on all three domains (cognitive, functional, and behavioral) is to be assessed by the primary care physician.

4. **What kind of dementia is it?** (Table 73–13).

a. **Alzheimer's disease (AD).** In patients in their mid 70s and older, a very slowly progressive dementia, of insidious onset and with no abrupt declines (unless it can be justified by concurrent illness or injury, relocation or some other disturbance), would appropriately lead to a "working" diagnosis of AD as the cause of the dementia. Features of the other primary dementing disorders can then be sought, at the initial visit, and at follow-ups.

b. **Dementia of Lewy body type (DLB)** is probably the second most common primary dementia and can start like AD in its earliest phases, or quite often has early features more suggestive of depression, but complex visual hallucinations may develop, with or without parkinsonian signs (e.g., bradykinesia, "pill rolling" tremor, flat facies, "cog wheel" rigidity, and the characteristic gait, with limited lifting of the feet while walking and a lack of spontaneous arm swing when doing so), which may be very subtle and may need to be specifically sought. Unfortunately, DLB patients are exquisitely sensitive to the extrapyramidal side effects of antipsychotic medications, even the more modern "atypical" ones, with the exception—generally—of quetiapine (Seroquel). Experts on DLB recommend against using antipsychotics at all for the psychotic features of DLB, because of the risk of long-term neurologic damage. Yet the patient will likely have been clinically regarded as having AD, and the clinician may well be tempted to use antipsychotics if the patient is frightened—and only then do the extrapyramidal parkinsonian signs start, with the extra possibility of their persistence after the medication is stopped. So the primary treatment for DLB remains a ChEI. DLB subsequently follows a less predictable, rather more rapid course than is generally seen in AD.

c. **Vascular dementia (VaD),** once regarded as the cause of a high proportion of dementias, is a group of dementias attributable to vascular disease, and includes multi-infarct dementia, Binswanger's disease (caused by small vessel changes) and poststroke dementia. However, **mixed dementia** (AD and VaD together) is very often seen. Stroke is a recognized risk factor for the development of AD (and therefore possibly other manifestations of cerebrovascular disease). So VaD is probably a less-frequent *primary* cause of dementia than it was considered to be in the

TABLE 73–13. **THE PRINCIPAL DEMENTIAS**

Primary Progressive Dementias	Common Secondary Dementias
Alzheimer's disease (AD)	Alcohol-associated
Dementia of Lewy body type (DLB)	Parkinson's-associated (subcortical)
Vascular dementia (VaD)	AIDS-associated
Frontotemporal dementia (including Pick's)	Postanoxic encephalopathy
Huntington's disease	Poststroke
Creutzfeldt-Jakob disease	Progressive supranuclear palsy

past. VaD is sometimes (inappropriately) diagnosed as a result of seeing vascular changes on a computerized tomography (CT) or magnetic resonance imaging (MRI) scan. Such findings are very common in patients at the typical age of onset of AD and in those in whom autopsy confirms AD. To diagnose VaD as the primary cause of a dementia requires a clear history of "stepwise" progression (not the smoothly inexorable progression of AD), or clinical (historical) as well as radiologic evidence of transient ischemic attacks (TIAs).

In practice, the primary care physician should always look for **vascular risk factors** in any patient with a progressive dementia and regard vascular changes on a CT or MRI scan simply as evidence of vascular disease and another cause of potential morbidity throughout the body. If there are vascular problems or risk factors, these must be addressed vigorously (blood pressure, aspirin, dysrhythmias—especially atrial fibrillation and heart block, sick sinus syndrome, and other bradycardic states—carotid bruits, and carotid ultrasound).

d. **Other, atypical dementias** are suspected because of features that are outside the range of symptoms characteristic of AD (e.g., the striking FH found in Huntington's disease (autosomal dominant inheritance); the early, disinhibited, personality changes—sometimes overshadowing the memory deficits—of the frontotemporal lobe dementias (such as Pick's disease). All of the "non-Alzheimer" dementias (Table 73–13) can look like AD at first. However, less harm results from mislabeling as AD and managing the situation, than in failing to even recognize and address the problem.

e. **Major depressive disorder (MDE).** "The dementia syndrome of depression" is now the preferred term to characterize the way in which MDE can, particularly in an older person, exhibit so much cognitive impairment that it looks like dementia. The term "pseudodementia" was previously used, but it does not express the actual diagnosis, which is depression. The history will be quite different from that of a dementia, and the clinical features are subtly different on interview, including the way questions are answered during mental status testing (Table 73–14). It has been suggested that prior depression, especially if prolonged, is a risk factor for the development of dementia, possibly because the depression is a sign of the brain's vulnerability

TABLE 73–14. **DEMENTIA AND DEPRESSION COMPARED**

Dementia	Depression
Insidious onset (maybe months)	Abrupt onset (maybe days)
Long duration	Short duration
No psychiatric history	Often psychiatric history
Conceals disability (often unaware)	Highlights disabilities (complains)
Near-miss answers	"Don't know" answers
Day-to-day fluctuation in mood	Diurnal variation in mood, mood more consistent day to day
Stable cognitive loss	Fluctuating cognitive loss
May try hard to perform, and be unconcerned about mistakes	Often does not try so hard, and more distressed by mistakes
Memory loss greatest for recent events	Memory loss for remote as well as recent events
Memory loss first (before mood)	Depressed mood first (before cognition)
Associated with unsociability, uncooperativeness, hostility, emotional instability, confusion, disorientation, reduced alertness	Associated with depressed/anxious mood, sleep disturbance, changed appetite, suicidal thoughts

TABLE 73–15. DELIRIUM AND DEMENTIA COMPARED

Delirium	Dementia
Precise onset (identifiable date)	Gradual onset (cannot date)
Acute, days to weeks	Chronic, over years
Usually reversible, often completely	Generally irreversible, often chronically progressive
Disorientation early	Disorientation later (months or years)
Variability moment to moment, hour to hour	Slight daily variation more characteristic
Prominent physiologic changes	Less physiologic changes
Clouded, altered, changing level of consciousness	Consciousness not clouded until terminal
Strikingly short-attention span	Attention span not characteristically reduced
Disturbed sleep–wake cycle, hour-to-hour variation	Disturbed sleep–wake cycle, day–night reversal
Marked psychomotor changes	Psychomotor changes less dramatic

or—more likely—that the physical changes of the brain during depression actually cause damage to the aging brain. This author recommends follow-up (even after the depression seems to have responded to an selective serotonin reuptake inhibitor (SSRI), for example) and screening for dementia 6 months or so down the road, as it frequently transpires that the apparent "depression" has in fact been the apathy which is such a characteristic symptom of early dementia.

    f. Differentiating delirium from dementia may be a dilemma when a patient presents acutely, without accompanying family members, in the emergency department. Delirium is a common complication of dementia and may be the presenting symptom of dementia. The greater moment-to-moment variability and the physiologic disturbance present in the patient with delirium helps the differentiation from dementia (Table 73–15). An acute change in mental status is an indication for urgent (even emergency) investigation because the acute delirium will, by definition, be a cerebral manifestation of an acute illness that may be life-threatening (e.g., evolving stroke, myocardial infarction, sepsis, pneumonia).

    g. It is necessary to rule out the **reversible causes of dementia;** however, it is very rare to find a true, "Alzheimer's-like" progressive dementia that is entirely caused by some treatable physical illness. Such "causes" are generally in fact concurrent to the dementia under investigation and may worsen the situation if untreated, but it will not *reverse* the dementia to treat such causes. This author has, over the years, modified the use of the well-known (anonymous) mnemonic "DEMENTIA" (Table 73–16) from being an aide-memoire for the "reversible causes of dementia" into its current version, a summary of the "aggravating factors of an apparent dementia," which form the basis for the workup of both a newly recognized dementia, and of an abrupt decline in a person with known dementia.

C. Laboratory tests. The choices of investigations are driven by the differential diagnosis described above and by the aggravating factors that must be sought (Table 73–17).

    1. Brain imaging. It is customary US practice to always obtain a CT scan or MRI of the brain in dementia as "rule out" only. A plain CT without contrast is sufficient in most cases. The test is usually noncontributory. In some radiologists' hands, an MRI may be more sensitive to vascular changes, but the primary care physician must be wary of overinterpretation of vascular changes, since they are risk factors for AD, and are not confirmatory of VaD, the diagnosis of which is based on the history and

TABLE 73–16. CAUSES AND AGGRAVATORS OF APPARENT DEMENTIA

D	Drugs
E	Emotional illness (including depression)
M	Metabolic/endocrine disorders
E	Eyes/ears/environment
N	Nutritional/neurologic
T	Tumors/trauma
I	Infections/impaction
A	Alcoholism/anemia/atherosclerosis
P	Pain ("postscript"!)

TABLE 73–17. **INVESTIGATIONS IN MEMORY DISORDERS**

All	Most	Some
TSH	Computerized tomography or magnetic	Neuropsychological
B$_{12}$	resonance imaging	testing*
Folate	(Comprehensive metabolic panel only	PET scan*
RPR/VDRL	if medical care compromised)	EEG*
(CBC/basic metabolic panel only if		LP*
medical care compromised)		HIV†

*Generally indicated only as part of specialty consultation.
† Dementia from HIV is virtually a terminal AIDS occurrence.

sometimes neurologic findings, as outlined above. Some patients with advanced dementia, presenting late in the illness with an uneventful history (no trauma) and no localizing neurologic signs, can forgo a scan. Some patients cannot tolerate either procedure; the risk/benefit of a long transfer from a remote area or sedation of the patient for the procedure may lead to a decision against a scan (although the family will need to know that the rare possibility of something intracranial has not been ruled out). It must be clarified to the family that scans are done to "rule out" space-occupying lesions such as an unsuspected brain tumor or metastases, an injury such as a subdural hematoma, or unsuspected cerebral infarction from stroke or TIAs, and not to confirm a diagnosis of the dementing illness.

The mere presence of cerebral atrophy on a scan should not be taken as evidence of the presence of a dementing process—atrophy can occur in individuals with no cognitive impairment. However, the fact that cerebral atrophy does occur in a proportion of elders makes a CT scan indicated in the emergency department when an elderly individual (especially a person with known dementia) has a head injury or is involved in a fairly high-speed car crash, for the movement of the atrophic brain within the skull increases the risk of subdural bleeding as well as a heightened risk of "*contra coup*" brain contusion.

2. **Required blood tests** are pretty standard: a TSH (thyroid-stimulating hormone), vitamin B$_{12}$ and folate levels, and a screen for syphilis (RPR or VDRL), and, if there is any clinical reason why they should be abnormal, electrolytes or renal function (Table 73–18).

III. **Treatment**

A. **Medications for the treatment of AD**

1. **Cholinesterase inhibitors (ChEIs).** These represent the first type of medication to be approved by the FDA specifically for the symptomatic treatment of mild to moderate dementia caused by AD. The ChEIs are underused in primary care, relative to the prevalence of AD, its terrible impact on families and economically, as well as in other ways, on society as a whole, and relative to the multiple double-blind, placebo-controlled trials in the United States (and internationally) that confirm that these medications, if given persistently, do—on average—postpone cognitive and functional decline and reduce the behavioral disturbances of AD and some other dementias. Patients on ChEIs will generally have a period of relatively little decline, quite frequently almost a "plateau,"

TABLE 73–18. **ACETYLCHOLINESTERASE INHIBITORS: THE "SECOND GENERATION"**

Name	Starting Dose	Titration Schedule	Recommended Dose Range
Donepezil (Aricept)	5 mg once daily	Increase to 10 mg after 4–6 wk	5–10 mg/d
Rivastigmine (Exelon)	1.5 mg twice daily	Increase by 1.5 mg per twice daily dose every 2+ wk to maximum 12 mg/d	6–12 mg/d
Galantamine (Razadyne)*	4 mg twice daily or 8 mg once daily	Increase by 4 mg per twice daily dose every 4+ weeks to maximum 24 mg/d	16–24 mg/d

and a very small proportion will actually improve (very exceptionally, and sometimes quite markedly and obviously for a time). However, families should not be led to expect improvement; rather, they should be counseled that a period of stability of the symptoms with "no change" in 6 months or a year should be regarded as a triumph in this otherwise inexorably progressive disease. They should also know that "slowed decline" is also a successful outcome of ChEI treatment. The cost of the medications is a consideration, since theoretically they should be given for at least several years. Therefore, the primary care physician should ensure that patients in need are made aware of the free programs that each of the three companies manufacturing these medications offer.

a. **Outcomes.** The data confirm that ChEIs are still keeping AD patients "ahead of the curve" at 3 to 5 years out (placebo-controlled, double-blind data) and even longer (up to 10 years: open-label, non–placebo-controlled data). Outcomes of recent trials in MCI (see above) are equivocal as to their effectiveness, but this author and many others would prescribe them for a patient with MCI that seems to be progressing, and/or if a patient with MCI had multiple risk factors for AD.

b. **When to start.** At present, the "standard of care" is that the ChEIs should be started as soon as a dementia with a clinical history supporting the typical insidious onset and smooth progression of AD is shown to be present. It is no longer ethically acceptable to "watch and wait" for decline as "proof" of the presence of AD. (SOR **C**)

c. **Which one to choose.** Of the four medications approved by the FDA, the first to be available, tacrine (Cognex) is virtually no longer used, in view of its frequent dosage and unacceptable side effects, plus its possible liver toxicity. The remaining three "second-generation" ChEIs (Table 73–18) are probably equally effective although donepezil (Aricept), being given once daily, started at a therapeutic dose and in use in the United States since 1997, has the advantage. Rivastigmine (Exelon) is a little more complicated to give, twice daily, and requiring dose titration. It also has FDA bolded warnings about its increased risk of gastrointestinal side effects, which are discouraging and uncomfortable for patients so afflicted; a percutaneous daily patch overcomes the latter problems. Galantamine (Razadyne, formerly Reminyl) has the same low side-effect profile as donepezil and is now available in a once a day form. A patient already receiving a ChEI should not be casually "swapped" to another. Such swapping can result in gaps in therapeutic level and can even lead to permanent loss of the ground already gained by the previous period on a ChEI. Donepezil should not be stopped for longer than 3 weeks if at all possible. Somewhere between 2 or 3 and 6 weeks off donepezil treatment, some patients will so completely lose efficaciousness that the previously acquired level of function cannot be regained when treatment is restarted. The shorter half-lives of rivastigmine and galantamine may give even less leeway. So the rule is "don't stop and don't swap." The exceptions to not swapping might be the patient who genuinely cannot tolerate a particular ChEI (usually because of persistent gastrointestinal symptoms, which are rare, e.g., diarrhea) and the patient who has continued to decline at the rate that would be expected without treatment (2–4 points on the MMSE per year in the mild to moderate stages), since theoretically the patient might respond to one medication in the group and not to another (although this has *not* been proved). In the latter case, it would be logical to swap to galantamine from rivastigmine or donepezil, or to donepezil or rivastigmine from galantamine, as galantamine works in a slightly different way from the other two. The only contraindication to ChEIs is an unstable bradycardia syndrome or complete heart block. Occasionally patients who develop this and yet need a ChEI are candidates for a pacemaker. Also, since theoretically existing peptic ulcer disease could be made worse by a cholinergic medication, questions about ulcer symptomatology should be asked, and should ulcer symptoms develop, they should be taken seriously and investigated and treated; in practice, peptic ulcer disease complications are extremely rare. Families should be warned that transient nausea or diarrhea may occur early on, particularly at increases of dosage during titration, and that either symptom generally resolves without stopping the ChEI (Table 73–18).

2. **Memantine (Namenda)** was introduced to the United States in January 2004. It is best used as addition to one of the ChEIs, when the patient reaches a moderate stage of dementia (Table 73–12) or first presents at the moderate or severe stage. The

available data indicate that though on average patients on memantine versus placebo, or on memantine and donepezil versus placebo and donepezil, do continue to decline cognitively and functionally, the average decline is significantly slowed on memantine, with some patients actually transiently improving. Clearly it should be used whenever (as is usually the case) even a very slight improvement relative to the untreated course would significantly reduce the burden on caregivers and support services and other personnel. Trials have included patients with VaD, but no indication has been FDA-approved for VaD for memantine or the ChEIs), although the ChEIs are often used "off label" in probably vascular dementias by experienced clinicians; this is justified by the slight diagnostic uncertainty that virtually always exists in primary care, the frequency of "mixed" dementia (VaD *and* AD), and because benefit from enhancing cholinergic neuronal function in cognitively impaired patients is anyway not exclusive to AD.

B. **Behavioral management.** A major advantage of early diagnosis, with naming of the illness, is that early training of the caregiving family in how to handle the patient with AD, in order to improve the quality of life for both caregiver and patient, and to minimize (or at least manage) the behavioral problems that will arise. The agency to teach all of this to the family is the Alzheimer's Association, many of whose chapters operate local instructional and support groups. The Alzheimer's Association itself can be accessed at its national headquarters toll-free (1–800-272-3900) or through their Web site (www.alz.org).

1. Many popular books have been written about how to handle AD patients. The classic text is still *The 36-Hour Day* by Mace and Rabins (4th ed., Johns Hopkins University Press, 2006).

2. Many simple techniques have evolved from caregiver experiences and formal research to make life easier, to keep the patient more functional and able to enjoy life. Such techniques include the following:

   a. Making choices for the patient, but doing it subtly: choosing the right clothes for today's weather and putting just those clothes in the patient's closet so that the right (and coordinated) clothes do not need to be chosen by the patient, who can thus still dress "without assistance"; reducing choices of food presented to the patient, which results in the foods being eaten rather than the patient being overwhelmed by choices and eating nothing; organizing reminiscence, such as family photographs, or finding CDs and tapes of music and films that are evocative for the person. ("The Honeymooners" on video—no commercials—is perfect for the present cohort of elders!)

   b. Families should be counseled that the characteristic early apathy of AD and lack of organizational capacity means that their patient will not have the initiative to start things, but once organized and started may well be able to continue, unsupervised. The caregiver's role becomes, then, to "organize" reminiscence and activities, which the patient and family alike can then enjoy.

      Table 73–19 summarizes common behaviors and the approaches that have been demonstrated to be useful.

IV. **Management Strategies**

A. **Advance directives.** As soon as a progressive dementia is diagnosed, the family should be given the appropriate paperwork to complete advance directives and a health care proxy, with or without a durable power of attorney for health care. Since the patient is likely to become confused as a result of any intercurrent illness, it is urgent to obtain this, so that the upsetting situation of trying to decide what the patient would have wanted in an extreme situation can be avoided. The family should realize that as long as the patient is competent, he or she will make the decisions, but once unable to do so, the health care proxy or the person holding the durable power of attorney for health care will have the power to make decisions "as the patient." They will be deciding what the patient would have wanted in the circumstances, not what they would personally choose.

TABLE 73–19. EFFECTIVE BEHAVIORAL APPROACHES IN DEMENTIA

Counter cognitive deficits (notebook, calendar, reminders, notices, clocks, orientation)
Improve function (limit choices, decide for the patient, simplify clothing, use finger foods, organize/start tasks)
Create the right environment (the right lighting, the right sounds, the right images)
Stimulate reminiscence (photos, videos, music, audios, including of absent family)
Organize pleasurable experiences (music, rides, pictures, conversations, social groups)

Advance directives and health care proxy documents can include details about desired and not desired aspects of medical management. This author advises against being too specific about such things, as medicine is continually advancing, and general attitudes (and people's own viewpoint) change over time. Some patients will incorrectly specify "no tube feeding," failing to recognize that this technique may be lifesaving if they are only temporarily unable to swallow (e.g., following a concurrent stroke). Forbidding the use of antipsychotic drugs and intravenous therapy may be similarly unwise.

B. **Nutrition** is an issue that should be addressed throughout the long course. Early in the disease patients will not eat if overwhelmed by choices. Later, they may need to be spoon-fed, as self-feeding becomes difficult. Later still, the issue comes up about maintenance with tube feeding. In most authorities' opinions, long-term tube feeding in the later stages of a dementing illness is inappropriate. However, individuals (or their families as surrogates) must make their own decisions; sometimes it may be reasonable to maintain an individual who has relatively early loss of appetite or dysphagia out of proportion to the degree of dementia.

C. **Health maintenance** activities will naturally not be sought by most patients with dementia. Depending on the progression and stage of the illness, preventive protocols should be somewhat modified (the issue being: "if the change sought *is* discovered, would treatment be undertaken?") Maintenance of range of movement, of the ability to walk, of ears clear of wax, a comfortable mouth, and painless feet represent more relevant "health maintenance" activities for a person with more severe dementia.

D. **Activities** which "exercise" the brain are receiving more attention, and "Maintain Your Brain" has become the Alzheimer's Association logo. This appeals to those who have realized that "use it or lose it" is true about the body, so why not exercise the brain and prevent Alzheimer's—at least until as late in life as possible? Crosswords exercise language and directional skills, and even a game show such as "Jeopardy" exercises the memory. One study carefully quantified "leisure activities" and showed that individuals who regularly did certain activities had a later onset of age-associated cognitive decline and subsequently a slower progression of cognitive symptoms. The four "top" activities showing this association were reading, playing a musical instrument, playing strategic games, such as bridge or chess, and dancing. This does not *prove* cause and effect of course, but it is enough to justify recommending these and similar activities to patients and families wishing to do all they can to postpone or slow cognitive decline.

E. **Driving** is a huge issue. Patients with an early AD can still drive with acceptable safety, provided they do not have too many other problems such as impaired vision, inability to turn the head, or a weak or stiff right leg, and provided there is an accompanying codriver who can take over if needed. Once an AD patient has had a crash to which he or she may have contributed, it is difficult to justify further driving. To avoid such an incident, the best approach is a formal driving assessment in simulated conditions, but this is rarely available. Second best is to have a family member drive with the person on a regular basis, looking critically at driving performance. If no one in the family is willing to drive with the patient, you know that sadly the patient needs to be off the road! If neighbors have warned the family that the person is not driving well, then this should be heeded. Otherwise sensible families sometimes take appalling risks. Sometimes a "copilot" truly increases safety, but the need to have one is a warning sign. Any older person should restrict their driving to quieter streets and daylight hours and should avoid driving in inclement weather (and turning left across a stream of traffic!).

F. **Depression** can occur at any stage. Decline in a patient with dementia rather abruptly, or over days, should signal a search for more characteristic symptoms of MDE: appetite change, loss of interest, worse mood in the morning, or the characteristic insomnia; even two such symptoms occurring concurrently justify a trial of an antidepressant (see Chapter 92). A selective serotonin reuptake inhibitor is first choice (Table 73–20). The dose should be started low, but should be raised to the normal therapeutic levels used in younger adults. Target symptoms for the family to observe and record should be defined. A trial is not over until at least 8 weeks at a normal therapeutic dose without relief of the target symptoms.

G. **Hallucinations and delusions** occur spontaneously, sometimes precipitated by intercurrent physical illness. Benign hallucinations are very frequent in the earliest stages of AD. They often involve children, and even if the patient realizes they are not quite "real," they are not particularly frightening, and therefore do not require treatment. However, if hallucinations become vivid and frightening, or directive, or start to foster a delusional

TABLE 73–20. FIRST LINE PSYCHOTROPICS IN DEMENTIA

Problem	Medications
Depression	SSRIs, bupropion occasionally
Persistent agitation, recurrent aggressiveness	Divalproex, quetiaprine
Persistent/recurrent frightening psychosis	Quetiapine
Anxiety	Lorazepam (short-term), buspirone (occasionally)
Agitation or anxiety with depression	SSRIs, short-term lorazepam (rarely)
Insomnia	Zolpidem and similar, or trazodone, or, if associated with depression, SSRI

SSRI, selective serotonin reuptake inhibitor.

system, then efforts should be made to ensure that the environment is not contributing to delusional activity (e.g., the patient may be misinterpreting noises they hear in the night, or shadows on the drapes), yet frequently, treatment with an antipsychotic is also justified. Quetiaprine (Seroquel) which has almost no extrapyramidal side effects is preferred. Much lower doses than are usually recommended for schizophrenic patients should be used (e.g., quetiaprine starting at 25 mg a day) with gradual, monitored increases (Tables 73–20 and 73–21).

H. **Sedation for procedures** such as dental care is usually achieved with lorazepam (Ativan) or some other relatively short-acting benzodiazepine. For lorazepam an oral dose of 0.25 mg may suffice; it can be tried, on a weekend perhaps, prior to a procedure such as dental work, to judge the individual response. If used intravenously (or intramuscularly if necessary), the dose (0.5–1.0 mg would be appropriate) can be titrated or repeated according to the patient's individual response. In any event, all involved should be prepared for the possibility of more prolonged sedation than would be expected in younger patients, with the obvious dangers of falling or other harm from the patient's temporarily impaired attention. Benzodiazepines should generally be avoided for longer-term use in AD patients because of this impaired perception and increased risk of falling.

I. **Sundowning** is a phenomenon whereby psychotic features or near psychotic states occur in the night, often starting in the early evening, and possibly associated with primitive fears of the dark. Symptoms can thus be sometimes relieved and/or prevented by lighting, familiar music, warmth, security, and company. However in patients with clearly psychotic, frightening symptoms, treatment with antipsychotic medications is indicated; the possibility of DLB (see above) must of course be considered prior to their use, and any sedating of a patient with dementia at night does increase the risk of falling when up in the night (as most elders are, e.g., for nocturia).

J. **Level of care.** As the dementia progresses, increased services will be indicated, in the home to relieve the burden of care. Unfortunately, most insurance does not pay for such services, and the cost must be found out of pocket by the family. The physician must counsel the family member or caregiver to spend wisely; the objective is to assist in them being able to persist in the caregiving role for as long it is safe (for them and the patient) to do so.

1. **Assisted living facilities** are a rapid-growth industry for the accommodation of moderately impaired dementia patients who can still manage most self-care and yet need meal preparation, medication management, etc.

2. **Skilled nursing facility (SNF)** care is indicated when the patient needs skilled care for a major portion of the day. Many SNFs now have specific Alzheimer's units, or

TABLE 73–21. INDICATIONS FOR ANTIPSYCHOTIC IN DEMENTIA (AFTER BEHAVIORAL METHODS HAVE FAILED)

Severe mental distress or fearfulness
Agitation with aggressiveness (consider divalproex)
Recurrent catastrophic reactions
Sundowning (if frightening psychotic features are present)
Frightening hallucinations (or if they are causing delusions)
Persistent paranoia (more than suspiciousness or accusation over lost items)
Frightening or directive delusions
Aggression or restlessness (if it prevents other necessary interventions)

have modified their facility to be more "Alzheimer friendly." However, some maintain an almost "hospital-like" environment, quite unsuitable for the needs of the patient with AD, who requires reminders, familiarity, reminiscence, and calm. This cannot be achieved in the increasingly busy and noisy atmosphere of some nursing home settings, as they are challenged by having more and more medically complex patients. In practice, most SNF placements follow some setback such as hospitalization for pneumonia, or hip fracture, or some complication that finally makes it clear that the person needs skilled care, at least in the short-term. The SNF admission is then rather precipitate and choices may be limited. It may also be a "trial of rehabilitation;" it generally becomes clear in a few weeks whether the patient will be able return home with increased services or should stay on in the SNF in the long-term.

3. **Nursing home care.** Once the patient with dementia is living in the nursing home, the environment and the care is increasingly regulated. If not clarified before, advance directives and decisions about intensity of treatment in certain circumstances, whether (or when) to hospitalize, as the terminal phase of the illness approaches, and whether to treat certain later complications (such as a relatively asymptomatic pneumonia) become considerations. Often the existing primary care physician does not/cannot continue to follow the patient, and a physician new to the situation takes over. The physician/patient/family relationships are very different from the long familiarity often achieved in office primary care. Difficulties over deciding on the appropriate intensity of treatment is a frequently contentious issue. Leadership by the physician, guiding decisions to do enough, but not too much, recognizing that quality rather than quantity of life is the priority in the late-stage patient. The physician should help families recognize when the patient's terminality is approaching, and appropriately involve the hospice, or at least hospice-type techniques of effective palliation, as the final months or year of the patient's life come to pass. Resuscitation must be addressed on admission to the facility because the outcomes of resuscitation of patients with dementia are much worse than the outcomes in other nursing home residents—the brain in dementia being even more vulnerable to hypoxic damage.

V. **Prognosis.** Patients with AD are frequently diagnosed as much as 3 to 4 years after the onset of typical symptoms, and the range of duration from diagnosis to death in AD is from approximately 10 to 20 years, although some studies have suggested that the lifespan is relatively on the short side of that range. However, individual cases lasting a couple of decades or more have certainly been seen and it is difficult to prognosticate for the individual case. Other dementias vary even more in terms of prognosis, and of course, in the affected age group, coexisting chronic illnesses, especially cardiovascular, determine the prognosis.

REFERENCES

Boustani MA, Callahan CM, Unverzagt FW, et al. Implementing a screening and diagnosis program for dementia in primary care. *J Gen Intern Med.* 2005;20(7):572-577.

Boustani MA, Ham RJ. Alzheimer's disease and other dementias. In: Ham RJ, Sloane PD, Warshaw GA, Bernard MA, Flaherty E, eds. *Primary Care Geriatrics: A Case-Based Approach.* 5th ed. Philadelphia: Mosby, Elsevier; 2007:Chap 16.

DeKosky ST. Pathology and pathways of Alzheimer's disease with an update on new developments in treatment. *J Am Geriatr Soc* 2003;51(5 suppl):S314-S320.

Petersen RC, Doody R, Kurz A, et al. Current concepts in mild cognitive impairment. *Arch Neurol.* 2001;58(12):1985-1992.

Sloane PD, Zimmerman S, Suchindran C, et al. The public health impact of Alzheimer's disease, 2000–2050: potential implication of treatment advances. *Annu Rev Public Health.* 2002;23:213-231.

74   Diabetes Mellitus

Mark B. Mengel, MD, MPH

KEY POINTS

- The prevalence of type 2 DM is increasing, mirroring the increase in the prevalence of obesity.
- All adults older than 45 years should be screened every 3 years using a fasting plasma glucose (FPG). (SOR **C**) The diagnosis of DM is made by 2 FPG values ≥126 mg/dL or one random ≥200 mg/dL.
- Instituting a healthy diet with just enough calories to maintain ideal body weight and engaging in regular exercise is the cornerstone of treatment for both type 1 and type 2 DM. (SOR **B**) Type 1 DM patients require insulin. Type 2 DM are usually started on an oral sulfonylureas, Glucotrol XL 5 mg po qd, or metformin 500 mg po qd to bid if obese, with other oral agents added as needed.
- Hemoglobin A_{1C} is the best measure of diabetic control, should be checked every 3 to 6 months, and should be kept under 7% to minimize complications. (SOR **A**) Control of blood pressure, lipids, and smoking cessation are also important to reduce the chance of macrovascular complications. (SOR **A**)
- Clinicians should also assess and reduce common barriers to care which prevent achievement of control goals, such as depression, family dysfunction, lack of financial resources and lack of health literacy.

I. **Introduction**
   A. Diabetes mellitus (DM) is a heterogeneous group of disorders caused by a relative or absolute insulin deficiency, resulting in abnormalities of carbohydrate and fat metabolism. The two principal forms of DM, type 1 and type 2, are the focus of this chapter.
   B. Type 1 DM, resulting form the destruction of pancreatic beta-cells, occurs in 5% to 10% of patients with DM, usually presenting between ages 10 to 15 years.
   C. Type 2 DM, resulting from insulin resistance, occurs in 90% to 95% of people with DM, usually presenting after age 40. As the prevalence of obesity has increased in the US over the past 20 years (two-thirds are now overweight or obese), so has the prevalence of type 2 DM (8%, in one-third the disease is undiagnosed). However, as the prevalence of obesity has increased in children and young adults, type 2 DM is increasingly being diagnosed in those populations as well. Major **risk factors** for type 2 DM include increasing age, being overweight, having a positive family history of DM, having a higher prediabetic fasting plasma glucose, being habitually physically inactive, and being a member of certain racial groups, specifically African Americans, Hispanics, Native Americans, Asian Americans, and Pacific Islanders.
II. **Diagnosis**
   A. **Symptoms and signs**
      1. **Type 1 DM.** Polyuria, polydipsia, polyphagia (the 3 Ps), weight loss, fatigue, and irritability are typical presenting complaints of patients with type 1 DM. Many type 1 DM patients are also in frank diabetic ketoacidosis at the time of diagnosis.
      2. **Type 2 DM.** Many patients with type 2 DM are relatively asymptomatic initially. Physicians should suspect type 2 DM in patients with symptoms (such as the 3 Ps), or with risk factors (see Section II.C), recurrent infections, visual difficulties, unexplained peripheral neuropathy, and signs of other insulin resistance states such as polycystic ovarian syndrome or the metabolic syndrome. Adults older than 45 years, particularly those with a BMI over 25, should be routinely screened every 3 years using a fasting plasma glucose. (SOR **C**)
      3. **Physical examination.** A search for complications should be instituted even in those patients with DM who are newly diagnosed, including: blood pressure, retinas, cardiac with peripheral pulses, and feet sensation. (SOR **C**)
   B. **Laboratory tests**
      1. **Urinalysis.** Most patients with diabetes "spill" sugar into their urine at the time of diagnosis. However, many substances, aging, and pregnancy affect the amount of

glucose in the urine. Thus, urine testing for glycosuria is not useful in diagnosing and following up on patients with diabetes. Urine testing for ketones in patients with diabetes is still advisable, however, particularly when the patient becomes ill, to monitor for the onset of diabetic ketoacidosis.

2. **Plasma glucose measurement.** This test is the preferred method of diagnosis. An elevated plasma glucose level should be confirmed with a subsequent fasting or postprandial value. (SOR **C**) Meeting any one of the following criteria establishes the diagnosis in nonpregnant adults:

   a. One random plasma glucose measurement of over 200 mg/dL (11.1 mmol/L) in a patient with classic diabetic signs and symptoms.

   b. Two fasting plasma glucose (FPG) levels of over 126 mg/dL (7.0 mmol/L).

   c. A glucose tolerance test (75-g load) in which any blood glucose value between time 0 and 2 hours exceeds 200 mg/dL.

   d. Those with non-normal FPG values that are not diagnostic for DM (110 mg/dL [6.1 mmol/L] ≤ FPG ≤ 126 mg/dL [7.0 mmol/L]), or a postload glucose tolerance test value of between 140 mg/dL (7.8 mmol/L) and 200 mg/dL (11.1 mmol/L) have impaired fasting glucose (if determined by a FPG), or impaired glucose tolerance (if diagnosed on an oral glucose tolerance test), and should be rescreened yearly.

III. **Treatment.** The goals of treatment are: (1) reduction of diabetic symptoms, (2) prevention of acute complications (e.g., diabetic ketoacidosis, hyperosmolar nonketotic coma, hypoglycemia), (3) encouragement of normal growth and development in children with DM, and (4) prevention of chronic complications.

A. **Dietary therapy**

   1. Consultation with a dietitian is recommended for all patients with type 1 DM to achieve balance between food consumption and insulin administration. An appropriate calorie, well-balanced meal plan combined with a high-fiber intake actually improves diabetic control.

   2. In type 2 DM, dietary therapy is often ineffective in restoring glucose control, since few patients are able to maintain significant weight loss. Obesity contributes to the insulin resistance found in type 2 DM; 80% of patients with type 2 DM are overweight or obese. Even modest reductions in weight can significantly improve diabetic control. Enrollment in behavior modification programs or support groups and involvement of the patient's family are necessary to increase the chances of weight loss success. (SOR **B**)

B. **Exercise**. Exercise has a glucose-lowering effect and is recommended for the improvement of diabetic control. (SOR **A**) Patients with type 2 DM who engage in an exercise program that is integrated with dietary therapy may lose weight, with subsequent improvement in diabetic control. Guidelines for planning an exercise program include the following:

   1. An exercise program should begin at low intensity and increase gradually to 30 to 45 minutes of moderate aerobic activity 3 to 5 days a week. Resistance training can then be added 3 times per week, progressing to 3 sets of 8 to 10 repetitions, exercising all major muscle groups by the end of the week. Consultation with a clinician is recommended to integrate exercise with the other aspects of the therapeutic regimen. Patients with DM whose plasma glucose values are over 300 mg/dL (16.7 mmol/L) should not exercise until their control has improved and their blood glucose levels have decreased. Vigorous exercise may be contraindicated in those with proliferative or severe diabetic retinopathy. Self-monitoring of blood glucose (see Section V.B) is useful during exercise. If blood glucose is low at the start of exercise (≤100 mg/dL), a carbohydrate snack is indicated.

   2. When possible, a patient with DM should exercise after meals to reduce postprandial hyperglycemia.

   3. Patients with DM should avoid exercise during peak insulin actions and should avoid exercising extremities in which insulin has recently been injected.

C. **Oral hypoglycemic agents** (Table 74–1). In patients with type 2 DM, oral hypoglycemic agents have become the mainstay of therapy, often using multiple oral agents as type 2 DM progresses. (SOR **A**) *These agents have no place in the treatment of patients with type 1 DM.*

   1. **Oral sulfonylureas** act by enhancing insulin secretion. There is little cost difference among first-generation agents, although generic brands are less expensive.

   2. **Second-generation oral sulfonylureas** are far more potent than first-generation agents, have a longer half-life allowing once- or twice-daily dosing, and thus these

TABLE 74–1. ORAL HYPOGLYCEMIC AGENTS

Drug	Starting Dose/ Maximum Daily Dose	Side Effects and Notes	Cost*
Sulfonylureas-first generation			
Acetohexamide	500 mg po qd/1500 mg	Hypoglycemia, wt gain, rash, increased LFTs	$
Chlorpropamide (Diabinese)	100–250 mg po qd/750 mg	Hypoglycemia, wt gain, rash, increased LFTs, disulfiramlike reaction, hyponatremia, extremely long-half life	$, (trade $ $)
Tolazamide (Tolinase)	100–250 mg po qd/1000 mg	Hypoglycemia, wt gain, rash, increased LFTs	$, (trade $ $)
Tolbutamide (Orinase, Tol-Tab)	250–500 mg po qd/3000 mg	Hypoglycemia, wt gain, rash, increased LFTs	$
Sulfonylureas-second generation			
Glimepiride (Amaryl)	1–2 mg po qd/8 mg	Hypoglycemia, wt gain, rash, increased LFTs	$
Glipizide (Glucotrol & Glucotrol XL)	5 mg po qd/40 mg, (20 mg for XL)	Hypoglycemia, wt gain, rash, increased LFTs	$
Glyburide (Diabeta, Micronase)	1.25–2.5 mg po qd/20 mg	Hypoglycemia, wt gain, rash, increased LFTs	$, (trade $ $)
Glyburide-micronized (Glynase PresTab)	1.5–3 mg po qd/12 mg	Hypoglycemia, wt gain, rash, increased LFTs	$
Alpha-Glucosidase Inhibitor			
Acarbose (Precose)	25 mg po tid before meals/ 300 mg	Bloating, flatulence, diarrhea/contraindicated in IBD	$ $ $
Miglitol (Glyset)	25 mg po tid with meals/ 300 mg	Bloating, flatulence, diarrhea/contraindicated in IBD	$ $ $
Biguanides			
Metformin (Glucophage & Glucophage XR)	500 mg po qd-bid/2550 mg/d (2000 mg/d for XR)	Nausea, vomiting, diarrhea, lactic acidosis/contraindicated if ethanol abuse, CHF, or renal insufficiency	$ $
Nonsulfonylureas secretagogues			
Nateglinide (Starlix)	60 mg tid before meals/360 mg	Hypoglycemia, wt gain, increased LFTs	$ $ $
Repaglinide (Prandin)	0.5 mg tid before meals/16 mg	Hypoglycemia, wt gain, increased LFTs	$ $ $
Thiazolidinediones			
Pioglitzone (Actos)	15 mg po qd/45 mg	Hepatitis, edema/monitor LFTs q 2 mo for first year	$ $ $ $
Rosiglitazone (Avandia)	4 mg qd to bid/8 mg	Hepatitis, edema/monitor LFTs q 2 mo for first year	$ $ $ $
DPP-4 inhibitors ("gliptins")			
Sitagliptin (Januvia)	100 mg qd/100 mg	URIs, headaches/lower dose in those with renal disease	$ $ $ $

* Cost: $, AWP, $ 0–$ 10; $ $, AWP, $ 10–25; $ $ $, AWP, $ 25–75; $ $ $ $, AWP, $ 75–150.
AWP, average wholesale price; CHF, congestive heart failure; IBD, irritable bowel disease; LFTs, liver function tests.

agents have become the drugs of choice for treating patients with type 2 DM. Second-generation agents lower hemoglobin A_{1C} levels by 1 to 2 percentage points on average, but can cause hypoglycemia and weight gain. All the sulfonylureas undergo hepatic metabolism and should be used with caution in patients with liver abnormalities. Glipizide is preferred in patients with renal abnormalities. Generic glipizide, glyburide, glimepiride (Amaryl), Glucotrol XL, and micronized glyburide are the most cost-effective agents in this class.

3. **Alpha-glucosidase inhibitors.** These agents inhibit the alpha-glucosidase enzyme that lines the brush border of the small intestine delaying absorption of simple sugars. These drugs must be taken with each meal in order to lower postprandial glucose levels. On an average, these agents lower hemoglobin A_{1C} by 0.5 to 1.0 percentage points. Patients taking these agents will have trouble treating hypoglycemic attacks with complex carbohydrates and so should have oral glucose tablets readily available. These agents are contraindicated in patients with bowel disease. These agents can be used in combination with other oral hypoglycemic agents.

4. **Biguanides. Metformin** (Glucophage) is the only biguanide available in the US and acts by decreasing hepatic glucose output and increases utilization of glucose in peripheral tissues. Endogenous insulin is required for metformin to work. Metformin does not stimulate insulin secretion. Clinical trials suggest that metformin is as effective as other oral agents in the treatment of patients with type 2 DM, with less weight gain noted when compared with patients taking sulfonylureas. Metformin is the agent of choice in type 2 DM patients who are obese or gain weight on other oral hypoglycemic agents, as they are associated with reduced risk of mortality compared with diet, sulfonylureas, or insulin aloneﬁn these patients. (SOR **B**) Adverse effects are mainly gastrointestinal and include nausea, vomiting, anorexia, diarrhea, and a metallic taste in the mouth. Lactic acidosis occurs rarely, but is potentially fatal. Since lactic acidosis usually occurs in the setting of renal failure, the drug should not be prescribed in patients with this condition. Metformin can be used with other oral hypoglycemic agents. Metformin has been used in patients with impaired glucose tolerance and shown to decrease the incidence of DM in that group (although a regimen of exercise and weight loss caused a greater decrease in the incidence of subsequent DM). Metformin is available in fixed combinations with sulfonylureas or thiazolidinediones.

5. **Non sulfonylureas secretagogues.** Meglitinides are rapid acting agents that stimulate insulin release postprandially, and thus must be taken before each meal. If a meal is missed, the drug should not be taken. Meglitinides lowing hemoglobin A_{1C} by 0.5 to 1 percentage points on average. These drugs are more expensive than oral sulfonylureas but may prove useful in patients with renal impairment or patients who eat sporadically. These agents should be used cautiously in patients with liver abnormalities.

6. **Thiazolidinedione** agents enhance insulin action via direct stimulation of receptors in the nucleus of hepatic and skeletal muscle cells, thus directly increasing insulin sensitivity. On an average, thiazolidinediones lower hemoglobin A_{1C} by 1 to 1.5 percentage points, over 6 months. These agents can be used as monotherapy or in combination with other oral hypoglycemic agents. Liver function tests should be monitored every 2 months for the first 12 months in patients on these agents and periodically thereafter. Weight gain because of fluid retention is also common and can lead to congestive heart failure. These agents are contraindicated in patients with class III or IV heart failure.

7. **Dipeptidyl peptidase-4 (DPP-4) inhibitors ("gliptins") slow the inactivation of incretin hormones, which increases insulin release and decreases glucagons release.** Gliptins lower hemoglobin A_{1C} by 0.5 to 1.0 percentage points, over 6 months, either as monotherapy or in combination with metformin or a thiazolidinedione. The dosage of these agents must be reduced in those with renal disease.

D. **Insulin therapy**
   1. **Indications**
      a. **All patients with type 1 DM require insulin therapy. (SOR Ⓐ)**
      b. Patients with type 2 DM may require insulin therapy if diet, exercise, and oral hypoglycemic agents do not control their DM sufficiently. (SOR **B**) Depending on the clinical situation, insulin may be added to oral hypoglycemics (for example, as a low dose of insulin glargine at bedtime [0.1 U/kg of body weight]), or oral hypoglycemics may be stopped and insulin started. Nocturnal insulin is then adjusted, based upon the results of a morning fasting plasma glucose value. Insulin may also be indicated

TABLE 74–2. INSULIN TYPES

Type	Onset of Action (h)	Maximum Action (h)	Duration of Action (h)
Rapid-acting			
Lispro (Humalog)			
Glulisine (Apidra)			
Aspart (Novolog)			
Inhaled insulin (Exubera)	0.2–0.5	0.5–1	3–5
Short-acting			
Regular	0.5–1	2–3	4–12
Intermediate-acting			
Neutral protamine hagedorn (NPH)	1–2	4–8	10–20
Long-acting			
Glargine (Lantus)	1–2	No peak	24
Detemir (Levemir)			

as initial therapy in patients with type 2 DM if the patient's initial fasting blood glucose value is greater than 400 mg/dL, particularly in young, nonobese, symptomatic patients. As glucotoxicity is reduced, these patients may be able to be switched to oral hypoglycemic agents. Premixed insulin preparations, such as humulin or Novolin 70/30 (70% NPH [Neutral protamine hagedorn], 30% regular), Humalog Mix 75/25 (75% insulin lispro protamine suspension and 25% lispro), Novalog Mix 70/30 (70 insulin aspart protamine suspension and 30% insulin aspart), work particularly well in type 2 patients, with improvements in diabetic control because of decreased mixing errors.

2. **Characteristics of insulin preparations.** Selection from available insulin preparation is based on **concentration** (usually U-100), **species source** (almost exclusively human insulin developed using recombinant DNA), **purity**, and **type** (Table 74–2). Recently rapid acting insulins, insulin lispro and insulin aspart, have been shown to more effective than regular insulin in controlling postprandial blood sugar. Very-long-acting insulins, insulin glargine and determir have no peak onset of action, are given once daily, and mimicking basal insulin secretion. In patients with type 1 and type 2 DM, use of insulin glargine (rather than twice a day NPH), has been shown to be associated with less hypoglycemia, less weight gain, and better glucose control. Recently, an inhaled insulin was released that is used before meals, similar to short-acting insulins. In studies, it has demonstrated similar efficacy to short-acting insulins, but better patient satisfaction and quality of life. As absorption is through the lungs, larger doses are needed, and the risks of pulmonary problems are still being assessed. Inhaled insulin shouldn't be used in smokers or those with lung disease.

3. **Initiating insulin therapy.** Patient newly diagnosed with type 1 DM either receive education and begin their insulin regimen while hospitalized or if not in ketoacidosis, can begin their insulin treatment as an outpatient. One injection of insulin per day rarely normalizes the glycemic response in such patients and often leaves type 1 DM patient hyperglycemic at night and in the morning. Therefore, patients with type 1 DM either typically receive a "split-dose" insulin regimen, consisting of a mixture of regular and NPH insulin before breakfast and in the late afternoon before supper, or now receive a once daily shot of insulin glargine with shots of rapid acting insulin prior to each meal. The amount of rapid acting insulin given can be tailored to the amount of carbohydrate that will be eaten during the meal and the preprandial blood glucose value. Two methods are general used to initiate insulin therapy as described below:

a. Patients with type 1 DM may first be placed on preprandial and nighttime injections of either regular insulin or rapid acting insulin based upon preprandial blood glucose values shown in Table 74–3. When glucose split-dose insulin therapy is going to be used, then two-thirds of the total amount of insulin is given in the morning and one-third in the evening. The morning and evening dosages can then be split into 75% NPH and 25% regular insulin. If insulin glargine with rapid acting insulin before each meal is used then 40% to 50% of the total dose is given as insulin glargine

TABLE 74–3. TYPICAL SLIDING SCALE USED TO INITIATE INSULIN THERAPY

Blood Glucose Value (mg/dL)	Amount of Regular Insulin to Be Given (U)
150–200	6–8
200–250	8–12
250–300	12–16
≥ 300	16–24

first thing in the morning or at bedtime with the other 50% to 60% split up and given as rapid acting insulin prior to each meal based upon preprandial glucose values.

   b. Alternatively, patients with type 1 DM can just be started on split-dose therapy or therapy with insulin glargine and a rapid acting insulin. Patients with type 1 DM should start with a total daily dose of 0.6 U/kg of body weight. Once again if split-dose therapy is used two-thirds of that is given in the morning and one-third in the evening. The morning and evening dosages are then split 75% NPH insulin and 25% regular insulin. If insulin glargine and rapid acting insulin are used 50% of the total daily dose is given as insulin glargine first thing in the morning and then the other 50% is given as rapid acting insulin split up prior to each meal based upon the results of preprandial glucose values. Self-blood glucose monitoring (see Section VI.B), can then be used to adjust insulin therapy (see Table 74–4).

4. **Intensive insulin therapy.** Three or more shots of insulin per day or the continuous subcutaneous insulin infusion (CSII) pump qualifies as intensive insulin therapy. Both methods require meticulous management including frequent self-blood glucose monitoring in order to reduce the risk of hypoglycemic attacks and ensure good diabetic control. While most primary care clinicians can manage three or more injections of insulin per day in their type 1 or type 2 DM patients, if four injections of insulin per day are not effective in achieving optimal glucose control, then patients should be referred to an endocrinologist for consideration of CSII pump therapy.

5. **Honeymoon period.** Soon after insulin therapy is initiated, a "honeymoon period" of 12 to 18 months occurs in nearly all patients with type 1 or type 2 DM. During this time patient's insulin requirements usually are drastically reduced. This phenomenon is thought secondary to reduced glucose toxicity. Therefore, patients should be encouraged to utilize self-blood glucose monitoring, and protocol should be designed so that they can reduce insulin therapy as their insulin requirements are reduced.

E. **Other injectables.**
1. **Exenatide (Byetta), an incretin mimetic, increases insulin release, lowers glucagons, delays gastric emptying, and suppresses appetite.** Exenatide is indicated in patients with type 2 DM who have not achieved glucose control goals while taking metformin or combination therapy with metformin. Exenatide should not be used in patients with type 1 DM. The initial dose of exenatide is 5 μg subcutaneously twice daily, 60 minutes before breakfast or dinner. The dose can be doubled after 1 month. Side effects include nausea and vomiting (usually at the start of treatment), and hypoglycemia.

2. **Pramlintide (Symlin)** is an analog of amylin that slows food absorption, inhibits glucagon, and reduces appetite. **Premlintide is injected along with premeal insulin,**

TABLE 74–4. ADJUSTMENT OF INSULIN DOSAGES BY SELF-MONITORING WITH A SPIT-DOSE REGIMEN

Measurement Time	Dosage to Adjust if Blood Glucose Out of Target Range
0700	Afternoon NPH
1200	Morning regular
1700	Morning NPH
2200	Afternoon regular
0300	Afternoon NPH

Protocol for all insulin dosages; If blood glucose ≤60 mg/dL, decrease appropriate dose by 2 U; If 60 mg/dL ≤ blood glucose ≤120 mg/dL, no adjustment; If 120 mg/dL ≤ blood glucose ≤150 mg/dL, increase appropriate dose by 2 U; If 150 mg/dL ≤ blood glucose ≤180 mg/dL, increase appropriate dose by 4 U; If blood glucose ≥180 mg/dL, increase appropriate dose by 6 U.

(separate syringes) and improves glucose control, while lowering body weight.
The starting dose is 15 μg, increased by 15 μg increments to 30 or 60 μg as tolerated
in patients with type 1 DM before each meal. The starting dose for patients with type
2 DM is 60 μg with the dose increasing to 120 μg twice a day if tolerated. Insulin
doses should be reduced by 50% when pramlintide is started. The main side effect
is nausea. Hypoglycemia occurs more commonly in patients with type 1 DM. Delayed
gastric emptying may delay the abosrption of orally administered medication.

IV. **Management Strategies.** Achieving optimal diabetic control, near normal hemoglobin A_{1C}
levels, while minimizing hypoglycemic episodes, is the clear goal of treatment in patients
with both type 1 and type 2 DM. Achieving near normal hemoglobin A_{1C} levels in both type 1
and type 2 DM patients has been shown to reduce micro- and macrovascular complications.
(SOR **Ⓐ**) Other risk factors for macrovascular complications, particularly in type 2 DM patients, should also be controlled including blood pressure, cholesterol and triglyceride levels,
and cessation of cigarette smoking. The American Diabetes Association recommends that
patients with DM strive for a hemoglobin A_{1C} of $\leq$ 7.0%, fasting plasma glucose of between
80 and 120 mg/dL, blood pressure $\leq$ 130/85 mm, an LDL cholesterol of $\leq$ 100 mg/dL, an
HDL cholesterol $\geq$ 40 mg/dL, triglycerides $\leq$ 150 mg/dL, and if smoking, patients should
quit.

A. **Hemoglobin A_{1C} (glycosylated hemoglobin)** is one of several forms of hemoglobin A
that result from the nonenzymatic attachment of glucose to hemoglobin A. Since the
percentage of hemoglobin A_{1C} depends on the average glucose concentration over
the life of a red blood cell (approximately 120 days), hemoglobin A_{1C} is a good measure of diabetic control over the previous 2 to 3 months. Falsely elevated levels of
hemoglobin A_{1C} occur in the presence of uremia, fetal hemoglobin, alcoholism, and aspirin
usage.

B. **Self-monitoring of blood glucose (SMBG).** This technique developed as the poor correlation between plasma glucose values and glycosuria became clear.
  1. SMBG is a reliable technique, providing patients receive proper instruction in the pro-
     cedure and potential problems. (SOR **Ⓑ**)
  2. Patients with diabetes who use SMBG determine their glucose values before meals, at
     bedtime, and occasionally in the middle of the night. They then adjust insulin dosages
     by using simple rules (Table 75–4). In addition, physicians can use the results of SMBG
     to adjust insulin dosages during regular follow-up visits. Patients with DM on intensive
     insulin regimens must use SMBG to adjust dosages of preprandial insulin. SMBG is
     also helpful if patients with DM become ill, allowing adjustment of insulin dosages so
     that control is maintained during sickness.

C. **Reducing barriers to care.** Certain nonmedical factors are associated with poor diabetic
control in patients with DM.
  1. **Patient-centered care.** Encouraging the involvement of patients with DM in decisions
     regarding goal setting and management options improves glucose control. Excellent
     clinician–patient relationship and communication skills, particularly in the area of ne-
     gotiation, are linked with improved control. (SOR **Ⓑ**)
  2. **Knowledge and self-management skills.** Patients with DM should be enrolled in an
     education program which discusses a wide range of topics pertinent to their care and
     encourages patient decision-making and self-management. A recent meta-analysis
     shows that such an approach increases knowledge about DM, increases the fre-
     quency and accuracy of SBMG, improves dietary habits, and improves glucose control.
     (SOR **Ⓐ**)
  3. **Psychosocial factors.** Clinicians should monitor for the following psychosocial factors
     which have been linked with poor diabetic control: pessimistic attitudes about DM, poor
     social support and social isolation, low self-efficacy skills, an external locus of control,
     excessive stress, being in precontemplation regarding necessary behavior change,
     and a passive pessimistic coping style. Screen all patients with DM periodically for de-
     pression and family dysfunction and recommend appropriate treatment. Determining
     use of complimentary and alternative therapies by patients and discussing the effica-
     cies of those therapies with patients have been shown to improve glucose control, as
     patients rely less on ineffective therapies.
  4. **Health literacy.** Clinicians often use medical terminology which is not understood by
     patients. Patients rarely admit their ignorance, as that would cause embarrassment.
     Health illiteracy is commonplace and associated with decreased adherence to treat-
     ment regimens, inability to keep appointments, and not understanding instructions

and education. If educational materials are utilized by clinicians, materials must be at a reading level and in a language understood by most patients.

   5. **Financial.** Even with health insurance, the cost of medications and supplies for DM can be prohibitive. In those situations, clinicians should make every attempt to use the most cost effective treatment options available.

D. **Prevention and early detection of complications.**

   1. **Achieving near normal diabetic control**. Design of an effective treatment regimen and the assessment and correction of factors associated with poor diabetic control and barriers to care, constitute the first step in preventing the onset of both microvascular and macrovascular complications of DM. Risk factor reduction for macrovascular complications is essential including smoking cessation, blood pressure control, and treatment of hyperlipidemia. Aspirin, 325 mg oral daily, to prevent macrovascular complications, is also indicated in all patients with type 2 DM.

   2. **Diagnosing complications as early as possible**. Periodic ophthalmologic, neurologic, vascular, renal (measurement of serum creatinine and microalbuminuria), and foot examinations aid early diagnosis of diabetic complications. The exact frequency of examinations, except for annual ophthalmologic examinations and annual tests for serum creatinine and microalbuminuria, has not been well studied; however, examining the feet of a diabetic patient at each visit has been associated with better diabetic control. Most clinicians follow patients with diabetes at least quarterly, with more frequent visits as necessary if diabetic control is poor.

   3. **Treating complications as they develop**. Once complications are diagnosed, risk factor reduction and symptomatic treatment remain the mainstays of complication management. Painful peripheral neuropathies can often be treated with a low dose of a tricyclic antidepressant, such as amitriptyline, 50 mg orally at bedtime, whereas the progression of diabetic nephropathy can be slowed with an angiotensin-converting enzyme inhibitor (even if the patient is not hypertensive) such as captopril, 25 to 50 mg orally twice daily or lisinopril, 10 mg orally daily.

E. **Immunizations.** Adult patient with DM should receive a yearly flu vaccine, a pneumococcal vaccine every 5 to 7 years, and a tetanus vaccine every 10 years.

F. **Office management.** An organized evidenced-based approach to the management of patients with DM in medical offices has been shown to improve diabetic control in patients visiting those offices. Use of multiple interventions has been associated with better control. Interventions include practitioner education through materials and meetings, developing a local consensus process regarding care protocols, auditing outcomes, and providing that feedback to practitioners, using reminders for clinicians regarding when to conduct certain interventions, such as annual ophthalmologic examinations, enhancing the professional role of nurses in the office, and utilizing case management and disease management for patients who need that additional support. A multidisciplinary treatment team is needed for many patients, particularly those on intensive insulin treatment regimens. Lastly, the Kaiser Permanente System has popularized group visits for patients with DM. During these visits approximately 20 patients with DM receive a group educational session, discuss supportive strategies among themselves, and receive a brief visit from the clinician. While the effects of these group visits have not been well studied, patients seem to be pleased with the camaraderie and social interaction.

V. **Prognosis.** The outcome of DM in a particular patient depends on several factors. These factors include the nature and severity of the disease in the patient, the simultaneous occurrence of other diseases, the presence of risk factors for diabetic complications (disease duration is the most important), genetic susceptibility to specific complications, and how well the patient responds to treatment. The patient's ability to adapt constructively to the disease also influences the course of the illness.

A. **The mean survival** of patients with type 1 DM diagnosed before age 30 is currently 10 to 15 years less than that of the general population. Death usually results from end-stage renal disease (40%–50%) or coronary artery disease, although ketoacidosis and hypoglycemic coma continue to cause significant mortality.

B. **Life expectancy** in type 2 DM patients is roughly one-third less than that of age-matched nondiabetic patients. Cardiovascular disease accounts for 75% of the deaths in patients with type 2 DM after age 60. Except for ketoacidosis, all the complications associated with type 1 DM occur in patients with type 2 DM. However, macrovascular complications are more common in type 2 DM patients. Hyperosmolar nonketotic coma, an acute complication, is seen almost exclusively in patients with NIDDM.

REFERENCES

American Diabetes Association website. www.diabetes.org/home.jsp. Accessed November 26, 2006. Clinical Practice Recommendation 2006. *Diabetes Care.* 2006;29:S1-S85.

Egede LE, Zheng D, Simpson K. Comorbid depression is associated with increased health care use and expenditures in individuals with diabetes. *Diabetes Care.* 2002;25:464-470.

Feit S. *Putting evidence into practice: Outpatient management of type 2 diabetes mellitus. Clinical Evidence.* A report funded by United Health Foundation. London: BMJ Publishing Group, summer 2006.

Peterson KA, Hughes M. Readiness to change and clinical success in a diabetes educational program. *JABFP.* 2002;15(4):266-271.

---

75   Dyslipidemias

Michael A. Crouch, MD, MSPH

KEY POINTS

- One-half of all American adults have **unhealthy blood lipid levels** (low-density lipoprotein [LDL] or high-density lipoprotein [HDL] cholesterol, or both, with or without triglycerides). Although higher cholesterol levels pose the greatest *relative* risk, more than one-half of all **myocardial infarctions** occur in those with suboptimal (100–129 mg/dL) or borderline (130–159 mg/dL) LDL cholesterol levels.
- Lowering intake of **dietary saturated fat, trans fats, and cholesterol** is the cornerstone for treating hypercholesterolemia and reducing risk for coronary heart disease. (SOR 🅐) Other useful dietary measures include regular intake of fiber, fish, or fish oil (omega-3 fatty acids), nuts, soy protein, and plant sterols or stanols. (SOR 🅑) Many patients with elevated LDL cholesterol require **medication** in addition to dietary modification to achieve **treatment target goals. (SOR 🅐)** Weight loss and exercise raise HDL cholesterol and lower triglycerides, but do not improve LDL cholesterol.
- **Dietary changes** maintained for 1 month lower LDL cholesterol all they are ever going to do. Prolonging dietary change yields no further reduction. It is not necessary to wait 6 months before initiating a trial of lipid medication.
- If 1 month of maintaining maximum achievable dietary change does not lower LDL cholesterol to ≤130 mg/dL in a high-risk patient (≥20% estimated 10-year coronary heart disease risk) or ≤160 in an intermediate-risk patient (10%–20% estimated 10-year risk), it is appropriate to urge a trial of lipid medication. (SOR 🅐)
- The most effective drugs for lowering LDL cholesterol are the HMG-CoA reductase inhibitors (**statins**). The usual daily starting dose is atorvastatin (Lipitor), 10 mg; rosuvastatin (Crestor), 5 mg; simvastatin (Zocor), 20 mg; pravastatin (Pravachol), 40 mg; lovastatin (Mevacor, Altocor), 40 mg; or fluvastatin (Lescol), 80 mg XL.
- The lowest dose of the combination drug Vytorin (simvastatin–ezetimibe) lowers LDL cholesterol as well or better than the maximum dose of any statin. Outcome study results, however, are not yet available to compare Vytorin's efficacy for reducing risk for heart attack and stroke with the proven efficacy of a statin alone.
- The **goal** of hypercholesterolemia treatment is to reduce risk for **myocardial infarction** and **stroke** by one-third or more, by lowering LDL cholesterol below **100 mg/dL** in those with diabetes or known coronary or carotid artery disease, or below **130 mg/dL** in high-risk patients not known to have diabetes or coronary or carotid artery disease.
- Long-term **adherence** is poor for **statin therapy**. Many patients are apprehensive about potential **adverse drug effects** and do not have a clear understanding of the **benefit/risk ratio.** Repetitive patient education in verbal, textual, and graphic formats, focused on specific patient concerns, may foster long-term statin compliance and maximize treatment benefit.

I. Introduction
  A. **Dyslipidemia** is a broad term that includes several lipid disorders with primary genetic, secondary metabolic, lifestyle, and iatrogenic contributing factors.

1. Primary lipid disorders are **familial**, being transmitted across generations by both genetic factors and learned behaviors.
2. **Secondary** causes of dyslipidemias include diabetes mellitus, hypothyroidism, pregnancy, nephrotic syndrome, obstructive jaundice, chronic renal failure, dysgammaglobulinemia, anorexia nervosa, porphyria, and glycogen storage disease.
3. **Recommendations** for screening, diagnosis, and treatment are detailed in the **National Cholesterol Education Program (NCEP) Adult Treatment Panel (ATP) III guidelines (2001).** Suggested modifications of the NCEP guidelines, published in 2004, advocate more aggressive LDL cholesterol target goals for high-risk patients. (SOR **Ⓐ**)
B. **Hyperlipidemia** refers to elevated total blood cholesterol, LDL cholesterol, or triglyceride (TG) levels (or both). **Familial combined (mixed) hyperlipidemia** is elevated LDL cholesterol and TGs.
C. **Hypercholesterolemia** is elevated total blood cholesterol (cutpoints below).
    1. Familial heterozygous and homozygous hypercholesterolemia display Mendelian dominant inheritance, but most cases of hypercholesterolemia are polygenic.
    2. The prevalence of hypercholesterolemia increases with age, peaking at age 55 to 65.
    3. If 240 mg/dL (6.2 mmol/L) is used as the cutoff for elevated total cholesterol, approximately 10% of adults have hypercholesterolemia.
    4. Given the designated cutoff value of 200 mg/dL (5.2 mmol/L) for borderline elevated total cholesterol, approximately 50% of adults in the United States have borderline elevated or high total cholesterol.
D. **Hypertriglyceridemia** is elevated fasting TGs.
    1. High TG is $\geq$200 mg/dL or 1.7 mmol/L.
    2. TGs of 150 to 199 mg/dL (1.3–1.7 mmol/L) are "borderline high."
    3. Elevated TGs are seen in 20% to 25% of American adults.
    4. Saturated fat and cholesterol are absorbed from the gut and packaged into TG-rich particles called chylomicrons. These chylomicrons are broken down into very low-density lipoprotein (VLDL) particles that are rich in TGs.
    5. Excessive **alcohol**, dietary **sugars**, and rapidly digested **starches** elevate TGs.
    6. **Physical inactivity** or being **overweight** or **obese** elevates TGs and VLDL cholesterol.
E. **Hyperbetalipoproteinemia** is elevated LDL cholesterol. LDL cholesterol is one of the main risk factors for coronary artery disease (CAD).
    1. High LDL cholesterol is $\geq$160 mg/dL (4.15 mmol/L). Approximately 30% of all myocardial infarctions occur in individuals with LDL cholesterol $\geq$160 mg/dL (4.15 mmol/L).
    2. "Borderline high" LDL cholesterol level is 130 to 159 mg/dL (3.35–4.15 mmol/L). Approximately 33% of all myocardial infarctions occur in individuals with LDL cholesterol in this range.
    3. "Above optimal" LDL cholesterol is 100 to 129 mg/dL (2.6–3.35 mmol/L). Approximately 33% of all myocardial infarctions occur in individuals with LDL cholesterol in this range.
    4. "Desirable" LDL cholesterol is $\leq$100 mg/dL (2.6 mmol/L).
    5. "Optimal" LDL cholesterol is $\leq$70 mg/dL (1.8 mmol/L).
    6. VLDL particles are metabolized (catalyzed by the enzyme lipoprotein lipase) into cholesterol-rich LDL particles. LDL particles attach to LDL receptors on cell membranes. Cholesterol from the LDL particles passes into cells. Influx of cholesterol into cells suppresses the activity of the rate-limiting enzyme in cholesterol synthesis, 3-hydroxy-3-methylglutaryl coenzyme A (HMG-CoA) reductase.
    7. Excessive dietary intake of **saturated fat** raises LDL and total cholesterol more than does excessive cholesterol intake.
    8. **Stress** and **coronary-prone (Type A) behavior** can markedly elevate LDL cholesterol and total blood cholesterol in susceptible persons.
    9. **Iatrogenic** causes of lipid problems are common.
        a. **Diuretics** raise LDL cholesterol transiently, but seldom have significant long-term effects.
        b. **Beta blockers** without intrinsic sympathomimetic activity (propranolol, etc.) lower HDL cholesterol and may raise LDL cholesterol.
        c. **Chenodiol,** a gallstone dissolver, lowers both HDL cholesterol and LDL cholesterol.
        d. **Oral contraceptives** with strong androgen/progestin effect lower HDL cholesterol, raise TGs, and sometimes raise LDL cholesterol.
        e. High-dose **steroids** and **disulfiram** (Antabuse) raise TGs.
F. **Hypoalphalipoproteinemia** is low HDL cholesterol.
    1. Low HDL cholesterol is $\leq$40 mg/dL or 1.0 mmol/L.

2. Borderline low HDL cholesterol is 40 to 49 mg/dL (1.0–1.3 mmol/L).
3. Five to ten percent of adults have low HDL cholesterol, mostly on an inherited basis.
4. HDL particles facilitate LDL metabolism, which results in cholesterol being carried back to the liver from peripheral tissues.
5. Patients with low HDL cholesterol and elevated TGs tend to have smaller, more dense LDL particles that are more atherogenic.
6. **Physical inactivity** or being **overweight** or **obese** decreases HDL_2 cholesterol.
7. **Cigarette smoking** decreases HDL_2 cholesterol.
8. **Alcohol** in moderation raises HDL_3 cholesterol, but not HDL_2 cholesterol.

G. **Metabolic syndrome** is a risk factor constellation seen in more than 25% of United States adults. It is associated with an extremely high risk for CHD. Metabolic syndrome is present if a patient has three or more of the following characteristics:
  1. Waist size greater than 40 in (102 cm) for men or greater than 35 in (89 cm) for women (NCEP criterion), or body mass index (BMI) $\geq$30 (WHO criterion).
  2. TG level at or above 150 mg/dL (1.7 mmol/L).
  3. Blood pressure at or above 130/85 mm Hg.
  4. Fasting glucose value at or above 100 mg/dL (5.55 mmol/L).
  5. HDL-C level less than 40 mg/dL (1.0 mmol/L) for men or less than 50 mg/dL (1.3 mmol/L) for women.

II. **Diagnosis**
  A. **Symptoms and signs.** Lipid problems are usually asymptomatic for several decades.
    1. **Arcus senilis, xanthelasma, tendon xanthomas, and eruptive xanthomas** are late or uncommon physical signs of lipid problems.
    2. **Retinal arteriovenous crossing changes** signal atherosclerosis.
    3. **Angina pectoris, intermittent claudication, and impotence** may develop as warning symptoms of advanced atherosclerosis.
    4. **Myocardial infarction, cerebrovascular accident (stroke), or sudden death** is often the first sign of a lipid problem.

  B. **Laboratory tests**
    1. **Screening** is recommended by the National Cholesterol Education Program (NCEP) every 3 to 5 years for most adults younger than age 70. (SOR ⓓ) Adults with LDL cholesterol levels $\leq$130 mg/dL (3.35 mmol/L) and HDL levels $\geq$50 mg/dL (1.3 mmol/L) probably do not need to be rescreened this often unless they experience major changes in weight, diet, or physical activity. Children and adolescents with a family history of severe dyslipidemia or early atherosclerotic disease should also be screened. (SOR ⓓ)
      a. A **random or fasting lipid profile** (with total, LDL, and HDL cholesterol and TGs) should be obtained initially to detect elevated LDL cholesterol or TGs and low HDL cholesterol. The more convenient random lipid profile increases compliance with screening, and it gives useful information about the extent of postprandial hyperlipidemia (considered to be a serious atherogenic factor).
      b. If a patient is at **high risk** for CAD and random LDL cholesterol levels are marginally or mildly elevated, a **fasting lipid profile** should be obtained to more accurately categorize the severity of elevated LDL cholesterol.
    2. **Interpreting cholesterol results**
      a. Blood lipids change acutely in response to food intake. The TG level is lowest in the fasting state, rises by an average of 50 mg/dL postprandially, and peaks 3 to 6 hours after a meal. As the TG level rises, total and LDL cholesterol each fall by an average of 5 to 15 mg/dL. Thus, total and LDL cholesterol tend to be higher when fasting. HDL cholesterol varies little between the fasting and postprandial states, averaging 45 mg/dL (1.16 mmol/L) for men and 55 mg/dL (1.42 mmol/L) for women.
      b. Blood lipids can fluctuate within minutes, days, or weeks in response to illness, emotional stress, or malnutrition.
      c. Blood lipid levels may fluctuate seasonally. In colder climates, cholesterol and TG levels tend to be somewhat higher in winter because of higher fat intake.
      d. Ranges of total blood cholesterol and LDL cholesterol that are preventive, permissive, or aggressive with respect to their risk for promoting atherosclerosis are shown in Figures 75–1 and 75–2.
    3. **Diagnosing lipid disorders**
      a. If a screening lipid profile shows elevated LDL cholesterol, low HDL cholesterol, or high TGs, a **second lipid profile** should be obtained (fasting) before starting treatment, to confirm elevation and establish an accurate baseline. (SOR ⓓ)

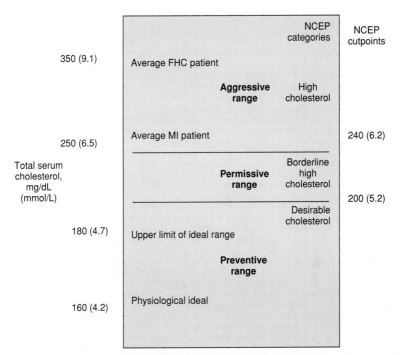

FIGURE 75–1. Prognostic range for total cholesterol. FHC, familial heterozygous hypercholesterolemia; MI, myocardial infarction; NCEP, National Cholesterol Education Program.

    b. **Excluding secondary causes.** If symptoms or signs are suggestive, the physician should consider ordering thyroid, renal, or liver function tests to rule out secondary causes of dyslipidemia.

    c. **Prognosis categorization** identifies those patients at highest risk. **Lipid ratios** summarize two or more lipid values into one number that correlates strongly with long-term prognosis; however, these ratios (total cholesterol:HDL cholesterol or LDL cholesterol:HDL cholesterol) predict outcome only marginally better than absolute HDL cholesterol and LDL cholesterol values.

        (1) At **highest risk** are patients who **smoke** or have **diabetes mellitus, the metabolic syndrome, left ventricular hypertrophy,** or moderately elevated **C-reactive protein** (CRP) levels (3.0–9.9 for the high-sensitive "cardiac" CRP).

        (2) Patients who have **low HDL** cholesterol levels are at some increased risk even if their LDL cholesterol levels are not elevated. Of the lipid values, HDL cholesterol is the best single predictor of adverse outcome. Above average or high HDL cholesterol levels ($\geq$60 mg/dL or 1.55 mmol/L), however, do not guarantee immunity from CAD. A pro-inflammatory form of HDL is present in the blood of some patients who have HDL levels $\geq$80 mg/dL (2.1 mmol/L); this form of HDL greatly increases the risk for atherosclerosis.

        (3) Patients with markedly elevated LDL cholesterol levels ($\geq$190 mg/dL, or 4.9 mmol/L) are at increased risk even if they have HDL cholesterol levels at or above average.

        (4) Patients with high fasting TG levels are at increased risk, especially obese females with diabetes mellitus.

    d. **Additional tests** sometimes can be helpful to refine a patient's estimated risk and adjust the aggressiveness of treatment, especially in those with a strong family history of CAD or stroke.

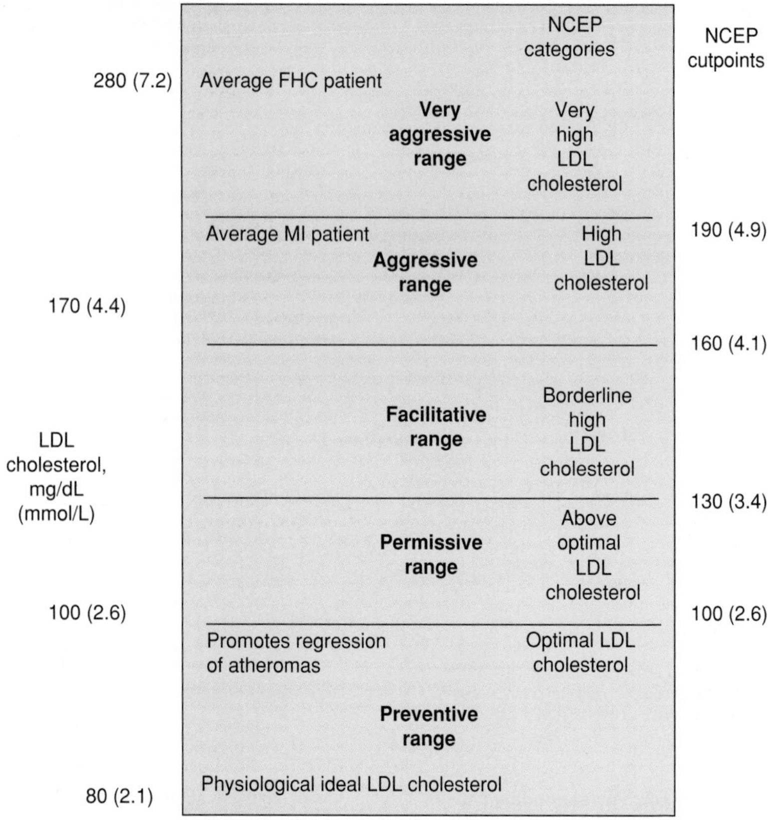

FIGURE 75–2. Prognostic range for LDL cholesterol. FHC, familial heterozygous hypercholesterolemia; LDL, low-density lipoprotein; MI, myocardial infarction; NCEP, National Cholesterol Education Program.

(1) **CRP** levels predict risk for myocardial infarction and stroke even better than LDL cholesterol levels do, when measured in healthy persons. CRP should be measured with the high-sensitivity cardiac method, not the older quantitative method. CRP is produced by the liver as an acute-phase reactant, quickly rising to exceed 10 mg/L with many acute infectious and inflammatory illnesses, and staying high with some chronic conditions (seen in approximately 5% of all patients screened). It falls rapidly to an individual's usual chronic level when illness resolves. Approximately 25% of patients have high-risk levels of 3.0 to 10.0 mg/L (Table 75–1). Approximately 50% of patients have "average risk" levels of 1.0 to 2.9 mg/dL, leaving 25% with low-risk levels ≤1.0 mg/dL. A CRP

TABLE 75–1. C-REACTIVE PROTEIN RISK PREDICTION RANGES

	C-Reactive Protein 2 Level (mg/L)	Prevalence (%)
Lowest risk	≤1.00	25
Average risk	1.00–2.99	45
High risk	3.00–10.00	25
Out of usual range	≥10.00	5

level of $\geq$10.0 mg/L usually indicates acute or chronic illness and should be repeated. A moderately elevated CRP should be repeated a few weeks later, at least once. It is unknown how often CRP should be retested for those with abnormal or normal results, and whether lowering CRP with aspirin or a statin is beneficial. While CRP testing provides potentially useful information, its cost (approximately $75) is not reimbursed by most healthcare insurance plans, so the patient pays for it out of pocket.

(2) Homocysteine elevation predicts risk for myocardial infarction and stroke. Elevated homocysteine ($\geq$10.0 mg/L) is seen in approximately 5% of adults. Intervention outcome study results, however, have shown no benefit from lowering homocysteine with folate, pyridoxine, and vitamin B_{12} when given together.

(3) Apolipoprotein levels predict outcome more accurately than does LDL cholesterol or HDL cholesterol, but their clinical usefulness has not been proved. Apolipoprotein levels can sometimes help the physician to decide how aggressively to treat patients with LDL cholesterol levels of 130 to 189 mg/dL (3.35–4.90 mmol/L) and patients with HDL cholesterol $\leq$40 mg/dL (1.0 mmol/L) whose LDL cholesterol is $\leq$130 mg/dL (3.35 mmol/L).

    (a) Prognosis is poor if the level of **apolipoprotein B**, the main apolipoprotein in LDL, is elevated.

    (b) A low level of **apolipoprotein A-I,** the main apolipoprotein in HDL, also indicates a poor prognosis.

(4) Lipoprotein (a) is a modified LDL moiety similar to plasminogen. Lipoprotein (a) elevation $\geq$50 mg/dL signals a bad prognosis, even if LDL cholesterol is $\leq$130 mg/dL (3.35 mmol/L). The test may be more useful than apolipoprotein levels for clarifying prognosis and adjusting treatment aggressiveness in marginal cases.

(5) PLAC is a newly available clinical test that measures the level of the enzyme **Lp-PLA2.** Lp-PLA2 combines with LDL and facilitates its movement into the arterial intima, where LDL becomes oxidized and accumulates in atheromatous plaque. Individuals with elevated Lp-PLA2 have a two-fold increased CAD risk. Those with elevated Lp-PLA2 and CRP have a three-fold increased risk.

(6) Pro-inflammatory HDL is measured by a test under development. This test may help clarify the risk status of those with high HDL levels who also have strong family histories of CAD.

III. Treatment

A. Treatment recommendations and treatment goals should be established based on the patient's clinical status, other risk factors (Table 75–2), and estimated 10-year risk for CHD (Table 75–3).

B. The estimated 10-year risk for CHD is a key step in evaluating candidacy for statin therapy for patients not known to have diabetes, CHD, or CHD-equivalent.

    1. Ten-year CHD risk can be estimated manually using the NCEP risk calculator sheet (see Section III.B.2.b, below).

    2. The 10-year risk for CHD can be estimated more quickly and easily by:

        a. Using any reliable Internet risk calculator online (http://hp2010.nhlbihin.net/atpiii/calculator.asp).

        b. Downloading a risk calculator program for local use with a computer or personal digital assistant from a Web site such as http://www.pdacortex.com/NCEP_ATPIII_CHD_Risk_Calculator_Download.htm.

C. With **clinical CAD** or CAD-equivalent (peripheral artery disease, abdominal aortic aneurysm, or symptomatic carotid artery disease, including transient ischemic attack and stroke), diabetes, or an estimated 10-year CHD risk above 20%, treatment goals are to lower LDL cholesterol to $\leq$**70** mg/dL (2.60 mmol/L). (SOR **A**) Treatment goals for other levels of risk are shown in Table 75–3.

D. For all hyperlipidemic patients, the **TG goal** is to lower fasting TG to $\leq$**150** mg/dL (1.3 mmol/L). (SOR **B**)

E. Hygienic approaches often improve lipid levels effectively. It is appropriate to encourage lifestyle changes in anyone with LDL cholesterol $\geq$130 mg/dL or HDL cholesterol $\leq$40 mg/dL (1.0 mmol/L). (SOR **A**) Those with HDL cholesterol levels in the 40- to 49-mg/dL (1.03–1.16 mmol/L) range may also be appropriate candidates for exercise counseling.

    1. Dietary modification. Depending on baseline diet, eating less saturated fat and cholesterol can often lower total blood cholesterol by 10% to 20%. Key dietary changes for lowering elevated cholesterol are listed below.

TABLE 75–2. OTHER RISK FACTORS FOR CORONARY ARTERY DISEASE

Factors cited by the National Cholesterol Education Program
Male gender
Cigarette smoking
Diabetes mellitus
Hypertension
Low HDL cholesterol
Obesity
Personal history of atherosclerotic disease
Family history of lipid disorder
Family history of atherosclerotic disease (especially men $\leq$55 years and
  women $\leq$65 years)

Other factors (not cited by the National Cholesterol Education Program)
C-reactive protein elevation
Homocysteine elevation
Lipoprotein (a) elevation
Apolipoprotein B elevation
Low apolipoprotein A-I level
Postmenopausal status for females
Lp-PLA2 elevation
Small, dense low-density lipoprotein particles
Pro-inflammatory high-density lipoprotein
Coronary-prone (Type A) behavior or personality
Old age (risk rises with increasing age)

    a. Eat **less beef and pork** (especially fatty cuts). (SOR **A**)
    b. Eat **cold-water fish** twice a week (salmon, tuna, herring, mackerel). Fish that tend
       to have high mercury content (e.g., swordfish) should be limited to once a month.
       (SOR **C**)
    c. Eat more **chicken** and **turkey** (white "skinless" meat). (SOR **C**)
    d. Eat 40 to 50 g of **soy protein** a day (tofu, soy burger, soy dog, soy milk). (SOR **A**)
    e. Drink **nonfat, $\frac{1}{2}$%, or 1% fat milk,** instead of 2% or whole milk (3.5% fat). Eat
       minimal amounts of other whole-milk dairy products such as cheese, butter, ice
       cream, and sour cream. (SOR **A**)
    f. Use **polyunsaturated oil products** (safflower, corn, soybean) or **monounsatu-
       rated oil products** (olive) for margarine and cooking oil (desired ratio of polyun-
       saturated to saturated fat is $\geq$1.5:1). **Avoid hydrogenated oils** present in **stick
       margarines;** instead use **tub margarines** (preferably small amounts). (SOR **A**)
    g. Minimize intake of commercial **fried fast foods,** which are the main source of **trans
       fats.** (SOR **C**)
    h. Eat **oat bran** as cereal or muffins, three to six servings per day. Oat bran can reduce
       total cholesterol and LDL cholesterol an average of 5% to 10% in some patients
       with elevated LDL cholesterol. (SOR **B**)
    i. Eat **nuts** (walnuts, pecans, almonds, peanuts, cashews) as a protein source, 1 oz a
       day. Nuts are high in alpha-linolenic acid, which is converted to omega-3 fatty acids
       in the body. Mounting evidence links nut intake with reduced risk for CAD events.
       (SOR **A**)

TABLE 75–3. LDL CHOLESTEROL TREATMENT GOALS

	Treatment Goal for LDL Cholesterol 2 or More CAD Risk Factors mg/dL (mmol/L)	$\leq$2 CAD Risk Factors mg/dL (mmol/L)
Known CAD or diabetes	$\leq$70 ($\leq$1.8)	$\leq$70 ($\leq$1.8)
No known CAD		
10-year risk, $\geq$20%	$\leq$100 ($\leq$2.6)	$\leq$100 ($\leq$2.6)
10-year risk, 10%–20%	$\leq$130 ($\leq$3.35)	$\leq$160 ($\leq$4.2)
10-year risk, $\leq$10%	$\leq$160 ($\leq$4.2)	$\leq$190 ($\leq$4.9)

CAD, coronary artery disease; LDL, low-density lipoprotein.

    j. Fish oil high in omega-3 fatty acids (i.e., eicosapentaenoic [EPA] and docosahex-aenoic [DHA]) has been shown to be beneficial. Fish oils decrease secretion of TGs by the liver, and reduce blood TGs, but there is little or no effect on total blood cholesterol level and HDL cholesterol. LDL-cholesterol level is unchanged or may increase with fish oil consumption. If regular intake of cold-water fish is ineffective or unacceptable, three capsules a day of fish oil provides close to the 1 g/d of EPA plus DHA that is recommended for preventive intake. To lower TGs, the recommended dose of is 2 to 4 g/d of EPA plus DHA daily. (SOR **Ⓐ**)

    k. Plant stanols or **sterols** can be beneficial as dietary supplements. Plant stanols derived from soybeans and corn are available in over-the-counter products (e.g., Benecol, Take Control). Stanols block absorption of dietary and biliary cholesterol in the intestine. Sterols work similarly but are absorbed more readily than stanols. Benecol costs approximately $5 per week when used as a food spread, like margarine. It has no significant medication interactions and no demonstrated side effects. At the recommended dose of 2 to 3 servings per day, plant stanols lower total cholesterol by 10% to 12% and reduce LDL-C by 14% to 17%. (SOR **Ⓐ**)

  2. Exercise. Regular aerobic exercise, at least 30 minutes at a time, 3 or more times a week, raises HDL cholesterol by 5 to 15 mg/dL, lowers TG and VLDL cholesterol, and sometimes lowers LDL cholesterol. Walking daily for several miles has been shown to have smaller favorable effects on lipids. (SOR **Ⓐ**)

  3. Weight loss lowers TG and VLDL cholesterol, raises HDL cholesterol by 5 to 10 mg/dL, but lowers LDL cholesterol only transiently during the weight reduction period. (SOR **Ⓐ**)

  4. Smoking cessation increases HDL cholesterol by 5 to 10 mg/dL, but does not affect LDL cholesterol, VLDL cholesterol, or TGs. (SOR **Ⓐ**)

  5. Behavioral modification for coronary-prone (Type A) behavior may lower LDL cholesterol in the absence of other interventions. (SOR **Ⓒ**)

F. Medications. The 2001 NCEP Adult Treatment Panel III recommends medical treatment if LDL cholesterol remains ≥190 mg/dL (4.9 mmol/L) despite hygienic management, regardless of the patient's clinical status and other CAD risk factors. For most patients with diabetes, coronary or carotid artery disease, or a 10-year estimated CHD risk greater than 20%, statin medication is now recommended, regardless of LDL cholesterol level. (Statins stabilize existing atherosclerotic plaque and reduce the risk of lesion rupture and thrombosis.) The guidelines for drug therapy with other combinations of risk factors and LDL cholesterol levels are shown in Table 75–4. (SOR **Ⓐ**)

  1. Over-the-counter drugs are sometimes the preferred choice for medical treatment because they are inexpensive and relatively safe, and some are fairly effective (Table 75–4).

    a. Psyllium hydrophilic mucilloid (Metamucil and other brands). Psyllium, which lowers LDL cholesterol and total cholesterol an average of 5% to 10%, is a logical choice to treat mildly elevated LDL cholesterol (130–159 mg/dL) when HDL cholesterol is ≥45 mg/dL, especially in elderly patients. (SOR **Ⓐ**) It promotes bowel regularity and sometimes causes flatulence, but causes no serious adverse effects.

    b. Niacin. Niacin is a logical first choice for treating the healthy patient with moderately elevated LDL cholesterol who also has either low HDL cholesterol (≤35 mg/dL) or

TABLE 75–4. LDL CHOLESTEROL DRUG THERAPY LEVELS

Risk Category	10-Year Estimated Risk for CHD	LDL Level for Considering Drug Therapy
CHD or CHD risk equivalent (diabetes, stroke)	≥20%	Regardless of LDL level*
2+ risk factors	10%–20%	≥130 mg/dL (3.35 mmol/L)
	≤10%	≥160 mg/dL (4.2 mmol/L)
0–1 risk factors (not diabetes)	Usually ≤10%	≥190 mg/dL (4.9 mmol/L) (160–189 mg/dL or 4.2–4.9 mmol/L: drug optional)

*Statins stabilize existing atherosclerotic plaque and reduce the risk of lesion rupture and thrombosis.

high TGs. Niacin has demonstrated value for preventing myocardial infarction and CAD death. (SOR **Ⓐ**)

(1) When taken in a dose of 1 to 3 g/d, niacin lowers LDL cholesterol by 15% to 20%, markedly lowers elevated TGs, and raises HDL cholesterol by 5 to 15 mg/dL. Patients should begin with a low dose of 100 to 200 mg of the regular release form or 250 to 500 mg of the sustained-release form (Slo-Niacin); then the dose should be gradually increased to a maximum of 2 to 3 g/d based on patient tolerance.

(2) Most patients experience minimal flushing and itching when taking sustained-release niacin. Patients who experience flushing and itching can block much of the adverse symptoms by taking 325 mg of aspirin daily before the first dose.

(3) Although it is sometimes well tolerated and usually safe, niacin can worsen diabetic hyperglycemia, exacerbate gout, precipitate serious arrhythmias in patients with heart disease, or cause severe reversible liver toxicity.

2. **Prescription drugs for modifying lipids** all are relatively costly, especially higher doses (Tables 75–5, 75–6, and 75–7).

   a. Cholestyramine (Questran). This resin sequesters bile acids in the gut. It is available as a powder to be mixed with water or food. Questran Light may be more palatable for long-term compliance. Cholestyramine is a logical choice for the patient with moderate LDL cholesterol elevation and HDL cholesterol levels ≥45 mg/dL who will tolerate its inconvenient form. (SOR **Ⓐ**)

   When two scoops or packs are taken 2 to 3 times a day, cholestyramine lowers LDL cholesterol and total cholesterol by 15% to 20%. Because more than 4 doses a day cause severe constipation, the maximal dose of six scoops/packs a day is poorly tolerated.

   b. Colestipol (Colestid) is very similar to cholestyramine in form, dose, efficacy, high cost, and poor patient tolerance, with no advantages.

   c. Colesevelam (Welchol) is another resin binder similar to cholestyramine and colestipol, with no demonstrated advantages.

   d. Gemfibrozil (Lopid) changes the hepatic metabolism of lipoproteins. Gemfibrozil is a logical choice for the patient with low HDL cholesterol and moderately or severely elevated TGs who has not tolerated or responded well to niacin. (SOR **Ⓐ**) The drug is well tolerated and appears to be relatively safe for long-term use.

   (1) Gemfibrozil lowers LDL cholesterol by 5% to 15%, markedly lowers TGs, and raises HDL cholesterol by 5 to 15 mg/dL. The usual dose is 600 mg twice a day; the maximum dose is 900 mg twice a day or 600 mg 3 times per day.

   (2) Gemfibrozil has been shown to lower CAD morbidity and mortality by 40% in patients with elevated LDL cholesterol, TGs, or both. It is most beneficial in patients with HDL cholesterol of ≤45 mg/dL. It may be used cautiously in combination with an HMG-CoA reductase inhibitor.

   e. Fenofibrate (Tricor) is similar to gemfibrozil and is appropriate for the same patients. (SOR **Ⓑ**) Its long-term safety is unknown.

   f. HMG-CoA reductase inhibitors (statins). This category is the rational choice for patients with moderately or severely elevated LDL cholesterol and for most high-risk patients. (SOR **Ⓐ**)

   (1) These agents lower LDL cholesterol by 30% to 60%—more than any other medication.

   (2) In controlled trials, statins have reduced heart attack, stroke, CHD death, and total mortality by 25% to 40%. Cost-effectiveness analyses of this class of agents have shown favorable cost–benefit ratios.

   (3) Depending on the patient's copayment situation, the cost-effectiveness of treatment may be improved by prescribing twice the intended dose and having the patient take one-half of a tablet. Table 75–6 shows recommended medications and doses for cost-effectively treating patients with different baseline LDL-C levels and different treatment goals.

   (4) All statins are usually well tolerated, and serious **adverse effects** are uncommon.

   (5) The most frequently reported side effects of statins are muscle aches, headache, flatulence, constipation, dyspepsia, insomnia, and mild harmless elevation of hepatic transaminases.

TABLE 75–5. HOW TO RECOMMEND AND PRESCRIBE LIPID-ALTERING MEDICATIONS

Medication	Retail Cost*
Over-the-counter medications	
Psyllium hydrophilic mucilloid (PHM)	$7–10/mo unsweetened/with sugar; artificially sweetened
Metamucil or equivalent	$15–21/mo; orange/lemon-line $11–21/mo
One heaping tsp (tbsp if with sugar) in 8 oz water/liquid, tid with meals	
Fiberall Fruit & Nut Fiber Wafer, 3.4-g	Metamucil Instant Mix $25/mo
1 to 2 wafers, tid with 8 oz+ liquid niacin/nicotinic acid	$35–40/mo if sole PHM source
(OTC, regular release 500/750-mg tab)	$8–14 for 100 tab; max 3 g/d
Sig: one to two 500-mg tab bid with meal	$10/20 mo for 1/2 g/d
one 750-mg tab bid with meal (med)	$12/mo for 1.5 g/d
Niacin (Slo-Niacin), 500-mg or 750-mg ER	$35/mo for 180 tab of 500/750-mg
Initial dose: 1 tab bid	$15/mo
Increase to 2 tab bid in wk 2	$30/mo
Prescription medications	
Atorvastatin (Lipitor), 10/20/40/80-mg tab	$240/330/335/355 for 90 tab 10/20/40/80
Sig: 10 mg qd evening (usual start dose)	$80/mo
20 mg qd evening (medium dose)	$110/mo
40 mg qd evening (high dose)	$110/mo
80 mg qd evening (very high dose)	$120/mo
Atorvastatin–amlodipine (Caduet), 5–10, 5–20, 10–20, 10–40 mg	$315/445/455/445 for 90 tab 5–10/5–20/10–20/10–40
Sig: 5–10 mg tab qd evening (low dose)	$105/mo
5–20 mg tab qd evening (low dose)	$115/mo
10–20 mg tab qd evening (medium dose)	$120/mo
10–40 mg tab qd evening (high dose)	$115/mo
Ceruvastatin (Crestor), 5/10/20/40-mg tab	$270/270/285/270 for 90 tab 5/10/20/40
Sig: 5 mg qd evening (small start dose)	$90/mo
10 mg qd evening (usual start dose)	$90/mo
20 mg qd evening (medium dose)	$95/mo
40 mg qd evening (high dose)	$90/mo
Cholestyramine (generic/Questran), powder (378 g/can or 4-g pks)	$170/$225 4 cans of cholestyramine powder or $210/365 for 3 cartons (180 pks)
Sig: one 4-g scoop or pack bid (start dose)	$30/40 mo gen/Questran can or $40/65/mo gen/Questran pk
two 4-g scoops or packs bid (maint)	$60/80/mo gen/Questran can or $800/130/mo gen/Quest pk
two 4-g scoops or packs tid (max dose)	$90/120/mo gen/Questran can or $120/195/mo gen/Quest pk
Cholestyramine (Questran Light), powd (210 g/can; 1 pk = 4 g)	$160/230, for 4 cans of generic or Questran Light
Sig: one 4-g scoop or pack bid (start dose)	$45/70 mo
two 4-g scoops or packs bid (maint)	$90/140/mo
two 4-g scoops or packs tid (max dose)	$135/210/mo
Colesevelam (Welchol), 625 mg,	$565 for 540 tabs
Sig: 3 tabs, bid	$190/mo
Colestipol (Colestid), flavored granules,	$360 for three 450-g cans
Sig: 1 scoops (5 g) bid	$80/mo
two scoops (10 g) bid	$160/mo
three scoops (15 g) bid	$240/mo
Colestipol (Colestid), 1-g tab	$750 for 900 one-g tabs
Sig: 5 tabs, bid (start dose)	$250/mo
10 tabs, bid (medium dose)	$500/mo
15 tabs, bid (max dose)	$750/mo
Colestipol (Colestid), 5-g powder pk	$450 for 180 five-g powder pks
Sig: 1 pk, bid (start dose)	$150/mo
2 pks, bid (medium dose)	$300/mo
3 pks, bid (max dose)	$450/mo
Colestipol (Colestid), 7.5-g flavored gran pk	$495 for 180 flavored granule pks
Sig: 1 pk bid (start dose)	$165/mo
2 pks bid (max dose)	$330/mo
Colestipol (Colestid), unflavored gran can	$255 for 900 g unflavored granules
Sig: 1 scoop (5 g) bid (start dose)	$85/mo
2 scoops (10 g) bid (medium dose)	$170/mo
3 scoops (15 g) bid (max dose)	$255/mo

(continued)

TABLE 75–5. (CONTINUED)

Medication	Retail Cost*
Ezetimibe (Zetia), 10-mg tab	$245 for 90 tab
Sig: 1 tab, qd (usually taken with statin)	$85/mo
Fenofibrate (Tricor), 48/145-mg tab	$120/$355 for 90 tab
one tab qd (usual dose)	$40/125/mo
Fluvastatin (Lescol), 20/40/80-mg tab	$250/250/275 for 90 tab of 20/40/80 mg
Sig: 20 mg qd evening (low dose)	$85/mo
40 mg qd evening (medium dose)	$85/mo
80 mg SR, qd evening (usual dose)	$90/mo
Gemfibrozil (generic/Lopid), 600-mg tab	$70/365 for 180 tab
Sig: 1 tab bid with meals (usual dose)	$25/120/mo (generic/Lopid)
Lovastatin (generic), 10/20/40-mg tab	$60/90/100 for 90 tab of 10/20/40 mg
Sig: 10 mg qd evening (low dose)	$20/mo
20 mg qd evening (usual start dose)	$30/mo
40 mg qd evening (medium dose)	$35/mo
two 40-mg tabs qd evening (high dose)	$70/mo
Lovastatin (Mevacor), 10/20/40-mg tab	$125/210/380 for 90 tab of 10/20/40 mg
Sig: 10 mg qd evening (low dose)	$45/mo
20 mg qd evening (usual start dose)	$70/mo
40 mg qd evening (medium dose)	$125/mo
two 40-mg tabs qd evening (high dose)	$250/mo
Lovastatin (Altoprev), 20/40/60-mg ER tab	$270/345/310 for 90 tab of 20/40/60 mg
Sig: 20 mg ER qd evening (low dose)	$90/mo
40 mg ER qd evening (medium dose)	$115/mo
60 mg ER qd evening (high dose)	$105/mo
Lovastatin–niacin (Advicor), 20–500/20–750/20–1000-mg tab	$275/270/335 for 90 tab of 20–500/20–750/20–1000-mg
Sig: one tab (20–500-mg), qd (low dose)	$75/mo
one tab (20–500-mg or 20–750-mg), bid	$90/mo
one tab (20–1000-mg), bid (high dose)	$110/mo
Niacin/nicotinic acid (Niaspan), 500/750/1000-mg XR tab	$465/550/630 for 180 tab of 500/750/1000-mg
Sig: one 500-mg tab bid with meal (start)	$155/mo
one 750-mg tab bid with meal (med)	$185/mo
one 1000-mg tab bid with meal (maint)	$210/mo
Pravastatin (generic), 10/20/40-mg tab	$170/125/205 for 90 of 10/20/40 mg
Sig: 10 mg qd evening (low dose)	$55/mo
20 mg qd evening (medium dose)	$40/mo
40 mg qd evening (high dose)	$70/mo
Pravastatin (Pravachol), 10/20/40/80-mg tab	$320/320/440/440 for 90 of 10/20/40/80 mg
Sig: 10 mg qd evening (low dose)	$105/mo
20 mg qd evening (usual start dose)	$105/mo
40 mg qd evening (medium dose)	$145/mo
80 mg qd evening (high dose)	$145/mo
Rosuvastatin (Crestor), 5/10/20/40-mg tab	$270/270/285/270 for 90 of 5/10/20/40 mg
Sig: 5 mg qd evening (low dose)	$90/mo
10 mg qd evening (usual starting dose)	$90/mo
20 mg qd evening (medium dose)	$95/mo
40 mg qd evening (high dose)	$90/mo
Simvastatin (generic), 5/10/20/40 mg	$125/155/250/250 for 90 of 5/10/20/40 mg
Sig: 5 mg qd evening (low dose)	$40/mo
10 mg qd evening (low dose)	$50/mo
20 mg qd evening (usual start dose)	$85/mo
40 mg qd evening (high dose)	$85/mo
Simvastatin (Zocor), 5/10/20/40/80 mg	$200/245/405/405/405 for 90 of 5/10/20/40/80 mg tabs
Sig: 1/2 a 10-mg or one 5-mg tab qpm (low dose)	$40/65/mo
1/2 a 20-mg or one 10-mg tab qpm (low dose)	$70/85/mo
1/2 a 40-mg or one 20-mg tab qpm (start dose)	$70/135/mo
1/2 an 80-mg or one 40-mg tab qpm (medium dose)	$70/135/mo
one 80-mg tab qd evening (high dose)	$135/mo

(continued)

TABLE 75-5. (CONTINUED)

Medication	Retail Cost*
Simvastatin–ezetimibe (Vytorin) 10–10, 10–20, 10–40, 10–80 mg	$300/300/300/300 for 90 tab of 10–10, 10–20, 10–40, 10–80 tabs
Sig: one 10–10-mg tab qd evening (low dose)	$100/mo
one 10–20-mg tab qd evening (usual start dose)	$100/mo
one 10–40-mg tab qd evening (medium dose)	$100/mo
one 10–80-mg tab qd evening (high dose)	$100/mo

*Quoted by on-line Walgreen's Pharmacy, June 22, 2007.
ER, extended release; Maint, maintenance dose; Start, starting dose.

(6) Rare side effects of statin therapy include pruritus, rashes, myopathy, rhabdomyolysis, and possibly lupus erythematosus or memory loss.

(7) Statin use is contraindicated in patients with active **hepatic disease** or significantly elevated serum transaminase levels (≥ 3 times normal upper limit). Because significant (but asymptomatic) elevation of alanine transferase (ALT) occurs in 1% to 2% and mildly elevated ALT (≤ 3 times normal) occurs in approximately 5% to 10% of treated patients, it is prudent to obtain a baseline ALT level and to recheck ALT 6 to 12 weeks after initiating treatment or after increasing the statin dose. It is not necessary to monitor aspartine transferase or other liver enzymes. No cases of serious or life-threatening liver toxicity have thus far been attributed to statin therapy.

TABLE 75-6. RETAIL MONTHLY COST* OF THERAPEUTIC EQUIVALENT DOSES OF HMG-CoA-REDUCTASE INHIBITORS (STATINS)†

Lovastatin	Pravastatin	Simvastatin	Simvastatin	Fluvastatin	Lovastatin ER	Pravastatin
Generic	Generic	Generic	Zocor	Lescol	Altoprev	Pravachol
20 mg	20 mg	10 mg	10 mg	40 mg	20 mg	20 mg
$30	$40	$50	$80	$85	$90	$105

Lovastatin	Pravastatin	Lovastatin–niacin	Atorvastatin	Simvastatin	Rosuvastatin
Generic	Generic	Advicor	Lipitor	Generic	Crestor
40 mg	40 mg	20–500 mg	10 mg	20 mg	5 mg
$35	$70	$75	$80	$85	$90

Simvastatin	Rosuvastatin	Lovastatin ER	Lovastatin–niacin	Atorvastatin	Simvastatin
Generic	Crestor	Altoprev	Advicor	Lipitor	Zocor
40 mg	10 mg	60 mg	20–1000	20 mg	40 mg
$85	$90	$105	$110	$110	$135

Rosuvastatin	Simvastatin–ezetimibe	Atorvastatin	Simvastatin
Crestor	Vytorin	Lipitor	Zocor
20 mg	10–10 mg	40 mg	80 mg
$95	$100	$110	$135

Rosuvastatin	Simvastatin–ezetimibe	Atorvastatin
Crestor	Vytorin	Lipitor
40 mg	10–20 mg	80 mg
$90	$100	$120

*Quoted by on-line Walgreen's Pharmacy, June 22, 2007, 3-Hydroxy-3-methylglutaryl coenzyme A (HMG-CoA) reductase inhibitors (statins).
† Based on taking whole tablets.

TABLE 75–7. COST-EFFECTIVE MEDICATION REGIMENS FOR TREATING ELEVATED LDL CHOLESTEROL

Baseline LDL-C (mg/dL)	LDL-C Treatment Goal ≤130 mg/dL	≤100 mg/dL	≤70 mg/dL
130–159	Lovastatin (generic), one 10-mg or one 20-mg qd, $15–20/mo; or pravastatin (generic), one 20 mg tab qd, $40/mo; or fluvastatin (Lescol), one-half a 40-mg tab qd, $45/mo; or simvastatin (generic), one-half a 10-mg, one 10 mg tab, or one-half a 20-mg tab, $25/50/60/mo	Lovastatin (generic), one 40-mg tab qd, $35/mo; or rosuvastatin (Crestor), one-half a 10-mg tab, $45/mo; or simvastatin (generic), one-half a 40-mg tab qd, $45/mo; or atorvastatin (Lipitor), one-half a 20-mg tab, $55/mo, or simvastatin (Zocor), one-half a 40-mg tab qd, $70/mo; or pravastatin (generic), one 40-mg tab qd, $70/mo	Rosuvastatin (Crestor), one-half a 20-mg tab qd, $50/mo; atorvastatin (Lipitor), one-half of a 40-mg tab qd, $60/mo; or simvastatin (Zocor), one-half an 80-mg tab qd, $70/mo; or simvastatin (generic), one 40-mg tab qd, $85/mo; or rosuvastatin (Crestor), one 10-mg tab qd, $90/mo
160–189	Lovastatin (generic), one 40-mg tab qd, $35/mo; or rosuvastatin (Crestor), one-half a 10-mg tab, $45/mo; or simvastatin (generic), one-half a 40-mg tab qd, $45/mo; or atorvastatin (Lipitor), one-half a 20-mg tab, $55/mo, or simvastatin (Zocor), one-half a 40-mg tab qd, $70/mo; or pravastatin (generic), one 40-mg tab qd, $70/mo	Rosuvastatin (Crestor), one-half a 20-mg tab qd, $50/mo; atorvastatin (Lipitor), one-half of a 40-mg tab qd, $60/mo; or simvastatin (Zocor), one-half an 80-mg tab qd, $70/mo; or simvastatin (generic), one 40-mg tab qd, $85/mo; or rosuvastatin (Crestor), one 10-mg tab qd, $90/mo	Rosuvastatin (Crestor), one 20-mg tab or one 40-mg tab qd, $90/95/mo; or simvastatin–ezetimibe (Vytorin), one 10–10, 10–20, 10–40, or 10–80 tab qd, $100/mo; or atorvastatin (Lipitor), one 40-mg or one 80-mg tab qd, $115/120/mo; or simvastatin (Zocor), one 80-mg tab qd, $135/mo
≥ 190	Rosuvastatin (Crestor), one-half a 20-mg tab qd, $50/mo; atorvastatin (Lipitor), one-half of a 40-mg tab qd, $60/mo; or simvastatin (Zocor), one-half an 80-mg tab qd, $70/mo; or simvastatin (generic), one 40-mg tab qd, $85/mo; or rosuvastatin (Crestor), one 10-mg tab qd, $90/mo; or simvastatin–ezetimibe (Vytorin), one 10–10 or 10–20-mg tab, $100/mo; or lovastatin (Altoprev), one 60-mg ER tab qd; $105/mo; or atorvastatin (Lipitor), one 20-mg tab qd, $110/mo	Rosuvastatin (Crestor), one 20-mg or one 40-mg tab qd, $90/95/mo; or simvastatin–ezetimibe (Vytorin), one 10–10, 10–20, 10–40, or 10–80 tab qd, $100/mo; or atorvastatin (Lipitor), one 40-mg or one 80-mg tab qd, $115/120/mo; or simvastatin (Zocor), one 80-mg tab qd, $135/mo	Rosuvastatin (Crestor), one 20-mg or one 40-mg tab qd, $90/95/mo; or simvastatin–ezetimibe (Vytorin), one 10–40, or 10–80 tab qd, $100/mo; or atorvastatin (Lipitor), one 80-mg tab qd, $120/mo; or simvastatin (Zocor), one 80-mg tab qd, $135/mo

LDL, low-density lipoprotein.

(8) **Myalgias** or muscle weakness occur in approximately 10% of patients, either early on or after prolonged treatment. Muscle symptoms caused by statins usually resolve within a few days to weeks after drug discontinuation. **Myopathy** occurs rarely, sometimes leading to **rhabdomyolysis** and **acute renal failure.** Muscle toxicity occurs somewhat more often when statins are used along with niacin, gemfibrozil, fenofibrate, and other drugs (Table 75–8). Taking coenzyme Q-10 (suggested dose of 100 mg twice a day) with a statin appears to prevent muscle symptoms in some patients complaining of myalgias.

(9) Renal failure is a risk factor for muscle side effects only with pravastatin.

TABLE 75–8. DRUGS THAT INTERACT WITH HMG-CoA REDUCTASE INHIBITORS (STATINS)*

Niacin—also called nicotinic acid (Slo-Niacin, Niacor, Niaspan, Nico-400,
   NIA delay, Endur-Acin)
Gemfibrozil (Lopid)
Fenofibrate (Tricor)
Itraconazole (Sporanox)
Amlodipine (Norvasc)
Diltiazem (Cardizem, Cartia, Dilacor, Diltia, Tiazac)
Verapamil (Calan, Covera, Isoptin, Verelan)
Amiodarone (Cordarone)
Cimetidine (Tagamet)
Erythromycin (EES, E-Mycin, EryC, PCE, Ery-Tab)
Clarithromycin (Biaxin)
Clindamycin (Cleocin)
Cyclosporine
Indinavir (Crixivan)
Nelfinavir (Viracept)
Ritonavir (Norvir)
Saquinavir (Invirase)
Tacrolimus (Prograf)

*Some statins (atorvastatin, simvastatin, and lovastatin, but not pravastatin, rosuvastatin, or fluvastatin) interact with other drugs metabolized by the cytochrome P-450 3A4 liver enzyme system.

(10) Numerous medications may interact with statins to increase their blood level and increase the risk for serious adverse effects. The medications in Table 75–8 should be avoided if possible when taking a statin, or the statin dose should be adjusted downward while they are being taken. Because they are metabolized differently from other statins, pravastatin, rosuvastatin, and fluvastatin are least likely to cause drug interactions.

(11) Grapefruit juice interferes with the metabolism of simvastatin, atorvastatin, and lovastatin (but not pravastatin, fluvastatin, or rosuvastatin) and raises their blood level, which can create an increased risk of adverse effects. Because this effect of grapefruit juice lasts 24 hours or more, it should be avoided or minimized by patients taking simvastatin, atorvastatin, or lovastatin.

(12) Supplemental intake of the antioxidant **vitamin E** does not appear to be advisable, since it interfered with the beneficial effects of statin therapy in the Heart Protection Study.

(13) Once started, statin therapy should be continued indefinitely, barring unacceptable side effects or allergic reactions.

(14) Perceived side effects from one statin can often be avoided by switching to a different statin. Because they are hydrophilic, pravastatin or fluvastatin may be least likely to cause side effects.

(15) Because of potential teratogenicity, statins should not be used in women of childbearing age unless contraception effectiveness is maximized and the potential benefits appear to exceed the risks.

(16) Statins are not approved by the US Food and Drug Administration for use in children younger than 14 years except for atorvastatin for homozygous familial hypercholesterolemia.

(17) Statin choices
   (a) Lovastatin (Mevacor) was the first available HMG-CoA reductase agent.
      (i) The 20-mg starting dose is well tolerated and often produces good results, lowering LDL cholesterol to an average of 25% to 30%.
      (ii) Newer formulations include generic (less expensive), sustained-release (Altocor), and in combination with niacin (Advicor).
   (b) Pravastatin (Pravachol) is similar to lovastatin, but is less costly.
      (i) The usual dose of 20 to 40 mg/d, taken 2 to 3 hours after the evening meal, lowers LDL cholesterol to an average of 25% to 35%.
      (ii) Pravastatin has reduced CHD events by 24% to 40% in primary and secondary prevention trials.

      (iii) Pravastatin is the only statin with prominent renal excretion (approximately 50% renal), so it should be used with caution, if at all, in patients with renal insufficiency or renal failure.

    (c) Simvastatin (Zocor) has a higher potency. (10 mg of simvastatin is equivalent to 20 mg of lovastatin or pravastatin.) It can be taken anytime in the evening.

      (i) Simvastatin, 20 to 80 mg/d, lowers LDL cholesterol by 35% to 50%.

      (ii) Simvastatin reduced acute myocardial infarction or death from CHD by 42% and reduced total deaths by 30% in a large secondary prevention trial.

      (iii) Simvastatin often raises HDL-C somewhat.

      (iv) Simvastatin's availability in generic form has lowered its cost substantially.

    (d) Fluvastatin (Lescol) costs substantially less than other trade name statins.

      (i) Higher doses (40–80 mg/d) lower LDL cholesterol by 23% to 33% (Tables 75–3 and 75–5).

      (ii) Outcome studies for fluvastatin have shown benefits similar to the other statins.

    (e) Atorvastatin (Lipitor) is one of the most effective statins for those with severely elevated LDL cholesterol.

      (i) Atorvastatin in the usual dose of 10 to 20 mg/d lowers LDL cholesterol by an average of 38% to 45% and TGs by 20% to 35%.

      (ii) Higher doses of 40 to 80 mg lower LDL cholesterol to an average of 50% to 55% and TGs by 35% to 50%.

      (iii) Atorvastatin outcome studies have demonstrated efficacy equal to or better than other statins.

    (f) Rosuvastatin (Crestor), the newest statin on the market, was approved in 2003.

      (i) Rosuvastatin lowers LDL cholesterol and raises HDL cholesterol more than any currently available statin. Treatment goals are reached substantially more often by rosuvastatin (10 mg/d) than atorvastatin (10 mg/d) or simvastatin (20 mg/d).

      (ii) Rosuvastatin has a similar side effect profile and fewer drug interactions than some other statins (Table 75–8).

      (iii) Proteinuria occasionally occurs (usually at the 40-mg dose), so periodic spot microalbumin/creatine ratio testing may be advisable.

    (g) Ezetimibe (Zetia), approved in 2002, lowers cholesterol by interfering with the absorption of cholesterol in the gut.

      (i) Used alone, ezetimibe lowers LDL cholesterol and TGs only modestly (15%–20%).

      (ii) When ezetimibe is added to the usual starting dose of a statin, the combination lowers LDL cholesterol as much or more than the maximum statin dose.

      (iii) Since ezetimibe is minimally absorbed, its combined use with low-dose statin may produce less adverse effects than high-dose statin therapy.

      (iv) Adding ezetimibe usually costs more than higher doses of a statin (two copayments instead of one for managed care patients, higher retail cost for other patients).

    (h) Statin combinations with other drugs

      (i) Vytorin (simvastatin–ezetimide), low dose (10 mg of each), lowers LDL cholesterol as much or more than the maximal dose of any statin by itself. Outcome studies are not yet available to compare Vytorin's efficacy for reducing risk for heart attack and stroke with the proven efficacy of a statin alone.

      (ii) Caduet (atorvastatin–amlodipine) combines a statin with a calcium channel blocker. It is a logical choice for patients with hyperlipidemia and hypertension.

G. Partial ileal bypass surgery, in conjunction with a low-fat diet, lowers LDL cholesterol by 40% to 50%. The operative and postoperative morbidity and mortality are low. This surgery is a reasonable option for patients with severely elevated LDL cholesterol that cannot be managed satisfactorily with any tolerable combination of lipid-altering medications. (SOR **B**)

IV. Management Strategies

A. **Long-term adherence** for hygienic measures and lipid-altering medications is quite poor. Many patients are reluctant to take preventive medications for asymptomatic conditions. Fear of potential adverse effects from chronic medications appears to be a major deterrent to adherence. A customized "informed choice" process might improve adherence by using a combination of textual and graphic materials to communicate treatment benefits and risks more effectively, and to allay patient fears and bolster confidence in the safety of statin therapy.

B. **Patient education** and discussions with key family members are vital in order to foster a thorough understanding of the importance of a lifelong commitment to hygienic and medical management of lipid problems. Explanations of important concepts need to be expressed in lay terms, accompanied by memory devices to help people remember them, such as drawing a "happy face" and characterizing HDL cholesterol as "healthy" cholesterol, and a "frown face" symbolizing LDL cholesterol as "lousy" or "lethal" cholesterol. Many good educational materials are available from the American Heart Association, the NCEP, and commercial sources.

C. **Family-oriented care** entails screening as many family members as possible and educating nuclear and extended families who have a member with an identified lipid problem. It is particularly important to work with the persons who buy and prepare the family's food, so that they thoroughly understand how to select and prepare "heart-healthy" foods.

D. **Elderly patients** are at a greatly increased risk for myocardial infarction or sudden death. Randomized controlled trials have shown that treating dyslipidemia in patients aged 65 to 85 years can decrease the risk of first and recurrent coronary events. Morbidity and mortality from cardiovascular disease was decreased by at least 29% in these studies. Data are limited for patients older than 85 years. The use of benign inexpensive medications such as psyllium seems prudent. Since outcome studies show similar benefits and no increase in adverse effects for elderly patients, the expense and small risk of statin therapy seems justified for those wishing to preserve their current quality of life as long as possible.

E. **Children and adolescents** with dyslipidemias should receive ongoing family-oriented education about diet, exercise, and weight control, as indicated. Extreme low-fat diets should be avoided in children younger than 6 years because of the risk of essential fatty acid malnutrition having deleterious effects on nervous system development. No information is available on the cost-effectiveness and long-term safety of lipid-altering medication treatment in children and adolescents. Children and adolescents with severe dyslipidemias should be treated with lipid-altering medications only with considerable caution and preferably with written parental informed consent detailing the limitations of what is known about benefits and risks.

F. **Secondary prevention** focuses on identifying and treating persons who have already developed clinical atherosclerosis. Many times the lipid problems of these patients are ignored or discounted, based on the faulty logic of "it is too late now to prevent atherosclerosis complications by modifying lipids." Persons with atherosclerosis have clearly demonstrated their high vulnerability to CAD death. They are the **most** likely to benefit from treatment to prevent further atheroma progression, prevent atheroma rupture, and regress existing atheromas. The lowering of LDL cholesterol has clearly demonstrated substantial benefit in secondary prevention trials. (SOR **A**) Long-term adherence is improved when statin therapy is started **prior** to hospital discharge for patients admitted with acute myocardial infarction or unstable angina pectoris. (SOR **C**)

G. **Systematic follow-up** at regular intervals is essential for effective long-term management of lipid problems. Initially monthly visits are advisable to monitor progress and sustain motivation. The interval can be gradually lengthened to every 6 to 12 months for dietary and medication management. A manual or computerized flowchart in the medical record documenting blood lipid results, dietary and exercise modifications, and medication regimens facilitates the evaluation and alteration of treatment for best results.

V. Prognosis.
The clinical course of lipid problems depends on the type and severity of lipid disorder and on other risk factors for atherosclerosis, especially cigarette smoking, diabetes mellitus, and hypertension. Other detrimental factors include abnormal levels of CRP, lipoprotein (a), small dense oxidized LDL particles, homocysteine, and probably other factors yet to be discovered.

A. Atherosclerotic disease. In childhood and adolescence, fatty streaks form on the lining of susceptible arteries and subsequently develop into atheromas. In adulthood, accumulation of cholesterol and fibrotic tissue causes atheromas to progress at variable rates. Atherosclerotic progression, plaque rupture, and thrombus formation may eventually block off crucial arteries, causing ischemic symptoms and necrosis in the tissue supplied by the arteries.

B. Acute pancreatitis can occur with severe TG elevation $\geq$1000 mg/dL (11 mmol/L). This serious lipid problem requires urgent treatment with intravenous heparin.

C. Other valuable measures for curtailing atherosclerosis or minimizing its damage include smoking cessation, good control of hypertension and diabetes, and daily aspirin (81 or 325 mg, enteric coated). Some studies indicate that getting a flu shot annually may lower risk for CAD events.

REFERENCES

AHA Scientific Statement. Fish consumption, fish oil, omega-3 fatty acids and cardiovascular disease, #71–0241. *Circulation.* 2002;106:2747-2757.

Ballantyne CM. Current and future aims of lipid-lowering therapy: changing paradigms and lessons from the Heart Protection Study on standards of efficacy and safety. *Am J Cardiol.* 2003;21:92(4B):3K-9K.

Food and Drug Administration. Mercury content of selected fish. U.S. Food and Drug Administration Center for Food Safety and Applied Nutrition, Office of Seafood. www.cfsan.fda.gov/~frf/ sea-mehg.html. Accessed May 15, 2001.

Grundy SM, Cleeman JI, Merz NB, et al. Implications of recent clinical trials for the National Cholesterol Education Program Adult Treatment Panel III guidelines. *Circulation.* 2004;110:227-239.

Heart Protection Study Collaborative Group. MRC/BHF Heart protection study of cholesterol lowering with simvastatin in 20,536 high risk individuals: a randomized placebo-controlled trial. *Lancet.* 2002;360:7-22M.

Hu FB, Willett WC. Optimal diets for prevention of coronary heart disease. *JAMA.* 2002;288:2569-2578.

Jones PH, Davidson MH, Stein EA, et al. Comparison of the efficacy and safety of rosuvastatin versus atorvastatin, simvastatin, and pravastatin across doses (STELLAR trial). *Am J Cardiol.* 2003;92(2):152-160.

Summary of the third report of the National Cholesterol Education Program (NCEP). Expert Panel on Detection, Evaluation, and Treatment of High Blood Cholesterol in Adults (Adult Treatment Panel III). *JAMA.* 2001;285:2486-2497.

---

76   Hypertension

Charles B. Eaton, MD, MS

KEY POINTS

- Multiple epidemiologic studies have shown a consistent, continuous, graded relationship between increasing systolic (SBP) and diastolic blood pressure (DBP) and cardiovascular disease (CVD) risk. For each incremental increase of 20 mm Hg in SBP, and 10 mm Hg in DBP, across the entire spectrum of blood pressures (115/75 mm Hg to 185/115 mm Hg), the rates of stroke, myocardial infarction, congestive heart failure, and end-stage renal disease double. (SOR **A**)
- Blood pressure levels. Taking these facts into account, the Seventh Report of the Joint National Committee (JNC 7) on Detection, Evaluation, and Treatment of High Blood Pressure has defined normal pressure as an SBP less than 120 mm Hg, and a DBP less than 80 mm Hg; prehypertension as an SBP of 120 to 139 mm Hg, or a DBP of 80 to 89 mm Hg; and hypertension as an SBP greater than, or equal to, 140 mm Hg, or a DBP greater than, or equal to, 90 mm Hg. These results should be based on the average of two or more readings, taken at each of two or more visits, after initial screening. (SOR **C**)
- Numerous studies have documented the benefits of lifestyle management in the treatment and prevention of hypertension, and the importance of antihypertensive medications in

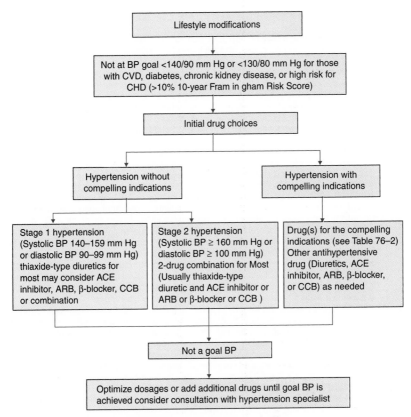

FIGURE 76–1. Hypertension treatment algorithm.

controlling blood pressure and preventing or improving the outcomes for coronary artery disease, myocardial infarction, heart failure, stroke, and chronic kidney disease. (SOR **A**)
- The most effective clinical strategy is to assess risk factors, target organ damage, and comorbidities, and to tailor treatment accordingly (Figure 76–1). All hypertensive patients should be treated to a BP goal of ≤140/90 mm Hg; (SOR **A**) patients with CHD, (SOR **B**) high CHD risk (Framingham risk score ≥10%),(SOR **C**) diabetes, or chronic kidney disease (GFR ≤60 mL/min) (SOR **A**) to a BP ≤130/80 mm Hg; and patients who have left ventricular dysfunction to a BP ≤120/80 mm Hg. (SOR **B**) The majority of patients will require two or more medications to reach their BP goal and will require lifelong therapy. In patients with elevated DBP and evidence of myocardial ischemia or who are at high risk for silent ischemia (diabetes, older than 60 years or with a wide pulse pressure), caution is advised in lowering DBP below 60 mm Hg because of concerns about the potential for underperfusion of the coronary arteries leading to symptomatic myocardial ischemia.(SOR **C**)

I. Introduction
   A. Epidemiology. Hypertension affects approximately 65 million people in the United States, or one in four adults. Another 25% of the population has prehypertension. According to recent surveys, 70% of Americans with hypertension are aware of the diagnosis, with 59% on treatment. However, only 34% of hypertensives are under good control, defined as a blood pressure of less than 140/90 mm Hg. Recent estimates from the Framingham heart study suggest that the lifetime risk of developing hypertension is close to 90%.

Those with prehypertension have twice the risk of developing hypertension as those with lower values.

B. Primary (essential) hypertension. Between 90% and 95% of individuals with hypertension do not have a known cause, and are therefore labeled as having essential hypertension.

C. Secondary, or identifiable, cause of hypertension. Approximately 5% to 10% of hypertension in the United States is owing to a secondary cause. In order for physicians to treat cost-effectively, secondary causes should be evaluated only in patients whose age, history, severity of presentation, or initial laboratory work-up suggests a secondary cause. Patients with sudden onset of hypertension, those with poorly controlled blood pressure, or those who were well controlled, yet suddenly worsen, should be evaluated for secondary causes.

Numerous independent processes are responsible for secondary causes of hypertension, including sleep apnea, drug-induced or -related causes, renal (polycystic kidney disease, glomerular and interstitial disease) or renovascular disease (renal artery stenosis accounts for 1%–2% of cases of hypertension), primary hyperaldosteronism (0.5%), increased intracranial pressure, chronic steroid therapy or Cushing syndrome, pheochromocytoma, coarctation of the aorta, hyperthyroidism, or primary hyperparathyroidism.

D. Resistant hypertension. Resistant hypertension is the failure to reach a BP goal in patients that are fully adherent to an appropriate 3-drug regimen including a diuretic. Common causes of resistant hypertension include improper BP measurement; excess dietary sodium; inadequate diuretic therapy; inadequate doses of medications; excess alcohol intake; and drug interactions, such as use of nonsteroidal anti-inflammatory drugs, illicit drugs, oral contraceptives, sympathomimetics, herbal supplements, and OTC preparations. Ruling out the secondary causes of hypertension mentioned above is crucial in evaluating resistant hypertension, if this has not already been done.

II. Diagnosis. The diagnostic work-up for hypertension should assess risk factors and cormorbidities, reveal identifiable causes of hypertension, and assess presence of target organ damage. This allows for appropriate risk stratification and tailoring of therapy. The major cardiovascular risk factors, besides hypertension, include cigarette smoking, obesity (BMI $\geq$ 30) especially truncal obesity, physical inactivity, dyslipidemia, diabetes mellitus, men older than 45 years, women older than 65 years, family history of premature CVD, and microalbuminuria (or estimated GFR $\leq$ 60 mL/min). (SOR Ⓐ) Target organ damage includes the heart (left ventricular hypertrophy, angina or prior myocardial infarction, prior coronary revascularization or heart failure); the brain (Stroke or TIA); the kidneys (chronic kidney disease); the peripheral arteries (PAD); and the retina (retinopathy).

A. Symptoms. Patients with hypertension usually remain asymptomatic, unless they have experienced severe blood pressure elevations (e.g., $\geq$220 mm Hg SBP, or $\geq$130 mm Hg DBP). Symptoms of hypertension can include fatigue, occipital and pulsating headaches in the early morning, light-headedness, flushing, epistaxis, chest pain, visual and speech disturbances, and dyspnea.

Specific symptoms of secondary causes can often aid in the diagnosis of hypertension: leg claudication from lower extremity ischemia (coarctation of the aorta); hirsutism; easy bruising (Cushing syndrome); excessive perspiration; sustained or intermittent hypertension, paroxysmal headaches, palpitations, anxiety attacks, pallor, tremor, nausea or vomiting (pheochromocytoma); hypokalemia, muscle weakness, cramps, polyuria, paralysis, nocturia (primary hyperaldosteronism); and flank pain (renal or renovascular disease).

B. Signs. Blood pressure measurement should be performed while the patient is sitting or supine, and standing on more than two occasions, to obtain an average for both systolic and diastolic readings. The patient should rest for 5 minutes prior to the reading, and should not smoke tobacco or ingest caffeine for a minimum of 30 minutes before measurement. The blood pressure cuff should be more than two-thirds the circumference of the arm and placed at heart level. The cuff should be inflated 30 mm Hg above where the radial pulse can no longer be felt. The systolic reading is made at the onset of Korotkoff sounds (phase I), and the diastolic reading is taken when the sounds completely disappear (phase V). The blood pressure should be measured in both arms; if there is a discrepancy in reading, the higher reading should be used.

C. Ambulatory blood pressure monitoring. Ambulatory blood pressure monitoring provides blood pressure readings during daily activities and sleep. Ambulatory BP measurements are usually lower than office readings. The level of BP using ambulatory measurements correlates with target organ damage better than office measurements.(SOR Ⓑ) Ambulatory BP measurements are indicated to evaluate "white-coat" hypertension in the absence of target organ damage, resistant hypertension, hypotensive episodes, and for suspected autonomic dysfunction. Awake BP readings averaging more than 135/85 mm Hg, or sleep BP readings averaging greater than 120/75 mm Hg, are consistent with the diagnosis of hypertension. Normally, there is a 15 mm Hg drop in the average SBP and a 10 mm Hg drop in the average DBP, between daytime BP ambulatory reading and sleeping BP readings. Failure to find this "nocturnal dipping" suggests that a secondary cause of hypertension is more likely, and is associated with an increased risk of CVD events. Besides aiding in the diagnosis, ambulatory blood pressure monitoring allows for the measurement of overall BP load, percentage of readings that are hypertensive, and the extent of nocturnal dipping to be evaluated.

  D. **Physical examination.** The initial physical examination of the hypertensive patient should include an assessment of target organ damage, identification of signs suggesting a specific secondary cause, and evaluation of metabolic syndrome.

   1. **Signs of target organ damage.** Signs of target organ damage include arteriolar narrowing, arteriovenous compression, hemorrhages, exudates, or papilledema on fundoscopic examination; carotid bruits and distended jugular veins in the neck; loud aortic second sound, precordial heave, arrhythmia, or early systolic click on cardiac examination; diminished or absent peripheral arterial pulses, peripheral edema of the extremities; aneurysm of the abdominal aorta; and abnormal neurologic assessment.

   2. **Signs of secondary hypertension.** Signs suggestive of secondary hypertension include abdominal or flank masses (polycystic kidneys); absence of femoral pulses (aortic coarctation); tachycardia, diaphoresis, orthostatic hypotension (pheochromocytoma); abdominal bruits (renovascular disease); truncal obesity, ecchymoses, pigmented striae (Cushing syndrome); and enlarged or nodular thyroid gland (hyperthyroidism).

   3. **Evaluation for metabolic syndrome.** Evaluation for metabolic syndrome is important in evaluating hypertension since it is associated with an insulin-resistant state and increased cardiovascular risk. (SOR **B**) Metabolic syndrome is defined as the presence of three or more of the following risk factors: abdominal obesity (waist circumference $\geq$40 inches in men, $\geq$35 inches in women); BP $\geq$130/85 mm Hg; glucose intolerance (FPG $\geq$100 mg/dL); and dyslipidemia (TG $\geq$150 mg/dL or HDL $\leq$40 mg/dL in men, or $\leq$50 mg/dL in women).

  E. **Laboratory tests.** Baseline screening is important to assess target organ damage, to identify patients at high risk for developing cardiovascular complications, to determine whether other cardiovascular risk factors exist, and to screen for possible secondary causes of hypertension.

   1. **Routine tests.** Routine tests on all newly diagnosed hypertensive patients include hemoglobin and hematocrit; potassium; creatinine; fasting glucose; calcium; a fasting lipid profile including total cholesterol, HDL cholesterol, LDL cholesterol, and triglycerides; urinalysis, and resting electrocardiogram. Obtaining a urinary microalbumin/creatinine ratio is optional. More extensive testing for identifiable causes is generally not indicated. (SOR **C**)

   2. **Laboratory tests to identify secondary causes.** The following laboratory tests may be helpful when specific secondary causes are suspected based on history, physical evaluation, and routine laboratory evaluation: (SOR **C**)

      a. Chest x-ray (coarctation of aorta)

      b. Angiotensin-converting enzyme (ACE) inhibitor renal scan or magnetic resonance angiogram of the kidneys to evaluate for renal artery stenosis

      c. Urinary metanephrine and vanillylmandelic acid levels (pheochromocytoma)

      d. Plasma renin activity levels (primary aldosteronism or renovascular disease)

      e. Cardiac echocardiography to evaluate for left ventricular hypertrophy, evidence of asymptomatic systolic dysfunction, or previous myocardial infarction.

III. **Treatment**

  A. **Goals of therapy.** Treatment of patients with elevated blood pressure or prehypertension focuses on the prevention or delay of hypertension through lifestyle modification, unless the patient has evidence of target organ damage. In this case, treatment with antihypertensive medications should begin immediately. If a patient has frank hypertension, then therapy is directed toward preventing cardiovascular and renal morbidity and mortality associated with hypertension. Since most persons with hypertension will reach the DBP goal once the SBP is at goal, the primary focus is to achieve a systolic BP goal.

  B. **Lifestyle modifications.** The lifestyle modifications are important in the treatment for all prehypertensive and hypertensive patients, no matter how severe the patient's

TABLE 76–1. LIFESTYLE MODIFICATIONS TO MANAGE HYPERTENSION*

Modification	Recommendation	Approximate Systolic BP Reduction, Range
Weight reduction	Maintain normal body weight (BMI, 18.5–24.9)	5–20 mm Hg/10-kg weight loss
Adopt DASH eating plan	Consume a diet rich in fruits, vegetables, and low-fat dairy products with a reduced content of saturated and total fat	8–14 mm Hg
Dietary sodium reduction	Reduce dietary sodium intake to no more than 100 mEq/L (2.4 g sodium or 6 g sodium chloride)	2–8 mm Hg
Physical activity	Engage in regular aerobic physical activity such as brisk walking (at least 30 minutes per day, most days of the week)	4–9 mm Hg
Moderation of alcohol consumption	Limit consumption to no more than 2 drinks per day (1 oz or 30 mL ethanol [e.g., 24 oz whiskey]) in most men and no more than 1 drink per day in women and lighter-weight persons	2–4 mm Hg

*For overall cardiovascular risk reduction, stop smoking. The effects of implementing these modifications are dose and time dependent and could be higher for some individuals.
BMI, body mass index calculated as weight in kilograms divided by the square of height in meters; BP, blood pressure; DASH, Dietary Approaches to Stop Hypertension.

hypertension. Not only are lifestyle changes effective, they reduce the number and dosage of medications needed to control hypertension. Evidence-based lifestyle modifications include weight reduction in those who are overweight, DASH diet, dietary sodium reduction, physical activity, and moderate alcohol consumption (Table 76–1).(SOR **A**)

1. **Weight loss.** A 10% weight loss in patients with a BMI $\geq$ 25 reduces SBP by 5 to 10 mm Hg. (SOR **A**) Weight loss is known to improve insulin sensitivity, decrease plasma norepinephrine and aldosterone levels, and decrease renin activity, which probably explains its benefits. Weight loss can be attained by a 500 to 1000 kcal dietary deficit, along with behavioral management that focuses on self-monitoring, goal setting, positive reinforcement, and promotes 30 minutes of daily moderate physical activity, such as walking (SOR **A**).

2. **DASH-diet eating plan.** Diets high in potassium, calcium, and magnesium have been individually shown to have modest benefits in lowering blood pressure. (SOR **A**) These minerals are found in abundance in fruits and vegetables. The recent landmark study, Dietary Approaches to Stop Hypertension (DASH), found that diets high in fruits and vegetables (8–10 servings of fruits and vegetables) significantly decreased both SBP and DBP in patients with hypertension, with results in only 2 weeks. The DASH-diet eating plan is now recommended for most prehypertensive and hypertensive patients. (SOR **C**) Recipes and patient education materials are available at http://www.nhlbi.nih.gov/health/public/heart/hbp/dash/index.htm.

3. **Sodium restriction.** While previous epidemiologic studies have been inconsistent in their findings of the relationship between sodium and hypertension, new randomized trials have now clearly shown the benefits of sodium restriction. (SOR **A**) The DASH-sodium study and the Trials of the Hypertension Prevention Collaborative collectively have shown that salt restriction successfully prevented hypertension in those with prehypertension and controlled BP in stage I hypertension. A restriction to 1500 mg/d or two-thirds of a teaspoon of salt led to a 2 to 8 mm Hg reduction in SBP. The degree of blood pressure lowering by sodium restriction appears to vary, with certain "salt sensitive" individuals experiencing a significant effect, and others receiving little apparent benefit. Therefore, if sodium restriction is burdensome for a patient, a trial of sodium restriction can be performed in order to tailor therapy.

4. **Physical activity.** A meta-analysis of trials has shown that physical activity is effective in lowering blood pressure in normal weight and overweight individuals, and in those with prehypertension and hypertension. (SOR **A**) Aerobic exercise is associated with a 3 to 5 mm Hg reduction in the SBP and a 2 to 3 mm Hg reduction in the DBP. Sedentary and unfit people with normal blood pressure have a 20% to 50% increased risk of

developing hypertension when compared with physically active peers. The PREMIER study showed that increasing physical activity could be successfully added to a DASH-sodium diet, with allowance for moderate alcohol consumption, to lower blood pressure. All sedentary prehypertensive and hypertensive patients should be encouraged to participate in 30 minutes of moderate or vigorous physical activity between 5 and 7 days per week.

5. **Moderate alcohol consumption.** Fifteen randomized clinical trials have shown that reduction in alcohol consumption results in a modest reduction in systolic (3 mm Hg) and DBP (2 mm Hg). All prehypertensive and hypertensive male patients should be encouraged to limit alcohol intake to two drinks per day, with female patients encouraged to limit alcohol intake to one drink per day; neither male nor female patients should consume more than five drinks in any 24-hour period.

C. **Pharmacologic treatment.** In clinical trials, antihypertensive drug therapy is associated with a 35% to 40% reduction in stroke, 20% to 25% reduction in myocardial infarction, and 50% reduction in heart failure in subjects with hypertension. (SOR Ⓐ) Reducing SBP by 12 mm Hg in stage I hypertension will prevent one death for every 11 patients treated, while treating those with target organ damage will prevent one death in every 9 patients treated. (SOR Ⓐ) Recently, it has been found in one study that treatment of prehypertension (SBP 130–139 and DBP 85–89) with an angiotensin receptor blocker (ARB) reduced the incidence of subsequent hypertension over a 2-year period, but this study was not designed or powered to evaluate cardiovascular outcomes. (SOR Ⓒ) Therefore, treatment of pre-hypertension with medication is not recommended.

1. **Initial drug therapy.** JNC 7 recommended low-dose diuretics are the most effective first-line treatment for preventing the occurrence of cardiovascular morbidity and mortality. (SOR Ⓒ) However, the recent AHA scientific statement stated that evidence supports the use of ACE inhibitor or ARB, calcium channel blockers (CCBs) or thiazide diuretics singly or in combination as first-line therapy. (SOR Ⓒ) JNC 7 suggested compelling reasons for use of nonthiazide diuretic therapy as first-line antihypertensive drugs include existing systolic congestive heart failure, S/P transmural myocardial infarction, diabetes mellitus, and chronic kidney disease. (SOR Ⓐ) Table 76–2, adapted from the JNC 7 and the recent AHA scientific statement, lists the indications and appropriate medications, based upon evidence gathered from clinical trials. Clinicians should avoid the use of doxazosin for hypertension control, as the ALLHAT trial showed a higher rate of congestive heart failure and combined CVD events for doxazosin when compared to diuretic therapy. (SOR Ⓐ)

   The precise target BP of antihypertensive therapy remains somewhat controversial, but there is increasingly clear evidence from both epidemiological, observational studies and clinical trials that subjects with known vascular disease and increased cardiovascular risk do better if treated to lower blood pressures. For this reason, BP goals of $\leq$130/80 and $\leq$120/80 have been recommended in the recent AHA scientific statement. (SOR Ⓑ)

2. **Drug regimens.** Drug regimens should be tailored based on multiple clinical factors, including age, cost, safety, effectiveness, disease severity, general lifestyle (diet and exercise) patterns, impact on the quality of life (physical state, emotional well-being, sexual and social functioning, and cognitive acuity), convenience, dosage frequency, possibility of other drug interactions, consideration of pathophysiologic mechanisms, concurrent risk factors and diseases, history of previous responses to other agents, and the potential use of the agent or agents for other medical problems. For instance, heart failure or hypertension complicated by diabetes mellitus with proteinuria can be treated with ACE inhibitors or ARBs. Hypertensive patients with a myocardial infarction can be treated with β-blockers (non-intrinsic sympathomimetic activity), ACE inhibitors, or ARBs. In the presence of systolic dysfunction, diuretics, β-blockers, ACE inhibitors or ARBs, and an aldosterone antagonist (if severe) are all recommended with a goal BP of $\leq$120/80 (Table 76–3).

3. **Effectiveness of drug regimens.** Even the most effective single agents are less than 70% effective on a long-term basis. However, 80% of compliant patients eventually achieve adequate control on one or two agents when BP goal is $\leq$140/90. If the initial agent does not control BP sufficiently, a second agent of a different class may be added. Keeping both agents at low doses will decrease side effects. (SOR Ⓑ) Combination treatment can be very effective, especially when a diuretic is added to monotherapy. For instance, the use of an ACE inhibitor with a diuretic can be effective for up to 85%

TABLE 76–2. SUMMARY OF TREATMENT RECOMMENDATIONS

Area of Concern	BP Target	Lifestyle Modification	Diuretic	β-Blocker	ACE Inhibitor	ARB	CCB	Aldosterone Antagonist	Comments
General	≤140/90	Yes	•	•	•	•	•	•	If SBP ≥160 mm Hg or DBP ≥100, then start two drugs
High-risk CAD	≤130/80	Yes	•	•	•	•	•	•	If SBP ≥160 mm Hg or DBP ≥100, then start two drugs
Stable angina	≤130/80	Yes	• can be added	• plus ACEI or ARB	• plus β-blocker	• plus β-blocker			If β-blocker contraindicated can substitute diltiazem or verapamil (but not if bradycardia or LVD is present)
Unstable angina/MI	≤130/80	Yes		If hemodynamically stable plus ACEI or ARB	• If hemodynamically stable add β-blocker	• If hemodynamically stable add β-blocker			
LVD	≤120/80	Yes	• plus	• plus	• or ARB	• or ACEI	•		
Diabetes	≤130/80	Yes	•	•	•	•	•		
Chronic kidney disease	≤130/80	Yes			•	•			
Recurrent stroke prevention	≤130/80	Yes	•		•				

TABLE 76–3. **ORAL ANTIHYPERTENSIVE DRUGS**

Class	Drug (Trade Name)	Starting Dose (mg)	Maximum Dose (mg)	Daily Frequency	Cost
Thiazide diuretics					
	Chlorothiazide (Diuril)	125	500	1	$
	Chlorthalidone (generic)	12.5	25	1	$$
	Hydrochlorothiazide (Microzide, HydroDIURIL)	12.5	50	1	$
	Polythiazide (Renese)	2	4	1	$$
	Indapamide (Lozol)	1.25	2.5	1	$
	Metolazone (Mykrox)	0.5	1.0	1	$$$
	Metolazone (Zaroxolyn)	2.5	5	1	$$$
Loop diuretics					
	Bumetanide (Bumex)	0.5	2	2	$$
	Furosemide (Lasix)	20	80	2	$
	Torsemide (Demadex)	2.5	10	1	$$
Potassium-sparing diuretics					
	Amiloride (Midamor)	5	10	1–2	$$–$$$
	Triamterene (Dyrenium)	50	100	1–2	$$$–$$$$
Aldosterone-receptor blockers					
	Eplerenone (Inspra)	50	100	1–2	$$$$
	Spironolactone (Aldactone)	25	50	1–2	$$–$$$
β-blockers					
	Atenolol (Tenormin)	25	100	1	$
	Betaxolol (Kerlone)	5	20	1	$$$
	Bisoprolol (Zebeta)	2.5	10	1	$$
	Metoprolol (Lopressor)	50	100	1–2	$$$–$$$$
	Metoprolol extended release (Toprol XL)	50	100	1	$$$
	Nadolol (Corgard)	40	120	1	$$–$$$
	Propranolol (Inderal)	40	160	2	$$$–$$$
	Propranolol long-acting (Inderal LA)	60	180	1	$$$–$$$$
	Timolol (Biocadren)	20	40	2	$$$
β-blockers with intrinsic sympathomimetic activity					
	Acebutolol (Sectral)	200	800	2	$$–$$$
	Penbutolol (Levatol)	10	40	1	$$$
	Pindolol (generic)	10	40	2	$$
Combined α- and β-blockers					
	Carvedilol (Coreg)	12.5	50	2	$$–$$$
	Labetalol (Normodyne, Trandate)	200	800	2	$$$
Ace inhibitors					
	Benazepril (Lotensin)	10	40	1–2	$$–$$$
	Captopril (Capoten)	25	100	2	$–$$
	Enalapril (Vasotec)	2.5	40	1–2	$–$$
	Fosinopril (Monopril)	10	40	1	$$$
	Lisinopril (Prinivil, Zestril)	10	40	1	$$–$$$
	Moexipril (Univasc)	7.5	30	1	$$$
	Perindopril (Aceon)	4	8	1–2	$$$–$$$$
	Quinapril (Accupril)	10	40	1	$$
	Ramipril (Altace)	2.5	20	1	$$$
	Trandolapril (Mavik)	1	4	1	$$
Angiotensin-receptor blockers					
	Candesartan (Atacand)	4	32	1	$$$
	Irbesartan (Avapro)	75	300	1	$$$
	Olmesartan (Benicar)	5	40	1	$$$
	Losartan (Cozaar)	25	100	1	$$$–$$$$
	Valsartan (Diovan)	40	320	1	$$$–$$$$
	Telmisartan (Micardis)	20	80	1	$$$
	Esprosartan (Teveten)	400	800	1	$$$$

Key: $, $0 to $10; $$, $10 to $25; $$$, $25 to $75; $$$$, $75 to $150.

of elderly patients. Common combinations include diuretic plus β-blocker, diuretic plus ACE inhibitor, diuretic plus CCB, CCB plus ACE inhibitor, and diuretic plus sympatholytic agent. With the newer BP goals of ≤130/80 or ≤120/80 for high CVD risk patients, three or more drugs may be required.

4. **Follow-up tests.** Serum potassium, sodium, blood urea nitrogen and creatinine, uric acid, and glucose levels should be measured periodically, especially if the patient has chronic renal disease, or diabetes mellitus, or is taking a diuretic agent. Fasting lipid profiles are indicated for most patients, given concomitant disease and the high prevalence of metabolic syndrome. The type and frequency of repeated laboratory tests should be based on the severity of target organ damage and the effectiveness of treatment. A periodic urinalysis or microalbumin/creatinine ratio is also indicated to monitor for subclinical vascular impairment.

IV. **Management Strategies**

Management strategies need to be individualized to take into consideration the severity of the patient's hypertension, the class or classes of pharmacologic agents being used for treatment, patient compliance, and cardiovascular risk factors or disease processes concurrent with hypertension. The three most common causes of uncontrolled hypertension are patient noncompliance (responsible for 50% of treatment failure), inadequate therapy, and inappropriate therapy.

A. **Patient education.** Patient education is an important part of the physician's management strategy. Education begins with the initial measurement of blood pressure. For a patient who has elevated pressures after three readings, the diagnosis of hypertension should be explained clearly, concisely, and completely. The beliefs of the patient regarding hypertension should be identified with respect to the effectiveness of treatment; the seriousness of the disease, if not treated; and personal susceptibility to complications that correspond to an increased risk of morbidity and mortality. Drug instructions should be written clearly and succinctly. Lifestyle barriers to compliance should be identified as early as possible. Family education should be provided when appropriate. Patient education by itself has been shown to be inadequate for chronic disease management including hypertension. It is important that the patient participates in the decision-making process when the goals of therapy are established, and strategies are delineated to reach these goals and achieve effective blood pressure control. For individuals with high blood pressure, the goal is a systolic BP consistently below 140/90 mm Hg, while the goal is 130/80 mm Hg for individuals with diabetes, chronic kidney disease, coronary artery disease or coronary artery disease equivalents (carotid artery disease, peripheral arterial disease, abdominal aortic aneurysm) or high cardiovascular risk (10-year Framingham risk score ≥10%).

B. **Self-monitoring.** Presently, only 34% of hypertensives are under good control. (SOR **B**) Recent studies have shown that this can be increased by self-monitoring. Having a record of blood pressures and receiving immediate individualized feedback has been shown to enhance blood pressure control significantly.

C. **Initial follow-up.** Monthly check-ups are recommended for the first 6 months of newly diagnosed hypertension, and should include an interval history to identify symptoms that may have developed, a discussion of health concerns and compliance problems, an evaluation of drug effects and possible drug reactions, and measurement of blood pressure and weight. Compliance can sometimes be improved by changing to an agent with a longer half-life, thereby reducing the number of doses. A memory-assist device, such as Medi-Set, is appropriate for patients receiving complex regimens, or with a memory disturbance.

D. **Early detection.** Early detection of complications is an important management strategy to identify potential morbidity from hypertension (retinopathy, coronary artery disease, renal disease, cerebrovascular disease, or nephropathy). Furthermore, people with hypertension may be at increased risk of having vascular disease, target organ damage, dyslipidemias, diabetes mellitus, obesity, arthritis, and liver and renal problems. Prevention, early identification, and treatment of these associated problems are important.

V. **Natural History and Prognosis.** Natural history and prognosis are directly related to the effectiveness of treatment, patient compliance, the presence of coexisting diseases, the age of the patient at diagnosis, and the ability of the patient to follow adjunctive therapy recommendations to make lifestyle and behavioral changes. Studies completed prior to the discovery of antihypertensive drugs revealed that 70% of hypertensive patients died of congestive heart failure or coronary artery disease, 15% from cerebral hemorrhage, and 10% from uremia.

Left ventricular hypertrophy (LVH) is a significant complication of hypertension. Progression of LVH can be prevented, and reversed, by good hypertension control. Development of LVH with strain is an ominous complication of hypertension, with a four- to eight-fold increase in mortality. Within 5 years of the development of LVH with strain, one-third of patients have a major cardiovascular event.

Patients with concurrent diabetes mellitus and hypertension are at greater risk for developing diabetic nephropathy. However, effective antihypertensive treatment (e.g., ACE inhibitors or ARBs) can reduce proteinuria and the rate of decline of the glomerular filtration rate, thus postponing end-stage renal failure. The likelihood of cardiovascular complications in elderly patients can best be predicted by SBP. Treatment has been shown to decrease cardiovascular events in patients up to the age of 80 years.

REFERENCES

ALLHAT Officers and Coordinators. Major cardiovascular events in hypertensive patients randomized to doxazosin vs chlothalidone: the Antihypertensive and Lipid-lowering Treatment to Prevent Heart Attack Trial (ALLHAT). *JAMA.* 2000;283:1967-1975.

ALLHAT Officers and Coordinators. Major outcomes in high-risk hypertensive patients randomized to angiotensin-converting enzyme inhibitor or calcium channel blocker vs diuretic: the Antihypertensive and Lipid-lowering Treatment to Prevent Heart Attack Trial (ALLHAT). *JAMA.* 2002;288:2981-2997.

Appel LJ, Champagne CM, Harsha DW, Cooper LS, Obarzanek E, et al. Effects of comprehensive lifestyle modification on blood pressure control: main results of the PREMIER clinical trial. *JAMA.* 2003;289:2083-2093.

Chobanian AV, Bakris GL, Black HR, et al. The seventh report of the Joint National Committee on Prevention, Detection, Evaluation, and Treatment of High Blood Pressure: the JNC 7 report. *JAMA.* 2003;289:2560-2572.

Hansson L, Hedner T, Lund-Johansen P, Kjeldsen SE, Lindholm LH, et al. Randomized trial of effects of calcium channel antagonists compared with diuretics and β-blockers on cardiovascular morbidity and mortality in hypertension: the Nordic Diltiazem (NORDIL) study. *Lancet.* 2000;356:359-365.

Hansson L, Lindholm LH, Ekborn T, Dahlöf B, Lanke J, et al. Randomized trial of old and new antihypertensive drugs in elderly patients: cardiovascular mortality and morbidity the Swedish Trial in Old Patients with Hypertension-2 study. *JAMA.* 2002;288(23):2981-2997.

Julius S, Nesbitt SA, Egan BM, et al; Trial Preventing Hypertension (TROPHY) Study Investigators. Feasibility of treating prehypertension with an angiotensin-receptor blocker. *N Engl J Med.* 2006;354:1685-1697.

Mancia G, Brown M, Castaigne A, deLeeuw P, Palmer CR, et al. Outcomes with nifedipine GITS or Co-amilozide in hypertensive diabetics and nondiabetics in intervention as a goal in hypertension (INSIGHT). *Hypertension.* 2003;41:431-436.

Psaty BM, Lumley T, Furberg CD, et al. Health outcomes associated with various antihypertensive therapies use as first-line agents: A network meta-analysis. *JAMA.* 2003;289:2534-2544.

Rogers MAM, Small D, Buchan DA, Butch CA, Stewart CM, et al. Home monitoring service improves mean arterial pressure in patients with essential hypertension: A randomized, controlled trial. *Ann Intern Med.* 2001;134:1024-1032.

Rosamond W, Flegal K, Friday G, et al. Heart disease and stroke statistics – 2007 update: A report from the American Heart Association Statistics Committee and Stroke Statistics Subcommittee. *Circulation.* 2007;115:e69-e171.

Rosendorff C, Black HR, Cannon CP, et al. Treatment of hypertension in the prevention and management of ischemic heart disease: a scientific statement from the American Heart Association Council for High Blood Pressure Research and the Councils of Clinical Cardiology and Epidemiology and Prevention. *Circulation.* 2007;115:2761-2788.

Sacks FM, Svetkey LP, Vollmer WM, Appel LJ, et al. Effects on blood pressure of reduced dietary sodium and the Dietary Approaches to Stop Hypertension (DASH) diet (DASH-Sodium). *N Engl J Med.* 2001;344:3-10.

Vasan RS, Larson MG, Leip EP, et al. Impact of high-normal blood pressure on the risk of cardiovascular disease. *N Engl J Med.* 2001;345:1291-1297.

Whelton S, Chin A, Xin X, He J. Effect of aerobic exercise on blood pressure: a meta-analysis of randomized, controlled trials. *Ann Intern Med.* 2002;136:493-503.

Xin X, He J, Frontini MG, et al. Effects of alcohol reduction on blood pressure: a meta-analysis of randomized controlled trials. *Hypertension.* 2001;38:1112-1117.

77   Ischemic Heart Disease & Acute Coronary Syndromes

Allen L. Hixon, MD, & Damon F. Lee, MD

KEY POINTS

- The highest priority in the evaluation of patients with chest pain is distinguishing cardiac from noncardiac causes.
- The clinical history including cardiac risk factors remains critical in the evaluation of each patient. Evidence-based primary and secondary prevention should be targeted at modifiable risk factors.
- A normal electrocardiogram result cannot be used to exclude ischemic heart disease. An exercise treadmill test remains the most valuable diagnostic tool.
- Consensus guidelines should be used to determine management of patients with chronic stable angina and acute coronary syndromes. Aspirin and beta-blockers should be considered in all patients with ischemic heart disease.

I. **Introduction**
   A. **Definition. Acute coronary syndrome (ACS)** is a cluster of clinical symptoms that are associated with acute myocardial ischemia. These symptoms typically result from the disruption of atherosclerotic plaques leading to obstruction of myocardial blood flow. The term ACS includes conditions with ST elevation and nonST elevation including both Q-wave and non Q-wave MI and unstable angina. Please see Figure 77–1.
   B. **Epidemiology**
      1. Cardiovascular disease is the leading cause of death in both men and women. It accounts for approximately half of all deaths in the developed world and one-quarter of all deaths in the developing world. More than 1 million men and women die annually in the United States alone from coronary artery disease or stroke. Fifty percent of postmenopausal women die of coronary artery disease or its sequelae. It is estimated that by the year 2020 cardiovascular disease will surpass infectious diseases as the leading cause of death and claim 25 million lives worldwide.
      2. Ischemic heart disease (IHD) has an enormous economic impact on medical care in this country. The cost of treatment is expected to rise with the aging of the United States population. In industrialized nations, economic loss, disability, and death from coronary artery disease exceeded any other cluster of illnesses.
      3. Unrecognized MIs are common and as lethal as symptomatic infarcts. At least 25% of MIs are silent and another 25% present with atypical chest pain. Only 20% of MIs are preceded by angina. Many MIs occur at rest and nearly as many occur during sleep as during heavy physical activity. Distressing life events reportedly occur with increased frequency in the months preceding an MI.
   C. **Pathogenesis.** The heart muscle functions almost exclusively as an aerobic organ, with little capacity for anaerobic metabolism. At rest, the heart extracts approximately 80% of the oxygen it receives, leaving it more susceptible to effects of decreased perfusion. ACSs arise from a mismatch of oxygen supply and demand to the myocardium. This mismatch is most often initiated by disruption of an atherosclerotic plaque, causing blockage to normal coronary blood flow. Partial or complete mechanical obstruction may result from thrombus or dynamic obstruction from coronary vasoconstriction. Inflammation as well as systemic hemodynamic factors also play a role in the development or severity of IHD. This process causing myocardial ischemia results in a variety of signs and symptoms. It is important for clinicians to recognize the many manifestations of this disease process. Chest pain is the foremost manifestation of myocardial ischemia and results from a disparity between myocardial oxygen demand and coronary blood flow.
II. **Diagnosis.** Chest pain is one of the common reasons for patients to visit primary care physicians. The major diagnostic considerations for chest pain are addressed in Chapter 10. The highest priority is generally given to distinguishing cardiac from noncardiac chest pain. Studies have demonstrated that 10% to 30% of patients with chest pain who undergo

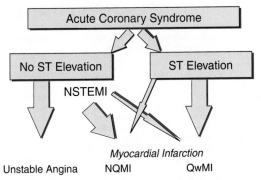

FIGURE 77–1. Schematic representation of the clinical diagnoses that comprise acute coronary syndromes. NSTEMI, nm ST elevation MI; NQMI, non Q-wave MI; QwMI, Q-wave MI. (Obtained from ACC/AHA 2002 Guidelines Update for the Management of Patients with Unstable Angina and Non-ST-Segment Elevation Myocardial Infarction.)

coronary arteriography have no arterial abnormalities. Of the many noncardiac causes of chest pain, gastrointestinal (esophageal), bronchopulmonary, and psychiatric (panic attacks and major depression) are common. Less common causes include chest wall (herpes zoster, costochondritis), aortic dissection, and referred pain from the abdomen.

A. **Risk factors.** Cigarette smoking, hyperlipidemia, hypertension, diabetes, older age, and male gender are commonly recognized risk factors for IHD. In addition, elevated homocysteine levels and markers of vascular inflammation such as highly sensitive C-reactive protein are associated with IHD. Mental stress has increasingly been recognized as related to IHD.

B. **Symptoms and signs**
   1. **Angina** is not simply one type of pain; it is a constellation of symptoms related to cardiac ischemia. The description of angina may fit several patterns.
      a. **Classic angina** presents as an ill-defined pressure, heaviness (feeling like a weight), or squeezing sensation brought on by exertion and relieved by rest. The location of classic anginal pain is most often substernal and left-sided. It may radiate to the jaw, interscapular area, or down the arm. Angina usually begins gradually and lasts only a few minutes. It is important to appreciate that the qualitative description of pain may be greatly influenced by socioeconomic status, education, culture, and personality.
      b. **Atypical angina.** The patient either experiences pain that is anginal in quality or has pain with exertional features. For example, this may be a sense of heaviness that is not consistently related to exertion or relieved by rest. Conversely, the pain may have an atypical character—sharp or stabbing—but the precipitating factors are anginal. This is the category of chest pain that is most prone to a diagnostic error. All presentations of chest pain should be taken seriously until proven to be benign.
      c. **Anginal equivalent.** The sensation of dyspnea may be the sole or major manifestation.
      d. **Nonanginal pain.** The pain has neither the quality nor precipitating characteristics of angina. Chest pain quality not consistent with IHD includes the following descriptive terms: needlelike, shooting, tingling, stabbing, jabbing, knifelike, and cutting.
      e. **Metabolic syndrome, insulin resistance, and diabetes**. IHD is the leading cause of death in adult diabetic patients. Hypertension, obesity, and hyperlipidemia cluster in patients with diabetes who have accelerated development of atherosclerotic vascular disease. Insulin resistance promotes atherosclerosis even before the diagnostic criteria for diabetes mellitus are met. Atypical clinical presentations have been thought to occur more frequently in diabetic patients; however, whether diabetic patients experience more "silent myocardial infarctions" (MIs) than the general population has recently been challenged.

TABLE 77–1. PRETEST PROBABILITY OF CORONARY ARTERY DISEASE BY AGE, GENDER, AND SYMPTOMS

Age (yr)	Gender	Typical/Definite Angina Pectoris	Atypical/Probable Angina Pectoris	Nonanginal Chest Pain	Asymptomatic
30–39	Men	Intermediate	Intermediate	Low	Very low
	Women	Intermediate	Very low	Very low	Very low
40–49	Men	High	Intermediate	Intermediate	Low
	Women	Intermediate	Low	Very low	Very low
50–59	Men	High	Intermediate	Intermediate	Low
	Women	Intermediate	Intermediate	Low	Very low
60–69	Men	High	Intermediate	Intermediate	Low
	Women	High	Intermediate	Intermediate	Low

(Data from Gibbons RJ, Balady GJ, Bricker JT, et al. ACC/AHA 2002 guideline update for exercise testing: summary article. A report of the ACC/AHA Task Force on Practice Guidelines (Committee to Update the 1997 Exercise Testing Guidelines). *Circulation.* 2002;106:1883-1892.)

    f. Women. Women are twice as likely as men to present with angina and less likely to present with infarction or sudden death. Diabetes in women increases both the risk and the mortality of myocardial infarction. Women are often overlooked as having significant IHD. Women older than 65 years are as vulnerable to IHD mortality as men. There is a precipitous increase in IHD in women after either natural or surgical menopause.

  2. Probability of IHD based on history. Despite the well-known problems experienced in determining the cause of chest pain, the clinical history remains critical in the evaluation of each patient. From the information gathered in the history, the physician should strive to categorize the patient's symptoms as nonanginal, atypical angina, or typical angina. Table 77–1 provides a guideline as to the likelihood of whether a patient has significant IHD based on the history. The Framingham Global Prediction model includes age, total cholesterol, LDL-C, HDL-C, blood pressure, diabetes, and tobacco use. It may be used to calculate the 10 years coronary heart disease risk. An online version is available at http://hp2010.nhlbihin.net/atpiii/calculator.asp.

  3. Use of nitrate and response to nitroglycerin. Response of the chest pain to sublingual nitroglycerin (NTG) may be used (with caution) as an adjunct for determining whether a patient's chest pain is from IHD. For example, a prompt response of ≤ 3 minutes increases the probability of IHD; however, esophageal spasm and biliary colic may also respond favorably to nitrate administration. Failure to respond to NTG should not be used to exclude the possibility of IHD.

  4. Signs. There are no reliable, consistent physical signs found on examination for IHD. The main purpose of the examination is to assess the patient for evidence of complications from atherosclerotic disease (e.g., peripheral vascular disease, cerebrovascular disease, congestive heart failure). The physician should pay attention to the vascular examination, such as peripheral artery bruits, retinal arteriolar changes, and the presence of an S_3 or S_4, and for the consequences of diminished myocardial contractility, such as lower extremity edema.

C. Diagnostic tests

  1. 12-Lead electrocardiogram (ECG) and serial cardiac enzymes are frequently used to rule out an MI. Several molecular markers and their sampling schedule are noted in Table 77–2.

TABLE 77–2. MOLECULAR MARKERS USED OR PROPOSED FOR USE IN THE DIAGNOSIS OF ACUTE MYOCARDIAL INFARCTION

Marker	Range of Times to Initial Elevation (h)	Mean Time to Peak Elevations (Nonthrombolysis)	Time to Return to Normal Range	Most Common Sampling Schedule
Myoglobin	1–4	6–7 h	24 h	Frequent; 1–2 h after CP
CTnI	3–12	24 h	5–10 d	Once at least 12 h after CP
CTnT	3–12	12 h–2 d	5–14 d	Once at least 12 h after CP
MB-CK	3–12	24 h	48–72 h	Every 12 h × 3*

*Increased sensitivity can be achieved with sampling every 6–8 h.
CP, chest pain; CTnI, cardiac troponin I; CTnT, cardiac troponin T; MB-CK, MB isoenzyme creatine kinase (CK).

2. The standard provocative test for IHD is the **exercise treadmill test (ETT).** The American College of Cardiology (ACC) and the American Heart Association (AHA) have developed consensus guidelines for exercise treadmill testing as follows:
    a. ETT is appropriate as a diagnostic test to determine the presence or absence of coronary artery disease in patients with an intermediate pretest probability (SOR **B**) (Table 77–1). This includes patients with complete right bundle branch block or less than 1 mm of resting ST depression.
    b. ETT may be useful for patients with known or suspected IHD who have experienced a change in clinical status. (SOR **C**)
    c. Low-risk unstable angina patients 12 hours after presentation who are free of ischemic symptoms or heart failure may be appropriate for stress testing. Similarly, intermediate-risk unstable angina patients 2 to 3 days after presentation and free of ischemic symptoms or heart failure may also be appropriate for stress testing.
3. Many protocols exist; however, the Bruce protocol has become the most widely used.
4. **Prognostic value of an ETT.** In addition to the diagnostic implications of an ETT, there are prognostic implications. The following are considered to be parameters associated with a poor prognosis or increased disease severity: failure to complete stage II of a Bruce protocol, failure to achieve a heart rate $\geq$120 beats per minute (off beta-blockers), onset of ST-segment depression at a heart rate of $\leq$120 beats per minute, ST-segment depression $\geq$2.0 mm, ST-segment depression lasting $\geq$6 minutes into recovery, ST-segment depression in multiple leads, poor systolic blood pressure response to exercise, angina with exercise, and exercise-induced ventricular tachycardia. Recently, heart rate recovery and the Duke treadmill exercise score have been determined to be independent predictors of mortality.
5. **Resting ECG.** A resting ECG, while important to do on all patients with suspected IHD, must be interpreted with caution. The ECG will be normal or show nonspecific changes in more than 50% of patients with IHD. A normal resting ECG may not be used to rule out IHD. The classic ECG changes of acute ischemia are peaked, hyperacute T waves, T-wave flattening or inversion with or without ST-segment depression, horizontal ST-segment depression, and ST-segment elevation.
6. **Angiography.** Cardiac catheterization is not routinely recommended for initial evaluation of patients with stable angina. Patients who warrant such an evaluation are those who exhibit evidence of severe myocardial ischemia on noninvasive testing (SOR **B**) or who have symptoms that are refractory to antianginal medications. (SOR **C**) In patients who undergo catheterization, the most important determinant of survival is left ventricular function, followed by the number of diseased vessels.

III. Prevention
   A. **Primary prevention** in symptomatic adults should target smoking cessation, blood pressure and cholesterol screening, maintaining a normal BMI, and discussing aspirin therapy. See Table 77–3 for the USPSTF screening guidelines and levels of evidence.
   B. **Secondary prevention** in those patients diagnosed with hypertension, dyslipidemia, or diabetes mellitus should focus on controlling blood pressure, cholesterol, and blood sugar in accordance with consensus guidelines such as the Seventh Report of the Joint National Committee on Prevention, Detection, Evaluation, and Treatment, of High Blood Pressure (JNC 7), the National Cholesterol Education Program (NCEP), and the American Diabetic Association, Standards of Medical Care in Diabetes. These and other important consensus guidelines may be found at the National Guideline Clearinghouse (www.guideline. gov)

IV. Treatment
   A. **Chronic stable angina.** Stable angina is characterized by no change in frequency, severity, duration, or precipitating factors for at least the past 2 months. The treatment of patients with stable angina includes identification and management of specific cardiovascular risk factors, aspirin, and antianginal drug therapy. Treatment goals include mortality reduction and symptom relief.
      1. **Risk factor modification.** Dietary modification, smoking cessation, and physical conditioning programs should be instituted.
      2. **Treatment of associated disease.** Diabetes, hypertension, hyperlipidemia. thyroid disease, anemia, congestive heart failure, valvular disease, and arrhythmias should

TABLE 77–3. USPSTF SCREENING RECOMMENDATIONS AND LEVEL OF EVIDENCE

Condition or Intervention	Demographic	Level of Evidence
Aspirin chemoprevention discussion	Adults with increased coronary heart disease risk	A
Tobacco cessation	All adults	A
Hypertension (HTN)	Age 18 and older	A
Intensive dietary behavioral counseling	Adults with hyperlipidemia and cardiovascular/diet-related chronic disease risk factors	B
Cholesterol	Men age 25–35 with coronary heart disease risk factors	B
	Men 35 and older	A
	Women 25–45 with coronary heart disease risk factors	B
	Women 45 and older	A
Obesity screening	Adults	B
Promotion of physical activity	Primary care settings	I
Type 2 diabetes screening	Asymptomatic adults	I
	Adults with HTN or hyperlipidemia	B
Screening EKG or ETT	Asymptomatic adults	D

Key: A = strongly recommends providing the service to eligible patients.
B = recommends providing the service to eligible patients.
D = recommends against providing the service.
I = insufficient evidence for or against routinely providing the service.
(Data from Agency for Healthcare Research and Quality, U.S. Preventive Services Task Force. The Guide to Clinical Preventive Services, 2006.)

be aggressively identified and managed. Lipid lowering: patients with high cholesterol should have their LDL cholesterol lowered to a target of ≤100 mg/dL with consideration of ≤70 mg/dL, according to ATP III guidelines (see Chapter 75). Blood pressure should be managed according to JNC 7 guidelines (see Chapter 76).

3. **Aspirin.** Most experts recommend a range of 75 to 325 mg of aspirin per day to decrease platelet aggregation. (SOR **A**)

4. **Antianginal drug therapy.** The goals are to abolish or reduce anginal attacks and myocardial ischemia and to promote a more normal lifestyle. The three classes of antianginal drugs commonly used are nitrates, beta-blockers, and calcium channel blockers. No greater efficacy in relieving chest pain or decreasing exercise-induced ischemia has been shown for one or another group of these drugs, although specific clinical indications may favor one over another (e.g., diastolic dysfunction, left ventricular hypertrophy, hypertension, asthma, depression, diabetes mellitus). Please reference Medication Table 77–4.

   a. **Beta-blockers.** Beta-blockade decreases heart rate, contractility, and arterial blood pressure, reducing myocardial oxygen demand and subsequently anginal symptoms. Beta-blockers are recommended as initial therapy for patients with chronic angina and prior myocardial infarction (SOR **A**) as well as for those without prior MI. (SOR **B**) All beta-blockers, regardless of their selective properties, are equally effective in patients with angina. Approximately 20% of patients do not respond to beta-blockers. Those who do not are more likely to have severe IHD. Contraindications to beta-blockers include heart block, sick sinus syndrome, severe bradycardia. Caution should be used in patients with asthma/obstructive lung disease, severe depression, or peripheral vascular disease. The dose of the beta-blocker should be adjusted to achieve a heart rate of 50 to 60 beats per minute.

   b. **Calcium channel blockers.** These are a diverse group of compounds that have different effects on the atrioventricular node, heart rate, coronary arteries, diastolic relaxation, cardiac contractility, systemic blood pressure, and afterload. Most studies show equal effects between beta-blockers and calcium channel blockers. Calcium channel blockers may be preferred in patients who cannot tolerate beta-blockers or have contraindications to their use. (SOR **B**) The most troublesome side effects are constipation, edema, headache, and aggravation of congestive heart failure. Studies suggest that short-acting dihydropyridine calcium channel blockers

TABLE 77–4. ANTIANGINAL MEDICATIONS

Drug	Usual Starting Dosage	Maximum Daily Dosage	Cost	Common Adverse Effects	Comments
Beta-blockers					
Noncardioselective					Beta-blockers are particularly useful in treating the following conditions that occur with IHD: hypertension, ventricular arrhythmia, supraventricular arrhythmias.
Propranolol	20 mg qid	320 mg/d divided bid–qid	$	Fatigue (dose-related), exacerbation of bronchospasm, bradycardia, AV conduction defects, left ventricular failure	
Propranolol (Long acting)	80 mg/d	320 mg/d	$		
Nadolol	40 mg/d	240 mg/d	$	Raynaud phenomenon, impotence, nightmares, mild increase in lipids; may block symptoms of hypoglycemia in diabetic patients.	There is no advantage in using a beta-blocker with ISA or alpha₁-sympathomimetic blockade. Cardioselectivity will be overcome as the dose is raised. Abrupt discontinuation may exacerbate angina.
Carvedilol	3.125 mg bid	25 mg bid (50 mg bid if ≥ 85 kg)	$$$	Edema, hypotension, bradycardia, AV block	Individualize dose. Consider in post MI with LVEF ≤ 40%. May titrate after 3–7 d. Monitor for bradycardia, hypotension, or fluid retention.
Carvedilol (extended release)	20 mg/d x 3–10 d	80 mg/d	$$$		
Cardioselective					
Atenolol	25–50 mg/d	100 mg/d	$		
Metoprolol	50 mg bid	400 mg/d	$		
Metoprolol (extended release)	100 mg/d	400 mg/d	$		

(continued)

TABLE 77–4. (CONTINUED)

Drug	Usual Starting Dosage	Maximum Daily Dosage	Cost	Common Adverse Effects	Comments
Calcium channel blockers					
Short-acting formulations				Edema, headache, nausea, dizziness, constipation, left ventricular failure, AV conduction defects. Use caution with combined use of beta-blockers or digitalis (may experience exacerbation of congestive heart failure or conduction delays). All calcium channel blockers have the potential to induce hypotension; it is important to titrate the dose especially in the elderly.	Calcium channel blockers are useful in treating the following conditions: IHD, hypertension, and supra-ventricular arrhythmias. Some consider them to be the drugs of choice in vasospastic (Prinzmetal) angina.
Diltiazem	30 mg qid	360 mg/d divided tid–qid	$		
Verapamil	40–80 mg tid–qid	480 mg/d	$		
Long-acting formulations					Dosage may vary by brand and formulation.
Diltiazem	120–180 mg/d	360–480 mg/d	$		
Nifedipine	30–60 mg/d	120 mg/d	$		Caution with doses ≥ 90 mg when treating angina.
Verapamil	180 mg/d	480 mg/d	$		
Second-generation calcium channel blockers (Dihydropyridines)					
Amlodipine	2.5–5 mg/d	10 mg/d	$$	Edema, hypotension, flushing, headache.	Plasma T½ 36 h, little negative inotropic effect, may be useful in treatment of angina associated with hypertension. Use lowest dose in elderly and with hepatic dysfunction.
Felodipine	2.5–5 mg/d	10 mg/d	$		
Nitrates					
Short-acting nitroglycerin					
Nitrostat	0.4 mg q 5 min ×3		$	Headache and hypotension. Potential for hypotension greater when used in combination with a calcium channel blocker.	Tolerance is the most significant issue in the use of nitrates. Oral nitrates are more effective given twice daily at a high dose than frequently at a low dose.
Nitrospray	400 µg 1–2 sprays q 5 min × 3		$		

Long-acting nitroglycerin				
Transderm NTG patch	0.2–0.4 mg/h for 12–14 h	0.8 mg/h	$$	Long acting nitrates should not be used for acute anginal attacks. Nitroglycerin patches should be removed at night to prevent tolerance. Nitrates work well with either beta-blockers or calcium channel blockers.
Isosorbide dinitrate				
Immediate-release				
Isordil	5–20 mg bid-tid	160 mg	$	Elderly start at low end of dosing range. Allow 14 h dose free interval. Caution in patients taking medications for erectile dysfunction; potential hypotension.
Longer-acting	40 mg bid	160 mg	$	Allow 18 h dose free interval. Severe hypotension may result.
Isordil SR				
Isosorbide mononitrate				
Immediate-release	20 mg bid		$	First dose on awakening and then 7 h later.
Extended release	30–60 mg/d	120 mg/d	$	

AV, atrioventricular; IHD, ischemic heart disease; ISA, intrinsic sympathomimetic activity.
$, least expensive; $$, moderately expensive; $$$, most expensive.

should be avoided because of increased risk of adverse cardiac events. There is no evidence of a similar effect with long-acting calcium antagonists.

    c. Nitrates. Nitrates improve myocardial blood flow and oxygen demand via endothelial vasodilatation. Short-acting nitroglycerin tablets or spray are useful for the immediate relief of angina. (SOR **B**) Long-acting nitrates are used for symptom prevention in patients with contraindications to beta-blockade. (SOR **B**) The most significant issue for this class of drugs is tolerance. Most studies show that tolerance develops rapidly when long-acting nitrates are given. Tolerance can develop within 24 hours. When prescribing a patch, it is important to have patch-free intervals of 10 to 12 hours to retain the antianginal effect. Patients should be warned about the potential for severe hypotension when sildenafil is taken within 24 hours after any nitrate preparation has been taken.

    d. Combination therapy. Calcium channel blockers or long-acting nitrates given with beta-blockers may provide greater antianginal effects than when used independently and may be considered when initial therapy with beta-blockers is unsuccessful. (SOR **B**) Calcium antagonists and nitrates may be used in combination therapy and substituted for beta-blockers as initial treatment in patients who cannot tolerate beta-blockers. (SOR **C**) Calcium channel antagonists and beta-blockers in combination should be used with caution because of the increased risk of extreme bradycardia or heart block.

  5. Angiotensin-converting enzyme (ACE) inhibitors. Studies such as the Heart Outcomes Prevention Evaluation (HOPE) trial have suggested that use of an ACE inhibitor substantially lowers the risk of death, MI, stroke, coronary revascularization, and heart failure in high-risk patients with preexisting vascular disease. ACE inhibition may have vasculoprotective effects. ACE inhibitors should be considered in all patients with IHD who also have diabetes or left ventricular systolic impairment. (SOR **A**)

  6. Antioxidants. Oxidized low-density lipoprotein particles are implicated in the development and progression of atherosclerosis. Recent studies have found no benefit of vitamin C, E or beta carotene supplementation with regards to mortality, myocardial infarction, and cardiovascular events.

  7. Vitamins B$_6$, B$_{12}$, and folate. Elevated homocysteine levels are associated with IHD. Although the mechanisms are not well understood, alteration in coagulation profile or endothelial damage is postulated to play a role. Supplementation with B$_6$, B$_{12}$, and folate reduce plasma homocysteine levels; however, the clinical significance of this remains under investigation.

  8. Hormone replacement therapy. The Women's Health Initiative (WHI) and the Estrogen/Progestin Replacement Study helped to clarify the role of hormone replacement therapy (HRT) in relation to IHD. HRT led to an increase in IHD events by 29%. Based on these studies, and consistent with ACC/AHA recommendations, HRT is not recommended for either primary or secondary prevention of IHD. (SOR **A**) The WHI trial of unopposed estrogen versus placebo in women who have undergone hysterectomy showed no increase in heart disease, but showed an increase in stroke in the treatment group.

B. Unstable angina (UA). UA manifests clinically as an abrupt onset of ischemic symptoms at rest or as an intensification or change in the pattern of ischemic symptoms as well as an increasing ease of provocation (symptoms at rest or with minimal effort). Acute management for UA includes hospitalization; bed rest with continuous ECG monitoring; ASA; NTG; supplemental oxygenation; morphine sulfate, if anginal symptoms persist despite NTG; and a beta-blocker, unless contraindicated. Clopidogrel may be considered in patients with UA who have contraindications to ASA including hypersensitivity and gastrointestinal side effects. (SOR **A**)

  1. Early invasive management. The ACC 2002 guidelines for the management of UA recommend work-up via angiography and treatment with revascularization, if indicated, for high-risk patients. High-risk patients are those who present with any of the following:

    a. Recurrent pain at rest or with minimal activity despite medical therapy

    b. Elevated troponin I or T

    c. New ST segment depression

    d. Angina with congestive heart failure symptoms, S3 gallop, pulmonary edema, or new or worsening mitral regurgitation

  e. High-risk findings on noninvasive stress testing
  f. Ejection fraction less than 0.40
  g. Hypotension/hemodynamic instability
  h. Sustained ventricular tachycardia
  i. Percutaneous coronary intervention within the past 6 months
  j. Prior coronary artery bypass grafting
  2. Early conservative management. Patients without the above high-risk features may be candidates for early conservative management, which includes medication management and noninvasive procedures (i.e., echocardiogram, stress test) to further identify those who may benefit from angiography and possibly revascularization (recurrent ischemia at rest or on a noninvasive stress test).
C. Percutaneous coronary interventions (PCI). PCI include percutaneous transluminal coronary angioplasty (PTCA) and stenting. General indications for PCI include patients with single- or double-vessel disease, excluding the proximal left anterior descending coronary artery. Patients with chronic IHD who have failed maximal medical management may also be considered for PCI. Restenosis after PTCA continues to be a complication; however, the long-term outcome after successful angioplasty has been reported to be excellent even when compared with patients undergoing bypass surgery. Stenting has become the most widely used PCI because of less associated closure and restenosis as compared with PTCA. Use of antithrombotic medications such as IIb/IIIa inhibitors and clopidogrel has improved short- as well as long-term outcomes following PCI. Drug eluting stents, coated with antiproliferative agents, have shown promise in further reducing the rates of restenosis and the need for repeat procedures as compared to bare metal stents; however, subacute and late stent thrombosis in drug eluting stents have recently been raised as possible causes for concern and further inquiry. Further research is needed in the areas of long-term outcome for multiple lesions, extensive disease, and avoidance of complications such as stent thrombosis.
D. Coronary artery bypass graft (CABG) surgery. Indications for CABG include significant ($\geq$50% stenosis) left main coronary artery disease, three vessel disease, or two vessel disease with significant proximal left anterior descending involvement and EF $\leq$50% or ischemia on noninvasive testing. (SOR **Ⓐ**) CABG may also be preferred over PCI for diabetic patients with multivessel disease. (SOR **Ⓑ**) Large randomized trials have shown that for patients in whom CABG is indicated, CABG provides better symptom relief, improved exercise tolerance, and decreased need for antianginal medications at 5 years when compared to medication management. Development of atherosclerosis in the graft resulting in angina generally occurs within 5 to 10 years. Improved survival with CABG versus medical therapy is seen only in the "sicker" subset of patients who are older and have more severe symptoms, particularly left main coronary artery disease, multivessel disease with left ventricular dysfunction or triple vessel disease including the left proximal LAD.
V. Prognosis
  A. The three major factors that determine the prognosis of patients with angina include the amount of viable but jeopardized left ventricular myocardium, the percentage of irreversibly scarred myocardium, and the severity of underlying coronary atherosclerosis. ETT has been used to establish the prognosis in patients with symptomatic IHD. The exercise parameters associated with poor outcome have been described above.
  1. Medical versus invasive management. Comparing medical management and PTCA, one randomized study of male patients with single-vessel disease found PTCA to be superior to medical management at 6 months, although 15% of patients required a second procedure. PTCA is superior to medical management in multivessel disease. The 2007 Clinical Outcomes Utilizing Revascularization and Aggressive Drug Evaluation (COURAGE) trial suggests that although PCI has been demonstrated to reduce death and MI in patients with ACS, for patients with chronic coronary artery disease, PCI does not reduce the incidence of death or MI as compared to medical management alone. For patients who have undergone CABG, approximately 75% can be predicted to be free from symptom recurrence, ischemic events, or sudden death after 5 years. Approximately 50% remain free after 10 years, and approximately 15% remain well after 15 years.

REFERENCES

Agency for Healthcare Research and Quality (AHRQ). *The Guide to Clinical Preventive Services: Recommendations of the U.S. Preventive Services Task Force.* 2006. Washington, DC: Agency for Healthcare Research and Quality; AHRQ Publication Number 06-0588.

Bodoen, William E, et al. Optimal medical therapy with or without PCI for stable coronary disease. (COURAGE TRIAL) *NEJM.* 2007;356(15):1503-1516.

Braunwald E. *Heart Disease: A Textbook of Cardiovascular Medicine.* 7th ed. Philadelphia, PA: Saunders; 2005.

78   Menopause

Tammy J. Lindsay, MD, & Mark Mengel, MD, MPH

KEY POINTS

- Menopause, and the perimenopausal period, is the natural transition from the reproductive years. It usually presents with a progressive lengthening of the menstrual cycle with irregular menses, hot flashes, and sleep disruption. Menopause can be confirmed when no menses have occurred for 12 months.
- A person's cultural preconceptions in a large part determine the general attitude, approach, and therefore smoothness by which this aging process occurs.
- Diagnostic testing is rarely indicated in women who are at an age when menopause is expected; however, in younger menopausal women determination of a follicle-stimulating hormone (FSH) level is warranted. Menopausal status is indicated by an FSH level of ≥30 MIU/mL.
- Menopause is associated with changes in many organ systems including skin, reproductive system and bones.
- Publication of the Women's Health Initiative (WHI) and Heart and estrogen/progestin Replacement Study (HERS) trials, revealing that synthetic estrogen/progesterone replacement therapy places women at greater risk for many significant illnesses, has resulted in a reversal of the previous widespread use of hormone replacement therapy. In postmenopausal women with debilitating symptoms at menopause, short-term use (less than 5 years) of hormone replacement therapy is appropriate, but long-term use to prevent chronic disease is no longer deemed acceptable. (SOR **A**)
- Certain drugs (clonidine, gabapentin, fluoxetine, paroxetine, and venlafaxine) and herbal treatments such as black cohosh, soy protein, and isoflavones have been shown in some studies to be modestly effective in reducing menopausal hot flashes. (SOR **B**)
- As women rapidly lose bone density once reproductive hormone secretion ceases, osteoporosis risk factor reduction, regular weight-bearing exercise, adequate intake of vitamin D and calcium, and routine use of bone density testing are indicated. (SOR **A**)

I. Introduction

A. Definitions. Menopause is the permanent cessation of menstruation caused by a loss of ovarian function. This condition can be confirmed after 12 months of amenorrhea. **Perimenopause** is the transitional period immediately prior to menopause. **Postmenopausal** is the term applied to the stage of life that involves all of the years a woman spends after menopause. **Premature menopause** is menopause that occurs before the age of 40.

B. Epidemiology

1. Between 0.2% and 1% of visits made to primary care physicians are for menopausal symptoms.

2. The mean age of menopause is 51.4 years, with a range of 41 to 59 years. A convincing risk factor associated with an earlier age of menopause is current smoking. Other factors that may play an important role include a family history of early menopause, nulliparity, and having a history of heart disease or type 1 diabetes mellitus. By 55 years of age, 95% of women are menopausal.

3. Disabling symptoms attributable to decline in estrogen production for which medical therapy is sought are estimated to occur in 10% to 15% of perimenopausal women. Current smoking and high body mass index were risk factors associated with the onset of hot flashes.

C. Pathophysiology. Menopause is associated with ovarian, hormonal, and target-organ changes. A progressive decrease in the number of ovarian follicles occurs from the 20th week of gestation in utero until the ovary is depleted of follicles at menopause. Levels of FSH dramatically increase during the perimenopausal period, while levels of plasma estradiol (the principal ovarian estrogen) decline at rates corresponding to the rise in FSH levels. Many organs have specific receptors for particular circulating steroid. Many

TABLE 78–1. END-ORGAN CHANGES RESULTING FROM ESTROGEN DEFICIENCY

Target Organ	Change or Symptom
Neuroendocrine organs (hypothalamus)	Hot flushes, flashes, or both Atrophy, dryness, pruritus
Skin/mucous membranes	Dry hair or loss of hair Facial hirsutism Dry mouth
Skeleton	Osteoporosis with related fractures Backache
Vocal cords	Lower voice
Breasts	Reduced size Softer consistency Drooping (loss of ligamentous support)
Heart	Coronary artery disease
Vulva	Atrophy, dystrophy, or both Pruritus vulvae
Vagina	Dyspareunia Vaginitis
Uterus/pelvic floor	Uterovaginal prolapse
Bladder/urethra	Cystoureteritis Ectropion Frequency and/or urgency Stress incontinence

(Adapted with permission from Utian WH. Overview on menopause. *Am J Obstet Gynecol.* 1987;156:1280.)

end-organ changes occur as a result of declining or absent circulating estrogen levels (Table 78–1).

II. **Diagnosis**

A. **Symptoms and signs.** Most women in their late 40s experience a progressive lengthening of the menstrual cycle with lighter menses. Irregular periods, caused by anovulation, are also common in the perimenopausal period.

1. **Vasomotor symptoms.** The hot flash and the flush are the two principal components of vasomotor symptomatology. Researchers believe that alterations in the hypothalamic set point because of estrogen withdrawal are responsible for the flush. Patients with such disorders as pheochromocytoma, hyperthyroidism, anxiety, excessive caffeine intake, hypoglycemia, and carcinoid syndrome usually present with vasomotor symptomatology in combination with other conditions, such as hypertension, tachycardia, and diarrhea. The presence of such concomitant conditions suggests a nonmenopausal origin.

a. The **hot flash** is the sudden onset of warmth lasting 2 to 3 minutes. Experienced by 75% to 85% of menopausal women, the hot flash begins approximately 1 minute before the flush and lasts approximately 1 minute after its onset.

b. The **flush** consists of visible redness of the upper chest, face, and neck and is followed by profuse sweating in these areas. The flush also lasts 2 to 3 minutes and is associated with a mean temperature elevation of 2.5° C (4.5°F). When left untreated, hot flushes are usually most intense and frequent in the first 1 or 2 years, after which severity gradually declines. On an average, vasomotor symptoms will last 4 years. However, 25% of women report a duration of hot flushes of more than 5 years, and occasionally symptoms persist into the seventh or eighth decade.

c. **Associated symptoms** commonly reported with the above vasomotor phenomena are heart palpitations, headache, throbbing in the head or neck, and nausea. Sleep disruption often occurs as a consequence because of the frequent nocturnal timing.

2. **Psychologic symptoms.** All the following symptoms have been reported during the perimenopausal period: fatigue, insomnia, anxiety, and depression. However, studies do not support menopause causing depression. It is felt that the sleep deprivation and possibility the many life changes (children leaving, retirement, aging parents) contributes the most to the mood fluctuations, not menopause as a state. (SOR **B**)

3. **Atrophy of the lower genital tract**
   a. **Vulvar pruritus** is common, especially in fair-skinned women.
   b. **Vaginitis and dyspareunia** from atrophy of vaginal mucosa are experienced by approximately 10% to 20% of women. Symptoms include dryness, burning, leukorrhea, itching, and bleeding.
   c. **Atrophy of the urethral mucosa,** which leads to frank urethritis, dysuria, urgency, and frequency, is less common.

4. **Signs.** The physical examination is usually normal during the early perimenopausal period, with characteristic findings evident after the onset of menopause, when the estrogen deprivation becomes visible.
   a. The **breasts** appear less firm and smaller, with a regression of glandular tissue and an increase in fatty tissue.
   b. The **pelvic examination** is most revealing in the postmenopausal period.
      (1) The **labia majora** are smaller, and hair in the perivulvar area is thin.
      (2) The **vaginal epithelium** appears pale, thin, and dry, with a loss of rugae and secretions.
      (3) The **cervical os** is often smaller and may be stenotic. The cervical epithelium is thinner and more easily traumatized.
   c. **Uterine size** is diminished. Reduced collagen in the supporting ligamentous structures of the pelvis can lead to uterine prolapse and pelvic relaxation. This relaxation occurs especially when there is a history of multiparity, prior birth trauma, a family history of uterine prolapse or pelvic relaxation, or chronic pelvic stress from coughing, constipation, or heavy work. This pelvic laxity often contributes to urinary incontinence.
   d. The **ovaries** should not be palpable after menopause. Palpable ovarian enlargement in a menopausal woman suggests ovarian carcinoma until proven otherwise.
   e. **Urethral prolapse** can occur because of atrophy of the urethral mucosa. A prolapsed urethra or caruncle appears as a red, friable mass within the urethra itself.
   f. **Dry, wrinkled, and more easily traumatized skin** is attributable to both menopause and age. Thinning of scalp hair and increased facial hair (hirsutism) may also be evident.

B. **Laboratory tests.** The presence of vasomotor symptoms, oligomenorrhea, and atrophy of the lower genital tract in women older than 45 years almost certainly confirms the onset of the perimenopausal period. Diagnostic testing (e.g., circulating estrogen and gonadotropin levels) is rarely, if ever, indicated in this circumstance.

A complete evaluation for premature ovarian failure is warranted in any woman younger than 40 years experiencing signs and symptoms of menopause. Specific causes of premature ovarian failure include genetic abnormalities, autoimmune disorders, and rare hormonal defects (see Chapter 3). FSH levels are the most sensitive indicator of ovarian failure. Menopausal status is indicated by FSH level ≥ 30 mIU/mL. As FSH levels are highly variable in the perimenopause, levels should be confirmed by a second test 1 to 3 months later.

Estradiol and progesterone are not reliably measured by single assays in perimenopausal women.

III. **Treatment.** The WHI and HERS findings have dramatically changed the use of hormone replacement therapy in postmenopausal women. (The WHI is a primary prevention trial in postmenopausal women; the HERS is a secondary prevention trial in postmenopausal women with coronary artery disease.) Both studies showed that the long-term risks of synthetic estrogen/progestin replacement therapy outweighed the benefit. Women on synthetic estrogen/progestin therapy were at greater risk for heart disease, strokes, invasive breast cancer, thromboembolic events, gallbladder disease, and dementia. Benefits included a reduction in fractures, osteoporosis, colorectal cancer, and diabetes (Table 78–2). However, given that the average age of women in both of these trials was older than 60 years and that many had risk factors for coronary artery disease, it is likely that younger women without any risk factors would have less risk of harm. Therefore, in postmenopausal women with debilitating symptoms of menopause, short-term use of hormone replacement therapy is appropriate. (SOR **A**)

A. **Indications for estrogen replacement therapy**
   1. Moderate to severe vasomotor instability.
   2. Moderate to severe genital atrophy.
   3. Diminished quality of life secondary to menopausal symptoms.

TABLE 78–2. HRT TRIALS SUMMARIES

Clinical Events	HERS Estrogen + Progestin	WHI Estrogen + Progestin	WHI Estrogen Alone
CHD events	0.99 (0.80–1.22)	1.29 (1.02–1.63)	0.91 (0.75–1.12)
Stroke	1.23 (0.89–1.70)	1.41 (1.07–1.85)	1.39 (1.1–1.77)
Pulmonary embolism	2.79 (0.89–8.75)	2.13 (1.39–3.25)	1.34 (0.87–2.06)
Breast cancer	1.30 (0.77–2.19)	1.26 (1.00–1.59)	0.77 (0.59–1.01)
Colon cancer	0.69 (0.32–1.49)	0.63 (0.43–0.92)	1.08 (0.75–1.55)
Hip fracture	1.10 (0.49–2.50)	0.66 (0.45–0.98)	0.61 (0.41–0.91)
Death	1.08 (0.84–1.38)	0.98 (0.82–1.18)	1.04 (0.88–1.22)
Global index*		1.15 (1.03–1.28)	1.01 (0.91–1.12)

CHD = coronary heart disease; HERS = Heart and estrogen/progestin Replacement Study; WHI = Women's health initiative
The global index was composed of the first occurrence of any of the events listed in the table.
Data are based on the intent-to-treat analyses.
For the primary CHD events outcome (myocardial infarction plus CHD death), the 3 trials had similar numbers of events and thus similar power. For other outcomes the smaller HERS trial has fewer events and less precise hazard ratios.
(Reproduced with permission from Hulley, SB, Grady D. The WHI estrogen-alone trial—do things look any better? *JAMA.* 2004;291:1769. Copyright © 2004 American Medical Association.)

   4. Osteoporosis prevention when other treatment options are contraindicated and patient is at significant risk for fracture.
B. **Contraindications to estrogen replacement therapy**
   1. Estrogen-dependent neoplasia (breast or endometrium).
   2. Undiagnosed vaginal bleeding.
   3. Past history of venousthromboembolism (deep venous thrombus, pulmonary embolus)
   4. Past history of arterial thromboembolism within 12 months (cerebral vascular accident or coronary artery disease).
   5. Liver disease.
   6. Caution, if several cardiovascular risk factors such as hypertension, hyperlipemia, tobacco abuse, or diabetes mellitus are present.
   7. Caution, if gallbladder disease is present.
   8. Caution, if age is above 65 years.
C. **Preparations available.** Estrogen is available as a pill, patch, topical gel and emulsion, vaginal ring, or cream.
   1. **Pills.** The oldest available and most widely prescribed oral estrogen preparation is equine conjugated estrogen (Premarin), 0.30 to 2.5 mg orally every day. The typical starting dose was 0.625 mg; however, lower doses of 0.45 and 0.3 mg are proving to be effective for both vasomotor symptoms as well as osteoporosis prevention. (SOR Ⓐ) Synthetic conjugated estrogen (Cenestin and Menest), 0.3 to 2.5 mg orally every day, micronized estradiol (Estrace and Gynodiol), 0.5 mg to 2 mg orally every day, ethinyl estradiol (Estinyl), 0.02 to 0.05 mg orally every day, and estropipate (Ogen or Ortho-est), 0.75 to 6 mg orally every day, are also available. Many women prefer the nonequine varieties of estrogen, fearing the effects of the metabolic breakdown products of that preparation. A 28-day supply of these preparations typically costs $25 to $40, with generic micronized estradiol being the least expensive, at under $10 for a 28-day supply.
   2. **Patches.** Transdermal estradiol patches are available at a dose of 25 to 100 μg/d. Many preparations are available, including Climera and Menostar (both one patch weekly), and Estraderm, Alora, Vivelle, Vivelle-dot, and Esclim (all one patch 2 times per week). Patches are typically more expensive, $40 to $50 for a 28-day supply. The advantage of patches is that they have a limited effect on hepatic function and preliminary evidence suggests that there is less risk of thromboembolic complications than with other estrogen preparations. (SOR Ⓑ) Unfortunately, approximately 24% of women who use this method have some form of skin irritation, which often can be managed by site rotation.
   3. **Vaginal rings.** An estradiol acetate vaginal ring (Femring) was recently approved by the US Food and Drug Administration at doses of 50 to 100 μg/d, lasting 90 days. Estring is a vaginal ring that provides 7.5 μg/d of estradiol, a very low dose, and is

used only for treating vaginal symptoms. The cost is approximate $110 to $130 each. Given that one is good for 3 months, the 28-day cost is comparable to other HRT methods.

4. **Topical gel and emulsion.** Estradiol can also be given topically in a gel form (Estrogel), 0.75 mg/pump, applied to the arms, and in an emulision form (Estrasorb), 0.025 mg/pouch, one pouch applied to each leg daily. The cost is higher, $50 to $120 for a 28-day supply of the gel and emulsion respectively.

5. **Vaginal creams.** Vaginal creams are most useful for those women with severe symptoms of atopic vaginitis but have mild vasomotor symptoms. Intervaginal creams, such as conjugated estrogen (Premarin), 0.625 mg/g, and estradiol (Estrace vaginal cream), 0.1 mg/g, may be helpful. Daily administration of 1.2 to 2.4 g is typically recommended on days 1 to 21 of the month, although continuous therapy on weekdays only is increasingly popular. Intervaginal estrogen creams do achieve some systemic absorption.

Vulvovaginal pruritus responds poorly to topical estrogens. Other treatments may be more helpful such as cotton underwear, adequate drying, loose fitting clothing, and steroid creams such as clobetasol proprionate titrated to the lowest effective dose. (SOR Ⓐ) Testosterone ointment is no longer recommended. (SOR Ⓑ)

D. **Progestins** have been shown to relieve vasomotor symptoms in postmenopausal patients either alone or in combination with estrogens. They are also useful in preventing endometrial hyperplasia in women on estrogen replacement therapy. (SOR Ⓐ)

1. **Progestin-only regimens.** Medroxyprogesterone acetate (Provera), 20 mg orally daily, is especially appealing for women for whom estrogen therapy is contraindicated or who have experienced intolerable side effects, such as breast tenderness, breakthrough bleeding, and nausea, on estrogen therapy. Other preparations include progesterone (Prometrium) and norethindrone acetate (Aygestin).

2. **Combination estrogen and progestin therapy.** Estrogen replacement alone may lead to endometrial hyperplasia which, in a small group of women, progresses to endometrial carcinoma. Maximal protection against endometrial hyperplasia occurs when progestin is prescribed for at least 10 days of each calendar month. Because that regimen usually results in periods continuing, continuous daily combination therapy is often preferred. There are several options available. In tablet form, Premarin and Provera are combined in two different options, Prempro (continuous) and Premphase (cyclic). Prempro is available in multiple dosing options 0.3 to 1.5 mg, 0.45 to 1.5 mg, 0.625 to 2.5 mg, 0.625 to 5 mg. Other options include ethinyl estradiol, norethindrone acetate (FemHrt), estradiol, norgestimate (Ortho-Prefest), and estradiol, norethindrone (Activella). Combination patch therapy is also available in estradiol, norethindrone acetate (Combipatch) and estradiol, levonorgestrel (Climara Pro).

Progestin use for women who have had a hysterectomy and are receiving estrogen replacement therapy is not indicated. (SOR Ⓐ)

E. **Effective nonhormonal treatments for menopausal symptoms.** Given the results of the WHI and HERS studies, nonhormonal treatments for menopausal symptoms have become more popular. Effective treatments include: (SOR Ⓑ for all)

1. Clonidine (Catapres), 0.1 to 0.2 mg/d.
2. Gabapentin (Neurontin), 300 mg orally 3 times daily.
3. Venlafaxine (Effexor), 37.5 to 150 mg orally every day.
4. Paroxetine (Paxil), 20 to 40 mg orally every day.
5. Fluoxetine (Prozac), 20 mg/d.
6. Black cohosh, 16 to 127 mg/d.
7. Soy and other isoflavones, 40 to 164 mg/d.

F. **Selective estrogen-receptor modulators.** Raloxifene, 60 mg orally every day, a drug that has both estrogen-agonist effects on bone, liver, and heart and estrogen-antagonist effects on breast and uterus, has been shown to reduce risks of breast cancer and osteoporosis in postmenopausal women. These effects make raloxifene an attractive alternative for those women concerned with estrogen's potential for cancer proliferation. Unfortunately, raloxifene has no effect on genital atrophy and may worsen the vasomotor symptoms of hot flashes and sweats. Like estrogen, the incidence of thrombophlebitis is increased compared with placebo. A 30-day supply costs $80 to $90.

G. **Complementary and alternative medicine treatments**

1. Regular exercise has proven effective in one small trial for hot flash prevention. Since the effects are helpful in general well being, important in the prevention of obesity,

TABLE 78–3. KEY QUESTIONS TO UNCOVER SEXUAL PROBLEMS DURING THE PERIMENOPAUSAL AND POSTMENOPAUSAL PERIODS

Are you sexually active?
Do you have a partner at the present time?
Has there been any change in your interest in or desire for sexual activity?
Is intercourse pleasurable?
Do you experience any discomfort during intercourse?
Have you noticed any change in lubrication when you become aroused?
Do you reach orgasm satisfactorily?
Does your partner have any problems with your sexual relationship?

(Adapted with permission from Iddenden DA. Sexuality during the menopause. *Med Clin North Am.* 1987;71:87.)

diabetes, hypertension, and osteoporosis, this recommendation goes beyond simple symptomatic treatment. (SOR **B**)

2. **Dong quai and ginseng appear not to work.** Wild yams are promoted as a "natural" precursor to hormones, but are not converted to reproductive hormones in the human body and have not proven more effective than placebo in one small trial. (SOR **B**)

3. **Bio-identical hormone replacement.** "Antiaging" advocates promote the use of bio-identical or natural estrogen, progestin, and testosterone replacement, feeling that natural hormone replacement will lack the risks and side effects of synthetic hormone replacement. The North American Menopause Society "does not recommend custom-compounded products over well-tested, government-approved proved products for the majority of women and does not recommend saliva testing to determine hormone levels." (SOR **C**)

IV. **Management Strategies**

A. **Patient education.** For many women, the worst thing about menopause is not knowing what to expect. Thorough evaluation of the woman's understanding of menopause and accurate education directed at identification of symptoms and management options will greatly reduce anxiety in many postmenopausal women. Many myths surround menopause, including that menopause signals the end of a woman's sexual experience and that menopause is associated with a high incidence of mental health problems, cancer, and heart disease. Risk factor reduction for heart disease and cancer, a discussion of the patient's sexual interest and activities, and pertinent patient education is a good starting point (Table 78–3). The final two references are available online and are a part of a growing body of patient oriented, web-based information.

B. **Patient follow-up**

1. **Periodic follow-up visits** are needed to monitor women on hormone replacement therapy. Women should be specifically questioned on known side effects of hormone replacement therapy at every visit. Hormone replacement therapy should be reduced as symptoms abate and stopped as soon as possible. It is recommended that after 1 to 2 years of treatment, that titration of HRT is attempted every 3 to 6 months. Current recommendations state that women should not be on hormone replacement therapy for longer than 5 years. (SOR **A**) The newer black box warnings associated with HRT should be reviewed with the patient. Dementia risk may go up after 4 to 5 years of therapy in those older than 65 years. (SOR **B**) Risk of heart disease, breast cancer, stroke, and pulmonary embolus are all small individually but increase with time. (SOR **A**) Current recommendations are that HRT is used at the lowest possible dose for the shortest amount of time. (SOR **A**)

2. **Endometrial biopsy.** Vaginal bleeding in a woman on hormone replacement therapy demands evaluation with either an endometrial biopsy and/or a vaginal ultrasound measuring the endometrial stripe. If the endometrial stripe on ultrasound is less than 5 mm, endometrial cancer is rare. Biopsies every 2 to 3 years for women at particularly high risk for endometrial cancer, even if asymptomatic, have been suggested as prudent.

3. **Osteoporosis management.** Women rapidly lose bone density once reproductive hormone secretion ceases. Risk factor reduction, weight-bearing exercise, adequate intake of vitamin D and calcium, and routine use of bone density testing are all indicated (see Chapter 81 on Osteoporosis).

REFERENCES

Armstrong C. NAMS updates recommendations on diagnosis and management of osteoporosis in postmenopausal women. *Am Fam Physician.* 2006;74:1631-1634, 1636, 1639.

Carroll DG. Nonhormonal therapies for hot flashes in menopause. *Am Fam Physician.* 2006;73:457-464, 467.

Freeman R, Lewis RM. The therapeutic role of estrogens in prostmenopausal women. *Endocrinol Metab Clin N Am.* 2004;33:771-789.

Grady D. Management of menopausal symptoms. *N Engl J Med.* 2006;355:2338-2347.

Harris D. *Menopause Guidebook.* 6th edition. Cleveland, OH: The North American Menopause Society; 2006.

National Heart, Lung, and Blood Institute. *Facts about menopausal hormonal therapy.* October 2002, revised June 2005 NIH publication 05-5200. www.nhlbi.nih.gov/health/woman/pht_facts.pdf. Accessed April 22, 2007.

Nelson HD, Haney E, Humphrey L, et al. *Management of Menopause-Related Symptoms.* Rockville, MD: Agency for Healthcare Research and Quality; 2005. Summary, Evidence Report/Technology Assessment No. 120. AHRQ publication 05-E016-1.

North American Menopause Society. Amended report from the NAMS Advisory Panel on Postmenopausal Hormone Therapy. *Menopause.* 2003;10(1):6.

Rossouw JE, et al. Risks and benefits of estrogen plus progestin in healthy postmenopausal women: Principal results from the Women's Health Initiative randomized controlled trial. *JAMA.* 2002;288(3):321.

U.S. Preventive Services Task Force. Postmenopausal hormone replacement therapy for the primary prevention of chronic conditions. Recommendations and rationale. *Am Fam Physician.* 2003;67(2):358.

---

79   Obesity

Radhika R. Hariharan, MD, MRCP (UK), Brian C. Reed, MD, & Sarah R. Edmonson, MD

KEY POINTS

- Obesity is diagnosed when the body mass index is ≥ 30 kg/m^2.
- The primary goal of treatment should be weight loss of at least 10% of initial body weight. Maintenance of this new weight is the next priority.
- Strategies for weight loss include a low-calorie diet, which is the cornerstone of management, along with exercise, behavioral therapies, and medications.
- Drug therapy is indicated when other therapies fail after 3 months of trial or when there is medical comorbidity indicating a need for more aggressive weight loss.
- Drug therapy should be viewed as long-term and the risks should be carefully considered in the individual patient.
- Bariatric surgery is an appropriate alternative for those patients who have failed conventional therapy; long- and short-term risks should be considered carefully before considering surgery.

I. Introduction
A. Definitions
1. **Obesity** is a disorder that occurs when a person has such an excess amount of body fat that they are at risk for adverse health conditions.
2. **Body mass index (BMI).** In 1997, the World Health Organization International Obesity Task Force recommended adoption of BMI as a standard for the assessment of body fat. (SOR **C**) BMI is calculated by dividing a person's weight in kilograms by one's height in meters squared. Based on these guidelines, one is considered **overweight** at a body mass index between 25.0 and 29.9 kg/m^2. A BMI ≥ 30 kg/m^2 meets the criteria for **obesity** (see Table 79–1).

TABLE 79–1. WORLD HEALTH ORGANIZATION CATEGORIZATION OF OBESITY

Body Mass Index (kg/m^2)	
Normal	18.5–24.9
Overweight	25–29.9
Obesity class I	30–34.9
Obesity class II	35–39.9
Obesity class III	$\geq$40

B. **Epidemiology**
  1. **Prevalence.** Over 97 million adults in the United States are overweight or obese. Data from the National Health and Nutrition Examination Survey (NHANES) conducted in 2003 and 2004 reveal that the prevalence of obesity among adults aged 20 years or older in the United States was 32.2%. The percentage of overweight adults in the United States is 66.3%.
  2. **Risk factors**
      a. **Race.** The most recent NHANES survey revealed that higher percentages of non-Hispanic blacks and Mexican Americans are either obese or overweight when compared to similar nonHispanic whites in similar age categories. Among nonHispanic blacks, 76.1% of individuals older than age 20 meet the criteria for being overweight and 45.0% meet the criteria for obesity. Data revealed that 75.8% of Mexican Americans met the criteria for being overweight and 36.8% of Mexican American adults met the criteria for being obese. Of nonHispanic whites older than 20 years, 64.2% meet the criteria for being overweight and 30.6% meet the criteria for being obese.
      b. **Age.** The prevalence of obesity increases with age and is particularly apparent between the ages of 40 and 60 years.
      c. **Inactivity.** The relative risk of obesity among children in the United States is 5.3 times greater for children who watch television for 5 or more hours a day compared with those who watched television for $\leq$2 hours. This is valid even after correcting for a wide range of socioeconomic variables.
      d. **Socioeconomic status.** In industrialized countries, a higher prevalence of obesity is seen in those with lower educational levels and low income.
      e. **Marital status.** A tendency to increase weight after marriage and parity exists.
  3. Current trends suggest that the prevalence of obesity will continue to increase.
C. **Etiology**
  1. Obesity represents a heterogeneous group of conditions with multiple causes. By definition, it results from imbalance between energy intake and expenditure. Energy expenditure is primarily derived from the resting metabolic rate and physical activity.
  2. **Environmental factors.** Migrant studies attest to the critical role of environment in the development of obesity. A marked change in BMI is frequently observed when populations with a common genetic heritage live under new circumstances of plentiful food and little exercise. Pima Indians in the United States, for example, are on average approximately 25 kg heavier than Pima Indians in Mexico.
  3. **Genetic factors**
      a. Evidence from several twin and adoption studies shows a strong genetic predisposition in obesity. Recently, specific mutations causing human obesity have been found in those rare children with extreme obesity with a clear evidence for monogenic inheritance. Genetic syndromes associated with severe obesity include Prader-Willi, Bardet-Biedl, Cohen, Alstrom, and Klinefelter's syndromes.
      b. The discovery of leptin, a novel adipocyte hormone, which is deficient in the obese ob/ob mouse, has significantly advanced the understanding of the neurobiology of obesity. Several mutations in leptin and leptin receptor have also been shown to cause monogenic human obesity.
      c. Genetic studies in the more common forms of obesity have shown a region of chromosome 2 that influences obesity-related phenotypes in several different racial groups. This region contains the pro-opiomelanocortin gene.
  4. **Gene–environment interaction.** Body weight is determined by an interaction between genetic, environmental, and psychosocial factors. Although obesity runs in families, the influence of the genotype on the etiology may be modified by nongenetic factors. The genetic influences seem to operate through susceptibility genes, which increase the

TABLE 79–2. RISK ASSESSMENT IN OBESITY

	Normal/ OverWeight	Obesity Class I	Obesity Class II	Obesity Class III
Waist circumference ≤40 inches (male) or ≤35 inches (female)	Low risk	Moderate risk	Moderate risk	High risk
Waist circumference ≥40 inches (male) or ≥35 inches (female)	Moderate risk		High risk	
Presence of comorbidities such as osteoarthritis, gallstones, stress incontinence, and menstrual irregularities		High risk		
Presence of comorbidities such as established coronary artery disease, other atherosclerotic disease, type 2 diabetes mellitus, and sleep apnea	High risk			

risk of developing obesity. The susceptible gene hypothesis is supported by findings from twin studies, in which pairs of twins were exposed to varying energy balance. The differences in the rate, proportion, and site of weight gain showed greater similarity within pairs than between pairs of twins.

5. **Other causes.** Medical conditions and some medications, such as long-term corticosteroid use, phenothiazines, and antidepressants, can also result in obesity, but such causes account for ≤1% of cases. Hypothyroidism and Cushing's syndrome are the most common diseases that cause obesity. Diseases of the hypothalamus can also result in obesity, but these are quite rare. Major depression, which usually results in weight loss, can occasionally present with weight gain. Consideration of these causes is particularly important when evaluating recent weight gain.

II. Diagnosis

A. **Assessment** of a patient's weight involves evaluation of **three key measures: BMI, waist circumference, and an individual's risk factors for diseases and conditions associated with obesity** (Table 79–2).

1. Assessing waist circumference is important because excess abdominal fat is an independent predictor of disease risk. Android obesity (excess fat located primarily in the abdomen or upper body) places an individual at greater risk for congestive heart disease, hypertension, lipid disorders, and type 2 diabetes mellitus, whereas gynoid obesity (excess fat located primarily in the lower extremities or hips) does not. A waist circumference of ≥40 inches in men and ≥35 inches in women signifies increased risk in those who have a BMI of 25 to 34.9.

2. Gross calculation of BMI is not an effective estimation of risk in the following subgroups:

   a. In children and adolescents, the appropriate ratio of weight to height differs from that for infants and toddlers; this ratio must be assessed on an age- and gender-specific table. Excessive calorie intake in children will usually manifest itself in additional height as well as excess weight. As such, children who demonstrate exceptional height should be evaluated for lifestyle factors that put them at risk for obesity.

   b. Individuals who are ≤4 feet tall, or ≥7 feet tall, cannot be evaluated with a BMI. For these individuals, secondary measures may be used, such as body fat analysis or fitness testing.

   c. Competitive athletes and bodybuilders may have misleadingly high-BMI levels. These patients often have low total body fat and excellent cardiovascular fitness. Although long-term survival data about this subgroup of patients is sparse, it seems likely that their excess muscle mass does not represent the same risk as in other overweight patients.

   d. Pregnant women should not use BMI to evaluate risk, particularly in the second or third trimester.

B. Screening for medical conditions that may promote obesity should be performed.

1. Endocrine disorders that promote weight gain, such as thyroid disease, hyperandrogenism or polycystic ovarian syndrome, and hypercortisolism, are generally accompanied by global symptoms such as skin changes, hair loss and distribution changes,

abnormal menstrual cycles, mood and energy derangement, gastrointestinal distress, and atypical fat distribution. In patients who demonstrate some or all of these symptoms, laboratory evaluation should precede weight-loss efforts.

2. Many medications are associated with weight gain, including corticosteroids, insulin or insulin secretagogues, antiepileptics, anxiolytics or antidepressants, and antipsychotics. Weight-loss plans are not necessarily contraindicated for patients on these drugs. However, changing therapy when possible will increase the patient's chance of successful weight loss.

3. Assess the patient for the presence of comorbid **psychiatric disease** that could affect their ability to understand and follow a dietary plan.

C. **Assess comorbidities**

1. Established coronary artery disease, other atherosclerotic disease, type 2 diabetes mellitus, and sleep apnea are considered to be very high-risk comorbidities. Patients with these conditions should be offered aggressive weight management.

2. Osteoarthritis, gallstones, stress incontinence, and menstrual irregularities, while also associated with obesity, are less life-threatening.

3. Other conditions that may increase mortality risk in association with obesity include hypertension, smoking, hyperlipidemia, elevated fasting glucose, and increased age.

D. **Dietary history.** Dietary history should include information about both typical daily intake and deviations from this routine. Information should be collected about family events, celebratory behavior, and binge eating behavior. The frequency and type of atypical behavior should be noted. Specifically inquire about high-calorie beverages, such as soda, juice, or milk. Alcohol intake should be noted and quantified.

E. **Exercise** history should include type, intensity, duration, and frequency. Encourage the patient to list informal physical activity at work or home in addition to deliberate attempts to exercise.

F. **Laboratory evaluation.** To rule out secondary causes and assess for comorbid conditions, an initial laboratory evaluation, including a fasting lipid profile, fasting chemistry panel including blood glucose, and a thyroid-stimulating hormone test, should be ordered.

III. **Treatment.** The aim of a treatment program should be to reduce weight and maintain lowered weight. The goals of treatment should be tailored to the individual. In general, the primary goal is a 10% reduction from the initial weight. Successful weight loss should be regarded as a loss of more than 5% of the initial weight while very successful weight loss would be that of greater than 20% of initial body weight. A loss of 10% of body weight is of major clinical benefit with associated changes such as lowered blood pressure, lowered total cholesterol and triglycerides, an increase in high-density lipoprotein (HDL) cholesterol, and a significant improvement in diabetic control. One appropriate treatment algorithm is described in Figure 79–1.

A. **Dietary interventions**

1. Diet control is the cornerstone of obesity management and its primary role should be emphasized to the patient. In order to successfully lose weight, one must create a deficit of 500 to 1000 kcal/d. There are several dietary approaches to achieve this goal.

a. Low-calorie diets consisting of approximately 1000 to 1200 kcal/d have been successfully demonstrated to result in weight loss and decreases of abdominal fat. (SOR **A**)

b. Very low-calorie diets that only permit 400 to 500 kcal/d promote initial weight loss between 13 and 23 kg. However, randomized controlled trials have shown that very low-calorie diets do not result in greater long-term weight loss when compared to low-calorie diets after 1 year. (SOR **A**)

2. In addition to the total caloric intake, the patient may benefit from changes in the dietary composition.

a. Lower-fat diets promote weight loss by limiting the percentage of daily calories from fat to 20% to 30%. Because dietary fat intake has been associated with cholesterol levels, heart disease, and increased risks for certain cancers, this approach may be desirable for patients with multiple comorbid conditions.

b. Low-carbohydrate diets such as the South Beach diet and the Zone diet are based upon the theory that overweight and obese people are efficient at converting excess carbohydrates into fat. Low-carbohydrate diets advocate restricting total daily carbohydrates to between 40 and 100 g/d. Currently there is insufficient evidence to make recommendations for or against such low-carbohydrate diets.

(1) The South Beach diet distinguishes itself from the Atkins diet using the glycemic index of foods to distinguish between "good" and "bad" carbohydrates and

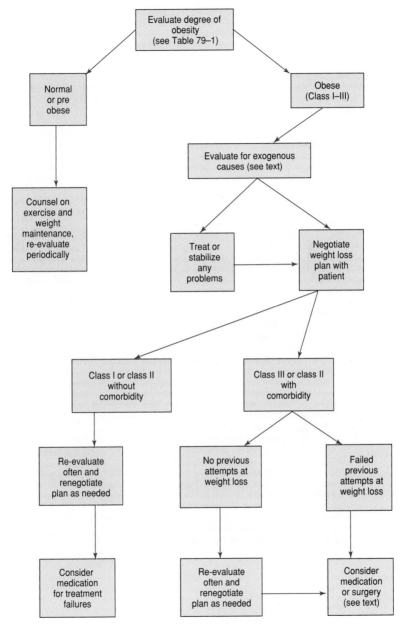

FIGURE 79–1. Treatment algorithm for obesity.

permitting moderate consumption of carbohydrates after the first 2 weeks. The South Beach diet seeks to also lower cholesterol and triglycerides by promoting heart healthy fats and whole grains.

(2) The Zone diet attempts to keep insulin levels at a steady state by adhering to a diet that consists of meals that are 40% carbohydrates, 30% protein, and 30% fat.

B. Behavioral therapy

1. Behavioral therapy refers to the application of psychologic techniques to treatment of obesity and is now an accepted modality of treatment. Behavioral weight programs seek to alter lifestyle and environment in order to effect a change in weight. They encourage the patient to become more aware of eating behavior and physical activity, and to focus on changing the behaviors that influence them. The chief feature of this form of treatment is that it emphasizes personal responsibility for the initiation and maintenance of treatment.

2. Behavior therapy is usually presented in an organized and comprehensive format and includes several components including stimulus control, self-reward, and cognitive restructuring.

3. Although the degree of weight loss achieved with behavioral techniques alone is modest, averaging less than 10 kg in most studies, the advantages include the lack of side effects and the low-attrition rate. (SOR **B**)

C. Exercise. While exercise alone results in only modest weight loss, randomized controlled trials consistently show the maintenance of weight loss for 2 years. (SOR **A**) A combination of diet and exercise generally produces more weight loss than diet alone. Regular exercise results in reduction in blood pressure and improvements in lipid profiles, glycemic control, and cardiovascular fitness. Persuading an obese patient to participate and maintain an exercise program is difficult. Less vigorous forms of activity such as brisk walking and swimming may also provide significant improvement in metabolic profiles.

D. Pharmacotherapy of obesity

1. **Indications, see Table 79–3.**

   a. **Strength of recommendations:** Obesity management guidelines differ on the utility of medications in the management of obesity.

      (1) The National Heart, Lung, and Blood Institute (NHLBI) of the National Institutes of Health issued a 1998 report recommending consideration of pharmacotherapy, in addition to lifestyle modification, for high-risk patients (Table 79–2) whose obesity has not responded to lifestyle modification alone. (SOR **C**)

      (2) The Canadian Task Force on obesity, on the other hand, concluded that there is insufficient data to evaluate the long-term effectiveness of pharmacotherapy in obesity treatment. (SOR **C**)

   b. Since weight loss with medications is maintained only for the duration of drug use, short-term use is generally unsuccessful. The long-term risks and benefits in the individual patient should be carefully weighed.

   c. At present, no medications have been approved for treatment of pediatric obesity.

   d. Weight loss drugs are not appropriate in pregnancy.

   e. **Combination therapy** in obesity treatment and maintenance is currently not recommended. While it is possible that safe combinations will eventually be developed, there are little data from large trials to support this at this time. (SOR **C**)

2. **Pharmacotherapeutic mechanisms**

   a. **Appetite suppressants (anorexiants)** decrease appetite or increase satiety. Currently approved anorexiants function primarily by increasing the level of anorexigenic neurotransmitters such as norepinephrine, dopamine, and serotonin

---

TABLE 79–3. NHLBI INDICATIONS FOR PHARMACOTHERAPY OF OBESITY

BMI ≥30

OR

waist circumference ≥35 "(women) or ≥40" (men)

OR

BMI ≥27 with presence of an additional risk factor for obesity-related disease (such as hyperlipidemia, diabetes, or hypertension)

in the central nervous system. Agents which selectively antagonize cannabinoid receptor-1 also suppress appetite. Many anorexiants also act as thermogenic agents, which increase energy expenditure.

  b. **Lipid-partitioning drugs** decrease energy intake by blocking absorption of dietary fat from the intestinal lumen.

  c. **Investigational targets for obesity pharmacotherapy** include beta-adrenergic receptor antagonists, which mediate catecholamine-stimulated thermogenesis in brown adipose tissue; and leptin, a catabolic hormone that plays a role in energy regulation.

3. **Medications approved for treatment of obesity**

  a. Table 79–4 compares the products that are currently approved in the United States for treatment of obesity, as well as one agent that is marketed outside of the United States and expected to receive domestic approval soon.

  b. None of these medications is effective at promoting weight loss in the absence of lifestyle change.

  c. There are no studies about the longer-term safety and efficacy of these medicines, or about whether weight loss achieved with them results in long-term decreases in obesity-related morbidity and mortality.

4. **Medications used off-label for obesity management**

  a. Some selective serotonin reuptake inhibitors, such as fluoxetine, fluvoxamine, and sertraline, have been shown to induce weight loss in short-term studies. In longer-term studies, outcomes are less consistent. (SOR **B**) These agents may be particularly helpful for patients with binge-eating disorder.

  b. Bupropion (Wellbutrin) has been associated with weight loss after 6 to 12 months use by depressed subjects. (SOR **B**) Prospective studies on nondepressed patients are not available.

  c. Insulin mediating agents such as metformin (Glucophage), Exenatide (Byetta), and Pramlintide (Amylin) have been associated with weight loss as a secondary effect in diabetic patients. (SOR **B**) Trials in nondiabetic patients are underway for metformin.

  d. The antiepilepsy drugs topiramate (Topomax) and zonisamide (Zonegran) have been demonstrated by randomized prospective trial (SOR **A**) to cause weight loss in nonepileptic patients, although trial results are quite heterogenous.

5. **Dietary supplements for obesity management**

  a. Agents such as chitosan, chromium picolinate, conjugated linoleic acid, and garcinia cambogia have been promoted for weight loss. Although some of these substances have mechanisms of action that could lead to weight loss, there are insufficient data at this time to indicate safety and efficacy.

  b. Ephedrine, an adrenergic agent with thermogenic and appetite suppressant properties, has been found in controlled studies to promote weight loss. Short-term randomized double-blind, placebo-controlled studies with herbal products containing ephedra alkaloids and caffeine have indicated efficacy in promoting weight loss. Dietary supplements with ephedra (ma huang) have unpredictable and unstandardized amounts of active ingredients and are not recommended. Side effects may be serious and include hypertension, arrhythmias, myocardial infarcts, seizures, stroke, and sudden death. In April of 2004, the FDA prohibited the sale of weight loss supplements that contain ephedrine.

6. **Drugs that are *not* recommended for obesity management**

  a. **Amphetamines** are associated with weight loss. However, because of the potential for abuse, amphetamines are not recommended for routine use.

  b. **Human growth hormone** has been suggested as a potential weight-loss agent, but prospective trials failed to show any effectiveness.

7. **No longer available**

  a. **Phenylpropanolamine**, the only over-the-counter appetite suppressant approved for obesity management, was recently withdrawn because of concerns about its association with hemorrhagic stroke in women.

  b. **Fenfluramine (Pondimin) and dexfenfluramine (Redux)**, both serotoninergic agents, were withdrawn in 1997 following association with pulmonary hypertension and valvular heart disease. Unlike the pure serotoninergic agents, sibutramine does not induce serotonin release and has not been associated with valvular heart disease.

TABLE 79–4. COMPARISON OF DRUGS CURRENTLY APPROVED IN THE UNITED STATES FOR PHARMACOTHERAPY OF OBESITY

	Lipid-Partitioning	Anorexiants		Rimonabant*
Generic	Orlistat (Xenical)	Phentermine† (Ionamin, Fastin);	Sibutramine (Meridia)	Rimonabant*
Mechanism	Gastrointestinal lipase inhibitor	Noradrenergic agonist	Mixed noradrenergic/serotonergic agonist	Cannabinoid receptor-1 antagonist
FDA approval	Long-term: up to 2 y	Short term: 3 mo	Long-term: up to 2 y	Pending
Dosing	120 mg 3 times daily with fatty meal	18.5–37.5 mg daily or split dose	5–15 mg daily	20 mg daily
Cost	$5–$6/d	$1–$2/d	$3–$4/d	n/a
Efficacy	9% preintervention weight; 2–3 kg better than placebo at 12 mo; 35% regain off meds (SOR Ⓐ)	Loss of 3–4 kg greater than placebo. Regain common. (SOR Ⓐ)	5%–8% preintervention weight; 4–5 kg better than placebo at 12 mo; 50% regain second year of therapy (SOR Ⓐ)	4–5 kg over placebo at 12 mo. Up to 100% regain off meds (SOR Ⓐ)
Other effects	Improvements in insulin levels, total cholesterol, LDL, hemoglobin A1 c, and blood pressure	No independent effects on obesity-related conditions reported.	Beneficial effects in glycemic control, insulin levels. Variable effects hyperlipidemia, hypertension	Improvement in waist circ., HDL, triglycerides, insulin resistance
Side effects	Oily or loose stools, flatulence, reduced absorption of fat-soluble nutrients such as vitamins E, D, K	Adrenergic stimulation, including insomnia, dry mouth, constipation, palpitations, and insomnia.	Dry mouth, constipation, drowsiness or insomnia, headache, elevated blood pressure, tachycardia	Nausea, dizziness, diarrhea, joint pain, depression, anxiety. May help smoking cessation.
Interactions	Cyclosporine, statins (potentiate effect), Warfarin, fat-soluble vitamin supplements	SSRIs, tricyclics, guanethidine, any sympathomimetic	Many interactions: includes common antibiotics, cold and pain medications, and antidepressants	No information yet available from FDA
		May be habit-forming.	May be habit-forming.	
Warnings	Use with caution in biliary, inflammatory bowel disease	Contraindicated in patients using sympathomimetics, MAOIs, furisolidone.	Use with caution with hypertension, stroke, heart disease, biliary, liver, or kidney disease.	No information yet available from FDA

*currently marketed under the trade name Acomplia in the United Kingdom and elsewhere; US FDA approval review scheduled for June 2007.
† Phendimetrazine (Bontril); Benzphetamine (Didrex) also available in the USA.

E. Surgical treatment of obesity may be very effective for a carefully selected group of morbidly obese adults. Recent advances have made these procedures safer and possibly more effective but very little data exists about the long-term safety and efficacy of bariatric surgeries. Recently developed laparoscopic approaches have reduced the complication rates of bariatric surgery, which has increased the popularity of these procedures in recent years.

1. Secondary effects. Bariatric surgery has been observed to improve insulin sensitivity, blood pressure, left ventricular ejection fraction, cholesterol and triglyceride levels, sleep apnea, fertility, menstrual irregularity, and urinary stress incontinence. These procedures have also been postulated to affect neuroendocrine feedback loops associated with satiety and food-seeking behavior as well as maintenance of metabolic rate, with variable results on long-term hunger levels and specific food cravings.

2. Selection criteria

   a. Bariatric surgery is indicated for the well-motivated, well-informed patient whose BMI is ≥ 40, or patients with a BMI of ≥ 35 who are experiencing significant obesity-related comorbid diseases such as type 2 diabetes mellitus. (SOR **C**) Patients should have failed at nonsurgical attempts at weight reduction.

   b. Bariatric surgery is contraindicated in patients with significant psychiatric disease or instability, alcohol or drug abuse, cardiac or other medical conditions that lead to high risk of intraoperative mortality, presence of endocrine disorders that promote obesity, inability to understand risks and benefits of surgery, children, and pregnant patients.

3. Types of surgery

   a. Procedures that limit intake include adjustable **gastric banding** and **stapled gastroplasty.** Stapled gastroplasty involves a partitioning of the stomach close to the gastroesophageal junction and creation of a small-caliber gastric outlet to the small intestine. In adjustable gastric banding, a diameter-limiting prosthetic device is placed about the gastric body; this device may be adjusted in size through a subcutaneous reservoir. Because of the reduced gastric capacity the patient reaches satiety earlier in the meal and presumably eats fewer calories.

   (1) Risks. Immediate postoperative complications may include surgical infection or wound dehiscence. Patients may develop severe gastroesophageal reflux or vomiting, chronic abdominal pain, obstructive disease, and incisional hernias. Up to 20% of patients may require reoperation for surgical correction of severe dysfunction, including stomal outlet stenosis. Gastric banding may cause foreign body reactions or gastric body erosions leading to emergency surgery.

   (2) Outcomes. Early weight-loss results from these procedures can be up to 60% of the preoperative excess weight. Many patients regain a substantial proportion of their lost weight within 5 years of surgery. By the tenth year after surgery, a nearly 80% failure rate is reported. (SOR **A**)

   b. Procedures that promote malabsorption include gastric bypass procedures that not only reduce the size of the stomach pouch but also bypass a portion of the small intestine, causing variable amounts of caloric malabsorption. The most popular procedure is the Roux-en-Y bypass, in which a small stomach pouch is anastomosed to the midjejunum; the bypassed sections of duodenum and jejunum are all or partially left as a blind-ended pouch. More recent techniques vary the anatomic arrangement of bypassed sections in order to maximize caloric malabsorption while preserving absorption of important nutrients. Other gastric bypass techniques include the biliopancreatic bypass, the distal Roux-en-Y, and the duodenal switch.

   (1) Risks. Perioperative complications, such as pulmonary embolus and gastrointestinal leakage, may be as high as 15% with a 1% mortality rate. Long-term morbidity is strongly linked to malabsorptive syndromes, including anemia, fat-soluble vitamin deficiencies, and protein-calorie malnutrition. Diarrhea is typical after these surgeries. Some patients may develop dumping syndrome, an intense physiologic reaction when poorly digested food is deposited lower in the digestive tract. Dumping syndrome causes nausea, bloating, diarrhea, colic, lightheadedness, palpitations, and sweating.

   (2) Outcomes. Initial weight-loss results are excellent, with a mean loss of 75% to 80% of excess weight. Longer-term efficacy is less well established, but appears to be better than volume restriction procedures.

4. **Long-term outcomes of bariatric surgery:** The Swedish Obese Subjects (SOS) study reports metabolic and cardiovascular effects of bariatric surgery up to 10 years after the procedure, in a nonrandomized prospective sample. This and other long-term studies provide the basis for predicting long-term outcomes of surgically-induced weight loss (SOR **B**).
   a. **Respiratory:** the majority of observed subjects had long-term improvement in symptoms of asthma and obstructive sleep apnea.
   b. **Cardiovascular:** Bariatric surgery has been demonstrated to result in short-term improvement of hypertension, hyperlipidemia, and hypertriglyceridemia. These improvements appear to diminish over time, and are indistinguishable from control groups at 10 years postsurgery.
   c. **Endocrine:** Bariatric surgery recipients have a reduced chance of developing insulin resistance and diabetes. Long-term, the degree of protection correlates to how well the weight loss is maintained.
   d. **Digestive:** After bariatric surgery, patients have a long-term increased risk of digestive problems including stenotic changes, fistula formation, bowel obstruction, incisional hernias, dumping syndrome, and chronic diarrhea. These patients may also develop nutritional deficiencies as a result of the disrupted digestive process.
F. **Complications of weight loss.** Weight loss, particularly rapid loss, has been associated with a variety of medical sequelae. Clinically, we often emphasize the positive effects of weight loss, but our patients also should be advised of the medical risks of weight loss. These include:
   1. **Biliary complications.** Rapid weight loss is associated with an increased prevalence of gallstones and cholecystitis. This complication has been observed in both low- and high-fat diets. Dietary supplementation with ursodeoxycholic acid has been proposed as a preventative tactic for this problem, but very little data supports its efficacy.
   2. **Ketosis.** Insufficient carbohydrate intake can promote production of large numbers of ketone bodies in the bloodstream. The long-term health impact of this phenomenon is controversial; speculation centers on the potential for renal damage or kidney stone formation in people following ketotic diets. Such complications have been well documented in children placed on ketotic diets for epilepsy control.
   3. **Dietary deficiencies.** Caloric restriction can lead to insufficient intake of vitamins, minerals, essential fatty acids, or protein. Long-term, this can cause protein-calorie malnutrition, vitamin deficiency, or osteoporosis.
   4. **Cosmetic issues.** Weight loss, particularly when rapid, may cause striae formation, which may be cosmetically offensive to the patient.
   5. **Psychiatric changes.** Slow or dramatic changes in body habitus may affect the patient's interaction with family, friends, and coworkers, as well as his own body image. Such changes are not always positive and may cause significant emotional distress.
IV. **Management Strategies**
   A. Obesity management should be an individually tailored approach.
   B. Although the goal of treatment is a 10% reduction from initial weight, weight loss of as little as 5% should be regarded as successful as there is considerable improvement in associated risk factors.
   C. Weight maintenance after initial weight loss is often difficult and requires an ongoing program of diet, exercise, and behavioral therapy.
   D. Regular physician contact is important to sustain maintenance efforts.
V. **Prognosis.** Obesity causes or exacerbates many disorders. It is, in particular, associated with the development of diabetes mellitus; coronary heart disease; congestive heart failure; obstructive sleep apnea; gallbladder disease; cancers such as breast, colon, and prostate; osteoarthritis of large and small joints; and premature death.

In the Framingham Heart Study, the risk of death within 26 years increased by 1% for each extra pound increase in weight between the ages of 30 and 42 years, and by 2% between 50 and 62 years.

REFERENCES

Lyznicki JM, Young DC, Riggs JA, Davis RM. Obesity: assessment and management in primary care. *Am Fam Physician.* 2001;63:2185-2196.

Mango VL, Frishman WH. Physiologic, psychologic, and metabolic consequences of bariatric surgery. *Cardiol Rev.* 2006;14(5):232-237.

National Institutes of Health. *The Practical Guide: Identification, Evaluation and Treatment of Overweight and Obesity in Adults.* Bethesda, MD: National Institutes of Health, National Heart, Lung, and Blood Institute, and North American Association for the Study of Obesity; 2000 NIH publication 00-4084.

Ogden CL, Carroll MD, Curtin LR, McDowell MA, Tabak CJ, Flegal KM. Prevalence of obesity and trends in obesity among U.S. adults 1999–2004. *JAMA.* 2006;295:1549-1555.

Palamara KL, Mogul HR, Peterson SJ, Frishman WH. Obesity: new perspectives and pharmacotherapies. *Cardiol Rev.* 2006;14(5):238-258.

Yanovski SZ, Yanovski JA. Obesity. *N Engl J Med.* 2002;346:591-602.

Li Z, Maglione M, Tu W, et al. Meta-analysis: pharmacologic treatment of obesity. *Ann Internal Med.* 2005;142(7):532-546.

80 Osteoarthritis

Charles Kodner, MD

KEY POINTS

- Osteoarthritis (OA) is no longer considered a normal process of aging and "wear and tear" on joints, but is a physiologically complex disorder involving physiologic and mechanical initiating events, joint and cartilage damage, synovial inflammation, and an imbalance of cartilage repair and destruction.
- Diagnosis is primarily on clinical grounds, emphasizing typical aching joint pain, crepitus, osteophyte formation, worsening pain with activity, and joint instability. Characteristic radiographic findings of joint space narrowing, osteophytes, irregular joint surfaces, and sclerosis of subchondral bone may assist in the diagnosis.
- Disease management should emphasize nonpharmacologic interventions, including regular exercise, physical therapy, weight loss, smoking cessation, physical pain relief modalities, gait support and other assistive devices, and patient education.
- Pharmacologic treatment should be initiated with adequate, scheduled doses of acetaminophen, starting at 500 mg twice daily up to 1 g 4 times daily. (SOR **B**)
- Other medication options include nonsteroidal anti-inflammatory drugs (NSAIDs), and other analgesics such as tramadol and narcotic analgesics. Details are available in Table 80–1, with a list of the most common medications and dosages including herbal compounds and other treatment options.
- COX-2 selective NSAIDs provide as effective pain relief as other agents (SOR **A**) with reduced gastrointestinal toxicity compared to traditional NSAIDs (SOR **A**) but should be used in selected patients in light of evolving concerns about cardiovascular risks
- Many patients require chronic opioid therapy for more advanced disease, and will require appropriate management of long-term opioid treatment. (SOR **C**)
- Topical capsaicin or oral glucosamine and chondroitin supplements may also provide pain relief.
- Joint injection with corticosteroids, hyaluronic acid injections, and acupuncture have been shown to be helpful in patients who have failed other treatment options or who are at risk of complications from NSAIDs or other therapy, though overall evidence for benefit is limited. (SOR **B**)
- Surgical joint replacement for hip or knee arthritis, or other surgical treatment options, should be considered for patients with disabling pain who have failed other treatment interventions.

I. Introduction

A. Definition. OA is characterized by slowly progressive joint pain, cartilage destruction, and functional instability, with typical radiographic findings of osteophytes and other characteristic changes. OA carries a significant potential for disability and reduced quality of life as the disease progresses. OA can be classified as primary (or idiopathic), involving the hands, feet, knees, hips, spine, and other joints; or secondary to trauma, obesity, congenital abnormalities affecting the limbs, other arthropathies (e.g., tophaceous gout,

TABLE 80–1. SELECTED ANTI-INFLAMMATORY ANALGESICS

Drug Class	Generic Name	Usual Effective Dose
Nonacetylated salicylates	Aspirin*	325–500 mg qd
	Diflunisal (Dolobid)	250–500 mg bid
	Salsalate (Disalcid)[†]	1500 mg bid
Propionic acids	Ibuprofen* (Motrin, Advil)	200–800 mg tid
	Naproxen (Naprosyn, Anaprox)	250–500 mg bid
	Ketoprofen (Orudis, Oruvail)	50 mg qid or 75 mg tid
	Oxaprozin (Daypro)[‡]	600–1200 mg qd
	Flurbiprofen (Ansaid)	200–300 mg/d divided bid–qid
Acetic acids	Indomethacin (Indocin)	25–50 mg bid–tid
	Sulindac (Clinoril)	150 mg bid
	Diclofenac (Voltaren)	50 mg bid–tid
	Tolmetin (Tolectin)	200–600 mg tid
	Etodolac (Lodine)	300–400 mg bid–tid
Fenamates	Mefenamic Acid (Ponstel)[‡]	250 mg qid
Oxicams	Piroxicam (Feldene)	20 mg once daily
	Meloxicam (Mobic)[‡]	7.5 mg qd–bid
Pyrrolizine carboxylic acid	Ketorolac (Toradol)	10 mg qid (not to exceed 5 d)
Naphthylalkanone	Nabumetone (Relafen)[‡]	1000 mg once daily
COX-2 selective agents	Celecoxib (Celebrex)[‡]	100–200 mg qd (or 50–100 mg bid)
	Meloxicam (Mobic)[‡]	7.5 mg qd–bid

*Available over-the-counter without prescription.
[†] The dose should be reduced in the elderly.
[‡] Not available generically.

rheumatoid arthritis, etc.), metabolic disorders (e.g., hemochromatosis), disorders of collagen, or other medical conditions. Some patients with rheumatoid arthritis, systemic lupus, gout, or other inflammatory conditions may develop degenerative changes in the joints that cause chronic symptoms without evidence of acute or active joint inflammation.

B. Epidemiology. OA is the most commonly encountered cause of joint pain and disability. Current estimates suggest that more than 40 million Americans have symptomatic OA; the prevalence increases with advancing age, and the prevalence of OA is expected to increase dramatically as the US population ages. The growing epidemic of obesity can be expected to dramatically increase the prevalence of OA as well. Many more people have radiographic or clinical evidence of OA than have symptomatic disease, with radiographic changes of knee OA in approximately half of the population older than 65 years.

C. Pathophysiology. OA is not solely because of expected "wear and tear" on aging joints related to activities, positioning, weight-related joint stresses, or other factors, though these do play an important role. Rather, OA is a complex disorder involving all joint structures, in which physical stresses act as disease initiating or aggravating factors, but the disorder primarily involves an imbalance between articular cartilage destructive and repair forces.

1. **Triggering factors** for OA appear to include excessive force applied to the joint, such as repetitive impact loading, or a genetic or metabolic defect in the articular cartilage or underlying subchondral bone. As a result of these triggering factors, chondrocytes multiply and become very metabolically active, initially overproducing articular cartilage to compensate for the triggering factors and maintain joint function. Over time, these factors lead to production of altered proteoglycans and collagen in the articular cartilage, which becomes subject to erosions, cracks, and other damage typical of OA.

2. **Synovial inflammation** appears to play an active role in the progression of OA and may lead to joint swelling and effusion, stiffness, pain, and other manifestations of OA. Established synovial inflammation eventually leads to production of cytokines and other agents that cause further degradation of articular cartilage.

3. **Metabolically active chondrocytes** appear to signal subchondral bone osteoblasts, which begin to form new bone tissue around the edges of the joints. The resulting "bone spurs" or osteophytes are characteristic clinical or radiographic findings and contribute to joint pain, instability, and loss of function as well as possible gross joint deformity in later stages of OA.

II. Diagnosis

In OA, the findings from the history and physical examination are key to the diagnosis and guide the intensity and nature of therapy. There is no gold standard for diagnosing OA, and clinical guidelines for diagnosis currently focus on typical pain symptoms, radiographic features, and absent evidence of inflammatory arthropathies.

A. Symptoms and signs

1. **History.** OA characteristically produces pain and stiffness in the joints, with the stiffness worsened by immobilization and resolving quickly with movement (generally in ≤30 minutes after arising in the morning). The pain is typically dull and aching in character and is aggravated by cold or damp weather and by increased activity. If activity-associated pain is present, it usually starts quickly when the joint is used but may last for hours after the activity has stopped. Often the history includes some minor injury leading to exacerbation of symptoms, though the true onset of OA symptoms is insidious in nature. Eventually, the pain becomes constant and wakes the patient from sleep.

   Many patients complain of instability or "giving way" in the case of OA involving the hips or knees and may have difficulty climbing or descending stairs. Some patients may actually fall as a result of knee or hip joint instability. Symptoms of crepitus—grinding, popping, catching, and clicking—may also be present.

2. **Physical examination.** Physical examination for OA should assess for features typical of OA, examine for evidence of other arthropathies, and assess the functional status of the joint. Specific findings to elicit include inspection for joint enlargement including osteophytes or nodules; examination for signs of inflammation including erythema, warmth, or "bogginess" of the joint; palpation for crepitus with passive range of motion; focal tenderness; and observation of instability with gait, squat-rise, or other movements.

   On examination of a normally mobile joint, crepitus may be noted when the joint is passively moved, and there may be localized tenderness. The range of movement of an osteoarthritic joint is limited. In testing the range of motion, the patient should move the joint actively first, because passive joint movement can be painful. In weight-bearing joints, it is important to assess joint stability and the status of the supporting musculature, which has therapeutic significance.

3. **Joint-specific signs and symptoms.** In addition to the above general findings on history and physical examination, OA involving specific joints may have additional clinical findings.

   a. **Knees.** In the knees, crepitus may be marked, with limitation of flexion and extension. Patients may complain of pain in the thighs, calves, or popliteal area related to compensatory muscle spasm. Osteophytes are sometimes actually palpable in the knee, and commonly, there are effusions.

   American College of Rheumatology (ACR) criteria for the diagnosis of OA of the knees include typical knee pain plus osteophytes on radiographs, or all of the following: morning stiffness ≤30 minutes, crepitus, and either age older than 40 years or synovial fluid suggestive of OA (2 of 3: clear, viscous, and less than 2000 polymorphonuclear leukocytes/cc). These criteria have a 77% positive predictive value (PPV) for patients meeting these criteria, based on 30% prevalence, and a 97% negative predictive value (NPV) for patients not meeting these criteria.

   b. **Hips.** In the hip, manifestations include changed gait, with a characteristically flexed, externally rotated hip, with the gait "sparing" the painful side. There may well be limb shortening because of subluxation of the head of the femur. Note that the pain from OA of the hip is often referred, with pain being felt in the groin, the buttocks, or even the knee. The first sign of OA in the hip is loss of rotation (since the hip is a ball-and-socket joint); this loss should be tested for in all older patients. Ultimately, there is limitation of all movements of the joint.

   ACR criteria for the diagnosis of OA of the hips include typical hip pain plus at least two of the following: erythrocyte sedimentation rate ≤20 mm/h; femoral or acetabular osteophytes on radiographs; or joint space narrowing on radiographs (52% PPV, 99% NPV).

   c. **Hands.** In the hands, typical joints affected by OA include the distal interphalangeal (DIP) joints, proximal interphalangeal (PIP) joints, and first carpometacarpal (CMC) joints. Heberden's nodes are a characteristic finding; these are firm, tender nodes on the dorsal aspect of the DIP joints, representing bony enlargement or osteophyte formation. Bouchard's nodes are similar lesions that occur over the PIP joints. Pain in the hands is worsened by fine motor or physical activities such as gardening, sports, hobbies, etc. Destructive joint changes are possible, but are not as common as in rheumatoid arthritis. ACR criteria for the diagnosis of OA of the hands include meeting all of the following: hand pain, aching, or stiffness; hard tissue enlargement of 2 or more of 10 selected joints (second and third DIP joints, second and third PIP joints, and first CMC joints on both hands); metacarpophalangeal joint swelling in fewer than three joints; and hard tissue enlargement of 2 or more DIP joints OR deformity of 1 or more of the 10 selected joints (99% PPV, 86% NPV).

  d. Cervical spine. Chronic neck pain from OA in the cervical spine may be related to work posture, repetitive athletic injuries, or other factors. Osteophytes in the spinal vertebrae can produce nerve root pressure, with resulting radicular symptoms.

  e. Lumbar spine. OA is common in the lumbar spine, but findings on examination or radiography do not correlate well with clinical symptoms. It is unclear where degenerative changes per se, facet joint changes, muscle spasm, disk herniation, soft tissue changes, or all of the above account primarily for lower back pain.

  f. Other joints. A number of other joints can be affected by OA, including the joints of the feet and ankles, the temporomandibular joint (TMJ), the true joint of the shoulder as well as the acromioclavicular joint, and the sternoclavicular joints. OA should be included in the differential diagnosis of pain in these areas, though other diagnoses (TMJ dysfunction, rotator cuff tendinitis, etc.) need to be considered.

B. Laboratory tests

  1. Radiographic findings. A number of radiographic features are common in OA, but especially in disease of the spine and hips, there may be relatively poor correlation between observed radiographic changes and symptoms. Approximately half of patients with radiographic changes of OA of the knees complain of persistent pain.

  a. Plain X-rays. Typical findings consistent with OA on plain radiographs include joint space narrowing because of destruction of articular cartilage, including narrowed intravertebral disk space; osteophyte formation at the margins of affected joints; irregular joint surfaces; sclerosis of subchondral bone; and bony cysts.

  b. MRI and CT. Computerized tomography (CT) and magnetic resonance imaging (MRI) are increasingly used, but have little role in diagnosing OA. These imaging modalities provide good visualization of soft tissues and subchondral bone changes, as well as of ligament and meniscal damage, and may be most useful to rule out other disorders causing joint pain, such as rotator cuff tear, knee ligament disruption, lumbar disc herniation, etc.

  2. Blood tests. There are no specific blood tests to order as part of the routine diagnosis of OA. "Rheumatologic tests" such as erythrocyte sedimentation rate, rheumatoid factor, and antinuclear antibodies are frequently ordered in patients with arthralgias, but these tests have poor predictive value in patients where the clinical suspicion is low for systemic lupus erythematosus or other connective tissue disorders. These tests should not be ordered as a "screening panel" in patients with arthralgias, and positive results in low-risk patients should be interpreted carefully. These tests should be ordered as confirmatory evidence in patients who are likely to have connective tissue disorders, rheumatoid arthritis, or similar conditions. Complete blood counts, uric acid levels, chemistry profiles, and other tests may be required to evaluate for septic arthritis, gout, renal osteodystrophy, or other disorders as the clinical picture dictates.

  3. Joint aspiration. When joint effusion is present, joint aspiration is usually desirable in order to provide symptomatic relief. Diagnostically, joint aspiration is typically indicated in a patient with a moderately inflamed, tender, and swollen joint with effusion, where it is important to definitively rule out septic arthritis, gout, pseudogout, or other disorders. Patients with septic arthritis may not present with characteristic findings of toxic appearance, fever, and marked joint tenderness and inflammation, but may only have focal joint inflammation early in the disease process.

  4. Arthroscopy. Arthroscopy also has a place in the diagnosis of arthritis, particularly in a joint that is "locking." Through the arthroscope, fragments of tissue can be removed and the fibrillar changes in the cartilages, which can contribute to early symptoms, can be planed off. The arthroscopic procedure itself is temporarily disabling, with a close risk/benefit balance, and should not be undertaken lightly.

III. Treatment

OA should be managed as any other chronic illness, with consideration of the patient's disease location and progression, the phase of the patient's illness, and attention to routine health maintenance and other medical comorbid conditions. Management of chronic pain can easily consume the time allotted to an outpatient office visit, and it is vital not to neglect these other management needs. The goals of therapy for OA include pain relief; improved or maintained joint function and mobility; prevention of destructive joint changes; minimization of disability and preserved functionality; and improved overall quality of life. An additional therapeutic goal is to educate patients and their families about the illness and enlist them as active participants in the management of the patient's illness.

A. Physical interventions. Nonpharmacologic interventions should be considered as primary therapy in OA, to accomplish therapeutic objectives listed above.

1. **Exercise.** At-home or supervised exercise programs have been shown to provide benefits in pain control, functionality, overall well-being, and prevention of disability, primarily for OA of the knees and hips. Exercise of weight-bearing joints must be of low impact, with avoidance of torsion, prolonged standing, and kneeling. Patients can be instructed in performing appropriate exercise by their physician, or should be referred to a physical therapist for instruction or supervision. Types of exercise programs include range-of-motion and flexibility exercises; instructions in joint positioning and posture; aerobic exercises, especially aquatic aerobics; fitness walking; and strength training, especially quadriceps strengthening since quadriceps weakness is common in OA. Nonweight-bearing exercise is preferred, and impact on the knees can be spared by shoes and surfaces that cushion the limb while walking; an indoor skiing machine can be very helpful in OA of the knees.

2. **Physical therapy.** The physical therapist can be helpful in instructing patients in the above exercises, supervising their correct and safe performance of exercise, and monitoring their therapeutic response. Therapists can also be helpful to assess patients' muscle weakness and gait, assist with the use of pain-control modalities, and assess patients for assistive devices. Occupational therapy evaluation can also provide support or assist devices for activities of daily living for patients with OA of the hands.

3. **Gait assist devices.** The use of canes (held in the hand contralateral to the affected knee or hip joint), crutches, walkers, or other devices may be helpful for some patients but should not supplant the role of muscle-strength training, range-of-motion exercises, and other measures to improve functionality. Shoe orthotics may also be helpful to preserve joint positioning and help prevent joint damage.

4. **Pain control modalities.** Persistent pain, particularly nerve root pain, may be relieved from other pain-relieving methods such as transcutaneous electrical nerve stimulation (TENS), ultrasonography, and other physical therapy techniques.

5. **Knee braces.** Some patients find relief of pain and improvement of joint stability through the use of knee bracing, patellar taping, or other interventions. These can be helpful in short term, but also should not replace other measures to maintain joint function and muscle strength. Neoprene knee braces with patellar cutouts may be most helpful in patients with early knee OA. Viscoelastic shoe inserts may also provide most relief early in the illness. Dynamic knee braces may be most helpful in patients with more advanced, or unicompartmental, knee OA. The evidence supporting all these interventions is limited.

6. **Foot care.** When the feet are affected, attention to the shoes and to podiatric health is vital. Orthotic devices can be of considerable help in correcting chronic foot deformities, which predispose to other musculoskeletal pain, not only in the feet themselves but also in the knee, hip, or lumbar spine. The use of cushioned athletic shoes may be beneficial. Women used to high heels who move rapidly to "flats" (including sneakers) may develop Achilles' tendinitis and other problems.

7. **Activities of daily living.** In all forms of arthritis of the hand, it is important to pay attention to the patient's routine tasks. Devices can assist in opening containers that require torsion strength and grip, functions that can chronically exacerbate and acutely precipitate arthralgia. Other methods of reducing joint stress and improving functionality, such as a raised toilet seat, grab bars, and tub seats or shower seats, can also reduce accidents.

B. Behavioral interventions

1. **Weight loss.** In the obese, weight must be reduced, if possible, where weight-bearing joints are involved. Patients should be enrolled in dedicated weight-loss programs

where possible, or advised regarding diet, exercise, and the role of weight-loss interventions if such programs are not available. Simple topics to address regarding diet include limiting portion size, avoiding high-carbohydrate drinks and snacks, and increasing the fruit and vegetable content of the diet. Aquatic aerobic exercises can be valuable in obese patients in terms of limiting the weight applied to the knees.

2. **Smoking cessation.** Cessation of tobacco use is important in improving patients' overall sense of well-being, reducing the risks of NSAID-induced gastropathy, maintaining joint blood flow and tissue healing, and reducing the risk of cardiovascular disease and other comorbidities. Patients who smoke should specifically be counseled regarding cessation methods as part of the overall management of their OA.

C. **Medications.** Most patients with OA use pharmacologic treatment for pain relief, though there is no evidence that treatment alters the natural history of the disease. Medications should be seen as adjuncts to preventive and protective therapy, as above, rather than the primary focus of intervention.

1. **Analgesics.** Acetaminophen remains first-line therapy for OA. Recent meta-analyses indicate that its efficacy is significantly superior to placebo, though somewhat less than NSAIDs in terms of pain relief; likewise, some surveys and measures of quality-of-life scores indicate that patients prefer NSAIDs. However, the safety profile and low cost for acetaminophen support its use as initial therapy in patients with OA; patients should be instructed that pain is best managed with daily, scheduled dosing rather than as-needed administration, as is the case with most pain-control regimens. Treatment should be initiated at 1 to 2 g total daily dose divided twice daily, with a maximum dose of 4 g daily divided into 4 doses (1 g 4 times daily). Safety issues with acetaminophen include hepatotoxicity with overdose or in patients with liver disease, or prolongation of the half-life of warfarin.

   a. **Tramadol.** Other analgesic agents include tramadol hydrochloride, a synthetic opioid; tramadol is unscheduled, is approved for moderate to severe pain in OA, and may be equivalent to moderate-strength narcotics such as codeine. It may be particularly useful in older patients or other patients at high risk of NSAID toxicity. Typical dosages are 200 to 400 mg daily, given as 4 divided doses; possible side effects include drowsiness, nausea, and constipation, with a low potential for addiction or tolerance. Seizures have been reported, but are rare and appear to have been in patients taking doses higher than recommended or in patients with epilepsy. Tramadol is marketed in formulations combined with acetaminophen and in extended-release formulations.

2. **Anti-inflammatory medications.** A variety of anti-inflammatory medications can be used to treat pain in patients who do not respond adequately to acetaminophen. These agents are effective in pain relief and are preferred to acetaminophen by many patients, highlighting the role of inflammation in OA. Issues to consider in prescribing NSAIDs include medication selection, dosage, and prevention of acute or chronic side effects.

   a. **Selecting a medication.** Meta-analysis studies have not shown any consistent difference in efficacy among the many available NSAIDs, including older nonacetylated agents as well as newer selective COX-2 inhibitor agents. Selection of agents should therefore be based primarily on cost or availability, side effects, and ease of dosing. For unknown reasons, some patients seem to find relief with different classes of NSAIDs, whereas other agents are less effective; if patients find one NSAID ineffective, it may be appropriate to switch to a medication in a different class. A selection of anti-inflammatory agents by class, including typical dosing regimens, is provided in Table 80–1. For reasons of ease of administration, efficacy, low cost, and lack of proven differences in side effects, older NSAIDs such as ibuprofen are usually recommended for patients at low risk of gastrointestinal or other side effects.

   b. **Dosage.** As with other analgesic regimens, it is appropriate to recommend that NSAIDs be dosed regularly to best affect the pain cycle rather than using these agents on an as-needed basis for a disorder that is chronic in nature. Dosing should therefore begin at low doses and titrate upward for therapeutic effect, given the high risk of toxicity with prolonged NSAID use.

   c. **Preventing side effects.** The primary side effects for NSAIDs are gastrointestinal bleeding, potentiation of renal insufficiency, and inhibition of platelet aggregation with prolongation of bleeding times. For the latter two complications, it is important to minimize the use and dosage of NSAIDs as much as possible in older patients or

TABLE 80–2. RISK FACTORS FOR NSAID-INDUCED GASTROPATHY

Definite risk factors
Age older than 65 y
Previous ulcer disease or upper gastrointestinal bleeding
Use of multiple NSAIDs or use of high dosage of one of these drugs
Concomitant oral corticosteroid therapy
Concomitant anticoagulant therapy
Duration of therapy (risk is higher in the first 3 mo of therapy)
Possible risk factors
Tobacco abuse
Alcohol abuse
Helicobacter pylori infection

those with other chronic medical conditions; specific risk factors for worsening renal function because of NSAIDs include age older than 65 years, hypertension, congestive heart failure, concomitant use of diuretics or angiotensin-converting enzyme inhibitors, or existing renal insufficiency. Hypersensitivity reactions and hepatotoxicity are also recognized NSAID side effects. However, the selection of agents is guided most by the effort to prevent gastrointestinal bleeding.

Among patients older than 65 years, approximately 25% of hospitalizations and deaths because of peptic ulcer disease are attributable to NSAIDs. Factors that place patients at high risk of NSAID-induced gastropathy are listed in Table 80–2. In patients at low risk of NSAID-induced gastropathy, there is no proven difference in safety profiles among the various anti-inflammatory medications; in these patients, drug selection should be based on cost, efficacy, and other factors, and physicians should attempt to minimize the dose, use, and duration of NSAID therapy. All patients should be advised to take NSAIDs following a meal or a snack and to limit or cease use of alcohol and tobacco products.

In patients at high risk, options to limit the risk of adverse gastrointestinal events include the use of COX-2 specific agents or use of a gastroprotective medication. In high-risk patients, COX-2 specific medications have a significantly lower incidence of gastrointestinal complications. In patients requiring additional medications for prevention of ulcers or gastritis, proton pump inhibitors are the preferred agents, though histamine$_2$ receptor antagonists, misoprostol, or Carafate (cost may be prohibitive) are other options (see Chapter 82 for dosages).

The uncertainty regarding the cardiovascular risks of the COX-2 specific agents necessitates additional care in selecting these for long-term management of OA. These agents should probably be reserved for patients who are at higher risk of gastrointestinal complications, lower risk of cardiovascular events, or who do not improve with nonselective NSAIDs.

3. **Narcotics.** Many patients with advanced OA do not respond adequately to acetaminophen, tramadol, or NSAIDs. Such patients can safely and effectively be treated with chronic opiates, including codeine, oxycodone, hydrocodone, and morphine (see Table 69–1). Some patients may require these agents only for short-term management of disease flares, though many will require chronic treatment with opioid medications, possibly during medical management to defer joint replacement. Sedation, respiratory depression, nausea, and vomiting are possible complications of these agents, though these are more likely to be problems in cases of inadvertent or intentional overdose. Addiction is a possible complication, but is unlikely in patients who do not display other propensities to drug misuse or addiction, and the risk of addiction in the general population is considered low.

Physical dependence is common, requires careful patient education about the difference between dependence and addiction, and may require slow escalation in dosage over time. There are, at present, very few guidelines regarding the timing of dosage adjustments for predictable physiologic tolerance.

Constipation and obstipation are more common complications, and patients on long-term narcotic therapy should be treated with an appropriate bowel regimen including walking, fluid intake, fiber supplementation, regular use of a stool softener, and as-needed use of laxatives. Many opiates are marketed in formulation with acetaminophen or aspirin. It is important to monitor for appropriate medication use, drug addiction, and drug diversion as described below.

4. **Topical analgesics.** Capsaicin cream is more effective than placebo for pain relief, especially for disease localized to the knee or hand, but requires 4 times daily application, which may limit its continued use by patients. Over-the-counter topical salicylates, and prescription topical lidocaine patches, may be effective alternatives in some patients, but there is little available evidence to guide their routine clinical use.

5. **Herbal preparations.** Glucosamine (1500 mg/d in 3 divided doses) and chondroitin (800–1200 mg/d in 3 divided doses) appear to provide some pain relief in meta-analyses and should be considered as adjunctive medications that may help limit the dose of NSAIDs or narcotics required to reduce pain. Patients should be advised that these agents are available over-the-counter and that different formulations may use lower doses, which may be less effective. Patients may be reluctant to continue paying out of pocket for these agents for a long term, but a trial of therapy for efficacy may be appropriate. Other herbal agents that may have some benefit include S-adenosylmethionine (SAMe), 400 to 1200 mg/d; topical dimethyl sulfoxide (DMSO), 25% gel; and avocado/soybean unsaponifiables, 300 mg/d.

D. **Joint injection.** In the presence of knee joint effusion and inflammation, corticosteroid injection has been shown to provide pain relief over 1 to 2 weeks but is not effective for long-term pain relief.

Viscosupplementation via intra-articular injection of hyaluronic acid provides pain relief superior to placebo and may be an option for patients who do not respond appropriately to medical therapy or who are at high risk for NSAID-induced gastropathy, narcotic addiction or side effects, or other complications. Patients with persistent pain and functional limitations who are not surgical candidates may also benefit, though the ideal candidate for injection therapy has not been defined, and the overall benefit is modest in meta-analyses. Weekly injections are given for 3 to 5 weeks, and this regimen may be repeated only twice per year. The cost of these medications may be prohibitive in some patients (approximately $600 for a treatment course).

Acupuncture likewise may provide relief in some patients with knee OA, but has not been directly compared to other treatment modalities.

E. **Surgical management.** Surgical options for OA of the knee include arthroscopic debridement, distal femoral osteotomy, unicompartmental knee replacement or hemiarthroplasty, or total knee arthroplasty. Indications for surgical intervention include pain, instability, or disability uncontrolled with physical and medical management. Given the likelihood of prosthesis loosening and the need for subsequent reoperation after approximately 10 years, it is usually appropriate to defer surgical intervention using conservative measures until patients are older and have more limited activity requirements. There is only limited evidence to support arthroscopic debridement for knee OA; this may be useful for some patients but should not be recommended as routine treatment.

IV. **Management Strategies**

It is very important for the family physician to manage the "whole patient" and not to focus solely on medications and formal physical therapy in treating OA. Patient-focused management includes educating the patient (and the caregiver if relevant) in the many techniques that can reduce symptoms by reducing the stress on diseased joints and addressing other social and medical dimensions of their care. These techniques thus reduce the impact of the arthritis on the patient's life and help address not only pain but also total quality of life.

A. **Patient education and support.** Patients and families must be educated about the pathophysiology of OA and should be able to identify significant symptoms and recognize inflammatory phases and other symptoms that may necessitate modifications in management. An understanding of the disease process may be especially important in younger patients with OA, who are forced to begin management of a chronic illness. Patients and families should be directed toward organizations such as the Arthritis Foundation, which has local chapters and extensive educational and support activities.

In older patients, arthritis and its many consequences (which can be devastating to the patient's overall health and function) are often tolerated as "normal" accompaniments of aging, and patients should understand the nature of their illness and the breadth of management options available. Some patients may benefit from more frequent, scheduled visits than from "follow-up as needed" to continue patient education and address other aspects of disease management. Topics for anticipatory counseling should include sexuality, including sexual position; posture, including chair height and style; toileting and bathing needs; exercise and activity habits; and driving, including entering and exiting the car.

B. Depression. Depression often accompanies chronic joint pain and then interferes with motivation and compliance as well as increasing the patient's awareness of the pain itself. Good clinical management thus involves seeing patients and their families in the entire context of their lives, functionality, and the rest of their health, since movement and every-day activities are inevitably affected by these illnesses. Counseling and medical treatment for depression may be appropriate in depressed patients; use of tricyclic antidepressants, if otherwise appropriate, may provide additional benefit in terms of pain relief and help with sleep.

C. Disability assessments. Patients with chronic pain and self-assessed disability often request assistance from their physicians in applying for disability benefits. Assessing for true disability in terms of overall "whole patient" disability or isolated disabilities of specific limbs and joints is complex. Rational disability assessment is further complicated by issues of credibility, secondary gain, and effort on the part of the patient, and lack of expertise or familiarity on the part of the physician. Guidelines on disability determination are available, and consultation with a physician trained in occupational medicine is recommended. Patients in general should not be determined to be fully disabled without a more thorough assessment of their true functional capacity.

D. Chronic narcotic therapy management. Routine management of patients who are on chronic narcotic therapy includes the following: explanation of appropriate drug use and refill patterns (obtain medications from only one physician and one pharmacy; take medications as prescribed; no early refills on medications will be given; medications will be discontinued if there is evidence of substance abuse; and patients need to follow up with their physician as instructed); periodic urine drug testing to help evaluate for drug diversion; and assessment for "doctor-shopping" or other evidence of drug addiction or "drug-seeking." Many physicians prefer to refer to specialists in pain management or to use "narcotic contracts" signed by the patient to address these requirements.

Management of patients on chronic opioids may require additional work and office protocols to ensure appropriate use of these medications and to prevent drug diversion; however, this management is well within the scope of practice for most family physicians, and management resting on an accurate diagnosis, an overall management plan, and appropriate monitoring and documentation is unlikely to lead to licensing or regulatory problems.

As above, physiologic tolerance or dependence is distinct from drug addiction, which is rare in patients with chronic pain who do not have a history of substance abuse.

E. Referral criteria. In general, patients with OA can be effectively managed by primary care physicians. Referral to physical therapists or occupational therapists is common, and joint management with therapists can be effective in overall patient care. Referral to rheumatologists should only be necessary to confirm the diagnosis of rheumatoid arthritis or other conditions, and referral to orthopedic surgeons should be undertaken when surgical intervention is required, or if the primary care physician is uncomfortable performing joint injections. Referral to pain management specialists, as above, may be helpful in patients requiring long-term narcotic therapy.

V. Prognosis.
Symptoms of OA can be expected to worsen over time, although improving muscular support and general fitness and continual attention to mobility and range of motion can keep symptoms at bay for years. Major interventions in OA, such as joint replacement (particularly the knee or hip), can be seemingly "curative" of that particular joint, provided that the patient can fully collaborate in the necessary rehabilitative process.

REFERENCES

American College of Rheumatology. Recommendations for the medical management of osteoarthritis of the hip and knee: American College of Rheumatology Subcommittee on Osteoarthritis Guidelines. *Arth Rheum.* 2000;43(9):1905-1915.

Easton BT. Evaluation and treatment of the patient with osteoarthritis. *J Fam Pract.* 2001;50(9):791.

Lo V. When should COX-2 selective NSAIDs be used for osteoarthritis and rheumatoid arthritis? *J Fam Pract.* 2006;55(3):260-262.

Nicholson B. Responsible prescribing of opioids for the management of chronic pain. *Drugs.* 2003;63(1):17-32.

Sisto SA. Osteoarthritits and therapeutic exercise. *Am J Phys Med Rehab.* 2006;85(suppl 11):S69-S78.

Stitik TP. Pharmacotherapy of osteoarthritis. *Am J Phys Med Rehab.* 2006;85(suppl 11):S15-S28.

van Dijk GM. Course of functional status and pain in osteoarthritis of the hip or knee: a systematic review of the literature. *Arthritis Rheum.* 2006;55(5):779-785.

Yonclas PP. Orthotics and assistive devices in the treatment of upper and lower limb osteoarthritis. *Am J Phys Med Rehab.* 2006;85(suppl 11):S82-S97.

---

81   Osteoporosis

Richard O. Schamp, MD, & William T. Manard, MD

KEY POINTS

- Fractures caused by osteoporosis affect 40% of women and 13% of men older than 50 years.
- Vertebral fractures remain under-recognized and undertreated and are associated with poor health outcomes.
- Patients at risk can be identified by clinical risk factors.
- Therapy should be started as soon as possible after presenting with a fragility fracture. (SOR **C**)
- Candidates for osteoporosis therapy:
  - All postmenopausal women who present with vertebral, wrist, or hip fractures. (SOR **A**)
  - All women with bone mineral density (BMD) T-scores below –2, in the absence of risk factors. (SOR **A**)
  - All men with BMD T-scores below –2. (SOR **C**)
  - All persons with BMD T-scores below –1.5, if other risk factors are present. (SOR **B**)
- Adequate calcium intake (total from diet and supplements):
  - 1200 mg/d in men and all premenopausal (starting in the second or third decade) women. (SOR **C**)
  - 1500 mg/d in postmenopausal women, especially if institutionalized. (SOR **A**)
  - Calcium carbonate is cheapest; maximum absorption occurs with 500-mg doses.
  - Calcium citrate has better absorption and is preferred in patients with achlorhydria, constipation, or gas with calcium carbonate, or history of renal stones. (SOR **C**)
- Adequate vitamin D intake:
  - 800 IU is the minimum recommended intake for persons at risk of fracture. (SOR **B**)
  - Higher initial doses may be required for persons who are vitamin D deficient. (SOR **A**)
  - Sunlight exposure and diet (e.g., fortified milk) are important sources of vitamin D (SOR **B**), but are often impractical in the population at risk.
- Drug therapy (always in conjunction with adequate calcium and vitamin D):
  - Most of these drugs feature a number needed to treat (NNT) of 12 to 30 over 3 years.
  - Alendronate (Fosamax), 10 mg every morning or 70 mg once a week on an empty stomach, sitting up for 30 minutes after dose to reduce risk of esophagitis. (SOR **A**)
  - Risedronate (Actonel), 5 mg every morning or 35 mg once a week on an empty stomach, sitting up as above. (SOR **A**)
  - Ibandronate (Boniva), 150 mg monthly, administered as above, or 3 mg intravenously once every 3 months. (SOR **A** for oral, SOR **B** for IV)
  - Calcitonin (Miacalcin nasal spray), 200 IU intranasally; one puff per day, alternating nostrils; or injectable calcitonin (Miacalcin), 100 IU subcutaneously every other day. (SOR **A**) (Calcitonin is alleged to reduce pain in acute compression fracture [SOR **C**].)
  - Raloxifene (Evista), 60 mg every day, with relative contraindications of hot flashes and history of thromboembolic conditions. (SOR **A**) Indicated in women only.

- Teriparatide (Forteo), 20 μg subcutaneously daily, for refractory or severe disease. (SOR **A**)
- Hormone replacement therapy (HRT) has been associated with increased bone density in randomized controlled trials, fewer fractures in observational studies, and fewer fractures in a recent meta-analysis of randomized controlled trials, but has essentially been abandoned except in unique cases because of risk–benefit ratio. (SOR **B**)

- Institutional care:
    - Inpatient care may be needed for acute back pain, especially for new vertebral fractures (bed rest and analgesia) and for acute treatment of upper femoral and pelvic fractures. (SOR **C**)
    - Nursing home or home health care may be needed following fracture. (SOR **C**)
    - Start supplement/drug therapy as soon as a diagnosis is made, because this often is neglected when patients are discharged from acute treatment. (SOR **C**)
- Lifestyle changes:
    - Use acute event or new diagnosis to assist patients' motivation in healthy lifestyle changes. (SOR **C**)
    - Both smoking cessation and avoiding excessive alcohol use reduce osteoporosis risk. (SOR **A**)
    - Weight-bearing exercise, such as walking 1 mile twice a day or dancing, is commonly recommended, but evidence is lacking to show fracture benefit, other than decreasing falls and modestly improving BMD. (SOR **B**)
    - Osteoporotic patients should avoid maneuvers that increase compressive forces on the spine. (SOR **C**)

I. Introduction

A. **Osteoporosis** is a heterogeneous group of metabolic bone diseases characterized by severe bone mineral loss, disruption of skeletal microarchitecture, and disturbed bone quality leading to enhanced bone fragility, chiefly manifested by atraumatic fractures of the vertebral column, upper femur, distal radius, proximal humerus, pubic rami, and ribs.

B. Osteoporosis is often defined (Table 81–1) as a BMD T-score $\geq$ 2.5 standard deviations (SDs) below mean or a fracture resulting from minimal trauma (fragility fracture). **Osteopenia** is defined as a BMD T-score between −1 and −2.5. **Osteomalacia** is characterized by abnormal bone, and is a potentially treatable metabolic bone disorder caused, for example, by inadequate vitamin D.

C. Bone constantly remodels through the process of resorption and formation. This process occurs at age-related rates, ranging from complete renewal of all bones in the first year of life to renewal of 15% to 30% of the skeleton per year in adults. Loss of BMD alone explains only approximately 60% to 80% of the variation in bone strength. Trabecular bone architectural changes contribute significantly to fracture risk but are not easily assessed clinically.

D. Bone mass reaches a peak by 35 years, with bone loss beginning by 40 years in both sexes. After menopause, the rate of bone resorption exceeds the rate of bone formation. Over her lifetime, a woman loses 35% of her cortical bone and 50% of her

TABLE 81–1. BMD DEFINITIONS OF BONE DENSITY*

Bone Status	BMD Description
Normal	BMD value within 1 SD of the young adult reference mean (T $\geq= -1.0$)
Osteopenia	BMD value of more than 1 SD below the young adult mean but less than 2.5 SD below this value ($-1.0 \geq T \geq -2.5$)
Osteoporosis	BMD value of 2.5 SD or more below the adult mean value (T $\leq= -2.5$)
Established osteoporosis	BMD value of 2.5 SD or more below the adult mean value (T $\leq= -2.5$) in the presence of one or more fragility fractures

*As established by WHO.
BMD, bone mineral density.

trabecular bone. Men lose only two-thirds of the bone that women lose as muscle mass decreases.

E. Five types of osteoporosis are recognized:

1. **Postmenopausal (type I).** The most common form in Caucasian and Asian women, because of acceleration of trabecular bone resorption in the first decade or two following menopause.

2. **Involutional (type II).** Occurs in both sexes older than 75 years and is because of a subtle, prolonged imbalance between rates of bone resorption and formation. Type II weakens cortical bone more than type I. Mixtures of types I and II are common, with additive effects.

3. **Idiopathic.** A rare form of primary osteoporosis occurring in premenopausal women and in men younger than 75 years. It is not related to secondary causes or risk factors predisposing to bone loss.

4. **Juvenile.** A rare form, with variable severity in prepubertal children and cessation of fractures at puberty.

5. **Secondary** (Table 81–2). Although secondary factors can cause osteoporosis, consider them as additive risk factors and treatable.

F. Osteoporosis affects approximately 28 million people in the United States ($\geq$15 million symptomatic cases) and thus is commonly seen in adult primary care practices. Seven percent of ambulatory postmenopausal women older than 50 years have osteoporosis already, and a 50-year-old white woman has lifetime risks of fracture of the spine, hip, and distal radius of 32%, 16%, and 15%, respectively. These risks greatly exceed her risk of developing endometrial or breast cancer combined. Age is a strong predictor of osteoporosis, which is 5 times more common in women older than 65 years than in women younger than 65 years.

G. Risk factors for osteoporosis are listed in Table 81–3. Factors associated with decreased risk for osteoporosis included higher body mass index, African American heritage, estrogen use, thiazide diuretic use, moderate exercise, and moderate alcohol consumption. Clinical risk factors have poorly validated roles in predicting fractures and in determining who should have BMD measurement.

TABLE 81–2. **CAUSES OF SECONDARY OSTEOPOROSIS**

Sex hormone deficiency
  Gonadal failure (hypogonadism including orchiectomy)
  Prolactin-secreting pituitary adenoma (prolactinoma)
  Smoking tobacco (decreases circulating estrogen)

Hormone excess
  Hyperthyroidism
  Hyperparathyroidism
  Corticosteroids, exogenous (not inhaled)
  Cushing's syndrome

Increased bone resorption/formation ratio
  Prolonged immobilization (localized osteoporosis)
  Space flight (lose 10% bone mass in 1 wk)
  Long-term heparin use
  Cancers (e.g., multiple myeloma, lymphoma, leukemia, breast cancer)
  Paget's disease
  Rheumatoid arthritis

Osteomalacia (defective bone mineralization)
  Vitamin D deficiency
  Anticonvulsants and chronic liver disease (25-hydroxylation of vitamin D)
  Malabsorption syndromes
  Eating disorders
  Alcoholism
  Calcium deficiency
  Renal calcium wasting (e.g., distal renal tubular acidosis)

Genetic abnormalities
  Osteogenesis imperfecta
  Ehlers-Danlos syndrome
  Homocystinuria

TABLE 81-3. **RISK FACTORS FOR OSTEOPOROSIS**

Nonmodifiable
  Most secondary causes (Table 81-2)
  Menopause (physiologic or surgical)
  Increasing age
  Female sex
  Family history of osteoporosis
  Personal history of fracture
  Caucasian, Hispanic, or Asian race
  Lean build, short stature, small bone, light weight

Modifiable
  Hyperathleticism
  Smoking
  Dietary excess of protein ($\geq$120 g/d) or vitamin A (retinol)
  Diet low in calcium, vitamin D, vitamin C, or magnesium
  Sedentary lifestyle or lack of exercise
  Alcohol excess

II. Diagnosis

A. Symptoms and signs, when present and not otherwise explained, indicate that significant bone loss, including fracture or microfracture, has already occurred, and thus establish the diagnosis of osteoporosis.

  1. Back pain may be caused by acute compression fractures or biomechanical changes resulting from previous fractures.

  2. Fractures of vertebra, hip, and forearm produce pain and disability. Fractures may result from such minimal trauma as bending, lifting, or getting out of bed.

  3. Loss of height is associated with loss of bone and fractures of the vertebrae and may be accompanied by disfiguring cosmetic changes.

  4. Poor dentition and premature tooth loss is associated with osteoporosis.

  5. Mechanical deformity (kyphosis, or dowager's hump) caused by vertebral compression fracture may interfere with both respiration and abdominal processes and may cause early satiety, bloating, decreased exercise tolerance, constipation, and loss of self-esteem.

  6. Signs of **secondary causes** may be observed if osteoporosis is suspected (e.g., moon facies, exophthalmos, etc.).

B. Be wary of the distinction between diagnosis (identification of the cause of symptoms and signs) and screening (case finding in a population at risk). The evidence supporting one process may not support the other. The following recommendations are diagnostic interventions for the patient with suspected or established osteoporosis. Diagnostic tests are considered not only to confirm the diagnosis of osteoporosis but also to rule out associated conditions.

C. Laboratory tests

  1. Testing of presumed healthy patients with osteoporosis may reveal bone and mineral metabolism disorders; retrospective chart review of 173 women in a referral population found 55 (32%) with previously undetected disorders including hypercalciuria, malabsorption, hyperparathyroidism, vitamin D deficiency, exogenous hyperthyroidism, Cushing's disease, and hypocalciuric hypercalcemia. (SOR **C**)

  2. Order CBC, ESR, CMP (for calcium, alkaline phosphatase, creatinine), serum phosphate, and thyroid-stimulating hormone (TSH) tests, which should be normal in primary osteoporosis. (SOR **C**)

  3. Consider 25-hydroxyvitamin D, especially for at-risk populations (home-bound, institutionalized, or other sunlight-deprived circumstances), intact parathyroid hormone (iPTH), serum protein electrophoresis (SPEP), testosterone (men), estradiol (women), and 24-hour urinary calcium excretion tests to rule out other secondary causes. (SOR **C**)

  4. Consider tests of bone metabolism in uncertain cases: (SOR **C**)

  a. Urine calcium/creatinine ratio.

  b. Tubular reabsorption of **phosphorus.**

  c. NTx assay (Osteomark) or pyridinium crosslinks (Pyrilinks-D). NTx and pyridinium crosslink assays are some type I collagen breakdown products in urine and serum and are used to assess osteoclast activity.

    d. Bone-specific alkaline phosphatase.

    e. Osteocalcin.

  5. Bone biopsy is rarely needed and requires a nondecalcified bone specimen with tetracycline labeling and a specialized laboratory for interpretation.

  6. Bone marrow aspiration and biopsy can rule out multiple myeloma, metastatic carcinoma, and lymphoma, if clinically indicated.

D. Imaging studies

  1. X-rays. By the time osteoporosis is evident on x-ray, 20% to 40% of bone is lost. The following changes can be seen on plain x-ray of the vertebral column: increased lucency, cortical thinning, increased density of end plate, anterior wedging and biconcavity of vertebrae, and loss of horizontal trabeculae.

  2. BMD testing. The decision to order BMD testing in the patient with suspected or established osteoporosis entails several considerations.

    a. Chief among these is whether the results will change the treatment. Patients who are at sufficiently high risk for osteoporotic fracture (e.g., those older than 70 years with multiple risk factors) will not likely benefit from BMD testing if treatment is indicated on clinical grounds anyway. (SOR **C**)

    b. Deciding which patients to consider for BMD measurement requires weighing risk factors on an individual basis. Table 81–4 identifies indications for BMD testing. (SOR **C**)

    c. Some clinicians will order serial studies to follow the effects of treatment on BMD, but there is little evidence to support this or to guide frequency of reassessment. (SOR **C**)

    d. Three imaging modalities are commonly available: dual-energy x-ray absorptiometry (DXA), quantitative computed tomography (QCT), and calcaneal ultrasonography. DXA measurements are the basis for WHO criteria, with other techniques being useful for screening in certain circumstances.

    e. DXA is the most precise technique, is used most widely for measuring BMD, and correlates best with the WHO criteria (Table 81–1). Measurements are typically taken from the lumbar spine and the proximal femurs.

    f. QCT results are less likely to be affected by degenerative spinal changes than spine DXA scanning. Also, unlike DXA, QCT allows for selective assessment of trabecular bone, which may show metabolic changes earlier. QCT can predict spinal fracture similarly to DXA scanning, but the costs and radiation exposure are higher.

    g. Ultrasonography measures the speed of sound (related to bone density) and broadband ultrasonic attenuation (related to bone architecture) of the calcaneus, typically. Fracture risk prediction is equivalent to that of DXA, especially for hip fracture. Ultrasound is available for in-office use and is portable, making evaluation in the long-term care facility feasible. Lower precision makes this technique not recommended for serial measurements. (SOR **C**)

    h. Deciding which bone imaging modality depends upon availability, age, site of interest, and costs. For example, vertebral fractures are of greater concern than hip fractures in women who are within 15 years of menopause. Any of the imaging modalities may be appropriate, especially those that include imaging of the spine. In women older than 65 years, hip fractures become more of a concern, so DXA of the hip or calcaneal ultrasound might be appropriate.

TABLE 81–4. INDICATIONS FOR BONE MASS MEASUREMENT TO DIAGNOSE OSTEOPOROSIS*

Strong indications

  Estrogen-deficient women in whom treatment decisions are based on BMD

  Patients receiving long-term steroids for treatment decisions

  Patients with vertebral abnormalities or incidental osteopenia on x-ray

  Patients with asymptomatic primary hyperparathyroidism or other disease associated with high risk of osteoporosis

Weaker indications

  Patients who have lost height or sustained a probable osteoporotic fracture

  Patients being treated for osteoporosis, to monitor changes

---

*Both males and females, unless stated.

(Data from the National Osteoporosis Foundation.)

TABLE 81–5. **DIETARY CALCIUM RECOMMENDATIONS**

Children 4–8 y—800 mg/d
Children 9–18 y—1300 mg/d
Adults 19–50 y (including pregnant and lactating women)—1000 mg/d
Adults older than 50 y—1200 mg/d
Postmenopausal women—1500 mg/d

(Data sources: Institute of Medicine, 1997. NIH, 1994.)

III. Treatment

A. The continuous distribution of BMD and current available evidence preclude an absolute "fracture risk threshold" to initiate treatment. Other factors such as skeletal architecture (presently difficult to measure), fall risk, exercise patterns, life expectancy, adverse side effects, patient preferences, and the constellation of risk factors (Table 81–3) must be considered in a manner analogous to the management of hyperlipidemia or hypertension, in which treatment thresholds may depend on other risk factors as well as lipid levels or blood pressure. An evidence-based, validated algorithm for the treatment of osteoporosis that includes patient-specific risk factors for fracture and BMD measure does not currently exist. Thus, current management has to be individualized.

B. **Primary prevention**

1. **Lifestyle.** Factors that can decrease calcium absorption, increase bone resorption, or impair bone formation, such as smoking, excessive alcohol intake, and medications associated with osteoporosis, should be avoided. (SOR **C**)

2. **Weight-bearing exercise.** Exercise should be weight bearing and skeletal stressing. Prolonged low-to-moderate physical activity is associated with higher BMD than either sedentary lifestyle or endurance-trained athletic activity. (SOR **B**)

3. **Calcium supplements.** The average American consumes ≤800 mg/d of calcium. Recommendations for calcium intake vary by age and a typical expert opinion is in Table 81–5. Calcium alone can prevent bone loss and fractures. (SOR **B**)

a. **Estimating calcium intake.** An estimation of the patient's dietary intake can be made quickly and easily with Repka's rules of 300: the basal diet contains 300 mg of calcium, and each serving of dairy products, such as 8 oz milk, 8 oz yogurt, 1.5 oz cheese, or 2 cups cottage cheese, provides 300 mg of calcium. Excellent sources of nondairy calcium include sardines (372 mg in 3 oz) and pink salmon (167 mg in 3 oz).

b. **General information.** There is little evidence favoring specific calcium supplements for efficacy in preventing osteoporotic fractures. Absorption is improved with doses ≤500 mg and when taken with food. Calcium can interfere with absorption of other minerals and many drugs (e.g., iron, zinc, quinolones, bisphosphonates, tetracycline). See Table 81–6 for typical supplements.

c. **Calcium carbonate.** Usually derived from oyster shells, this is the least expensive oral form of calcium supplement available and requires fewest tablets per day. It may

TABLE 81–6. **COMPARISON OF TYPICAL CALCIUM SUPPLEMENTS**

Calcium Supplement	Trade Name	Elemental Calcium (mg)	Vitamin D (IU)	Tablets Per Day	Relative Cost
Calcium carbonate	Generic	500	200	2	$
	Os-Cal 500 + D	500	200	2	$
	Caltrate + D	600	200	2	$$
	Tums 500	500	0	2	$
	Viactiv (chewable)	500	100	2	$$
Calcium citrate	Citrus Cal D	315	200	3	$$
	Cal Citrate 950	200	0	5	$$
	Citracal D	200	200	5	$$
Calcium lactate	Generic 650 mg	100	0	10	$$
Calcium glubionate liquid	Calcionate liquid	115/5 cc	0	45 cc	$$$
Calcium complex (carbonate, lactate, gluconate)	Calcet	150	100	7	$$
Calcium phosphate	Posture-D 1500	600	125	2	$$
Calcium acetate	Phos-lo	169	0	6	$$$
Calcium gluconate	Generic 650 mg	60	0	17	$$

cause more gastrointestinal upset (constipation, bloating, gas) than other preparations. Stomach acid is required for absorption, which may limit effectiveness in patients who are elderly, taking proton pump inhibitors, or have achlorhydria. Excess dosing can cause milk–alkali syndrome.

    d. Calcium citrate is best absorbed, has fewest side effects, need not be taken with meals in order to maximize absorption, and costs more than calcium carbonate. If carbonate forms are poorly tolerated, this option can be helpful. Theoretically, lower doses may be as effective because more is absorbed, but this has not been well studied. (SOR **C**)

    e. Absorption of all calcium products is improved with adequate vitamin D, with supplemental magnesium salts, and with thiazide diuretics. Sodium restriction reduces urinary excretion of calcium, but has unclear effects on bones.

    4. Vitamin D is traditionally recommended in supplemental form since intake or endogenous production is frequently suboptimal. This vitamin is manufactured variably in the skin following direct exposure to sunlight. Exposure of 10 to 15 minutes for the hands, arms, and face 3 times per week is enough for fair-skinned persons. Vitamin D production is decreased by dark skin, sunscreen, window glass, clothing, air pollution, aging, and lack of sun exposure (northern latitude, homebound persons, or cultural dressing habits).

    a. In combination with adequate calcium intake, 700 to 800 IU vitamin D can reduce fractures significantly, up to 50% in nursing home patients. NNT = 45/y to prevent one fracture. (SOR **B**)

    b. Potential (3%–5%) for hypercalcemia exists with high doses of vitamin D.

    c. Calcium and vitamin D together is strongly recommended for all patients taking long-term corticosteroids.

    5. Secondary causes of osteoporosis should be sought and treated (Table 81–2).

    6. Risks factors for fracture, such as orthostatic hypotension, lower limb dysfunction, drug use, and visual impairment especially in the frail, elderly patient, should be sought and reduced (Table 81–3). A home safety evaluation should be considered to prevent falls.

C. Secondary prevention attempts to detect disease early and minimize the risks in patients discovered to have asymptomatic osteoporosis, usually through screening or clinical suspicion. **Primary prevention strategies remain in force.** Drug therapy is often indicated. Agents shown to prevent vertebral fractures in postmenopausal women include alendronate, risedronate, ibandronate, teriparatide, and raloxifene, although only alendronate, risedronate, and teriparatide also prevent hip fractures (Table 81–7). Large trials with fracture outcomes are lacking regarding estrogen and calcitonin.

    1. Bisphosphonates inhibit bone resorption and have the best evidence for efficacy. (SOR **A**)

    a. Because calcium supplements or food taken at the same time as a bisphosphonate reduce already low (0.5%–1%) absorption of the drug, it should be taken on an empty stomach (usually before breakfast) with a full glass of water and without eating or lying down for 30 minutes. Bisphosphonates may cause heartburn, esophageal irritation, esophagitis, abdominal pain, and diarrhea. In spite of black box warning, a causal relationship between bisphosphonate therapy and osteonecrosis of the jaw has not been established.

TABLE 81–7. MEDICATIONS INDICATED TO TREAT OSTEOPOROSIS

Generic Name (Trade Name)	Class	Dosage	Frequency	Approximate Cost Annually ($)*
Alendronate (Fosamax)	Bisphosphonate	70 mg	Weekly	1058.20
		10 mg	Daily	1032.00
Risendronate (Actonel)	Bisphosphonate	35 mg	Weekly	935.87
		5 mg	Daily	1051.56
Boniva (ibandronate)	Bisphosphonate	150 mg (oral)	Monthly	940.92
		3 mg (IV)	Quarterly	1575.00
Raloxifene (Evista)	Selective estrogen receptor modulator (SERM)	60 mg	Daily	1095.96
Calcitonin (Miacalcin)	Calcitonin	200 units	Daily	1346.64
Teriparatide (Forteo)	PTH analog	20 μg (SQ)	Daily	7850.51

(*Price information Data from http://www.drugstore.com. Accessed June 22, 2007.)

    b. Alendronate (Fosamax), 10 mg orally every day or 70 mg orally once weekly, has an NNT of 45 to 140/y for symptomatic fracture prevention in women with known osteoporosis (previous vertebral fractures). Alendronate prevents bone density loss after discontinuation of HRT. Benefits of treatment with alendronate persist after discontinuation of therapy if treated for 5 years.

    c. Risedronate (Actonel), 5 mg orally every day or 35 mg orally weekly, has an NNT of 90/y for nonvertebral fracture prevention in women with preexisting vertebral fracture.

    d. Ibandronate (Boniva), 150 mg orally once monthly, has NNT of 120/y for prevention of clinical vertebral fracture. It is also available as 3 mg intravenously once every 3 months; efficacy appears equivalent to oral administration.

    e. Zoledronic acid (Zometa) is a bisphosphonate with indications for use in myeloma and metastatic bone disease and hypercalcemia of malignancy. Infusions given at intervals of up to 1 year produce effects on bone turnover and bone density as great as other bisphosphonates, suggesting that an annual infusion of zoledronic acid might be an effective treatment for postmenopausal osteoporosis. More study is underway as the FDA does not yet approve it for the treatment of osteoporosis.

2. Raloxifene (Evista) is an example of a selective estrogen receptor modulator (SERM). These agents may provide the beneficial effects of estrogen replacement therapy without some of its potentially serious side effects.

    a. Raloxifene reduces risk of recurrent vertebral fracture in postmenopausal women with known osteoporosis (NNT 90/y for 60 mg/d; 64/y for 120 mg/d).

    b. The benefit of preventing hip fractures is yet unproven.

    c. Adverse effects include venous thromboembolism (NNH 440/y).

    d. No increased risk of heart disease or breast cancer mortality is found with raloxifene so far.

3. Calcitonin (Miacalcin) intranasally one nasal puff (200 U) every day, alternating nostrils, is shown to reduce bone loss and decrease vertebral fracture risk (NNT 65/y).

    a. No studies are available on clinical or nonvertebral fractures.

    b. Calcitonin appears to preserve bone mass in steroid-induced osteoporosis, but fracture prevention is not established.

    c. The drug must be kept refrigerated.

    d. Decreased bone pain in acute vertebral fracture is reportedly because of the increase in endorphins stimulated by calcitonin.

    e. The intranasal form has largely replaced use of subcutaneous calcitonin 100–200 U 3 times per week, although the subcutaneous form prevents more bone loss than intranasal calcitonin. The subcutaneous form is associated with nausea and occasional allergic reaction.

4. HRT. Estrogen alone or in combination with progestins had been previously prescribed for prevention of postmenopausal osteoporosis. Accumulated evidence is variable regarding the fracture benefits of this practice (NNT ranges from 132/y to 1429/y for vertebral fracture prevention and NNT 2000/y for hip fracture prevention). The risks of estrogen supplementation are significant in regard to cancer, heart disease, and other conditions. Estrogens and combined estrogen–progestin products should only be considered for women with significant risk of osteoporosis that outweighs the risks of the drug. (SOR **B**)

5. Teriparatide (Forteo) is *N*-terminal fragment (1–34) recombinant human PTH and the first FDA-approved agent that stimulates new bone formation for osteoporosis in postmenopausal women and men with primary or hypogonadal osteoporosis.

    a. Teriparatide increases BMD.

    b. In high-risk patients with established osteoporosis, it prevents new vertebral fracture (NNT 10–11), new nonvertebral fractures (NNT 30), and new nonvertebral fragility fractures (NNT 35). So, teriparatide may be more effective than bisphosphonates. (SOR **A**)

    c. It is supplied as an injector pen with 750 μg/3 mL, given as 20 μg subcutaneously into the thigh or abdominal wall once daily.

    d. The black box warning states that teriparatide should not be use if increased baseline risk for osteosarcoma, Paget's disease of bone, unexplained alkaline phosphatase elevations, open epiphyses, prior radiation therapy of skeleton, metastases, history of skeletal malignancies, metabolic bone diseases (other than osteoporosis), or preexisting hypercalcemia.

    e. Adverse effects include pain, arthralgia, asthenia, nausea, rhinitis, dizziness, headache, hypertension, increased cough, pharyngitis, constipation, diarrhea, and dyspepsia.

6. Fluoride therapy

    a. Most authorities are not recommending fluoride therapy currently. Some form of fluoride may have a role in osteoporosis therapy in the future. (SOR **C**)

7. Ipriflavone is a synthetic flavonoid (isoflavone) available over-the-counter (OTC). Ipriflavone promotes the incorporation of calcium into bone and inhibits bone resorption.

    a. Isoflavones are approved in European and Asian countries for osteoporosis prevention and treatment.

    b. It does not possess intrinsic estrogenic activity and behaves more like a SERM without significant adverse side effects.

    c. Studies are controversial regarding efficacy, but ipriflavone appears to prevent postmenopausal bone loss. No studies yet show a reduction in fracture rates. (SOR **C**)

    d. Unregulated manufacture of OTC products in the United States limits the reliability of OTC product purity and potency.

8. Hydrochlorothiazide in low doses (up to 25 mg/d) was associated with preservation of BMD in one randomized trial. In doses of 50 mg/d, thiazides may be beneficial in treating the high urine calcium of patients with idiopathic hypercalciuria via improving gastrointestinal absorption of calcium. Thiazides should be used only in conjunction with other therapies for osteoporosis. (SOR **C**)

9. Secondary causes of osteoporosis should be sought and treated. (SOR **C**)

D. Tertiary prevention involves the care of established symptomatic osteoporosis, with attempts made to restore to highest function, minimize the negative effects of disease, and prevent disease-related complications. Since the disease is now established, primary prevention activities may have been unsuccessful. Early detection through secondary prevention may have minimized the impact of the disease.

    1. Pain relief is of primary importance in the patient with acute fracture and often will require hospital or nursing home admission. The nature of the fracture will guide specific therapeutic options.

        a. Vertebral compression fractures are commonly treated with bed rest, prevention of further injury and, occasionally, spinal bracing. (SOR **C**)

        b. A long period of therapeutic exercises may be required to regain full function.

        c. As stated above, calcitonin may reduce pain acutely. (SOR **C**)

        d. Analgesics may be used liberally as the clinical situation dictates, and nonsteroidal anti-inflammatory drugs are often suitable if no contraindications exist. Beware of the pitfalls of using analgesics and NSAIDs in the elderly.

    2. If bed rest is prolonged, consider deep vein thrombosis prophylaxis.

    3. Percutaneous procedures

        a. In vertebroplasty, polymethylmethacrylate cement is injected into the compressed vertebral body. Balloon kyphoplasty uses a balloon inflated inside the compressed vertebral body before the cement is injected.

        b. Vertebroplasty and kyphoplasty are associated with reduced pain and improved function in uncontrolled studies.

        c. These procedures, typically performed by orthopedic surgeons, interventional radiologists, and pain management specialists, are now becoming more widely used. Long-term outcomes remain uncertain because of lack of good studies and inability to adequately control/blind to intervention.

    4. Risks factors for fracture, such as orthostatic hypotension, lower limb dysfunction, drug use, and visual impairment especially in the frail, elderly patient, should be sought and reduced. A home safety evaluation should be considered to prevent falls. (SOR C)

E. Screening

    1. The US Preventive Services Task Force (USPSTF) recommends that women aged 65 years and older be screened routinely for osteoporosis. (SOR **C**)

    2. The USPSTF recommends that routine screening begin at 60 years for women at increased risk for osteoporotic fractures. (SOR **C**)

    3. National Osteoporosis Foundation (NOF) urges bone density tests for all women older than 65 years + postmenopausal women with additional risk factor for osteoporotic fracture. (SOR **C**)

    4. The National Institutes of Health Osteoporosis Consensus Panel claims that there is no evidence that widespread screening will decrease important clinical outcomes (e.g., fracture rates).

5. Who should be screened? Current evidence suggests that measurement of BMD can predict fracture risk in populations but not in individuals. Four risk indices all performed well in identifying postmenopausal women with low bone density (T score ≤ −2.5). They may be most useful in selecting women to screen who are between 60 and 65 years old. Osteoporosis Self-assessment Tool (OST) is simplest since it is based on only age and weight: (weight in kilograms) minus (age in years) ≤10 in women or ≤3 in men suggests increased risk, thus a possible indication for screening. Screening tools in common use were primarily developed in Caucasian western populations and are not well validated in other ethnic groups. (SOR **C**)

6. If one is going to screen, DXA scans of the femoral neck seem to be the best predictor of hip fracture. Since treatment of osteoporosis has been shown to decrease hip fractures, this indirectly supports the routine (every 2–3 years) screening of older women. (SOR **B**)

7. Heel ultrasound has some utility in screening because of its portability and availability. Compared to DXA, a combination of risk factors or ultrasound had 90% sensitivity, 38% specificity, 22% positive predictive value, and 95% negative predictive value in detecting osteoporosis by BMD criteria.

IV. **Management Strategies**

A. **Patient education**

1. **Counseling** should be offered to all women regarding universal preventive measures related to fracture risk, calcium and vitamin D intake, weight-bearing exercise, smoking cessation, fall prevention, avoidance of excess alcohol intake, and the risks and benefits of HRT. (SOR **C**)

2. The National Resource Center on Osteoporosis is a federally funded clearing house for the latest risks, prevention, and treatment of and information on osteoporosis (National Osteoporosis Foundation; http://www.nof.org).

B. **Compliance** with pharmacotherapy is improved when patients are given BMD testing. (SOR **C**) This may be because of the objectification of the disease when viewed as a laboratory report.

C. **Follow-up** after diagnosis or fracture includes the following:

1. Schedule office visits bimonthly initially, then every 6 months. (SOR **C**)

2. Promote periodic multiphasic screening, annual physical examination, and preventative screenings. (SOR **C**)

3. Every 2 or 3 years, obtain BMD using the same technique and the same facility if possible. (SOR **C**)

4. Repeat x-rays for acute pain or suspected fractures. (SOR **C**)

V. **Prognosis**

A. **Risk**

1. 1 vertebral fracture at baseline = fivefold risk of more vertebral fractures.

2. ≥1 vertebral fracture at baseline = 12-fold risk of more vertebral fractures.

3. 1 symptomatic vertebral fracture at baseline = twofold risk of hip fractures.

4. 1 SD decrease in hip BMD = two- to three-fold increase in hip fracture.

B. **Life expectancy**

1. Hip fractures—50% of patients never fully recover; 25% require long-term care.

REFERENCES

Campion JM, Maricic MJ. Osteoporosis in men. *Am Fam Physician*. 2003;67:1521-1526.

Fitzpatrick LA. Secondary causes of osteoporosis. *Mayo Clin Proc*. 2002;77(5):453-468. [Commentary in *Mayo Clin Proc*. 2002;77(9):1005-1006].

Poole KES, Compston JE. Osteoporosis and its management. *BMJ*. 2006;333:1251-1256.

South-Paul JE. Osteoporosis: Part I. Evaluation and assessment. *Am Fam Physician*. 2001;63:897-904, 908; and Osteoporosis: Part II. Nonpharmacologic and pharmacologic treatment. *Am Fam Physician*. 2001;63:1121-1128.

Tannenbaum C, Clark J, Schwartzman K, et al. Yield of laboratory testing to identify secondary contributors to osteoporosis in otherwise healthy women. *J Clin Endocrinol Metab*. 2002;87:4431-4437.

Wagman RB, Marcus R. Beyond bone mineral density—navigating the laboratory assessment of patients with osteoporosis [editorial]. *J Clin Endocrinol Metab*. 2002;87:4429-4430.

Zizic TM. Pharmacologic prevention of osteoporotic fractures. *Am Fam Physician*. 2004;70:1293-1300.

82   Peptic Ulcer Disease

Carol Stewart, MD, Lesley Wilkinson, MD, & Nancy Tyre, MD

KEY POINTS

- Peptic ulcer disease (PUD) is primarily caused by *Helicobacter pylori* infection or by non-steroidal anti-inflammatory drug (NSAID) use.
- Many patients present complaining of epigastric pain. Most have gastroesophageal reflux disease (GERD) or functional dyspepsia; generally 15% or less have PUD. Initial endoscopy is reserved for patients with "alarm" symptoms (weight loss, anemia, bleeding, dysphagia or odynophagia, prior PUD, persistent vomiting) suggesting bleeding, perforation, or cancer. (SOR **C**)
- All patients at higher risk for *H pylori* deserve a "test and treat" approach. (SOR **A**) Many younger patients can be empirically treated with acid suppression. (SOR **A**) Rarely, one needs to consider more obscure causes such as Zollinger–Ellison syndrome.
- The first step in treatment is stopping any NSAIDs or aspirin, starting acid-blocking medication, and initiating treatment for *H pylori* if infection is present.

I. Introduction
   A. **Definitions.** PUD is present when acid–peptic injury to the gastrointestinal mucosa results in defects (ulcerations) through the epithelial layer. GERD is usually defined as predominant or frequent (at least once a week) heartburn or acid regurgitation. Dyspepsia is chronic or recurrent pain or discomfort in the upper abdomen.
   B. **Pathophysiology.** PUD is predominantly caused by one or both of two underlying causes: (1) *H pylori* infection or (2) use of NSAIDs. Less common causes are (3) idiopathic and (4) acid hypersecretory conditions (e.g., Zollinger–Ellison syndrome). A small but growing percentage of disease is now associated with nonNSAID medication use, including potassium chloride, nitrogen-containing bisphosphonates and immunosuppressants. Infrequently, PUD is caused by Crohn disease, systemic mastocytosis, alcoholism, malignancy, viral infections (herpes simplex, cytomegalovirus), tuberculosis, syphilis, and cocaine usage. Acid is necessary, but not sufficient by itself, to develop PUD lesions.
      1. ***H pylori*** is a gram-negative microaerophilic, urease-producing bacterium that has adapted to the environment of the gastric mucosa. It causes persistent inflammation in the stomach with a vigorous immune response that rarely eliminates *H pylori*. (Children clear the infection up to 20% of the time.) *H pylori* gastritis is variable in clinical expression, and often asymptomatic. The lifetime risk of PUD in a patient infected with *H pylori* is 3% in the United States and 25% in Japan.
      2. **NSAIDs** have a different mechanism of ulceration. They do not cause a diffuse gastritis. They primarily induce mucosal injury by disrupting prostaglandin-mediated cell protection and proliferation. Gastroprotective mechanisms that are disrupted include inhibition of acid secretion, bicarbonate production, gastric mucus production, and promotion of mucosal growth and repair. Many NSAIDs are also weak acids themselves and directly injure epithelial cells in the acid stomach environment.
   C. **Epidemiology.** PUD results in approximately 3 million patient visits per year in the United States, with a current lifetime prevalence of up to 10%. US mortality owing to PUD is approximately 3500 per year.
      1. Patients usually present with dyspepsia (epigastric pain), not "PUD." Dyspepsia accounts for 2% to 5% of all symptomatic ambulatory care visits in the United States. Up to 15% of patients with dyspepsia have PUD. Of the remainder, 1% to 2% have cancer, 6% to ±25% have GERD, and more than 60% have functional dyspepsia with normal endoscopies. Most patients with typical PUD symptoms do not have PUD.
      2. The diagnosis and treatment of PUD have been transformed over the last 25 years by the development of medications that suppress acid formation and by the discovery that one of the primary etiologies of PUD is a curable infectious disease—*H pylori*.

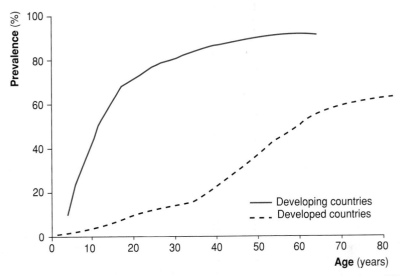

FIGURE 82–1. Prevalence of *Helicobacter pylori* infection by age. (Reproduced with permission from Logan RPH, Walker MM. ABC of the upper gastrointestinal tract: epidemiology and diagnosis of *Helicobacter pylori* infection. *BMJ*. 2001;323:920.)

    a. *H pylori* is extremely common in the developing world (prevalence more than 80%), but rates in the industrialized world have been dropping as hygiene and public health have improved. Infection occurs almost exclusively before age 10 in the industrialized world, so current prevalence rates by age reflect a cohort effect. The adult infection rate is approximately 0.5% per year (Figure 82–1).

    b. *H pylori* is transmitted by fecal/oral or oral/oral routes. Its prevalence correlates strongly with socioeconomic conditions. Risk factors in the United States include birth in another country, older age, lower socioeconomic status, domestic crowding, and unsanitary conditions; these conditions are currently more common in nonwhite populations. US *H pylori* prevalence in individuals younger than 30 is <10%, so the incidence and etiology of PUD have already begun changing, and will be shifting more in the future.

  3. NSAIDs are a major cause of PUD, primarily because of the huge number of patients utilizing them. At least 30 billion over-the-counter tablets and 70 million prescriptions for NSAIDs per year are purchased just in the United States. Nearly 40% of elderly Americans are prescribed NSAIDs each year, and NSAID use is gradually increasing because of the aging of the population and increasing use of aspirin prophylaxis. Since symptoms cannot reliably point to PUD with NSAIDs, it is important to be aware of preexisting risk factors for PUD when initiating NSAID treatment (Table 82–1).

  4. A minor number of cases, currently 1% to 5%, are now attributed to the other factors listed under pathophysiology. This is an emerging list, explaining some of the previous idiopathic cases. This list is likely to take on increasing importance as the incidence of *H pylori* continues to decline.

II. Diagnosis

  A. History. Epigastric distress is the most common presentation of PUD. Patients usually describe this as a midline gnawing discomfort or feeling of hunger. Sometimes it is painful with aching or burning, or a patient may have nausea with or without actual emesis. An acid taste is more common with GERD. The discomfort typically occurs 1 to 3 hours postprandially and overnight, classically during 1 to 2 AM. Food, antacids, or vomiting may relieve the symptoms within minutes. Minor weight loss may occur in up to 50% of patients with benign gastric ulcers. Significant weight loss is a red flag for malignancy. Patients with duodenal ulcers who eat to control their pain are more likely to present

TABLE 82-1. RISK FACTORS FOR NSAID GASTROINTESTINAL COMPLICATIONS

Helicobacter pylori infection, even if asymptomatic
Older age, more risk with higher age
History of peptic ulcer disease
Alcoholism
Female at advanced age
Poor health
Smoking
Use of steroids, chemotherapy, anticoagulation, or alendronate
High-dose or prolonged course of NSAID use, or both

NSAID, nonsteroidal anti-inflammatory drug.

with weight gain. **ALARM SYMPTOMS** may indicate complicating diagnoses (Table 82–2). The presence of alarm symptoms is an indication for immediate endoscopy in the dyspeptic patient. (SOR **⊙**)
   B. **Physical examination.** The physical examination is usually nonspecific; epigastric tenderness is the most common finding.
   C. **Tests**
      1. Definitive diagnosis of PUD requires endoscopy. Barium studies can also confirm the diagnosis, but do not allow for biopsy. Treatment with proton pump inhibitors (PPIs) significantly decreases the sensitivity of endoscopy. Ideally, endoscopy should take place prior to treatment, or PPIs should be discontinued for at least 4 weeks before endoscopy. Even cancer may partially heal with PPI treatment despite its malignant nature, and it can be deceptive even for skilled endoscopists.
      2. Blood counts should be checked if there is any concern about a bleeding ulcer. Concerns about acute bleeding should prompt stool guaiacs and gastric aspiration.
      3. Histology of tissue from at least two different sites remains the gold standard for diagnosis of *H pylori* infection, but many other methods are available (Table 82–3). Serology is the most common method used for diagnosis, but it is unsuitable for following up eradication. Stool antigen tests and urea breath tests generally revert to negative 1 month after effective treatment. Stool antigen tests are insensitive in the setting of PPI use.
   D. **Differential diagnosis.** As noted above, most patients with PUD symptoms actually have functional dyspepsia or GERD. The differential does include serious illnesses that require a high index of suspicion to diagnose: bleeding ulcer, perforated ulcer, gastric or esophageal cancer (duodenal ulcer is almost never malignant), severe GERD with stricture, as well as pancreatitis, cholecystitis, and cardiac or pulmonary etiologies.
III. **Treatment.** The overall treatment algorithm is outlined in Figure 82–2. (Applicable only to geographic locations with low levels of *H pylori* infection—not developing countries, or Russia, China, Japan, and others.)
   A. **Test and treat.** Current expert consensus is that patients presenting with dyspepsia, but NO alarm symptoms, should first be managed with acid suppression or a "test and treat" approach, without obtaining a definitive diagnosis. (SOR **Ⓐ**) Patients can be considered

TABLE 82-2. ALARM SYMPTOMS FOR PEPTIC ULCER DISEASE

Age older than 55 years (incidence of cancer increases with age, <1% younger than age 50)
Unintentional weight loss or anorexia/early satiety
Anemia (iron deficiency)
Gastrointestinal bleeding (either hematemesis or hematochezia)
Dysphagia (difficulty swallowing)
Odynophagia (pain on swallowing)
Vomiting (persistent)
Epigastric mass
Prior gastric surgery or peptic ulcer disease
Family history of gastric cancer
Severe or penetrating pain, or both

TABLE 82-3. DIAGNOSTIC TESTS FOR *HELICOBACTER PYLORI*

Diagnostic Tests	Sensitivity (%)	Specificity (%)
Histology (specialized stains)	93–96	97–99
Bacterial culture (of gastric contents)	80–94	100
Urea breath tests	90–96	90–98
Stool antigen tests	88–95	90–98
Rapid urease assays	88–95	95–99
Lab serology tests	85–94	80–95
Office whole blood tests	70–88	75–90

(Data from Smoot DT, Go MF, Cryer B. Peptic ulcer disease. *Prim Care; Clin Office Practice* 2001;28(3):487.)

for treatment without testing for *H pylori* if they are young (<55) and not in a group or family suggestive of increased *H pylori* risk, such as immigrants from high-prevalence countries (less than 10% prevalence cutoff for empiric treatment, SOR **Ⓒ**). Noninvasive testing for *H pylori* should be performed if needed and treatment initiated if positive. If the patient is on an NSAID, it should be stopped if at all possible. Treatment with acid suppression should begin. If these treatments fail to control symptoms, then referral for endoscopy is indicated.

B. Acid suppression promotes ulcer healing, and *H pylori* treatments require higher pH to be successful. An empiric trial of 4 to 8 weeks of acid suppression is indicated for young people with low *H pylori* risk. (SOR **Ⓐ**) If symptoms are not controlled, then the "test and treat" approach is indicated, with endoscopy if it fails also. If initial treatment is successful, but symptoms recur after medication is discontinued, then a repeat trial of acid suppression is acceptable before any testing. (SOR **Ⓒ**)

1. PPIs are the most effective medications. (SOR **Ⓐ**) They significantly raise gastric pH by disabling active hydrogen ("proton") pumps in the parietal cells. It takes 3 to 4 days to reach full activity because all the pumps are not normally turned on at one time. All PPIs are similarly effective, but differ somewhat in drug interactions (Table 82–4).

2. H_2 receptor antagonists (H_2 blockers) quickly decrease acid secretion by blocking histamine stimulation of parietal cell activity (Table 82–5). They are effective, but tolerance develops, and they are not as potent as PPIs for acid suppression or healing. Although

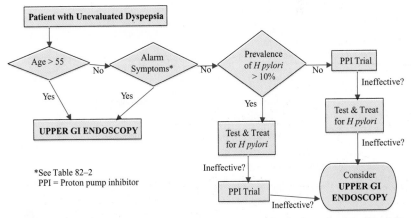

FIGURE 82–2. Work-up of dyspepsia. (Data from Talley NJ, Vakil N; the Practice Parameters Committee of the American College of Gastroenterology. Guidelines for the management of dyspepsia. *Am J Gastroenterol.* 2005;100: 2324-2337.)

TABLE 82–4. **MEDICATIONS FOR TREATMENT OR PREVENTION OF PEPTIC ULCER DISEASE, PART I**

Drug	Dose	Notes	Cost
Proton pump inhibitors (PPIs)			
Esomeprazole magnesium (Nexium)	20–40 mg qd	Maint: 20 mg qd ♀ (Pregnancy category) B	$$$$$
Lansoprazole (Prevacid)	DU: 15 mg qd GU: 30 mg qd	Maint: 15 mg qd for DU Hypersecretory conditions: 60 mg qd, adjust up to max 90 mg bid; ♀ B	$$$$$
Omeprazole (Prilosec)	DU: 20 mg qd GU: 40 mg qd OTC: 20 mg qd	Maint: 20 mg qd Hypersecretory conditions: 60 mg qd, adjust up to max 120 mg tid Available OTC, ♀ C; more potential drug interactions than the other PPIs*	$$ trade $$$$$
Pantoprazole sodium (Protonix)	40 mg qd	Maint: 40 mg qd Hypersecretory conditions: 40 mg bid, adjust up to max 240 qd; ♀ B	$$$$
Rabeprazole sodium (Aciphex)	20 mg qd after morning meal	Maint: 20 mg qd Hypersecretory conditions: 60 mg qd, adjust max up to 100 mg qd or 60 mg bid, Swallow whole. Caution with severe hepatic impairment; ♀ B	$$$$$

*All PPIs have a risk rating of category D (consider therapy modification) for concomitant use with systemic antifungals (imidazoles) and atazanavir. This is because of decreased absorption of these medications in a nonacidic environment. For category C (monitor therapy) interactions, omeprazole has more potential problems, especially with warfarin and benzodiazepines. All seizure medications, digoxin, statins, methotrexate, and their effects should be monitored if given with any PPI. Lansoprazole and rabeprazole are less effective if taken with St. John's wort.
DU, duodenal ulcer; GU, gastric ulcer; OTC, over the counter. ♀, pregnancy class. (Cost: $, <$25; $$, $25–49; $$$, $50–99; $$$$, $100–199; $$$$$, >$200 for a month or a course.)

TABLE 82–5. **MEDICATIONS FOR TREATMENT OR PREVENTION OF PEPTIC ULCER DISEASE, PART II**

Drug	Dose	Notes	Cost
H₂ blockers			
Cimetidine (Tagamet)	300 mg qid OR 400 mg bid OR 800 mg hs OTC 100 mg	Maint: 400 mg qhs Hypersecretory conditions: 300 mg qid up to 2400 mg qd. Many drug interactions; may induce confusional states, particularly in the elderly. ♀ B	$ $ $$
Famotidine (Pepcid)	40 mg qhs OR 20 mg bid OTC 10 mg	Central nervous system adverse effects reported with moderate to severe renal insufficiency. Few drug interactions. ♀ B	$ $
Nizatidine (Axid)	300 mg qhs OR 150 mg bid OTC 75 mg	Maint: 150 mg qhs False-positive for urobilinogen with Multistix. ♀ C	$$ $$ $$
Ranitidine (Zantac)	150 mg bid OR 300 mg qhs OTC 75 mg	Maint: 150 mg qhs Hypersecretory conditions: 150 mg bid Bradycardia reported with rapid infusion. Few drug interactions. ♀ B	$ $ $
Other Medications for PUD treatment/prevention			
Misoprostol (Cytotec)	200 μg qid, or if not tolerated, 100 μg qid	For prevention of NSAID-induced ulcers in patients at risk. ♀ X	$$$
Sucralfate (Carafate)	1 g qid ac and hs	Maint: 1 g bid on empty stomach, adheres to ulcer crater; ♀ B	$$$

OTC, over the counter; NSAID, nonsteroidal anti-inflammatory drug. ♀, pregnancy class. (Cost: $, <$25; $$, $25–49; $$$, $50–99; $$$$, $100–199; $$$$$, >$200 for a month or a course.)

they work to an extent, they are not the primary treatment for PUD in the United States at this point.

3. All other drugs are inferior at acid suppression and healing (Table 82–5). Patients can, of course, use antacids for symptom relief. Sucralfate is helpful, but is inferior to H_2 blockers. Misoprostol (Cytotec) is fairly effective at preventing NSAID-induced ulceration, but has a high (up to 30%) rate of diarrhea, is very expensive, and is inferior to PPIs.

C. **Therapy for *H pylori***

1. All diagnosed *H pylori* should be treated (even if PUD is ultimately ruled out). A drug regimen of at least two antibiotics and an acid suppressor is required (Table 82–6). Multiple regimens have been tried because none is ideal; all suffer from potential side effects, potential poor adherence, expense, and significant failure rates. (There is significant antibiotic resistance of approximately 40% to metronidazole and approximately 10% to clarithromycin.)

2. To confirm eradication after *H pylori* treatment for PUD, the patient should ideally be retested for active *H pylori* 4 to 8 weeks after treatment, with either the urea breath test or stool antigen test. Treatment failure requires a second regimen, generally quadruple therapy with alternative antibiotics. A second treatment failure requires specialty referral with endoscopy, and culture for sensitivities. (*Note:* It is fairly common for patients to resolve their *H pylori* and PUD, but still require symptomatic PPI treatment for GERD or functional dyspepsia.)

D. **Therapy for NSAID-related ulcers.** The primary treatment is to stop the NSAID if at all possible and initiate acid suppression, usually with a PPI. Generally, treatment is rapid and effective if the NSAID can be stopped. Unfortunately, many patients need continuing NSAID treatment or aspirin prophylaxis. Under those circumstances, the NSAID dose should be minimized, and prophylaxis begun with a PPI. Previous consideration of the use of COX-2 specific NSAIDs in these patients has fallen in popularity as the increased risk of cardiovascular side-effects with these agents has become more apparent. Also, the improved GI benefits may be ameliorated if the patient needs aspirin for cardiac prophylaxis.

E. **Relapse.** If NSAIDs are discontinued and *H pylori* is cured but the patient clinically relapses, then referral to a specialist is indicated, and PPIs should be reinitiated. Consider unusual causes, particularly acid hypersecretory states. A fasting gastrin level is indicated for multiple ulcers, ulcers resistant to therapy, ulcer patients awaiting surgery, ulcers associated with severe esophagitis, and patients with a family history of similar ulcer problems or other endocrine tumors.

F. **Idiopathic PUD.** If all treatable etiologies for PUD are ruled out, then treatment focuses solely on acid suppression. The percentage of idiopathic ulcers is increasing as the percentage of all ulcers from *H pylori* is decreasing.

G. **Surgery.** Operative treatment is indicated for patients with acute complications or refractory PUD. Rates of surgery for PUD have plummeted.

IV. **Management Strategies.** The goal of ulcer therapy is complete healing without relapse. The most important aspects of management are reviewed in the Treatment section (Section III). Prior to the appreciation of the role of *H pylori,* many lifestyle issues were thought to be important in the pathogenesis and treatment of PUD. Now, they are largely understood to be secondary or even unrelated.

A. **Smoking** does promote ulcerogenesis, at least in patients with *H pylori.* Smoking adversely affects ulcer development, healing, and complications. However, if *H pylori* is eradicated, smokers do not appear to be at continued increased PUD risk. It is considered appropriate to recommend smoking cessation to ulcer patients who smoke, but primary treatment remains that appropriate for the primary ulcer etiology (e.g., *H pylori* or NSAIDs).

B. **Alcohol** has long been considered a cause of PUD. In fact, it is usually not a significant contributor. In large doses, it does damage the stomach epithelium directly. In patients who consume more than 20 drinks a week, ulcer rates are significantly increased, especially in the presence of cirrhosis.

C. **Emotional stress** may affect ulcer frequency to some extent. Severe societal stressors (such as major earthquakes) cause an increase in PUD rates in the affected areas. Severe physiologic stressors (such as surgery or intensive care unit admissions) are well known to predispose patients to ulcers. Emotional stress may be one of the factors that causes patients exposed to *H pylori* or NSAIDs to become part of the small percentage that

TABLE 82-6. TREATMENT OPTIONS FOR *HELICOBACTER PYLORI*

Regimen	PPI	Antibiotic #1	Antibiotic #2	Bismuth	Number of Days	Efficacy (%)
Triple therapy—usual initial regimen	PPI* bid	Amoxicillin 1 g bid (*If PCN allergic*: metronidazole 500 mg bid or quadruple therapy)	Clarithromycin 500 mg bid (*If macrolide allergic*: metronidazole 500 mg bid or quadruple therapy)	N/A	14	70–85
Cost §	‡	$	$$			
Quadruple therapy—for resistant infections or primary therapy in: (1) allergic patients or (2) those recently exposed to triple component antibiotics	PPI* bid (*H₂ blocker possible if must*)	Tetracycline 500 mg qid	Metronidazole 500 mg qid	Bismuth subsalicylate† 525 mg qid	14	75–90
Cost §	‡	$	$	$		
Sequential therapy—promising primary therapy but not re-confirmed for the USA	PPI* bid	**Days 1–5** Amoxicillin 1g bid	Days 6–10 Clarithromycin 500 mg bid PLUS Tinidazole 500 mg bid	N/A	10	85–90
Cost §	‡	$	$ + $			
Salvage therapy for cont infection after 1 or 2 regimens—no studies USA	PPI* bid	Amoxicillin 1 g bid	Levofloxacin 500 mg daily	N/A	10	87
Cost §	‡	$	$$$$			

*Any PPI can be used: omeprazole (Prilosec), 20 mg; esomeprazole (Nexium), 20 mg; lansoprazole (Prevacid), 30 mg; pantoprazole (Protonix), 40 mg; rabeprazole (AciPhex), 20 mg, see table 82-4.
† Pepto-Bismol.
‡ PPI, proton pump inhibitor, costs, see Table 82-4.
§(Cost: $, <$25; $$, $25–49; $$$, $50–99; $$$$, $100–199; $$$$$, >$200 for a month or a course.
(Data adapted from Chey WD, Wong BCY. American College of Gastroenterology guideline on the management of *Helicobacter pylori* infection. *Am J Gastroenterol.* 2007;102(8):1808.)

actually develop an ulcer. However, emotional strain does not interfere with treatment. Although conventional wisdom is that all ulcers are directly caused by "stress," reduction in stress is not necessary for adequate healing. Treatment should be directed at the primary etiology.

D. Diet does NOT contribute to PUD, and no special diets are needed during treatment. Patients may perceive diet as significant because it can affect symptoms of dyspepsia, but it does not affect ulcer healing.

E. Alternative treatments for PUD are unproven. Listed are a few of the most common strategies.

1. Acupuncture may decrease epigastric pain, acid secretion, or both.
2. Chinese herbal treatments include Xao Yao Wan at 8 tablets 3 times daily for soothing stress and gastric upset.
3. Naturopathic remedies include aloe vera juice 1 to 2 tablespoons twice daily or "stomach formula" as directed.
4. Homeopathic remedies are individualized by nonWestern parameters.

V. Prognosis. The prognosis of PUD has improved dramatically. Although the mortality of acute upper GI bleed is approximately 5%, PUD can usually be cured or controlled for most of the patient population.

A. NSAIDs. Up to 4% of NSAID users develop serious complications such as frank PUD with bleeding or perforation each year. Between 5% and 20% of long-term NSAID users have peptic ulcers at any given time. Of NSAID users with PUD, there is a 400% to 500% increase in complications. However, even for patients who must continue NSAIDs, continuous treatment with PPIs causes relapse rates for PUD to decrease to 5%.

B. *H pylori*. Eradication of *H pylori* dramatically alters the natural history of PUD. Previously, the natural history of PUD was chronic and relapsing, with more than 75% recurrence of ulcers. Now patients cured of *H pylori* often require no further treatment, with relapse rates for PUD decreased to 5%.

VI. Prevention. The American College of Gastroenterology has identified risk factors for PUD that should be considered when starting someone on an NSAID.

A. Prior history of a gastrointestinal event (ulcer, hemorrhage)

B. Age > 60

C. High dosage of an NSAID

D. Concurrent use of glucocorticoids

E. Concurrent use of anticoagulants

Use of a PPI for prophylaxis should be considered for these patients, especially if more than one risk factor is present, and particularly if the use of NSAIDs will be longer term. (SOR **⊙**) Which NSAID is employed does make a small difference in the risk of PUD, but the dosage and length of use are greater factors.

Concurrent *H pylori* infection is a risk factor for PUD with NSAIDs, so testing and treating for *H pylori* in older patients or those otherwise at higher risk of *H pylori* infection is also appropriate when starting long-term NSAID therapy, even though not every study supports this. (SOR **⊙**)

Evidence is weaker on the association of PUD and the concomitant use of NSAIDs and SSRIs (selective serotonin reuptake inhibitors). Some studies show a 12- to 15-fold increase in UGI bleeding with the combined use of NSAIDs and SSRIs, but more work needs to be done. In the meantime, high-risk patients such as the elderly and patients with a history of PUD may benefit from a course of PPIs with their NSAIDs and antidepressants. (SOR **⊙**)

REFERENCES

Arents NLA, Thijs JC, Kleibeuker JH. A rational approach to uninvestigated dyspepsia in primary care: review of the literature. *Postgrad Med J.* 2002;78:707-716.

Chey WD, Wong BCY. American College of Gastroenterology guideline on the management of *Helicobacter pylori* infection. *Am J Gastroenterol.* 2007;102(8):1808-1825.

Smoot DT, Go MF, Cryer B. Peptic ulcer disease. *Prim Care.* 2001;28(3):487-503.

Suerbaum S, Michetti P. *Helicobacter pylori* infection. *N Engl J Med.* 2002;347(15):1175-1186.

Talley NJ, Vakil N; the Practice Parameters Committee of the American College of Gastroenterology. Guidelines for the management of dyspepsia. *Am J Gastroenterol.* 2005;100:2324-2337.

83   Premenstrual Syndrome

Lt Col Heather R. Pickett, DO, & Maj Michael Michener, MD

KEY POINTS

- Premenstrual syndrome is a group of symptoms affecting many women of reproductive age. Sharing many features of depression and anxiety disorders, premenstrual syndrome represents a distinct entity characterized chiefly by its occurrence exclusively in the luteal phase of the menstrual cycle.
- Symptoms occur only within approximately 2 weeks before the onset of menses, and subside with the onset of bleeding. They may occur in either ovulatory or nonovulatory cycles.
- Symptoms usually include one or more of the following clusters:
  - Anxiety, irritability, or mood swings.
  - Weight gain, swelling, bloating, or breast tenderness.
  - Appetite change, food cravings, and fatigue.
  - Depression, sleep disturbance, or cognitive difficulty.
  - Pain, including headache and general muscular pains.
- Major depressive disorder with suicide risk must be ruled out, and hypothyroidism may present some of the same symptoms.
- Lifestyle modification includes the following:
  - A diet high in protein and complex carbohydrate-rich foods/beverages that is also low in fat, salt, and refined sugar (SOR **B**) (see the Food Guide Pyramid www.eatright.org/pyramid/).
  - Supplementing the diet with magnesium, 200 to 400 mg; vitamin E, 400 mg; vitamin B6, 50 to 100 mg; and calcium, 1000 mg/d. (SOR **B**)
  - Getting regular aerobic exercise. (SOR **C**)
  - Avoiding caffeine, tobacco, and excess alcohol. (SOR **C**)
- Education and cognitive therapy can also help. (SOR **C**)
- Medication, if necessary in addition to the above, starting approximately on day 12 to 14 of the menstrual cycle, can include the following:
  - A selective serotonin reuptake inhibitor. (SOR **A**) *The following have been studied and found effective for* premenstrual syndrome/*premenstrual dysphoric disorder:* fluoxetine, 20 to 60 mg/d; sertraline, 50 to 100 mg/d; citalopram, 10 to 20 mg/d.
  - Consider buspirone, 30 mg/d in divided doses, if the selective serotonin reuptake inhibitor is not tolerated or if complaints are mostly anxiety-related or pain symptoms. (SOR **B**)
  - Alprazolam—similar indications as for buspirone. (SOR **B**)
  - GnRH agonists and surgical oophorectomy—side effects can limit their usefulness. (SOR **B**)
  - Oral contraceptives may improve some of the physical symptoms. (SOR **B**)

I. Introduction

  A. **Definition.** Premenstrual syndrome (PMS) is the cyclic recurrence in the luteal phase of the menstrual cycle of a combination of distressing physical, psychological, and behavioral changes of severity that results in deterioration of interpersonal relationships or interference with normal activities. Premenstrual dysphoric disorder (PMDD) is a more severe variant of PMS that has primarily psychiatric symptoms with specific DSM-IV-R criteria (Table 83–1).

  B. **Epidemiology.** Most women report at least some minor physical and emotional symptoms in the postovulatory phase of the menstrual cycle. Thirty to forty percent have symptoms of moderate intensity, and it is estimated that 3% to 5% of women of reproductive age have PMS of an intensity that is temporarily disabling.

   1. **Age.** Symptoms of PMS may occur at any age in the reproductive years; incidence of presenting for care peaks in the mid-30s. Some women experience cyclic symptoms even after menopause.

   2. **Social class.** No clinically useful differences have been defined.

TABLE 83-1. RESEARCH CRITERIA FOR PREMENSTRUAL DYSPHORIC DISORDER

In most menstrual cycles during the past year, five (or more) of the following symptoms were present for most of the time during the last week of the luteal phase, began to remit within a few days after the onset of the follicular phase, and were absent in the week postmenses, with at least one of the symptoms being either (1), (2), (3), or (4):

(1) Markedly depressed mood, feelings of hopelessness, or self-deprecating thoughts
(2) Marked anxiety, tension, or feeling of being "keyed up" or "on edge"
(3) Marked affective lability (e.g., feeling suddenly sad or tearful or having increased sensitivity to rejection)
(4) Persistent and marked anger or irritability or increased interpersonal conflicts
(5) Decreased interest in usual activities (e.g., work, friends, or hobbies)
(6) Subjective sense of difficulty in concentrating
(7) Lethargy, easy fatigability, or marked lack of energy
(8) Marked change in appetite, overeating, or specific food cravings
(9) Hypersomnia or insomnia
(10) A subjective sense of being overwhelmed or out of control
(11) Other physical symptoms, such as breast tenderness or swelling, headaches, joint or muscle pain, a sensation of "bloating," or weight gain

The disturbance must seriously interfere with work or usual social activities or relationships, and not be merely an exacerbation of the symptoms of another disorder, such as major depression, panic disorder, dysthymia, or a personality disorder (although it may be superimposed on any of these).

The criteria must be confirmed by prospective, daily self-ratings during at least two cycles.

(Adapted with permission from American Psychiatric Association (APA). *Diagnostic and Statistical Manual of Mental Disorders.* 4th ed. APA; 1994.)

3. **Race.** PMS is reported to occur in all ethnic groups. Cultural variation in the prevalence rates and patterns of symptoms occur, but no clinically useful diagnostic or therapeutic differences have yet emerged.

4. **Reproductive factors.** Women with regular (ovulatory) menstrual cycles, as well as those with longer cycles and heavier menstrual flow, report symptoms of swelling, mood swings, and depression more than other women. PMS may occur in spontaneous anovulatory cycles and following oophorectomy or hysterectomy. More than half of severe PMS patients have a history of preeclampsia or postnatal depression.

5. **Genetics.** A majority of studies have supported a strong genetic component to PMS and PMDD.

C. **Pathophysiology.** No single theory currently accounts for all the clinical and pathophysiologic features of PMS. The similarity of PMS to depressive illness, as well as its response to antidepressant therapy, suggests shared metabolic abnormalities. Metabolic differences between the two entities have been found, however. The interaction of several pathways may result in the development of PMS. Research seems to point toward an interaction of hormones, neurotransmitters (serotonin being the most often implicated), nutrients, and behavioral or environmental factors in the development of significant symptoms. Because of the differences in response to treatment for women with similar symptoms, subtypes of PMS have been postulated. Multiple physiologic alterations may coexist that yield the same symptomatic outcomes; correction of single abnormalities without normalizing others (as is likely to happen in a clinical trial) may explain the variability in reported effectiveness of various treatments in different studies.

One study concluded that the symptoms of PMS represent an abnormal response to normal cyclic hormone changes. Twenty women with PMS and twenty without PMS were given leuprolide versus placebo for 3 months. There were no differences in women without PMS, but there was a significant decrease in symptoms in the women with PMS who were given leuprolide. Leuprolide responders were then given estradiol and progesterone, which were associated with a return of symptoms. Evidence also supports a role for serotonin in PMS. Cyclic fluctuations in estrogen and progesterone can have effects on the serotonin system. Patients with PMS have lower blood serotonin levels.

II. **Diagnosis.** For the woman who presents with symptoms of PMS, beginning the diagnostic process with an open-ended inquiry will provide tremendously useful information. Symptoms commonly noted (Table 83–1 and Figure 83–1) include depressed mood or feelings of hopelessness or self-deprecation; anxiety; affective lability; irritability; anger; feelings of difficulty concentrating; decreased energy; change in sleep, appetite, or both (increase or decrease); feelings of being out of control; and physical symptoms of bloating, breast tenderness,

Name: _____ Month: _____

Write the date in the first now, starting with today. Circle the days of your menstrual period.
Each day, rate the severity of your symptoms: 1 = no symptoms; 2 = mild symptoms; 3 = moderate symptoms;
4 = severe symptoms.

Date																															
Day of the month	1	2	3	4	5	6	7	8	9	10	11	12	13	14	15	16	17	18	19	20	21	22	23	24	25	26	27	28	29	30	31
Irritability or tension																															
Anger or short temper																															
Anxiety or nervousness																															
Depression or sadness																															
Crying or tearfulness																															
Relationship problems																															
Tiredness or lack of energy																															
Insomnia																															
Changes in sexual interest																															
Food cravings or overeating																															
Difficulty concentrating																															
Feeling overwhelmed																															
Headaches																															
Breas tenderness or swelling																															
Back pain																															
Abdominal pain																															
Muscle and joint pain																															
Weight gain																															
Nausea																															
Other (please specify)																															
Other (please specify)																															

FIGURE 83–1. Take home patient chart for tracking of symptoms.

muscle or joint aches, and headache. These symptoms must interfere with usual daily activities. The National Institute of Mental Health has recommended that, for a diagnosis of PMS, there must be a marked change in intensity (at least 30%) of symptoms measured from cycle days 5 to 10 compared to the 6-day interval prior to menses for at least two consecutive cycles.

In some studies, up to 50% of women presenting to PMS clinics did not meet diagnostic criteria for that disorder, but instead were assigned another diagnosis: most frequently, major depression, followed in frequency by dysthymia, anxiety disorder, menopause, or another gynecologic or medical disorder (e.g., hypothyroidism). "PMS" may be a diagnosis that is more acceptable to the patient than is depression or anxiety. By starting the evaluation in an unstructured manner, the clinician can avoid a premature (and possibly erroneous) diagnosis.

Once an overview of the symptoms has been obtained, the patient's symptoms can be rated to establish a baseline (Table 83–2 and /Figure 83–2), and other essential information can be requested, including: Is there a previous diagnosis of PMS? What criteria were used to

TABLE 83-2. SHORTENED PREMENSTRUAL ASSESSMENT FORM

The patient is asked to consider the changes currently experienced with regard to her menstrual period: pain, tenderness, enlargement, or swelling of breasts
Feeling unable to cope or overwhelmed by ordinary demands
Feeling under stress
Outbursts of "irritability" or bad temper
Feeling sad or blue
Backaches, joint and muscle pain, or stiffness
Weight gain
Relatively steady abdominal heaviness, discomfort, or pain
Edema, swelling, puffiness, or "water retention"
Feeling bloated
Patients may rate each change on this list on a scale from 1 (not present or no change from usual) to 6 (extreme change, perhaps noticeable even to casual acquaintances)

(Adapted with permission from Allen SS, McBride CM, Pirie PL. The shortened premenstrual assessment form. *J Reprod Med.* 1991;36:769.)

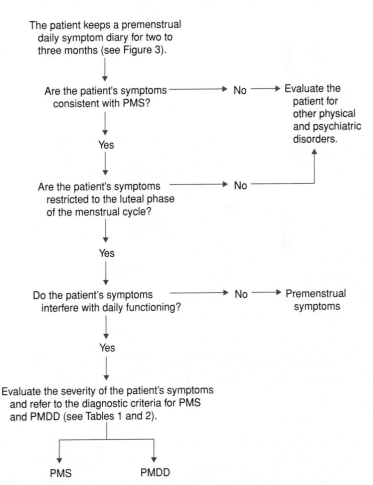

FIGURE 83-2. Algorithm for use in differentiating premenstrual symptoms, premenstrual syndrome (PMS), and premenstrual dysphoric disorder (PMDD).

make the diagnosis? Have the symptoms changed over time? What previous treatments have been successful or unsuccessful? Many patients will self-diagnose PMS from information found in the lay literature. Other important questions include the following:

A. **Is there a history of treatment for an affective disorder?** As many as 10% of women with PMS may report suicidal ideas and death wishes and thoughts.

   Are there vegetative symptoms of depression? (See Chapter 92.) Of women with major depression, more than half will have exacerbation of symptoms in the premenstrual phase, including increased severity of usual symptoms or the appearance of new symptoms such as increased aggression, suicidal tendencies, or depersonalization.

B. **Is there seasonal variation of the depressive symptoms?** Seasonal and nonseasonal PMDD have been shown to improve with phototherapy. (SOR **B**)

C. **Does she consider her general health to be good, or is there chronic disease?** PMS must be differentiated from symptoms arising from other chronic disorders, but which are exacerbated during the premenstrual phase of the cycle ("premenstrual magnification"). Some patients experience exacerbation or precipitation of other medical problems, such as asthma, migraine, epilepsy, or bipolar illness just prior to menstruation.

D. **Are her menses regular? Has she had pelvic inflammatory disease, surgery, or endometriosis? What contraceptive method does she use?** A primary complaint of pain may be related to gynecologic disease. By suppression of ovulation, oral contraceptives may provide relief of PMS (SOR **B**), but studies have been inconsistent in this regard. Marked relief of symptoms was noted in a majority of women treated with depot medroxyprogesterone acetate in one study. Suggest keeping a symptom diary (see Figure 83–1) for 2 to 3 months and charting basal body temperature (or other method) to reliably identify ovulation.

E. **Has she been pregnant? What was the outcome? Were her symptoms present during pregnancy? Did she have postpartum depression?** PMS is not present during pregnancy. Current affective symptoms could relate to a pregnancy outcome, such as abortion, other fetal loss, or abnormality. Postpartum depression is frequently found in patients with PMDD.

F. **Is the patient taking medications? Is she taking vitamin or mineral supplements, and on whose advice? What alternative therapies has she tried?** Diuretic therapy can result in paradoxical water retention, especially in "idiopathic edema." Large amounts of dairy products may interfere with magnesium absorption, leading to chronic deficiency, which has been noted in PMS. High phosphate intake (e.g., from colas) can cause relative deficiency of calcium, especially when coupled with low intake of dairy products. Some women will take large amounts (200 mg or more) of vitamin B_6 in an attempt to relieve PMS symptoms, without understanding the risk of peripheral neuropathy. However, some supplements, in the correct amounts, can be therapeutic for PMS. Women, in the search for PMS treatment, may have encountered clinicians who were less than empathetic toward their complaints. Many seek care from alternative practitioners, who may provide some relief of their symptoms, and this alternative treatment may be continued along with the traditional prescription obtained from the clinician. An understanding of all current treatments is necessary to avoid adverse interactions.

G. **Is there a personal history of alcohol or drug abuse?** Compared with the general population, women seeking treatment for PMS are more likely to have lifetime histories of depression, anxiety disorder, suicide attempts, panic disorder, and substance abuse.

H. **Is there a history of smoking?** Women who smoke are more likely to experience PMS symptoms.

I. **Is there evidence of bulimia? Does she have food cravings? Does she follow any particular diet regimen?** Electrolyte imbalances from frequent vomiting can yield behavioral symptoms, especially fatigue. Ingestion of large amounts of sugar can exacerbate symptoms in at least two ways: refined sugar increases the urinary excretion of magnesium (as do diuretics) and also interferes with renal clearance of sodium and water. In response to a large sugar load, the production of keto acids is suppressed by an insulin surge. The resulting impairment in excretion of sodium and water causes expansion of the extracellular fluid volume with resultant edema, bloating, and breast tenderness. This sodium retention is resistant to aldosterone inhibitors. Table salt enhances the intestinal absorption of glucose, which enhances this insulin response and contributes to the edema. Alcohol may play a role in reactive hypoglycemia of PMS.

J. **Was there early victimization and trauma?** Up to 40% of patients diagnosed with PMS have a history of sexual abuse.

K. Is there a family history of PMS, affective disorders, substance abuse, or alcoholism? Familial occurrence is documented.

L. Symptom clusters. PMS symptoms may fall into "clusters," which may be helpful in choosing therapy. Some women experience more anxiety, irritability, or mood swings. For some, the primary symptoms are weight gain, swelling, and bloating; for others changes in appetite or cravings, fatigue, and headache are most troublesome. Still others have depression, sleep disturbance, or cognitive difficulties. Some women experience any or all of these, with variations in severity and symptoms from cycle to cycle. Treatment success is not contingent upon identifying a particular symptom cluster.

M. Timing of symptoms. Patients should be encouraged to keep a prospective calendar of symptoms experienced relative to phase of the menstrual cycle (Figure 83–3) to help confirm that they are indeed premenstrual; (SOR **Ⓐ**) some women experience erratic symptom patterns and incorrectly attribute them to PMS. Basal temperature measurements can help rule out disorders of ovulation and provide further confirmation of the premenstrual timing of symptoms.

N. Physical examination. General physical and pelvic examinations are indicated to exclude rheumatologic disease, anemia, electrolyte imbalance, neoplasms, endometriosis, or menopause.

O. Laboratory tests. There are no specific laboratory tests for PMS at this time. Other laboratory or physiologic tests may be necessary in individual cases to rule out other potential causes of symptoms. Tests that are *not* likely to be useful in the diagnosis of PMS include follicle-stimulating hormone, luteinizing hormone, estrogen, progesterone, or testosterone unless other conditions are suspected. Tests to consider include:

1. **A complete blood cell count** if there is chronic fatigue or menorrhagia.
2. **SMA-18 chemistry profile** if there is chronic fatigue or suspicion of electrolyte disorder.
3. **Thyroid-stimulating hormone** (unless done within the last 3 months), as the prevalence of thyroid disease is high for women in this age group.
4. **Serum prolactin** in patients with galactorrhea, an irregular menstrual cycle, history of infertility, decreased libido, or atypical presentations of mastalgia.
5. **Chlamydia and gonorrhea testing** if there is high-risk behavior, cervicitis, or pain upon pelvic examination.

III. Treatment

A. Patient education. Patients are exposed to information about PMS from many medical and nonmedical sources and may have strong convictions about the condition and its treatment. Some express the fear that their symptoms represent an untreatable

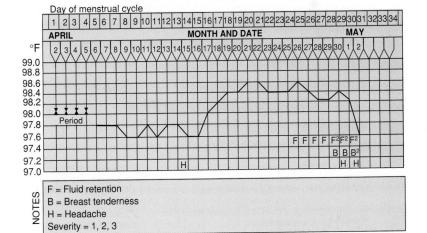

FIGURE 83–3. Premenstrual syndrome symptom diary. A minimum of two symptomatic cycles must be included to establish the diagnosis.

condition. Uncertainties about PMS causes in the literature notwithstanding, the likelihood of successful treatment of PMS is high, and reassurance of this fact is the first step to successful treatment. Empathy and affirmation are particularly useful in dealing with PMS.

Patient education alone may lead to a dramatic reduction in symptoms during the 3 months when the patient is completing the symptom diary. In addition, such general advice builds patient's self-esteem and ability to cope with symptoms. In controlled trials of PMS treatment, the placebo response rate is typically greater than 20% and sometimes as high as 50%, emphasizing the significant therapeutic value of discussing symptoms with a caring clinician. (SOR **C**)

B. Symptomatic treatments

1. Encourage proper diet with adequate composition according to the current US Recommended Daily Allowances and Dietary Guidelines for healthy adults. Instruct the patient to follow the Food Guide Pyramid (http://www.nal.usda.gov/fnic.html) with specific emphasis on avoiding salt, high loads of refined sugar, and animal fats. This will often provide symptom relief and potentially confer general health benefits as well. A diet high in complex carbohydrate-rich foods may improve mood symptoms and reduce food cravings. (SOR **B**)

   a. Supplementation may be necessary to ensure adequate amounts of certain nutrients, including calcium (1000 mg of elemental calcium per day) (SOR **B**), vitamins (vitamin E, 400 IU/d; (SOR **B**) vitamin B$_6$, – 50–100 mg/d (SOR **B**)) Higher doses have been linked to peripheral neuropathy.

   b. Trace minerals (magnesium, 200-400 mg/d SOR **B**) have primarily been shown to help decrease fluid retention.

   c. High intake of calcium (1200 mg/d) and Vitamin D (700 IU/d) has been associated with lower risk of developing PMS over a 10-year period.

2. Regular aerobic exercise (SOR **C**) and elimination or reduction of adverse health habits, such as tobacco and alcohol use, may directly improve PMS through the pathophysiologic mechanisms previously described.

3. Teaching women to take control of symptoms through reduction of negative emotions by cognitive restructuring, improving problem-solving skills, and developing responsible assertiveness to deal with discomforts has been shown to provide significant relief of both physical and emotional symptoms. If there is suboptimal improvement after 2 to 3 months of the treatments described above or if symptoms are severe, secondary treatment modalities may be considered.

   a. **Anxiety, irritability, and mood swings.** Several selective serotonin reuptake inhibitor (SSRI) antidepressants have been found effective for both the depressive as well as the anxiety symptoms of PMS. (SOR **A**) Fluoxetine and sertraline have been the most extensively studied. SSRIs reduce both the physical and behavioral symptoms of PMS, and are equally effective if prescribed continuously or intermittently (during luteal phase only). Fluoxetine and sertraline are FDA approved for treatment of PMDD. The effective doses for SSRIs are: fluoxetine, 20 to 40 mg/d; sertraline, 50 to 100 mg/d; and citalopram, 10 to 20 mg/d. Paroxetine has previously been recommended, but was made pregnancy category D in 2005 because of increased concern for cardiac malformations if exposed in the first trimester. If SSRIs are ineffective or cannot be used, buspirone, 30 mg/d (10 mg 3 times a day) for 12 days prior to menses, is effective not only for social dysfunction but also for fatigue, cramps, and general aches and pains. (SOR **B**) Clonidine (0.1 mg twice a day) and verapamil (80 mg 3 times a day or one 240-mg sustained-release capsule once a day) have also been reported to have beneficial effects on mood in PMS. The anxiolytic alprazolam, 0.25 mg tid, (SOR **B**) has been shown to be effective for some patients who meet the strict criteria of PMDD; however, side effects and risk for addiction limit its use to a second-line therapy. TCAs, MAOIs, and lithium are not effective in treating PMS/PMDD.

   b. **Weight gain, swelling, and bloating.** Spironolactone, 25 mg orally 4 times a day, has produced significant reduction in somatic and affective symptoms. (SOR **A**) Diuretic therapy should only be prescribed after two or three cycles of restriction of intake of simple sugars and salt, as the edema from these is diuretic-resistant, and other benefits accrue from their restriction.

   c. **Breast tenderness.** Vitamin E, 400 IU twice daily, may reduce mastodynia if lower doses are ineffective. Treatment is usually continued for 4 to 6 months and resumed if symptoms recur.

     d. Changes in appetite, cravings, and fatigue. Adherence to dietary guidelines, achievement of adequate sleep, and management of the environment to minimize exposure to added stress may offer some mitigation of symptoms.

     e. Depression, sleep disturbance, and cognitive difficulty. Antidepressant therapy with SSRIs has been shown to be significantly more effective than placebo. (SOR **A**)

     f. Pain syndromes. Isolated headaches and general muscular pains are best treated with simple analgesics, such as acetaminophen and ibuprofen. Migraine headaches occurring as part of PMS may be alleviated by daily treatment beginning approximately 10 days prior to menstruation. Possible preventive measures and treatment of migraine attacks are described in Chapter 34.

  C. Treatments based on presumed hormonal cause

    1. Progesterone. An ineffective treatment.

    2. Contraceptives. Combination oral contraceptive pills may reduce physical symptoms of PMS. (SOR **B**) A shortened pill-free interval (4 days instead of 7) may be helpful. Two recent studies have shown efficacy for the OCP Yaz, and it is the first FDA approved OCP for PMDD.

    3. Gonadotropin-releasing hormone analogues. Leuprolide has been shown to be effective in reducing symptoms of PMS, but causes side effects and symptoms and sequelae of menopause (bone loss, vaginal dryness), which may be equal to or more troubling than PMS. (SOR **B**)

  D. Complementary and alternative therapies. Massage therapy has been shown to decrease general pain symptoms in women with PMS or dysmenorrhea. In studies of depression, hypericin 300 mg 3 times a day (the principal active component of St. John's wort) was found to be as effective as TCAs, with fewer side effects and at lower cost, but with considerably slower onset. Photosensitivity may occur, and information about potential adverse interactions of hypericin with other medication is lacking. L-Tryptophan (2 g 3 times daily with meals, from day 14 through day 3 of the cycle) has been a useful adjunct to antidepressant therapy. *Silix Donna,* a yeast-based dietary supplement, was found effective in improving mood symptoms in mild to moderate PMS. Chasteberry (20 mg/d) was found to be significantly effective in reducing symptoms of PMS. (SOR **B**) A meta-analysis of complementary medicine approaches included 27 trials, and it was determined that there was insufficient evidence to recommend any of the treatments.

  E. Treatments likely NOT to be of help

    1. Progesterone/progestins. Although in the past this has been a commonly used therapy, the bulk of evidence now shows that this is an ineffective therapy. (SOR **A**)

    2. Primrose oil. Evidence does not support the use of primrose oil for PMS. (SOR **A**)

    3. Free fatty acids.

    4. Ginkgo Bilboa extract.

IV. Management Strategies. An approach to PMS management is diagrammed in Figure 83–4.

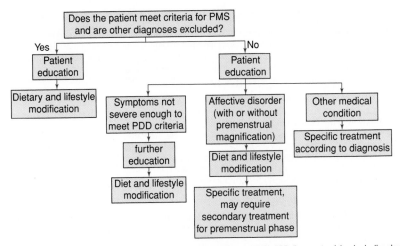

FIGURE 83–4. An approach to the management of premenstrual syndrome (PMS). PDD, Premenstrual dysphoric disorder.

V. Prognosis. PMS ceases in most patients around the time of menopause. Many therapies have been found to provide significant relief to a proportion of patients; therefore, the prognosis for improvement of symptoms in PMS is excellent. The medical team must be empathetic, creative, patient, and persistently willing to try different or multiple therapies. Other comorbid conditions, such as memory of past trauma, may surface during treatment for PMS and indicate the need for further treatment or referral. In the rare refractory case of severe PMDD, surgery (usually a bilateral salpingo-oophorectomy with hysterectomy) can be considered, and has been shown to be effective in multiple observational studies. (SOR **B**) Strict guidelines should be followed for selecting a patient who may be appropriate for surgical therapy.

REFERENCES

Casper RF, Yonkers KA. Clinical manifestations and diagnosis of premenstrual syndrome and premenstrual dysphoric disorder, Version 15.1, 2007. www.utdol.com. Accessed August 5, 2008.

Casper RF, Yonkers KA. Epidemiology of pathogenesis of premenstrual syndrome and premenstrual dysphoric disorder, Version 15.1, 2007. www.utdol.com. Accessed August 5, 2008.

Casper RF, Yonkers KA. Treatment of premenstrual syndrome and premenstrual dysphoric disorder, Version 15.1, 2007. www.utdol.com. Accessed August 5, 2008.

National Guideline Clearinghouse. Premenstrual syndrome. www.guidelines.gov. Current as of Dec 2005.

Premenstrual Syndrome (PMS). www.dynamed.com. Updated May 20, 2008. Accessed August 6, 2008.

Schellenberg R. Treatment for the premenstrual syndrome with agnus castus fruit extract: prospective, randomized, placebo controlled study. *BMJ.* 2001;322:134-137.

Schmidt PJ, Nieman LK, Danaceau MA, Adams LF, Rubinow DR. Differential behavioral effects on gonadal steroids in women with and in those without premenstrual syndrome. *N Engl J Med.* 1998;338:209-216.

Stevinson C, Ernst E. Complementary/alternative therapies for premenstrual syndrome: a systematic review of controlled trials. *Am J Obstet Gynecol.* 2001;185:227-235.

Premenstrual syndrome recommendations. www.essentialevidenceplus.com. Accessed August 6, 2008.

---

84   Renal Failure

Terrence T. Truong, MD

KEY POINTS

- Prerenal disease may be distinguished from ischemic or nephrotoxic acute tubular necrosis by the recovery of renal function within 24 to 72 hours after fluid repletion.
- For patients with systolic heart failure, inotropic agents and vasodilator should be initiated when serum creatinine and blood urea nitrogen (BUN) rise with diuretic therapy. Calcium channel blocker or β-adrenergic blockers are indicated if diastolic heart failure is present.
- Treatment of hypertension in patients with polyarteritis nodosa and renal disease may require calcium channel blocker if angiotensin-converting enzyme (ACE) inhibitors worsen renal function.
- ACE inhibitors and angiotensin II receptor blockers are efficacious in treating hypertension and confer renal protection in patients with benign hypertensive nephrosclerosis. However, thiazide diuretics provide greater cardioprotective effects.
- Radiocontrast media-induced renal failure may be prevented by the use of lower dose low- or iso-osmolal nonionic agents, maintenance of normovolemia, and avoidance of concomitant use of nonsteroidal anti-inflammatory drugs (NSAIDs).
- Bladder catheterization, performed to rule out bladder neck obstruction, may also be therapeutic in bladder and urethral obstruction.

I. Introduction

A. Definition. Renal failure is a syndrome describing disturbances in renal function resulting in impaired or loss of maintenance of extracellular homeostasis, systemic and renal hemodynamics, calcium and bone metabolism, and erythropoiesis. Renal failure is defined as an acute failure when there is recent increase of serum creatinine concentration of at least 0.5 mg/dL with baseline concentration of <3.0 mg/dL, and at least 1.0 mg/dL when the baseline is higher. Acute failure may occur in patients with previously normal renal function or preexisting stable renal impairment.

B. Etiology. Renal diseases can be characterized by the anatomic location primarily affected by the underlying pathology.

1. **Prerenal disease** occurs with glomerular hypoperfusion secondary to decreased circulating volume or relative hypotension, leading to acute decline of glomerular filtration rate. Etiologies include acute hemorrhage, gastrointestinal, urinary, or cutaneous fluid losses, congestive heart failure, hepatorenal syndrome, sepsis, and shock.

2. **Vascular disease** may cause acute or chronic renal failure.
   a. **Acute.** Malignant hypertension, thromboemboli, scleroderma, and systemic vasculitides cause acute disease.
   b. **Chronic.** Hypertensive nephrosclerosis and bilateral renal artery stenosis are the major causes of chronic renal failure.

3. **Glomerular disease** is caused by entities that result in focal nephritis, diffused nephritis, or nephrosis. Overlap of these patterns may occur.
   a. **Focal glomerulonephritis.** Etiologies include postinfectious glomerulonephritis, Henoch-Schönlein purpura, IgA nephropathy, thin basement membrane disease, hereditary nephritis, mesangial proliferative glomerulonephritis, and systemic lupus erythematosus.
   b. **Diffused glomerulonephritis.** Etiologies include postinfectious glomerulonephritis, membranoproliferative glomerulonephritis, rapidly progressive glomerulonephritis, vasculitides, and fibrillary glomerulonephritis.
   c. **Nephrotic syndrome.** Etiologies include diabetic nephropathy, IgA nephropathy, minimal change disease, focal glomerulosclerosis, mesangial proliferative glomerulonephritis, and membranous nephropathy.

4. **Tubular or interstitial disease** can lead to acute or chronic renal failure.
   a. **Acute.** Acute tubular necrosis, acute tubular nephritis, and cast nephropathy are the major causes of acute renal failure.
   b. **Chronic.** Polycystic kidney disease, vesicoureteral reflux, autoimmune disorders, and analgesic abuse cause chronic disease.

5. **Obstructive uropathy** may occur secondary to urinary flow obstruction anywhere along the urinary tract.
   a. **Adults.** Prostatic disease, urinary calculus, and pelvic or retroperitoneal neoplasm are major causes in adults. Bilateral obstruction is obligatory to produce renal insufficiency in patients with otherwise normal renal functions.
   b. **Children.** Urethral valves and strictures, and ureterovesicular and ureteropelvic stenosis are major causes in children.

II. Diagnosis

A. Symptoms and signs

1. **Prerenal disease.** Symptoms and signs are related to fluid loss and the resultant electrolyte abnormalities. Response to fluid administration with recovery of renal function within 24 to 72 hours is highly suggestive, though not diagnostic, of prerenal disease.

2. **Vascular disease**
   a. **Acute.** Aside from characteristic, systemic symptoms, systemic vasculitides produce renal function impairment and hypertension. Patients with thromboemboli typically present with flank pain, nausea, vomiting, fever, and hypertension. Renal atheroemboli, in contrast, may present with acute marked renal impairment, progressive renal impairment interspersed with episodes of relatively stable function over periods of weeks, or chronic stable renal impairment. Typically, there is preceding aortic or other large artery manipulation.
   b. **Chronic.** Patients with benign hypertensive nephrosclerosis have no specific symptom. They present with slowly progressive, worsening renal function, and mild proteinuria with a history of preexisting mild to moderate hypertension. Chronic renal failure secondary to bilateral artery stenosis should be considered in patients who have systemic atherosclerosis, hypertension that is severe or refractory, elevation of serum creatinine with ingestion of ACE inhibitor, or asymmetric renal size.

3. **Glomerular disease**
   a. **Focal nephritic patients** may be asymptomatic. They have normal blood pressure and no edema. They typically have hematuria and proteinuria with no significant renal impairment.
   b. **Diffused nephritic patients** have hypertension, edema, and usually renal insufficiency.
   c. **Nephrotic syndrome patients** may present with malaise, anorexia, edema, weight gain, and frothy urine. By definition, nephrotic syndrome requires the presence of proteinuria ≥3 g/d serum albumin <3.0 g/dL, and peripheral edema.

4. **Tubulointerstitial disease**
   a. **Acute tubular necrosis** typically produces no specific symptoms or signs. There is usually a history of exposure to nephrotoxic agent or medical conditions leading to ischemia. Differentiating acute tubular necrosis from prerenal acute renal failure can be difficult, and may require serial BUN and serum creatinine measurements.
   b. **Acute interstitial nephritis,** most commonly induced by medications such as NSAIDs, antibacterials, and sulfonamides, occurs within 3 days to months after exposure to the offending agent. Symptoms and signs include fever and skin rash associated with an acute rise in the serum creatinine concentration related to drug exposure, generalized aches and pains, or history of recent infection. Additionally, signs of Fanconi syndrome may be observed.
   c. **Cast nephropathy** occurs with multiple myeloma secondary to tubular injury and intratubular cast formation and obstruction. Symptoms and signs, secondary to the underlying multiple myeloma, include weakness, bone pain, anemia, lytic bone lesions, and hypercalcemia. Renal failure can be acute or chronic. Radiocontrast media exposure may precipitate acute renal failure in this setting.

5. **Postrenal disease.** Obstructive uropathy may cause acute or chronic renal failure. Pain may or may not be present, depending on the location and rate of the developing obstruction. Normal urine volume is maintained except in complete bilateral obstruction and shock. Hypertension may also be present. Bladder catheterization should be performed to rule out bladder neck obstruction.

B. **Laboratory tests**
   1. **Serum creatinine concentration** estimates glomerular filtration rate. A rise in serum creatinine concentration represents a reduction in glomerular filtration rate.
   2. **Creatinine clearance** is obtained from a 24-hour urine collection. It is more accurate than serum creatinine concentration in estimating glomerular filtration rate. Creatinine clearance may be estimated by the Cockcroft-Gault equation in patients with stable serum creatinine concentration.
   3. **Urinalysis** is an essential test to evaluate renal failure. Urinary sediment patterns may be indicative of the underlying renal disease.
      a. **Normal or near normal with few cells and little or no cast** indicates prerenal disease, obstruction, hypercalcemia, multiple myeloma, acute tubular necrosis, or vascular disease.
      b. **Hematuria with red cell casts and heavy proteinuria** indicates glomerular disease or vasculitis.
      c. **Renal tubular epithelial cells with granular and epithelial cell casts** indicate acute tubular necrosis.
      d. **Pyuria with white cell and granular or waxy casts and no or mild proteinuria** indicates tubular or interstitial disease or obstruction.
      e. **Hematuria and pyuria with no or variable casts or proteinuria** indicates glomerular disease, vasculitis, infection, obstruction, renal infarction, or acute, usually drug-induced, interstitial nephritis.
      f. **Hematuria alone** indicates vasculitis or obstruction.
   4. **Urinary sodium concentration** is useful in differentiating acute tubular necrosis from volume depletion as the cause of renal failure.
   5. **Fractional excretion of sodium** eliminates the effect of urine output on urinary sodium concentration.

C. **Entity specific tests**
   1. **Prerenal disease.** An elevated BUN to serum creatinine ratio, often greater than 20:1, occurs in the absence of increased urea production. However, a normal ratio may be observed with concomitant liver disease or decreased protein intake. Urinalysis is normal, though hyaline casts may be present. Urinary sodium concentration is

typically <20 mEq/L, with fractional excretion of sodium <1% and urinary osmolality >500 mOsm/kg.

2. **Vascular disease**
   a. **Acute**
      (1) **Systemic vasculitides.** Urinalysis reveals an active sediment with red cells, red cell and granular casts, and nonnephrotic range proteinuria. Classic polyarteritis nodosa, on the other hand, may only produce glomerular ischemia, and thus, a relatively normal urinalysis. Renal biopsy with histologic, immunofluorescence, and electron microscopic evaluation would be confirmatory.
      (2) **Thromboemboli.** One-third of patients have gross or microscopic hematuria. Serum lactate dehydrogenase levels are often elevated with no significant change of serum transaminases. Radioisotope renogram is confirmatory.
      (3) **Renal atheroemboli.** Urinalysis reveals few cells or casts. Proteinuria is usually in the nonnephrotic range. Eosinophilia, eosinophiluria, and hypocomplementemia may be present.
   b. **Chronic**
      (1) **Hypertensive nephrosclerosis.** Proteinuria is typically minimal unless an underlying renovascular disease is also present. Urinary sediments are relatively normal. Renal biopsy is rarely indicated, except in instances when there is no clear history of hypertension preceding the development of proteinuria and renal function impairment.
      (2) **Bilateral renal artery stenosis.** Serum creatinine is increased with exposure to ACEI. Renal size may be asymmetric. Doppler ultrasonography may be confirmatory.

3. **Glomerular disease**
   a. **Focal nephritic.** Urinalysis reveals red cells, occasionally red cell casts, and proteinuria <1.5 g/d. Renal function is preserved. Light microscopy reveals inflammatory lesions in less than half of the glomeruli.
   b. **Diffused nephritic.** Urinalysis is similar to that of focal nephritic patients, although proteinuria may be in nephrotic range. Light microscopy reveals lesions in most or all of the glomeruli.
   c. **Nephrotic syndrome.** Few cells or casts are observed in the urine. Proteinuria is at least 3 g/d and serum albumin <3.0 g/dL. Hyperlipidemia and hyperlipiduria may also be present.

4. **Tubulointerstitial disease**
   a. **Acute tubular necrosis.** The BUN: serum creatinine ratio remains normal, with the rate of rise of serum creatinine >0.3 to 0.5 mg/dL/d. Additionally, urinary sodium concentration is >40 mEq/L. Fractional excretion of sodium is >2% in the absence of chronic prerenal states such as cirrhosis. Urine-to-serum creatinine concentration is <20. Muddy brown, granular, and epithelial cell casts and free, epithelial cells are usually, though not universally, present on urinalysis. Urinary osmolality, usually <450 mOsm/kg, and urine flow rate are of limited value in distinguishing acute tubular necrosis from prerenal disease.
   b. **Acute interstitial nephritis.** Eosinophilia and eosinophiluria are also present except in NSAID exposure in which there is no fever, rash, or eosinophilia. Urinalysis reveals pyuria, hematuria, and white cell casts. Minimal proteinuria, <1 g/d is present except in the elderly patients, who can excrete up to 3 g/d and NSAID exposure cases in which nephrotic syndrome can be concurrent. Renal biopsy is the only definitive diagnostic tool.
   c. **Cast nephropathy.** Urinalysis reveals minimal or no albumin by dipstick, though is markedly positive with sulfasalicylic acid testing indicating the presence of light chains. Diagnosis is confirmed by bone marrow examination.

5. **Postrenal disease.** Urinalysis may be normal. Plain film x-ray of the abdomen, renal ultrasonography, or computerized tomography (CT scan) scanning is diagnostic in most cases. Intravenous pyelogram is of limited value except when staghorn calculus or multiple renal or parapelvic cysts are suspected, when CT scan cannot identify the level of obstruction, and when an obstructing calculus is suspected in the absence of collecting system dilatation.

III. **Treatment.** Careful history-taking and physical examination with judicious use of the laboratory will frequently identify the processes that require prompt intervention. Supportive measures are initiated to correct fluid balance and electrolyte abnormalities and to maintain optimum nutritional status. Medications are reviewed and withdrawn or adjusted accordingly. Dialysis is indicated when fluid overload, acidosis, or electrolyte imbalance develops despite medical therapy, or when uremia ensues.

A. Prerenal disease

1. **Hypovolemia.** Fluid repletion is necessary to restore circulating volume. The tonicity of the fluid is dependent on the serum sodium concentration. Blood transfusion is required if the underlying abnormality is acute hemorrhage.

2. **Hypotension.** As hypotension may occur with hypovolemia, cardiac dysfunction, or sepsis, treatment would be directed at the underlying entity. Additionally, hypotension may be the result of therapy of chronic severe hypertension. Unless an ACE inhibitor is given in the presence of underlying bilateral renal artery stenosis, renal function will improve without discontinuing the antihypertensive agent.

3. **Heart failure.** Enhancing cardiac output will improve renal function. Diuretic therapy reduces pulmonary and peripheral edema, thus increases cardiac output. However, when serum creatinine and BUN levels rise with diuresis, inotropic agents and vasodilators should be started unless there is underlying diastolic dysfunction, in which case the nondihydropyridine calcium channel blockers, verapamil and diltiazem, or β-adrenergic blockers would be indicated to improve ventricular filling (Table 84–1). Verapamil or diltiazem may be started at 120 to 240 mg orally every day or in divided doses. Atenolol or metoprolol may be initiated at 12.5 to 25 mg orally every day. Carvedilol, a nonselective β-receptor and α_1 antagonist receptor with an evidence of decreased cardiovascular mortality (SOR **B**), is given 12.5 mg orally twice daily. Careful monitoring for hemodynamic compromise and drug accumulation is mandatory with titration.

4. **Cirrhosis.** Hepatorenal syndrome treatment is aimed at reversing hepatic failure to recover renal function. Medical therapy and shunting procedures only provide short-term benefits. (SOR **B**) Definitive treatment is liver transplantation.

B. Vascular disease

1. **Acute**

   a. **Vasculitides.** Corticosteroids and immunosuppressive agents are used in the treatment of the underlying disease. Treatment of hypertension in polyarteritis nodosa may require the use of a calcium channel blocker such as amlodipine, at 2.5 to 5 mg orally every day, if ACE inhibitors worsen renal functions (Table 84–1).

   b. **Thromboemboli.** Intravenous heparin and oral warfarin is the standard treatment. Thrombolytic therapy may be beneficial if treatment is instituted within 2 hours. Treatment of hypertension, which may be transient, can be effected with ACE inhibitors such as captopril at 12.5 to 25 mg orally twice daily; enalapril (5 mg) or lisinopril (10 mg) orally every day (Table 84-2). Monitoring for first-dose hypotension is advisable for patients who have not been previously exposed to ACE inhibitors or who are currently on diuretics.

   c. **Atheroemboli.** There is no effective medical therapy.

2. **Chronic**

   a. **Hypertensive nephrosclerosis.** Blood pressure control is essential and may necessitate utilization of multiple agents from different classes. ACE inhibitor and angiotensin II receptor blockers are drugs of choice for renal protection (Table 84–2). However, thiazide diuretics, such as hydrochlorothiazide (12.5–25 mg orally every day), provide greater cardioprotective effects. (SOR **A**)

   b. **Bilateral renal artery stenosis.** ACE inhibitors can control blood pressure in most patients. However, revascularization, whether by renal artery bypass grafting or percutaneous angioplasty, would be indicated with severe or refractory hypertension and progressive renal function decline.

C. Glomerular disease.
Treatment involves corticosteroids and immuno-suppressive agents directed at the underlying pathology.

D. Tubulointerstitial disease

1. **Acute tubular necrosis.** As the process is short-lived, supportive measures are instituted and any offending agent is discontinued. Radiocontrast media-induced renal failure may be prevented by the use of lower-dose, low- or iso-osmolal nonionic agents, maintenance of normovolemia, and avoidance of concomitant use of NSAIDs. Treatment includes hydration with normal saline.

2. **Acute interstitial nephritis.** Withdrawal of the responsible agent in drug-induced cases is the primary treatment. Corticosteroids may also be indicated.

TABLE 84–1. ANTIHYPERTENSIVE AGENTS: CALCIUM CHANNEL BLOCKERS AND β-BLOCKERS

Agent Name	Starting/Max Dosage	Renal Impairment Dose	Side Effects/Benefits/Notes	Cost
Calcium channel blocker				
Amlodipine (Norvasc)	5 mg po qd/10 mg		Jaundice, elevated LFTs 2.5 mg po qd in hepatic dysfunction	$$
Diltiazem (Cardizem CD)	180 mg po qd/540 mg		Elevated LFTs	$$$
Felodipine (Plendil)	5 mg po qd/10 mg		Elevated level in elderly and hepatic dysfunction	$$
Isradipine (DynaCirc CR)	5 mg po qd/20 mg		Elevated level in elderly and hepatic dysfunction Elevated level in mild renal impairment	$$
Nicardipine (Cardene SR)	30 mg po bid/120 mg		Maximum BP effect 2–6 h after dose	$$$
Nifedipine (Procardia XL, Adalat CC)	30 mg po qd/120 mg		Giddiness, heat sensation, muscle tremor, positive Coombs'	$$
Nisoldipine (Sular)	20 mg po qd/60 mg		Elevated level in elderly and hepatic dysfunction	$$
Verapamil (Calan SR)	180 mg po qd/480 mg		Elevated LFTs	$$$
β-adrenergic blocker				
Acebutolol (Sectral)	200 mg po bid/1200 mg	Total daily dosage reduction	Selective β_1-receptor blocker Reduce dose 50% when GFR <50, 75% GFR <25	$
Atenolol (Tenormin)	50 mg po qd/100 mg	Max 50 mg/d GFR <35 Max 25 mg/d GFR <15	Selective β-receptor blocker Indicated for angina pectoris	$
Carvedilol	6.5 mg po bid/50 mg		Decreased mortality with CHF, overall mortality	$$$$
Labetalol (Normodyne, Trandate)	100 mg po bid/2400 mg		Nonselective β- and α_1-receptor blocker Jaundice, elevated LFTs Elevated levels in elderly and hepatic dysfunction	$$$
Metoprolol (Lopressor, Toprol XL)	100 mg po qd/400 mg		Long-acting agent decreased mortality in CHF Indicated for angina pectoris	$$
Nadolol (Corgard)	40 mg po qd/320 mg	Q36 h dose GFR ≤50 Q48 h dose GFR ≤30 Q72 h dose GFR <10	Nonselective β-receptor blocker Indicated for angina pectoris	$
Propranolol (Inderal, Inderal LA)	80 mg po qd/640 mg		Nonselective β-receptor blocker Reduction of CV mortality and reinfarction Indicated for angina pectoris	$$
Timolol (Blocadren)	10 mg po bid/60 mg		Nonselective β-receptor blocker Reduction of CV mortality and reinfarction	$

BP, blood pressure; CHF, congestive heart failure; CV, cardiovascular; GFR, glomerular filtration rate; LFTs, liver function tests. $, least expensive; $$$$, most expensive.

TABLE 84–2. **ANTIHYPERTENSIVE AGENTS: ANGIOTENSIN-CONVERTING ENZYME INHIBITORS (ACEI) AND ANGIOTENSIN RECEPTOR BLOCKERS (ARB)**

Agent Name	Starting/Max Dosage	Renal Impairment Dose	Side Effects/Benefits/Notes	Cost
ACEI				
Benazopril (Lotensin)	10 mg po qd/40 mg	5 mg/d if CrCl <30 mL/min	Reduces progression to renal failure	$$
Captopril (Capoten)	25 mg po bid–tid/ 450 mg	Reduce initial dose	Neutropenia, nephritic syndrome, rash Reduces mortality in MI Slows progression of diabetic nephropathy	$
Enalapril (Vasotec)	5 mg po qd/40 mg	2.5 mg/d CrCl <30 mL/min	Reduces mortality in NYHA II–IV CHF Reduces renal function decline in type 2 diabetics	$
Fosinopril (Monopril)	10 mg po qd/80 mg	5 mg/d	Impaired LFT increases unchanged plasma level Lower risk of MI, CVA than amlodipine	$$$
Lisinopril (Prinivil, Zestril)	10 mg po qd/40 mg	5 mg/d CrCl 10–30 mL/min 2.5 mg/d CrCl <10 mL/min	Reduces mortality in MI Reduces renal function decline in type 2 diabetics	$
Moexepril (Univasc)	7.5 mg po qd/40 mg	3.75 mg/d CrCl ≤30 mL/min	Food decreases bioavailability Dosage reduction in hepatic dysfunction	$
Perindopril (Aceon)	4 mg po qd/16 mg	2 mg/d CrCl >30 mL/min	Safety not known CrCl <30 mL/min	$$
Quinapril (Accupril)	10 mg po qd/80 mg	5 mg/d CrCl 30–60 mL/min 2.5 mg/dCrCl 10–30 mL/min	Reduces tetracycline absorption Not removed by dialysis	$$
Ramipril (Altace)	2.5 mg po qd/20 mg	1.25 mg/d CrCl <40 mL/min 5 mg/d maximum	Impaired LFT increases unchanged plasma level Reduces mortality in MI with CHF; CVA, CVD, MI and mortality in patients at high risk for CVD	$$$$
Trandolapril (Mavik)	1 mg po qd/4 mg	0.5 mg/d CrCl <30 mL/min	Reduce dosage to 0.5 mg/d in hepatic cirrhosis No data on removal by hemodialysis	$$$
ARB				
Candesartan (Atacand)	16 mg po qd/32 mg		Reduces microalbuminemia in type 2 diabetes mellitus	$$$
Eprosartan (Teveten)	600 mg po qd/800 mg			$$
Irbesartan (Avapro)	150 mg po qd/300 mg			$$$
Losartan (Cozaar)	50 mg po qd/100 mg		Decreased CHF morbidity and mortality Decreased CHF morbidity and mortality after MI	$$$
Olmesartan (Benicar)	20 mg po qd/40 mg			$$
Telmisartan (Micardis)	40 mg po qd/80 mg			$$
Valsartan (Diovan)	80 mg po qd/320 mg			$$$

CHF, congestive heart failure; CrCl, creatine clearance; CVA, cerebrovascular accident; CVD, cardiovascular disease; LFT, liver function tests; MI, myocardial infarction; NYHA, New York Heart Association. $, least expensive; $$$$, most expensive.

   3. **Cast nephropathy.** Vigorous hydration, corticosteroids, and cyclophosphamide decrease light-chain production. Loop diuretics may be administered if hypercalcemia is present. Plasmapheresis (SOR **Ⓒ**) and dialysis are other modalities that may be considered.
   E. **Postrenal disease.** Treatment, directed at restoration of urinary flow by relieving the underlying obstruction, may include bladder catheterization, percutaneous nephrostomy, lithotripsy, ureteral stenting, and urethral stenting.
IV. **Management Strategies.** Effective management of renal failure begins with the evaluation and diagnosis of the underlying disease process. Proper management includes preventing, monitoring for, treating complications, and maintaining nutritional support with protein restriction.
   A. **Acute renal failure.** Prerenal disease and acute tubular necrosis are the most common etiologies in the inpatient setting. If there is difficulty in differentiating between the two, fluid replacement may be initiated, in the absence of heart failure and hepatorenal syndrome, and potentially offending agents are withheld while the work-up is ongoing. Recovery of renal function in the ensuing 24 to 72 hours would point to prerenal disease. Other acute causes will have their characteristic history, physical findings, or urinalysis findings. Their management would be specific to the underlying pathology.
   B. **Chronic renal failure.** While treatments of chronic renal failure are determined by the primary diagnosis, supportive measures and treatment of hypertension are initiated to prevent in many instances further deterioration of renal function. Additionally, monitoring for, preventing and managing metabolic, fluid balance, hematologic, and nutritional complications are of paramount importance. Metabolic surveillance should include periodic assessment of serum potassium, calcium, phosphorus, albumin, and acidemia. Nephrology consultation is beneficial to assist in diagnosis of the renal disease, comanage complications, initiate dialysis, and prepare the patient for kidney replacement as indicated. Comprehensive patient care consists of clear communication and concise coordination of care with the nephrologist and other specialists during the predialysis, dialysis, and transplantation period.
      1. **Hypertension** is common once chronic renal failure develops. Often blood pressure responds well to ACE inhibitors or angiotensin II receptor blockers (Table 84–2). The goal blood pressure is <130/80. In the ACE inhibitor naïve or frail patient, captopril, with its short half-life and thus quicker clearance once discontinued should class-related side effects be detected, may be initiated at 6.25 mg orally two to 3 times daily and titrated up to 50 mg orally 3 times daily. Alternatively, longer-acting agents such as enalapril, 5 mg, or lisinopril, 10 mg orally every day, with titration up to 40 mg orally every day, would improve compliance without incurring significant cost. For patients who cannot tolerate an ACE inhibitor, losartan (50 mg) or irbesartan (150 mg) orally every day may also be used, with target doses of 100 mg and 300 mg orally every day, respectively. No dosage reduction for renal impairment is necessary. However, patient cost for these agents is approximately doubled. Up to a 35% increase in serum creatinine is acceptable in the course of therapy, unless hyperkalemia develops. Once glomerular filtration rate drops below 30 mL/min, increased doses of loop diuretics and the addition of other classes of medications are typically necessary to control blood pressure.
      2. **Potassium metabolism**
         a. **Hyperkalemia** occurs commonly secondary to decreased tubular secretion, medications, volume depletion, dietary intake, and hypoinsulinemia. Specific treatments are dependent on the severity of hyperkalemia and may include removing offending medications, restoring fluid balance, maintaining a strict low-potassium dietary regimen, initiating thiazide or loop diuretics, and using sodium polystyrene, such as Kayexalate 15 to 30 g orally every 6 hours.
         b. **Hypokalemia** results from diuresis or renal disease itself. Each mEq/L decrease represents a 200-mEq reduction in total body potassium. Oral replacement with potassium chloride, 40 to 100 mEq/d may be initiated for mild hypokalemia. Intravenous replacement is reserved for severe cases. Judicious replacement, 10 mEq/h, is coupled with frequent assessment of serum levels.
      3. **Calcium metabolism**
         a. **Hypocalcemia** is observed with renal disease when glomerular filtration rate is <30 mL/min or when there is secondary hypoparathyroidism or hypoalbuminemia. Serum ionized calcium and mathematical correction for hypoalbuminemia confirm

hypocalcemia. Elemental calcium, 500 mg to 2 g, is given 3 to 4 times daily with meals. Replacement strategy, utilizing carbonate or acetate salt, is contingent on the presence of hyperphosphatemia. Calcium carbonate contains 40% elemental calcium. Though more expensive, calcium acetate, containing 25% elemental calcium, is preferred over calcium carbonate when serum phosphorus is >4.5 mg/dL.

    b. Hypercalcemia in renal failure occurs with multiple myeloma, malignancy, sarcoidosis, and calcium replacement therapy. Treatment is targeted at the underlying pathology. Calcium replacement is halted or decreased. When calcium × phosphate products exceeds 70, aluminum hydroxide, 300 to 600 mg orally 3 times daily with meals, can be used for no more than 10 days.

4. **Phosphorus metabolism** is impaired in renal failure. Phosphate retention leads to hyperphosphatemia and consequently secondary hyperparathyroidism. Treatment begins with dietary restriction of 0.8 to 1.2 g/d of phosphorus. Binders such as calcium carbonate or calcium acetate are then added if hyperphosphatemia persists. Aluminum hydroxide, 1.9 to 4.8 g orally 2 to 4 times daily, may also be used for short duration, though not concurrent with citrate-based binders.

5. **Serum albumin and prealbumin,** though of limited value in the presence of inflammation, can estimate nutritional status. Dialysis patient mortality rate increases with decreasing albumin levels.

6. **Metabolic acidosis** exists in renal failure secondary to the accumulation of organic acids and impaired renal acidification. Treatment, aimed at raising serum bicarbonate level to 20 mEq/L, is effected by providing 0.5 mEq/kg/d of bicarbonate in divided doses. Each 650-mg tablet provides 7.6 mEq of bicarbonate.

7. **Volume overload** commonly occurs with chronic renal failure secondary to progressive renal impairment, excess salt load, inadequate diuresis, and medication side effects. Treatment initially includes weight monitoring and dietary salt restriction. A loop diuretic is then administered daily or twice daily if euvolemia is not achieved. A thiazide diuretic may be added if twice daily loop diuretic therapy is unsuccessful. Refractory volume overload is best treated with dialysis.

8. **Anemia** requires work-up when hemoglobin is <11 g/dL in premenopausal and prepubertal females and <12 g/dL in adult males and postmenopausal females. Evaluation should include iron studies, reticulocyte count, red blood cell indices, and occult stool blood test. Gastrointestinal blood loss is treated in consultation with a gastroenterologist. Oral iron replacement therapy, ferrous sulfate (325 mg orally 3 times daily without food or other medicines), begins when ferritin is <200 ng/mL and is maintained for 6 months or until iron deficiency anemia resolves. Intravenous iron, iron dextran, may be given if ferritin is <100 ng/mL or percent transferrin saturation is <20%. If hemoglobin remains <10 g/dL despite identification and adequate treatment of all causes of anemia, epoetin alfa should be considered. Treatment then should be coordinated with a hematologist/oncologist and a nephrologist. Red blood cell transfusions are necessary for patients with severe symptomatic anemia or those with epoetin resistance and chronic blood loss.

9. **Nutritional imbalance** is common in renal failure. Nutritionist consultation should be arranged early in the course of the disease. Assessment should include evaluation of general nutritional and energy status, electrolyte modification requirements, and lipid status. The daily caloric requirement is 35 kcal/kg body weight for patients younger than 60 years, and 30 to 35 kcal/kg body weight for those older than 60 years. A low-protein diet, 0.6 g/kg/d may slow the progression of renal impairment. (SOR **B**) A very low-protein diet, 0.3 g/kg, supplemented by 10 g/d of essential amino acids, is even more efficacious. (SOR **B**) However, compliance may be of issue. Additionally, this must be balanced with protein malnutrition that may result from adherence to a very low-potassium-restricted diet in the treatment of persistent hyperkalemia.

10. **Dialysis** indications include metabolic derangement unresponsive to medical therapy, refractory volume overload, uremic symptoms unmanageable by dietary manipulation, or advanced uremia.

V. **Prognosis.** Generally, the prognosis for recovery of renal function depends on the underlying pathology, presence of coexisting diseases, and complications associated with renal failure.

    A. **Prerenal disease.** Recovery of renal function is generally expected when there is prompt resolution of glomerular hypoperfusion. Residual impairment may persist with prolonged ischemia. Patients with hepatorenal syndrome tend to have a poor prognosis overall.

B. Vascular disease. The prognosis is contingent on response to treatment of the underlying vascular disease. Patients with atheroembolic disease tend to have a very poor prognosis, though this may be related to the severity of the associated cardiac and vascular disease.

C. Glomerular disease. The prognosis depends on the underlying pathologic process. Children with poststreptococcal glomerulonephritis typically recover fully from the initial renal failure. Some, however, may develop hypertension, proteinuria, and renal insufficiency later in life.

D. Tubulointerstitial disease

    1. Acute tubular necrosis. Recovery of function occurs within 3 weeks except in those with preexisting renal disease and repeated ischemia or exposure to nephrotoxic agents.

    2. Acute interstitial nephritis. Though renal function may not return to baseline, most patients recover after withdrawal of the offending agent or treatment of the underlying infection.

    3. Cast nephropathy. The prognosis is dependent on tumor mass and light-chain production rate. Improvement is expected in treated individuals.

E. Postrenal disease. Recovery of renal function is inversely related to the severity and duration of the obstruction, as well as the presence of any preexisting renal disease and infection. Full recovery is expected in complete obstruction of <1 week's duration. It is much more variable in incomplete obstruction.

REFERENCES

ALLHAT Officers and Coordinators for the ALLHAT Collaborative Research Group. Major outcomes in high-risk hypertensive patients randomized to angiotensin-converting enzyme inhibitor or calcium channel blocker vs. diuretic: the Antihypertensive and Lipid-Lowering Treatment to Prevent Heart Attack Trial (ALLHAT). *JAMA.* 2002;288:2981-2997.

Chobanian AV, Bakris GL, Black HR, et al. The Seventh Report of the Joint National Committee on Prevention, Detection, Evaluation, and Treatment of High Blood Pressure: The JNC 7 Report. *JAMA.* 2003;289(19):2560-2572.

K/DOQI clinical practice guidelines on hypertension and antihypertensive agents in chronic kidney disease. *Am J Kidney Dis.* 2004;43:5(suppl 1):S1.

Palevsky PM. Acute renal failure. *Neph SAP.* 2003;2(2):41-76.

Veterans Health Administration, Department of Defense. VHA/DoD *Clinical Practice Guideline for the Management of Chronic Kidney Disease and Pre-Esrd in the Primary Care Setting.* Washington, DC: Department of Veterans Affairs (U. S.), Veterans Health Administration; 2001.

---

85   Seizure Disorders

Shawn H. Blanchard, MD, & William L. Toffler, MD

KEY POINTS

- A seizure is a clinical sign of an underlying condition and does not necessarily warrant treatment acutely.
- Epilepsy is a condition of recurrent seizures requiring definitive diagnosis and treatment.
- Status epilepticus is an acute state of continued or frequent seizures for greater than 5 to 30 minutes without a return to consciousness or alertness and requires emergent treatment.
- Should the patient be seizing, ascertain the duration of the seizure, ensure airway, breathing and circulation, and protect the patient from physical harm. (SOR **B**)
- A seizure continuing past 5 minutes warrants loading with 2 to 4 mg Ativan IV or 5 to 10 mg of Valium IV (see Table 85–1). (SOR **A**)
- Obtain a brief history from third-party witnesses shortly after the patient is stabilized so as to determine etiology. Follow with an examination and studies as predicated by the patient presentation.

TABLE 85–1. STATUS EPILEPTICUS TREATMENT

1. Ensure airway—assist ventilation, if necessary
2. IV with normal saline
3. Dextrostix, or give 50 mL of 50% dextrose solution
4. Diazepam IV, 0.25–0.4 mg/kg (up to 10 mg) at a maximum rate of 1 mg/min; may need to repeat in 20–30 min
5. If seizures continue, phenobarbital IV, 10–15 mg/kg; 20% of total dose every 5–10 min at a rate of less than 50 mg/min; preferred over phenytoin especially in very young children
6. Phenytoin, loading dose of 15 mg/kg, undiluted, at a rate of 0.5–1.5 mg/kg/min; an additional 5 mg/kg can be given after 12 h
7. General anesthesia can be considered and given

I. **Introduction**
   A. **Definition.** A seizure is a sudden change in cortical electrical activity, manifested through motor, sensory, or behavioral changes, with or without an alteration in consciousness.
   B. **Classification.** A seizure first needs to be defined as an epileptiform or nonepileptiform seizure (NES).
   C. Nonepileptiform seizures are further defined as physiologic NES or psychogenic NES.
      1. Physiologic NES require acute evaluation and treatment with respect to the root cause (see Table 85–2).
      2. Psychogenic NES, formerly pseudoseizures, require psychotherapy and possibly pharmacotherapy with antidepressant and/or anxiolytic drugs (SOR Ⓒ) (see Table 85–2).
   D. The Seizure is then further defined by classical description.
      1. **Simple partial (focal) seizures** occur without loss of consciousness and involve one hemispheric epileptogenic focus. These may have motor, sensory, psychic, and autonomic characteristics and may progress toward a generalized seizure.
      2. **Complex partial seizures** cause loss of consciousness and maintain a hemispheric cerebral focus. This category includes absence (loss of consciousness or posture), myoclonic (repetitive muscle contractions), and tonic-clonic (a sustained contraction followed by rhythmic contractions of all four extremities) seizures.
      3. **Generalized seizures** involve alteration of consciousness, both hemispheres of the cerebral cortex, and have a nonfocal origin. These include absence seizures, tonic-clonic seizures, tonic seizures, and atonic seizures.
   E. **Febrile seizures** are one or more generalized seizures occurring between 3 months and 5 years of age associated with fever and that are without evidence of any other apparent cause.
   F. **Status epilepticus** is a neurologic emergency involving repetitive generalized seizures without return to consciousness between seizures (see Table 85–1).

TABLE 85–2. CLASSIFICATION OF NONEPILEPTIC SEIZURES

Physiologic	Psychogenic
Cardiac arrhythmias	Misinterpretation of physical symptoms
Complicated migraines	Psychopathologic processes
Dysautonomia	Anxiety disorders
Effects of drugs and toxins, overdose, and withdrawal	Posttraumatic stress disorder
Hypoglycemia, Natrena	Conversion disorder
Movement disorders	Dissociative disorder
Sleep disorders	Hypochondriasis
Syncopal episodes	Psychoses
Transient ischemic attacks	Somatization disorders
Vestibular symptoms	Reinforced behavior patterns in cognitively impaired patients
Hyperthyroidism	Response to acute stress without evidence of psychopathology
Hypoglycemia	Panic attacks
Nonketotic hyperglycemia	
Hyponatremia	
Uremia	
Porphyria	
Hypoxia	

II. Epidemiology

A. Each year four million people in the United States have at least one seizure. The risk of recurrence after a single unprovoked seizure is approximately 35%.

B. 2.7 million, or roughly 1% of people in the US have a diagnosis of epilepsy.

C. The risk increases to 10% for children with mental retardation, or cerebral palsy, and to 50% with both conditions.

D. There is no significant difference in prevalence between genders.

E. Approximately 1 in 15 children will have a seizure during their first 7 years of life. The prevalence of seizures in children delivered breech is 3.8% as compared with a prevalence of 2.2% in children delivered vertex.

F. Febrile seizures occur in 3% to 4% of all children. Fifty percent of febrile seizures occur during the second year of life and almost 90% before the third birthday. Sixty-four percent of children with febrile seizures will have only one episode. The earlier the age of onset, the more likely the child is to have more febrile seizures. No evidence exists that would suggest recurrent febrile seizures increase the risk of epilepsy.

G. More than 10,000 episodes of status epilepticus occur in the United States each year.

III. Diagnosis

A. Symptoms. The patient's history, often by a family member, detailing the episode including antecedent events, auras, progression, duration, ictal period, and any prolonged neurologic impairment are vital toward an accurate diagnosis.

B. The possible causes of a seizure can be grouped into the following categories; the age of the patient may help find a cause (Table 85–3).

TABLE 85–3. **POSSIBLE CAUSES OF RECURRENT SEIZURES BASED ON AGE**

Age at Onset (Y)	Most Likely Causes
Infancy (0–2)	Perinatal hypoxia
	Birth injury
	Congenital abnormality
	Metabolic
	Hypoglycemia
	Hypocalcemia
	Hypomagnesemia
	Vitamin B_{12} deficiency
	Phenylketonuria
	Acute infection
	Febrile seizure
	Idiopathic
Childhood (2–10)	Acute infection
	Trauma
	Idiopathic
Adolescent (10–18)	Trauma
	Drug and alcohol withdrawal
	AV malformations
	Idiopathic
Early adulthood (18–25)	Drug and alcohol withdrawal
	Tumor
Middle age (25–60)	Drug and alcohol withdrawal
	Trauma
	Tumor
	Vascular disease
Late adulthood (older than 60)	Vascular disease, Atrioventricular disease
	Tumor
	Degenerative disease
	Metabolic
	Hypoglycemia
	Uremia
	Hepatic failure
	Electrolyte abnormality
	Drug and alcohol withdrawal

1. **Focal brain disease,** including cerebrovascular events (e.g., stroke), head trauma, and neoplasm.
2. **Infection,** such as meningitis, encephalitis, and abscess.
3. **Drug-related causes,** such as cocaine, amphetamines, and alcohol withdrawal.
4. **Metabolic derangements,** including uremia, hyponatremia, hypoglycemia, and deficiency states such as phenylketonuria.
5. **Subacute conditions,** such as Creutzfeldt-Jakob disease and subacute sclerosing panencephalitis.
6. **Toxins,** such as lead poisoning (especially in children) and mercury poisoning in adults.
7. **Conditions causing syncope,** including vasovagal episodes, postural hypotension, and arrhythmias.
8. **Asphyxia** from hypoxia, carbon monoxide poisoning, or birth injury.
9. **Idiopathic seizures,** in which no clear etiology is found.

C. **Signs**
1. **Fever** may indicate an infectious cause such as meningitis or encephalitis, or it may directly trigger a febrile seizure.
2. **Focal neurologic findings** may indicate a possible tumor or a localized injury to the brain.
3. **Papilledema** indicates increased intracranial pressure that may be caused by an intracranial hemorrhage or tumor.
4. **Hemorrhagic eye grounds** suggest underlying high blood pressure and may be a cause of seizure associated with hypertensive intercranial bleeding.
5. **Stiff neck (meningismus)** may be present with inflamed meninges.
6. **Headache** is a nonspecific complaint compatible with infection or hemorrhage.

D. **Laboratory tests**
1. The following laboratory tests should be considered for all patients with a new seizure and for those with recurrent seizures if indicated by the history and physical examination.
   a. **Serum tests** (glucose, sodium, potassium, calcium, phosphorus, magnesium, blood urea nitrogen, and ammonia levels) generally should be ordered, especially in any clinical situations associated with dehydration, nausea, vomiting, alteration in consciousness, or drug ingestion.
   b. **Antiepileptic drug (AED) levels.** The most common cause of recurrent seizures in children as well as many adults is a subtherapeutic Antiepileptic drug level. Drug levels should be considerred in all individuals already taking an antiepileptic drug who present with recurrence of their underlying seizure disorder.
   c. **Drug and toxic screens,** may be indicated if an adequate history cannot be obtained.
   d. **A complete blood count** can assist in the evaluation of a possible underlying infection.
   e. **Brain imaging** is useful unless the physician can confidently attribute the seizure to a metabolic cause.
      (1) **Computerized tomography (CT scan).** A head CT scan scan is helpful in detecting mass effect or hemmorage.
      (2) **Magnetic resonance imaging (MRI).** A MRI of the head is superior to CT scan in evaluation of temporal lobe lesions.
2. The following tests should be ordered only if the results might alter management.
   a. **Electroencephalogram (EEG).** The diagnosis of epilepsy is not made on the basis of an EEG, unless the EEG captures a clinical seizure. The sensitivity, specificity, and predictive value of this test depend on the underlying cause and anatomic location of a seizure focus. EEG and video EEG are becoming increasingly valuable in diagnosing epilepsy, particularly in patients having difficulty with monotherapeutic control. (SOR **B**)
      (1) **Delta waves** (less than three waveforms per second) are an indication of a disturbance of cerebral function.
      (2) **Generalized slowing** is related to an acute disturbance such as encephalitis, encephalopathy, anoxia, a metabolic disturbance, or drug effect. Generalized slowing may occur with hyperventilation, sleep, and drowsiness, and is more common in young patients.
      (3) **Focal slowing** implies acute local disturbance, such as contusion, stroke, local infection, or tumor. Focal slowing may occur as a postictal phenomenon that

may last hours or days after a focal seizure. Slowing also varies with age and state of arousal.

    (4) Spikes generally represent an old disturbance seen after brain damage, but they may take years to develop. Spikes are less of an indication for further evaluation than focal slowing. A spike wave, defined as three spikes per second, is noted in absence seizures.

  b. 24-Hour ambulatory EEG may be very helpful in identifying "events" and is useful in separating psychogenic NES for epileptic seizures, especially where the two coexist.

  c. Video monitoring may be coupled with a continuous EEG. It may be useful in localizing seizures such as a frontal seizure or a temporal seizure, when the physician is considering surgical correction. This method may also be useful in evaluating suspected psychogenic nonpileptiform seizures and other paroxysmal behaviors. The evaluation is generally performed with the patient as an inpatient.

  d. Skull x-rays are not usually helpful except in the evaluation of severe head trauma.

  e. Lumbar puncture is not routinely indicated in children older than 12 months with a first febrile seizure. In infants younger than 12 months, it should be strongly considered because clinical seizures and symptoms of meningitis may be subtle.

  f. Positron emission tomography (PET) scans are used primarily in research but are becoming increasingly useful when recalcitrant epilepsy leads to surgical consideration.

IV. Treatment

A. Acute treatment
1. The patient's airway must be protected.
2. No medication is usually necessary.
3. If seizure activity persists longer than 5 minutes, intravenous medication may be given (Table 85–1).

B. Drug therapy
1. Only one drug should be prescribed (see Table 85–4). A specific side effect, such as decrease in cognitive function), might lead the physician to select a particular drug (e.g., phenytoin over phenobarbital) in certain circumstances.
2. Dosage should be increased as tolerated to achieve a therapeutic blood level. However, clinical response is a more reliable therapeutic indicator than blood levels. (SOR **C**)
3. Another drug can be substituted if therapy is ineffective. Only after failure of each single agent should combination therapy be considered.

C. Treatment during pregnancy
1. Drug metabolism may be drastically altered during pregnancy.
2. There is about a twofold risk of congenital malformation (predominantly facial cleft and neural tube defects) in mothers who take anticonvulsants to control seizures. Malformations are most strongly associated with trimethadione and valproic acid.

D. Converting from polytherapy to monotherapy
1. The single agent most likely to be successful should be chosen. The dosage of the agent should be slowly increased while the undesirable drug is slowly withdrawn. Long-acting drugs should be discontinued slowly over 1 to 3 months by halving the dose once per week. (SOR **B**)
2. The plan, including the alternatives and the risks, should be fully discussed with the patient. It should be modified if control of seizures is diminished.

E. Febrile seizures
1. In general, anticonvulsants are not indicated for a patient with febrile seizures. Anticonvulsant prophylaxis for febrile seizure can be considered in some cases. For example, if the neurologic examination is abnormal; if the seizure activity lasts for more than 15 minutes; if a transient or permanent neurologic defect is present; or if there is a family history of nonfebrile seizures. (SOR **C**)
2. Phenobarbital or other anticonvulsant therapy is effective in preventing recurrence of febrile seizures. (SOR **B**) Treatment does not affect the percentage of individuals who will develop epilepsy in the future.

V. Management Strategies are dependent on the type of seizure the patient has experienced.

A. Seizures beginning early in life may be caused by developmental defects, perfusion defects of the brain, intrauterine hypoxemia, or fetal infection. Assisting the patient with developmental problems such as learning deficits is as important as controlling the seizures.

TABLE 85–4. POSSIBLE CAUSES OF RECURRENT SEIZURES BASED ON AGE

Drug of Choice for Particular Type of Seizure	Adult Dose (mg/d)	Pediatric Dose (mg/kg/d)	Adult Starting Dose	Side Effects	Therapeutic Range (μg/mL)	Cost
Generalized—tonic-clonic						
Phenytoin (Dilantin)	300–400	4–7	100 mg bid–tid	Decrease in cognitive function, sedation, ataxia, diplopia, gingival hyperplasia	10–20	$
Phenobarbital	120–250	4–6	30–60 mg bid	Respiratory depression, hyperactivity, sedation	15–40	$
Carbamazepine (Tegretol)	600–1200	20–30	200 mg bid–qid	Sedation, diplopia, ataxia, aplastic anemia, hypo-osmolality	6–12	$
Valproic acid (Depakene)	1000–3000	10–60	250 mg tid	Sedation, nausea, vomiting, weight gain, hair loss, GI hematologic toxicity	50–100	$$$
Primidone (Mysoline)	750–1500	10–25	250 mg tid–qid	Sedation, vertigo, nausea, ataxia, change in behavior	6–12	$
Generalized—absence						
Ethosuximide (Zarontin)	250–1000	20–40	250 mg bid	Nausea, vomiting, lethargy, hiccups, headache blood dyscrasias	40–100	$$$
Valproic acid (Depakene)	1000–3000	10–60	250 mg tid	Sedation, nausea, vomiting, weight gain, hair loss, GI hematologic toxicity	50–100	$$$
Clonazepam (Klonopin)	1.5–20	0.01–0.3	0.5 mg tid	Drowsiness, ataxia, change in behavior	0.013–0.072	$$$
Generalized—myoclonic						
Valproic acid (Depakene)	1000–3000	10–60	250 mg tid	Sedation, nausea, vomiting, weight gain, hair loss, GI hematologic toxicity	50–100	$$$
Clonazepam (Klonopin)	1.5–20	0.01–0.3	0.5 mg tid	Drowsiness, ataxia, change in behavior	0.013–0.072	$$$
Phenytoin (Dilantin)	300–400	4–7	100 mg bid–tid	Decrease in cognitive function, sedation, ataxia, diplopia, gingival hyperplasia	10–20	$
Partial						
Carbamazepine (Tegretol)	600–1200	20–30	200 mg bid–qid	Sedation, diplopia, ataxia, aplastic anemia, hypo-osmolality	6–12	$
Phenobarbital (Dilantin)	120–250	4–6	30–60 mg bid	Respiratory depression, hyperactivity, sedation	15–40	$
Valproic acid (Depakene)	1000–3000	10–60	250 mg tid	Sedation, nausea, vomiting, weight gain, hair loss, GI hematologic toxicity	50–100	$$$$
Primidone (Mysoline)	750–1500	10–25	250 mg tid–qid	Sedation, vertigo, nausea, ataxia, change in behavior	6–12	$
Oxcarbazepine (Trileptal)	1200 bid max	300–450 bid	600 mg bid	Hyponatremia, rash, dizziness, visual changes, speech impairment, behavioral changes	—	$$$$
Topiramate (Topamax)	200 bid	200 bid	25 mg bid	Metabolic acidosis, behavioral problems, kidney stones, diabetes, rash, speech changes	—	$$$$
Levetiracetam (Keppra)	1000 bid	1000 bid	500 mg qd	Depression, headache, pancytopenia, alopecia, behavioral change	—	$$$$
Gabapentin (Neurontin)	1200 tid max	50 mg/kg/d	300 mg qd	Rash, thrombocytopenia, leucopenia, dizziness, edema, blurred vision, headache	—	$$$$
Status epilepticus						
Lorazepam (Ativan)	0.05 mg/kg IV	0.05 mg/kg IV	2–4 mg q20–30 min	Respiratory depression, sedation	—	$$$
Diazepam (Valium)	0.25–0.5 mg/kg IV	0.25–0.5 mg/kg IV	5–10 mg q20–30	Respiratory depression, sedation	—	$
Phenytoin (Dilantin)	15–20 mg/kg IV drip at 30–50 mg/min	15–20 mg/kg IV drip at 0.5–1.6 mg/min	—	Decrease in cognitive function, sedation, ataxia, diplopia, gingival hyperplasia	10–20	$
Phenobarbital	300–800 mg IV drip at 25–50 mg/min	20 mg/kg IV drip at 25–50 mg/min	—	Respiratory depression, sedation	15–40	$

GI, gastrointestinal. $, least expensive; $$$$, most expensive.

B. In 80% of childhood seizures, no clear cause is found despite an exhaustive work-up. If the seizures are controlled, normally no impairment in development occurs. If seizures are poorly controlled, difficulties with scholastic, emotional, and social development may arise.

C. New onset of seizures in adolescence generally has no adverse effect on the patient's development as long as the seizures are controlled. Compliance with treatment may prove a significant problem in this age group.

D. New onset of seizures in adults may indicate serious disease, including alcoholism or drug abuse. Patients in early adulthood or middle age must be screened carefully regarding the use of alcohol and "recreational" drugs, as well as the appropriate use of prescription drugs. Identification and intervention may prevent an extensive work-up.

E. Onset of seizures late in life indicates possible cerebral vascular disease or tumor. If the cause of the seizures is not investigated, a potentially correctable problem may be missed and control of the seizures may be difficult to achieve.

VI. Prognosis

A. With time, seizure activity may become quiescent. Withdrawal of therapy should be considered after the patient has been seizure-free for 2 years. The relapse rate of patients who have been medication-free for 3 years is approximately 33%. Relapse is related to seizure type. Patients with complex partial seizures with generalization have the worst prognosis, and those with partial seizures without generalization have the best prognosis.

B. Prognosis also is dependent on the cause of the seizure and whether the patient can change their seizure provocative behavior.

REFERENCES

Alsaadi Taoufik M, Marquez Anna V. Psychogenic nonepileptic seizures. *Am Fam Physician.* 2005;72:849-856.

Gelb DJ. *Introduction to Clinical Neurology.* 2nd ed. Woburn, MA: Butterworth-Heinemann; 2000:129-151.

National Institute for Clinical Excellence (UK). Newer drugs for epilepsy in adults, full guidance. Technology appraisal guidance 76. ; 2004. www.nice.org.uk/guidance/TA76. Accessed August 15, 2008.

Reuber M, Elger C. Psychogenic nonepileptic seizures: review and update. *Epilepsy Behav.* 2003;4(3):205-216.

www.epilepsy.org – at International League Against Epilepsy. Accessed August 7, 2008.

www.epocrates.com. Accessed August 7, 2008.

---

86   Stroke

Michael P. Temporal, MD

KEY POINTS

- Rapid evaluation (including noncontrast computerized tomography of the head) and use of intravenous recombinant tissue plasminogen activator (rtPA) within 3 hours of onset of symptoms of ischemic stroke can improve outcome.
- Immediate stroke management should include monitoring of oxygen and cardiac rhythm status as well as management of fever, agitation, and tight glucose control.
- Blood pressure control during the acute ischemic stroke syndrome may be detrimental and should be treated only if systolic blood pressure is ≥ 220 or diastolic blood pressure is ≥ 120. Aggressive treatment of blood pressure may be required in the setting of hemorrhagic stroke, postthrombolytic therapy, and postoperative carotid endarterectomy or subdural hematoma evacuation.
- Secondary prevention should be based on stroke etiology and may include warfarin (for cardiac embolic source or intracranial disease) or an antiplatelet agent (aspirin, 325 mg/d; clopidogrel, 75 mg/d, ticlopidine 250 mg twice daily, or aspirin/dipyridamole twice daily) for stroke with an atherosclerotic etiology.

- Chronic anticoagulation is indicated in patients with a stroke caused by cardiogenic emboli.
- Modifiable risk factors including smoking cessation, blood pressure control, alcohol consumption, reduction of elevated cholesterol, and diabetes management are important to decrease future stroke risk.

I. Introduction
  A. **Stroke** is a clinical syndrome consisting of the sudden or rapid onset of a constellation of neurologic deficits that persist for more than 24 hours secondary to a vascular event. "Brain attack" is a term used to alert health care providers, patients, and their families and friends of the emergency condition that threatens the life and function of irreplaceable brain tissue.
  B. Stroke and cerebrovascular disease is the third leading cause of death in the United States, the most common cause of disability, and the most frequently cited reason for patients needing long-term care. Nearly 500,000 Americans have new (75%) or recurrent (25%) stroke each year. Although one-third of stroke survivors will have permanent disability requiring help to care for themselves, up to one-half of the 4.4 million survivors of stroke have no or little disability.
  C. **Transient ischemic attacks (TIA)** can be reversible neurologic defects and should prompt the clinician to aggressively evaluate. Following first TIA, 10% to 25% will have a cerebrovascular accident in the next 90 days; up to half of these within the 48 hours following the TIA.
  D. **Types of stroke.** In adults, 80% of strokes are **ischemic:** atheroembolic/atherothrombotic stroke (60%–70% of strokes), cerebral embolic, and lacunar (small vessel occlusive). The rest of strokes in adults are **hemorrhagic** and are classified by location: intracerebral or subarachnoid.
  E. The **differential diagnosis for stroke** includes mass lesions (e.g., subdural hematoma or neoplasm), metabolic abnormalities (e.g., hypoglycemia, hyponatremia, or hypernatremia), infectious processes (e.g., meningitis or cerebral abscess), inflammatory processes (e.g., temporal arteritis), and idiopathic processes (e.g., epilepsy, migraine headache). Syncope and acute cardiac events or arrhythmia may also present like a stroke. Illicit drug use may be a consideration.
II. Diagnosis. The presentation of stroke represents a continuum from TIA (with quickly resolving neurologic deficit) to acute stroke syndrome with progression (worsening deficits, most common with large vessel thrombosis, lacunes, or emboli) to completed stroke (static neurologic deficits). Early presentation, rapid imaging, and prompt treatment are key goals for health care providers and the communities they serve. Evaluation and management in dedicated stroke centers can improve outcomes. (SOR **A**)
  A. **Symptoms** and **signs** of stroke reflect the cerebrovascular territory affected by the stroke process. The vessels most often involved are listed in Table 86–1. Sudden onset of weakness, numbness, or problems with speech or vision or the sudden development of dizziness, trouble walking, or headache are early warning signs of stroke. The initial history must document time of onset of symptoms, associated activities or trauma, other neurologic symptoms (headache, seizure, vomiting, alteration of consciousness) as well as present and past illnesses and surgeries, medications taken, illicit drug use, and allergies. Identifying stroke risk factors and contraindications to thrombolytic therapy are also essential.
  B. **Physical examination** The NIH Stroke Scale **(NIHSS) (Table 86–2)** provides a rapid and relatively comprehensive neurologic assessment that can facilitate communication among health care professionals. (SOR **B**) The general physical examination should identify trauma, infection, or comorbid cardiac, respiratory, and abdominal disorders.
  C. **Brain imaging studies** are used to detect the presence of hemorrhage and exclude other causes (tumor, abscess, or subdural hematoma). The initial study should be obtained and interpreted within 3 hours of onset of symptoms, and ideally within 60 minutes of presentation to an emergency setting to facilitate decisions on thrombolytic therapy. (SOR **C**) Advances in brain imaging promise early distinction of the core area of ischemic tissue with severely compromised cerebral blood flow (CBF) from the "penumbra," that is, the surrounding rim of moderately ischemic brain tissue with impaired electrical activity but preserved cellular metabolism and viability.

TABLE 86–1. CLINICAL PRESENTATION OF STROKE

Stroke Type/Artery or Site Involved	Clinical Presentation	Special Considerations
Atherothrombotic stroke Internal carotid artery (mostly extracranial) Vertebral artery (mostly intracranial) Basilar artery	Stuttering onset, can occur upon waking; cerebellar infarction causes severe edema/brain stem compression	Preceded by TIA in 50% of cases
Embolic stroke Middle cerebral artery Anterior cerebral artery Posterior cerebral artery	Sudden onset of maximal deficit	
Lacunar infarction (penetrating arteries) Middle cerebral perforator–lenticulostriate Posterior cerebral perforator Basilar artery perforating branches	Develops suddenly or over several hours; headache, loss of consciousness, and emesis do not occur	Lacunar syndromes: pure motor hemiparesis, pure sensory loss, crural paresis, and ataxia/dysarthria (clumsy hand syndrome)
Intracerebral hemorrhage Deep cerebral hemisphere (putamen) Subcortical white matter (lobar intracranial hemorrhage) Cerebellar Thalamic Midbrain	Smooth onset, although can be sudden; emesis and loss of consciousness do occur	Selective surgical clot evacuation; unpredictable course in cerebellar ICH; most midbrain ICHs improve with supportive care
Subarachnoid hemorrhage (ruptured aneurysm) Circle of Willis Internal carotid artery Anterior communicating artery Middle cerebral artery	Sudden onset ("brutal" headache, emesis, loss of consciousness then awakening with headache and stiff neck); *note:* aneurysms are rarely symptomatic before rupture	Complications: rerupture, obstruction of spinal fluid flow (communicating hydrocephalus), vasospasm 3–14 d postevent

ICH, intracerebral hemorrhage; TIA, transient ischemic attack.

1. **Computerized tomography (CT)** gives reliable differentiation of hemorrhagic from ischemic stroke with scanning obtained during the first 72 hours of the stroke. All rtPA-administration protocols call for pretreatment noncontrast CT scan within 3 hours of onset of symptoms to rule out hemorrhagic events. (SOR **A**) CT san will show a subarachnoid hemorrhage with 95% sensitivity if performed within 5 days of the event. Normal CT scans are frequently obtained in lacunar or brain stem infarctions when the lesions are small. Early in the course of an ischemic infarction, plain CT scan results are usually negative unless edematous changes are present. The diagnostic yield of plain CT scanning in ischemia is greatest 7 days after the event.

   Indent Multimodal imaging can include perfusion or angiography studies and provide additional information. While they may improve the diagnosis of ischemia, their roles have not been established in the acute stroke setting. Whole brain perfusion CT can identify regions of hypoattenuation and may differentiate thresholds of reversible and irreversible ischemia. Dynamic perfusion CT can be used to measure blood flow and blood volume but provides incomplete visualization of selected vascular territories. Spiral CT angiography can rapidly and noninvasively evaluate the intracranial and extracranial vasculature in the acute, subacute, and chronic stroke setting. (SOR **A**)

2. **Magnetic resonance imaging (MRI)** is more sensitive than CT in detecting ischemic stroke. Multimodal MRI techniques for assessing acute cerebral infarction provide more functional information about the status of the brain on presentation of stroke symptoms: fluid-attenuating inversion recovery imaging, diffusion-weighted imaging (DWI), perfusion-weighted imaging (PWI), functional MRI, and magnetic resonance spectroscopy. These techniques promise ever-increasing delineation of infarcted (irreversibly damaged) tissue from "stunned" (at-risk, potentially reversibly ischemic) tissue. Abnormalities often appear within hours of stroke onset. (SOR **A**)

D. **Laboratory tests.** The following blood tests are recommended for all patients with a suspected acute ischemic stroke: **basic metabolic panel, glucose, complete blood**

TABLE 86–2. NATIONAL INSTITUTES OF HEALTH STROKE SCALE*

Item	Description	Scoring Response
	Level of Consciousness	0—alert 1—drowsy 2—obtunded 3—coma/unresponsive
	Orientation Questions (2)	0—answers both correctly 1—answers one correctly 2—answers neither correctly
	Response to Commands (2)	0—performs both tasks correctly 1—performs one task correctly 2—performs neither correctly
	Gaze	0—normal horizontal movements 1—partial gaze palsy 2—complete gaze palsy
	Visual Fields	0—no visual field defect 1—partial hemianopia 2—complete hemianopia 3—bilateral hemianopia
	Facial Movements	0—normal 1—minor facial weakness 2—partial facial weakness 3—complete unilateral palsy
	Motor Function (arm) R L	0—no drift 1—drift before 5 s 2—drift before 10 s 3—no effort against gravity 4—no movement
	Motor Function (leg) R L	0—no drift 1—drift before 5 s 2—drift before 10 s 3—no effort against gravity 4—no movement
	Limb Ataxia	0—no ataxia 1—ataxia in 1 limb 2—ataxia in 2 limbs
	Sensory	0—no sensory loss 1—mild sensory loss 2—severe sensory loss
	Language	0—normal 1—mild aphasia 2—severe aphasia 3—mute or global aphasia
	Articulation	0—normal 1—mild dysarthria 2—severe dysarthria
	Extinction or Inhibition	0—absent 1—mild (loss 1 sensory modality) 2—severe (loss 2 sensory modalities)

*http://www.ninds.nih.gov/doctors/NIH_Stroke_Scale.pdf

count and platelets, prothrombin time (PT) and international normalized ratio (INR), and cardiac enzymes. (SOR **B**) In selected patients additional acute tests may include liver function tests, toxicology and blood alcohol level, pregnancy test, and arterial blood gas.

Subsequent tests can be helpful after the acute stroke including lipid profile, and specific coagulation factors (proteins C, S, and antithrombin III). (SOR **B**) Elevated homocysteine levels have been associated with increased stroke risk and may be improved with vitamin B complex supplementation. (SOR **C**)

E. Additional studies

1. An initial **electrocardiogram** is obtained in all stroke patients to identify arrhythmia or other cardiac conditions. Routine **chest radiographs** are indicated only if underlying lung pathology is suspected. (SOR **B**)

2. **Imaging of the extracranial and intracranial vessels.** The initial evaluation of patients with symptoms of acute cerebrovascular ischemia includes **carotid noninvasive testing** (carotid duplex ultrasonography and color Doppler flow imaging), looking for significant lesions of the carotid arteries. **Transcranial Doppler ultrasonography (TCD)** detects middle cerebral and distal (intracranial) internal carotid artery stenosis with a sensitivity of 92% and a specificity of 100%. However, this technique is insufficient to detect stenosis or occlusion in the posterior circulation, and the middle cerebral artery cannot be seen in up to one-fourth of patients. TCD is capable of detecting microembolic material of both gaseous and solid states within intracranial cerebral arteries. **Spiral computed tomographic angiography** provides definition of vascular lesions; however, the preferred technique for screening patients for extracranial carotid and intracranial artery disease (including the posterior circulation) is **magnetic resonance angiography. Cerebral angiography,** the gold standard of vascular imaging, is performed on a case-specific basis, primarily when surgical intervention is considered or when angiographic confirmation of stenosis detected by other techniques is required. **Digital subtraction angiography** is another technique. **Oculoplethysmography** offers an indirect measure of carotid arterial blockage by measuring arterial pulsations in the retinal artery.

3. **Echocardiography** (transthoracic or transesophageal) and **24-hour Holter monitoring** are performed when an embolic process is suspected, when surgical intervention is planned, or when the stroke patient has significant risk factors for emboli (e.g., atrial fibrillation, suspected infective endocarditis, prosthetic heart valve, dilated cardiomyopathy, or recent anterior myocardial infarction).

4. A **lumbar puncture** is useful when brain imaging is normal and subarachnoid hemorrhage or meningitis is suspected. Although cerebrospinal fluid is usually bloody in ventricular extension of a hypertensive hemorrhage, vascular malformation, and ruptured aneurysm, a clear tap does not guarantee absence of hemorrhage. Leukocytosis in the cerebrospinal fluid suggests infection.

5. **Electroencephalography** may show slow waves in strokes involving the cortex and is performed when seizure activity has occurred or is suspected.

III. Treatment.

A. **Brain attack is a medical emergency.** The first step is patient education directed at encouraging patients to seek medical care as soon as symptoms develop. Initiation of diagnosis and treatment within the first few hours of onset enhances the very real chances to minimize irreversible ischemic damage and thus improve outcomes. Care in specialized stroke units has been shown to improve outcomes. Attention to rehabilitation goals begins as soon as possible after the acute event.

1. **Stabilization of the patient** involves blood pressure (BP) control, arrhythmia detection and treatment, airway protection, and, if needed, ventilatory assistance and correction of hypoxemia. Proper positioning to avoid pressure sores, diligent correction of metabolic disturbances, and skilled monitoring of stroke progression via repeated neurologic examinations are important. Continuous cardiac monitoring during the first 24 hours is advised because of the high risk of cardiac arrhythmias.

2. **Blood pressure (BP) control.** The prevention of neurologic and cardiovascular compromise caused by the extremes of BP poses a unique clinical challenge in the stroke patient. Poststroke BP elevation usually declines spontaneously by approximately 10% in the first 24 hours. In fact, elevated BP can be a physiologic response to acute brain ischemia. Normalization of BP often occurs when specific effects of stroke are controlled: pain, nausea, agitation, bladder distention, increased intracranial pressure, stress of stroke, and underlying hypertension. Furthermore, exaggerated responses to antihypertensive drugs can cause sudden drops in BP that compromise cerebral perfusion and thus worsen neurologic status. Pharmacologic therapy for hypertension associated with **ischemic stroke** is only for specific indications (e.g., myocardial infarction or arterial dissection) or for systolic BP $\geq$220 mm Hg or diastolic BP $\geq$120 mm Hg on repeated measurements over a 30- to 60-minute period. (SOR **B**) Treatment options include intravenous labetalol (10–20 mg), nitropaste (1–2 inches), or nicardipine infusion (5 mg/h). The approach to BP control must take into account

whether the preevent BP was known to be normotensive or not. Additionally, patients with **hemorrhagic stroke,** after **thrombolysis** and in the **postoperative period** (e.g., carotid endarterectomy or hematoma removal) require more aggressive treatment of hypertension. Long-term antihypertensive therapy can be considered 24 hours after the acute event. (SOR **C**)

B. Reverse ischemia

1. **Reperfusion** therapy aimed at recanalization of the affected vessel(s) in the acute stroke is a very recent advancement. Pharmacologic, angioplastic, and surgical re-canalization are the current options.

   a. **Pharmacologic agents** are infused during the initial 3 hours after onset of stroke symptoms. rtPA is approved by the US Food and Drug Administration (FDA) for treatment of CT-proved nonhemorrhagic stroke within the first 3 hours of onset of symptoms. Studies show the sooner the intervention, the greater the chance of a good outcome. Uncontrolled blood pressure greater than $\geq 185/110$ is a contraindi-cation to rtPA. After evaluation for inclusion or exclusion criteria for its use (Table 86–3), rtPA is administered at 0.9 mg/kg (up to 90 mg) intravenously; the first intra-arterial administration of rtPA is recommended for patients with occlusions of the internal carotid, main stem middle cerebral, and basilar arteries. Intravenous rtPA is best for patients with intracranial circumferential branch artery occlusions. The greatest risk of thrombolysis in acute stroke is intracerebral hemorrhage (ICH). In-tensive care unit monitoring after thrombolysis includes attention to signs of ICH: decreased consciousness, headache, nausea, vomiting, and increased neurologic focal deficits. The risk of ICH is decreased by lowering BP (treat for systolic ≥ 185 and diastolic ≥ 110). Neither aspirin nor anticoagulation is given for the initial 24 hours after thrombolysis, and neither is initiated after that until a repeat CT scan shows no hemorrhage.

   b. **Carotid endarterectomy (CEA)** for ipsilateral severe (70%–99%) carotid artery stenosis in symptomatic patients with recent nondisabling carotid artery ischemic events (TIA or stroke) is clearly beneficial. The NASCET (North American Symptom-atic Carotid Endarterectomy Trial) has demonstrated highly significant ($p \leq 0.001$) benefit for severe lesions, and significant ($p = 0.045$) in moderate (50%–69%) stenosis in recurrent ischemic events compared to medical therapy. (SOR **A**)

   Recommendation for prophylactic CEA in **asymptomatic** patients based on the AHA guidelines for CEA is related to surgical risk. The surgeon's specific morbidity and mortality statistics are a significant factor in estimating this risk. Patient selec-tion and postoperative management of modifiable risk factors apply as well. For asymptomatic patients with a life expectancy of at least 5 years and a surgical risk

TABLE 86–3. RECOMBINANT TISSUE PLASMINOGEN ACTIVATOR (rtPA) USE IN PATIENTS WITH STROKE

Inclusion criteria
  Stroke onset of ≤ 3 hours prior to drug administration
  Patient age ≤ 75 years
  Normal blood glucose
  Normal coagulation assays

Exclusion criteria
  Recent major surgery or trauma in past 14 days
  Intra-arterial needle-sticks in noncompressible sites
  Computerized tomography (CT) results showing involvement of more than one third of the distribution of the
    major carotid artery
  Infective endocarditis
  Seizure at onset of stroke
  Any evidence of blood on CT imaging
  Abnormal platelet counts ($\leq 100,000/mm^3$)
  Elevated International normalized ratio (≥ 1.7) or partial thromboplastin time (PTT)
  Administration of heparin in the past 24 hours
  Chest compression
  Gastrointestinal or urinary tract hemorrhage in past 21 days
  Recent myocardial infarction
  Recent lumbar puncture in past 7 days
  Pregnancy
  Uncontrolled hypertension: systolic ≥ 185 mm Hg; diastolic ≥ 110 mm Hg

≤6% ipsilateral, CEA is considered a proven benefit when stenosis is greater than 59%, regardless of plaque characteristics (e.g., ulceration), contralateral carotid status, or antiplatelet therapy. (SOR **B**) Unilateral CEA is acceptable at the time of indicated coronary artery bypass grafting in asymptomatic patients whose ipsilateral carotid artery stenosis is ≥59%. Those whose surgical risk is ≥3% have no proven indication. (SOR **B**)

  c. Other endovascular interventions are being evaluated and are showing favorable outcomes. All of these have been in association with intra-arterial thrombolytic therapy and limited to comprehensive stroke centers. Angioplasty with stenting may be considered in the higher risk surgical candidate. Emergency angioplasty with stent in conjunction with intra-arterial thrombolysis has been helpful. (SOR **C**) Mechanical clot disruption of the middle cerebral artery and the internal carotid artery can improve the success of recanalization. (SOR **C**) A clot extraction device (MERCI) has obtained FDA approval for intracranial clot removal. (SOR **B**)

2. Acute **anticoagulation.** There is no standard of care for the use of **heparin** in the acute phase of stroke and should not be a substitute for patients otherwise eligible for thrombolytic therapy. (SOR **A**) Studies from the International Stroke Trial showed that while the risk of early recurrent stroke was lowered, excess major bleeding complications negated any benefits. Likewise, trials using low-molecular-weight heparins or danaparoid for acute stroke have not demonstrated benefit. (SOR **A**) Heparin as an adjunctive therapy should not begin within 24 hours of thrombolytic therapy. (SOR **B**)

3. Cerebral edema is a leading cause of death in the first week of stroke. Treat or avoid conditions that tend to increase intracranial pressure (ICP): fever, pain, hypoxia, agitation, fluid overload, hypercarbia, and drugs that dilate intracranial vessels. Corticosteroids are ineffective in managing brain edema secondary to stroke. The two medical modalities used to treat cerebral edema are **osmotherapy** (e.g., mannitol and glycerol) and **hyperventilation therapy** in patients with markedly increased ICP. (SOR **C**) Surgical intervention (e.g., decompression hemicraniectomy) is sometimes necessary to control increasing ICP. (SOR **B**)

4. Nimodipine is a dihydropyridine calcium channel blocker that affects mainly the central nervous system vasculature. Approved for treating cerebral ischemia associated with subarachnoid hemorrhage, nimodipine is initiated within 96 hours of bleeding at a dosage of 60 mg orally every 4 hours for 21 days (the period of time during which neurologic deficit from vasospasm is most likely). (SOR **B**)

C. Prevention of stroke recurrence through secondary risk reduction is key to continued reduction of morbidity and mortality of stroke.

1. Nonmodifiable risk factors for stroke include age (risk doubles each decade beyond 55 years), family history, male gender, ethnicity (African American and Hispanic). The greatest risk factor however, is previous stroke: Stroke begets stroke.

2. Modifiable risk factors. General lifestyle modification should be encouraged for healthy weight, smoking cessation, and alcohol consumption. (SOR **C**) **Weight** goal is body mass index between 18.5 and 24.9 kg/m^2. Moderate intensity **physical activity** of at least 30 minutes almost daily is desireable. **Tobacco** and street drug use is highly discouraged. Moderate **alcohol** consumption (≤2 drinks per day) can be allowed; binge drinking, particularly in young adults, has been associated with increased stroke risk. **Diabetes** control remains glycohemoglobin ≤7.0%. (SOR **B**)

3. Antihypertensive treatment is associated with a 30% to 40% stroke risk reduction. (SOR **A**) The benefit of treatment should be considered for all patients following TIA and the acute stroke period, both with or without a history of hypertension. (SOR **B**) BP goal should aim for below 130 mm Hg/80 mm Hg with at least an average reduction of 10 mm Hg/5 mm Hg. (SOR **B**) Lifestyle modification is always encouraged (see Chapter 76). A meta-analysis demonstrated significant reduction of recurrent stroke with the use of diuretics, diuretics combined with ACE inhibitors (ACEI). The same reduction was not seen in beta-blockers nor ACEI alone, but may have been related to the degree of BP reduction achieved. (SOR **B**) Angiotensin II blockade has been helpful for protecting against vascular occlusive disease. The Heart Outcomes Prevention Evaluation (HOPE) study demonstrated a 32% relative risk reduction for any stroke, and 61% reduction in fatal stroke with the use of ramipril. (SOR **B**) The Perindopril Protection Against Recurrent Stroke Study (PROGRESS) used a flexible regimen of perindopril plus indapamide if necessary, versus placebo. A 28% relative reduction was noted. (SOR **B**) The Losartan Intervention for endpoint Reduction in

Hypertension (LIFE) study showed favorable (25%) relative risk reduction in stroke compared to atenolol. (SOR **B**)

4. Cholesterol management should follow National Cholesterol Education Program Adult Treatment Panel (NCEP-ATP III) recommendations. Low density lipoprotein (LDL-c) goal should be less than 100 mg/dL in those with CHD or symptomatic atherosclerotic disease, and ≤70 mg/dL for very high risk persons with multiple risk factors. (SOR **A**) Even those with no preexisting indication for statins are reasonable candidates for treatment with statins to reduce the risk of vascular events. (SOR **B**)

5. The role of **CEA** has been discussed in Section III.B.1.b.

6. **Anticoagulation therapy** with warfarin may be indicated for the 20% of ischemic strokes caused by cardiogenic emboli. For patients with persistent or paroxysmal **atrial fibrillation**, anticoagulation is recommended; (SOR **A**) if unable to take oral anticoagulants, Aspirin 325 mg/d is recommended. (SOR **A**) In the setting of **acute myocardial infarction and left ventricular thrombus,** anticoagulation may be used for at least 3 months and up to 12 months. (SOR **B**) Concomitant enteric coated aspirin for coronary artery disease should be used. (SOR **A**) Patients with **dilated cardiomyopathy** may be offered warfarin or antiplatelet therapy. (SOR **C**) For patients with **rheumatic mitral valve disease**, warfarin is reasonable. Routine addition of concomitant enteric coated aspirin is not recommended, but 81 mg/d may be added if there is recurrent embolism on warfarin. (SOR **C**) Likewise, for patients with **prosthetic heart valves** who have ischemic stroke on warfarin, aspirin 81 mg/d is reasonable. (SOR **B**)

7. Antiplatelet therapy. For patients with noncardioembolic ischemic stroke or TIA, antiplatelet agents rather than oral anticoagulation are recommended to reduce the risk of recurrent stroke and other cardiovascular events. (SOR **A**) In meta-analyses, a 28% relative odds reduction in nonfatal strokes and a 16% reduction in fatal strokes has been demonstrated.

   a. Aspirin 325 mg/d for secondary prevention following stroke may begin 24 to 48 hours after the acute event. (SOR **A**) While the acute initation of aspirin or the glycoprotein IIb/IIIa inhibitors may be helpful in acute coronary syndromes, they are not recommended in the management of acute stroke outside of clinical trials (SOR **B**).

   b. Clopidogrel (Plavix), 75 mg/d, is a potent, noncompetitive inhibitor of adenosine diphosphate induced platelet aggregation. It can be used in patients allergic to aspirin. The Clopidogrel versus Aspirin in Patients at Risk of Ischemic Events (CAPRIE) trial included patients with stroke, MI or peripheral vascular disease and was marginally better than aspirin for stroke risk reduction. (SOR **B**) It may have relatively more stroke risk benefit in those with diabetes and MI. The combination of aspirin with clopidogrel has been advocated for up to 12 months following acute coronary syndromes, but a similar risk benefit was not demonstrated in stroke or TIA in the Management of Atherothrombosis with Clopidogrel in High-Risk Patients with TIA or Stroke (MATCH) trial.(SOR **B**) Also, the risk of bleeding is increased. Diarrhea and rash are common side effects, and while neutropenia is not a problem, thrombotic thrombocytopenic purpura has been reported.

   c. Extended release dipyridamole and aspirin (Aggrenox), 200 mg/20 mg twice daily, also inhibits platelet activation and aggregation. The combination has been shown to decrease the risk of stroke by 37% compared to aspirin (18%) or dipyridamole (18%) alone in the European Stroke Prevention Study (ESPS-2). (SOR **B**) Headache is the most common side effect; no additional bleeding risk compared to that by aspirin was noted.

   d. Ticlopidine (Ticlid), 250 mg twice daily, works same as clopidogrel and is offered as 21% relative risk reduction for recurrent stroke compared to aspirin in the Ticlopidine/Aspirin Stroke Study. (SOR **B**) As with Clopidogrel, diarrhea and rash are the reported side effects. Additionally, initial weekly monitoring for neutropenia is warranted. Thrombotic thrombocytopenic purpura has also been described.

IV. **Management Strategies.** Stroke indicates generalized vascular disease; it is one event in a prolonged and ongoing process. Management strategies center on prevention of further manifestations of the disease and maximization of poststroke function during the three stages of stroke.

   A. **Stage I.** The **acute stage** of stroke spans the first week. Attention to evaluation, maintenance, and return of function includes passive range of motion of extremities, proper positioning, frequent turning, and maintenance of good hygiene. (SOR **C**) Evaluation of swallowing function should be done before starting eating and drinking. (SOR **B**)

B. **Stage II.** The **subacute stage** of stroke usually lasts 3 months. Return of neurologic function is greatest during this interval. **Rehabilitation** involves interdisciplinary assessment and treatment by a team of nurses, physical therapists, occupational therapists, speech therapists, a dietitian, and the physician to maximize functional return and independence. Selection of the site of rehabilitation (e.g., a formal rehabilitation unit, a skilled nursing home, the patient's home with home health care agency coordination, or outpatient facilities) depends on the patient's medical condition, the family situation (supports and weaknesses), financial considerations, and available resources. To benefit from any kind of rehabilitation, the patient must be able to communicate (verbally or nonverbally), follow a two- to three-step command, and remember what is learned. Rehabilitation units require that a patient's cardiopulmonary endurance allows 2 to 3 hours of intense therapy daily. Patients with marked dementia, severe chronic obstructive pulmonary disease, marked limitation of cardiovascular reserve, or severely debilitating multiple joint disease are not likely to benefit from acute inpatient rehabilitation, although such patients may receive benefit from skilled or subacute care in the immediate posthospitalization period.

C. **Stage III.** The **chronic stage** of stroke recovery begins after 3 months. Neurologic return may continue for as long as 1 year after an event and functional recovery can occur for as long as 2 years. Maintenance of the functional gains achieved in the subacute stage is important.

TABLE 86–4. BARTHEL INDEX

A score above 60 usually means that ≤ 2 hours of personal care assistance is required each day. A score of 60 or less indicates that 4 or more hours of personal care assistance is needed daily. A score of 0 is given when a criterion cannot be met.

Functional activity

1. Feeding
     5—Dependent
     10—Independent
2. Transfer from bed to wheelchair, back to bed (includes sitting up in bed)
     5—Assisted out of bed only
     10—Needs some help/cueing
     15—Independent
3. Grooming (wash face; comb hair; shave, including preparing razor; clean teeth; and apply own make-up if worn)
     0—Dependent
     5—Independent
4. Toileting (transfer on/off toilet, handling clothing, wiping, and flushing)
     5—Dependent
     10—Independent
5. Bathing (tub, shower, or complete sponge bath)
     0—Dependent
     5—Independent
6. Ambulation, 50 yards, level surface
     0—Totally dependent
     5—Dependent on wheelchair but able to propel
     10—Able to walk with assistive device
     15—Able to walk without assistive device
(5) Unable to walk (e.g., wheeled walker or wheelchair required)
7. Ascending/descending stairs (mechanical assistive devices allowed)
     5—Dependent
     10—Independent
8. Dressing (includes tying shoes and donning assistive devices; excludes nonprescribed girdles or bras)
     5—Dependent
     10—Independent
9. Bowel continence (suppository, enema allowed)
     5—Dependent
     10—Independent
10. Urinary continence
     5—Dependent
     10—Independent

(Modified with permission from Mahoney FI, Barthel DW: Functional evaluation: The Barthel index. *Md State Med J.* 1965;14:61.)

1. **Involvement of the family or caregiver** in the acute and intermediate phases of stroke care enhances their knowledge and expectations regarding the patient's condition. Careful coordination of patient and family involvement, including discharge planning, and involving the family or caregiver in teaching sessions with the patient and with each of the patient's regular therapists and team nurse is helpful.
2. **Home health care agency involvement** allows for smooth transition and capable problem solving as the patient returns home.
3. **Monitoring of the patient by the physician** at regular intervals is important to assess and promote risk management strategies, identify and treat complicated illness (e.g., depression), evaluate recurrence of symptoms, assess functional status (Barthel index [Table 86–4]), negotiate potential blocks to maintenance of function, and facilitate the patient's acceptance of disability.

V. **Prognosis.** Overall, the vast majority of initially alert patients survive the acute phase of stroke. Acute-phase deaths are generally due to cerebral causes related to irreversible failure of vital function of the brain stem. Pulmonary embolism and cardiac events contribute to early mortality in stroke patients. Systemic causes (e.g., pneumonia, pulmonary embolism, ischemic heart disease, or recurrent stroke) are the usual causes of death in the subacute and chronic phases. The risk of recurrence of stroke is substantial. The major complications of stroke are aspiration, infection (e.g., urinary tract infection or pneumonia), pressure sores, corneal abrasion, and depression. Third-nerve palsy (signaling uncal herniation), increased age of the patient, and hemorrhagic events are associated with grave immediate prognoses. In hemorrhagic events, the prognosis for total unilateral motor deficit and coma is poor. Brain stem infarctions such as pontine hemorrhages have an extremely poor prognosis. Lacunar infarctions involve subcortical small vessels and have the lowest mortality rate of all strokes.

REFERENCES

Adams HP, del Zoppo G, Alberts MJ, et al. Guidelines for the early management of adults with ischemic stroke. *Stroke.* 2007;38:1665-1771.
Bravata DM, Kim N, Concato J, Krumholz HM, Brass LM. Thrombolysis for acute stroke in routine clinical practice. *Arch Intern Med.* 2002;162:1994-2001.
Sacco RL, Adams R, Albers G, et al. Guidelines for prevention of stroke in patients with ischemic stroke or transient ischemic attack. *Stroke.* 2006;37:577-617.

ELECTRONIC RESOURCES

http://www.ninds.nih.gov/ is the Web site for the National Institute of Neurologic Disorders and Stroke with links to multiple organizations. Accessed August 15, 2008.
http://stroke.ahajournals.org/ is the Web site of the American Heart Association with links to consensus statements and journal articles. The parent site is www.strokeassociation.org. Accessed August 15, 2008.
http://www.stroke.org is the Web site of the National Stroke Association with excellent resources for patients, providers, and caregivers. Accessed August 15, 2008.
http://www.strokecenter.org is the clinical Web site of Washington University in St. Louis also with clinical updates and useful tools. Accessed August 15, 2008.

---

87   Thyroid Disease

Jeri R. Reid, MD & Stephen F. Wheeler, MEng, MD

KEY POINTS

- A sensitive thyroid-stimulating hormone assay (sTSH) is the best single screening test for both hypothyroidism and hyperthyroidism.
- Levothyroxine, usually begun at the full estimated replacement dose (1.6 μg/kg) in patients younger than 65 years without cardiac disease, is the treatment of choice for hypothyroidism. (SOR **B**) In older patients and those with known or suspected cardiac disease, an initial dose of 25% of the calculated replacement dose is indicated. (SOR **C**)

- Radioactive iodine (^{123}I) uptake scanning can help clarify hyperthyroidism of uncertain etiology.
- Oral radioactive iodine (^{131}I) is the treatment of choice for most patients with hyperthyroidism in the United States, but antithyroid drugs and surgery are appropriate in selected patients.
- The evaluation of a thyroid nodule usually begins with sTSH, ultrasound, and a fine needle aspiration biopsy.

I. Introduction

A. Physiology. Thyrotropin-releasing hormone, secreted by the hypothalamus, stimulates the anterior pituitary to produce thyroid-stimulating hormone (TSH). The major hormone released by the thyroid gland in response to TSH is thyroxine (T_4), which is converted peripherally to triiodothyronine (T_3), a more potent hormone. T_4 and T_3 are both highly but reversibly bound to plasma thyroid-binding globulin (TBG) and, to a lesser extent, to albumin and prealbumin. Only the minute unbound (free) fractions are metabolically active. The most sensitive indicator of thyroid status is the level of TSH, which is controlled in classic negative-feedback fashion by the concentration of unbound thyroid hormones.

B. Diagnostic evaluation. Diagnosis of thyroid disease depends on symptoms, clinical signs, and laboratory tests.

1. Table 87–1 lists the most common symptoms and signs of hypothyroidism according to frequency.
2. Table 87–2 lists the most common clinical findings of hyperthyroidism according to frequency.
3. The single most important diagnostic test is the **highly-sensitive serum TSH (sTSH).** The accepted range of normal sTSH is between 0.45 and 4.5 mIU/L.
   a. A **normal** sTSH level rules out thyroid dysfunction in most cases. However, a normal level coupled with signs and symptoms of hypothyroidism should prompt further testing for central hypothyroidism,
   b. A **suppressed** sTSH occurs in hyperthyroidism but can also be decreased by severe nonthyroidal illness, use of dopamine, and glucocorticoid therapy. Also, sTSH may be suppressed in some euthyroid elderly patients.
   c. An **elevated** sTSH is usually an indication of hypothyroidism but it may be mildly elevated during recovery from severe nonthyroidal illness, by various drugs, including lithium and amphetamines, and in some euthyroid elderly patients.
   d. **Free thyroxine (T_4)** measured directly, is now commonly used for the routine diagnostic evaluation of thyroid disease. Direct measurement of free T_3 is also available. These tests decrease the need for more traditional tests such as total T_4, total T_3, and T_3resin uptake.

TABLE 87–1. COMMON SIGNS AND SYMPTOMS OF HYPOTHYROIDISM*

Sign or Symptom	Affected Patients (%)
Weakness	99
Skin changes (dry or coarse skin)	97
Lethargy	91
Slow speech	91
Eyelid edema	90
Cold sensation	89
Decreased sweating	89
Cold skin	83
Thick tongue	82
Facial edema	79
Coarse hair	76
Skin pallor	67
Forgetfulness	66
Constipation	61

*Only signs and symptoms that occur in 60% or more of patients with hypothyroidism are listed in this table. (Adapted with permission from Larsen PR, Davies TF, Hay ID. The thyroid gland. In: Wilson JD, Foster DW, Kronenberg HM, Larsen PR, eds. *Williams Textbook of Endocrinology.* 9th ed. Philadelphia, PA: Saunders; 1998:461. Copyright © Elsevier.)

TABLE 87–2. COMMON SIGNS AND SYMPTOMS OF HYPERTHYROIDISM

Signs and Clinical Symptoms	Patients Older Than 70 y (%)	Patients Younger Than 50 y (%)	P Value
Tachycardia	71	96	.01
Fatigue	56	84	.01
Weight loss	50	51	.87
Tremor	44	84	<.001
Dyspnea	41	56	.20
Apathy	41	25	.20
Anorexia	32	4	<.001
Nervousness	31	84	<.001
Hyperactive reflexes	28	96	<.001
Weakness	27	61	.01
Depression	24	22	87
Increased sweating	24	95	<.001
Polydipsia	21	67	<.001
Diarrhea	18	43	.02
Confusion	16	0	.01
Muscular atrophy	16	10	.52
Heat intolerance	15	92	<.001
Constipation	15	0	.01
Increased appetite	0	57	<.001

(Trivalle C, Doucet J, Chassagne P, et al. Differences in signs and symptoms of hyperthyroidism in older and younger patients. *J Amer Geriatr Soc.* 1996;44:51. With permission from Wiley-Blackwell Publishing, Ltd.)

C. **Screening** for thyroid disease in the general population, except newborns, is controversial. A consensus conference, made up of members of the most prominent endocrine societies, recently recommended screening for all women aged 60 or older and all persons with previous thyroid surgery or neck radiation, type 1 diabetes or other autoimmune disease, atrial fibrillation, or a family history of thyroid disease. They also recommended screening patients with any signs or symptoms of thyroid disease, including thyroid enlargement or nodules. Another panel, made up of members of the same societies, countered with the recommendation that all adults should be screened, including pregnant woman and those contemplating pregnancy. (SOR **C**)

II. **Hypothyroidism**

A. **Introduction.** Hypothyroidism results from insufficient production of thyroid hormones. Overt hypothyroidism is found in 0.3% to 2% of the general population. It is at least twice as common in females as in males and prevalence increases progressively with age.

   1. **Primary hypothyroidism,** most commonly from chronic autoimmune (Hashimoto's) thyroiditis, radioactive iodine therapy, or surgery, accounts for the overwhelming majority of hypothyroidism cases. A high sTSH and a low free T_4 are indicative of primary hypothyroidism.

   2. **Secondary hypothyroidism** results from decreased pituitary secretion of TSH. This condition is usually accompanied by other manifestations of pituitary hyposecretion. Causes include postpartum pituitary necrosis (Sheehan's syndrome) and pituitary tumors.

B. **Diagnosis**

   1. In a patient with suggestive signs and symptoms, a high sTSH (>4.5 μU/mL) and a low free T_4 are diagnostic of primary hypothyroidism. When autoimmune thyroiditis is the presumptive cause, confirmation with a serum antithyroid peroxidase level (formerly called antimicrosomal antibody) may be helpful.

   2. In the setting of signs and symptoms of hypothyroidism, a sTSH that is normal or only mildly elevated suggests secondary hypothyroidism. Concurrent amenorrhea, galactorrhea, postural hypotension, loss of axillary and pubic hair, and visual field deficits may be present to suggest a central cause.

C. **Treatment**

   1. **Levothyroxine** is preferred for routine replacement therapy. Interchangeability studies of levothyroxine products have not shown significant fluctuations in hormone levels when switching among name-brand or generic preparations. (SOR **B**) Current

evidence does not support the use of combinations of levothyroxine and T_3 for re-placement therapy. (SOR **C**)

2. Adults require approximately 1.8 μg/kg/d for full replacement. Older patients may re-quire only 0.5 μg/kg/d. Therapy is usually initiated with the full replacement dose in patients younger than 65 years. (SOR **B**) In patients older than 65 years, or in younger patients with known or suspected cardiac disease, a lower initial dose of 25% of the calculated replacement dose, with gradual titration, is indicated. (SOR **C**)

3. Clinical and biochemical **re-evaluation** at 6- to 8-week intervals is necessary until the levothyroxine dose has been titrated to produce a normalized sTSH. Subsequently, an interim history and physical examination pertinent to thyroid status and a sTSH should be performed at least annually.

4. **Drugs** such as cholestyramine, ferrous sulfate, sucralfate, and antacids containing aluminum hydroxide may interfere with levothyroxine absorption. Other drugs, such as phenytoin, carbamazepine, and rifampin, may accelerate levothyroxine metabolism, necessitating higher replacement doses.

D. **Subclinical hypothyroidism**

1. **Introduction.** Subclinical hypothyroidism is distinguished by an elevated sTSH, a nor-mal free T_4, and few, if any, hypothyroid symptoms. This condition is estimated to occur in 4% to 8% of the general population and in as many as 20% of women aged 60 or older. Approximately 20% of patients taking thyroid replacement medication have subclinical hypothyroidism.

2. **Clinical course.** Subclinical hypothyroidism progresses to clinical hypothyroidism at a rate of 2% to 5% per year. Risk factors for progression include the presence of thy-roid autoantibodies, age older than 65 years, female gender, and a higher sTSH level ($\geq$10 μU/mL). Patients who do not progress are considered to be euthyroid with a reset thyrostat, probably because of a subtle insult to the thyroid gland. Subclinical hypothy-roidism has been linked to adverse cardiac events, elevations in total and low-density lipoprotein (LDL) cholesterol, and the development of systemic and neuropsychiatric symptoms.

3. **Treatment.** Levothyroxine is recommended for patients with sTSH levels above 10 mIU/L since these patients are more likely to show an improvement in symptoms and a possible lowering of LDL cholesterol. A trial of levothyroxine for symptomatic patients with sTSH between 4.5 and 10 mIU/L can be considered, but it should be discontinued if symptoms do not improve. Women who are pregnant or contemplating pregnancy should be treated at all TSH levels regardless of symptoms since adverse outcomes affecting the fetus or the mother have been associated with untreated subclinical hy-pothyroidism in this group. Patients who are **not treated** should be monitored clinically and biochemically at yearly intervals for evidence of progressive thyroid dysfunction. (SOR **C**)

III. **Hyperthyroidism**

A. **Introduction.** Hyperthyroidism results from elevated levels of thyroid hormones. Hyper-thyroidism is less common than hypothyroidism in the general population. Community-based studies have found prevalences of 2% in women and 0.2% in men. Approximately 15% of cases occur in persons older than 60 years. Graves' disease accounts for approxi-mately 60% to 80% of hyperthyroidism. Hyperthyroidism encompasses a heterogeneous group of disorders.

1. **Graves' disease** is an autoimmune disease that results from the action of thyroid-stimulating immunoglobulin G antibody (TS Ab) on thyroid gland TSH receptors. It demonstrates a familial predisposition.

2. **Toxic multinodular goiter (Plummer's disease),** the most common cause of hyper-thyroidism in those older than 40 years, occurs when a patient with nontoxic multin-odular goiter develops one or more autonomous hyperfunctioning nodules.

3. **Toxic adenoma,** the least common cause of hyperthyroidism, is produced by one or more hyperfunctioning thyroid adenomas capable of functioning independently of TSH or other thyroid stimulators.

4. **Thyroiditis** may produce transient hyperthyroidism as hormone leaks from an inflamed gland. Transient hypothyroidism often follows as the intrathyroidal stores of hormone are depleted.

B. **Diagnosis**

1. The **history** and the **physical examination** are critical to distinguish among the causes of hyperthyroidism (Table 87–3).

TABLE 87–3. COMMON ETIOLOGY AND CLINICAL DIAGNOSIS OF HYPERTHYROIDISM

Cause	Pathophysiology	Gland Size*	Nodularity	Tenderness
Toxic adenoma	Autonomous hormone production	Decreased	Single nodule	Nontender
Toxic multinodular goiter	Autonomous hormone production	Increased	Multiple nodules	Tender
Subacute thyroiditis	Leakage of hormone from gland	Increased	None	Tender
Lymphocytic thyroiditis, postpartum thyroiditis, medication-induced thyroiditis	Leakage of hormone from gland	Moderately increased	None	Nontender
Graves' disease (thyroid-stimulating antibody)	Increased glandular stimulation (substance causing stimulation)	Increased	None	Nontender
Iodine-induced hyperfunctioning of thyroid gland (iodide ingestion, radiographic contrast, amiodarone [Cordarone])	Increased glandular stimulation (substance causing stimulation)	Increased	Multiple nodules or no nodules	Nontender
Functioning pituitary adenoma (TSH); trophoplastic tumors (human chorionic gonadotropin)	Increased glandular stimulation (substance causing stimulation)	Increased	None	Nontender
Factitial hyperthyroidism	Exogenous hormone intake	Decreased	None	Nontender
Struma ovarii; metastatic thyroid cancer	Extraglandular production	Decreased	None	Nontender

*In most cases.
(Reproduced with permission from Reid JR, Wheeler SF. Hyperthyroidism: diagnosis and treatment. *Am Fam Physician.* 2005;72:623–630.)

2. A **diagnostic approach** to patients who present with signs and symptoms of hyperthyroidism is summarized in Figure 87–1. A suppressed sTSH and an elevated free T_4 level are diagnostic of hyperthyroidism. In a clinically hyperthyroid patient with a suppressed sTSH and a normal free T_4 level, T_3 or free T_3 should be measured to evaluate for possible T_3 thyrotoxicosis.

3. **Radioactive iodine (^{123}I) uptake** can help clarify hyperthyroidism of uncertain origin. Diffused increase in ^{123}I uptake is consistent with Graves' disease, whereas nodular concentration indicates toxic adenoma or multinodular goiter. If ^{123}I uptake is decreased, a serum **thyroglobulin** measurement can distinguish between exogenous (factitious) hyperthyroxinemia (thyroglobulin decreased) and thyroiditis, iodine-induced thyrotoxicosis, or extraglandular production of thyroid hormone (thyroglobulin increased).

C. Treatment

1. **Antithyroid drugs (ATDs)** are the preferred first-line treatment for Graves' disease in Europe, Japan, and Australia. Methimazole and propylthiouracil (PTU), the two agents available in the United States, work by inhibiting thyroid hormone synthesis. PTU also inhibits peripheral conversion of T_4 to T_3. ATDs suppress thyroid autoantibodies, decrease TS Ab, and lead to remission in up to 60% of patients with Graves' disease treated for 2 years. The addition of levothyroxine to ATD therapy has not been shown to improve remission rates.

a. Methimazole is the drug of choice in nonpregnant patients because of its lower cost, longer half-life, and lower incidence of hematologic side effects. The usual starting doses are 15 to 30 mg/d for methimazole. PTU is the preferred treatment for pregnant patients since methimazole has been associated with a rare congenital anomaly. The starting dosage is 100 mg 3 times daily. If there is no decrease in free T_4 in 4 to 8 weeks, the dose should be increased. Doses as high as 60 to 90 mg/d of methimazole and 300 mg 3 or 4 times daily of PTU may be required to

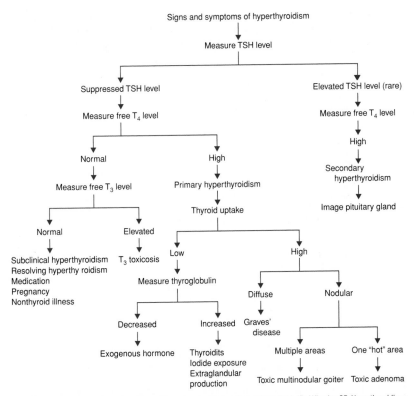

Signs and symptoms of hyperthyroidism

Measure TSH level

Suppressed TSH level

Measure free T$_4$ level

- **Normal**

  Measure free T$_3$ level

  - **Normal**

    Subclinical hyperthyroidism
    Resolving hyperthyroidism
    Medication
    Pregnancy
    Nonthyroid illness

  - **Elevated**

    T$_3$ toxicosis

- **High**

  Primary hyperthyroidism

  Thyroid uptake

  - **Low**

    Measure thyroglobulin

    - **Decreased**

      Exogenous hormone

    - **Increased**

      Thyroidits
      Iodide exposure
      Extraglandular
      production

  - **High**

    - **Diffuse**

      Graves' disease

    - **Nodular**

      - Multiple areas

        Toxic multinodular goiter

      - One "hot" area

        Toxic adenoma

Elevated TSH level (rare)

Measure free T$_4$ level

High

Secondary hyperthyroidism

Image pituitary gland

FIGURE 87–1. Diagnosing hyperthyroidism. (Reproduced with permission from Reid JR, Wheeler SF. Hyperthyroidism: diagnosis and treatment. *Am Fam Physician.* 2005;72:623–630.)

normalize thyroid function. TSH may remain suppressed for several months after thyroid hormone levels normalize.

b. Once euthyroidism is achieved (usually within 6–8 weeks), the dose can be titrated down to maintain euthyroidism. Typical maintenance doses are 100 to 200 mg PTU or 5 to 10 mg methimazole daily.

c. Most clinicians treat patients for 12 to 24 months before attempting to withdraw antithyroid therapy. Before discontinuing therapy, the patient should be clinically and biochemically euthyroid and have an undetectable TS Ab level. Relapse can occur in up to 50% of patients and is more likely to occur in smokers, patients with large goiters, and patients with persistently elevated TS Ab levels. Relapse is more likely in the first 3 to 6 months after ATD discontinuation. (SOR **A**)

d. Major side effects of ATDs include polyarthritis (1%–2%) and agranulocytosis (0.1%–0.5%). Agranulocytosis usually occurs within 3 months of starting therapy. PTU has a higher dose-related risk of this reaction, and it is very rare with methimazole doses less than 30 mg daily. Patients should be warned to discontinue the drug if they experience a sudden fever or sore throat. Routine monitoring of leukocyte counts is controversial, but may be beneficial in the early detection of agranulocytosis. Other adverse reactions associated with ATDs include rash, fever, arthralgias, and hepatic abnormalities, but these generally occur in less than 5% of patients and do not result in discontinuation of therapy.

2. **Radioactive iodine (RAI, ^{131}I),** usually administered orally, concentrates in the thyroid gland, where it destroys follicular cells. It is the treatment of choice for Graves' disease in the United States, as well as for multinodular goiter, toxic nodules in patients older than 40 years, and relapses from ATDs.

   a. An ablative RAI dose, rather than a lower gland-specific dosage, is recommended, especially in elderly or cardiac patients, and results in permanent remission in approximately 80% of patients. If symptomatic hyperthyroidism persists 3 to 6 months after therapy, a second ^{131}I treatment may be given. (SOR **A**)
   b. RAI exerts its full effect over a 2- to 6-month period. Follow-up at 4- to 6-week intervals to measure free T_4 and assess clinical response is appropriate until thyroid function stabilizes within the normal range or hypothyroidism ensues.
   c. Permanent hypothyroidism occurs in 82% of patients at 25 years regardless of the RAI dosage used. Hypothyroidism occurs earlier with higher-dose therapy, allowing for prompt diagnosis and treatment during frequent follow-up visits. Hypothyroidism is less likely in patients with toxic nodules or multinodular goiter since the rest of the gland may start to function normally after treatment. Thyroid replacement therapy should be initiated as the free T_4 and sTSH pass from normal into the hypothyroid range.
   d. RAI is contraindicated during pregnancy, and it is usually advised that pregnancy should be postponed 6 to 12 months following therapy. Otherwise, there are no contraindications to the use of RAI in women of child-bearing age, since it has not been shown to cause cancer, infertility, or to produce ill effects in subsequent children of those so treated. Breastfeeding women should avoid RAI because it appears in breast milk. The use of RAI in children is controversial, but is becoming more accepted as data emerges about its long-term safety.
 3. Surgery for hyperthyroidism has declined in popularity because of the effectiveness of ATDs and RAI. Subtotal thyroidectomy is the usual procedure performed.
   a. Specific indications include patients unwilling or unable to take ATDs or to be treated with ^{131}I, as well as those with neck obstruction, large goiters that may be relatively resistant to ^{131}I, or cosmetic concerns. Total thyroidectomy may be indicated for patients with severe disease or very large goiters.
   b. Patients should be rendered euthyroid with ATDs and/or iodides preoperatively to avoid thyrotoxic crisis.
   c. Complications include temporary or permanent hypoparathyroidism and/or recurrent laryngeal nerve paralysis. The mortality rate for elective surgery is close to 0% with experienced surgeons, and the rate of complications is reported to be 3%.
   d. Recurrent hyperthyroidism occurs in 8% of patients who are treated surgically. Permanent hypothyroidism occurs in 25% of patients undergoing subtotal thyroidectomy. Total thyroidectomy is 100% effective, but carries a 100% risk of permanent hypothyroidism. (SOR **A**)
 4. Adjunctive medical therapies are useful for relieving symptoms in patients undergoing definitive therapy with other agents or in those with transient forms of hyperthyroidism.
   a. **β-adrenergic antagonists** provide prompt symptomatic relief of the hyperadrenergic manifestations of hyperthyroidism. Propranolol is the most widely used beta-blocker for this purpose. Initial doses of 10 to 20 mg 4 times daily are adjusted to control tachycardia and symptoms. In most cases, a dose of 80 to 320 mg/d is sufficient.
   b. **Calcium channel blockers** such as diltiazem or verapamil may be used in patients who cannot tolerate, or have contraindications to, beta-blockers.
D. Choice of therapy
 1. Graves' disease
   a. RAI is the treatment of choice for most elderly patients.
   b. For children and adolescents, ATDs have commonly been recommended for initial therapy, with surgery or RAI reserved for patients who either fail ATD therapy or experience complications. However, the high-failure rate of ATDs and the efficacy and apparent safety of RAI have prompted increasing use of RAI in this age group.
   c. The treatment of young adults is also controversial. Specific patient characteristics, along with the risks and benefits of each treatment, should be considered. In young women with this condition who are anticipating pregnancy, RAI is often preferred to obviate future concern about ATDs causing fetal goiter or hypothyroidism.
   d. RAI therapy may exacerbate **ophthalmopathy** in 15% of patients with Graves' disease, especially smokers. This exacerbation can be prevented or improved in

two-thirds of patients by prednisone (40–80 mg/d, with the dose tapered to 0 over a period of 3 months). Although it is controversial, some physicians substitute ATDs or lower-dose RAI to treat patients with active eye disease, since posttreatment hypothyroidism has been associated with worsening Graves' ophthalmopathy. Aggressive treatment with high-dose glucocorticoids, in consultation with an ophthalmologist experienced in the treatment of orbital disease, can also be considered for progressive and severe ophthalmopathy.

2. Toxic multinodular goiter. There are no spontaneous remissions of hyperthyroidism resulting from nodular thyroid disease. RAI is usually the treatment of choice. Surgery may be appropriate for very large goiters, if there is concern about thyroid cancer, or in children, adolescents, or young adults. ATDs are valuable as pretreatment before thyroid surgery and before or after RAI in elderly patients and those with concurrent health problems.

3. Toxic adenoma. RAI is usually the treatment of choice. Surgical removal may be appropriate in patients younger than 40 years.

4. Thyroiditis (subacute, lymphocytic, and postpartum) may produce a transient hyperthyroidism that usually resolves within 8 months. Treatment focuses on symptom control with beta-blockers and other adjunctive medical therapies such as nonsteroidal anti-inflammatory drugs. Severe symptoms respond to prednisone, 20 to 40 mg/d. Transient hypothyroidism may follow the initial hyperthyroid phase and may be symptomatic enough to warrant levothyroxine therapy.

E. Subclinical hyperthyroidism

1. Introduction. Subclinical hyperthyroidism is distinguished by a low or undetectable sTSH (<0.45 mIU/L) and normal free T_4 and free T_3 in an asymptomatic person.

a. Subclinical hyperthyroidism is much less common than subclinical hypothyroidism. Excluding patients receiving thyroid hormone therapy, the prevalence is 2% and is more common in women, the elderly, and in patients with low-iodine intake.

b. Excessive thyroid hormone replacement is the most common cause (14%–21%). Other important causes include nodular thyroid disease, subclinical Graves' disease, thyroiditis, and ingestion of iodine-containing drugs such as amiodarone. A radioiodine scan can be useful in determining the etiology.

c. Factors that can suppress sTSH levels, such as severe illness, high-dose glucocorticoids, dopamine, and pituitary dysfunction, should be excluded.

d. Laboratory findings consistent with subclinical hyperthyroidism can be a normal variant in the elderly.

2. Clinical course. Subclinical hyperthyroidism often disappears, and progression to overt hyperthyroidism is uncommon in patients with a sTSH between 0.1 and 0.45 mIU/L. However, in patients with a sTSH lower than 0.1 mIU/L, the risk of developing overt hyperthyroidism is 1% to 2% per year. The condition has been associated with atrial fibrillation and other cardiac abnormalities and with increased cardiac mortality in patients older than 60 years. The incidence of atrial fibrillation is increased by threefold in patients with sTSH <0.1 mIU/L. Bone density is also decreased with prolonged subclinical hyperthyroidism but no link to increased fractures has been demonstrated.

3. Treatment

a. If excessive hormone replacement is the cause, the dose should be reduced.

b. If subclinical hyperthyroidism is associated with nodular thyroid disease, subclinical Graves' disease, heart disease, osteoporosis, or is found in patients older than 60 years, antithyroid treatment should be seriously considered. (SOR **G**)

c. In patients not meeting the above criteria, careful follow-up is acceptable.

IV. Thyroid Nodules

A. Introduction

1. Palpable nodules are present in 3% to 7% of adults in North America. However, physical examination is relatively insensitive, and, with the increase in the use of ultrasonography over the past 20 years, thyroid nodules are now estimated to occur in 20% to 76% of the general population. In addition, many patients with solitary nodules on examination are found to have multiple nodules on ultrasound. Approximately 5% of all thyroid nodules are carcinomas.

2. Thyroid nodules are found more commonly in the elderly, in women, and in patients with iodine deficiency or exposure to radiation. Prior radiation exposure increases the rate of development of both benign and malignant new nodules to approximately 2% per year. Peak incidence is 15 to 25 years after exposure.

     3. Since similar frequencies of cancer have been found in patients who have solitary or multiple nodules on palpation, dominant nodules in multinodular glands should also be considered for diagnostic evaluation.

B. Thyroid cancer risk factors

     1. Family history of benign or malignant thyroid disease, especially familial medullary thyroid carcinoma and multiple endocrine neoplasia 2.

     2. Personal history of prior head and neck radiation exposure. Childhood exposures increase thyroid cancer risk 10-fold.

     3. Physical findings suggestive of cancer are progressive or rapid growth, firmness, fixation to surrounding structures, local lymphadenopathy, and persistent hoarseness, dysphonia, dysphagia, or dyspnea.

     4. Other risk factors include age younger than 20 years or older than 70 years and male gender.

C. Diagnostic and management strategies

     1. A thorough **history** and **physical examination** should focus on thyroid cancer risk factors.

     2. High-resolution ultrasound with **Doppler capability** should be performed in all patients with thyroid cancer risk factors, regardless of physical examination. Ultrasound

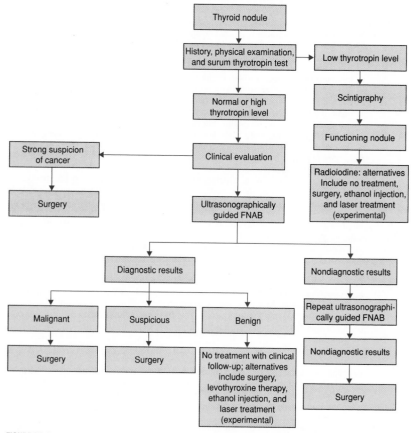

FIGURE 87–2. Flowchart indicating scheme for the diagnosis and management of palpable thyroid nodules. (Reproduced with permission from Hegedus L. The thyroid nodule. *N Engl J Med.* 2004;351(17):1764-1771. Copyright © Massachusetts Medical Society. All rights reserved.)

should also be part of the work-up of all palpable thyroid nodules or multinodular goiter. Ultrasound and color-flow Doppler criteria such as margins, shape, vascularity, content, and echogenicity are used to stratify the malignant potential of a nodule. (SOR **C**)

3. Serum **sTSH** identifies patients with unsuspected thyroid dysfunction. If the sTSH is normal, no further laboratory testing is warranted. An elevated sTSH should prompt testing of free thyroxine levels and antithyroperoxidase antibodies to rule out hypothyroidism. Decreased sTSH levels should be followed by testing of free thyroxine and triiodothyronine levels to rule out hyperthyroidism. Basal serum calcitonin is indicated only if there is a family history of medullary thyroid cancer or multiple endocrine neoplasia 2.

4. **Fine needle aspiration (FNA) biopsy** plays an integral role in the evaluation of thyroid nodules. Ultrasound-guided FNA (US-FNA) is more accurate than direct FNA and is recommended for all nodules in patients with a high-risk history or at least two suspicious ultrasound findings. (SOR **B**) Biopsy specimens should be interpreted by an experienced cytopathologist.

5. **Cytologic diagnosis** should be specified as inadequate, benign, suspicious, or malignant. US-FNA should be repeated after an inadequate sample is obtained. Suspicious, malignant, or repeatedly nondiagnostic specimens are an indication for surgery. Cytologically benign nodules should be followed clinically every 6 to 12 months. (SOR **C**)

6. An algorithm for the evaluation and management of nodular thyroid disease is displayed in Figure 87–2.

7. **Thyroid hormone suppression** is not recommended in most cases of nodular thyroid disease. It may be considered in iodine deficient patients, young patients with small nodules, or nodular goiters with no evidence of functional autonomy. However, clinically significant reduction in nodule volume with suppressive therapy is rare and the risks of prolonged subclinical hyperthyroidism must be included in the risk-benefit analysis. (SOR **C**)

REFERENCES

American Association of Clinical Endocrinologists (AACE) Thyroid Task Force. AACE medical guidelines for clinical practice for the evaluation and treatment of hyperthyroidism and hypothyroidism. *Endocr Pract.* 2002;8(6):457-469.

American Association of Clinical Endocrinologists (AACE) and Associazione Medici Endocrinologi (AME) Task Force on Thyroid Nodules. AACE/AME medical guidelines for the diagnosis and management of thyroid nodules. *Endocr Pract.* 2006;12:63-102.

Gharib H, Tuttle M, Baskin HJ, et al. Subclinical thyroid dysfunction: a joint statement on management from the American Association of Clinical Endocrinologists, the American Thyroid Association, and the Endocrine Society. *Endocr Pract.* 2004;10:497.

Reid JR, Wheeler SF. Hyperthyroidism: diagnosis and treatment. *Am Fam Physician.* 2005;72(4): 623-630.

Roberts CG, Ladenson PW. Hypothyroidism. *Lancet.* 2004;363:793.

Surks MI, Ortiz E, Daniels GH, et al. Subclinical thyroid disease: scientific review and guidelines for diagnosis and management. *JAMA.* 2004;291:228-238.

SECTION III. Psychiatric Disorders

88   Alcohol & Drug Abuse

Robert Mallin, MD, & D. Todd Detar, DO

KEY POINTS

- The diagnosis of substance use disorders is most typically begun with a screening test that identifies a user at risk. The CAGE questionnaire (Table 88–1) is perhaps the most widely used screening tool for the identification of patients at risk for substance use disorders. When answering yes to two or more questions on the CAGE, the sensitivity is 60% to 90% and the specificity 40% to 60% for substance use disorders. (SOR **Ⓐ**) Because a screening test is more predictive when applied to a population more likely to have a disease, clinical clues (Table 88–2) to substance use disorders may be useful to determine whom to screen. Once the patient screens positive for a substance use problem, the question becomes: Is it abuse or dependence?

- Substance abuse is a pattern of misuse during which the patient maintains control, whereas in substance dependence, control over use is lost. Physiologic dependence, evidenced by a withdrawal syndrome, may exist in either state (see Tables 88–3 and 88–4 for the diagnostic criteria for substance abuse and dependence). The primary means by which the diagnosis of substance abuse or dependence is made, then, is a careful history. Although substance-disordered patients may be consciously less truthful in their history, more often the defense mechanism of denial is what prevents the patient from seeing the connection between substance use and consequences.

- Biochemical markers may help support the diagnostic criteria gathered in the history, or can be used as a screening mechanism to consider patients for further evaluation (Table 88–5).

- There is a strong relationship between the time and intensity spent in alcohol and drug treatment and success at remaining abstinent.

- The prognosis for professionals who participate in a monitoring program after treatment is better than nonprofessionals. (SOR **Ⓑ**)

I. Introduction

A. The prevalence of alcohol and drug disorders in primary care outpatients is between 23% and 37%. The high prevalence of these disorders in primary care outpatients suggests that family physicians are confronted with these problems daily. These disorders rarely present overtly, however. Patients in denial about the connection between their substance use and the consequences caused by it frequently minimize the amount of their use and often do not seek assistance for their substance problem.

B. The epidemiology of alcohol and drug disorders has been well studied and is most often reported from data of the National Institute of Mental Health Epidemiologic Catchment Area Program (ECA). Lifetime prevalence rates for alcohol disorders from the ECA survey data were 13.5%. For men, the lifetime prevalence was found to be 23.8%, and for women, 4.7%. The National Comorbidity Survey revealed lifetime prevalence of alcohol abuse without dependence to be 12.5% for males and 6.4% for females. For alcohol

---

TABLE 88–1. CAGE QUESTIONS ADAPTED TO INCLUDE DRUGS

1. Have you felt you ought to **C**ut down on your drinking or drug use?
2. Have people **A**nnoyed you by criticizing your drinking or drug use?
3. Have you felt **G**uilty about your drinking or drug use?
4. Have you ever had a drink, or used drugs first thing in the morning to steady your nerves or to get rid of a hangover or to get the day started? (**E**ye-opener)

Two or more yes answers indicate a need for a more in-depth assessment. Even one positive response should raise a red flag about problem drinking or drug use.
(Data adapted from Schulz JE, Parran T, Jr. Principles of identification and intervention. In: Graham AW, Shultz TK, eds. *Principles of Addiction Medicine*. 2nd ed. Chery Chase, MD: American Society of Addiction Medicine; 1998:249.)

TABLE 88-2. CLINICAL CLUES TO ALCOHOL AND DRUG PROBLEMS

Social History	Medical History
Arrest for driving under the influence	History of addiction to any drug
Loss of job or sent home from work for alcohol or drug reasons	Withdrawal syndrome
	Depression
Domestic violence	Anxiety disorder
Child abuse/neglect	Recurrent pancreatitis
Family instability (divorce, separation)	Recurrent hepatitis
Frequent, unplanned absences	Hepatomegaly
Personal isolation	Peripheral neuropathy
Problems at work/school	Myocardial infarction <age 30 (cocaine)
Mood swings	Blood alcohol level >300 or >100 without impairment
	Alcohol on breath or intoxicated at office visit
	Tremor
	Mild hypertension
	Estrogen mediated signs (telangiectasias, spider angiomas, palmer erythema, muscle atrophy)
	Gastrointestinal complaints
	Sleep disturbances
	Eating disorders
	Sexual dysfunction

TABLE 88-3. DSM-IV CRITERIA FOR SUBSTANCE ABUSE

A maladaptive pattern of substance use, leading to clinically significant impairment or distress, as manifested by one (or more) of the following occurring at any time within a 12-month period:

1. Recurrent substance use resulting in failure to fulfill major role obligations at work, school, or home (e.g., repeated absences or poor work performance related to substance use; substance-related absences, suspensions, or expulsions from school; neglect of children or household).
2. Recurrent substance use in situations in which it is physically hazardous (e.g., driving an automobile or operating a machine when impaired by substance use).
3. Recurrent substance-related legal problems (e.g., arrests for substance-related disorderly conduct).
4. Continued substance use despite having persistent social or interpersonal problems caused or exacerbated by the effects of the substance (e.g., arguments with spouse about consequences of intoxication, physical fights).

The symptoms have never met the criteria for Substance Dependence for this class of substance. (Modified with permission from American Psychiatric Association *Diagnostic and Statistical Manual of Mental Disorders IV.* American Psychiatric Press; 1994:182.)

TABLE 88-4. DSM-IV CRITERIA FOR SUBSTANCE DEPENDENCE

A maladaptive pattern of substance use, leading to clinically significant impairment or distress, as manifested by three (or more) of the following occurring at any time in the same 12-month period:

1. Tolerance as defined by either of the following:
   a. A need for markedly increased amounts of the substance to achieve intoxication or the desired effect.
   b. Markedly diminished effect with continued use of the same amount of the substance.
2. Withdrawal, as manifested by either of the following:
   a. The characteristic withdrawal syndrome for the substance.
   b. The same (or closely related) substance is taken to relieve or avoid withdrawal symptoms.
3. The substance is often taken in larger amounts or over a longer period than was intended.
4. There is a persistent desire or unsuccessful efforts to cut down or control substance use.
5. A great deal of time is spent in activities necessary to obtain the substance, use the substance, or recover from its effects.
6. Important social, occupational, or recreational activities are given up or reduced because of the substance use.
7. The substance use is continued despite knowledge of having a persistent or recurrent physical or psychological problem that is likely to have been caused or exacerbated by the substance.

(Modified with permission from American Psychiatric Association *Diagnostic and Statistical Manual of Mental Disorders IV.* American Psychiatric Press; 1994:181.)

TABLE 88–5. **BIOCHEMICAL MARKERS OF SUBSTANCE USE DISORDERS**

Marker	Substance	Sensitivity (%)	Specificity (%)	Predictive Value (%)
Mean corpuscular volume (MCV)	Alcohol	24	96	63
γ-Glutamyl transferase (GGT)	Alcohol	42	76	61
Carbohydrate-deficient transferrin (CDT)	Alcohol	67	97	84

dependence, males' lifetime prevalence as 20.1% and females' 8.2%. The ECA data yield an overall prevalence of drug use disorders to be 6.2%. As with alcohol use disorders, drug use disorders occur more frequently in men (lifetime prevalence 7.7%) than in women (4.8%). Characteristics known to influence the epidemiology of substance use disorders include gender, age, family history, marital status, employment status, and occupation/educational status. Males have a higher risk than females, substance use disorders become less frequent with age, the risk of alcoholism for the child of an alcoholic is approximately 50%, single persons have a higher risk than married, and the unemployed and less educated have a higher risk.

C. The difference between abuse and dependence is an important one. With substance abuse, the patient retains control of their use. This control may be affected by poor judgment and social and environmental factors and mitigated by the consequences of their use. When patients become dependent (addicted), they no longer have full control of their drug use. The brain has been "hijacked by a substance that affects the mechanism of control over the use of that substance." This addiction is far more than physical dependence. The need to use the drug becomes as powerful as the drives of thirst and hunger. The evidence that the brains of addicted individuals are different from those of nonaddicted persons is enormous. Many of these abnormalities predate the use of the substance and are thought to be inherited. In genetically predisposed individuals, substances of abuse cause changes in the dopaminergic mesolimbic system that result in a loss of control over substance use. These changes are mediated by a number of neurotransmitters: dopamine, γ-aminobutyric-acid (GABA), glutamate, serotonin, and endorphins. The different classes of substances of abuse act through one or more of these neurotransmitters, ultimately affecting the level of dopamine in the mesolimbic system, otherwise known as the reward pathway. These changes in the brain are permanent and are the primary reason for relapse in the addicted patient trying to maintain abstinence, or control of use.

II. Diagnosis
  A. **Differential diagnosis.** Because substance abuse is a behavioral disorder, when one thinks of a differential diagnosis, psychiatric disorders often come to mind. There is a high comorbidity of substance use disorders with psychiatric disorders. Patients with psychiatric disorders have a high rate of substance abuse. Approximately 50% of psychiatric patients have a substance use disorder. (SOR **Ⓐ**) When one looks at patients with addictions, however, the rates of psychiatric disorders are similar to those in the general population. Problems, such as substance-induced mood disorders (frequently noted in alcohol, opiate, and stimulant abuse) and substance-induced psychotic disorders (most frequently associated with stimulant abuse), complicate differentiating the primary psychiatric disorders from those that are primarily substance use disorders. Most clinicians agree that psychiatric disorders cannot be reliably assessed for patients who are currently or recently intoxicated. Thus, detoxification and a period of abstinence are necessary before evaluation for other psychiatric disorders may effectively be done. (SOR **Ⓑ**)
  B. **Symptoms and signs.** The symptoms and the signs of substance abuse are varied and often subtle. Most patients do not recognize their substance use as the cause of their problems and are often quite resistant to that interpretation. Signs, such as those described in Table 88–2 as potential clues to substance abuse, should lead the clinician to obtain a full substance use history (Table 88–6) from the patient. While physical dependence is not always seen with substance abuse, its presence suggests abuse unless the patient is on long-term, prescribed addictive medicines.
  C. **Symptoms and signs of withdrawal.** In dealing with sedative hypnotic, alcohol, or opiate withdrawal, assessment of the degree of withdrawal is important to determine appropriate use and dose of medication to both reduce symptoms and, in the case of sedative hypnotic drugs including alcohol, prevent seizure and mortality. The Clinical Institute Withdrawal

TABLE 88-6. ELEMENTS OF THE SUBSTANCE USE HISTORY

1. Determine the type, frequency, route of administration, and amount of substance use
   a. Alcohol
   b. Tobacco
   c. Other drugs
      i. Cocaine
      ii. Marijuana
      iii. Others
2. Determine consequences of substance use; ask about
   a. Legal problems
      i. Arrests (driving under the influence, public intoxication, disorderly conduct, etc.)
      ii. Civil suits for financial problems, bankruptcy, etc.
   b. Social problems
      i. Social isolation
   c. Family problems
      i. Marital problems
      ii. Parenting problems
      iii. Domestic violence
      iv. Family members with depression
      v. Divorce
   d. Work or school problems
      i. Frequent absences
      ii. Poor performance
      iii. Frequent job changes
   e. Financial problems
      i. Significant debt
      ii. Selling personal possessions
      iii. Stealing and selling possessions of others
   f. Psychological problems
      i. Agitation
      ii. Irritability
      iii. Anxiety
      iv. Panic attacks
      v. Mood swings
      vi. Hostility
      vii. Violence
      viii. Sleep disturbance
      xi. Sexual dysfunction
      x. Depression
      xi. Blackouts
   g. Medical problems
      i. Gastritis
      ii. Peptic ulcer
      iii. Abdominal pain
      iv. Hypertension
      v. Peripheral neuropathy
      vi. Nasal septum perforation
      vii. Vasospasm
      viii. Dysrhythmias
      xi. Weight loss
      x. HIV
      xi. Skin abscesses
      xii. Trauma

Assessment Scale (Table 88–7) allows quantification of the symptoms and signs of withdrawal in a predictable fashion that allows clinicians to discuss the severity of withdrawal for a given patient and thus choose intervention strategies that are effective and safe. (SOR **Ⓐ**)

D. Laboratory tests
   1. **γ-Glutamyl transferase (GGT).** GGT is an enzyme produced in the liver and induced by heavy alcohol consumption. In addition, damage to the hepatic cells during chronic heavy alcohol consumption results in leakage of GGT into the serum. It has a sensitivity that is higher than mean corpuscular volume, but its specificity remains low secondary

TABLE 88–7. CLINICAL INSTITUTE WITHDRAWAL ASSESSMENT SCALE

Patient _____ Date _____ Time _____ BP ___/___
Age _____ Race/Sex _____ Drugs of choice (Primary) _____ Other _____

1. Autonomic hyperactivity
   Pulse rate/minute
   0   <80
   1   81–100
   2   101–110
   3   111–120
   4   121–130
   5   131–140
   6   141–150
   7   >150

      Sweating (observation)
   0   No sweating
   1   Barely perceptible sweating, palms moist
   2
   3
   4   Beads of sweat obvious on forehead
   5
   6
   7   Drenching sweats

2. Hand tremor: arms extended and fingers spread apart:
      Observation
   0   No tremor
   1   Not visible
   2
   3
   4   Moderate with patients arms extended
   5
   6
   7   Severe, even with arms not extended

3. Anxiety: Ask, "Do you feel nervous or anxious?"
      Observation
   0   No anxiety, at ease
   1   Mildly anxious
   2
   3
   4   Moderately anxious
   5
   6
   7   Severe equivalent to panic
   Total Score ___ Max Score = 56
   Rater's initials ___

4. Transient tactile auditory or visual disturbances: Ask, "Have you any itching, pins and needle sensations, any burning or numbness, or do you feel bugs crawling on or under your skin" Are you more aware of sounds around you and are they harsh? Are you hearing things that you know are not there? Does the light appear too bright? Does it hurt your eyes? Are you seeing anything that is disturbing to you?"
      Observation
   0   Not present
   1   Present but minimal
   2
   3   Moderate
   4   Frequent
   5
   6
   7   Hallucinations almost continuous

5. Agitation:
      Observation
   0   Normal activity
   1   Somewhat more than normal activity
   2
   3
   4   Moderately fidgety and restless
   5
   6
   7   Paces back and forth during most of the interview, or constantly thrashes about

6. Nausea or vomiting: Ask, "Do you feel sick to your stomach or have you vomited?" Include recorded vomiting since last observation
      Observation
   0   Not present
   1   Very mild
   2
   3
   4   Moderate
   5
   6
   7   Severe

7. Headache: Ask, "Does your head feel full? Does it feel like there is a band around your head?" Don't rate for lightheadedness.
      Otherwise rate severity
   0   Not present
   1   Very mild
   2
   3
   4   Moderate
   5
   6
   7   Severe

to nonalcoholic liver disease, diabetes, pancreatitis, hyperthyroidism, heart failure, and anticonvulsant and anticoagulant use, all of which may cause it to be elevated. (SOR **Ⓐ**)

2. Other liver functions that may be elevated during heavy alcohol consumption include aspartate aminotransferase (AST) and alanine aminotransferase (ALT). These markers are also elevated as the result of hepatic cellular damage caused by heavy alcohol consumption. Sensitivity of these markers is low, because there must be significant

liver damage before these markers rise. Specificity is compromised because non alcoholic liver disease also causes increases. Differences in the ratio of AST/ALT may help to distinguish between alcohol and non-alcohol-related liver disease. A ratio of >2 is highly suggestive of alcohol-related liver disease. (SOR **A**)

3. **Carbohydrate-deficient transferrin (CDT).** CDT has recently become available in clinical settings to screen for excessive alcohol consumption. Consumption of four to seven drinks daily for at least a week results in a decrease in the carbohydrate content of transferrin. Sensitivity and specificity of CDT is high with regard to differentiating heavy drinkers from those who drink very little or not at all. When used in larger, more heterogeneous populations, it appears less sensitive, and is less sensitive in females than in males. (SOR **A**)

Urine drug screening is a sensitive test for common substances of abuse. Knowledge of drug half-life and the importance of confirmation of positive tests by gas chromatography are essential for interpretation of results.

4. **Ethyl glucuronide testing of the urine (EtG).** EtG has recently become a popular test for detecting recent alcohol consumption. Unlike CDT, the presence of EtG in the urine only confirms that the patient has recently consumed alcohol, and says nothing about the level of the consumption. Consequently, its greatest usefulness is in the monitoring of those patients who are committed to abstinence from alcohol. (SOR **B**)

III. **Treatment.** Many substance use disorders resolve spontaneously, or with brief interventions on the part of physicians or other authority figures in the workplace, legal system, family, or society. This resolution occurs because the patient with a substance abuse disorder continues to maintain control over their use, and when the consequences of that use outweigh the benefits of the drug, they choose to quit. Patients with substance dependence disorders, on the other hand, have impaired control by definition. They rarely get better without assistance.

Substance use disorders can be treated successfully. Brief interventions and outpatient, inpatient, and residential treatment programs reduce morbidity and mortality associated with substance abuse and dependence. Detoxification, patient education, identification of defenses, overcoming denial, relapse prevention, orientation to 12-step recovery programs and family services are the goals of substance abuse treatment. (SOR **B**)

A. **Formal process.** The traditional intervention for alcohol or drug addiction is a formal process, best accomplished by an addictions specialist trained in this process. This approach is often effective, resulting in positive results in approximately 80% of cases. Although effective, the traditional, formal model of intervention is often less than ideal for the primary care provider. Specialist involvement and orchestration of significant relationships of the patient is sometimes difficult to achieve. In addition, if the intervention fails, the physician's relationship with the patient may become difficult if not impossible to continue.

B. **Brief interventions.** This highly effective approach to intervention is based on the work of Miller and Rollnick on motivational interviewing and Prochascka and DiClementi's work on stages of change. Presenting the diagnosis of a substance use disorder by itself may be viewed as a brief intervention. As many as 70% of patients are in the precontemplation or contemplation stage when presented with the diagnosis. The resistance associated with these stages tends to force the clinician into one of two modalities, that of avoiding the diagnosis, or confronting and arguing with the patient, generally both futile approaches. One approach in presenting the diagnosis is to use the SOAPE glossary (Table 88–8) for positive suggestions to use when talking to patients about their addiction.

Even when the patient is in the precontemplative stage at presentation of the diagnosis, continued use of the brief intervention strategy will ultimately reduce the amount of drug use if not result in abstinence. Brief interventions should include some of the elements of motivational interviewing. These elements include offering empathetic, objective feedback of data, meeting patient expectations, working with ambivalence, assessing barriers and strengths, reinterpreting past experience in light of current medical consequences, negotiating a follow-up plan, and providing hope.

C. **Detoxification.** Detoxification, treatment of withdrawal, and any medical complications must have first priority. Alcohol and other sedative hypnotic drugs share the same neurobiological withdrawal process. Chronic use of this class of drugs results in downregulation of the GABA receptors throughout the central nervous system (GABA is an inhibitory neurotransmitter). Abrupt cessation of sedative hypnotic drug use results in an upregulation of GABA receptors and a relative paucity of GABA for inhibition. The result is stimulation of the autonomic nervous system.

TABLE 88–8. SOAPE GLOSSARY FOR PRESENTING THE DIAGNOSIS

Support: Use phrases such as "We need to work together on this," "I am concerned about you and will follow-up closely with you," and "As with all medical illnesses, the more people you work with, the better you will feel." These words reinforce your physician–patient relationship, strengthen the collaborative model of chronic illness management, and help to convince the patient that the physician will not just present the diagnosis and leave.

Optimism: Most patients have controlled their alcohol or drug use at times and may have quit for periods of time. They may expect failure. By giving a strong optimistic message, such as "You can get well," "Treatment works," and "You can expect to see improvements in many areas of your life," the physician can motivate the patient.

Absolution: By describing addiction as a disease and telling the patients that they are not responsible for having an illness, but that now only they can take responsibility for their recovery, the physician can lessen the burden of guilt and shame that often is a barrier to recovery.

Plan: Having a plan is important to the acceptance of the illness. Using readiness to change categories can help you design a plan that takes the patient's willingness to move ahead. Indicating that abstinence is desirable, but recognizing that all patients will not be able to commit to that goal immediately, can help prevent a sense of failure early in the process. Ask "What do you think you will be able to do at this point?"

Explanatory model: Understanding your patient's beliefs about addiction may be important. Many patients believe this is a moral weakness and that they lack willpower. An explanation that willpower cannot resolve physical illnesses like diabetes mellitus, hypertension, or alcoholism may go a long way to reassure the patient that recovery is possible.

(Modified with permission from Clark WD: Alcoholism: Blocks to diagnosis and treatment. *Am J Med.* 1981;71:285.)

1. **Withdrawal seizures.** These are a common manifestation of sedative hypnotic withdrawal. They have been described to occur in 11% to 33% of patients withdrawing from alcohol. Alcohol withdrawal seizures are best treated with benzodiazepines and by addressing the withdrawal process. Lorazepam is a good choice because it can be given intravenously or intramuscularly, 2 to 4 mg every 1 to 4 hours as needed for seizure activity. Patients should be on a cardiac monitor and may need to be intubated to protect their airway if seizure activity is persistent. Long-term treatment for alcohol withdrawal seizures is not recommended, and phenytoin should not be used to treat seizures associated with alcohol withdrawal. (SOR **A**)

2. **Other withdrawal symptoms.** The cornerstones of treatment for alcohol withdrawal syndrome are the benzodiazepines. All drugs that provide cross-tolerance with alcohol are effective in reducing the symptoms and sequelae of alcohol withdrawal, but none has the safety profile and evidence of efficacy of the benzodiazepines (see Table 88–9 for recommendations in the treatment of alcohol withdrawal).

3. **Opiate withdrawal.** This may not be life-threatening, but the symptoms are significant enough that without supportive treatment most patients will not remain in treatment (see Table 88–10 for recommendations for the treatment of opiate withdrawal). The symptoms of cocaine and other stimulant withdrawal are somewhat less predictable and much harder to improve. Despite multiple studies with many different drug classes, no medications have been shown to reliably reduce the symptoms and craving associated with cocaine withdrawal.

TABLE 88–9. TREATMENT REGIMENS FOR ALCOHOL WITHDRAWAL

Using the Clinical Institute Withdrawal Assessment (CIWA) for monitoring

Do CIWA scale every 4 h until score is below 8 for 24 h

For CIWA >10

Give Chlordiazepoxide 50–100 mg

or   Diazepam 10–20 mg

or   Oxazepam 30–60 mg

or   Lorazepam 2–4 mg

Repeat CIWA 1 h after dose to assess need for further medication.

Non-symptom-driven regimens

For patients likely to experience withdrawal:

Chlordiazepoxide, 50 mg every 6 h for four doses, followed by 50 mg every 8 h for three doses, followed by 50 mg every 12 h for two doses, and finally by 50 mg at bedtime for one dose.

Other benzodiazepines may be substituted at equivalent doses.

Patients on a predetermined dosing schedule should be monitored frequently for breakthrough withdrawal symptoms as well as excessive sedation.

TABLE 88–10. TREATMENT FOR OPIOID WITHDRAWAL

Methadone: A pure opioid agonist restricted by federal legislation to inpatient treatment or specialized outpatient drug treatment programs. Methodone 15–20 mg for 2–3 d then tapered by 10% –15% reductions daily, guided by patient's symptoms and clinical findings.

Clonidine: An α-adrenergic blocker, 0.2 mg every 4 h to relieve symptoms of withdrawal, may be effective. Hypotension is a risk and sometimes limits the dose. It can be continued for 10–14 d and tapered by the third day by 0.2 mg/d.

Buprenorphine: This partial μ receptor agonist can be administered orally or sublingually, in doses of 2, 4, or, 8 mg every 4 h for the management of opioid withdrawal symptoms.

Naltrexone/clonidine: A rapid form of opioid detoxification involves pretreatment with 0.2–0.3 mg of clonidine followed by 12.5 mg of naltrexone (a pure opioid antagonist). Naltrexone is increased to 25 mg on the second day, 50 mg on day three, and 100 mg on day four, with clonidine given at 0.1–0.3 mg three times daily.

D. **Patient education.** Patient knowledge and understanding of the nature of substance use disorders is key to recovery. For patients still in control of their use, education about appropriate substance use will help them to choose responsibly if they continue to use. For patients who meet the criteria for substance dependence (addiction), abstinence is the only safe option. Once having made the transition to addiction, one can never use addictive substances reliably again. The neurobiologic changes in the brain are permanent, so loss of control may occur at any time when the brain is presented with an addictive substance. Unfortunately, this occurrence of loss of control can be unpredictable. Consequently, the addicted patients may find that they can use a drug (or alcohol) for a variable period of time with control. This sense of control gives them the false impression that they were never addicted, in the first place, or perhaps that they have been cured. Invariably if they continue to use addictive substances they will lose control of their use and begin to experience consequences at or above the level that they did before. Understanding addiction as a chronic disorder for which there is remission but not cure becomes essential. The question then becomes not if one should remain abstinent, but rather how one remains abstinent.

E. **Identification of defenses/overcoming denial.** During this phase of treatment, patients typically work in a group therapy setting and are encouraged to look at the defenses that have prevented them from seeking help sooner. Denial can best be defined as the inability to see the causal relationship between drug use and its consequences. Thus the patients who believe they drank because they lost their job may be encouraged to consider that they lost their job because they drank.

F. **Pharmacologic treatment of addiction**
1. These drugs attempt to have an impact on drug use by one of the several mechanisms: (1) sensitizing the body's response to result in a negative reaction to ingesting the drug, causing an aversion reaction, such as with disulfiram and alcohol; (2) reducing the reinforcing effects of a drug, such as the use of naltrexone, or acamprosate in alcoholism; (3) blocking the effects of a drug by binding to the receptor site, such as the use of naltrexone for opiates; (4) saturating the receptor sites by agonists, such as the use of methadone in opioid maintenance therapy; and (5) using unique approaches, such as the creation of an immunization to cocaine. Drug therapy for addiction holds promise. As our understanding of the neurobiology of addiction improves, so does the chance that we can intervene at a molecular level to prevent relapse. At the current level, however, pharmacotherapy to prevent relapse must be relegated to an adjunctive position. No drug alone has provided sufficient power to prevent relapse to addictive behavior. Still, in some patients the use of appropriate medication may give them the edge necessary to move closer to recovery.

2. Disulfiram is a drug that is not often initiated by family physicians but is frequently continued and monitored in the primary care setting. The usual dose of this medication is 250 to 500 mg every morning. It works as a deterrent to drinking alcohol. When a patient who is taking disulfiram ingests alcohol (in any form), a severe negative reaction occurs that is manifested by flushing, nausea, and vomiting. Disulfiram's record in achieving abstinence is mixed and is enhanced by taking the medication in an observed fashion. It must be avoided in patients who are hypersensitive to its use, those who have drunk alcohol in the past 12 hours, or those with psychosis or severe coronary artery disease. The cost is approximately $40/month, retail. (SOR **A**)

3. Naltrexone, an opiate antagonist, has been shown to be effective in reducing the craving to drink in alcoholics. At doses of 50 mg daily, this medication may reduce the patient's desire to drink. It is contraindicated with opiate use, liver failure,

or acute hepatitis. Its cost is considerable—$147.20/month. This medication is less effective when not accompanied by a comprehensive recovery program. (SOR Ⓑ)

4. Acamprosate, recently released and FDA approved for treatment of alcoholism, has been shown to be an effective medication for the reduction of the craving to drink alcohol. Currently, it is prescribed at 333 mg three times daily. It too is costly at $138.98/month, and is not effective in the absence of a comprehensive recovery program. (SOR Ⓑ)

IV. Management Strategies

A. Relapse prevention. Once patients are educated to the nature of their disease and have identified destructive defense mechanisms, relapse prevention becomes the primary goal. Identification of triggers for alcohol and drug use, plans to prevent opportunities to relapse, and new ways to deal with problems help patients to maintain their abstinence. In most treatment programs, a relapse prevention plan will be developed and individualized for each patient. The most effective way that the family physician can support relapse prevention is to be aware of the relapse prevention plan that the patient has developed in treatment and reinforce its application. For example, it is useful, when seeing the patients who are new to recovery, to ask them about their 12-step meeting attendance, sponsor contacts, and whether they have been able to remain abstinent since your last meeting. For patients who have not had the benefit of treatment, identification of triggers followed by cognitive strategies to avoid these triggers may enhance their recovery. These are usually relatively simple to create. For example, for patients who report that they drink after an argument with their spouse, consideration of alternative means of coping, such as calling a friend, exercising, or engaging in relaxation techniques, may be helpful. (SOR Ⓑ)

B. Orientation to 12-step recovery. Despite millions of dollars in research, and the efforts of a large segment of the scientific community, there has been no treatment, medication, or psychotherapy that has taken the place of the 12 steps of Alcoholics Anonymous (AA) (see Table 88–11).

Other important 12-step programs for patients with substance use disorders include Al-Anon, for friends and family of alcoholics; Narcotics Anonymous, for those with drug problems other than alcohol; and Cocaine Anonymous, for those with cocaine addiction.

At the heart of each of these fellowships is the program of recovery outlined in the 12 steps. AA and related 12-step programs are spiritual, not religious, in nature. No one is told they must believe in anything, including God. Agnostics and atheists are welcome in AA and are not asked to convert to any religious belief. Newcomers in AA are encouraged to go to meetings regularly (daily is wise initially), get a sponsor, and begin work on the 12 steps. A sponsor is someone of the same sex who is in stable recovery and has worked the steps. The sponsor helps guide the newcomer through the steps and provides a source of information and encouragement. At meetings members share their experience, strength, and hope around topics of their recovery. In this fashion, storytelling often becomes the means by which information about strategies for recovery is relayed. AA meetings vary in their composition and structure, given that one of the traditions of AA is that each group

---

TABLE 88–11. THE TWELVE STEPS OF ALCOHOLICS ANONYMOUS

We:

1. Admitted we were powerless over alcohol—that our lives had become unmanageable;
2. Came to believe that a Power greater than ourselves could restore us to sanity;
3. Made a decision to turn our will and our lives over to the care of God *as we understood Him;*
4. Made a searching and fearless moral inventory of ourselves;
5. Admitted to ourselves, and to another human being the exact nature of our wrongs;
6. Were entirely ready to have God remove all these defects of character;
7. Humbly asked Him to remove our shortcomings;
8. Made a list of all persons we had harmed, and became willing to make amends to them all;
9. Made direct amends to such people wherever possible, except when to do so would injure them or others;
10. Continued to take personal inventory and when we were wrong promptly admitted it;
11. Sought through prayer and meditation to improve our conscious contact with God *as we understand Him,* praying only for knowledge of His will for us and the power to carry that out;
12. Having had a spiritual awakening as the result of these steps, we tried to carry this message to alcoholics, and to practice these principles in all our affairs.

(From Alcoholics Anonymous World Service.)

is autonomous. Consequently, if a patient feels uncomfortable at one meeting, another may be more acceptable. There are meetings for women or men only, for young people, and for physicians or lawyers; virtually any special-interest group is represented in large cities. (SOR **B**)

There is often a great deal of confusion about what AA does and does not do. AA is not treatment. Despite the close connection many treatment programs have with 12-step recovery fellowships, these fellowships are not affiliated with treatment centers by design.

C. **Effectiveness of AA.** From multiple sources, it appears clear that AA and other 12-step recovery programs are among the most effective tools we have to combat substance disorders. Approximately 6% to 10% of the population has been to an AA meeting during their lives. This number doubles for those with alcohol problems. Although, one-half of those who come to AA leave; of those who stay for a year, 67% stay sober; of those who stay for 2 years, 85% stay sober; and of those who stay sober for 5 years, 90% remain sober indefinitely. Outcome studies of 8087 patients treated in 57 different inpatient and outpatient treatment programs showed that those attending AA at 1 year were 50% more likely to be abstinent than those not attending. Adolescents studied were found to be

TABLE 88–12. **MEDICAL COMPLICATIONS OF SUBSTANCE ABUSE**

Drug	Medical Complication
Alcohol	Trauma
	Hypertension
	Cardiomyopathy
	Dysrhythmias
	Ischemic heart disease
	Hemorrhagic stroke
	Esophageal reflux
	Barrett's esophagus
	Mallory–Weiss tears
	Esophageal cancer
	Acute gastritis
	Pancreatitis
	Chronic diarrhea malabsorption
	Alcoholic hepatitis
	Cirrhosis
	Hepatic failure
	Hepatic carcinoma
	Nasopharyngeal cancer
	Headache
	Sleep disorders
	Memory impairment
	Dementia
	Peripheral neuropathy
	Fetal alcohol syndrome
	Sexual dysfunction
	Substance-induced mood disorders
	Substance-induced psychotic disorders
	Immune dysfunction
Cocaine (other stimulants)	Chest pain
	Congestive heart failure
	Cardiac dysrhythmias
	Cardiovascular collapse
	Seizures
	Cerebrovascular accidents
	Headache
	Spontaneous pneumothorax
	Noncardiogenic pulmonary edema
	Nasal septal perforations
Injection drug use	Hepatitis C, B
	HIV infection
	Subacute endocarditis
	Soft tissue abscesses

four times more likely to be abstinent if they attended Alcoholics Anonymous/Narcotics Anonymous, when compared to those who did not. Finally, in an effort to identify what groups in AA did better than others, studies of involvement in AA (defined as service work, having a sponsor, leading meetings, etc.) found that those who were involved, as compared to those just attending meetings, did better in maintaining abstinence.

D. Contacts. Having a list of AA members willing to escort potential new members to meetings is a powerful tool for physicians to help patients into recovery. Generally in every AA district, there is a person identified as the chair of the Cooperation with Professional Community Committee who can help physicians identify people willing to perform this service. Al-Anon and Narcotics Anonymous have similar contacts. The telephone numbers for most of these 12-step groups can be found in the phone book. These contacts can often supply the physician with relevant literature to help dispel some of the myths patients may hold regarding 12-step recovery. Patients will often use these myths as excuses for why AA will not work for them.

V. Prognosis. Alcohol causes approximately 100,000 deaths yearly and is associated with motor vehicle accidents, other accidents, homicides, cirrhosis of the liver, and suicide. Injection drug use is responsible for the fastest-growing population of human immunodeficiency virus infection. See Table 88–12 for common medical complications from substance abuse.

REFERENCES

Enoch MA, Goldman D. Problem drinking and alcoholism: Diagnosis and treatment. *Am Fam Physician.* 2002;65(3):441-448. [Summary in Am Fam Physician 2002;65(3):449-450; PMID: 11858628].

USPTF. Screening and behavioral counseling interventions in primary care to reduce alcohol misuse: Recommendation statement. *Ann Intern Med.* 2004;140:554-556.

Saitz R. Clinical practice. Unhealthy alcohol use. *N Engl J Med.* 2005;352:596-607.

Gomez A, Conde A, Santana JM, Jorrin A. Diagnostic usefulness of brief versions of Alcohol Use Disorders Identification Test (AUDIT) for detecting hazardous drinkers in primary care settings. *J Stud Alcohol.* 2005;66:305-308.

Beich A, Thorsen T, Rollnick S. Screening in brief intervention trials targeting excessive drinkers in general practice: Systematic review and meta-analysis. *BMJ.* 2003;327:536-542.

Kenna GA, McGeary JE, Swift RM. Pharmacotherapy, pharmacogenomics, and the future of alcohol dependence treatment, part 1. *Am J Health Syst Pharm.* 2004;61:2272-2279.

---

89   Anchiety

Anxiety

John C. Rogers, MD, MPH

KEY POINTS

- More than 19 million adult Americans aged 18 to 54 years have anxiety disorders. Anxiety disorders encompass several clinical conditions:

  Generalized anxiety disorder: Exaggerated worry and tension over everyday events and decisions.

  Panic disorder: Feelings of extreme fear and dread strike unexpectedly and repeatedly for no apparent reason, accompanied by intense physical symptoms.

  Phobias: Fear of an object or situation or fear of extreme embarrassment.

  Posttraumatic stress disorder: Reaction to a terrifying event that keeps returning in the form of frightening, intrusive memories and brings on hypervigilance and deadening of normal emotions.

- There is extensive evidence that cognitive-behavioral therapies are useful treatments for a majority of patients with anxiety disorders. (SOR **Ⓐ**) The hallmarks of cognitive-behavioral therapies are evaluating apparent cause-and-effect relationships between thoughts, feelings, and behaviors as well as implementing relatively straightforward strategies to lessen symptoms and reduce avoidant behavior.

- Medications typically used to treat patients with anxiety disorders are antidepressants, benzodiazepines, and buspirone (see Table 89–5 later in this chapter for drug-prescribing information).
  - –Most antidepressant medications have substantial antianxiety and antipanic effects in addition to their antidepressant action. Current practice guidelines rank the tricyclic antidepressants below the selective serotonin reuptake inhibitors (SSRIs) for treatment of anxiety disorders because of the SSRIs' more favorable tolerability and safety profiles. (SOR ♠) Other antidepressants are effective as well: serotonin norepinephrine reuptake inhibitors (SNRI), serotonin antagonist and reuptake inhibitors, and noradrenergic and serotonin selective antagonists. When effective in treating anxiety, antidepressants should be maintained for at least 6 months, then tapered slowly to avoid discontinuation-emergent activation of anxiety symptoms (SOR ♠) (starting doses: sertraline, 25 mg/d; paroxetine, 10 mg/d; escitalopram, 10 mg/d).
  - –Four benzodiazepines widely prescribed for treatment of anxiety disorders are diazepam (starting dose, 2 mg 2–4 times daily); lorazepam (1 mg 2 or 3 times daily); clonazepam (0.25 mg twice daily); and alprazolam (0.25 mg 3 times daily). Each is now available in generic formulations. Benzodiazepines have the potential for producing drug dependence (i.e., physiologic or behavioral symptoms after discontinuation of use). Shorter-acting compounds have somewhat greater liability because of more rapid and abrupt onset of withdrawal symptoms.
  - –Buspirone is most useful for treatment of generalized anxiety disorder, and it is now frequently used as an adjunct to SSRIs. Buspirone (starting dose, 5 mg 3 times daily) takes 4 to 6 weeks to exert therapeutic effects, like antidepressants, and it has little value for patients when taken on an "as-needed" basis.

I. Introduction
  A. One or more fearful experiences prime a person to respond excessively to situations in which most people would experience no fear or only moderate nervousness. Deeply etched memory results in hypervigilance, making it hard to focus, leading to feelings of anxiety in many situations.
  B. Recent research suggests that anxiety disorders may be associated with activation of the amygdala.
    1. Studies suggest that memories stored in the amygdala are relatively indelible. Research aims to develop therapies that increase cognitive control over the amygdala so that the "act now, think later" response can be interrupted.
    2. Cognitive factors play a significant role in the onset of anxiety disorders. People at risk tend to be overly responsive to potentially threatening stimuli.
    3. Research evidence points to genetics as a factor in the origin of anxiety disorders. Studies of twins found that genes play a role in panic disorder and social phobia.
  C. **Generalized anxiety disorder** is a syndrome of excessive or unrealistic anxiety or worry about two or more life circumstances for 6 months or longer.
    1. Generalized anxiety disorder is the fourth most common mental disorder, following substance abuse, major depressive disorder, and phobias. Two to five percent of the US population exhibits this disorder in any given year.
      a. The mean age at onset of symptoms is in the mid-20s, with most cases developing between the ages of 16 and 40. The mean duration of symptoms before treatment is approximately 5 years.
      b. In the general medical care setting, the female–male ratio is 2–3:1, but among psychiatric patients, the sex ratio is 1:1. First- and second-degree relatives of a person affected by generalized anxiety disorder have at least a threefold increased risk of being affected.
      c. Comorbidity with depression is frequent (just more than 50% of depressed patients have concurrent generalized anxiety disorder).
  D. **Panic disorder** is the recurrence of episodic periods of intense fear or apprehension accompanied by at least any of four somatic symptoms, such as diaphoresis, dyspnea, faintness, paresthesias, or flushing.
    1. Panic disorder occurs in 1.4% of the US population.
      a. The mean age at presentation is 25 years, with onset generally between ages 17 and 30 years.

      b. The female–male ratio is 2.5–3:1. This disorder has a familial tendency, with first-degree relatives having a twofold increased risk of being affected compared to control subjects.

      c. Comorbidity with depression occurs (nearly 10% of depressed patients have panic disorder) and leads to more frequent and severe symptoms.

  E. A **phobia** is a persistent fear of an object, activity, or situation that is out of proportion to the objective danger.

    1. Phobia is the most common anxiety disorder. Fifteen to twenty percent of the population may be affected by phobias.

      a. Social phobia usually begins during the early to late teens. Simple phobias can begin at any age, however, depending on typical exposure to the object or situation. The most common objects of simple phobia are, in descending order and frequency, animals, storms, heights, illness, and death.

      b. Social phobia is reportedly more frequent in males than in females, whereas simple phobias are more frequent in females than in males.

      c. Comorbidity with depression is common (more than 20% of depressed patients have concurrent phobia).

Posttraumatic stress disorder develops after an individual experiences emotionally or physically distressing events that are outside the range of usual human experience and would be extremely traumatic for virtually any person. Examples include combat experience, natural catastrophes, assault, rape, serious threat or harm to one's family members, or sudden destruction of one's home or community.

    1. The cause of this disorder is related to the severity of stressor, the social environment of the victim and availability of social supports, the personality traits of the victim, and the victim's premorbid biologic vulnerability.

    2. Posttraumatic stress disorder affects 0.5% of men and 1.2% of women in the general population. Onset may be at any age, but because of the types of precipitating situations that are most common, this disorder is most common in young adults. The initiating trauma for men is usually combat experience. The initiating trauma for women is most often assault or rape.

II. Diagnosis

  A. Generalized anxiety disorder. Diagnostic criteria are specified in Table 89–1. Diagnoses that must be ruled out include medical disorders and diagnosable mental disorders.

TABLE 89–1. DIAGNOSTIC CRITERIA FOR GENERALIZED ANXIETY DISORDER

A. Excessive anxiety and worry (apprehensive expectation), occurring more days than not for at least 6 months, about a number of events or activities (e.g., work or school performance)

B. The person finds it difficult to control the worry

C. The anxiety and worry are associated with three or more of the following six symptoms (with at least some symptoms present for more days than not for the past 6 months). *Note*: Only one item is required in children

  (1) Restlessness or feeling keyed up or on edge

  (2) Being easily fatigued

  (3) Difficulty concentrating or mind going blank

  (4) Irritability

  (5) Muscle tension

  (6) Sleep disturbance (difficulty falling or staying asleep, or restless, unsatisfying sleep)

D. The focus of the anxiety and worry is not confined to features of an axis I disorder; for example, the anxiety or worry is not about having a panic attack (as in panic disorder), being embarrassed in public (as in social phobia), being contaminated (as in obsessive–compulsive disorder), being away from home or close relatives (as in separation anxiety disorder), gaining weight (as in anorexia nervosa), having multiple physical complaints (as in somatization disorder), or having a serious illness (as in hypochondriasis), and the anxiety and worry do not occur exclusively during posttraumatic stress disorder

E. The anxiety, worry, or physical symptoms cause clinically significant distress or impairment in social, occupational, or other important areas of functioning

F. The disturbance is not caused by the direct physiologic effects of a substance (e.g., a drug of abuse or a medication) or a general medical condition (e.g., hyperthyroidism) and does not occur exclusively during a mood disorder, psychotic disorder, or pervasive developmental disorder

---

(Adapted with permission from American Psychiatric Association (APA). *Diagnostic and Statistical Manual of Mental Disorders.* 4th ed. Washington, DC: APA; 1994.)

TABLE 89–2. DIAGNOSTIC CRITERIA FOR PANIC DISORDER WITHOUT AGORAPHOBIA

A. Both (1) and (2):
  (1) Recurrent, unexpected panic attacks (see below)
  (2) At least one of the attacks has been followed by 1 month (or more) of one or more of the following:
    (a) Persistent concern about having additional attacks
    (b) Worry about the implications of the attack or its consequences (e.g., losing control, having a heart attack, or "going crazy")
    (c) A significant change in behavior related to the attacks
B. Absence of agoraphobia
C. The panic attacks are not caused by the direct physiologic effects of a substance (e.g., a drug of abuse or a medication) or a general medical condition (e.g., hyperthyroidism)
D. The panic attacks are not better accounted for by another mental disorder, such as social phobia (e.g., occurring upon exposure to feared social situations), specific phobia (e.g., on exposure to a specific phobic situation), obsessive–compulsive disorder (e.g., upon exposure to dirt in someone with an obsession about contamination), posttraumatic stress disorder (e.g., in response to stimuli associated with a severe stressor), or separation anxiety disorder (e.g., in response to being away from home or close relatives)
E. Criteria for panic attack: A discrete period of intense fear or discomfort, in which four or more of the following symptoms developed abruptly and reached a peak within 10 minutes
  (1) Palpitations, pounding heart, or accelerated heart rate
  (2) Sweating
  (3) Trembling or shaking
  (4) Sensations of shortness of breath or smothering
  (5) Feeling of choking
  (6) Chest pain or discomfort
  (7) Nausea or abdominal distress
  (8) Feeling dizzy, unsteady, lightheaded, or faint
  (9) Derealization (feelings of unreality) or depersonalization (being detached from oneself)
  (10) Fear of losing control or going crazy
  (11) Fear of dying
  (12) Paresthesia (numbness or tingling sensations)
  (13) Chills or hot flushes

(Adapted with permission from American Psychiatric Association (APA). *Diagnostic and Statistical Manual of Mental Disorders.* 4th ed. Washington, DC: APA; 1994.)

  1. Biomedical disorders may include thyrotoxicosis, paroxysmal atrial tachycardia, mitral valve prolapse, hyperventilation, caffeine intoxication, stimulant abuse, alcohol withdrawal, and sedative or hypnotic withdrawal.
  2. Mental disorders may include panic disorder, phobias, obsessive–compulsive disorder, adjustment disorder with anxious mood, depression, dysthymia, somatization disorder, and schizophrenia.
 B. Panic disorder. Diagnostic criteria are displayed in Table 89–2. Panic attacks, which are spontaneous, unexpected episodes that occur in the absence of any apparent precipitant, generally last no more than 20 to 30 minutes, with attacks of 1 hour being rare. Fear without any apparent source and an impending sense of death and doom are characteristic. Such thoughts are associated with somatic symptoms, typically tachycardia, palpitations, dyspnea, and sweating. As many as 20% of patients may experience syncope during panic attacks.
 C. Phobia. Diagnostic criteria are listed in Table 89–3.
  1. The most common biomedical disorders are intoxication with hallucinogens, sympathomimetics, and other drugs of abuse; small cerebral tumor; and cerebrovascular accidents.
  2. The most common mental disorders in the differential diagnoses are depression, schizophrenia, obsessive–compulsive disorder, and personality disorders (schizoid, avoidance, or paranoid).
 D. Posttraumatic stress disorder. Diagnostic criteria are specified in Table 89–4.
  1. Biomedical conditions to be ruled out include head injury and alcohol and drug abuse. Psychiatric conditions include generalized anxiety disorder, panic disorder, depression, adjustment reaction, factitious disorder, malingering, borderline personality disorder, and schizophrenia.
III. Treatment
 A. Generalized anxiety disorder treatment is directed toward reduction in symptoms so that patients can function in relationships and work. To achieve this goal, the physician

TABLE 89–3. DIAGNOSTIC CRITERIA FOR SPECIFIC PHOBIA

A. Marked and persistent fear that is excessive or unreasonable, cued by the presence or anticipation of a specific object or situation (e.g., flying, heights, animals, receiving an injection, or seeing blood).

B. Exposure to the phobic stimulus almost invariably provokes an immediate anxiety response, which may take the form of a situationally bound or situationally predisposed panic attack. *Note*: In children, the anxiety may be expressed by crying, tantrums, freezing, or clinging.

C. The person recognizes that the fear is excessive or unreasonable. *Note*: In children, this feature may be absent.

D. The phobic situation(s) is avoided or else is endured with intense anxiety or distress.

E. The avoidance, anxious anticipation, or distress in the feared situation(s) interferes significantly with the person's normal routine, occupational (or academic) functioning, or social activities or relationships, or there is marked distress about having the phobia.

F. In individuals under age 18 years, the duration is at least 6 months.

G. The anxiety panic attacks, or phobic avoidance associated with the specific object or situation, are not better accounted for by another mental disorder, such as obsessive–compulsive disorder (e.g., fear of dirt in someone with an obsession about contamination), posttraumatic stress disorder (e.g., avoidance of stimuli associated with a severe stressor), separation anxiety disorder (e.g., avoidance of school), social phobia (e.g., avoidance of social situations because of fear of embarrassment), panic disorder with agoraphobia, or agoraphobia without history of panic disorder. Specify type.

  (1) Animal type

  (2) Natural environment type (e.g., heights, storms, or water)

  (3) Blood–injection–injury type

  (4) Situational type (e.g., airplanes, elevators, or enclosed places)

  (5) Other type (e.g., phobic avoidance of situations that may lead to choking, vomiting, or contracting an illness; in children, avoidance of loud sounds or costumed characters).

(Adapted with permission from American Psychiatric Association (APA). *Diagnostic and Statistical Manual of Mental Disorders*. 4th ed. Washington, DC: APA; 1994.)

must provide patience, realistic reassurance, education about the condition, and encouragement to socialize and assume work and family responsibilities.

1. Interventions with longest duration of effect are (in descending order): psychological therapy, pharmacologic treatment (antidepressants), and self-help. (SOR **A**)

   a. Psychological therapy

      (1) Cognitive behavioral therapy (CBT) should be used and delivered only by those trained in and following established treatment protocols. (SOR **A**) Two-thirds of patients are clinically improved by 6 months. (SOR **A**)

      (2) The optimal range of CBT is 16 to 20 hours, (SOR **A**) typically 1 to 2 hours per week over 4 months. (SOR **B**)

      (3) Briefer CBT should be supplemented with information and tasks. (SOR **A**)

   b. Pharmacologic therapy

      (1) Short-term treatment

         Benzodiazepines are appropriate pharmacologic treatment for immediate management of this disorder (SOR **A**) but should not be used for more than 2 to 4 weeks. (SOR **B**) The pharmacologic properties of common benzodiazepines are displayed in Table 89–5. Patients respond best to anxiolytic agents with short half-lives. Use of rapid-acting benzodiazepines as needed may be superior to routine dosing. The problems with the use of these drugs are that 20% to 30% of patients fail to respond to these agents, tolerance and dependence may occur, and impaired alertness and increased risk of accidents are possible.

         The sedating antihistamine hydroxyziune 50 mg/day is effective for immediate management as well. (SOR **A**)

         Beta-blockers can be used to treat peripheral somatic symptoms such as tremor or palpitation. Propranolol can be started at 60 to 80 mg/day in divided doses and gradually increased to optimum response or a maximum dose of 240 mg/day. Combination of a beta-blocker and a benzodiazepine is more effective than a benzodiazepine alone.

         Azepirones are superior to placebo but not benzodiazepines in the short-term. (SOR **A**) It is unclear if the azepirones are superior to antidepressants. Long-term effectiveness is not known. These medications act on the serotoninergic system and do not act through the γ-aminobutyric acid–benzodiazepine

TABLE 89–4. DIAGNOSTIC CRITERIA FOR POSTTRAUMATIC STRESS DISORDER

A. The person has been exposed to a traumatic event in which both of the following were present:
   (1) The person experienced, witnessed, or was confronted with an event or events that involved actual or threatened death or serious injury, or a threat to the physical integrity of self or others
   (2) The person's response involved intense fear, helplessness, or horror. *Note*: In children, this may be expressed instead by disorganized or agitated behavior

B. The traumatic event is persistently re-experienced in one or more of the following ways:
   (1) Recurrent and intrusive distressing recollections of the event, including images, thoughts, or perceptions. *Note*: In young children, repetitive play may occur in which themes or aspects of the trauma are expressed
   (2) Recurrent distressing dreams of the event. *Note*: In children, there may be frightening dreams without recognizable content
   (3) Acting or feeling as if the traumatic event were recurring (includes a sense of reliving the experience, illusions, hallucinations, and dissociative flashback episodes, including those that occur upon awakening or when intoxicated). *Note*: In young children, trauma-specific re-enactment may occur
   (4) Intense psychological distress at exposure to internal or external cues that symbolize or resemble an aspect of the traumatic event
   (5) Physiologic reactivity upon exposure to internal or external cues that symbolize or resemble an aspect of the traumatic event

C. Persistent avoidance of stimuli associated with the trauma and numbing of general responsiveness (not present before the trauma), as indicated by at least three or more of the following:
   (1) Efforts to avoid thoughts, feelings, or conversations associated with the trauma
   (2) Efforts to avoid activities, places, or people that arouse recollections of the trauma
   (3) Inability to recall an important aspect of the trauma
   (4) Markedly diminished interest or participation in significant activities
   (5) Feeling of detachment or estrangement from others
   (6) Restricted range of affect (e.g., unable to have loving feelings)
   (7) Sense of a foreshortened future (e.g., does not expect to have a career, marriage, children, or normal life span)

D. Persistent symptoms of increased arousal (not present before the trauma), as indicated by two or more of the following:
   (1) Difficulty falling or staying asleep
   (2) Irritability or outbursts of anger
   (3) Difficulty concentrating
   (4) Hypervigilance
   (5) Exaggerated startle response

E. Duration of the disturbance (symptoms in B, C, and D) is more than 1 month.

F. The disturbance causes clinically significant distress or impairment in social, occupational, or other important areas of functioning. Specify if:
   Acute (if duration of symptoms is less than 3 months)
   Chronic (if duration of symptoms is 3 months or more)
   Specify if:
   With delayed onset (if onset of symptoms is at least 6 months after the stressor)

(Adapted with permission from American Psychiatric Association (APA). *Diagnostic and Statistical Manual of Mental Disorders*. 4th ed. Washington, DC: APA; 1994.)

receptor complex, so problems of tolerance, dependence, and impaired alertness are avoided. Buspirone should be started at 5 mg 3 times a day for 3 to 7 days and then increased to 10 mg 2 or 3 times daily, the usual maintenance dose. The dose should not exceed 60 mg/day.

   (2) Long-term treatment. Antidepressants are first-line agents over benzodiazepines for long-term treatment. (SOR **A**) SSRIs should be offered first unless there are other considerations. (SOR **B**) Number-needed-to-treat is approximately 5. The SSRI paroxetine is effective compared with placebo, as is the SNRI venlafaxine. (SOR **A**) Nefazadone (serotonin antagonist and reuptake inhibitor) and mirtzapine (noradrenergic and serotonin selective antagonist) are effective as well. (SOR **B**) Imipramine can be used as well. (SOR **C**) Imipramine starts at 50 to 75 mg/day and is increased every 2 weeks, depending on response, to a maximum of 150 mg/day in divided doses.

c. Self-help
   (1) Bibliotherapy based on CBT should be offered. (SOR **A**)
   (2) Regular exercise may help reduce symptoms. (SOR **B**) Elimination of caffeine and other stimulants may help as well.

TABLE 89–5. DRUG TREATMENT OF ANXIETY DISORDERS

Drug	Starting Dosage (mg)	Usual Daily Dosage (mg)	Maximum Daily Dosage (mg)	Rate of Onset	Half-life (hr)	Common Side Effects	Cost for #30
Selective Serotonin Reuptake Inhibitors							
Fluoxetine (Prozac)	5 mg qd	10–20	40	Delayed	Days	Insomnia, agitation, anorgasmia	20 mg $12 (trade $141)
Sertraline (Zoloft)	25 mg qd	50–100	200	Delayed	26	Insomnia, nausea, sexual dysfunction	100 mg $68 (trade $88)
Paroxetine (Paxil)	10 mg qd	20–40	50	Delayed	21	Drowsiness, fatigue, delayed ejaculation	30 mg $36 (trade $103)
Fluvoxamine (Luvox)	25 mg bid	100–150	300	Delayed	15	Drowsiness, nausea, anorgasmia	100 mg $62 (trade $97)
Escitalopram (Lexapro)	10 mg qd	10–20	20	Delayed	27–32	Nausea, insomnia, delayed ejaculation, somnolence, increased sweating, fatigue	20 mg (trade $75)
Citalopram (Celexa)	20 mg qd	20–60	60	Delayed	35	Nausea, dry mouth, somnolence, increased sweating	40 mg $39 (trade $92)
Tricyclic antidepressants							
Imipramine (Tofranil, Janimine)	75 qd or hs	50–150	200	Delayed	11–25	Sedation, anticholinergic effects, orthostatic hypertension	50 mg $17 (trade $180)
Desipramine (Norpramin, Pertofrane)	50 qd	100–200	300	Delayed	12–24		100 mg $18 (trade $101)
Benzodiazepines							
Alprazolam (Xanax)	0.25 tid	0.5–4	10	Intermediate	12–15	Transient drowsiness, alexia, confusion, depression	0.5 mg $7 (trade $40)
Chlordiazepoxide (Librium, Lipoxide, Mitran, etc.)	5 tid or qid	15–80	100	Intermediate	5–30	Withdrawal symptoms upon abrupt discontinuation	10 mg $10 (trade $75)
Clonazepam (Klonopin)	0.25 tid	0.5–1.5	4	Rapid	18–50	Withdrawal symptoms upon abrupt discontinuation	0.5 mg $10 (trade $40)
Clorazepate (Tranxene)	7.5 qd or bid	15–30	60	Rapid	30–100		7.5 mg $28 (trade $93)
Diazepam (Valium, Vazepam)	2 bid or qid	4–40	40	Very rapid	20–80		5 mg $7 (trade $64)
Lorazepam (Alzapam, Ativan)	1 bid or tid	2–4	10	Intermediate	10–20		1 mg $14 (trade $51)
Oxazepam (Serax)	10–15 tid or qid	30–90	120	Intermediate to slow	5–20		15 mg $15
Azepirone							
Buspirone (BuSpar)	5 tid	20–30	60	Delayed	2–3	Dizziness, nervousness, nausea, headache	5 mg $16 (trade $58)
Beta-blockes							
Propranolol (Inderal)	40 bid	80–120	320	Rapid	3–5	Bradycardia, dizziness, fatigue, depression, impotence	40 mg $5 (trade $28)

B. Panic disorder treatment is directed toward control of symptoms so that the patient may be as functional as possible.

   1. Interventions with evidence of longest duration of effect in descending order are psychological treatment, pharmacologic treatments, and self-help.

   a. Psychological treatments

   (1) CBT is psychological treatment of choice. (SOR **Ⓐ**) Combined psychological and pharmacologic in acute treatment is superior to either treatment alone. After acute active treatment, combined treatment is better than antidepressant treatment alone and equal to psychological treatment. Either psychological or pharmacologic treatments are acceptable as first-line treatments. (SOR **Ⓐ**)

   b. Pharmacologic treatments

   (1) *SSRIs* are considered first-line pharmacologic treatment. (SOR **Ⓐ**) They are as effective as benzodiazepines in improving anxiety, have fewer side effects than the alternatives, have no interference with CBT, and provide treatment of concurrent depression. Fluoxetine, 5 to 40 mg/day, is recommended as a single morning dose. The starting dose is 5 mg (2 mg if there is significant insomnia or agitation) with increases each week. The dose for sertraline is 25 mg/day to start, with a maximum of 200 mg/day. The starting dose for paroxetine is 10 mg/day, with a maximum of 50 mg/day. Fluvoxamine starts at 25 mg twice a day, with a maximum of 150 mg twice a day. The dose of escitalopram is most often 10 mg/day with 20 mg/day used infrequently. The starting dose of citalopram is 20 mg/day, with a maximum of 60 mg/day. Full response occurs after 4 weeks, and perhaps 8 to 12 weeks. Relapse is common. (SOR **Ⓐ**) Treatment should continue for at least 6 months (SOR **Ⓐ**) and up to 12 to 24 months (SOR **Ⓑ**) with slow discontinuation over 4 to 6 months.

   (2) *Tricyclic antidepressants.* Imipramine and clomirpamine are effective agents. (SOR **Ⓐ**) Imipramine, 150 to 300 mg/day, is recommended as a single bedtime dose. The starting dose is 50 to 100 mg/day, which can be increased every 2 weeks until an optimum response or maximum dose is reached. Desipramine is sometimes better tolerated by patients than is imipramine.

   (3) *Benzodiazepines.* Alprazolam and clonazepam provide effective rapid relief, but relapse is high when discontinued. (SOR **Ⓐ**) Benzodiazepine produce long-term outcomes that are less effective than those of the antihistamines and should not be prescribed routinely. (SOR **Ⓐ**) Another disadvantage of using benzodiazepines is that nearly half of patients with panic disorder have concurrent major depression that is not helped by benzodiazepines, abuse can be a potential problem, and benzodiazepines are more difficult to taper than are tricyclic antidepressants. Gradual tapering of the dose is recommended when discontinuing treatment. (SOR **Ⓐ**) CBT may facilitate tapering. (SOR **Ⓐ**)

   c. Self-help

   (1) Bibliotherapy based on CBT principles is effective. (SOR **Ⓐ**)

   (2) Exercise may help control symptoms. (SOR **Ⓑ**)

C. Treatment of phobia requires commitment on the part of the patient and clear identification of the phobic object or situation.

   1. Behavioral treatment techniques are the most effective, with systematic exposure therapy to the feared situation/object. (SOR **Ⓐ**) A cognitive strategy of suggesting new ways of thinking about the phobic object or situation may be used in addition to muscle relaxation techniques. CBT, exposure to feared situation, and group approaches are effective for social phobia. (SOR **Ⓐ**)

   2. Pharmacologic therapy

   a. Beta-blockers such as propranolol may be useful for specific performance anxiety (SOR **Ⓑ**) just prior to direct challenge to the phobic situation. Propranolol, 10 to 20 mg, 45 to 60 minutes before exposure to the phobic object, or up to 40 mg, should be effective.

   b. SSRIs are effective first-line treatments for social phobia (SOR **Ⓐ**) with paroxetine studied the most. Fluvoxamine and sertraline may be of use, particularly in patients with social phobia.

D. Posttraumatic stress disorder treatment consists primarily of psychotherapy, but there is growing evidence for a role of pharmacotherapy when the patient has symptoms of depression or a panic-like disorder.

1. Trauma-focused CBT, stress management, and group trauma-focused CBT are effective (SOR **A**) and should be continued for 6 months. (SOR **A**) Treatment should not be initiated and continued only in the primary care setting. (SOR **C**) Time-limited psychotherapy uses cognitive and supportive approaches to minimize the risk of dependency and chronicity. The patient is encouraged to garner support from friends and relatives; to review emotional feelings associated with the event; to consciously re-enact the event through imagination, words, or actions; and to plan for future recovery. Group and family therapies have been particularly effective.

2. SSRIs are effective (SOR **A**) and should be continued at least for 12 months. (SOR **A**)

IV. Management Strategies

A. Generalized anxiety disorder. Physician time and involvement need not be extensive. Education of the patient about the disorder and the scheduling of frequent, short office visits are the physician's primary responsibilities. Listening carefully to the patient's account of problems is very beneficial. Specific management techniques include being supportive of patient choices, expanding coping strategies, normalizing symptoms through reassurance, encouraging confrontation of anxiety-provoking situations, and being available for brief clinical encounters.

B. Panic disorder. Patients with panic disorder should be reassured that they have a treatable condition. The patient's somatic symptoms should be discussed in such a way as to avoid the attachment of any stigma to the patient. Eliciting the patient's explanation of the symptoms and goals for treatment is crucial. Panic-focused CBT and medications are effective treatments for panic disorder. There is no evidence that one is superior to the other, so the choice between psychotherapy and pharmacotherapy depends on the efficacy, benefits, risks, and the patient's personal preferences.

C. Phobias. The goal of therapy is for the affected person to discover that the feared situation is not as much of a threat as previously thought. Avoidance should be discouraged, and behavioral techniques should be used until the phobic object or situation has been fully confronted. Hypnosis may be used as an adjunct method of relaxation and as a method of offering alternative cognitive appraisals of the phobic object. Family therapy may be particularly useful in this condition.

D. Posttraumatic stress disorder. Physicians caring for patients with this disorder must deal effectively with suspicion, paranoia, and mistrust on the part of the patient. Gentle confrontation is necessary to overcome the patient's denial of the traumatic event and to encourage the individual to remain in the treatment program of therapy and medications. Groups of individuals suffering similar events, such as assault self-help groups, may also be useful. Hospitalization may be necessary if the patient is suicidal or a danger to others.

V. Prognosis

A. Generalized anxiety disorder is a chronic condition with a typical duration of illness just more than 10 years. Affected individuals usually respond to treatment, but relapse after withdrawal of treatment may occur in as many as 80% of patients, nearly 25% of whom may go on to develop panic disorder.

B. Panic disorder is a chronic, remitting, and relapsing condition that is often precipitated by stressful life events. In one study, at 5-year follow-up, 30% of affected patients were moderately to severely impaired and 50% were mildly impaired; at 20-year follow-up, 15% had moderate to severe symptoms and 70% had mild symptoms with no disability. Between 30% and 70% of patients experience a major depressive disorder subsequent to the onset of the panic attacks. These individuals are at increased risk for suicide, alcohol and drug dependence, and obsessive–compulsive disorder. Once an effective drug dose is achieved, the medication should be continued unchanged for 6 to 12 months. At that time, the medication is slowly tapered. Drug treatment should be reinstituted if symptoms return. Patients with good function prior to development of symptoms of brief duration tend to have a better prognosis.

C. Phobias beginning in childhood may resolve without treatment, but others may become chronic. Those that are chronic in nature seem to increase after middle age. Most affected individuals experience little disability, since the phobic object or situation can usually be easily avoided.

D. Posttraumatic stress disorder. The full syndrome usually develops sometime after the traumatic event, and delay can be from 1 week to as long as 30 years. Symptoms fluctuate with exacerbations during periods of stress. Individuals with a good prognosis usually have rapid onset of symptoms, symptoms of less than 6 months' duration, good functioning before the onset of the syndrome, strong social support, and the absence of any other medical or emotional disorders. Over time, 10% of affected patients remain unchanged or become worse, 20% have moderate symptoms, 40% have mild symptoms, and 30% recover.

REFERENCES

Bisson J, Andrew M. Psychological treatment of post-traumatic stress disorder (PTSD). *Cochrane Database Syst Rev.* 2005; (2). Art. No.: CD003388. doi: 10.1002/14651858.CD003388.pub2.

Borkovec TD, Newman MG, Castonguay LG. Cognitive-behavioral therapy for generalized anxiety disorder with integrations from interpersonal and experiential therapies. *CNS Spectr.* 2003;8(5):382-389.

Bruce S, Vasile RG, Goisman RM, et al. Are benzodiazepines still the medication of choice for patients with panic disorder with or without agoraphobia? *Am J Psychiatry.* 2003;160(8):1432-1438.

Chessick CA, Allen MH, Thase ME, et al. Azapirones for generalized anxiety disorder. *Cochrane Database Syst Rev.* 2006; (3). Art. No.: CD006115. doi: 10.1002/14651858.CD006115.

Furukawa TA, Watanabe N, Churchill R. Combined psychotherapy plus antidepressants for panic disorder with or without agoraphobia. *Cochrane Database Syst Rev.* 2007; (1). Art. No.: CD004364. doi: 10.1002/14651858.CD004364.pub2.

Hambrick JP, Weeks JW, Harb JC, Heimberg RG. Cognitive-behavioral therapy for social anxiety disorder: Supporting evidence and future directions. *CNS Spectr.* 2003;8(5):373-381.

Kapczinski F, Lima MS, Souza JS, Cunha A, Schmitt R. Antidepressants for generalized anxiety disorder. *Cochrane Database Syst Rev.*2003; (2). Art. No.: CD003592. doi: 10.1002/14651858. CD003592.

Lepola U, Arato M, Zhu Y, Austin C. Sertraline versus imipramine treatment of comorbid panic disorder and major depressive disorder. *J Clin Psychiatry.* 2003;64(6):654-662.

Pollack MH. New advances in the management of anxiety disorders. *Psychopharmacol Bull.* 2002;36 (4 Suppl 3):79-94.

Quilty LC, Van Ameringen M, Mangni C, et al. Quality of life and the anxiety disorders. *J Anxiety Disord.* 2003;17(4):405-426.

Rayburn NR, Otto MW. Cognitive-behavioral therapy for panic disorder: A review of treatment elements, strategies, and outcomes. *CNS Spectr.* 2003;8(5):356-362.

Resick AP, Nishith P, Griffin MG. How well does cognitive-behavioral therapy treat symptoms of complex PTSD? An examination of child sexual abuse survivors within a clinical trial. *CNS Spectr.* 2003;8(5):340-355.

Rose S, Bisson J, Churchill R, Wessely S. Psychological debriefing for preventing post traumatic stress disorder (PTSD). *Cochrane Database Syst Rev.* 2002; (2). Art. No.: CD000560. doi: 10.1002/14651858.CD000560.

Solvason HB, Ernst H, Roth W. Predictors of response in anxiety disorders. *Psychiatr Clin North Am.* 2003;26(2):411-433.

Stein DJ. Algorithm for the pharmacotherapy of anxiety disorders. *Curr Psychiatry Rep.* 2003;5(4):282.

Stein DJ, Ipser JC, Seedat S. Pharmacotherapy for post traumatic stress disorder (PTSD). *Cochrane Database Syst Rev.*2006; (1). Art. No.: CD002795. doi: 10.1002/14651858.CD002795.pub2.

CLINICAL GUIDELINES

American Psychiatric Association (APA). *Practice Guideline for the Treatment of Patients with Panic Disorder.* American Psychiatric Press; 1998:86.

Institute for Clinical Systems Improvement (ICSI). Major depression, panic disorder and generalized anxiety disorder in adults in primary care. Bloomington, MN: Institute for Clinical Systems Improvement (ICSI); May 2002:55.

Practice guideline for the treatment of patients with panic disorder. Work Group on Panic Disorder. American Psychiatric Association (APA). *Am J Psychiatry.* May 1998;155(5 Suppl):1-34.

WEB SITES

http://www.nlm.nih.gov/medlineplus/anxiety.html
http://www.nlm.nih.gov/medlineplus/panicdisorder.html
http://www.nlm.nih.gov/medlineplus/phobias.html
http://www.nlm.nih.gov/medlineplus/posttraumaticstressdisorder.html
http://www.surgeongeneral.gov/library/mentalhealth/chapter4/sec2.html

90   Attention-Deficit/Hyperactivity Disorder

H. Russell Searight, PhD, MPH, Jennifer Gafford, PhD,
& Stephanie L. Evans, Pharm D, BCPS

KEY POINTS

- Attention-deficit/hyperactivity disorder (ADHD) has three core symptom clusters: inattention, hyperactivity, and impulsivity.
- Among US children, current prevalence rates are 6% to 8%, and the results of non-US studies reveal prevalence rates that are at least as high as those in US studies.
- Approximately 80% of children diagnosed with ADHD continue to manifest symptoms in adolescence, with 60% meeting diagnostic criteria in adulthood. (SOR **B**)
- Common comorbid psychiatric conditions include oppositional defiant and conduct disorder.
- Evaluating suspected ADHD includes a history and physical, detailed clinical interview, behavioral ratings, and on occasion, referral for specialized assessment.
- Stimulant pharmacotherapy continues to be the most common treatment. However, there are several nonstimulant medication options.

I. Introduction

A. Overview of condition. ADHD is a common neurobehavioral disorder beginning in childhood that typically continues through adulthood, and is characterized by chronic, pervasive inattention, hyperactivity-impulsivity, or both, that is inconsistent with the child's developmental level and affects cognitive, academic, behavioral, emotional, and social functioning.

1. The initial diagnosis is typically made between the ages of 6 and 10 years, when symptoms of hyperactivity and impulsivity tend to peak. Inattention remains stable through the lifespan.

2. Although children may begin to develop symptoms of ADHD as early as age 3, diagnoses of ADHD made during the very early years are unreliable. Approximately 50% of these individuals will no longer meet criteria by later childhood. (SOR **C**) However, diagnoses made between ages 4 and 6, particularly of more severe forms of the condition, are associated with persistent symptoms later in childhood.

3. Approximately 50% to 75% of children with ADHD continue to exhibit symptoms into adulthood. (SOR **B**)

4. ADHD is often comorbid with other conditions, including learning disabilities, speech and language disorders, oppositional defiant disorder, conduct disorder, mood disorders, anxiety disorders, and Tourette syndrome.

5. Additionally, ADHD is often associated with substantial impairments such as low self-esteem, rejection by peers and adults, school difficulties, and academic underachievement.

B. Etiology. The etiology of ADHD is not entirely clear. However, at least seven genes, coding for proteins contributing to the neurotransmitters dopamine, serotonin, and norepinephrine are likely diatheses. Other contributing factors include subtle central nervous system anomalies, psychophysiologic variables, and psychosocial factors. Allergens and environmental toxins do not appear to play a role in the development of the disorder.

C. Risk factors. A number of risk factors have been identified for the development of ADHD.

1. Family history of ADHD is a major risk factor for the development of the disorder. Based on numerous studies of twins, the mean heritability for ADHD was shown to be 77%.

2. **Pre- and perinatal risk factors include maternal smoking and/or alcohol use during pregnancy, premature delivery, and other delivery complications.** (SOR **B**)

3. Children with ADHD who are very active and demanding, coupled with maternal psychological distress and family dysfunction, exhibit symptoms of ADHD that are more persistent into later childhood and often comorbid with oppositional behaviors.

II. Diagnosis

A. Primary features of ADHD include inattention, hyperactivity, and impulsivity (behavioral disinhibition). Deficient rule-governed behavior and variability in task performance may be considered core features as well.

1. Inattention refers to problems with alertness, arousal, selectivity, sustained attention, and distractibility, which tend to be most evident in situations in which children are required to sustain attention to repetitive and monotonous tasks. Children with attentional problems are commonly described by parents and teachers as "not listening to instructions," "not finishing assigned work," "daydreaming," and "becoming bored easily." In addition, they may be perceived as forgetful, careless, or lazy because of failing to follow through on tasks, losing things, or making mistakes.

2. Hyperactivity across multiple settings is the most classic, distinguishing feature of ADHD. Described by parents and teachers as "in constant motion," "driven by a motor," and "talks excessively," ADHD children are thought to be deficient in their ability to regulate their activity level to the particular setting or task demands. They tend to be more active, restless, and fidgety than normal children throughout the day and even during sleep. In addition to heightened motor activity, ADHD children are characterized by excessive speech and commentary. Hyperactivity tends to be the most socially problematic feature for children with ADHD because it tends to be disruptive in situations such as the classroom.

3. Impulsivity, or behavioral disinhibition, is also socially problematic for ADHD children, especially in situations in which cooperation, sharing, and restraint with peers is required. Clinically, these children appear to respond quickly to situations without waiting for instructions or considering consequences. They are characterized by poor delay of gratification, poor behavioral inhibition, and high risk-taking behavior.

B. Other core features

1. Difficulty with rule-governed behavior may be another primary deficit of children with ADHD. Failing to follow through with instructions or to comply with rules is a common problem for ADHD children, particularly in situations in which directions are not repeated or when there is no adult present. ADHD children do not necessarily refuse to follow rules and directions; it is more a problem of behavioral self-regulation, or sustaining response to rules or commands.

2. Children with ADHD also tend to show high variability in task performance. While all children display a certain amount of behavioral inconsistency, children with ADHD exhibit this fluctuation to a much greater degree.

C. ADHD tends to be associated with a variety of other problems in addition to the primary features of inattention, hyperactivity, and impulsivity.

1. Children with ADHD often experience behavior problems such as noncompliance, argumentativeness, and temper outbursts.

2. Emotional functioning tends to be impaired in children with ADHD, including low self-esteem, reduced tolerance for frustration, and symptoms of depression or anxiety (or both).

3. Academic performance and cognitive and language abilities represent other areas of difficulty for these children. They are typically underachievers in school and frequently exhibit learning disabilities and language problems. (SOR **B**) As a whole, children with ADHD score lower on standardized intelligence tests as compared to normal controls and exhibit more difficulty on complex problem solving tasks.

4. Children with ADHD tend to experience medical and health problems more commonly than normal controls. These include physical injuries, minor physical anomalies, sleep disturbances, and ear and respiratory infections. (SOR **B**)

D. DSM-IV-TR criteria for ADHD require that six or more symptoms of inattention, hyperactivity–impulsivity, or both are present for at least 6 months, and that the symptoms are severe, maladaptive, and inconsistent with the child's developmental level. By definition, some symptoms must have been present before the age of 7 years. Additionally, symptoms must be present in two or more settings and result in clinically significant impairment in social, academic, or occupational functioning. The symptoms should not be better accounted for by another mental disorder.

1. Inattention

   a. Often fails to give close attention to details or makes careless mistakes in schoolwork, work, or other activities.

   b. Often has difficulty in sustaining attention in tasks or play activities.

    c. Often does not seem to listen when spoken to directly.

    d. Often does not follow through on instructions and fails to finish schoolwork, chores, or duties in the workplace (not because of oppositional behavior or failure to understand instructions).

    e. Often has difficulty organizing tasks and activities.

    f. Often avoids, dislikes, or is reluctant to engage in tasks that require sustained mental effort (such as schoolwork or homework).

    g. Often loses things necessary for tasks or activities (e.g., toys, school assignments, pencils, books, or tools).

    h. Is often easily distracted by extraneous stimuli.

    i. Is often forgetful in daily activities.

2. Hyperactivity–impulsivity

    a. Often fidgets with hands or feet or squirms in seat.

    b. Often leaves seat in classroom or in other situations in which remaining seated is expected.

    c. Often runs about or climbs excessively in situations in which it is inappropriate (in adolescents or adults, may be limited to subjective feelings of restlessness).

    d. Often has difficulty in playing or engaging in leisure activities quietly.

    e. Is often "on the go" or often acts as if "driven by a motor."

    f. Often talks excessively.

    g. Often blurts out answers before questions have been completed.

    h. Often has difficulty in awaiting his or her turn.

    i. Often interrupts or intrudes on others (e.g., butts into conversations or games).

E. The DSM-IV-TR describes three different subtypes: predominantly inattentive, predominantly hyperactive/impulsive, or combined.

    1. ADHD, **combined type** represents the most common diagnosis of the three subtypes, accounting for 50% to 75% of ADHD individuals. Youths with the combined type have features of both inattention and hyperactivity-impulsivity; they also exhibit more co-occurring psychiatric and substance abuse disorders and are the most impaired overall compared to the other subtypes. Children with this subtype are commonly diagnosed at 6 to 7 years of age when symptoms of hyperactivity and impulsivity begin to peak.

    2. The **predominantly inattentive subtype** is the next most common group, accounting for 20% to 30% of individuals with ADHD. Symptoms of inattention are present without associated hyperactivity and impulsivity. This diagnosis is often made somewhat later, at the age of 9 or 10 years, when symptoms of inattention typically become more noticeable. In fact, in the DSM-IV field trials, only 57% of the inattentive type became symptomatic before age 7. Compared with the other subtypes, individuals with predominant inattention are more likely to be female and have fewer other emotional and behavioral problems. However, they tend to have greater academic impairment than those with only hyperactivity/impulsivity.

    3. ADHD, **predominantly hyperactive-impulsive type** accounts for <15% of ADHD diagnoses and describes a subset of individuals with symptoms of hyperactivity and impulsivity without the inattention. Children with this subtype are also often diagnosed at approximately 6 to 7 years of age.

F. Limitations of DSM-IV criteria

    1. A major difficulty with the criteria is that they are most applicable to children between the ages of 7 and 12. Applying the criteria to young children, adolescents, and adults can be problematic since inattention, hyperactivity, and impulsivity are exhibited differently across the lifespan.

    2. There is little evidence supporting the requirement of six symptoms for a diagnosis. Authors have suggested that developmentally sensitive criteria would require more than six symptoms to be present for a diagnosis in preschool, and fewer symptoms (e.g., four) for a diagnosis in adolescence and adulthood. (SOR **C**)

    3. Determining whether symptoms are present in two or more settings is often difficult because of different interpretations of behavioral characteristics by different observers. Inter-rater agreement coefficients for behavior ratings between parents and teachers, for example, are often <0.50. (SOR **A**) Ratings between parents differ as well, with coefficients typically <0.6 or 0.7.

    4. The diagnostic process is heavily weighted toward meeting a specified number of symptoms with far less attention paid to the degree of functional impairment. As a result, patients demonstrating long-standing, pervasive inattention and

distractibility that substantially impairs social and work relationships, but no other symptoms, would not, by DSM-IV standards, receive the diagnosis.

5. Finally, the symptoms of ADHD overlap with many other disorders, making it often difficult to determine whether symptoms of other disorders are mimicking ADHD or comorbid with ADHD.

G. **Epidemiology.** ADHD is among the leading reasons school-age children in the United States are referred to mental health practitioners. As one of the most widespread childhood psychiatric disorders, the rate of ADHD in the general population is estimated to be 9% of males and 3% females. (SOR **B**) Rates vary, however, depending on the population studied, the geographic region under investigation, the definition of ADHD employed, and the degree of agreement required among parents, teachers, and professionals. In fact, prevalence estimates range from between 1% and 20% depending on these factors.

1. ADHD occurs two to four times more commonly in boys than girls for the predominantly inattentive and predominantly hyperactive-impulsive subtypes, respectively. (SOR **A**) In clinical populations, the ratio of males to females is estimated to be as high as 9:1 because of referral biases.

2. Based on current childhood rates, it appears that between 2% and 10% of the adult population experiences ADHD symptoms.

3. Rates of ADHD appear to vary as a function of socioeconomic status (SES), with women from lower-SES groups having a slightly higher incidence of ADHD in their offspring.

H. **Variations in symptom presentation through the lifespan.** Symptoms of inattention, hyperactivity, and impulsivity peak at different ages, decline with age at different rates, and manifest differently depending on the individual's level of development. As a result, ADHD presents differently from preschool through adulthood.

1. **Preschool.** Many children begin to exhibit symptoms of ADHD in preschool, as early as 3 to 4 years of age. However, it is often difficult to differentiate ADHD in preschool children from other discipline problems at this age; some children have simply never learned limits, rules of behavior, or empathy. Preschool children with ADHD tend to show predominantly features of hyperactivity and impulsivity. Symptoms of inattention tend to peak several years later and are less apparent during the preschool years.

2. **Late childhood/adolescence.** By adolescence, features of hyperactivity have declined steadily while symptoms of inattention and impulsivity continue to be problematic. Individuals with the predominantly inattentive subtype may have only recently been diagnosed with ADHD because of the later symptom expression. Comorbidity increases dramatically in adolescents with ADHD, to the extent that "pure" ADHD may be the exception rather than the rule by this age. (SOR **B**) Problems that tend to be associated with ADHD include poor academic performance, affective disorders, school suspensions, expulsions, cigarette and alcohol use, illicit drug use, aggressive behavior, and conduct problems. Adolescents with ADHD who are untreated, poorly supervised, and in an environment in which alcohol and other illicit substances are readily available appear to be at highest risk for negative outcome. (SOR **C**)

3. **Adults.** The symptom picture is likely to be more subtle in adults than in children. Deficits in executive function tend to be most salient, including poor organization, poor time management, and memory disturbance, which can be associated with academic and occupational failure. The "hyperactivity" of childhood may be replaced by experiences of restlessness, difficulty relaxing, and feeling chronically "on edge." Patients with impulsivity, or behavioral disinhibition, may be unable to prevent immediate responding and have deficits in their capacity for monitoring their behavior and modulating emotional intensity.

I. **Differential diagnosis**

1. **Medical conditions.** While psychiatric conditions are more common differential diagnoses, some medical conditions may present with ADHD-like symptoms. Vision and hearing should be routinely screened among children. Elevated lead levels may be associated with cognitive impairment and hyperactivity. An audiologic condition that may appear similar to the inattentive subtype of ADHD-inattentive type is auditory processing disorder (APD). **APD,** typically diagnosed by audiologists, is a deficit in comprehending or tracking information presented through auditory channels despite normal hearing. APD may arise from deficits in underlying functions such as auditory discrimination, pattern recognition, and management of competing input. Cognitive deficits may also be attributable to mental retardation and fetal alcohol or drug syndrome.

Thyroid disturbance may affect activity and secondarily, attention, and concentration. Cognition and motor activity may also be altered pharmacologically. For example, anabolic steroids commonly used by athletes are associated with impulsive aggression while the anticonvulsant, phenytoin, often results in cognitive inefficiency. Seizure disorders, particularly convulsive status epilepticus, produce cognitive impairment similar to the inattention seen in ADHD. Among adolescents and adults, obstructive sleep apnea may impair attention, concentration, and short-term recall. Adults with other sleep disorders such as narcolepsy and idiopathic hypersomnia commonly report impaired attention. Further complicating the picture is that children and adults with ADHD have a particularly high incidence of sleep disorders.

2. **Psychiatric conditions.** Many pediatric and adult psychiatric conditions feature impulsivity and impaired attention, concentration, and short-term memory as commonly associated symptoms. The diagnosis of ADHD is complicated by conditions appearing similar to ADHD that also are part of the differential diagnosis. These psychiatric disorders are challenging because they are often comorbid with ADHD. Pediatric and adult patients will be discussed separately.

   a. **Pediatric conditions.** Table 90–1 summarizes common psychiatric conditions that are part of the differential diagnosis of childhood ADHD, including features shared with ADHD as well as distinguishing symptoms.

      Childhood ADHD is a risk factor for developing other psychiatric conditions. More than 40% of children with ADHD have at least one other disorder, with approximately 30% having two comorbid psychiatric conditions. (SOR **B**) Developmentally, rates of comorbidity increase with age. For example, up to half of ADHD adolescents may also have oppositional-defiant disorder.

   b. **Adult conditions.** While the differential diagnosis of adult ADHD includes some of the same conditions as in childhood, symptoms of both ADHD and other psychiatric syndromes vary with age. Adult ADHD symptoms are more subtle than those in children. While some ADHD adults will have an established diagnosis from early childhood, many patients will be seeking assistance for the first time as adults. Up to two-thirds of adults self-referred for inattention, distractibility, and impulsivity actually have a different primary psychiatric condition (SOR **C**) (Table 90–2.).

J. **Process of diagnosis in primary care** (Table 90–3)

   1. **Thorough diagnostic interview.** Parents should be encouraged to describe their concerns about their child in an open-ended manner. Physicians should carefully listen for core symptoms of ADHD versus those of other psychiatric conditions. Examples of specific behavior concerns should be elicited. The duration and degree of functional impairment should also be assessed. To meet DSM-IV criteria, the patient should be exhibiting significant deficits in at least two life domains (school, work, and family relationships). Parents should be asked when they initially noticed symptoms. Fluctuation or variability in symptoms according to time of day or setting should also be noted. A detailed developmental history is also important, with particular attention to specific milestones and the initial appearance and course of ADHD symptoms.

   2. **Medical history and physical examination.** A history of ADHD symptoms in all biological relatives should be elicited. During the physical examination, the physician may

TABLE 90–1. DIFFERENTIAL DIAGNOSIS OF PEDIATRIC ADHD

Condition	Commonly Shared Features	Distinctive Features
Conduct disorder	Disruptive, impulsive behavior	Severe rule violations; illegal acts; significant aggression
Oppositional-defiant disorder	Disruptive behavior annoying to others; noncompliant with adult requests	Argumentative; negativistic; irritable
Learning disabilities	Poor academic performance; may appear off task in classroom.	Academic skills significantly below level expected for IQ.
Major depression	Impaired attention and concentration; initial insomnia	Hypersomnia/terminal insomnia; appetite/weight disturbance; pervasive dysphoric/irritable mood; suicidal ideation
Bipolar disorder	High activity level; distractability cyclic mood variation	Delusions, pronounced insomnia, widely fluctuating mood

TABLE 90–2. DIFFERENTIAL DIAGNOSIS OF ADULT ADHD

Condition	Commonly Shared Features	Distinctive Features
Major depression	Subjective report of poor concentration, attention, and memory (often not supported by objective data); difficulty with task completion	Enduring dysphoric mood or anhedonia; sleep and appetite disturbance
Bipolar disorder	Hyperactivity, difficulty with maintaining attention; distractibility	Enduring dysphoric or euphoric mood; insomnia; delusions
General anxiety	Fidgetiness; difficulty concentrating	Exaggerated apprehension and worry; somatic symptoms of anxiety
Substance abuse or dependence	Difficulties with attention, concentration, and memory; mood swings	Pathologic pattern of substance use with social consequences; physiologic and psychologic tolerance and withdrawal
Personality disorders, particularly borderline and antisocial personality	Impulsivity; affective lability	Arrest history (antisocial personality); repeated self-injurious or suicidal behavior (borderline personality); lack of recognition that behavior is self-defeating

(Data adapted from Searight HR, Burke JM, Rottnek F. Adult AD/HD: Evaluation and treatment in family medicine. *Am Fam Physician*. 2000;62:2077, 2091.)

note multiple scars and abrasions among ADHD children because of their impulsivity. Histories of prematurity and otitis appear to be risk factors for developing AD/HD.

3. **Laboratory tests.** Blood chemistry should be obtained with particular attention to abnormal thyroid function and elevated serum lead levels. While most ADHD children do not exhibit abnormal laboratory values, these tests can exclude other causes of symptoms.

4. **Behavioral rating forms.** Standardized behavioral rating forms should be given to the parents and teachers to complete. Commonly used pediatric scales are classified into broad-band measures, assessing a number of psychiatric conditions, versus narrow-band instruments, assessing only externalizing behavioral problems such as ADHD, oppositional-defiant disorder, and conduct disorder. The Child Behavior Check List (CBCL) and the longer Connors Parent and Teacher Rating Scales assess a wide range of psychiatric symptoms. More narrowly focused instruments include the Connors-Short Forms, the Disruptive Behavior Disorder (DBD) Scale, and the NICHQ Vanderbilt Assessment Scale. The Vanderbilt Scale is included in the National Initiative for Children's Healthcare Quality (NICHQ) ADHD toolkit and includes depressive symptoms along with externalizing behaviors.

With adults, the Brown, the Connors Adult ADHD Rating (CAARS), and the Adult Self Report Scale (ASRS-v1.1) are used to assess current symptoms. Both the CAARS and the Brown scales are self-report measures, but can also be administered to a collateral informant such as a spouse, parent, or close friend. The Brown Scale is based on five dimensions: organization/activation, attention and concentration, sustained energy and effort, management of emotionality, and working memory/access to previously learned material. The CAARS assesses hyperactivity, impulsivity, emotional

TABLE 90–3. EVALUATION PROCESS FOR SUSPECTED ADHD

Typically at initial office visit
1. Diagnostic interview
2. Medical history and physical examination
3. Any indicated laboratory tests
4. Behavioral rating forms to teachers, parents, other collateral informants, and with adults, to patients themselves
5. Review of behavior ratings and other relevant documents (e.g., report cards)

Typically at follow-up office visit
6. Mental status evaluation (possible continuous performance testing)
7. If indicated, referral for specialized psychological or educational testing
8. If ADHD, institute treatment
9. If other conditions are present, refer for mental health or educational intervention (or both)

lability, attention/memory, and self-concept. The ASRS, developed through the World Health Organization, assesses the 18 DSM-IV-TR AD/HD symptoms. A six-item version, intended for brief screening in primary care, was derived from the items most predictive of an ADHD diagnosis.

In reviewing completed rating scales, the physician should distinguish core symptoms of ADHD such as inattention, distractibility, and impulsivity from other problem behaviors. Extreme ratings—particularly when they suggest significant levels of broadband symptomatology—should be viewed with caution. While these extreme profiles suggest a significant degree of disruptive behavior, they may have limited value in making a specific diagnosis. Comparing teacher and parent ratings may be helpful. Agreement rates are likely to better with narrow- versus broad-band instruments. In general, when parent ratings suggest high levels of perceived problems at home with few symptoms reported at school, a diagnosis of ADHD is less likely. (Sources for scales are provided at the end of the reference section. Most of those instruments are proprietary.)

5. **Office mental status examination.** Brief cognitive screening conducted in the office, focusing on short-term memory and attention and concentration, while not adequate for diagnosis, does provide useful clinical data. Immediate recall and attention may be assessed by orally presenting progressively longer strings of random digits and asking the patient to repeat them. Attention may also be assessed through vigilance tasks such as asking the patient to hold up a finger whenever the physician says the letter "A" in a series of random letters. A slightly more demanding task involving a higher level of concentration and attentional focus is asking patients to repeat digits in reverse order. Both children and adults may be asked to remember four words and queried about their recall at 5, 10, and possibly 15 minutes. Adolescents' and adults' short-term recall may be further assessed by reading them a short paragraph and asking them to verbally present it back to the examiner.

6. **Continuous performance tasks.** There are several computer-based tests of attention, concentration, and ability to manage distractions such as the Gordon Diagnostic System, the Test of Variable Attention (TOVA), and the Conners Continuous Performance Task. These tests are brief and provide a useful source of data that can be obtained in a standard office visit. The computer program typically calculates the number of omission errors—an index of inattention; and commission errors—a measure of impulsivity. While these tests provide useful information, there is no single task that is diagnostic of ADHD.

7. **Diagnosis and referral.** The evaluation process typically leads to one of four outcomes:
   a. **ADHD is not present.** Symptoms are attributable to another medical or psychiatric condition.
   b. **Clear, unequivocal evidence of ADHD.** Pharmacotherapy will likely be initiated.
   c. **Diagnosis of ADHD and a comorbid condition.** The physician initiates pharmacotherapy for ADHD and refers the patient to a mental health provider for further assessment and treatment of comorbid conditions, such as oppositional-defiant disorder or learning disability.
   d. **Diagnosis remains unclear.** In cases of an ambiguous diagnostic picture, the patient may be referred for more in-depth testing. For example, when a learning disability is suspected, the physician may refer the patient to the school district for a psychoeducational evaluation. Concerns about APD would lead to referral to a clinical audiologist. The results of these consultations may lead the physician to exclude ADHD or diagnose ADHD with a comorbid condition or ADHD alone.

III. **Treatment.** The goal of treatment is to decrease the core symptoms of ADHD—inattentiveness, hyperactivity, and impulsiveness—without causing adverse effects.
   A. **Pharmacotherapy** (Table 90–4). Stimulant medications (e.g., methylphenidate [MPH], D-amphetamine, D,L-amphetamine) are first-line pharmacologic agents in conjunction with behavioral techniques, if appropriate. (SOR **C**) If a patient does not respond to stimulant medications or there are contraindications, then alternative nonstimulant medications such as atomoxetine, antidepressants (tricyclics and bupropion), or antihypertensives (clonidine and guanfacine) may be used. (SOR **C**).
      1. **Stimulants** reduce symptoms of hyperactivity, impulsivity, and inattentiveness. Inhibition of dopamine and norepinephrine reuptake is the principle mechanism. Children and adolescents demonstrates a response rate of approximately 70% for a specific

TABLE 90–4. DOSE AND TITRATION OF MEDICATIONS USED IN ADHD

Medication	How Supplied	Usual Initial Dose	Titration Schedule	Maximum Dose/d	Dosage Schedule	Duration	Cost *
Stimulants							
Methylphenidate Preparations							
Short Acting							
Ritalin, Methylin[†]	Tablet: 5, 10, and 20 mg Chewable: 2.5, 5, and 10 mg Oral Solution: 5 mg/5 mL and 10 mg/5 mL	5 mg bid	Increase 5–10 mg weekly	60 mg	bid–tid 30 min before breakfast and lunch; after school, if needed	3–6 h	$ $$ $$$
Focalin[†]	Tablet: 2.5, 5, and 10 mg	2.5 mg bid	Increase 2.5–5 mg weekly	20 mg	bid	4–5 h	$$
Intermediate Acting							
Metadate ER[†]	Tablet: 10, 20 mg	10 mg qd	Increase by 10 mg at weekly intervals	60 mg	qd–bid	5–8 h	$$
Methylin ER[†]	Tablet: 10, 20 mg	10 mg qd	Increase by 10 mg at weekly intervals	60 mg	qd–bid	5–8 h	$$
Ritalin SR[†]	Tablet: 20 mg	20 mg qd	Increase by 20 mg at weekly intervals	60 mg	qd–bid	5–8 h	$$
Metadate CD	Capsule: 10, 20, 30, 40, 50, and 60 mg	20 mg qd	Increase by 10–20 mg at weekly intervals	60 mg	qd	8 h	$$$
Ritalin-LA	Capsule: 10, 20, 30, and 40 mg	20 mg qd	Increase by 10 mg weekly	60 mg	qd	8 h	$$$
Long Acting							
Concerta	Tablet: 18, 27, 36, and 54 mg	6–12 years old: 18 mg qd 13–17 years old: 18 mg qd	Increase by 18 mg weekly	54 mg 72 mg not to exceed 2 mg/kg/d	qd	12 h	$$$
Focalin XR	Capsule: 5, 10, 15, and 20 mg	5 mg qd	5 mg increments weekly	20 mg	qd	8–10 h	$$$
Daytrana	Transdermal Patch: 10, 15, 20, and 30 mg/9 h (in trays of 10 or 30)	10 mg qd	Increase by next patch strength weekly until response is maximized	30 mg	Apply to hip area 2 h before effect is needed, then remove patch 9 h after applying	12 h	$$$$

(Continued)

671

TABLE 90-4. (*Continued*)

Medication	How Supplied	Usual Initial Dose	Titration Schedule	Maximum Dose/d	Dosage Schedule	Duration	Cost *
Amphetamine Preparations							
Short Acting							
Adderall[†] (dextroamphetamine/ amphetamine)	Tablet: 5, 7.5, 10, 12.5, 15, 20, and 30 mg	3–5 years old: 2.5 mg qd ≥ 6years old: 5 mg qd-bid	Increase 2.5 mg weekly Increase 5 mg weekly	40 mg	qd-tid	6–8 h	$$
Dexedrine[†] (dextroamphetamine)	Tablet: 5 mg	2.5 mg bid	Increase 5–10 mg weekly	40 mg	bid-tid	4–6 h	$
DextroStat[†] (dextroamphetamine)	Tablet: 5 and 10 mg	2.5 mg bid	Increase 5–10 mg weekly	40 mg	bid-tid	4–6 h	$
Long Acting							
Adderall XR (dextroamphetamine/ amphetamine)	Capsule: 5, 10, 15, 20, 25, and 30 mg	10 mg qd	Increase 5–10 mg weekly	30 mg	qd	10–12 h	$$$
Dexedrine Spansule[†] (dextroamphetamine)	Capsule: 5, 10, and 15 mg	5 mg qd	Increase 5–10 mg weekly	40 mg	qd-bid	6–10 h	$$
Vyvanse (lisdexamfetamine)	Capsule: 20, 30, 40, 50, 60, and 70 mg	30 mg qd	Increase by 10–20 mg weekly	70 mg	qd	12 h	$$$
Nonstimulant Medications							
Atomoxetine (Strattera)	Capsule: 10, 18, 25, 40, 60, 80, and 100 mg	<70 kg—0.5 mg/kg/d >70 kg—40 mg qd	Increase to 1.2 mg/kg/d after 3 d Increase to 80 mg after 3 d; may increase to 100 mg after 2–4 wk	1.4 mg/kg/d or 100 mg (whichever is less)	qd-bid	24 h	$$$
Bupropion (Wellbutrin)[†, ‡]	IR Tablet: 75 and 100 mg	3 mg/kg or 150 mg, whichever is less	Increase 50 to 100 mg every 7–10 d	6 mg/kg or 300 mg, whichever is less	bid-tid (Separate doses by at least 6 h. No single dose should exceed 150 mg.)		$$
	SR Tablet: 100, 150 and 200 mg						$$
	XL Tablet: 150 and 300 mg				bid (Separate doses by at least 8 h) qd		$$$

Drug	Formulations	Starting dose	Titration	Maximum dose	Dosing schedule	Cost*
Clonidine†,‡ (Catapres)	Tablet: 0.1, 0.2 and 0.3 mg	0.05 mg qd	Increase in increments of 0.05 or 0.1 mg per dose every 3–7 d, usually starting with hs dose	0.3 mg	bid–qid (unless dosing at hs to decrease insomnia)	$
Guanfacine†,‡ (Tenex)	Tablet: 1 and 2 mg	Children: 0.5 mg qd Adolescents: 1 mg qd	Increase every 3 or 4 d in increments of 0.5 to 1 mg until benefit noted	4 mg	qd–qid	$
Imipramine†,‡ (Tofranil)	Tablet: 10, 25, and 50 mg Capsule: 75, 100, and 150 mg	0.5–1 mg/kg/d	Increase every 7–10 d by 10, 20, or 25 mg increments (or 1 mg/kg/wk) until improvement noted	200 mg or 4 mg/kg, whichever is less	bid (to prevent excess sedation)	$
Nortriptyline†,‡ (Pamelor)	Capsule: 10, 25, 50, and 75 mg Oral Solution: 10 mg/5 mL	0.5 mg/kg/d	Increase every 7–10 d by 10, 20, or 25 mg increments (or 1 mg/kg/wk) until improvement noted	100 mg or 2 mg/kg, whichever is less	bid	$$

*Generic cost given when generic formulation is available.
† Generic available.
‡ Non-FDA approved indication.

stimulant, and approximately 90% will respond if a second stimulant is tried. One stimulant agent is not preferred over another, but if a child does not respond to one stimulant medication, then another one may be tried. Currently there is no method to predict which stimulant a patient will respond to best. Providers may use a long-acting version first rather than switching the patient from a short-acting medication to a long-acting version once the dose has been titrated. Long-acting MPH may improve adolescent driving performance compared to short-acting agents. Short-acting stimulants are the preferred treatment in very small children (<16 kg). Since many of the long-acting versions are not yet available in a generic preparation, it may be prudent to confirm which stimulant is formulary to decrease cost issues for the parents or caregivers. The dose may be increased every 1 to 3 weeks. The medication should be titrated until maximum dosage is reached, symptoms of ADHD subside, or unbearable adverse effects occur, whichever occurs first. A positive response to a stimulant is not diagnostic of ADHD since children with comorbid conditions such as narcolepsy and depression may show a positive response as well. Additionally, children and adults without ADHD who ingest stimulants demonstrate improvement in attention, concentration, and memory tasks.

a. **Methylphenidate** preparations are available in various dosages and delivery systems, including a transdermal patch. Immediate release (IR) forms (e.g., Ritalin, Methylin) should be dosed two to three times daily. A third dose may be added after school to help children with homework and after-school activities. Metadate CD and Ritalin LA are extended release (ER) capsules with a bimodal release profile. Metadate CD's capsules contain a mixture of IR and ER beads in a 30:70 ratio; whereas Ritalin LA's capsules are in a 50:50 ratio. Both capsules' contents may be emptied and sprinkled over a spoonful of applesauce. Ritalin SR is composed of a wax matrix that provides a sustained release (SR) of MPH. It is not widely used by clinicians because of its erratic absorption, delayed onset of action, and lower plasma peak concentrations. Concerta is dosed once daily and uses osmotic pressure to deliver MPH at a constant rate. Table 90–5 includes conversions of IR and SR MPH to Ritalin LA, Metadate CD, and Concerta. Daytrana is the first transdermal system introduced for ADHD treatment, and it provides several advantages to oral medications: patients who have difficulty taking oral medications may prefer the patch; caregivers can visually monitor compliance; and therapy can be tailored to the patient—Daytrana provides a constant release of medicine yet can be removed early to minimize adverse effects late in the day. The patch should be placed 2 h before an effect is needed, and it is applied to alternating hips daily for a period of 9 hours. Once removed, the patch continues to deliver medication for approximately three more hours. When switching from another form of MPH to the patch, the same titration schedule should be followed (Table 90–4) as the initial titration because of differences in bioavailability.

TABLE 90–5. **CONVERSION OF IMMEDIATE-RELEASE TO EXTENDED-RELEASE PREPARATIONS**

Previous Methylphenidate (MPH) Dose	Recommended Dose
MPH IR 5 mg bid-tid	Concerta 18 mg qam
MPH-SR 20 mg qd	
MPH IR 10 mg bid-tid	Concerta 36 mg qam
MPH-SR 40 mg qd	
MPH IR 15 mg bid-tid	Concerta 54 mg qam
MPH-SR 60 mg qd	
MPH IR 5 mg bid	Ritalin LA 10 mg qd
MPH IR 10 mg bid	Ritalin LA 20 mg qd
MPH-SR 20 mg qd	
MPH IR 15 mg bid	Ritalin LA 30 mg qd
MPH IR 20 mg bid	Ritalin LA 40 mg qd
MPH-SR 40 mg qd	
MPH IR 30 mg bid	Ritalin LA 60 mg qd
MPH-SR 60 mg qd	
MPH IR 10 mg bid	Metadate CD 20 mg qd
MPH IR 20 mg bid	Metadate CD 40 mg qd

b. **Dexmethylphenidate (Focalin)** is composed of the d-threo-enantiomer of MPH. It is available as an IR and ER formulation. Focalin XR is a 50:50 mixture containing one-half the dose as IR beads and the other one-half as enteric coated, delayed release beads. As with Ritalin LA and Metadate CD, Focalin XR can be sprinkled over applesauce. When converting a patient from MPH to dexmethylphenidate, only one-half of the total daily MPH dose is used (e.g., MPH IR 5 mg bid = dexmethylphenidate 2.5 mg bid.)

c. **D-Amphetamine** is also available in IR and ER forms. It is as effective as MPH, but may be preferred for those who do not tolerate or do not respond to MPH. The IR formulation, Dexedrine and Dextrostat, is dosed two to three times a day, with a third optional dose in late afternoon. Dexedrine Spansule is a SR preparation that lasts for 8 to 10 hours and is consistently absorbed. When switching a patient from MPH to dextroamphetamine, approximately one-half of the MPH total daily dose is used.

d. **D,L-Amphetamine (Adderall)** has a longer half-life than IR MPH, but not as long as the Dexedrine Spansule. Adderall XR is a capsule composed of IR and delayed-release beads in a ratio of 50:50 and may be sprinkled over food.

e. **Lisdexamfetamine (Vyvanse)** is the first stimulant prodrug introduced for the treatment of ADHD. It is pharmacologically inactive until it is absorbed in the gastrointestinal tract where it is converted to D-amphetamine. It was designed to reduce the potential for abuse, overdose toxicity, and drug tampering. The capsule's contents may be opened and dissolved in water for ease in administration.

f. **Adverse effects.** Common adverse effects include anorexia or appetite disturbance, insomnia, headache, and weight loss. Less common side effects include social withdrawal, nervousness, irritability, and tics. In controlled studies, MPH has not been shown to worsen motor tics in patients with comorbid Tourette syndrome and ADHD and has shown no increase in motor tics in children without Tourette syndrome. Studies have shown no conclusive evidence that stimulants suppress growth during treatment or affect ultimate adult height. The transdermal patch can also cause application site irritation. Table 90–6 discusses possible management strategies for adverse effects caused by stimulants.

g. **Contraindications.** Concomitant use of monoamine oxidase (MAO) inhibitors, psychosis, agitation, glaucoma, or history of recent stimulant drug abuse or dependence.

h. **Drug interactions.** Stimulants should not be used in combination with MAO inhibitors because of the risk for developing a hypertensive crisis. The effectiveness of medications to treat hypertension may be decreased while taking stimulants. Methylphenidate and amphetamines may decrease the metabolism of warfarin, anticonvulsants (e.g., phenobarbital, phenytoin), and tricyclic antidepressants (TCAs) (e.g., imipramine, desipramine). The doses of these medications may need to be decreased while given concomitantly with a stimulant. Antacids can alter the release of bimodal release preparations of Metadate CD, Ritalin LA, and Focalin XR by altering gastrointestinal pH.

TABLE 90–6. HOW TO MANAGE ADVERSE EFFECTS OF STIMULANT MEDICATIONS

Adverse Effect	Management
Anorexia	– Bedtime snack – Reduce dose
Dyspepsia	– Take with food
Insomnia	– Add clonidine or diphenhydramine – Eliminate last dose or adjust time last dose of medication given (IR formulations) – Take off patch earlier (Daytrana) – Recommend sleep hygiene protocol – If enuresis, add imipramine
Emotional lability, nervousness, irritability	– Reduce or adjust dose – Switch to another medication
Tics	– Switch to another medication – Add α_2-agonist

i. **Cardiovascular Concerns**. Patients with preexisting structural cardiac abnormalities or other serious heart problems should generally not be prescribed stimulant medication. Sudden death, stroke, and myocardial infarction have been reported in patients taking stimulant drugs for ADHD. Even though a causal relationship has not been established, prescribers should be aware of the risk when prescribing this class of drugs.

j. **Abuse of Stimulants**. Currently all available stimulant medications for ADHD are a schedule II controlled substance. While it is true that these drugs may be abused or diverted, prescription stimulants fail to produce a euphoric sensation via the oral route. Abuse or diversion is more common with IR preparations that can be crushed and snorted rather than with ER forms. Reports have shown that treating ADHD in adolescents actually decreases the risk of substance abuse compared to those not treated for ADHD. Alternatives for prescribers who have patients and/or patient's family members with a history of substance abuse include using the ER formulations, atomoxetine, the MPH patch, or lisdexamfetamine. ER formulations may be used to prevent diversion since it can be taken once daily at home and not taken to school. The transdermal patch has limited abuse potential since it is difficult to extract MPH from the patch and is difficult to reapply a used patch. Lisdexamfetamine is a prodrug that is not therapeutically active until it is metabolized in the body, thus limiting its abuse potential.

k. **Miscellaneous.** When writing a prescription for multiple daily doses, it is helpful to write for a separate labeled bottle that may be taken to school by the child that only has the school dose on it. ER preparations may be used to help increase compliance since many children may be uncomfortable taking a dose at school or may forget the second or third daily doses. When writing a prescription for the transdermal patch during the titration stage, it may be cost-effective to only write for the 10 count tray, if titrating the dose weekly, until a stable dose is reached since some insurance companies may not pay for more than a 1-month supply, even if it is a dose change.

2. **Nonstimulant medications,** such as atomoxetine, antidepressants, and antihypertensives, should be considered when stimulants have failed or patients have contraindications or significant adverse effects to stimulants. Except for atomoxetine, nonstimulant medications usually do not demonstrate benefit for all three core ADHD symptoms—hyperactivity, inattention, or impulsivity. The antidepressants, tricyclics and bupropion, decrease hyperactivity and inattention; however, they do not reduce impulsivity. Antihypertensives, such as the α_2 agonists, are more effective in decreasing impulsivity and hyperactivity than improving inattentiveness. These alternative medications require closer patient monitoring than stimulants, but may be dosed less frequently.

a. **Atomoxetine** is the first nonstimulant medication to be approved by the Food and Drug Administration (FDA) for treatment of both pediatric and adult ADHD. Similar to stimulants, atomoxetine inhibits norepinephrine reuptake. Advantages of atomoxetine include low risk for diversion or abuse; no known adverse effects on tic disorders; and no known long-term effects on growth suppression.

   (1) **Adverse effects.** In clinical trials, decreased appetite, nausea, vomiting, fatigue, dyspepsia, dizziness, and mood swings were the most common adverse effects reported by children and adolescents. In adults, dry mouth, insomnia, nausea, decreased appetite, constipation, erectile disturbances, dysmenorrhea, dizziness, and decreased libido were the most commonly reported adverse effects.

   (2) **Contraindications.** Use with MAO inhibitors or narrow angle glaucoma.

   (3) **Drug interactions.** Atomoxetine is a CYP-2D6 substrate; therefore, its levels may increase when used with CYP-2D6 inhibitors such as fluoxetine and paroxetine. For patients using atomoxetine concomitantly with strong CYP-2D6 inhibitors, atomoxetine should only be increased up to 1.2 mg/kg/d after 4 weeks if the patient weighs <70 kg and only increased to 80 mg/d after 4 weeks if the patient weighs >70 kg. Concomitant use with albuterol can increase heart rate.

   (4) **Cardiovascular Concerns.** As with stimulant medications for ADHD, sudden death has been reported in adults, children, and adolescents with structural cardiac abnormalities or other serious heart problems. In adults, stroke and myocardial infarction have also been reported. In patients with known structural cardiac abnormalities, atomoxetine is generally not recommended. Additionally,

the manufacturer recommends using atomoxetine with caution in patients with hypertension, tachycardia, or cardiovascular or cerebrovascular disease.

(5) Severe Liver Injury. Two reports of severe liver injury have been reported in patients treated with atomoxetine. Based on these reports, the FDA has mandated a bolded warning to be added to the package insert to warn prescribers of the potential danger. The medication should be discontinued in patients who develop jaundice or laboratory evidence of liver injury. Currently routine liver enzyme testing is not recommended.

(6) Suicidal Ideation in Children and Adolescents. In short-term studies, an increased risk of suicidal ideation in children and adolescents was reported. While no suicides occurred, the average risk was 0.4% (5/1397 patients) in patients treated with atomoxetine compared to 0% in placebo-treated patients. Although the number of patients affected was low, physicians, parents, and caregivers should closely monitor patients during the initial months of treatment and after any dose change. Patients and caregivers should report occurrences of agitation, irritability, unusual changes in behavior, and any suicidal ideations to the provider immediately. All events occurred during the first month of treatment and a similar analysis of adult ADHD patients using atomoxetine did not reveal an increased risk of suicidal ideation.

b. Antidepressants

(1) Tricyclic antidepressants inhibit the reuptake of norepinephrine and serotonin. When using TCAs, blood pressure, pulse, complete blood count, electrocardiograms (ECGs), and serum blood levels should be carefully monitored. Desipramine should be used with extreme caution since there have been case reports of sudden cardiac death in young adolescents. While there is no clear explanation for these events, it is recommended that ECGs be performed at initiation of treatment and after each dose increase. Blood pressure should not exceed 130/85 mm Hg and resting pulse should be less than 100 beats per minute. Serum blood levels do not correlate with the therapeutic effect in the treatment of ADHD, but rather with the incidence of adverse effects. Serum levels for depression for imipramine are 180 to 240 ng/mL; for desipramine, 100 to 300 ng/mL; and for nortriptyline, 50 to 150 ng/mL. Routine serum levels to determine efficacy are not recommended, but may be drawn once a stable dose is reached to assess for toxic levels or if adverse effects are noticed.

(a) Adverse effects. Dry mouth, constipation, blurred vision, and sedation. (Nortriptyline is the least sedating of the three, while imipramine is the most sedating.)

(b) Contraindications. Concomitant use with an MAO inhibitor. Use with extreme caution in children with cardiac conduction abnormalities.

(2) Bupropion inhibits the reuptake of dopamine and norepinephrine. Although safety has not been formally established in children younger than 18 years, bupropion has been studied in children and adolescents. Results were better in adolescents than in children. Bupropion appears to be particularly beneficial in adolescents with comorbid psychiatric conditions.

(a) Adverse effects. Nausea, headache, and insomnia.

(b) Contraindications. History of seizure disorder, history of anorexia/bulimia, and concomitant use with MAO inhibitors.

(3) MAO inhibitors, while an effective alternative treatment, are limited by food and drug interactions.

(4) Selective Serotonin Reuptake Inhibitors (SSRIs) have not been found to reduce the symptoms associated with ADHD, but may be used in combination with stimulants to treat comorbid depression.

(5) Venlafaxine possesses both noradrenergic and serotonergic properties. Several studies have shown promising results, but further investigation is needed.

c. Antihypertensives—α_2 agonists, such as **clonidine** and **guanfacine**—can be useful in children not responding to MPH alone, or those with posttraumatic stress disorder or significant aggression. Sedation may limit the use of these drugs, but a bedtime dose of clonidine may be beneficial in children with sleep disturbances. α_2 agonists do not worsen tics, but may be used with a stimulant to help decrease unwanted tics. Guanfacine is preferred by many practitioners over clonidine because of its longer duration of action, possibly fewer sedative effects, and reduced likelihood of inducing hypotension. α_2 agonists should not be used in children with preexisting cardiac or vascular disease without consultation with a cardiologist. Blood pressure and pulse should be measured when initiating therapy, increasing the dose, and periodically while taking the medication. Clonidine and guanfacine should be tapered more than 7 to 14 days to avoid rebound hypertension. Adverse effects include sedation and dry mouth.

B. Discussing pharmacotherapy with patients

1. Listen to the parents' concerns and dispel any myths. Reassure parents that the child will not become addicted to the stimulant medication, final adult height will not be affected, and that stimulant safety and efficacy have been demonstrated in numerous studies and years of clinical practice. Set realistic behavioral goals with the parent and child. Emphasize the benefits of treatment, such as decreased hyperactivity, improved concentration, impulse control, and decreased disruptive behavior. Educate the parents about the potential consequences of untreated ADHD, such as poor school performance, grade retention, relationship difficulty, and increased risk of adolescent substance use, psychiatric disorders (major depression and personality disorders), traffic violations, and delinquency. (SOR **B**)

2. Educating the parents about the most common adverse effects of stimulants such as appetite suppression (with weight loss), sleep difficulties, rebound moodiness, and irritability will reduce their anxiety if these symptoms occur. Parents should periodically assess their child's nutritional status. It may be helpful to have the child eat breakfast before taking their morning dose. Children who eat little at lunch will usually eat a hearty snack in the afternoon as their medication is wearing off. Difficulty falling asleep may be addressed by delaying the child's bedtime to after 9 PM or adding a sedating medication such as clonidine. Recent research suggests that ADHD children fall asleep more quickly when a sleep hygiene protocol is implemented. (SOR **B**) Rebound moodiness and irritability may occur for approximately 30 to 60 minutes as the medication is wearing off. Adding a small, short-acting dose immediately after school or allowing the child some quiet time before beginning homework may help alleviate these symptoms.

3. Between 50% and 75% of individuals diagnosed with ADHD as a child will continue to have symptoms persisting into adulthood. As in other chronic health conditions, pharmacotherapy may be lifelong.

4. Although drug holidays have been advocated in the past, many children will require drug therapy year-round to maintain attention and decrease hyperactivity—symptoms that frequently disrupt family, recreational, and social activities.

5. Children who have been responding well to medication treatment for many months may return to the physician with complaints by parents and teachers that the medication is no longer "working." While adjustments of medication dosages may be indicated, other causes should be considered. The physician should very specifically inquire about the types of behavior that are of concern. Issues such as lying, talking back, and angry outbursts may reflect development of comorbid conditions. Adults' point of reference for the ADHD child may have unconsciously shifted over time. Initially, children treated with medication are compared with themselves prior to medication initiation. However, over time this reference point may change and the ADHD child may be implicitly compared to school-aged peers or siblings. Most ADHD children continue to manifest some symptoms of the disorder even when on an optimal regimen of medication. When questions of medication effectiveness arise, a new set of behavioral ratings may clarify the clinical picture.

C. Special issues in pharmacotherapy with adults. Stimulants are effective in adults, but must be used with caution in patients with a history of drug abuse. Even though patients will not become "high" from oral MPH because of its slow release to the brain, patients can become "high" from injecting a liquid form of MPH. This "high" is similar to that of cocaine. For adults who do not respond to stimulants or have contraindications for their use, bupropion, TCAs, and atomoxetine are suitable alternatives. Bupropion and TCAs are used more often in adults and may be beneficial in patients with comorbid psychiatric conditions.

D. Nonpharmacologic treatment for children and adolescents with ADHD

1. Pharmacotherapy is clearly the treatment of choice for ADHD and is beneficial for the vast majority of patients. In head-to-head comparisons with behavioral therapies, medications yield a greater effect on problem behavior.

2. Nevertheless, two psychosocial treatments have received empirical support: behavioral parent training and behavioral modification in the classroom. They are clearly superior to no-treatment conditions and can be helpful for children with ADHD who cannot tolerate medication or who do not respond well. Additionally, some evidence exists that combining systematic behavior therapy with well-delivered medication can yield better outcomes than medication alone.

   a. **Behavioral parent training** typically involves 8 to 30 sessions in which the therapist guides the parents through a structured behavioral program designed to enhance the parents' understanding of ADHD and of behavioral principles. The therapist teaches the importance of specifying target behaviors, providing consistent and regular rewards for positive behavior, involving teachers in the behavioral plan, and generalizing the skills to a variety of situations.

   b. Clinicians perform **behavioral modification in the classroom** by teaching the regular- or special-education teachers how to implement the behavioral strategies that are taught in parent training (e.g., specific target behaviors and regular rewards), with modifications for classroom settings. Teachers may do any or all of the following: seat the child with ADHD closer to the front of the classroom; encourage attention through prompting; implement a reward system; and complete a daily behavioral report card.

3. Additional psychosocial treatments include psychoeducation, special education services, and child interventions.

   a. **Psychoeducation** provides the child, parents, family, and school with information about ADHD, its treatment, and its impact on learning, behavior, self-esteem, social skills, and family functioning. Educating the family also allows the physician an opportunity to correct misperceptions. For example, the child may feel that s/he is "dumb," or the parents may fear that the child is going to become a "drug addict" as a result of the stimulant medication. Family physicians should inform families of appropriate sources for ADHD information, such as Children and Adults with Attention Deficit/Hyperactivity Disorder (CHADD) (www.chadd.org), The Society for Developmental and Behavioral Pediatrics (www.dbpeds.org/handouts), and the American Academy of Child and Adolescent Psychiatry (AACAP) (www.aacap.org/publications/factsfam/noattent.htm).

   b. **Special education services** are often important in the treatment and monitoring of ADHD symptoms.

     (1) ADHD is included as a disability under the Individuals with Disabilities Education Act (IDEA [PL-101-476]). Therefore, children with ADHD may qualify for special education services or appropriate accommodations within the regular classroom setting under Section 504 of the Rehabilitation Act of 1973. Patients may also be eligible for reasonable accommodations in secular private schools and postsecondary education under The Americans with Disabilities Act.

     (2) Classroom accommodations may include changes in the child's educational programming, such as tutoring, resource room support, extended time to complete tasks, and decreased workload.

   c. Most **child interventions** for ADHD such as social skills training, cognitive behavioral therapy, and study/organizational skills do not have solid empirical support for the treatment of ADHD, and the gains achieved in the treatment setting typically do not transfer into the classroom or home settings. However, child interventions may be indicated when there are comorbid disorders, particularly internalizing symptoms, that are also the focus of treatment. Additionally, computer-aided training of working memory has recently shown promise with parent-reported improvement in attention and hyperactivity maintained at follow-up.

E. **Psychotherapy, organizational skills, and environmental modification for the ADHD adult.** Cognitive-behavioral therapy was recently found to be a beneficial adjunct to medication and improved AD/HD symptoms and global symptom severity to a greater extent than medication alone. (SOR **B**) In addition, these strategies are helpful:

1. To foster **self-management skills**, organizers such as calendars, day planners, and Palm Pilots, when consistently employed may prompt recall and improve personal organizational skills.

2. **Reducing distractions in the workplace** is helpful. For ADHD adults with flexible work times, going into work before most coworkers arrive is valuable. This "quiet time" may help the ADHD adult get organized and accomplish tasks before distractions increase.

Similarly, this strategy of early awakening is also useful in managing a household. The patient's immediate workplace itself should be free of clutter and other distractions such as family photos and personal mementos.

3. For adults in an ongoing relationship, conjoint counseling can address **communication issues** and help educate both spouses about the impact of ADHD in their daily lives. Formal documentation of an ADHD diagnosis is typically required.

4. For adults involved in a formal educational program such as college or professional school, accommodations may be available. Examples include **extended time for tests and the option of taking tests alone** in a special resource room rather than in a traditional classroom with other students.

F. **Complementary and alternative medicines.** Complementary and alternative treatments are used by up to 60% of parents with ADHD children. (SOR **Ⓑ**) Neurofeedback, attention training, progressive relaxation, meditation, iron supplements, diet, homeopathy, herbal medicines, and dietary supplements have all been used in the treatment of ADHD.

1. **Neurofeedback** is believed to improve attentiveness and impulsivity. While it may have some success in reducing symptoms, the long-term effects are not known.

2. **Attention training** often uses laboratory vigilance tasks in which children receive reinforcement for correct responses. While ADHD children demonstrate improvement on laboratory tasks, there has not been consistent evidence of improved attention and reduced hyperactivity in daily functioning.

3. **Progressive relaxation and meditation have demonstrated some benefit for reducing hyperactivity.** (SOR **Ⓒ**) **However, the clinical significance and durability of this improvement has, so far, been limited.**

4. **Iron supplements** are based on the belief that children with ADHD have an iron deficiency. If iron-deficiency is suspected, hematologic testing should be performed; otherwise, routine use of iron supplementation should not be used in nondeficient children.

5. **Diet** for children has been altered in several different ways to attempt to decrease the symptoms of ADHD. Despite popular myths, sugar does not exacerbate or cause hyperactivity. Elimination of food dye from food and drinks has yielded inconclusive evidence.

6. **Homeopathic** treatments such as Cina and Hyoscyamus Niger have been used to decrease symptoms. Despite potential use for these products, additional evaluation is needed to determine efficacy and place in therapy.

7. **Herbal medicines,** such as ginkgo, evening primrose, valerian, lemon balm, and more have been used to decrease symptoms of hyperactivity. Parents should be reminded that herbal medications are not regulated by the FDA and may not contain standardized doses.

8. **Dietary supplements.** There is no evidence to support that ADHD children benefit from megadoses of vitamins.

Until more controlled studies are done to determine efficacy of complementary and alternative treatments, proven pharmacological therapies should remain first line.

IV. **Prognosis.** ADHD is a chronic neurologic condition with many symptoms persisting into adolescence and adulthood in up to 70% of diagnosed children. Developmentally, specific symptoms may change, with marked reductions in hyperactivity and impulsivity beginning at age 9. However, inattention typically persists through adolescence and into adulthood.

The relatively few prospective ADHD studies suggest that adolescents and adults with ADHD histories are at risk for legal problems, traffic accidents, noncompletion of formal education, substance abuse, and other psychiatric disorders. (SOR **Ⓒ**) However, in counseling parents about the prognosis for ADHD children, available ADHD research has several limitations. Diagnostic standards have changed during the past 15 years, with current DSM-IV criteria identifying milder forms of ADHD than previously. These changing diagnostic criteria are likely to be a major factor in recent increased ADHD prevalence rates than previously reported. Adults with ADHD, if diagnosed as children, were likely to have had particularly severe symptoms.

ADHD's longitudinal course is further complicated by increased comorbidity through the lifespan. Comorbidity rises to at least 50% during adolescence and may be as high as 70% in adulthood. A consistent research finding is the particularly poor psychiatric and legal outcomes for ADHD with comorbid conduct disorder.

With these caveats, adolescents with an ADHD history are two to four times more likely to be arrested, two to four times more likely to be diagnosed with antisocial personality, and four times more likely to have nonalcohol substance abuse problems. While severity of substance use is greater for ADHD with comorbid conduct disorder, young adults with ADHD alone are more likely than non-ADHD controls to smoke cigarettes. Primary care risk counseling should be particularly thorough with ADHD teenagers.

Among adults, an ADHD history is associated with a greater likelihood of receiving both inpatient and outpatient psychiatric treatment. These adults are more likely to be fired from or quit jobs and have lower SES than non-ADHD adults. ADHD is also a risk factor for relationship conflict, including separation and divorce.

While data are scarce, ADHD treatment during childhood appears to reduce the incidence of later adverse outcomes. A common parental fear is that stimulant pharmacotherapy during childhood may lead to substance abuse. A recent meta-analysis concluded that stimulant treatment actually protected against later adolescent and young adult drug and alcohol abuse.

REFERENCES

Biederman J. Practical considerations in stimulant drug selection for the attention-deficit/hyperactivity disorder patient—efficacy, potency and titration. *Today's Therapeutic Trend.* 2002;20(4):311-328.

Biederman J, Mick E, Faraone SV. Age-dependent decline of symptoms of attention-deficit/hyperactivity disorder. Impact of remission definition and symptom type. *Am J Psychiatry.* 2000;157:816-818.

Clinical Practice Guideline. Treatment of school-aged child with attention-deficit/hyperactivity disorder. *Pediatrics.* 2001;108(4):1033-1044.

Greydanus DE, Sloan MA, Rappley MD. Psychopharmacology of ADHD in adolescents. *Adolesc Med.* 2002;13(3):599-624.

Nass RD. Evaluation and assessment issues in the diagnosis of attention deficit hyperactivity disorder. *Semin Pediatr Neurol.* 2005;12:200-216.

Osterloo M, Lammers GJ, Overeem S, de Noord I, Kooij S. Possible confusion between primary hypersomnia and adult attention-deficit/hyperactivity disorder. *Psychiatry Res.* 2006;143:293-297.

Pliszka S. Practice parameter for the assessment and treatment of children and adolescents with attention-deficit/hyperactivity disorder. *J Am Acad Child Adolesc Psychiatry.* 2007;46(7):894-921.

Rickel AU, Brown RT. *Attention-Deficit Hyperactivity Disorder in Children and Adults.* Cambridge, MA: Hogrefe & Huber; 2007.

Spencer TJ, Biederman J, Mick E. Attention-deficit/hyperactivity disorder: Diagnosis, lifespan, comorbidities, and neurobiology. *Ambulat. Pediatr.* 2007;7:73-81.

Voeller KKS. Attention-deficit/hyperactivity disorder (ADHD). *J Child Neurol.* 2004;19(10):798-814.

Weiss MD, Wadell MB, Bomben MM, Rea KJ, Freeman RD. Sleep hygiene and melatonin treatment for children and adolescents with ADHD and initial insomnia. *J Am Acad Child Adolesc Psychiatry.* 2006;45:512-519.

Wilens TE, Faraone SV, Binderman J, Gunawardene S. Does stimulant therapy of attention-deficit/hyperactivity disorder beget later substance abuse? A meta-analytic review of the literature. *Pediatrics.* 2003;111:179-185.

SOURCES FOR RATING SCALES

Achenbach System of Empirically Based Assessment. www.aseba.org. Accessed August 12, 2008.

Adult Self Report Scale (ASRS v1.1). http://www.med.nyu.edu/psych/assets/adhdscreen18.pdf. Accessed October 10, 2008.

Brown Attention Deficit—Disorder Scales for Adolescents and Adults. http://pearsonassess.com. Accessed October 10, 2008.

Child Behavior Checklist (CBCL). www.aseba.org. Accessed October 10, 2008.

Conners Rating Scales. Revised http://www.pearsonassessments.com/tests/crs-r.htm. Accessed October 10, 2008.

Disruptive Behavior Disorders Rating Scale. Comprehensive Treatment for Attention Deficit Disorder. http://ccf.buffalo.edu/pdf/DBD_rating_scale.pdf. Accessed October 10, 2008.

National Initiative for Children's Healthcare Quality. Vanderbilt Parent and Teacher Scales. American Academy of Pediatrics. http://www.ncpeds.com/ADHD/05.pdf. Accessed October 10, 2008.

91   Family Violence: Child, Intimate Partner, & Elder Abuse

F. David Schneider, MD, MSPH, Nancy D. Kellogg, MD, &
Melissa A. Talamantes, MS

KEY POINTS

- Know the laws in your state regarding mandatory reporting of family violence, including child abuse, intimate partner violence (IPV), and elder abuse. Most states have mandatory reporting laws for both those younger than 18 years and older than 64 years.
- Ask about family violence as a routine part of your history taking. This gives patients permission to talk about it when they feel comfortable.
- Assess the situation for lethality—use of guns or knives by the perpetrator or escalating violence may require immediate intervention by police.
- Learn about your community resources for support of victims of family violence, and use them when appropriate with your patients.

I. Child Abuse and Neglect

A. Introduction

1. Definitions

a. **Child physical abuse** is any intentional injury resulting in tissue damage, including bruises, burns, lacerations, fractures, and organ or blood vessel rupture. In addition, any inflicted injury that lasts more than 24 hours constitutes significant injury. Physical abuse comprises approximately 25% of the four types of abuse and neglect.

b. **Child sexual abuse** encompasses a variety of interactions that adults or adolescents use to take advantage of vulnerable children in a sexual manner, including both sexual contact and exploitation for pornography or prostitution. Another form of sexual abuse involves solicitation through the computer; almost one in five children who go "online" regularly is approached by strangers for sex. Approximately 15% of abuse and neglect is sexual abuse.

c. **Neglect** is the inadequate nutrition, shelter, or care (or all of these) necessary to meet the basic needs of a child, allowing him to grow and develop. Medical neglect occurs when the caretaker ignores important medical or dental treatment plans. Neglect is most common of the four types and comprises 50% of the total.

d. **Emotional abuse** includes rejecting a child's worth or needs, constant berating or belittlement, or making the child engage in destructive behavior. While accounting for 10% of all types, emotional abuse commonly accompanies physical abuse, sexual abuse, and neglect.

2. Epidemiology

There are more than 3.5 million reported cases of child abuse and neglect in United States annually; 2000 to 4000 children die of abuse or neglect each year. Eighty percent of child abuse fatalities occur in children younger than 5 years, and 40% occur during a child's first year of life. Neglect most often involves preverbal children, whereas sexual abuse is reported during school-age and adolescent years. Despite large numbers of reported cases, child abuse and neglect remains an under-detected and under-reported problem. It has been estimated that 20% of children will sustain an abusive injury during childhood, and 14% to 40% of females will be sexually abused before reaching adulthood.

B. Diagnosis

1. Barriers to diagnosis

Since child abuse only recently became a recognized subspecialty of Pediatrics, many physicians lack the knowledge and training to recognize the signs and symptoms of abuse and neglect. Detection is also compromised by the following: the child or family may attribute injuries to discipline rather than abuse; physicians typically rely on a caretaker's history, which may be untruthful if abuse has occurred; victims may be preverbal and unable to provide important information; verbal victims may be reluctant to disclose

TABLE 91–1. INJURIES (BRUISES, BURNS, AND FRACTURES) THAT SHOULD BE CAREFULLY EVALUATED FOR PHYSICAL ABUSE

1. Age 0–6 mo: *Any injury.*
2. Age 6 mo or older:
   a. Bruises, lacerations, or burns to protected, fleshy, or flexor surfaces—*for example,* inner thighs, abdomen, neck, face (other than frontal prominence), pinna, and genitalia.
   b. Bruises, lacerations, or burns showing an object pattern—*for example,* belt loop, cigarette burn, and curling iron.
   c. Oral injuries, *especially* frenulum and palate lacerations.
   d. Third-degree burns or large second-degree burns, *especially* scald burns.
   e. Fractures, *especially* metaphyseal fractures, complex or wide skull fractures, rib fractures, spiral fractures of humerus or femur, and scapula fractures.
   f. Significant head injury, *especially* subdural hematoma, retinal hemorrhage, subgaleal hematoma, avulsed hair, complex, or wide skull fracture. Head injury should be considered whenever a child presents with vomiting or altered consciousness, or bloody spinal fluid is found on lumbar puncture, but an infectious process cannot be readily diagnosed.
   g. Intra-abdominal injury, *especially* rupture or hematoma of internal organ.
3. Age 0–10 y: Positive urine or blood screen for alcohol or drugs of abuse.

Findings that should be carefully evaluated for *sexual abuse:*
1. Any injury to the genitalia (*especially* to the hymen or vestibule in girls) or anus.
2. Identification of an STD: Chlamydia, gonorrhea, HSV, HPV, HIV, HBV, HCV, *Trichomonas,* syphilis.
3. Positive pregnancy test.
4. Any history or statement or witnessed incident consistent with sexual abuse.

Findings that should be carefully evaluated for *neglect*:
1. Growth parameters below expected for age.
2. Lack of medical care for a significant health problem—*for example,* no medications for asthma, diabetes; no care for severe dental caries.
3. Lack of normal bonding with parent/guardian.
4. Disregard of one or more basic child care needs—*for example,* soft drink in baby bottle, child found in street, failure to place child in auto safety seat or belt.

Note: A child may have findings suggesting more than one form of abuse or neglect.
HBV, hepatitis B virus; HCV, hepatitis C virus; HIV, human immunodeficiency virus; HPV, human papilloma virus; HSV, herpes simplex virus; STD, sexually transmitted disease.
(Excerpted with permission from the Texas Pediatric Society Committee on Child Abuse. Clinical Practice Resource for Hospitals and Emergency Departments.)

abuse out of fear, guilt, or shame; and injuries may be old, indistinct, or nonexistent. In addition, the physician must have an index of suspicion to make the diagnosis.

2. **Physical abuse**
   The diagnosis of physical abuse and neglect typically begins with "what you see." Bruises are the most common manifestation of physical abuse, yet most bruises of childhood are accidental rather than inflicted. Patterned bruises, and location of bruises (such as buttocks, neck, and side of face) help distinguish nonaccidental from accidental causes. In addition, any unexplained injury in a younger child is suspicious for abuse; as one study suggests, "if you don't cruise (developmental milestone achieved around 8 months of age), you don't bruise." Table 91–1 lists injuries and conditions that are suspicious for abuse and neglect.
   a. **Explanation consistency.** Once a suspicious injury or condition is identified, the physician must establish whether the explanation is consistent with the characteristics of the injury or condition. Vague or no explanation for a severe injury is suspicious for nonaccidental trauma or criminal neglect. An explanation that is inconsistent with the severity, age, or pattern of the injury(s) constitutes a suspicion of abuse. The physician should listen carefully and respectfully to the caretaker's statements, maintain a nonjudgmental demeanor, and document all explanations, including discrepancies. Caretakers should be interviewed separately, gathering detailed information about the child's injury, developmental capabilities, food intake, and behavior and activity prior to the injury or deterioration in condition. If the child is 4 years or older, the physician may question the child out of the presence of the parent. The physician must remain unbiased, and ask questions that are not leading or suggestive. For example, "What happened to your arm?" is preferable

to "Who hurt your arm?" or "Did Daddy hurt you?" Physicians should remain emotionally neutral, and strive to earn, not assume, the child's trust. Physicians should also refrain from making statements to family members about the probability of abuse or neglect since further investigation or referral to child abuse specialists may alter the final diagnosis.

    b. Tests. Serious injuries warrant further laboratory and radiologic testing to rule out coagulopathies, bone disorders, and other conditions that may mimic abuse and to assess for additional occult liver (liver function tests), bone (skeletal survey), and intracranial (magnetic resonance imaging or computerized tomography of the head) injuries. In addition, a dilated ophthalmologic examination is indicated to look for retinal hemorrhages, which may be attributable to abusive head trauma. When abuse is strongly suspected in a child younger than 4 years, a repeat skeletal survey 2 weeks after the initial evaluation is recommended. In evaluating suspected nutritional neglect, complete electrolyte and hematologic profiles may establish the severity and chronicity of malnutrition, but a comprehensive history, including social and family factors, will establish the diagnosis in most cases.

3. Sexual and emotional abuse

These forms of abuse begin with "what you hear." More than 90% of child sexual abuse is first discovered when the child tells someone about the abuse. Emotional abuse is typically detected when a child's behavioral or emotional state causes concern and questioning confirms the diagnosis. The diagnosis of sexual abuse is based on the history from the child. Forensic evidence, genital or anal injury, and sexually transmitted diseases are each detected in fewer than 15% of sexual abuse or assault victims. When forensic evidence is gathered, approximately 25% of such kits will yield useful evidence; however, a minority (fewer than one-third) of children present within 72 hours of their assault, the time frame within which such evidence is recoverable. Injuries due to acute sexual assault occur less than 25% of the time and are most likely to heal completely within a week. While most examinations are normal, "normal" does not mean "nothing happened." One study of 36 pregnant adolescents found that 82% had normal hymens. Documentation of the child's history, preferably in quotes, is critically important, and may be read during civil or criminal court proceedings. In addition, photo-documentation of physical or sexual abuse injuries, as well as visible signs of neglect, is a standard of care for abuse evaluations.

C. Treatment strategies and intervention

Once a physician has established that the child may have been abused, laws in all 50 states require that the physician report to Child Protective Services or law enforcement. Centralized or local reporting procedures are established in each state. The physician is not required to prove that abuse has occurred to report; failure to report suspected abuse is a criminal offense. The decision to inform the family of reporting depends on whether sharing such information could potentially jeopardize the child's safety until reporting agencies can intervene.

    Many areas have established specialized child abuse assessment programs that include trained medical professionals. A primary care physician may opt to conduct a limited medical assessment once abuse is suspected and refer such cases to specialized child abuse programs, when available. Children's Advocacy Centers and Sexual Assault Nurse Examiner programs are found in most states and can provide assistance to physicians regarding resources, services, and assessments for abused children.

D. Prognosis

Abused children are at greater risk for psychiatric disorders, learning disabilities, eating disorders, and low school functioning. Abused and neglected children are also more likely to become teenage mothers, substance abusers, runaways, and delinquents. Affective, anxiety, and personality disorders often persist into adulthood. Obesity, posttraumatic stress disorder, and chronic pelvic pain are frequently seen in adult survivors of child sexual abuse. Child abuse and neglect clearly compromise children's abilities to become productive, healthy members of society.

    Without effective intervention, child abuse becomes an intergenerational cycle. An abused child is more likely to become an abuser, an adult partner of a child abuser, or an abused adult.

II. Intimate Partner Violence

  A. Definition

Wife or spouse abuse is often used interchangeably with *domestic violence* or **intimate partner violence (IPV)**. IPV is used more often today because it is more inclusive of all kinds of intimate relationships, including dating, sex partners, and same-sex relationships. IPV includes verbal harassment or threats, sexual assault, financial or physical isolation of the victim, and physical attacks. The battering syndrome, which includes all of these forms of abusive behavior, is used to gain control of the victim's behavior. Examples of these forms of abuse include:

1. Verbal abuse
Verbal abuse ranges from repeated insults or insinuations up to threats to hurt or kill the victim or loved ones.

2. Sexual assault
Sexual assault is any form of nonconsensual sexual activity, it occurs in approximately 35% to 40% of battered women.

3. Physical abuse
Physical abuse includes harming an intimate partner by punching, kicking, choking, use of a knife or a gun, or any other method.

B. Epidemiology
A minimum of 2 to 4 million women are abused annually by their male partners. More than 1.8 million of these women are seriously assaulted. The abuse can become lethal; domestic violence causes one-third of the female murders in the United States. Ninety percent of these cases are the result of males' violently assaulting their female partners. Although mutual battering exists, studies have shown that men are more likely than women to perform more severe acts of violence. Men who admit to acts of violence often cite a desire to control or alter their victim's behavior. On the other hand, women who admit to violence indicate that they are responding to a perceived threat.

C. Violent relationships
Within an abusive relationship, there is usually a typical pattern of tension building, violence, and reconciliation. Over the duration of an abusive relationship, this cycle recurs many times, often with the violence increasing in severity.

1. Tension building
Characterized by frequent hostile verbal attacks, heightened surveillance of the victim, and escalating demands. This part of the cycle is actually the most destructive to the woman's ego and self-esteem.

2. Outburst
Violence occurs after a build-up of days or months of increasing tension. This can be precipitated by a particular event or can come without warning. Some women have been awakened by beatings.

3. Honeymoon
The reconciliation phase quickly follows. The attacker is often remorseful and promises never to be physically abusive again.

4. Abusive partners exert control over their partners using many common techniques: financial control, isolation, coercion and threats, intimidation, male privilege, guilt, shame, and using their children.

D. Diagnosis
1. Awareness
The key to identification by the primary care physician is the realization that anyone could be a battered woman. Stereotypes regarding poor, uneducated, minority women, or the woman who somehow "provokes" her partner to attack her must be dispelled. A heightened awareness is necessary to consider battering when evaluating women. Victims of abuse commonly present with multiple somatic complaints, including headache, abdominal pain, muscle aches, joint pain, fatigue, vaginal or pelvic complaints, anxiety disorders, or depression. Battered women often go from physician to physician and are frequently identified as "difficult patients." Feelings of guilt, shame, and low self-esteem, and patients' perceptions that physicians do not want to know about abuse are the primary reasons that many battered women are hesitant to discuss the abuse.

2. Screening versus case finding
This has become a controversial issue with respect to IPV. Most professional medical organizations recommend that physicians should ask about abuse routinely as part of any history and physical examination. However, the United States Preventive Health Services Task Force recently reviewed IPV screening and found they could not recommend for or against screening. Their rationale was that there is no evidence that screening leads to improved health outcomes and no evidence that screening does not lead to harm.

By asking about abuse, the physician lets the patient know that he or she is approachable and willing to help. Battered women who do not reveal abuse at an initial visit may discuss it later if they feel safe and that their physician is receptive. A nonjudgmental statement such as "I often see depression in women who have been hurt by someone close to them. Has this ever happened to you?" is a good screening question for partner abuse. This statement lets the patient know that her physician is willing and able to help. Additionally, literature in a safe place, such as the restroom, gives the patient the knowledge that their physician is open to discussing IPV.

E. Management strategies

Physicians are often reluctant to elicit a history of abuse because they are unsure about how to proceed if abuse is reported. Consider the following in offering treatment to victims of domestic violence:

1. Acknowledge the abuse

The therapeutic process has already begun when the patient talks to the physician about the abuse. The physician needs to convey:

a. There are many women who have had similar experiences
b. It is not their fault,
c. Abuse is wrong,
d. They are not crazy.

It is normal for them to feel overwhelmed and in need of support. It is also important that the patient understands that her symptoms are a reaction to the abuse. Reassurance helps decrease the sense of isolation and helplessness.

2. Assess for potential lethality

The level of continuing danger must be assessed. If there is imminent danger of serious harm or death, arrangements for a shelter should be made before the patient leaves the office.

It is important to ask about the following indicators of potential lethality:

a. Change in severity/frequency of violence
b. Drug or alcohol use
c. Possession of a firearm
d. Threats of suicide/homicide
e. Recent break-up
f. Threats or assault with weapon
g. Attempted strangulation
h. Stalking behavior

If children are involved in the abuse, by law this must be reported to your state's child protection agency. In some states (Utah, for example) domestic violence in the presence of children constitutes child abuse. Every physician should be aware of your state's laws concerning abuse. If there is no shelter in your area, encourage the patient to report the abuse to the police. Most police agencies have a Victims Assistance Unit or equivalent.

3. Provide resources

The patient needs to know what resources are available, even if she is not yet ready to leave an abusive relationship. Group sessions with women who had similar experiences are especially helpful. The patient should be given the telephone number of a women's shelter or other resources in the area before she leaves the office. If you are not familiar with your area's resources for victims of domestic violence, contact your local police department and ask.

4. Documentation

Objective documentation including as many details as possible in the history and physical examination is very helpful. Drawing figures or diagrams, depicting exact areas of ecchymoses, swelling, lacerations, etc., further documents the abuse. Taking photographs may contribute evidence if this were to go to court and is helpful to the victim. Record the name and badge number of any police officer who comes to your office, and any legal action that ensues.

5. Remember your role

The physician may feel frustrated because the patient cannot or will not leave an abusive relationship. The physician cannot make this decision for the patient. The role of physician is that of facilitator, helping the woman work through the process of recovery.

F. Prognosis

Effects on the victim vary, but certain emotional and behavioral sequelae are commonly seen in an abused partner.

1. Depression

Depression is one of the most common manifestations suffered by battered women. Depression can come from anger at the abuser turned inward, and feelings of guilt or self-blame for "allowing the abuse to happen." Additionally, survivors of abusive relationships often end up lacking financial resources, which adds to their depression. Suicide attempts are not uncommon. Depression can persist after the victim has left the abusive relationship.

2. Anxiety disorders and PTSD

Living in an abusive relationship produces high levels of anxiety, and even after the relationship has terminated, many women will still have environmental triggers that can provoke panic attacks. Anxiety, posttraumatic stress disorder, and depression are common ways battered women will present to the primary care physician. Victims and survivors are often substance abusers, self-treating their undiagnosed psychiatric disorders. Other self-destructive behavior is common and can manifest itself as smoking, or failure to use safety items such as seat belts.

3. Somatic complaints and chronic pain

Somatic symptoms such as abdominal or pelvic pain, headaches, or chronic musculoskeletal pain are also common in patients with histories of victimization. Patients' understanding of this connection often helps ameliorate the severity of the pain. These patients are also more likely to enter into future abusive relationships, thus monitoring for this is important.

III. Elder Abuse

Abuse occurs as a result of underlying family problems. Treatment must include the family system as well as the victim of abuse. The physician cannot treat elder abuse alone; a team approach, using social workers, mental health professionals, case managers, and lawyers, is more likely to be successful.

A. Definitions

The term *elder abuse* is used interchangeably with *elder mistreatment* and includes many types of abuse against older adults. The National Aging Resource Center on Elder Abuse (NARCEA) has developed working definitions for elder abuse and neglect. The types of elder abuse include physical, psychological, and sexual abuse; psychological and physical neglect; violation of rights; and financial or material exploitation. Neglect, physical, and psychological abuse may also be self-inflicted.

1. Physical abuse

Physical abuse is the act of causing physical pain or injury resulting in bruising, fractures, dislocations, abrasions, burns, welts, lacerations, and other multiple injuries. Physical abuse can be intentional or unintentional and includes at least one act of violence including beating, slapping, burning, cutting, inappropriate use of physical restraints, and intentional overmedicating.

2. Physical neglect

Physical neglect is the failure of a caregiver to meet care obligations such as providing goods and services including food, clothing, shelter, medical, and personal care. Indicators of neglect may include malnutrition, dehydration, decubitus ulcers, poor hygiene, and lack of caregiver compliance with medical regimens.

3. Psychological neglect

Psychological neglect is the failure of a caregiver to provide a dependent elder with meaningful social contact or stimulation. Examples of this type of neglect include isolating or ignoring the elder for long periods. This commonly results in depression, anxiety, extreme withdrawal, or agitation.

4. Psychological abuse

Psychological abuse includes the infliction of mental anguish through intimidation, threats, verbal assaults, berating, deprivation, infantilization (treating the older adult like an infant), humiliation, or the provocation of internal fear. The end result of this type of abuse is similar to that of psychological abuse in which the elder is depressed, withdrawn, or fearful, and can present with symptoms of "failure to thrive."

5. Sexual abuse

Sexual abuse is defined as molestation or forced sexual activity. Although this type of abuse is the most underreported, it may occur more often than previously suspected.

6. Violation of personal rights

Violation of personal rights includes preventing elders from making their own decisions regarding housing arrangements, financial matters, and personal decisions such as marriage, divorce, and medical treatment. Physicians can observe for signs of violation of personal rights through observation of the caregiver–elder interaction. Does the caregiver insist on being present for the examination? Does the caregiver interrupt the elder's conversation, never allowing the elder to respond to the physician's questions? Does the caregiver deny the elder the right to make health-care decisions?

7. Material or financial abuse

Material or financial abuse refers to the illegal exploitation of monetary or material assets. This type of abuse includes control of the elder's income and assets by the caregiver; coercion in signing contracts or making changes in a will or durable power of attorney; or the theft of money or property. Specific indicators include a caregiver's refusal to release funds to purchase needed care or patient complaints that they have inadequate funds to buy medication.

8. Self-neglect

Self-neglect refers to the behavior of an elderly person that threatens his/her own health or safety. Self-neglect occurs when an older person refuses or fails to provide himself/herself with adequate food, water, clothing, shelter, personal hygiene, medication (when required), and safety precautions.

Signs and symptoms of self-neglect include but are not limited to: dehydration, malnutrition, untreated or improperly attended medical conditions, and poor personal hygiene; hazardous or unsafe living conditions/arrangements (e.g., improper wiring, lack of indoor plumbing, heat, or running water); unsanitary or unclean living quarters (e.g., animal/insect infestation, fecal/urine contamination, or odor); inappropriate and/or inadequate clothing, lack of the necessary medical aids (e.g., eyeglasses, hearing aids, and dentures); and grossly inadequate housing or homelessness.

Self-neglect excludes any situations whereby a mentally competent older person makes a conscious and voluntary decision to engage in acts that threaten his/her health or safety as a matter of personal choice.

B. Epidemiology

1. Prevalence and incidence

The NARCEA estimates that between 1.5 and 2 million older adults in the United States suffer from physical abuse or neglect annually. Elder abuse occurs in all communities, regardless of gender, ethnicity or race, socioeconomic status, or religious affiliation. Because of the variation in state reporting requirements, it is difficult to determine the actual rate of elder abuse; however, the majority of state adult protective and regulatory agencies responsible for the identification, investigation, and prevention of elder abuse report an increase in reported cases over the last decade. Because of the absence of a nationalized tracking system for elder mistreatment prevalence and incidence studies are based on individual researchers and various statewide studies. Estimates on the frequency of elder mistreatment range from 2% to 10% based on various sampling methods and case studies.

2. Identity and background of the perpetrators

Physical abuse is perpetrated most often by spouses with acute or chronic health problems or responsibilities for providing companionship, financial resources, or property maintenance for their dependent spouse. Adult children may psychologically abuse and neglect their parents as well as financially exploit them. These children are often financially dependent on the parent and have a history of mental illness or substance abuse. Pillemer and Suitor found that 64% of abusers were financially dependent on their victims and 55% were dependent on them for housing needs.

3. Risk factors for abuse

Increased life expectancy, functional or psychological dependency, learned helplessness, poor physical health, and stress and burnout experienced by the caregiver are primary risk factors for abuse. Other risk factors include living arrangements, caregivers with mental illness or substance abuse, or a family history of violence. Lachs et al found that mistreated elders were likely to live with someone and have fewer social networks. Potential predictors of elder mistreatment include poverty, race, and cognitive impairment.

C. Diagnosis

Clinicians and researchers are in agreement with the protocol regarding assessing potential cases of elder mistreatment. A physical examination assessing the patient's general appearance, hygiene, functional status, and mannerisms should be part of the preliminary assessment phase followed by examining skin for bruising, lesions, abrasions, decubitis ulcers, bite marks, and dehydration. Examination of the head and neck areas for trauma, scalp hematomas, traumatic alopecia, or other evidence of direct physical violence should be part of the physical examination. An examination of the musculoskeletal system should reveal any new or old fractures, lesions on wrists or ankles, gait difficulties, cigarette, or other burns. In the genitourinary tract area attention should be paid to poor hygiene, vaginal or rectal bleeding, inguinal rash, and impaction of feces or infestations. Thorough neurologic/psychiatric evaluation to assess mental status, depressive symptoms, anxiety, or other psychiatric symptoms including hallucinations or delusions is essential in the evaluation process. Cognitive impairment and depression have been shown to be risk factors for elder mistreatment. Finally, based on clinical findings, specific laboratories should include albumin, blood urea, nitrogen, creatinine levels, toxicological screening, and assessment for other deficiencies.

D. Management

The American Medical Association (AMA) recommends that all physicians ask their patients about family violence regardless of whether there is clinical evidence or suspicion of abuse or neglect. If the elderly patient is not cognitively impaired, a thorough interview, separate from the caregiver, should occur to assess whether the patient is safe. Non-threatening questions should be asked, such as (1) "Do you feel safe in your home?," (2) "Who helps you with your personal care, such as bathing, taking your medications, preparing your meals?," (3) "What happens if your family member becomes tired or cannot help you?," (4) "What happens if you have a disagreement?," and (5) "Who helps you pay your bills?" If the patient has cognitive impairment, history and screening questions must be obtained from the caregiver or family member if available.

If the elder does not feel safe and accepts physician intervention, hospitalization should be considered. If hospitalization is not an option, the physician should discuss other placement options with Adult Protective Services (APS). APS has several emergency, court-ordered options available, and can facilitate this process. The following approach with the caregiver facilitates the interview process and reduces some of the tension that may exist: "It must be very difficult to care for your mother with this type of illness. Do you find yourself feeling tired, frustrated, and unable to deal with the situation?" Advising the family member that you will be making a report to APS to help reduce some of the stress that the caregiver may be experiencing may be less threatening to the caregiver. The caregiver should be informed of available resources such as adult day care, respite care, home health care, senior companion programs, caregiver support groups, and individual counseling.

E. Ethical and legal obligations

Physicians play a critical role in the assessment of elder abuse and neglect, as well as in the intervention process. In long-term physician–patient relationships in which trust has been established, the process may be easier to facilitate.

Physicians have a legal responsibility to report suspected cases of abuse or neglect. Mandatory reporting laws exist in most states. Designated state agencies are responsible for conducting investigations and interventions. APS is the agency assigned to investigate and intervene with elder abuse cases. Persons who are licensed, registered, or certified to provide health care, education, and social, mental health, and other human services are required to report abuse. Anonymous reports can be made. Physicians usually are granted immunity from civil suits in reporting cases of suspected abuse or neglect. Failure to report suspected abuse can result in civil liability and fines for any subsequent damages that may occur. Failure to follow state guidelines for reporting abuse may result in criminal prosecution, professional delicensure, or other penalties.

REFERENCES

Adams JA. Evolution of a classification scale: medical evaluation of suspected child sexual abuse. *Child Maltreat.* 2001;6:31-36.

Bonnie RJ, Wallace RB, Eds. *Elder Mistreatment: Abuse, Neglect and Exploitation in an Aging America.* Washington DC: National Research Council Panel to Review Risk and Prevalence of Elder Abuse and Neglect. National Academies Press; 2003.

Christian CW, Lavelle JM, De Jong AR, Loiselle J, Brenner L, Joffe M. Forensic evidence findings in prepubertal victims of sexual assault. *Pediatrics* 2000;106(1):100.

Fisher JW, Dyer CB. The hidden health menace of elder abuse. Physicians can help patients surmount intimate partner violence. *Postgrad. Med.* 2003;113:21.

Kellogg ND, American Academy of Pediatrics Committee on child abuse. The evaluation of child sexual abuse. *Pediatrics*. 2005;116:506-512.

Kellogg ND, American Academy of Pediatrics Committee on Child Abuse. The evaluation of suspected child physical abuse. *Pediatrics*. 2007;119:1232-1241.

Lachs, MS, Pillemer, K. Elder abuse. *The Lancet.* 2004:364:1192-1263.

Mitchell KJ, Finkelhor D, Wolan J. Risk factors for and impact of online sexual solicitation of youth. *JAMA.* 2001;285:3011.

National Center on Elder Abuse. http://www.elderabusecenter.org/default.cfm. Accessed November 15, 2007.

Rodriguez MA, Wallace SP, Woolf NH, Mangione CM. Mandatory reporting of elder abuse: between a rock and a hard place. *Ann. Internal Med.* 2006;4:403.

Schindeler-Trachta RE, Schneider FD. Interpersonal violence in Texas: a physician's role. *Texas Med.* 2007;103:43.

Shugarman LR, Fries BE, Wolf RS, Morris JN. Identifying older people at risk of abuse during routine screening practices. *J Am Geriatr Soc.* 2003;51:24.

Taliaferro E. Screening and identification of intimate partner violence. *Clin Fam Pract.* 2003;5:89.

U.S. Preventive Services Task Force. Screening for family and intimate partner violence: recommendation statement. *Ann Intern Med.* 2004;140:382.

Wathen CN, MacMillan HL. Interventions for violence against women. *JAMA.* 2003;289:589.

---

92   Depression

Rhonda A. Faulkner, PhD, Martin S. Lipsky, MD, & Michael Polizzotto, MD

KEY POINTS

- Depression is the most common psychological disorder that primary care practitioners will encounter. According to recent studies, depression is more common than any other disorder (with the exception of hypertension) and is the seventh most common outpatient diagnosis in family medicine. While depression is a common disease with substantial morbidity and mortality, it is often undiagnosed and under-treated. Approximately 5% of the population has major depression at any given time, with men at 7% to 12% risk of experiencing MDD and women at 20% to 25% risk over the course of a lifetime. The point prevalence of MDD in primary care patients is 4.8% to 8.6%; 14.6% of adult medical inpatients meet criteria for MDD. Annual economic consequences of depression have been estimated at 83 billion dollars in the United States and 11.5 billion euros in the United Kingdom.

- Most adults with major depression never see a mental health professional and will receive most or all of their care through primary care physicians. Depressed patients frequently present to their primary care provider with somatic complaints as opposed to complaining of depressed mood. (SOR Ⓑ) The US Preventive Services Task Force (USPSTF) recommends that all clinicians routinely screen adults for depression. They recommend asking the following two simple questions regarding mood and anhedonia: (1) "Over the past 2 weeks, have you felt down, depressed, or hopeless?" and (2) "Over the past 2 weeks, have you felt little interest or pleasure in doing things?"

- There are several types of depressive illnesses classified by diagnosable symptoms as defined by the American Psychological Association's *Diagnostic and Statistical Manual of Mental Disorders* (DSM-IV; Table 92–1). It is recommended that primary care providers be familiar with the distinctive classifications of depression. In particular, since approximately 1% of patients with depression may have bipolar disease, the family physician should be alert for manic episodes that might be precipitated by treatment with an antidepressant.

- Physicians have a variety of treatment options for depression. Among the choices, selective serotonin reuptake inhibitors (SSRIs) offer simpler dosing schedules and fewer side effects than some of the older antidepressants (Table 92–2). ***The combination of antidepressant medications with psychotherapy has proven to demonstrate the best outcomes in treatment of depression.*** (SOR **A**) Patients starting a course of antidepressant therapy should be advised that symptoms will not subside for 2 to 6 weeks, with a trial of 6 to 8 weeks at maximum dose necessary to confirm treatment success or failure. To prevent the risk of relapse, a treatment period of 6 to 9 months is recommended. (SOR **A**) No one particular antidepressant agent has proven superior over another in regards to efficacy; therefore, side effect profiles, presence of medical and psychiatric comorbidities, and prior treatment response are used as guidelines in selecting antidepressant medications. (SOR **A**)

- The prognosis for patients who receive treatment for depression is generally favorable, with 50% to 60% of patients responding to the first trial antidepressant. (SOR **A**) Patients who do not respond to one particular type of medication may respond well to another. At least 80% of patients will respond to at least one antidepressant medication. Studies show that patients respond best when antidepressant medications are combined with counseling. (SOR **A**) Patients treated with antidepressants should be closely monitored for potential worsening of depression or suicidal ideation at the onset of therapy and during any change of dosage. (SOR **C**)

I. Introduction
  A. Definitions
     1. **Major depressive disorder (MDD),** the most severe form of depression, is a mood disorder characterized by at least 2 weeks of five or more of the following symptoms: (1) depressed mood; (2) loss of interest or pleasure in daily activities; (3) weight loss or gain; (4) insomnia or hypersomnia; (5) psychomotor agitation or retardation; (6) fatigue or loss of energy; (7) feelings of guilt or worthlessness; (8) inability to concentrate; and (9) thoughts of death or suicidal ideation.
     2. **Dysthymia** is a milder, chronic disorder that is diagnosed when patients experience depressed mood and at least two other DSM-IV criteria of depression for at least 2 years. Patients with dysthymia may be thought of as having a depressive personality or character style. Although depressive symptoms in dysthymia are not as severe as those of major affective disorder, they are too prolonged to be thought of as adjustment responses. While antidepressants have been found somewhat less efficacious in treatment of dsythymic disorder as compared to MDD, a substantial proportion of patients will respond to antidepressants and psychotherapy. (SOR **B**)

TABLE 92–1. DSM-IV CRITERIA FOR MAJOR DEPRESSIVE EPISODE

Five (or more) of the following symptoms have been present during the same 2-week period and represent a change from previous functioning; at least one of the symptoms is either (1) depressed mood or (2) loss of interest or pleasure.

Note: Do not include symptoms that clearly result from a general medical condition or mood-incongruent delusions or hallucinations.

(1) Depressed mood most of the day, nearly every day, as indicated by either subjective report (e.g., feels sad or empty) or observation made by others (e.g., appears tearful). **Note:** In children and adolescents, can be irritable mood

(2) Markedly diminished interest or pleasure in all, or almost all, activities most of the day, nearly every day (as indicated by either subjective account or observation made by others)

(3) Significant weight loss when not dieting or weight gain (e.g., a change of > 5% of body weight in a month) or decrease or increase in appetite nearly every day. **Note:** In children, consider failure to make expected weight gains

(4) Insomnia or hypersomnia nearly every day

(5) Psychomotor agitation or retardation nearly every day (observable by others, not merely subjective feelings of restlessness or being slowed down)

(6) Fatigue or loss of energy nearly every day

(7) Feelings of worthlessness or excessive or inappropriate guilt (which may be delusional) nearly every day (not merely self-reproach or guilt about being sick)

(8) Diminished ability to think or concentrate, or indecisiveness, nearly every day (either by subjective account or as observed by others)

(9) Recurrent thoughts of death (not just fear of flying), recurrent suicidal ideation without a specific plan, or a suicide attempt or a specific plan for committing suicide

---

(Data from American Psychiatric Association (APA). *Diagnostic and Statistical Manual of Mental Disorders.* 4th ed (DSM-IV). Washington, DC: APA; 2000.)

TABLE 92–2. ANTIDEPRESSANTS

Drug	Starting Dose	Therapeutic Daily Dose	Cost	Sedation	Anticholinergic	Orthostatic Hypotension	Cardiac Conduction	Insomnia
						Adverse Effects		
Tricyclics								
Amitriptyline (Elavil)	50 mg qhs*	75–300 mg	$	High	High	High	High	Very low
Doxepin (Sinequan)	50 mg qhs*	75–300 mg	$	High	Moderate	Moderate	Moderate	Low
Imipramine (Tofranil)	50 mg qd*	75–300 mg	$	Moderate	Moderate	High	High	Very low
Nortriptyline (Pamelor)	25 mg qd*·†	40–200 mg	$$	Low	Low	Low	Moderate	Low
Heterocyclics								
Bupropion (Wellbutrin)	100 mg bid‡	200–450 mg	$$	Low	Very low	Very low	Very low	Moderate
Trazodone (Desyrel)	150 mg qhs*	75–300 mg	$$	High	Very low	Moderate	Very low	Very low
Selective serotonin reuptake inhibitors								
Citalopram (Celexa)	20 mg qd	20–60 mg qd	$$$	Low	Very low	Very low	Very low	Very low
Escitalopram (Lexapro)	10 mg	20 mg qd	$$$	Very low	Very low	Very low	Very low	Very low
Fluoxetine (Prozac)	10–20 mg qam	10–80 mg	$$$	Very low	Very low	Very low	Very low	High
Paroxetine (Paxil)	10–20 mg qd	10–60 mg	$$$	Low	Low	Very low	Very low	Low
Sertraline (Zoloft)	50 mg qd	50–200 mg	$$$	Very low	Low	Very low	Very low	Low
Serotonin/norepinephrine reuptake inhibitor								
Venlafaxine (Effexor)	37.5 mg bid	75–300 mg	$$	Very low	Low	Very low	Very low	Moderate
Duloxetine hydrochloride (Cymbalta)	20 mg bid	40–60 mg	$$$	Very low	Low	Very low	Very low	Moderate
Other antidepressants								
Mirtazapine (Remeron)	7.5–15 mg qhs	30–45 mg qhs	$$$	High	Low	Low	Low	Low
Nefazodone (Serzone)	50–100 mg bid	100–300 mg bid	$$$	High	Low	Low	Low	Low
Trazodone (Desyrel)	50 mg qhs	100–300 mg bid	$	High	Low	Moderate	Low	Low

*May be better tolerated if given in divided doses.
† Begin at lower dose in the elderly, titrate to serum level of 50 to 150 ng/mL.
‡ Not to exceed 150 mg/dose to minimize seizure risk.
$, least expensive; $$, moderately expensive; $$$, most expensive.

3. **Adjustment disorder with depressed mood** is a type of mood disorder readily attributable to a recent psychosocial stressor such as a loss of a loved one or employment and should resolve as the stressor decreases. It is distinguished from an MDD by its milder severity and shorter time course. Some bereaved patients manifest primarily psychological symptoms and seek counseling, while others develop somatic symptoms and seek medical attention. Unfortunately, many individuals with MDD have stressors that may be identified as the cause of their depression, and thus their illness may be overlooked.

4. **Depressive disorder not otherwise specified (NOS)** is a depressive illness that lasts longer than 6 months. This diagnosis is used to describe mixed states of anxiety and depression that do not meet the criteria for other anxiety or depressive diagnoses.

5. **Mood disorder due to a general medical condition (or substance).** This condition is diagnosed when a prominent mood disturbance can be attributed to a direct physiological consequence of a general medical condition (i.e., hypothyroidism, AIDS), substance abuse (i.e., alcohol withdrawal), or medication (i.e., beta-blockers, levodopa, steroids, reserpine, and oral contraceptives).

6. **Bipolar disorder** (also known as manic-depressive illness), a condition with a strong genetic predisposition, occurs in approximately 1% of the population. These patients experience symptoms of depression along with mania.

7. **Other psychiatric disorders.** Depressive symptoms may also be present in other psychiatric disorders, although they are not predominant. In particular, depression and anxiety are highly comorbid conditions. Therefore, the evaluation of depressive symptoms should include a psychiatric history and a brief review of systems, looking for psychotic features, phobias, panic attacks, somatization, and personality disorders.

8. **Seasonal affective disorder (SAD).** This condition has similar features to MDD and occurs on a cyclical basis related to ambient light deprivation particularly during winter months. Phototherapy has been found to offer modest though promising antidepressive efficacy, especially when administered in the mornings during the first week of treatment. (SOR **A**) Antidepressant medications are also used in the treatment of SAD.

9. **Premenstrual Dysphoric Disorder (PMDD).** This severe premenstrual syndrome affects 3% to 5% of women of reproductive age. Such severe PMS is classified under the Diagnostic and Statistical Manual of Mental Disorders as premenstrual dysphoric disorder, PMDD. Selective serotonin reuptake inhibitors (SSRIs) are increasingly being used as a front-line therapy for PMDD. (SOR **B**)

B. **Epidemiology.** At any one time, at least 5% of the US population suffers from chronic depression. More than 17% of the population has had a major depressive episode in their lifetime, and more than 10% have experienced an episode within the past 12 months. Epidemiologic studies indicate that a lifetime prevalence of major depression in 7% to 12% of men and 20% to 25% of women. Studies report a 5% to 10% prevalence of major depression in primary care settings with 20% to 40% prevalence in patients with coexisting medical problems.

1. A depressive disorder may begin at any age, but the average age at onset is the late 20s. Psychosocial events or stressors may play a significant role in precipitating the first or second episode of MDD, but may play little or no role in subsequent episodes.

2. Multiple studies support the finding that major depression is more common in women than in men. This gender difference is found in community samples and is not the result of higher rates of help-seeking behavior by women. Recent studies have disproved the belief that the incidence of depression in women increases during the climacteric. Prevalence rates for MDD are unrelated to race, education, or income.

3. Certain individuals are at increased risk for depression, including alcohol and drug abusers, hypochondriacs, patients with a life-threatening disease such as a stroke or myocardial infarction, individuals recovering from major surgery, women in the postpartum state, and patients with a family history of depression. Screening for postpartum depression is particularly important, as recent data demonstrates that between 50% and 80% of women experience this "normal" reaction within 1 to 5 days after childbirth, lasting up to 1 week. This condition should be distinguished from postpartum psychosis, which occurs in 0.5% to 2% of women, with symptoms beginning 2 to 3 days after delivery. (SOR **A**)

C. **Etiology**

1. **Genetic factors.** A combination of biological and environmental factors causes depression. Multiple lines of research point to a genetic or inherited predisposition for

MDD that may be activated or precipitated by psychosocial or physiologic stressors. The general understanding of how these stressors interact with a genetic predisposition to produce clinical depression is limited.

2. **Psychosocial factors.** Psychosocial stressors such as death of a spouse, divorce, or developmental life course transitions (e.g., empty nest syndrome) may make patients more vulnerable to experiencing depression. The presence of social support is a mitigating factor for depression; therefore, primary care providers should assess social support and facilitate mobilization of these resources.

3. The interaction among these environmental and genetic factors is postulated to culminate in the final common pathway of limbic–hypothalamic dysfunction, which is clinically manifested as a depressive illness. It was originally believed that a depletion of neurotransmitters, including norepinephrine, serotonin, and γ-aminobutyric acid, in hypothalamic centers of the brain contributed to the symptom complex of depression. More recent studies suggest a dysregulation hypothesis rather than depletion of a single neurotransmitter.

II. **Diagnosis.** Recent studies have documented improvements in the recognition and treatment of MDD in primary care settings, with two-thirds of patients recognized and nearly half prescribed antidepressants.

A. **Symptoms and signs**

1. The clinical diagnosis of depression depends on recognition of an identifiable cluster of signs and symptoms suggesting the disorder. See Table 92–1 for a list of criteria for diagnosing MDD according to the DSM-IV. Any of the symptoms listed may represent the leading edge of a cluster of depressive symptoms. For example, a recent study found that 80% of patients with the chief complaint of fatigue go on to be diagnosed with an affective disorder. The DSM-IV requires that five or more symptoms be present during the same 2-week period and that at least one be either a depressed mood or loss of interest or pleasure. It is important to note that the DSM-IV includes a loss of interest in all, or almost all, activities as an alternative to depressed mood as the primary symptom. It is not uncommon for a depressed patient to deny feeling sad, but instead admit to "not caring anymore."

2. Although the DSM-IV is useful in evaluating the possibility of depression in a patient, it was designed primarily by and for psychiatric researchers and was validated on a psychiatric population. DSM-IV criteria may not be as applicable to a primary care population.

3. The wide application of the term *depression* often leads to confusion about its diagnosis. The following guidelines are suggested to distinguish bereavement or dysphoric symptoms from clinical depression.

   a. Patients with established clinical depression usually need more treatment than positive changes in the psychosocial environment.

   b. Clinical depression is usually incapacitating and interferes with work performance and relationships.

   c. Diurnal variation of symptoms, which become worse in the morning, is more common with clinical depression.

   d. Psychomotor retardation, which may be associated with depression, is almost never observed with bereavement.

   e. Recurrence is especially characteristic of a mood disorder. A prior history of a similar episode is strong evidence for clinical depression. More than half of all patients with depression will experience a recurrence in their lifetime and therefore should be advised of this risk.

   f. Finally, a positive family history of a similar disorder is characteristic of a primary mood disorder.

4. **Age-specific features** in the diagnosis of depression.

   a. Elderly patients with psychomotor retardation, slow thinking, and indecisiveness may be misdiagnosed as having dementia (see Chapter 73).

   b. Prepubertal children often present with somatic complaints, irritable mood, or a psychomotor agitation that may manifest itself as a marked drop in school performance.

   c. In adolescents, similar findings may occur. Antisocial behavior, restlessness, agitation, **substance abuse,** aggression, poor school performance, withdrawal from social activities, and increased emotional sensitivity are also common. Children and adolescents are often unable to recognize these changes or to associate them with depression. Tricyclic drugs do not seem useful for treating children before puberty, and are of moderate benefit at best for adolescents. (SOR **B**)

   d. Patients with depression may present with vague physical symptoms without organic diseases or with symptoms out of proportion to the physical examination. Complaints such as fatigue and dizziness that result in multiple visits without a specific diagnosis should alert the clinician to consider depression.

B. Laboratory tests

   1. The clinical interview remains the most effective method for detecting depression. No reliable biochemical markers for depression exist. Only a limited number of laboratory tests should be conducted to detect potential general medical causes of depressive symptoms. No standard "screening" work-up can be used to rule out potential underlying organic causes for depressive symptoms. The evaluation should be directed by demographic and historical clues. For example, hypothyroidism should be considered in an older patient who presents with depressive symptomatology. Medications known to be associated with depressive symptoms should be stopped, especially if recently prescribed.

   2. Several **self-administered questionnaires and depression screening tools** are available for use across the lifespan and are designed to help identify patients with depressive symptomatology. (Please see the following website for access to screening tools: http://www.aafp.org/afp/20020915/1001.html.) These tests, which are more useful as case-finding instruments than as screening tests, possess sensitivities in the 70% range and specificities in the 80% range. They are easily administered and well accepted by patients. Widely used tests include the following:

   a. Beck Depression Inventory, including the short-form version with 13 items.

   b. The National Institute of Mental Health (NIMH) Center for Epidemiologic Studies Depression Scale (CES-D), which has 20 items.

   c. The Zung Self-Rating Depression Scale (SDS), which also has 20 items.

III. Treatment. Primary care physicians, not mental health professionals, treat most patients with symptoms of depression. The objectives of treatment are (1) to resolve all signs and symptoms of the depressive syndrome, (2) to restore occupational and psychosocial functioning to baseline, and (3) to reduce the likelihood of relapse and recurrence. Treatment may be divided into three phases: acute, continuation, and maintenance.

A. Acute phase treatment. In primary care, the most common acute treatment modalities are medication, psychotherapy or counseling, or a combination of medication and psychotherapy. Mild depression may be treated effectively with either medication or psychotherapy, while the combination approach of medication and psychotherapy together, yields best treatment outcomes for moderate to severe depression. (SOR **A**)

   1. Medication

   a. Medications have been shown to be effective in all forms of MDD and should be considered first-line therapy in moderate to severe MDD. (SOR **A**)

   b. Medication selection should be based on side effect profiles; history of prior response; and patient symptoms, concurrent medical conditions, and concurrently prescribed medications (Table 92–2). Although there are no clinically significant differences in the effectiveness of antidepressant medications, SSRIs are usually preferred over tricyclic antidepressants (TCAs) and monoamine oxidase inhibitors (MAOIs) due to simpler dosing schedules and fewer side effects. No single medication results in remission for all patients.

   c. To be proficient in the treatment of depression, the primary care physician should learn how to use at least three or four antidepressants well and become familiar with dosages, side effects, and serum levels. The chosen medications should have varying side effect profiles and be applicable to different types of presenting symptomatologies.

   d. Suggested guidelines for selection include the following:

   (1) If the patient has insomnia and early morning awakening, a more sedating medication (for example a TCA such as amitriptyline or imipramine) should be chosen.

   (2) If patient's symptoms are characterized by an excessive need for sleep, then a more stimulating and less sedating medication should be selected. Patients with hypersomnia and motor retardation may benefit from bupropion or venlafaxine and should avoid using nefazodone and mirtazapine.

      (3) If anxiety is a major component of the symptom complex, then a medication with a lower index of insomnia or agitation side effects is recommended. For patients with generalized anxiety and insomnia, nefazodone and mirtazapine are good choices.

      (4) For patients in whom weight gain is a goal, mirtazapine is a good choice.

      (5) For patients in whom smoking cessation is also a goal, bupropion can work well.

      (6) Elderly patients are especially sensitive to the orthostatic and anticholinergic side effects of some antidepressants. As a result, the SSRIs have replaced TCAs as first-line therapy in the elderly. Careful observation of cardiac function, vital signs, cognitive functioning, and physical complaints will often help identify potential problems early.

      (7) If the medication is relatively sedating, compliance can be improved by having the patient take the entire dosage either at bedtime or a few hours before.

   e. Contraindications for specific antidepressants:

      (1) Nefazodone should not be used in patients with liver disease.

      (2) Bupropion is contraindicated for patients with seizure disorder.

      (3) For patients who have experienced sexual dysfunction prior to depression, SSRIs **should** be avoided.

      (4) Hypertension is a relative contraindication to venlafaxine.

      (5) Patients experiencing hypersomnia and motor retardation should avoid nefazodone and mirtazapine.

      (6) For patients experiencing agitation and insomnia, bupropion and venlafaxine should be avoided.

      (7) Mirtazapine and TCAs are *less* preferred for patients with obesity.

2. Psychotherapy

   a. Studies have shown that the combination of medication with psychotherapy provides a better response than either form of treatment used alone. (SOR **A**)

   b. Depression rarely occurs independent of psychosocial issues. It is vital that the patient begin to address these issues if true recovery is to occur. If relationships within the family, such as a poor marital relationship, prove to be a precipitating factor, then involvement of other family members in counseling may be important.

   c. Psychotherapy alone may be preferable in patients with milder forms of MDD who do not desire medication, who have unacceptable side effects to medication, and who have medical conditions limiting medication options.

   d. Physicians may find it useful to use the **BATHE** technique in order to help focus the counseling encounter. The acronym "BATHE" stands for the following: B = *background*: "What is going on in your life?"; A = *affect*: "How do you feel about that?"; T = *trouble*: "What about this situation or problem troubles you the most?"; H = *handling*: "How are you handling that?"; and E = *empathy*: "That must be very difficult for you."

      (1) Often, the patient needs only a sympathetic listener to be able to work through the conflicts he or she is experiencing.

      (2) Encounters need not be lengthy. Ten or 15 minutes is enough time to allow the patient to explore problems in a therapeutic way, with the physician facilitating this process by asking open-ended questions.

      (3) It is not important that the physician produce a final answer to all of the patient's questions, doubts, or problems, but help the patients to set goals and decrease negative thoughts about their life.

   e. Many physicians establish a good working relationship with a local psychiatrist, psychologist, or family therapist to whom they can refer patients for counseling or psychotherapy.

3. Patient education

   a. A key element in acute phase treatment is the provision of adequate information to both the patient and his or her family about the condition. In addition, the provision of support, advice, reassurance, and hope is critical for depressed patients who are experiencing fatigue, low mood, and poor concentration. Several studies have found that patient education improves adherence to treatment in depressed outpatients.

   b. An important point to make with many patients is that antidepressant medication is not habit-forming or addictive. Many patients are fearful of "nerve pills" because of friends or relatives who may have developed a drug dependence.

    c. Nearly half of all patients will stop taking their antidepressant medication within the first month of treatment. Patients should be educated in advance about the side effects of the medications, such as dry mouth, constipation, sexual side effects, and sedation. Patients should be reassured that most will resolve with time.

    d. Patients should be told not to expect overnight results. It often takes 4 to 6 weeks for noticeable improvement to occur. It is often helpful to remind patients that their symptoms developed over a similar, if not longer, time interval. (SOR **Ⓐ**)

  4. Herbal products. Many patients may attempt to use herbal remedies, such as St. John's wort (*Hypericum perforatum*), for treatment of their depression without consulting their physician. A multisite, large-scale clinical trial of St. John's wort, conducted by The National Institutes of Health found that St. John's wort is no more effective for treating major depression of moderate severity than placebo, and may also influence adverse effects of other drugs. (SOR **Ⓑ**)

  5. Alternative treatment modalities. Studies indicate there is a growing preference among patients to pursue self-help and complementary/alternative therapies in the treatment of depression. Exercise is often promoted as an active strategy to prevent and treat depression and has been shown to report decreased depression scores when compared to no intervention in a small number of treatment trails. While additional alternative approaches to the treatment of depression such as acupuncture, yoga, tai-chi, and meditation are of interest to some patients, there is currently insufficient evidence to determine whether or not these alternative modalities are effective in the management of depression.

B. Continuation and maintenance treatment

  1. The goal of continuation treatment is to decrease the likelihood of relapse (a return of the current episode of depression).

    a. Patients who respond well to acute treatment should be continued on the same dosage for at least 6 to 12 months after they have resolved their depressive symptoms. There is very strong evidence that continuation of treatment for this time interval is effective at preventing relapse and recurrence. (SOR **Ⓐ**)

    b. Those patients who experience a second episode of depression will have an 80% chance of additional recurrences and should continue with antidepressant medications for 1 to 2 years. Patients experiencing a third episode of depression have a 90% chance for recurrence and will require indefinite treatment maintenance. (SOR **Ⓑ**)

IV. Management Strategies

A. Overcoming patient resistance

  1. Depression is often difficult for the primary care physician to treat because the diagnosis itself is often socially unacceptable and culturally invalid for many patients. A survey of 350 family practice physicians revealed that the major obstacle to treatment of depressed patients was patient resistance to the diagnosis.

  2. Many physicians find it useful to approach an explanation of the illness in terms that are better understood by the patient.

    a. Such an explanation often begins by explaining how the human body responds to stress and then defining the illness as an imbalance of chemical messengers in the nervous system.

    b. Patients are often more accepting of the diagnosis of depression and more willing to address the psychosocial precipitants, as well as use medication properly, when such an explanation is given.

  3. It is often useful, if not crucial, to involve the family in such an explanation, since their support is vital to a successful outcome.

B. Suicide. Suicide potential and prevention must always be considered when the diagnosis of depression is made.

  1. Many physicians are leery of asking about suicide out of fear that it may precipitate a suicide attempt. Such fears are unfounded. The evidence to date suggests that patients appreciate the concern demonstrated by such questioning. Many physicians find it useful to ask a patient who has considered suicide to form a suicide pact or agreement. The patient agrees to call the physician or another health provider before taking any action. No studies exist to support the efficacy of this arrangement, however.

  2. Those individuals at highest risk for suicide attempt are young females. These attempts are usually gestures and are often not successful. Medication overdose is a common method of suicide in females. If suicide is judged to be a risk, it is prudent to limit the amount of medication prescribed to <1500 mg of an antidepressant at any one time.

3. Those persons at highest risk for successful suicide are middle-aged to older men. Other high-risk factors include social isolation and substance abuse.

C. Referral or hospitalization. Even though most depressed patients who present to primary care settings can be managed as outpatients, some will need hospitalization in an inpatient psychiatric unit or referral to a psychiatrist. General recommendations are given below.

1. The patient who presents with suicide ideation and specific suicide plans is at serious risk, and hospitalization should be strongly considered.
2. The patient whose depression is severe enough to interfere with activities of daily living, such as dressing and feeding, should probably be hospitalized.
3. Referral should be considered if the patient has a history suggestive of bipolar disorder.
4. Referral should be sought if evidence of a thought disorder or psychotic features of the depression itself, such as fixed delusions, are present.
5. If the patient fails to respond to treatment after 3 months, referral to a psychiatrist should be considered.

D. Frequency of office visits

1. Follow-up should be scheduled at 2 weeks after the initial diagnosis for most mild to moderate depression. Patients with more severe forms of MDD should be seen weekly for the first 4 to 6 weeks of treatment. Subsequent visits may be scheduled at 4- to 12-week intervals, depending on the degree of response and the need for office counseling.
2. Therapeutic blood levels of antidepressant drugs have been established. Nortriptyline, imipramine, and amitriptyline have well-established minimal therapeutic blood levels. Drug levels should be obtained in the following instances.
   a. When an adequate response is not achieved on full therapeutic doses. Nonresponsiveness to a medication cannot be established unless the steady-state serum level is within the therapeutic range for 2 to 4 weeks.
   b. When serious side effects occur at normal doses. Similarities exist between depressive and toxic symptoms in patients who are clinically deteriorating.

E. Screening. The US Preventive Services Task Force (USPSTF) found evidence that screening improves the accurate identification of depressed patients in primary care settings and that treatment of depressed adults identified in primary care settings decreases clinical morbidity. Based on these findings, the USPSTF made a grade B recommendation that primary care practitioners routinely screen their adult patients for depression. *There was insufficient evidence to support a recommendation for routine screening of child and adolescent patients, although primary care physicians should use their clinical judgment about screening their younger patients.* They recommend asking the following two simple questions regarding mood and anhedonia: (1) "Over the past 2 weeks, have you felt down, depressed, or hopeless?" and (2) "Over the past 2 weeks, have you felt little interest or pleasure in doing things?" Additionally, eight of the DSM-IV symptoms (all but depressed mood) may be readily recalled using the mnemonic "SIG: E CAPS" (i.e., "prescribe energy capsules") to assess Sleep, Interest, Guilt, Energy, Concentration, Appetite, Psychomotor, Suicide.

V. Prognosis

A. Prognosis without treatment

1. An untreated episode of depression typically lasts 6 months or more. A remission of symptoms then occurs, and functioning often returns to the premorbid level.
2. Of those patients with recurrent episodes, 5% will have a manic attack at a later date, resulting in a change in their diagnosis to a bipolar mood disorder.
3. The toll in lives lost is high; half of all suicide victims are thought to have had a major depression. Suicide occurs in 1% of patients with an acute episode of depression and in 25% of patients with a chronic depression.

B. Prognosis with treatment

1. Most antidepressants are effective in approximately 50% to 60% of patients with MDD. Patients who do not respond to one particular type of medication may respond well to another. At least 80% of patients will respond to at least one antidepressant medication. (SOR **Ⓐ**)
2. In severe cases of MDD, electroconvulsive therapy has a high rate of therapeutic success, including speed and safety, and may be the treatment of choice for the elderly or acutely suicidal patients. However, this is not administered as a first-line treatment and

patients requiring this form of treatment should be referred for psychiatrist consultation. (SOR **A**)

REFERENCES

Feldman MD, Christensen JF. *Behavioral Medicine in Primary Care: A Practical Guide.* 2nd ed. New York, NY: McGraw-Hill; 2003.

Hypericum Depression Trial Study Group. *Effect of Hypericum perforatum* (St. John's wort) in major depressive disorder: a randomized, controlled trial. *JAMA.* 2002;287:1807-1814.

Pinquart M, Duberstein PR, Lyness JM. Treatments for later-life depressive conditions: a meta-analytic comparison of pharmacotherapy and psychotherapy. *Am J Psychiatry.* 2006;163:1493-1501.

Sharp LK, Lipsky MS. Screening for depression across the lifespan: a review of measures for use in primary care settings. *Am Fam Physician.* 2002;66:1001-1008.

Stuart MR, Lieberman JA. *The Fifteen Minute Hour: Practical Therapeutic Interventions in Primary Care.* 3rd ed. Philadelphia, PA: Saunders; 2002.

Sutherland JE, Sutherland SJ, Hoehns JD. Achieving the best outcome in treatment of depression. *J Fam Pract.* 2003;52:201-209.

U.S. Preventive Services Task Force. Screening for depression: recommendations and rationale. *Ann Intern Med.* 2002;136:760-764.

---

93   Eating Disorders

Brian C. Reed, MD

KEY POINTS

- Individuals with anorexia nervosa or bulimia nervosa have altered perceptions of their body weight or shape and often engage in a mixture of food restriction or purging behaviors.
- Weight and cardiac status are the most important components of the physical examination of individuals with eating disorders. Individuals with abnormal vital signs or fail to gain weight in highly structured outpatient programs should be hospitalized. (SOR **A**)
- Psychotherapy and nutritional rehabilitation are the mainstay of the treatment of eating disorders. (SOR **A**) Adjunctive treatment with antidepressants may provide additional benefit during the weight maintenance phase of treatment of patients with anorexia nervosa and may decrease binge eating behavior in patients with bulimia nervosa. Examples of medication doses are as follows:
  - **Fluoxetine (Prozac).** This drug is typically dosed at 40 mg/d during the weight-maintenance phase of anorexia or 60 to 80 mg/d in the treatment of bulimia nervosa.
  - **Tricyclic antidepressants.** These drugs are typically dosed at the same levels for the management of depression. Doses are imipramine (Tofranil), between 50 and 300 mg/d; amitriptyline (Elavil, Endep), 50 and 300 mg/d; or nortriptyline (Pamelor, Aventyl), 50 and 150 mg/d.
  - **Monoamine oxidase inhibitors (MAOIs).** Phenelzine or isocarboxazid dosed between 30 and 45 mg/d reduces binge eating behavior in patients with bulimia.

I. Introduction
    A. **Definition.** Eating disorders are psychological disorders characterized by an altered perception of body weight or shape and serious disturbances in eating behavior.
        1. **Anorexia nervosa** (Table 93–1). Individuals may have anorexia nervosa if they concurrently exhibit the following behaviors or characteristics:
            a. **Criterion A** show a refusal to maintain a minimally normal body weight for age and height. As a guideline, an individual fails to maintain a minimally normal weight if he or she weighs <85% of the weight that is considered normal for that individual's age and height based on published Metropolitan Life Insurance Tables or pediatric growth charts. The use of a body mass index equal to or below 17.5 kg/m^2 serves as alternative guideline in determining when an individual is underweight.
            b. **Criterion B.** Has an intense fear of gaining weight or becoming fat.

TABLE 93–1. DIAGNOSTIC CRITERIA FOR EATING DISORDERS

Anorexia nervosa
A. Refusal to maintain body weight at or above a minimally normal weight for age and height (e.g., weight loss leading to maintenance of body weight less than 85% of that expected; or failure to make expected weight gain during period of growth, leading to body weight less than 85% of that expected).
B. Intense fear of gaining weight or becoming overweight, even though the patient is underweight.
C. Disturbance in the way in which one's body weight or shape is experienced, undue influence of body weight or shape on self-evaluation, or denial of the seriousness of the current low body weight.
D. Amenorrhea in premenopausal females (i.e., the absence of at least three consecutive menstrual cycles. A woman is considered to have amenorrhea if her periods occur only with hormone administration.)
E. Type
    1. Restricting type: During the current episode, the patient has not regularly engaged in binge eating or purging (i.e., self-induced vomiting or the misuse of laxatives, diuretics, or enemas).
    2. Binge eating/purging type: During the current episode, the patient has regularly engaged in binge eating or purging.
Bulimia nervosa
A. Recurrent episodes of binge eating. An episode of binge eating is characterized by both of the following:
    1. In a discrete period of time (e.g., within any 2-h period), eating an amount of food that is larger than what most people would eat during a similar period of time and under similar circumstances.
    2. A sense of lack of control over eating during the episode.
B. Recurrent inappropriate compensatory behaviors to prevent weight gain, such as self-induced vomiting; misuse of laxatives, diuretics, enemas, or other medications; fasting; or exercising excessively.
C. The binge eating and inappropriate compensatory behaviors both occur, on average, at least twice a week for 3 mo.
D. Self-evaluation is unduly influenced by body shape and weight.
E. The episode does not occur exclusively during episodes of anorexia nervosa.
F. Specify type
    1. Purging type: During the current episode, the patient has regularly engaged in self-induced vomiting or the misuse of laxatives, diuretics, or enemas.
    2. Nonpurging type: During the current episode, the patient has used inappropriate compensatory behaviors, such as fasting or exercising excessively, but has not regularly engaged in self-induced vomiting or the use of laxatives, diuretics, or enemas.

(Reprinted with permission from the American Psychiatric Association. *Diagnostic and Statistical Manual of Mental Disorders.* 4th ed. text revision. American Psychiatric Association; 2000:589, 594.)

    c. **Criterion C.** Possesses a distorted perception of body weight and shape.
    d. **Criterion D.** Has amenorrhea if the individual is a postmenarcheal female.
    e. Two subtypes of anorexia nervosa exist: restricting type and binge eating/purging type. An individual with the restricting type of anorexia nervosa accomplishes weight loss through dieting, fasting, or excessive exercise. An individual who has the binge eating type of anorexia nervosa regularly engages in binge eating and purging.
  2. **Bulimia nervosa** (Table 93–1). An individual may have bulimia nervosa if they concurrently display the following behaviors or characteristics:
    a. **Criterion A.** Has recurrent episodes of binge eating.
    b. **Criterion B.** Shows recurrent use of inappropriate compensatory behaviors such as self-induced vomiting or misuse of laxatives to prevent weight gain.
    c. **Criterion C.** Performs these binge eating and inappropriate compensatory behaviors at least twice a week for the duration of 3 months.
    d. **Criterion D.** Possesses a distorted perception of body weight or shape.
    e. **Criterion E.** Displays these behaviors not exclusively during an episode of anorexia nervosa.
    f. Like anorexia nervosa, two subtypes of bulimia nervosa exist: purging type and nonpurging type. Individuals with the purging subtype regularly engage in self-induced vomiting, laxative abuse, and misuse of diuretics and enemas. A person with the nonpurging type of bulimia nervosa employs fasting or excessive exercise as a means of compensating for an episode of binge eating.
  3. **Eating disorder not otherwise specified.** This category describes disorders of eating that fail to meet the criteria for either anorexia nervosa or bulimia nervosa. Examples include females who display all of the behaviors consistent with anorexia nervosa except that they have regular menstruation or someone who engages in binge eating and inappropriate compensatory behaviors at a frequency of less than twice a week for 3 months. Two conditions that fall within this category are:

    a. Binge eating disorder
- **(1)** Binge eating disorder features recurrent episodes of binge eating similar to bulimia nervosa.
- **(2)** Since individuals with binge eating disorder do not regularly employ inappropriate compensatory behaviors such as purging or fasting, this disorder differs from bulimia nervosa.

    b. Female athlete triad
- **(1)** When associated with athletic training, the combination of disordered eating, amenorrhea, and osteoporosis is known as the female athlete triad.
- **(2)** Usually these athletes do not meet the criteria for anorexia nervosa.
- **(3)** Amenorrhea in female athletes results from intense training, fluctuations in weight, and low levels of estrogen.
- **(4)** Prolonged low levels of estrogen may lead to osteoporosis and fractures.

B. Epidemiology

1. Anorexia nervosa

    a. Prevalence. Studies estimate that the lifetime prevalence of anorexia nervosa ranges between 0.5% and 3.7% of women. Among men, the prevalence of anorexia nervosa is approximately one-tenth that among females. More than 90% of the individuals with anorexia nervosa are women.

    b. Because of the typical age of onset, anorexia nervosa is most commonly encountered in adolescents and young women. Anorexia nervosa usually begins in mid-to-late adolescence (age 14–18 years). The disorder rarely occurs in women older than 40 years.

    c. When comparing women of different ethnic origins, anorexia nervosa is more common among Caucasians, Native Americans and Hispanic women and less common among African American and Asian American women in the United States.

2. Bulimia nervosa

    a. Prevalence. The lifetime prevalence of bulimia nervosa ranges between 1.1% and 4.2% among women. Like the prevalence of anorexia nervosa, the prevalence of bulimia nervosa among men is one-tenth that of women. Bulimia nervosa usually begins in late adolescence or early adulthood.

    b. When comparing women of different ethnic origins, bulimia nervosa is most common among Caucasians. However, studies reveal that African American women are more likely to develop bulimia nervosa than anorexia nervosa and are much more likely to engage in purging with laxatives instead of vomiting.

3. Risk factors

    a. Cultural factors. Women and adolescents who are preoccupied with their weight and experience social pressure to be thin are at an increased risk for developing an eating disorder. Such societal pressures are found more commonly in industrialized nations such as the United States, Canada, Western Europe, and Japan.

    b. Familial factors. Studies reveal that a hereditary component in the development of eating disorders, especially anorexia nervosa, may exist.
- **(1)** First-degree female relatives of individuals with anorexia nervosa have higher rates of both anorexia nervosa and bulimia nervosa. They also have higher rates of eating disorders that do not fully meet the diagnostic criteria for anorexia or bulimia.
- **(2)** Studies of the identical twin siblings of individuals who have anorexia nervosa or bulimia nervosa reveal that they have higher prevalence of eating disorders.
- **(3)** However, the studies of first-degree relatives of patients with bulimia nervosa do not conclusively demonstrate a hereditary transmission of bulimia nervosa.

    c. History of sexual abuse. Differing studies report that between 20% and 50% of individuals with anorexia nervosa and bulimia nervosa have been victims of sexual abuse.

    d. Psychiatric illness. High rates of comorbid psychiatric illness, such as major depression or dysthymia, have been reported to exist among 50% to 75% of individuals with anorexia nervosa and bulimia nervosa. The estimated prevalence of bipolar disorder among patients with anorexia or bulimia is between 4% and 6%. Reports indicate that obsessive–compulsive disorder has the lifetime prevalence as high as 25% among patients with anorexia. Personality disorders are also common among patients with eating disorders.

TABLE 93–2. SUGGESTED MEDICAL EVALUATION OF PATIENTS WITH EATING DISORDERS

Evaluation	Anorexia Nervosa Restricting Type	Binge/Purge Type	Bulimia Nervosa Purging Type	Nonpurging Type
Weight for height	X	X	X	X
Temperature, pulse, blood pressure	X	X	X	X
Physical examination	X	X	X	X
Dental examination		X	X	
Electrocardiogram	X	X	X	
Complete blood cell count	X	X	X	X
Urinalysis	X	X	X	X
Blood urea nitrogen				
Creatinine	X	X	X	X*
Amylase		X*	X*	X*
Electrolytes	X	X	X	X*
Magnesium	X	X	X*	
Calcium	X	X	X*	
Phosphate	X		X	X*
Albumin	X	X	X*	
Bone mineral densitometry†	X*	X*	X*	X*
LH/FSH/estradiol†	X*	X*	X*	X*
Liver enzymes	X	X	X	
TSH, T₄	X	X	X	X
Cholesterol	X	X	X	X
Glucose	X	X	X	X
Blood/urine screen for drugs/alcohol, laxatives/diuretics	X*	X*	X*	X*

*May be indicated, depending on the patient's clinical circumstances.
†In patients with long-standing amenorrhea.
FSH, follicle-stimulating hormone; LH, luteinizing hormone; TSH, thyroid-stimulating hormone.

C. **Pathophysiology.** Although a conclusive origin of eating disorders has yet to be discovered, several theories exist regarding their etiology of anorexia nervosa and bulimia nervosa.
   1. Some studies suggest a neuroendocrine etiology in anorexia nervosa and bulimia nervosa. Some researchers have noted impaired serotonin transmission among individuals with eating disorders. Other studies have observed alterations in serum leptin levels, an important regulator of weight gain and loss.
   2. A genetic etiology has been postulated. Refer to Section I.B.3.b for further detail.
   3. Cultural influences and a history of dieting are also thought to be a component in the development of eating disorders.
II. **Diagnosis.** One must meet the diagnostic criteria mentioned in Section I.A to have either anorexia nervosa or bulimia nervosa. See Table 93–2 for a suggested medical evaluation.
   A. **Symptoms and signs**
      1. Patients with eating disorders may **present with nonspecific complaints** such as fatigue, dizziness, and general lack of energy. Additional complaints include symptoms associated with starvation or purging behaviors such as abdominal pain, constipation, amenorrhea, sore throat, and palpitations. Since patients with anorexia rarely possess insight into their illness, they rarely present with complaints about weight loss. Concerned family members and friends may bring patients with eating disorders.
      2. When obtaining a history, it is important to **establish rapport and obtain a thorough diet history**. Questions should include inquiries about number of diets used within the past year and questions about the patient's perception of their weight.
      3. **Weight and cardiac status are the most important components of the physical examination of individuals with eating disorders**.
      4. During treatment, one must closely monitor the weight of patients. Patients with eating disorders may wear extra layers of clothing, place weights in their pockets, and drink extra fluids prior to being weighed.

5. Early in the disorder, the physical examination may be normal.
6. As the severity of the eating disorder worsens, complications may cause several abnormal findings on physical examination. Listed below are some physical examination findings:
   a. **Cardiac.** Bradycardia, orthostatic hypotension, and acrocyanosis are among the cardiac abnormalities.
   b. **Dental.** Erosion of dental enamel and salivary gland enlargement are signs of purging behavior.
   c. **Gastrointestinal.** Patients may have significant abdominal distention secondary to decreased bowel motility.
   d. **Skin.** Patients may develop lanugo, dry skin, or loss of subcutaneous fat. Repeated induction of vomiting may cause calluses or scarring on the dorsum of the hand (Russell's sign).

B. **Laboratory findings**
   1. Among individuals with eating disorders, laboratory testing may be normal until complications develop.
   2. Because of complications, testing may reveal abnormal electrolytes, renal functioning, complete blood cell counts, thyroid function test abnormalities, and osteopenia. See Section V.A (medical complications) for further detail.

C. **Differential diagnosis**
   1. **General medical conditions.** When evaluating an individual for anorexia nervosa or bulimia nervosa, one must consider other possible causes of weight loss and binge eating.
      a. Gastrointestinal disorders, endocrine diseases, occult malignancies, and acquired immunodeficiency syndrome (AIDS) are among the medical conditions that should be considered.
      b. Individuals with the neurologic disorder Kleine–Levin syndrome may experience binge eating similar to a person with bulimia nervosa.
      c. However, patients who experience weight loss because of a medical condition usually do not experience the distortion of body image that individuals with anorexia nervosa display.
   2. **Psychiatric disorders.** Several psychiatric disorders can cause severe weight loss.
      a. **Major depressive disorder** may cause decreased appetite and weight loss.
      b. Patients with **schizophrenia** may display odd eating behaviors and experience weight loss.
      c. **Social phobia** may provoke feelings of humiliation or embarrassment while eating in public.
      d. **Body dysmorphic disorder** can cause altered perception of body image.
      e. Some individuals with **obsessive–compulsive disorder** may experience obsessions and compulsions related to food.

III. **Treatment**
  A. **Goals**
   1. **Anorexia nervosa.** Goals in the treatment of anorexia nervosa include the restoration of a healthy weight, management of physical complications, treatment of comorbid psychiatric conditions, restoration of healthy eating patterns, correction of maladaptive thoughts regarding food, building of a support network, and prevention of relapse.
   2. **Bulimia nervosa.** A reduction in binge eating and purging are the primary goals in the treatment of bulimia nervosa. Since most individuals with bulimia nervosa have a normal body weight, weight restoration is not a primary goal.
  B. **Treatment location** (Table 93–3). Weight and cardiac and metabolic status are the most important physical parameters in the determination of treatment location.
   1. **Inpatient hospitalization**
      a. Indications for immediate hospitalization are marked orthostatic hypotension with an increase in pulse of >20 beats per minute or >20 mm Hg drop in standing blood pressure, bradycardia <40 beats per minute, tachycardia >110 beats per minute, or inability to sustain body core temperature. (SOR **Ⓐ**)
      b. Severely underweight individuals (usually those patients who weigh <75% of their individually estimated healthy weights) and adolescents and children with rapid weight loss will also require 24-hour hospitalization. (SOR **Ⓐ**)
      c. Failure of outpatient treatment, persistent weight loss, and declines in oral intake despite participation in outpatient treatment programs, and the presence of additional

TABLE 93-3. LEVEL-OF-CARE CRITERIA FOR PATIENTS WITH EATING DISORDERS

Characteristic	Level 1 Outpatient	Level 2 Intensive Outpatient	Level 3 Full-day Outpatient	Level 4 Residential Treatment Center	Level 5 Inpatient Hospitalization
Medical complications	Medically stable to the extent that more extensive monitoring as defined in levels 4 and 5 is not required			Medically stable (not requiring NG feeds, IV fluids, or multiple daily laboratories)	Adults: HR < 40 beats/min, BP < 90/60 mm Hg; glucose < 60 mg/dL (3.3 mmol/L); K^+ < 3 mg/dL (0.8 mmol/L); temperature < 36.1°C (97°F); dehydration; renal, cardiovascular, or hepatic compromise. Children and adolescents: HR < 50 beats/min; BP < 80/50, orthostatic BP, hypokalemia, hypophosphatemia.
Suicidality	No intent or plan			Possible plan but no intent	Intent and plan
Weight, as percent of healthy body weight	>85%	>80%	>70%	<85%	Adults < 75%. Children and adolescents: acute weight decline with food refusal.
Motivation to recover (cooperativeness, insight, ability to control obsessive thoughts)	Good to fair	Fair	Partial, preoccupied with ego-syntonic thoughts more than 3 h/d; cooperative.	Fair to poor; preoccupied with ego-syntonic thoughts 4–6 h/d; cooperative with highly structured environment.	Poor to very poor; preoccupied with ego-syntonic thoughts, uncooperative with treatment or cooperative only with highly structured environment.
Comorbid disorders (substance abuse, depression, anxiety)	Presence of comorbid condition may influence choice of level of care				Any existing psychiatric disorder that would require hospitalization.
Structure needed for eating/gaining weight	Self-sufficient		Needs structure to gain weight	Needs supervision at all meals or will restrict eating	Needs supervision during and after all meals, or NG/special feeding
Impairment and ability to care for self, ability to control exercise	Able to exercise for fitness; fitness; able to control obsessive exercise		Structure required to prevent excessive exercise	Complete role impairment, cannot eat and gain weight by self; structure required to prevent patient from compulsive exercise	

Purging behavior	Can greatly reduce purging in nonstructured settings; no significant medical complications such as ECG abnormalities or others suggesting the need for hospitalization	Can ask for and use support or skills if desires to purge	Needs supervision during and after all meals
Environmental stress	Others able to provide adequate emotional and practical support	Others able to provide at least limited support and structure	Severe family conflict, problems or absence so as unable to provide structured treatment in home, or lives alone without adequate support system and structure
Treatment availability/living situation	Lives near treatment setting		Too distant to live at home

BP, blood pressure; ECG, electrocardiogram; HR, heart rate; IV, intravenous; K$^+$, potassium level; NG, nasogastric.
(Adapted with permission from Practice guideline for the treatment of patients with eating disorders (revision) American Psychiatric Association Work Group on Eating Disorders. *Am J Psychiatry.* 2000;157(suppl 1):1-39.)

physical stressors such as concurrent viral illnesses or psychiatric disturbances are indications for inpatient treatment. (SOR **Ⓐ**)

  d. Most patients with uncomplicated bulimia do not require inpatient hospitalization. Bulimic patients may require inpatient treatment they have serious concurrent medical problems, suicidality, severe psychiatric disturbances, concurrent substance abuse, or failed trials of outpatient therapy. (SOR **Ⓐ**)

  e. Evidence suggests that patients with eating disorders have better outcomes when treated on inpatient units that specialize in the treatment of these disorders than when treated in general inpatient hospitals. (SOR **Ⓐ**)

2. Outpatient treatment

  a. Highly structured outpatient programs are often necessary for individuals with anorexia nervosa who weigh <85% of their individually estimated healthy weight.

  b. The more successful programs require patients participate in treatment at least 8 hours a day for 5 days a week. (SOR **Ⓐ**)

  c. Partial hospitalization and day hospital programs are being increasingly used in the treatment of eating disorders.

C. Nutritional rehabilitation

  1. A program of nutritional rehabilitation should be established for those who are markedly underweight. The program should seek to restore weight, achieve normal eating patterns, correct maladaptive thoughts about hunger, and correct sequelae of malnutrition. (SOR **Ⓐ**)

  2. Typical goals for weight gain are 2 to 3 lbs per week for patients in the inpatient setting and 0.5 to 1 lb/wk in the outpatient setting. Initial intake levels should begin at 30 to 40 kcal/kg/d and should be gradually advanced. During the weight-gain phase, daily food intake may be increased 70 to 100 kcal/kg/d. (SOR **Ⓑ**)

  3. During refeeding, solid foods are preferable to liquid diets.

  4. In life-threatening situations, nasogastric feeding and parenteral feedings may be necessary.

  5. During nutritional rehabilitation or refeeding, medical monitoring of vital signs, electrolytes, edema, and volume overload is essential.

  6. Since many patients with bulimia nervosa have a normal weight, restoration of weight is often not necessary. In these patients, nutritional counseling should focus on reducing dysfunctional eating behaviors and correcting nutritional deficiencies.

D. Psychosocial interventions

  1. For patients with anorexia nervosa, the goals of treatment are to encourage patient cooperation during their physical and nutritional rehabilitation, change dysfunctional behaviors related to their eating disorder, address comorbid psychopathology, and improve their social functioning.

  2. Systematic trials, case series, and expert opinions suggest that a well-conducted regimen of psychotherapy helps to improve symptoms of anorexia nervosa and prevent relapse. (SOR **Ⓐ**) One meta-analysis that compared behavioral psychotherapy programs to treatment with medication alone revealed that behavioral therapy resulted in more consistent weight gain and shorter hospital stays. Clinical consensus favors individual psychotherapy during the acute phase of treatment for anorexia nervosa.

  3. Structured inpatient and partial hospitalization programs have been demonstrated to produce good short-term therapeutic effects. These behavioral programs often employ nonpunitive reinforcers such as empathic praise and privileges for achieving weight goals.

  4. Individual psychotherapy and family psychotherapy have been proved to be helpful in the management of anorexia nervosa. (SOR **Ⓐ**)

  5. Cognitive behavioral therapy has been proven to be the single most effective intervention in the treatment of bulimia nervosa. (SOR **Ⓐ**)

  6. Additionally, studies have demonstrated that group treatment, family therapy, and individual psychotherapy have been proved helpful in the treatment of bulimia nervosa. (SOR **Ⓐ**)

E. Medications

  1. Antidepressants. Although antidepressants do not augment the benefits of psychotherapy during the acute management phase of patients with anorexia, antidepressants have been demonstrated to be effective in the weight maintenance phase of treatment plans. (SOR **Ⓐ**) Additionally, antidepressants have been proved to be effective in the acute treatment of bulimia nervosa. Studies have demonstrated 50%

to 75% reductions in binge eating and vomiting with antidepressant medications. (SOR **Ⓐ**)

  a. Selective serotonin reuptake inhibitors (SSRIs). Selective serotonin reuptake inhibitors, or SSRIs, such as fluoxetine are commonly considered for patients with anorexia nervosa who have depressive, obsessive, and compulsive symptoms. Fluoxetine is typically dosed at 40 mg/d in the weight-maintenance phase of anorexia. Doses of fluoxetine up to 60 mg/d may help prevent relapse among patients with anorexia. Similarly, a 60- to 80-mg daily dose of fluoxetine has been proved beneficial in the treatment of bulimia nervosa. Presently, fluoxetine (Prozac) is the only medication to be approved by the US Food and Drug Administration (FDA) for the treatment of bulimia nervosa.

  b. Bupropion. The FDA has issued a black box warning against the use of bupropion in patients with eating disorders because of increased risk of seizures.

  c. Tricyclic antidepressants and MAOIs: tricyclic antidepressants, bupropion, and MAOIs have been demonstrated to be effective in the treatment of bulimia nervosa. The MAOIs phenelzine or isocarboxazid dosed between 30 and 45 mg/d may reduce binge eating behavior in patients with bulimia. Dosing of the tricyclic antidepressants usually starts at 50 mg/d. MAOI and tricyclic antidepressants should be avoided in malnourished patients because of greater risk of adverse reactions.

  2. Psychotropic medications. Antipsychotic medications such as olanzapine, risperidone, and quetiapine have demonstrated some usefulness in anorexic patients with severe, unremitting resistance to gaining weight, severe obsessional thinking and extreme denial. (SOR **Ⓒ**) Thus far, controlled studies have yet to demonstrate efficacy of psychotropic medications such as neuroleptics in the treatment of anorexia nervosa or bulimia nervosa.

  3. Other medications

  a. Treatment of osteoporosis. Calcium (500 mg 2–3 tablets daily), estrogen replacement, and bisphosphonates have been used in the treatment of patients with anorexia nervosa to prevent osteopenia and osteoporosis. Usually oral contraceptives are used as a means of hormone replacement and restoration of menstruation. Presently, no evidence has proved the effectiveness of these interventions.

  b. Management of abdominal pains. Metoclopramide, 10 mg with meals, has been used in the treatment of gastroparesis and early satiety.

IV. Management Strategies

  A. Establish a therapeutic relationship. The idea of gaining weight for an individual with an eating disorder or discontinuing binge eating patterns can be anxiety provoking. Without patients having a trusting relationship with their physician, such goals will never be achieved.

  B. Collaborate with other health professionals. Nutritional counseling, group psychotherapy, and medical consultation with specialists may be necessary to fully restore the health of an individual with bulimia nervosa or anorexia nervosa.

  C. Monitor dysfunctional eating behaviors. The careful assessment of a patient's perceived food intake and the anxiety provoked by eating is necessary. Having a meal with a patient may allow the clinician further insight into the patient's disordered patterns of eating.

  D. Monitor the patient's general medical condition and psychiatric status.

  E. Assess the family and provide treatment. Parents often struggle with denial, feelings of guilt, anger, and feelings of rejection. Family assessment and family therapy is usually a significant part of comprehensive care.

V. Prognosis

  A. Medical complications. Patients with anorexia nervosa and bulimia nervosa are susceptible to serious medical complications as a result of starvation and purging.

  1. Cardiovascular complications. Cardiovascular complications include orthostatic hypotension, palpitations, and arrhythmias such as bradycardia. Cardiomyopathy may result from low weight or syrup of ipecac abuse. Additionally, severe electrolyte imbalances may lead to sudden cardiac death.

  2. Dental complications. Multiple dental caries and dental enamel erosions can occur after several years of induced vomiting in anorexia nervosa. Patients may also develop enlarged salivary glands.

  3. Gastrointestinal complications. Vomiting related to the compensatory purging behavior in patients with anorexia nervosa and bulimia nervosa may eventually cause gastritis, esophagitis, or Mallory–Weiss tears. Patients may develop esophageal dys-motility disorders like gastroesophageal reflux. Individuals who repeatedly use lax-atives as a means of purging may develop melanosis coli and other problems with colonic motility. Chronic constipation and bloating may occur in laxative abusers. Cases of rectal prolapse have been reported in the literature.

4. **Endocrine complications.** Patients with anorexia nervosa may develop elevated serum cortisol levels and decreased levels of serum thyroxine (T_4) and triiodothyronine (T_3).

5. **Hematologic complications.** Nutritional deficits and changes associated with starva-tion may cause normochromic normocytic anemia, neutropenia, and thrombocytope-nia. Rarely patients with anorexia nervosa may experience clotting disorders.

6. **Metabolic complications.** Because of starvation and purging, patients may develop serious electrolyte imbalances. Laxative abusers may develop a metabolic acidosis, hypomagnesemia, and hypophosphatemia. Metabolic alkalosis (elevated serum bi-carbonate levels, hypochloremia, and hypokalemia) and hyperamylasemia can result from repeated induced vomiting.

7. **Musculoskeletal complications.** Musculoskeletal complications include osteoporo-sis and arrested skeletal growth. Young female athletes with amenorrhea and altered eating behaviors are particularly at risk for the development of stress fractures. Bone mineral density testing for osteoporosis and osteopenia should be considered in pa-tients with chronic amenorrhea.

8. **Renal complications.** Renal abnormalities are seen in up to 70% of patients with anorexia nervosa. Complications include decreased glomerular filtration rate, in-creased blood urea nitrogen, and pitting edema. Monitoring of renal function during treatment is strongly recommended.

9. **Reproductive complications.** Reproductive complications include amenorrhea and infertility. Amenorrhea occurs in women secondary to low estrogen levels. Males with anorexia nervosa may have low serum testosterone levels. Both males and females with eating disorders may have loss of libido and infertility. Adolescents and young women may experience arrest of sexual development or regression of secondary sex-ual characteristics.

10. **Skin complications.** Repeated manual stimulation of the gag reflex to induce vomiting may cause callus development and scarring on the dorsum of the hand. This is known as Russell's sign.

11. **Suicide.** Suicide is a major cause of death among patients with anorexia nervosa.

B. **Outcomes**

1. **Anorexia nervosa**

   a. Approximately 44% of patients with anorexia nervosa fully recover and successfully restore their weight to within 15% of recommended weight for height. Approximately 24% of patients never restore their weight and between 2.5% and 5% of patients with anorexia nervosa die.

   b. Worse prognosis is associated with lower minimum weight, earlier age of onset, and disturbed family relationships.

   c. Follow-up studies conducted more than 10 to 15 years reveal that it may take be-tween 57 and 79 months to achieve full recovery.

2. **Bulimia nervosa**

   a. Approximately 25% to 30% of patients with bulimia demonstrate spontaneous im-provement within a 1- to 2-year period.

   b. With interventions such as medication and psychosocial intervention, between 50% and 70% of patients have some significant reductions in binge eating and purging.

REFERENCES

American Psychiatric Association. *Diagnostic and Statistical Manual of Mental Disorders.* 4th ed., text revision. American Psychiatric Association; 2000:583-595.

Hobart JA, Smucker DR. The female athlete triad. *Am Fam Physician.* 2000;61:3357, 3367.

The McKnight Investigators. Risk factors for the onset of eating disorders in adolescent girls: Results of the McKnight Longitudinal Risk Factor Study. *Am J Psychiatry.* 2003;160:248.

Practice guideline for treatment of patients with eating disorders (third edition). American Psychiatric Association Work Group on Eating Disorders. *Am J Psychiatry.* 2006;163(suppl 7):1.

Pritts SD, Susman J: Diagnosis of eating disorders in primary care. *Am Fam Physician.* 2003;67:297, 311.

94 Somatization

Laura B. Frankenstein, MD, & Ryan M. Niemiec, PsyD

KEY POINTS

- Approximately 90% of the 10 most common problems that present in primary care settings have no identifiable medical etiology.
- Diagnosis involves recognizing positive criteria (Table 94–1) before ruling out specific diseases with tests and procedures.
- Treatment is multifaceted but relies most heavily on active listening, education, self-regulation strategies, and developing a therapeutic contract that includes both supportive care and setting limits.

I. **Introduction**
   A. **Definition.** Somatization is a process by which persons experience and express emotional discomfort or psychosocial stress through physical symptoms. There is an absence in disease or tissue damage.
   B. **Epidemiology**
      1. **Prevalence**
         a. Between 60% and 80% of healthy persons experience somatic symptoms in any given week. About one-third of all primary care patients have ill-defined symptoms not attributable to physical disease, and 70% of those with emotional disorders present a somatic complaint as the reason for their office visit.
         b. The prevalence of **somatization disorder**, as defined in the *Diagnostic and Statistical Manual of Mental Disorders,* 4th edition (DSM-IV) (Table 94–2), is <1% in community-based studies, 5% among primary care outpatients, and 9% among hospitalized medical and surgical patients. The great majority of these patients are female. Clinical somatization is more common than these percentages suggest. For example, a diagnosis of **undifferentiated somatoform disorder** requires one or more unexplained physical symptoms that cause clinically significant distress in the person's functioning.
         c. The prevalence of **psychogenic pain disorder** is unknown, but the disorder appears to be quite common in medical settings.
         d. In primary care practice, the prevalence of **hypochondriasis**, a preoccupation with the fear or belief that one has serious illness, may be as high as 10%. Full-blown somatization disorder is rare in men, but hypochondriasis appears in both sexes with equal frequency.
         e. **Conversion symptoms** (e.g., sudden blindness or paralysis), while apparently common several decades ago, are now infrequent.
      2. **Risk factors**
         a. **Personal characteristics** associated with somatization include female gender, older age, currently unmarried state, lower level of education, lower socioeconomic class, and urban residence.
         b. **Cultural factors.** Somatization occurs throughout the world but is more prevalent in cultures in which emotional distress is generally couched in nonpsychological terms. In the United States, somatization appears to be particularly frequent among Hispanic and Asian populations. People exposed to war trauma and torture often present with unexplained symptoms that are often very troubling.
   C. **Pathophysiology.** Multiple theories have been proposed to explain somatization (Table 94–3). These are not mutually exclusive, and it is likely that somatization is a complex phenomenon with multiple risk factors playing a role in its causation.
II. **Diagnosis.** Somatization is a complex, multifactorial process. It is perhaps best to think of somatization as a spectrum that ranges from occasional functional somatic symptoms to full-blown DSM-IV somatoform disorders.

TABLE 94–1. POSITIVE CRITERIA FOR DIAGNOSIS OF PSYCHOGENIC SYMPTOMS

1. The patient's descriptions of symptoms are vague, inconsistent, or bizarre.
2. Symptoms are in excess of objective findings.
3. There are multiple symptoms in different organ systems.
4. Symptoms persist despite apparently adequate medical therapy.
5. The illness began in the context of a psychologically meaningful setting (e.g., death of relative, conflict with spouse, work injury, or job promotion).
6. The patient denies that any emotional distress or psychological factors play a role in symptom development.
7. The patient has visited several physicians or has had several operations.
8. There is evidence of an associated psychiatric disorder.
9. Discussion reveals that the patient attributes an idiosyncratic meaning to symptom.
10. Alexithymia (i.e., difficulty describing emotions or inner processes in words) is present.

A. **Differential diagnosis**
   1. **Poorly understood conditions** in which somatization might play a role or which might be confused with somatization include **fibromyalgia, irritable bowel syndrome, dysphagia, chronic fatigue syndrome, multiple chemical sensitivity,** and **temporomandibular joint dysfunction.** Other disorders with vague, multiple, and confusing symptoms (e.g., hypothyroidism, multiple sclerosis, porphyria, systemic lupus erythematosus, or musculoskeletal and neuropsychiatric manifestations of Lyme disease) must also be considered, although, except for hypothyroidism, the prevalence of these conditions in the primary care setting is quite low.
   2. **Amplified symptoms** of underlying organic disease may also be involved in somatization.
   3. **Psychiatric disorders** in which somatization is not the primary process may be "masked" by an array of somatic complaints. These disorders include **major depression** (see Chapter 92), **alcohol and substance abuse** (see Chapter 88), and **generalized anxiety** and **panic disorders** (see Chapter 89). Physician recognition of psychiatric distress is decreased when patients present with high levels of somatization. Among somatizers in one primary care study, 24% had major depression, 17% had dysthymia, and 22% had generalized anxiety disorder.
   4. **Somatoform disorders**
      a. Somatization disorder (Table 94–2).
      b. Conversion disorder (Table 94–4).
      c. Hypochondriasis (Table 94–5).
      d. Psychogenic pain disorder (Table 94–6).
      e. Body dysmorphic disorder (Table 94–7).
   5. **Factitious disease** occurs when a patient feigns physical or psychological symptoms in order to assume the sick role. Less than 5% of patients referred to psychiatrists

TABLE 94–2. DIAGNOSTIC CRITERIA FOR SOMATIZATION DISORDER

A. A history of many physical complaints beginning before the age of 30, occurring over a period of several years and resulting in treatment being sought or significant impairment in social or occupational functioning.
B. Each of the following criteria have been met at some time during the course of the disorder. To count a symptom as significant, it must not be fully explained by a known general medical condition, or the resulting complaints or impairment is in excess of what would be expected from the history, physical examination, or laboratory findings.
   1. Four pain symptoms: a history of pain related to at least four different sites or functions (e.g., head, abdomen, back, joints, extremities, chest, rectum, during sexual intercourse, during menstruation, or during urination).
   2. Two gastrointestinal symptoms: a history of at least two gastrointestinal symptoms other than pain (e.g., nausea, diarrhea, bloating, vomiting other than during pregnancy, or intolerance of several different foods).
   3. One sexual symptom: a history of at least one sexual or reproductive symptom other than pain (e.g., sexual indifference, erectile or ejaculatory dysfunction, irregular menses, excessive menstrual bleeding, or vomiting throughout pregnancy).
   4. One pseudoneurologic symptom: a history of at least one symptom or deficit suggesting a neurologic disorder not limited to pain (conversion symptoms such as blindness, double vision, deafness, loss of touch or pain sensation, hallucinations, aphonia, impaired coordination or balance, paralysis or localized weakness, difficulty swallowing, difficulty breathing, urinary retention, or seizures; dissociative symptoms such as amnesia or loss of consciousness other than fainting).

TABLE 94–3. THEORIES OF SOMATIZATION ETIOLOGY

1. **Neurobiological.** Abnormal central nervous system regulation of incoming sensory information leads to an impairment in attentional processing.
2. **Psychodynamic.** Somatization is a defense mechanism.
3. **Behavioral.** Somatization is a learned behavior in which environmental reinforcers maintain abnormal illness behavior.
4. **Sociocultural.** "Correct" ways of dealing with emotions and feelings are culturally determined.

TABLE 94–4. DIAGNOSTIC CRITERIA FOR CONVERSION DISORDER

A. One or more symptoms or deficits affect voluntary motor or sensory function, suggesting a neurologic or general medical condition.
B. Psychological factors are judged to be associated with the symptom or deficit because the initiation or exacerbation of the symptom or deficit is preceded by conflicts or other stressors.
C. The symptom or deficit is not intentionally produced or feigned (as in factitious disorder or malingering).
D. The symptom or deficit cannot, after appropriate investigation, be fully explained by a neurologic or general medical condition and is not a culturally sanctioned behavior or experience.
E. The symptom or deficit causes clinically significant distress or impairment in social, occupational, or other important areas of functioning or warrants medical evaluation.
F. The symptom or deficit is not limited to pain or sexual dysfunction, does not occur exclusively during the course of somatization disorder, and is not better accounted for by another mental disorder.

TABLE 94–5. DIAGNOSTIC CRITERIA FOR HYPOCHONDRIASIS

A. Preoccupation with fears of having, or the idea that one has, a serious disease based on the person's misinterpretation of bodily symptoms.
B. The preoccupation persists despite appropriate medical evaluation and reassurance.
C. The belief in A is not of delusional intensity (as in delusional disorder, somatic type) and is not restricted to a circumscribed concern about appearance (as in body dysmorphic disorder).
D. The preoccupation causes clinically significant distress or impairment in social, occupational, or other important areas of functioning.
E. The duration of the disturbance is at least 6 months.
F. The preoccupation does not occur exclusively during the course of generalized anxiety disorder, obsessive–compulsive disorder, panic disorder, a major depressive episode, separation anxiety, or another somatoform disorder.

TABLE 94–6. DIAGNOSTIC CRITERIA FOR PSYCHOGENIC PAIN DISORDER

A. Pain in one or more anatomic sites is the predominant focus of the clinical presentation and is of sufficient severity to warrant clinical attention.
B. The pain causes clinically significant distress or impairment in social, occupational, or other important areas of functioning.
C. Psychological factors are judged to have an important role in the onset, severity, exacerbation, or maintenance of the pain.
D. The pain is not better accounted for by a mood, anxiety, or psychotic disorder and does not meet criteria for dyspareunia.

TABLE 94–7. CRITERIA FOR BODY DYSMORPHIC DISORDER (BDD)

Preoccupation with an imagined defect in appearance. If a slight physical anomaly is present, the person's concern is markedly excessive. [As with all the somatoform disorders, the preoccupation causes significant distress or impairment in functioning; the preoccupation is not better accounted for by another mental disorder.]

for evaluation of unexplained somatic symptoms have factitious disease. Patients who persistently exhibit factitious disease have **Munchausen syndrome.** Diagnostic tests and medical interventions often lead to additional symptoms (e.g., drug side effects), clinical findings (e.g., surgical scars), and dysfunction (e.g., intestinal adhesions) in these patients. **Malingering** occurs when a patient feigns symptoms in order to receive external incentives or secondary gain (e.g., avoid legal responsibility or economic gain).

B. Symptoms and signs

1. Symptoms favoring somatization are presented in Table 94–2. The presence of several of these characteristics strongly suggests somatization, even though evidence of organic disease may also be present.

2. **Pain** is the most frequent single complaint, present in more than 80% of patients with somatization.

3. **Three symptom clusters suggestive of somatization secondary to depression, anxiety, or panic disorder are described below.**

   a. Atypical chest pain, palpitations, tachycardia, or difficulty catching one's breath (sighing, not true dyspnea), or all of these.

   b. Headache, dizziness, lightheadedness, presyncope, or paresthesias.

   c. Dyspepsia, heartburn, "gas," flatulence, or other gastrointestinal symptoms, or all of these.

4. **Globus hystericus,** the sensation of a lump in the throat that interferes with swallowing, is a frequent symptom of anxiety or conversion.

C. Laboratory tests. Laboratory and imaging studies serve only to rule out organic disease, although evidence of a disease entity does not exclude the diagnosis of somatization. Abnormalities unrelated to the patient's symptoms may be discovered with sophisticated diagnostic technology that are not particularly helpful. For example, the presence of minimal mitral valve prolapse on echocardiography cannot explain an array of somatic symptoms. Avoid tests with low yields that may create new problems for the patient, either increased anxiety or side effects from the procedure itself.

III. Treatment. Appropriate treatment for any underlying problems is the first priority. Treatment is not likely to be effective unless maintaining factors are addressed and minimized.

A. Basic treatment principles

1. Never say, "It's all in your head" or "There's nothing wrong with you": The patient's problem should be considered as deserving of attention. This requires attentive listening, empathic responses, and validation of patient's distress.

2. Give a clear explanation of symptoms presented in functional or physiologic terms. Explain the sympathetic nervous system's "fight or flight" stress response, the science of how emotions reside in the physical body, and the interaction (not cause) of cognitions and the body. The physician should describe the problem in terms the patient can understand and in a way that fits in with his or her belief system about health and illness. Disease labels should be avoided as much as possible. When you do not understand and cannot explain a symptom, tell the patient that with empathy.

3. Initiate a well-defined treatment program: Regular, brief appointments every 4 to 8 weeks are often recommended over "as needed" appointments. Treatment may consist of a combination of explanation, reassurance, observation, and symptomatic measures. The physician should provide relatively definite information about how to proceed, how long the symptoms might last, and what to do next. Ambiguity increases anxiety.

4. Engage the patient's active participation: Encourage the patient to keep a log or diary of factors that influence symptoms, such as emotion, daily stressors, and activities they are involved in; this may serve to make the problem appear less unpredictable and out of control. General behavior change techniques also may be initiated. For example, an exercise program to enhance "muscle tone" or a diet for weight reduction, if successful, generally enhances the patient's sense of control and self-mastery.

B. Multifaceted treatment approach

1. **Pharmacotherapy.** There are no adequate clinical trials of drug treatment for primary somatization per se. However, drugs may be effective in the following situations.

   a. Specific intractable symptoms such as headaches, myalgias, and other forms of chronic pain may be ameliorated by **selective serotonin reuptake inhibitors** or **tricyclic antidepressants** (see Chapter 92 for starting dosages). (SOR **B**)

   b. Even when DSM-IV criteria for depression are not present, patients who demonstrate somatic symptoms of depression often benefit from adequate doses of serotonin reuptake inhibitors. Likewise, anxious patients may experience relief of somatic symptoms in response to **benzodiazepine therapy,** even though they do not fulfill DSM-IV criteria for panic or anxiety disorders (see Chapter 89 for starting dosages).

   c. Because patients who somatize often have a low tolerance for the side effects of medications, symptomatic medications (e.g., analgesics or antispasmodics) should be used sparingly and in the minimal effective doses.

   d. There is rarely, if ever, a place for opioids in treating somatization symptoms.

  2. Consultation with a psychiatrist or psychologist. While integrated care or collaborative care in which a psychologist is a part of the primary care team is ideal, this does not always work out practically. Consultation or referral to behavioral medicine programs, psychiatry, or cognitive behavior therapy has been shown to be effective with this population. Psychiatric consultation has been shown over the short term (i.e., 1 year) to be effective in reducing hospitalizations and overall medical costs of patients with somatization disorder. (SOR **B**) In one study, a single consultation report to the primary physician was associated with a 12% reduction in costs. A course of cognitive behavioral therapy has been associated with improvements in functioning and decreases in health care utilization for up to 18 months. (SOR **B**) Many patients with somatization disorder are skeptical of referrals to mental health professionals, therefore, care should be taken to explain that their suffering is "real" and that this is a "part" of their treatment plan, not a "physician replacement" or rejection of future treatment.

  3. Patients with severe chronic somatization may benefit from intensive, multidisciplinary treatment programs that include individual, group, and family therapy; educational programs; physical and occupational therapy; biofeedback; and vocational rehabilitation.

IV. Management Strategies. Optimal management of somatizing patients requires relief of symptoms, treatment of underlying medical or psychiatric disorders, and avoidance of the pathologic cycle of intervention (medical treatment, temporary improvement, renewal of symptoms, disappointment, and patient and physician anger).

  A. The **therapeutic contract** should be emphasized and its parameters defined. While recognizing the reality of the patient's symptoms, one should attempt to develop a broader framework for physician–patient interaction by following the guidelines described below.

    1. Tolerate symptoms and scale down the goals of therapy. Speak in terms of reduction, lessening, and coping, rather than complete symptom alleviation. Evaluate new symptoms as they occur, but do so conservatively in a stepwise fashion. Openly discuss the risks of medication side effects and the possibility of complications with invasive procedures.

    2. Discuss psychiatric or psychosocial issues not as direct causes of symptoms, but rather as possible aggravating factors or as unfortunate results of physical symptoms.

    3. Promote stability in the physician–patient relationship by scheduling office visits at regular intervals, thereby diminishing the patient's need for a "ticket of admission." Increase the length of office visits to allow relatively unrushed attention. Schedule visits at times when interruptions will be minimal, not on "emergency-prone" days such as Mondays or Fridays.

    4. Explicitly discourage dependent behaviors, such as unscheduled phone calls or drop-in visits. Prearranged follow-up phone calls may allow a reduction in the frequency of office visits. Ask the patient not to "doctor shop" or to seek specialist care without consulting the primary care physician.

  B. Somatization may be a sign of **family dysfunction** in which the identified patient's symptoms may serve to stabilize a pathologic family situation. It may be necessary to enlist family members in behavioral strategies to "wean" the patient from secondary gain (e.g., using somatization to avoid household tasks, to require special meals, or to excuse irritability and angry outbursts).

  C. While remaining supportive of the symptomatic person, the physician should attempt to avoid certifying the person as **permanently and totally disabled.** The label of *disability* can be viewed as another "medical intervention" with adverse consequences as well as benefits. Nonetheless, the physician should realize that severe and chronic somatization is a disabling condition. Chronic pain syndrome, for example, may qualify under Medicare guidelines as a cause of total disability. While perhaps not desirable in terms of "curing" the somatization, disability may, in certain cases, for economic and social reasons be the best palliative option.

   D. Physicians develop a great deal of **anger** and **frustration** when treating patients who
   somatize. To maintain equanimity, the physician may use the following strategies.
   1. Make the diagnosis of somatization and modify treatment objectives accordingly, rather
      than wallowing in frustration over the absence of objective findings of disease.
   2. Set up firm and explicit guidelines as described above, and review them frequently with
      the patient. Arrange office appointments so that somatizers are not clustered together.
   3. Develop an informal relationship with a psychiatrist or a psychologist to whom feelings
      about these patients can be ventilated and with whom treatment problems can be
      discussed.
V. Prognosis
   A. A large proportion of patients with functional somatic symptoms recover without specific intervention. Favorable prognostic factors include acute onset and short duration of
   symptoms, younger age, higher socioeconomic class, absence of organic disease, and
   absence of personality disorder.
   B. The long-term prognosis for patients with somatization disorder is guarded, and usually
   lifelong supportive treatment is required. If somatization is a mask for another psychiatric
   disorder, its prognosis depends on that of the primary problem. In one study of patients
   with psychiatric disorders presenting with a recent onset of physical symptoms, 40%
   subsequently developed chronic somatoform disorders.
   C. If hypochondriasis is conceptualized as an "amplifying somatic style," patients who exhibit
   this condition are likely to have recurrent physical complaints and require frequent medical
   intervention. Appropriate treatment for somatization should minimize these complaints by
   providing education and reassurance, by reducing anxiety, and by enhancing the patient's
   coping skills.
   D. Discrete conversion symptoms have a better prognosis. They may resolve spontaneously
   when no longer "required" or may respond to specific psychotherapy.

REFERENCES

Coulehan JL, Block MR. Seal up the mouth of outrage: interactive problems in interviewing, Chapter
   12. In: The *Medical Interview: Mastering Skills for Clinical Practice.* Philadelphia, PA: FA Davis;
   2001:195-219.
Dickinson WP, Dickinson LM, deGruy FV, et al. The somatization in primary care study: a tale of three
   diagnoses. *Gen Hosp Psychiatry.* 2003;25:1-7.
Escobar JI, Hoyos-Nervi C, Gara M. Medically unexplained symptoms in medical practice: a psychiatric
   perspective. *Environ Health Perspect.* 2002;110(suppl 4):631-636.
Hiller W, Fichter MM, Riet W. A controlled treatment study of somatoform disorders including analysis
   of healthcare utilization and cost-effectiveness. *J Psychosomatic Res.* 2003;54:369-380.
Maynard CK: Assess and manage somatization. *Nurse Pract.* 2003;28:20-29.
Stanley IM, Peters S, Salmon P. A primary care perspective on prevailing assumptions about persistent
   medically unexplained physical symptoms. *Int J Psychiatry Med.* 2002;32:125-140.

95   Contraception

Marjorie Guthrie, MD

I. **Introduction:** Contraception is an important topic to discuss with all sexually active women of child-bearing age.
  A. The demand for birth control is great; an estimated 41 million women in the United States are sexually active.
  B. Half of all pregnancies in the United States are unintentional, as are 92% of pregnancies in adolescents aged 15 to 19 years.
  C. Three million women in this country between the ages of 15 and 44 years do not use contraception.
  D. Unintentional pregnancies occur either because contraceptives are not used or because they are used sporadically or incorrectly.
  E. Numerous contraceptive options are available, so the choice of a particular option should take place after a review of the risk and benefits of all choices and through education on the option chosen so correct use is assured.
  F. The only 100% effective method of birth control is abstinence. Correct use of any contraceptive device does not guarantee protection. Up to 20% of women who experienced unintended pregnancy used their selected methods consistently and properly.
II. **Choosing a Birth Control Method.** Consideration of the following factors will help patients and physicians make the best possible choices: efficacy, safety, and acceptability. It is important to take the time also to educate patients about the risks and benefits of their birth control options. Desirable properties of contraceptives are a high rate of effectiveness, prolonged duration of action, rapid reversibility, privacy of use, protection against sexually transmitted infections (STIs), and easy accessibility.
  A. **Efficacy**
    1. **Theoretical efficacy rates** are defined as the number of unintended pregnancies per 100 women that occur during the first year of use of a given contraceptive method (if the method is used correctly).
    2. **Actual efficacy rates** reflect the percentage of women who become pregnant during the first year of contraceptive use. The efficacy of a given contraceptive method is influenced by the fertility, individual motivation, and risk-taking attitude of each partner; the frequency of intercourse; the ability of the patient to master the method; and the theoretical efficacy rate of the method.
    3. **Safety concerns** include risks of morbidity and mortality as well as noncontraceptive safety benefits, such as protection from STIs or the resolution of menstrual problems.
    4. **Acceptability** of a method depends on a number of factors.
       a. **Cost.** What is the cost of the method? Does insurance cover the method?
       b. **Individual preferences.** Does the patient have any ethical or religious concerns regarding the method?
       c. **Duration**. How long until it is the method effective? How often is the method used?
       d. **Reversibility.** After stopping the method how long until the patient is able to conceive?
       e. **Privacy**. Does the method afford the patient enough privacy?

      f. Availability. Does the method require office visits, prescription, or any other special situation to obtain?

   B. Patient education. When a physician can educate their patient about the method of birth control, efficacy can be increased and discontinuation can be minimized. As many as 50% of users stop taking the pill in the first year secondary to side effects. When discussing the possible side effects and use of a particular method of birth control with patients, the physician should explain how problems can be minimized and point out the benefit and risks of the method. When a patient reports breakthrough bleeding while taking the medication, use this as an opportunity to see if she is taking the pill daily, since spotting may reflect missed pills.

  III. Hormonal Contraception. This method works by suppressing ovulation, changing cervical mucus so that sperm are less effective, and making the endometrium less receptive to implantation.

   A. Oral combination. This birth control method, used by 18 million women, is the most popular reversible form of contraception in the United States. Oral contraceptive pills have different doses of two types of estrogen and nine types of progestin. Biphasic and triphasic oral contraceptives contain different amounts of hormone throughout the menstrual cycle in an attempt to more closely mimic natural hormone production. Choosing among the many oral contraceptives can be done on the basis of characteristics of both the patient and the contraceptive. See Table 95–1 for common characteristics and recommendations for use.

    1. Failure rates (number of pregnancies expected per 100 women per year): 1 to 2 .

    2. Risks: Dizziness, nausea, change in menstruation, mood, and weight.

     a. Contraindications

      (1) Women older than 35 years who smoke.

TABLE 95–1. **CHOOSING AMONG ORAL CONTRACEPTIVES (OCPS)**

Characteristic	Oral Contraceptive	Comment
Nursing women	Ovrette Micronor	Progesterone-only pills will not interrupt milk supply
Nausea or breast tenderness when taking OCPs	Ovrette Micronor	Progesterone-only or lower estrogenic activity pills
No prior use of OCPs	Ortho Novum 1/35 Tri-Norinyl Ortho Novum 7/7/7 Ortho Tri-cyclen Ortho cyclen Alesse Loestrin 1/20	Lower-dose pills minimize side effects
Acne, hirsutism, or obesity	Demulen Desogen/Ortho-Cept Ovcon 35 Ortho Tri-Cyclen	Less androgenic activity pills
Hypertension, hyperlipidemia, or diabetes mellitus	Desogen/Ortho-Cept Ortho Cyclen Ortho Tri-cyclen Ovocon-35	All produce favorable cholesterol pattern
Scanty or absent withdrawal bleeding	Increase estrogen component or lower progestin	Build up endometrium
Spotting (over 3 mo)	Increase estrogen and progestin in monophasic combinations	Stabilize endometrium
Minimize risk of thrombosis	Loestrin 1/20 Alesse	Less estrogen
Use of rifampin or dilantin	Ovral Ovcon 50 Demulen Ortho-Novum/Norinyl 1/50	Increase estrogen

(2) Women with cardiovascular problems, such as a history of thromboembolic disease, cerebrovascular disease, and ischemic heart disease. Other conditions, such as breast cancer, liver tumor, or undiagnosed vaginal bleeding, preclude oral contraceptive use. (SOR **B**)

(3) Lactating women <6 weeks postpartum because oral contraceptives can diminish breast milk production. Progesterone-only pills are acceptable.

3. **Benefits:**
   a. **Protection from endometrial cancer** after 1 year of use.
   b. **Reduction in the risk of ovarian cancer** after 6 months of use.
   c. **More regular and *less painful* menstrual periods** with less bleeding and iron deficiency anemia. Premenstrual syndrome is less common and less severe in women using oral contraceptives, as are benign breast disease and benign ovarian cysts, endometriosis, acne, hirsutism, and anovulatory bleeding.
   d. **Pelvic inflammatory disease (PID)** caused by *Chlamydia* occurs less often because of the effects oral contraceptives have on the menses, cervix, and mucus.
4. **Acceptability**
   a. **Convenience:** Must be taken daily.
   b. **Availability:** Must have prescription.
B. **Oral contraception progestin only.** These medications contain only progestin and are most often used when combinations pills are contraindicated. They work by reducing and thickening cervical mucus to prevent sperm from implantation.
   1. **Failure rates** (number of pregnancies expected per 100 women per year): 2.
   2. **Risks:** Irregular bleeding, weight gain, and breast tenderness
   3. **Benefits:**
      a. Ability to use during lactation.
      b. Does not carry the cardiovascular risks of combination pills.
   4. **Acceptability**
      a. **Convenience:** Must be taken daily.
      b. **Availability:** Must have prescription.
C. **Injectable hormones.** Depo-Provera (depo-medroxyprogesterone acetate) has been used safely by more than 10 million women worldwide. It has been approved in over 90 countries, including the United States. It is given as a deep intramuscular injection of 150 mg every 12 weeks.
   1. **Failure Rate** (number of pregnancies expected per 100 women per year): <1.
   2. **Risks:** Irregular bleeding, weight gain, breast tenderness, and headaches.
      a. **Contraindications.**
         (1) This method should not be used in women who are at significant risk for breast cancer or who have been treated for this type of cancer.
         (2) This method should be used with caution in patients at increased risk for osteoporosis. (SOR **C**)
   3. **Benefits**
      a. **Amenorrhea** is a consequence that many women enjoy.
      b. **Lactation** is not adversely affected if the hormone is given immediately postpartum; trace amounts are detectable in breast milk without adverse outcome to infants.
      c. **Women with epilepsy** have fewer seizures.
   4. **Acceptability**:
      a. **Convenience:** One injection every 3 months.
      b. **Availability**: Must have prescription.
D. **Injectable combination hormones:** Lunelle is an injectable form of progestin and estrogen.
   1. **Failure rates** (number of pregnancies expected per 100 women per year): 1.
   2. **Risks:** Changes in menstrual cycle, weight gain, and otherwise similar to other combination hormones.
   3. **Benefits:** Similar to other combination hormone.
   4. **Acceptability**
      a. **Convenience:** Injection given once a month.
      b. **Availability:** Must have a prescription.
E. **Ortho Evra** is a combination contraceptive that is provided in a transdermal system. Patches containing 6.00 mg norelgestromin and 0.75 mg ethinyl estradiol are placed on the skin of the buttocks, abdomen, and upper torso or upper outer arms weekly. Each

patch releases 150 μg of norelgestromin and 20 μg of ethinyl estradiol daily. It functions in the same manner as combination oral contraceptives, but is more convenient in a transdermal route for some women.

1. **Failure rates** (number of pregnancies expected per 100 women per year): 1 to 2 (less effective in women weighing more than 198 lbs).
2. **Risks:** Similar to oral combination pills, may be associated with increased risk of thromboembolic disease. (SOR **B**)
   a. **Contraindications:** Same as those for oral contraceptives.
3. **Benefits** are the same as for oral contraceptives.
4. **Acceptability** is enhanced over that of oral contraceptives because of the weekly transdermal route of administration.
   a. **Convenience:** Patch is applied once a week for three weeks. Patch is not worn during the fourth week, and woman have a menstrual cycle.
   b. **Availability:** Must have a prescription.

F. **Nuvaring** is another alternative route of administration for combination hormonal contraceptives. It is a flexible ring impregnated with etonogestrel and ethinyl estradiol. It delivers 0.120 mg of etonogestrel and 0.015 mg ethinyl estradiol daily. The ring is placed weekly in the posterior fornix of the vagina. Because of the "local" administration of hormones, lower doses can be used.

1. **Failure rates** (number of pregnancies expected per 100 women per year): 1 to 2
2. **Risks:** Vaginal discharge virginitis, irritation, and otherwise similar to combination pills.
   a. **Contraindications** are the same as those for oral contraceptives.
3. **Benefits:** Similar to that of oral combination hormones. May be associated with less prolonged bleeding or spotting. (SOR **B**)
4. **Acceptability:** It is also a good choice for women who desire a lower dose of hormones.
   a. **Convenience:** Inserted by the woman, remains for 3 weeks, then removed for 1 week. If out of place for more than 3 hours an alternative method is required.
   b. **Availability:** Must have a prescription.

G. **Postcoital Contraceptives** (Emergency Contraceptives) The hormones that make up the medication appear to inhibit ovulation if it has not occurred. They also may impact gamete transport, function of the corpus luteum, and implantation of a conceptus.

1. **Failure rates** (number of pregnancies expected per 100 women per year): Almost 80% reduction in risk of pregnancy for a single act of unprotected sex.
2. **Risk:** Nausea, vomiting, abdominal pain, fatigue, and headache.
   a. Pregnancy is the only contraindication to its use.
3. **Benefits:** Emergency use.
4. **Acceptability**
   a. **Convenience:** Taken within 72 hours of unprotected intercourse. The earlier the method is used the more effective.
   b. **Availability:** A prescription is required at this time.
5. **Special note:** It is important to discuss this method of birth control with female victims of sexual assault. When this method is chosen it is also important to discuss STI screening and choosing a method with a lower failure rate.
6. **Administration.** All forms of ECP are administered as the first dose, then the second identical dose is given 12 hours later. Women should expect their menses within 3 weeks of taking ECP; otherwise, they need a pregnancy test.

IV. **Barrier Methods.** These methods prevent contraception by providing a mechanical barrier to sperm. Avoid using oil-based lubricants and medications (Femstat, Monistat, estrogen, and Vagisil creams), because they cause the latex in condoms to deteriorate.

A. **Male condoms** are made of latex, the cecum of lambs ("skins"), or polyurethane (for latex-sensitive individuals). Most condoms have a shelf life of 5 years if stored properly in a cool place.

1. **Failure rates** (number of pregnancies expected per 100 women per year): 11.
2. **Risks:** Irritation and allergic reactions
   a. **Contraindications.** Condoms should not be used if one or both partners are allergic to them.
3. **Benefits:** include protection from STIs for latex and polyurethane condoms; skin condoms are too porous.
4. **Acceptability:** Limited if a couple finds using condoms distracting or embarrassing.

        a. Convenience: Applied before intercourse, one time use.

        b. Availability: No prescription needed.

    B. Female condom: This method provides coverage of the external genitalia and lines the vagina entirely. They can be inserted 6 hours before intercourse.

      1. Failure rates (number of pregnancies expected per 100 women per year): 21.

      2. Risks: Irritation and allergic reaction.

      3. Benefits: Some protection from STI.

      4. Acceptability

        a. Convenience: Inserted before intercourse, one time use.

        b. Availability: No prescription needed.

V. Chemical Methods. These methods inactivate the sperm by interfering with motility. Spermicides are available in the form of gels, creams, foams, suppositories, and film.

    A. Lea's shield. A dome-shaped rubber disk with a valve and loop that is held in place by the vaginal wall, covering the upper vagina and cervix so that sperm cannot reach. Used with spermiacide.

      1. Failure rates (number of pregnancies expected per 100 women per year): 15.

      2. Risks: Skin irritation, spotting, and discomfort (female and male), urinary tract infection. Theoretical risk of toxic shock.

      3. Benefits: Privacy of use.

      4. Acceptability

        a. Convenience: Inserted before intercourse and left in place at least 8 hours after, can be left in place for up to 48 hours with additional spermicide for repeated intercourse.

        b. Availability: Must have a prescription.

    B. Diaphragms are dome-shaped, rubber cups with arching, or coiled rims. Additional spermicide inserted before intercourse.

      1. Failure rate (number of pregnancies expected per 100 women per year): 17.

      2. Risks: Irritation and allergic reaction, urinary tract infection.

        a. Contraindications. A history of toxic shock syndrome.

      3. Benefits: Privacy of use.

      4. Acceptability

        a. Convenience: Inserted before intercourse and left in place at least 6 hours, can be left in place for 24 with additional spermicide for repeated intercourse.

        b. Availability: Must have prescription.

    C. Cervical Cap: Soft rubber cup with a round rim, which fits snugly around the cervix, used with spermicide.

      1. Failure rates (number of pregnancies expected per 100 women per year): prentiff Cap-17 FemCap 23.

      2. Risks: irritation and allergic reaction, abnormal Pap test and toxic shock.

      3. Benefits: Privacy.

      4. Acceptability:

        a. Convenience: May be difficult to insert, can remain in place for 48 hours without reapplying spermicide for repeated intercourse.

        b. Availability: Must have a prescription.

    D. Spermicide alone: A foam, cream, jelly, film suppository, or tablet that contains nonoxynol-9

      1. Failure rates (number of pregnancies expected per 100 women per year): 20 to 50.

      2. Risks: irritation and allergic reaction and urinary tract infection.

      3. Benefits: Privacy of use.

      4. Acceptability:

        a. Convenience: inserted between 5 and 90 minutes before intercourse and usually left in place at least 6 to 8 hours after.

        b. Availability: No prescription needed.

VI. Intrauterine Devices (IUDs). IUDs immobilize sperm, prevent implantation of the fertilized ovum, and dislodge the blastocyst from the endometrium. Both IUDs that are available are T-shaped; the ParaGard T380A has copper wound around the base, and the Progestasert is impregnated with progesterone. Both have fine, nylon tails that hang through the cervix, which allows women to check for the presence of the IUD.

    A. Failure rates (number of pregnancies expected per 100 women per year): <1.

    B. Risks: Cramping, bleeding, pelvic inflammatory disease, infertility, and perforation of uterus.

    1. Contraindications
      a. Women who are not in mutually monogamous relationships, who are at risk of acquiring STIs for other reasons, or who have acute pelvic infections should not use IUDs.
      b. Pregnancy is a contraindication.
      c. Preexisting severe dysmenorrhea will become worse with the copper IUD.
  C. Benefits. The Progestasert decreases the volume of menstrual blood and dysmenorrhea in symptomatic women.
  D. Acceptability.
    1. Convenience: Must be placed by a physician.
    2. Availability: Must have a prescription.
  E. Special notes. Always read the manufacturer's instructions for the specific kind of IUD to be used. The insertion and removal of an IUD are office procedures. A consent form must be signed. Both types of IUDs come with lengthy forms that take considerable time for women to complete.
    1. One size of both IUDs discussed above fits all women.
    2. One dose of a nonsteroidal anti-inflammatory drug such as Anaprox or Motrin is helpful if taken 1 hour prior to insertion or removal.
    3. Insertion is easiest during menses because the cervix is slightly dilated, although the incidence of expulsion and infection is slightly higher if the IUD is inserted at this time. Any time during the cycle is acceptable for insertion. The preferred time for removal is at the menses, both for comfort and to insure that recent exposure will not result in pregnancy.
    4. Leave a tail of at least 4 cm to allow the patient to check for expulsion of her IUD and to allow for easy removal. Let her feel the remnant of string so that she knows what to feel for monthly after her menses.

VII. Natural Family Planning
  A. Periodic abstinence depends on avoidance of intercourse during fertile days. These can be determined by many different methods. The Billings method of family planning relies on changes in cervical mucus. Other methods use the length of past menstrual cycles or a combination of basal body temperature and cervical mucus changes (sympto-thermal method). These methods rely heavily on motivated patients, but can enhance awareness of a woman's body and cycles. Two newer methods are the Creighton model NaProEducation system and the newer Standard Days Method from Georgetown. Abstinence is usually required for 6 to 9 days during the cycle. Some couples use barrier methods during the fertile time.
    1. Failure rates (number of pregnancies expected per 100 women per year): 20.
    2. Risks: There are no risks.
      a. There are no contraindications to the use of natural family planning. The calendar method alone should not be used in women with irregular menstrual cycles (as in lactating or nearing menopause).
    3. Benefits: Self-knowledge of a woman's cycles, which can be helpful if desiring pregnancy as well. This information also enhances both partners' awareness and involvement in family planning.
    4. Acceptability
      a. Convenience: Requires frequent monitoring of body functions.
      b. Availability: Requires special instructions.
    5. Special notes: Patient instructions are complex initially and take some time to master. A course with a trained instructor is necessary. More information is available through Natural Family Planning Practitioners, Couple to Couple League, or Georgetown University Institute for Reproductive Health.
  B. Lactational Amenorrhea Method (LAM) is based on the normal time of infertility after pregnancy. If a woman breast-feeds exclusively, the average length of infertility is 14 months. If a woman has given birth in the past 6 months, is exclusively breast-feeding (no solids, water, juice, or pacifier), and has not yet menstruated, she has approximately 98% effectiveness for breast-feeding alone. The longest time between feedings is the strongest factor leading to the return of fertility. Few women nurse exclusively on demand; thus, this is rarely effective or used in the western world today.
  C. Coitus interruptus, or the withdrawal method, depends on withdrawal of the penis from the vagina before ejaculation occurs. While risks are low for this method, the failure rate is high.

VIII. Sterilization. Sterilization is a permanent form of birth control resulting from obstruction of the vas deferens in males (vasectomy) or the fallopian tubes in females (tubal ligation). It is the most widely relied-on form of birth control in the United States. It is used by about one-third of women to prevent pregnancy.

A. **Vasectomy:** Sealing, tying, or cutting the vas deferens inhibiting sperm travel.
  1. **Failure rates** (number of pregnancies expected per 100 women per year): <1.
  2. **Risks:** Swelling, bruising, pain, and hematoma epididymitis.
  3. **Benefits:** Pertinent.
  4. **Acceptability:**
     a. **Convenience:** Surgical procedure.
     b. **Availability:** Surgery.

B. **Sterilization implants:** Small metallic implant that is placed into the fallopian tubes. The device causes scaring blocking fallopian tubes.
  1. **Failure rates** (number of pregnancies expected per 100 women per year): <1.
  2. **Risks:** Pain and ectopic pregnancy.
  3. **Benefits:** Pertinent.
  4. **Acceptability:**
     a. **Convenience:** Surgical procedure
     b. **Availability:** Surgery

C. **Transabdominal surgical sterilization:** Fallopian tubes are blocked, so the egg and sperm cannot meet.
  1. **Failure rates** (number of pregnancies expected per 100 women per year): <1.
  2. **Risks:** Pain bleeding, infection, surgical complications, and ectopic pregnancy.
  3. **Benefits:** Pertinent.
  4. **Acceptability:**
     a. **Convenience:** Surgical procedure
     b. **Availability:** Surgery

D. **Special notes:**
  1. Informed consent is critical for a surgical procedure and must describe the methods as irreversible, yet acknowledge a small risk of failure and pregnancy (possibly ectopic for the tubal ligation).
  2. It is important for patients to think carefully about whether any change such as death or separation from a partner or from a child would make them regret the choice. A good question to ask is "If anything were to happen to your current spouse and children, would you want to have another child?"

REFERENCES

Hatcher RA, Zieman M, Cwiak C, et al. *Managing Contraception.* Tiger, Georgia: Bridging the Gap Foundation; 2002.

Herndon EJ. New Contraceptive Options. *Am Fam Physician.* 2004;69(4):853-860.

Kippley JF, Kippley SK. *The Art of Natural Family Planning.* 4th ed. Couple to Couple League International; 2000.

Lesnewski R. Initiating hormonal contraception. *Am Fam Physician.* 2006;74(1):105-112.

www.fda.gov/fdac/features/1997/babytabl.html. Accessed August 19, 2008.

---

96   Infertility

Keith A. Frey, MD, MBA, & Andrea L. Darby-Stewart, MD

KEY POINTS

- Infertility occurs in approximately 15% of couples, many of whom present to their primary care physician for initial evaluation.
- A thorough evaluation of both partners is necessary, as 25% of couples have more than one etiologic factor.
- Emotional support for the couple is an important aspect of their care.

I. **Introduction**

  A. Definition. Infertility is defined as 1 year of unprotected intercourse in which a pregnancy has not been achieved. Fifteen percent of couples in the United States are infertile.

  B. Common diagnoses. The causes of infertility include abnormalities of any portion of the male or female reproductive system. Although infertility results from a single cause in the majority of couples, more than one factor contributes to infertility in as many as 25% of couples. "Unexplained" infertility, in which no specific cause is identified, occurs in approximately 28% of infertile couples. The following causes of infertility have been identified.

    1. Male factors (24%).

    2. Ovulatory dysfunction (21%).

    3. Tubal pathology (14%).

    4. Other problems including endometriosis, uterine or cervical factors and unusual problems (13%).

  C. Pathophysiology

    1. Male factors. The most commonly encountered cause of male infertility is oligo- or azoospermia secondary to varicocele. Other causes of male infertility include primary hypogonadism (e.g., congenital or acquired testicular disorders, orchitis), altered sperm transport (e.g., absent vas deferens), and secondary hypogonadism (e.g., androgen excess or pharmacologic effects). These disorders manifest as oligospermia or azoospermia, disorders of sperm function or motility (asthenospermia), and abnormalities of sperm morphology (teratospermia).

    2. Ovulatory dysfunction. Ovulation disorders account for 40% of female factor infertility. The possible causes of anovulation may be grouped into the following major categories:

      Aging

      Diminished ovarian reserve

      Endocrine disorders (e.g., hypothalamic amenorrhea, hyperprolactinemia, thyroid disease, adrenal disease)

      Polycystic ovary syndrome

      Premature ovarian failure

      Tobacco use

    3. Tubal and pelvic pathology. Infertility may be associated with tubal damage or adnexal adhesions. Tubal obstruction may result from scarring secondary to acute salpingitis, although many cases of tubal occlusion are encountered in which no episodes of salpingitis are recalled. Anatomic distortion of adnexal structures may also be caused by endometriosis. The chronic inflammation associated with endometriosis may disrupt normal conception by causing tubal damage or by secretion of toxic substances.

    4. Unusual problems. Cervical mucus abnormalities occur if at the time of ovulation the mucus is either insufficient in quantity or poor in quality. Factors contributing to the formation of such unreceptive cervical mucus include cervical infections, previous cervical surgery or cautery, and clomiphene therapy.

II. **Diagnosis.** The physician should arrange a meeting with the couple early in the diagnostic work-up. This provides an important opportunity to review reproductive biology and the rationale for subsequent laboratory test results.

  A. Signs and symptoms. Since infertility may arise from one or more areas of the reproductive system, it requires a comprehensive diagnostic evaluation. The initial assessment of both the male and the female partner consists of a thorough history and physical examination. Specific areas requiring extra attention are noted in Table 96–1.

  B. Laboratory tests (Tables 96–2 and 96–3). In addition to a comprehensive history and physical examination, each couple must be evaluated by a series of routine laboratory tests and appropriately timed studies to evaluate each major reproductive factor that may be the cause of infertility. This comprehensive diagnostic survey should be completed for most couples in 6 to 12 months. Each couple's evaluation must be individualized based on the findings of the history and the physical examination. However, an initial survey of each major reproductive factor is necessary in *all* couples and can be coordinated by the primary care physician.

    1. Male factors. Evidence of oligospermia after two or more semen analyses will require further diagnostic evaluation. The initial evaluation includes blood levels for follicle-stimulating hormone (FSH) and testosterone. If the testosterone level is low, a pituitary

TABLE 96–1. THE INFERTILITY WORK-UP IN OUTLINE: HISTORY (MALE, FEMALE, OR BOTH)

Marriage
Duration of infertility
Fertility in previous relationships
Frequency of intercourse
Sexual potency and techniques
Use of coital lubricants

Adult illnesses
Acute viral or febrile illness in past 3 mo
Mumps orchitis
Renal disease
Radiation therapy
Sexually transmitted disease
Stress and fatigue
Tuberculosis

Occupation and habits
Exposure to radiation, chemicals, and excessive heat (saunas, hot tubs, etc)

Childhood illness
Cryptorchidism
Timing of puberty

Surgery
Herniorrhaphy
Retroperitoneal surgery
Vasectomy
Female pelvic surgery

Drug use
Alcohol, tobacco, marijuana, and cocaine
Alkylating agents
Anabolic steroids
Nitrofurantoin
Sulfasalazine
Cimetidine

Review of systems
Focus on endocrine conditions (diabetes, thyroid disorders)

Gynecology
Contraceptive use
Diethylstilbestrol use by mother
Menarche
Menses (regularity and flow)
Mittelschmerz

Genetic diseases
Cystic fibrosis
Tay–Sachs
Sickle cell disease
Others

etiology may be evaluated by luteinizing hormone (LH) and prolactin levels. Testicular biopsy may be required, particularly if azoospermia is discovered.

2. **Ovulatory dysfunction.** Anovulation or inconsistent ovulation may be diagnosed by the history (irregular menses), a nonbiphasic basal body temperature (BBT) pattern, absence of LH surge during at-home ovulation predictor kit testing, abnormally low serum progesterone levels during the luteal phase, or endometrial biopsy.

3. **Tubal factors.** The female partner must undergo an evaluation for tubal patency. If the history or the physical examination shows no clear evidence of tubal damage, proceed with a hysterosalpingogram; otherwise, refer the patient for laparoscopy (especially if there are other indications for laparoscopy, such as possible endometriosis).

TABLE 96–2. THE INFERTILITY WORK-UP IN OUTLINE: PHYSICAL EXAMINATION/ROUTINE LABORATORY TESTS (MALE AND FEMALE)

Male		Female	
Physical Examination	**Routine Laboratory Tests**	**Physical Examination**	**Routine Laboratory Tests**
Hair pattern	CBC	Breast formation	CBC, RPR, Rubella titer
Genitalia	Semen analysis	Distribution of body	Pap smear
Meatus size and location	Abstinence of 2–8 d	fat	Urinalysis and urine
Prostate and seminal	Masturbation into sterile	Galactorrhea	culture if indicated
vesicles	vessel	Hair pattern	Day 3 FSH and Estradiol
Scrotum	To laboratory (warm) within	(virilization)	(for age ≥ 30 y)
Testicular size (≥4 cm in	1 h	Height and weight	TSH and Prolactin (if
long axis)	Results	Neurology	oligoovulation or
Varicocele (standing and	Volume: 2–5 mL	Anosmia	anovulation)
Valsalva's maneuver)	Liquelaction: complete	Visual fields	At-home test
Neurology	within 30 minutes	Pelvis	Basal body temperature
Anosmia	Sperm count: >20	External genitalia	Home ovulatory kit
Visual fields	million/mL	Retrovaginal area	
	Sperm motility: 50%	(endometriosis)	
	Morphology: 50% normal	Uterus and adnexa	
	forms	Vagina and cervix	
	Repeat testing if		
	azoospermia or severe		
	oligospermia		
	Urinalysis and urine		
	culture if indicated		
	RPR		

CBC, complete blood cell count; RPR, rapid plasma reagin; TSH, thyroid-stimulating hormone.

III. **Treatment.** Generally, treatment should not be initiated until the diagnostic evaluation is completed. The male and female partners should be treated as a couple whenever possible. Therapy should proceed at a rate that the couple finds comfortable.

A. **Male factors.** Specific antibiotics are used to treat infections such as prostatitis and epididymitis (see Chapter 61). Consultation with an urologist will generally be required to complete the evaluation and coordinate treatment. It should be noted that varicocele repair has not been shown to increase the likelihood of conception. (SOR **A**)

B. **Ovulatory dysfunction.** Underlying causes of ovulatory dysfunction such as thyroid abnormalities or hyperprolactinemia should be corrected. If anovulation is diagnosed, consider treatment with clomiphene.

1. **Clomiphene treatment.** A careful evaluation for galactorrhea and a prolactin level should precede treatment. Chronic anovulation and unexplained infertility patients attempting to conceive are among the patients best suited for clomiphene. (SOR **A**) The usual starting dose is 50 mg/d orally on days 5 to 9 of the menstrual cycle. The dose may be increased to 100 mg/d in the second and third cycles. (SOR **C**)

TABLE 96–3. THE INFERTILITY WORK-UP IN OUTLINE: FURTHER DIAGNOSTIC TESTS

Hysterosalpingography
Preferred test of tubal patency
Performed 2–6 days after cessation of menstrual flow
May enhance fertility temporarily

Laparoscopy
Performed if hysterosalpingography is unproductive
Permits examination of pelvic contents

Serum progesterone
May be an alternative to endometrial biopsy
Sample drawn 5–7 days after supposed ovulation
Serum level 6 ng/mL is compatible with ovulation

Common side effects include vasomotor flushes (10%), abdominal or pelvic discomfort (5.5%), nausea (2.2%), and breast tenderness (2%). Ovarian hyperstimulation and twinning may occur in patients who receive clomiphene therapy. Polycystic ovary syndrome (PCOS) patients are at highest risk for these complications. Consider referral to an infertility specialist if pregnancy is not achieved within 6 months of clomiphene therapy.

2. **Expected results.** Ovulation should be expected 5 to 10 days after the treatment ends; this should be confirmed by biphasic BBT or positive ovulation predictor kit and an elevated level of serum progesterone on day 21. If ovulation does not occur despite clomiphene therapy, consultation with a reproductive endocrinologist is recommended.

3. **Metformin treatment.** Metformin has been found to increase the rate of ovulation in patients who have anovulation secondary to PCOS. However, there was no increase in the rate of pregnancy in women who received metformin alone. Clomiphene plus metformin may increase the rate of pregnancy in women with resistant PCOS compared to clomiphene alone. (SOR **A**)

C. **Tubal and pelvic pathology.** Tubal blockage or deformity may necessitate surgical correction. The management of endometriosis in a woman desiring to achieve pregnancy depends on the degree and location of endometrial deposits. Conservative surgical treatment may enhance fertility potential by destroying endometrial implants and endometriomas. Laparoscopic conservative surgical treatment should be considered as a treatment option for mild endometriosis-associated infertility. Patients with endometriosis may also benefit from ovulation induction with or without other assisted-reproduction techniques. (SOR **A**) For patients with more severe tubal and pelvic pathology, referral for assisted reproductive technologies is warranted.

D. **Unusual problems.** For cervical mucus abnormalities, antibiotics should be used to treat the specific bacterial cause of the problem. Low-dose estrogens can be used for poor cervical mucus that does not result from infectious causes. However, intrauterine insemination (IUI) is the best treatment option for a cervical factor.

IV. **Management Strategies.** The work-up, diagnosis, and treatment of infertility can precipitate intense emotional reactions. The sensitive physician should discuss such emotions as anger, guilt, self-doubt, depression, and grief with the couple. The actions described below may also prove beneficial.

A. Help the couple understand their motives for parenting, which may include desires (1) to parent, (2) to experience a pregnancy, (3) to meet the expectations of others, and (4) to promote genetic continuity.

B. Assist the couple in the development of mutual support and an adaptive "couple-coping" style. Discuss sexual issues, and encourage the couple to nurture their intimacy; they will need its strength to deal with the problems associated with infertility. Periodic meetings with the couple to review diagnostic progress provide further opportunity to reinforce coping skills.

C. Help the couple broaden their support systems, including self-help groups, such as Resolve, Inc.

V. **Prognosis.** The exact prognosis of infertility is difficult to define because of the multiple potential causes. For most of these, conception will not be achieved without specific treatment. However, with specific therapy, subsequent pregnancy rates have been studied and the results are favorable. "Unexplained" infertility is the persistent inability to conceive after a comprehensive diagnostic assessment of the couple fails to establish a specific diagnosis. If a comprehensive diagnostic work-up fails to identify a cause, or if the appropriate treatment is unsuccessful, the physician should discuss adoption options with the couple.

REFERENCES

Al-Inany H. Female Infertility. *BMJ Clin Evidence.* Accessed on April 19, 2007 from http://www. clinicalevidence.com/ceweb/conditions/woh/0819/0819.jsp

Frey KA, Patel KS. Initial Evaluation and Management of Infertility by the Primary Care Physician. *Mayo Clin Proc.* 2004;79(11):1439-1443.

Jose-Miller AB, Boyden JW, Frey KA. Infertility. *Am Fam Physician.* 2007;75:849-856.

ELECTRONIC RESOURCE

RESOLVE National Home Page. http://www.resolve.org. Accessed July 24, 2008.

97   Preconception & Prenatal Care

Kirsten Vitrikas, MD

KEY POINTS

- Preconception care that offers smoking cessation, folic acid supplementation, (SOR **Ⓐ**) excellent glycemic control in patients with diabetes mellitus, (SOR **Ⓐ**) monotherapy for seizures and avoidance of phenytoin and valproic acid, (SOR **Ⓑ**) immunization against rubella, and alcohol cessation has been shown to improve subsequent pregnancy outcome.
- Comprehensive prenatal care, particularly if begun early in pregnancy, has been shown to improve pregnancy outcomes. (SOR **Ⓑ**) Clinicians should follow specific evidence-based protocols and monitor women for signs of obstetric emergencies, particularly late in pregnancy.
- Women older than 35 years should be offered genetic counseling and testing. All women who present for care prior to 20 weeks should be offered Down syndrome screening in the first trimester. (SOR **Ⓑ**)
- To prepare for labor and delivery, all women and their partners should be enrolled in prenatal classes. A great majority of women deliver in hospitals utilizing family-centered birthing, focusing on safety for the mom and child, and fostering a positive experience for the woman and her family.

I. Introduction

A. Antenatal care refers to a comprehensive approach to medical care and psychosocial support of the family that ideally begins prior to conception and ends with the onset of labor.

B. Preconception care is the physical and mental preparation of both parents for pregnancy and childbearing prior to conception in order to improve pregnancy outcomes.

C. Prenatal care formally begins with the initial diagnosis of pregnancy and includes ongoing risk assessment, education, and counseling to promote health as well as identification and management of problems.

II. Preconception care

A. Medical history. Nearly half of all pregnancies are unintended; therefore all women of childbearing age, particularly those not using contraception effectively, are candidates for preconception evaluation. Identifying conditions and risks that could adversely affect a future pregnancy, followed by appropriate interventions and counseling to improve the outcome of pregnancy are the primary tasks of the preconception evaluation.

1. **Chronic medical conditions** should be evaluated both for potential effects on pregnancy and for effects that pregnancy may have on the medical condition. Significant chronic illnesses include diabetes mellitus, hypertension, thyroid disorders, anemias, coagulopathies, seizure disorders, asthma, human immunodeficiency virus (HIV)/acquired immunodeficiency syndrome, and cardiovascular diseases. Also notable are a past history of recurrent urinary tract infections and phlebitis.

2. Note **previous surgeries**, particularly abdominal and pelvic procedures.

3. A thorough review of **prescription and over-the-counter medications** currently being taken is helpful to anticipate and minimize adverse effects, particularly during the period of organogenesis from the 4th to the 10th weeks of gestation. The US Food and Drug Administration's Pregnancy Categories and other reviews such as the Teris classifications are useful in determining risk versus benefit and teratogenic risk. Drugs clearly proven to have significant teratogenic risk in humans include alcohol, chemotherapeutic agents, anticonvulsants, androgens, warfarin, lithium, and isotretinoin.

4. Note **allergies and sensitivities** to medications and anesthetics.

5. **Current methods of contraception.** Ideally, methods should be discontinued several menstrual cycles prior to conception to assist with accurate dating.

6. **Genetic risk assessment** performed in the preconception period, as opposed to the prenatal period, allows women and their partners to consider a greater number of options in family planning. The background incidence of congenital malformations is approximately 3%. Genetic causes account for approximately 20% of anomalies. Genetic counseling and further testing may be beneficial when the following conditions are identified: advanced maternal (older than 35 years) or paternal (older than 55 years) age; family history of or previous child with neural tube defect (NTD), congenital heart disease, hemophilia, thalassemia, sickle cell disease, Tay–Sachs disease, cystic fibrosis, Huntington's chorea, muscular dystrophy, mental retardation, Down syndrome, or other inherited disorders; maternal metabolic disorders; recurrent pregnancy loss (three or more); use of alcohol, recreational drugs, and medications; and environmental or occupational exposures.

7. **Obstetric and menstrual history.** Review the number, date, length, and outcome of prior pregnancies. Record any history of significant pregnancy-related health concerns, such as gestational diabetes, intrauterine growth retardation (IUGR), preterm labor, or hemorrhage. Make note of any complications during labor and delivery. A detailed menstrual history is helpful, paying particular attention to irregular menses and infertility.

B. **Psychosocial history.** This is a critical area of the history, since significant risks may be identified that may be addressed prior to pregnancy. A potential pregnancy may also serve as an incentive to the patient to alter certain unhealthy habits. Unhealthy habits include tobacco use, alcohol consumption, illicit drug use, and poor nutrition. Psychosocial risks include a past history of mental illness, inadequate personal supports and coping skills, high stress, exposure to domestic violence or abuse, single marital status, inadequate housing, low income, and less than high school education.

C. **Immunization history.** Rubella, varicella, and hepatitis B immunity are best addressed prior to conception.

D. **Physical examination**
   1. **Height and weight.** Patients who weigh >200 lbs or <90 lbs may be at greater risk for problems in pregnancy.
   2. **Blood pressure**
   3. **Breast examination**
   4. **Pelvic examination,** including clinical pelvimetry (although pelvimetry is unlikely to affect the outcome of the pregnancy).

E. **Laboratory tests**
   1. **Recommended laboratory tests** include hemoglobin or hematocrit, rubella titer, Pap smear, screening for gonorrhea and Chlamydia, hepatitis B surface antigen, and syphilis serology. Counseling regarding HIV testing should occur with all patients. Urine dipstick for protein and glucose is controversial as to usefulness.
   2. Additional screening with the following may be appropriate for women who are identified to be at greater risk: tuberculosis, toxoplasmosis, cytomegalovirus, herpes simplex, varicella, and hemoglobinopathies.

F. **Health promotion**
   1. Optimize management of preexisting medical conditions such as diabetes mellitus and hypertension.
   2. Administer appropriate immunizations (see Chapter 101).
   3. The US Public Health Service recommends that all women of childbearing age should consume 0.4 mg of folic acid per day to reduce the risk of NTDs. (SOR **A**)
   4. Provide counsel and educate regarding the following topics.
      a. **Pregnancy planning.** Accurate recording of menstrual cycles is helpful. Oral contraceptives should be discontinued and a barrier method should be used to establish regular cycles prior to attempting pregnancy.
      b. **Nutrition and weight correction, if necessary.** Obese women (BMI > 30) are at increased risk for adverse perinatal outcomes and operative complications. (SOR **A**) They should be encouraged to lose weight prior to attempting pregnancy.
      c. **Smoking cessation** (SOR **A**) **and avoidance of alcohol** (SOR **A**) **and illicit drugs.** (SOR **C**)
      d. **Genetic risks, if any.**
      e. **Avoidance of teratogens, including prescription and nonprescription medications, and occupational and environmental exposures.**

    f. Preparation of the family for pregnancy and enhancement of social support. Domestic violence may begin or escalate during pregnancy. It is more prevalent than any condition in pregnancy with the exception of preeclampsia.

    g. Proper exercise. Current recommendations are for 30 minutes or more of exercise on most if not all days of the week in the absence of contraindications. (SOR **C**)

III. Prenatal Care

A. Initial diagnosis of pregnancy

    1. Symptoms include cessation of menses, breast tenderness and enlargement, nausea, fatigue, and frequent urination.

    2. Signs such as uterine enlargement and a dark bluish coloring of the cervix and vaginal mucosa (Chadwick's sign) are present.

    3. Urinary tests for elevated levels of β-human chorionic gonadotropin (β-hCG) are generally positive at about the time of the first missed menses and have a sensitivity of 98% and a specificity of 99%.

B. The **first prenatal visit** should occur before 8 weeks' gestation, as it is critical for determining an accurate delivery date, evaluating risk status, and providing essential patient education. The visit may be abbreviated if a recent preconceptual visit has occurred.

    1. Patient history (see Section II). A detailed menstrual history as well as the last contraceptive method used is important for establishing dates. The estimated date of delivery (EDD) should be established before 20 weeks' gestation, when techniques for dating are most accurate. The date of the start of the last menstrual period is used to determine EDD. A first-trimester ultrasound can confirm gestational age within ±4 days and is considered more accurate than last menstrual period, although routine use for dating is controversial. (SOR **B**) In addition, a history of illnesses, medications, and exposures since the LMP should be obtained. A patient's questions concerning common symptoms in early pregnancy can be answered at this time.

    2. Complete physical examination. This should include evaluation of fetal heart tones (usually heard by hand-held Doppler between 11 and 13 weeks).

    3. Routine laboratory work. In addition to testing recommended during the preconception visit (see Section II.E), blood and Rh type, antibody screen, microscopic urinalysis, and urine culture are recommended.

    4. Patient education early in pregnancy is critical. Important issues to be addressed are described below.

        a. High-risk behaviors

            (1) Smoking has been associated with IUGR, prematurity, placenta previa, placental abruption, and preterm rupture of membranes. Brief counseling during visits has been shown to be effective in reducing number of cigarettes smoked per day. (SOR **B**) If nonpharmacologic therapy fails, nicotine replacement with patches or gum should be considered.

            (2) Alcohol use is linked to fetal alcohol syndrome (craniofacial abnormalities, limb and cardiovascular defects, and growth and mental retardation) and other childhood behavioral problems such as learning disabilities and attention-deficit/hyperactivity disorder. There is no known safe amount of alcohol consumption during pregnancy.

            (3) Cocaine is associated with increases in spontaneous abortions, placental abruption, preterm labor and delivery, low birth weight, neonatal withdrawal syndromes, and central nervous system damage. To reinforce or encourage abstinence from illicit drugs, consider periodic questioning or random drug screens.

            (4) Opiates may cause IUGR, preterm delivery, and an increased rate of intrauterine hypoxemia and fetal distress.

            (5) Daily consumption of more than 300 mg of **caffeine** (about three cups of coffee) has been associated with an increased risk of IUGR and low birth weight.

        b. Nutrition and weight gain. Total weight gain of 25 to 35 lbs is recommended for women at an appropriate weight at the time of conception. Women at <90% or >120% of ideal body weight should gain 30 to 35 lbs or 15 to 25 lbs, respectively, to minimize risks. A weight gain of <10 lbs at 20 weeks' gestation is associated with increased complications.

            (1) The average pregnant woman needs approximately 1900 to 2750 kcal/d (300 kcal more than nonpregnant patients). The best clue to adequate caloric intake is maternal weight gain.

(2) The diet should include increased amounts of calcium (1200 mg/d, equivalent to 3–4 milk servings), iron (30 mg essential iron), vitamins C and D, and folic acid (0.4–0.8 mg/d) and consist of 50% to 60% complex carbohydrate, up to 20% protein, and no more than 30% fat. A prenatal multivitamin and mineral supplement is recommended when dietary intake is inadequate. Vegetarians require additional iron, vitamin B_{12}, and zinc. Excessive doses of vitamins, particularly vitamins A, C, and D, can be harmful to the fetus.

c. **Patient expectations,** the benefits of childbirth education classes, and family issues should be discussed.

d. **Sexual intercourse** during pregnancy is contraindicated only for patients with placenta previa and for those at risk for abortions or premature labor.

e. **Physical activity** should not be significantly increased during pregnancy; however, regular, low-intensity exercise (walking, swimming, and bicycling) should be encouraged. Contact sports, activities requiring repeated Valsalva maneuvers or rapid changes in direction, or those involving unpredictable risk should be discouraged.

f. **Symptoms for which patients need to promptly contact their physician** should be clearly outlined. These include any vaginal bleeding or escape of fluids from the vagina, swelling of the face and fingers, severe continuous headache, dimness or blurring of vision, abdominal pain, persistent vomiting, chills or fever, dysuria, and change in frequency or intensity of fetal movements.

C. Common symptoms

1. **Nausea and vomiting,** which usually begin at approximately 6 weeks and disappear by 14 to 16 weeks, are commonly worse in the morning and occur in up to 70% of pregnant women. Hyperemesis gravidarum occurs in 0.5% to 2% of pregnancies. Non pharmacologic therapies include having frequent, small meals; avoiding greasy, spicy foods; having a protein snack at bedtime; eating dry crackers before getting out of bed in the morning; and avoiding drinking liquids on an empty stomach. (SOR **C**) Purposeful stimulation of the P6 (Neiguan) acupuncture point located three fingerbreadths proximal to the distal wrist crease and between the two central flexor tendons of the forearm, via pressing firmly with the fingers for 5 minutes every 4 hours while awake or via use of Seabands, can be quite helpful. (SOR **B**) Women who consume a daily multivitamin at the time of conception have reduced severity of nausea and vomiting. Ginger capsules have shown promise in alleviating symptoms. (SOR **B**) American College of Obstetricians and Gynecologists (ACOG) recommends pyridoxine (vitamin B6) 25 mg two or three times daily or in combination with doxylamine 10 mg as first-line pharmacologic treatment. (SOR **A**) Other medications include promethazine 12.5 to 25 mg oral or rectally every 4 hours, dimenhydrinate 50 to 100 mg every 4 to 6 hours, metoclopramide 5 to 10 mg every 6 to 8 hours. (SOR **B**) For severe cases, ondansetron or even steroid tapers may be considered. Early treatment is important to prevent progression to hyperemesis. Reassurance that symptoms may be related to higher levels of maternal estrogens and an associated improved pregnancy outcome may also be useful.

2. **Headache** is common before 20 weeks' gestation and is usually benign, although in most cases no specific cause can be found. This symptom may be safely treated with acetaminophen. Relaxation and use of warm compresses may help. The pattern of migraine may change during pregnancy. The physician must consider preeclampsia, particularly later in pregnancy.

3. **Gastrointestinal symptoms common during pregnancy**

   a. Heartburn occurs in approximately one-half of pregnant women at some time. This condition has been attributed to a number of factors, including decreased tone in the lower esophageal sphincter, displacement and compression of the stomach by the uterus, and decreased gastric motility. Treatment consists of having frequent small meals and avoiding bending over or lying flat soon after eating. Low-sodium liquid antacids are helpful and safe; however, those agents that contain magnesium or aluminum hydroxides impair absorption of iron. Over-the-counter H_2-blockers such as ranitidine are also considered safe for use in the second and third trimesters.

   b. Constipation is common in pregnancy because of steroid-induced changes in bowel transit time. Dietary measures are the mainstay of treatment and include high-fiber foods, liberal consumption of water and other liquids, and regular, low-intensity exercise. Mild laxatives, such as milk of magnesia, stool softeners, and bulk laxatives, are safe and effective.

    c. Abdominal pain may occur in pregnancy and warrants evaluation. The physician should consider the same causes for abdominal pain that occur in the nonpregnant state. However, these conditions may present differently in pregnant patients. Types of abdominal pain specific to pregnancy are described below.

        (1) Ectopic pregnancy should be ruled out in women with lower abdominal or pelvic pain early in pregnancy (see Chapter 51).

        (2) Preeclampsia may be associated with upper abdominal pains in the epigastrium or the right upper quadrant.

        (3) Placental abruption should be considered when pain is associated with bleeding, particularly in the third trimester.

        (4) Urinary tract infections (see Chapter 21).

        (5) Other, less significant causes include round ligament or broad ligament discomfort, which results from increased tension on these structures as the uterus enlarges.

4. Urinary complaints, such as increasing frequency and stress incontinence, are often noted, especially during the first and third trimesters, because of uterine pressure on the bladder. Decreasing nighttime fluid intake (without any overall restrictions) and Kegel's exercises can be helpful. Infection, however, is common and should be considered when frequency is associated with dysuria.

5. Increased **vaginal discharge (leukorrhea)** is common, often with no pathologic cause. This physiologic discharge is related to increased estrogen. Infectious causes should be ruled out (see Chapter 64) in the presence of associated symptoms of itching, burning, foul odor, or labial swelling.

6. Vaginal bleeding may occur at any time during pregnancy and should always be considered significant enough to warrant further evaluation, including pelvic examination, appropriate cultures, and pelvic ultrasound.

    a. Bleeding in the first trimester is a relatively frequent occurrence. Causes range from physiologic bleeding as a result of implantation to life-threatening conditions. Extrauterine pregnancy should be considered when bleeding occurs during this time, even in the absence of pain. Any bleeding occurring in the first half of pregnancy, particularly with cramping, may be associated with spontaneous abortion.

    b. Bleeding in the latter half of pregnancy occurs less frequently and may be associated with cervical trauma during coitus. Painless bleeding may suggest placenta or vasa previa, whereas painful bleeding is classically associated with placental abruption.

7. Edema in the feet and the ankles is common, particularly during the third trimester. This edema is secondary to sodium and water retention combined with increased lower extremity venous pressure. Edema should raise concerns of preeclampsia when it is accompanied by hypertension and proteinuria. Benign edema normally responds to leg elevation, avoidance of long periods of sitting or standing, and use of support stockings.

8. Backache is relatively common during pregnancy and is partially related to increased joint laxity as well as compensatory postural changes that occur as the uterus enlarges. Avoiding excessive weight gain, wearing flat or low-heeled shoes, and improving posture may provide some relief. Chiropractic care may be effective and is safe during pregnancy.

9. Varicose veins are aggravated by pregnancy, prolonged standing, and advancing age. This condition usually worsens as pregnancy advances, because of increased femoral pressure. Treatment is limited to periodic rest with leg elevation and elastic stockings; more definitive treatment is delayed until after pregnancy.

10. Hemorrhoids are the result of increased pressure on hemorrhoidal veins by the uterus and by the tendency toward constipation during pregnancy. Effective treatments include sitz baths with warm water for 20 minutes followed by local application of witch hazel, topically applied anesthetics, and stool softeners (see Chapter 52).

D. Additional prenatal care. Traditionally, prenatal visits should occur every 4 weeks through the 28th week of pregnancy, every 2 to 3 weeks through the 36th week, and then weekly until delivery. The frequency of visits may be altered based on the risk status of the patient. Decreasing the frequency of visits has not been shown to affect maternal or fetal outcomes, but may decrease the satisfaction level of the patient. (SOR Ⓐ) Measurement of weight, blood pressure, and fundal height; assessment of edema; and documentation of fetal heart rate should occur at every visit. Some providers check a urine dipstick for protein and glucose at each visit. Other tests and interventions may be needed at specific times during pregnancy, as noted below.

1. **Care prior to 14 weeks (first trimester).** Initial care during the first trimester can prepare both clinician and patient for a healthy pregnancy.

   a. Review initial laboratory work and define maternal risk status more precisely.

   b. Counsel patients regarding the initial troubling symptoms of pregnancy, such as nausea, fatigue, and emotional changes. Encourage good nutrition. Review signs of miscarriage. Inquire about the partner's adjustment.

   c. All patients who present for care before 20 weeks gestation should be offered first trimester screening for Down syndrome. (SOR **B**) Screening that assesses nuchal translucency in addition to serum markers is equivalent to the quadruple screen in detection of Down syndrome and allows for early intervention. There are several ways this can be accomplished.

      (1) **Integrated screening.** Measurement of nuchal translucency and serum PAPP-a levels at 10 to 13 weeks combined with serum levels of hCG, estriol, AFP, and inhibin at 15 to 20 weeks.

      (2) **Serum integrated screening.** Serum testing as above, no nuchal translucency.

      (3) **Sequential screening.** First trimester testing as above with second trimester testing only in those at intermediate risk based on calculations. Those at high risk based on screening should be offered diagnostic testing in the first trimester.

   d. Offer early prenatal diagnostic studies to all patients with genetic risk factors (see Section II.A.6). Chorionic villus sampling (CVS) is performed between 9 and 12 weeks' gestation, which allows for earlier termination of pregnancy with less maternal morbidity. Amniocentesis is usually performed after 15 weeks, but can be done as early as 13 weeks' gestation. Unlike amniocentesis, CVS cannot be used for prenatal diagnosis of NTDs and may be associated with limb reduction defects. Amniocentesis carries a 0.5% to 1% risk of fetal loss. The risk from CVS is slightly higher. A detailed ultrasound scan performed in the second trimester can also assist in the evaluation of fetal anomalies but is not recommended as a screening test.

   e. Fetal heart tones are first heard with Doppler ultrasound between 11 and 13 weeks' gestation and sometimes as early as 8 weeks in multigravidas.

2. **Care between 14 and 28 weeks' gestation (second trimester).** An obviously pregnant body and the first sensations of fetal movement often lead to an increased appreciation of being pregnant. The second trimester is an excellent time to schedule a joint visit with the patient and her partner to discuss expectations about parenting.

   a. **Confirmation of the estimated date of delivery.** At approximately 20 weeks' gestation, the uterine fundus is at the level of the umbilicus, and fetal heart tones can usually be heard with a fetoscope. The sensation of fetal movement (quickening), which may first be a fluttering sensation, is usually felt at 16 to 20 weeks.

   b. **Routine prenatal screening for neural tube defects and chromosomal abnormalities** such as Down syndrome (trisomy 21) are offered during this time for women who do not present early enough for first trimester screening. NTDs occur in 4 per 10,000 live births. Screening involves measuring the **maternal serum α-fetoprotein (MSAFP)** between 16 and 18 weeks' gestation. Approximately 50 of 1000 women will have an elevated (>2.5 multiples of the median) MSAFP, indicating the possibility of an NTD. Most will be falsely positive, resulting from inaccurate dating, multiple gestation, or other anomalies. An elevated MSAFP in the absence of other anomalies is associated with poor pregnancy outcomes. A targeted anatomic ultrasound to confirm dates can detect 90% to 95% of NTDs in addition to other defects associated with elevated MSAFP (omphalocele, gastroschisis, and cystic hygroma).

   Reduced levels of MSAFP (<0.7 multiples of the median) indicate an increased risk of Down syndrome. An association with reduced levels of estradiol and elevated levels of hCG and inhibin-A (the more recently available quadruple screen) has a false-positive rate of 5% and will identify approximately 76% of cases. (The older "triple screen" has a similar false-positive rate but a lower detection rate of 60%–69%.) Amniocentesis offers the only definitive diagnosis, once dating is confirmed by ultrasound. Parents should be carefully advised of the benefits and risks of these screening tests, with documentation of the discussion and their decision recorded in the chart.

    c. Universal screening for gestational diabetes between 24 and 28 weeks is widely recommended and practiced. Testing based on risk factors excludes only few women. Recent evidence indicates that treatment of gestational diabetes decreases pregnancy complications such as macrosomia and subsequent birth trauma. (SOR **Ⓐ**) Measurement of plasma blood glucose 1 hour after ingesting a 50-g oral glucose load is most commonly done, and fasting is not required. Levels >140 mg/dL require further evaluation with a 3-h oral glucose tolerance test. Women with borderline levels between 130 and 140 may benefit from repeat testing in several weeks. Some physicians advocate earlier screening (prior to 24 weeks) when conditions increasing risk for gestational diabetics are present. Such conditions include a past history of gestational diabetes or a macrosomic infant (>4000 g), family history of type II diabetes, or a maternal weight >200 lbs.

    d. The hemoglobin or hematocrit can be repeated at the same time as screening for diabetes, along with antibody screening for D (Rh)-negative women.

    e. D (Rh)-negative women should be given D (Rh) immune globulin at 28 weeks' gestation if the antibody screening is negative. D (Rh) immune globulin should be given earlier if an event has occurred exposing the patient to fetal blood (e.g., CVS, amniocentesis, or significant trauma). A repeat dose given within 72 hours after delivery is also necessary.

    f. Influenza vaccine should be offered to all pregnant women during the flu season.

3. Care beyond 28 weeks of gestation (third trimester). This is often a period of increasing discomfort for the patient, with sleep disturbances, dyspnea, urinary frequency, and fatigue being common. The incidence of complications such as preeclampsia, maternal hypertension, and malposition of the fetus lead to a need for more frequent and intensive monitoring. Allow time to discuss expectations and wishes regarding labor and delivery, and review indications for calling the office. Prepared childbirth education can have beneficial effects on performance in labor. (SOR **Ⓐ**)

    a. Blood pressure should be carefully monitored. Systolic blood pressures ≥140 mm Hg or diastolic blood pressures ≥90 mm Hg are diagnostic of gestational hypertension and warrant further evaluation for preeclampsia, particularly when associated with proteinuria.

    b. Fetal position should be regularly assessed. Most babies are vertex by the final month of pregnancy. For other presentations, external version is often successful and increases the chances of a vaginal delivery.

    c. Testing for **sexually transmitted diseases** in high-risk women, if appropriate, should be repeated at 36 to 38 weeks' gestation. Testing allows for treatment prior to delivery.

    d. The Centers for Disease Control and Prevention (CDC) revised guidelines for **screening for group B streptococcal (GBS) infection** in 2002, based on findings that universal screening was >50% more effective in preventing GBS infection in newborns than basing treatment on risk factors. The CDC now recommends that all pregnant women (except for those with a history of GBS bacteriuria or a past history of an infant with invasive GBS disease) be screened with vaginal and rectal swabs for GBS between 35 and 37 weeks' estimated gestational age. Intrapartum antibiotic prophylaxis is then offered to all women who test positive, as well as to those women with a history of GBS bacteriuria in the current pregnancy or a past history of an infant with invasive GBS disease. Antepartum prophylaxis is not recommended.

    e. Patients who wish a trial of labor after cesarean section should be counseled on the risks and benefits. In addition obese women should receive consultation with anesthesia providers prior to presenting in labor.

    f. Women should be counseled on the nutritional and immunological benefits of breastfeeding. (SOR **Ⓑ**)

E. Medications in pregnancy. Most drugs should be used only when benefits clearly outweigh risks, particularly in the first trimester. Patients need to understand that taking any medication during pregnancy involves some small degree of risk.

    1. Antihistamines are generally acceptable when used in normal therapeutic doses, with the possible exception of brompheniramine.

    2. Antiemetics may be used safely if other conservative measures are not effective.

    3. Decongestants. Pseudoephedrine (30 mg every 6 hours) is relatively safe to use for limited periods, but large doses should be avoided, as they may negatively influence uterine perfusion. Decongestants are contraindicated when uteroplacental insufficiency is suspected. Try recommending the substitution of saline nose spray or irrigation or judicious use of topical decongestants.

4. **Oral analgesics and anti-inflammatory agents**

   a. Acetaminophen is the drug of choice for mild analgesia and antipyresis. Continuous high doses may cause maternal anemia and fatal kidney disease in the newborn (case report).

   b. Low-dose aspirin has been used to lower the risk of preeclampsia in high-risk women. Although there is no clear consensus regarding the benefits related to preeclampsia, aspirin has proved to be a relatively safe drug, although there does seem to be an increased risk of placental abruption. Caution should be used in the second half of pregnancy.

   c. Nonsteroidal anti-inflammatory drugs (NSAID), such as ibuprofen and naproxen, have a theoretical risk of prenatal closure of the ductus arteriosus when used near term. They also cause a reversible decrease in amniotic fluid levels. Indomethacin, if used after 34 weeks' gestation, may lead to persistent pulmonary hypertension of the newborn, inhibition of labor, and prolongation of pregnancy. NSAIDs have been shown to block blastocyst implantation and are associated with and increased risk of spontaneous abortion.

   d. Codeine is not absolutely contraindicated, although association with malformations has been reported. Neonatal withdrawal has been documented. Hydrocodone–acetaminophen combinations (Vicodin) may be safer in pregnancy than codeine.

5. **Antibiotics**

   a. Penicillins (with or without clavulanate) and cephalosporins are among the most effective and least toxic of available antibiotics and can be used at any time during pregnancy.

   b. Erythromycin has not been reported to be of harm to the fetus, except as the estolate salt, which is contraindicated in pregnancy.

   c. Tetracyclines and quinolones are contraindicated in pregnancy because of adverse effects on developing teeth and bones.

   d. Sulfonamides may be used in the first two trimesters. Use near term and during nursing should be avoided, since sulfonamides may cause significant jaundice or hemolytic anemia in the newborn.

   e. Oral metronidazole is considered safe, although some prefer to wait until after the first trimester for its use. (SOR **C**) Topical metronidazole is safe throughout pregnancy.

   f. Nitrofurantoin should be used with care in late pregnancy since it has the ability to induce hemolysis in neonatal red blood cells.

6. **Antidepressants and benzodiazepines**

   a. Tricyclic antidepressants should be used with caution, as no extensive studies of their use in the first trimester are available.

   b. Selective serotonin reuptake inhibitors, particularly fluoxetine, have generally been proved to be relatively safe during pregnancy. However, recent evidence has associated paroxetine with congenital cardiac defects. Use in the third trimester may require caution, as there is some evidence for a neonatal withdrawal that may include irritability and seizures in rare cases.

   c. Lithium is contraindicated during pregnancy.

   d. Benzodiazepines should be used cautiously, if at all, as there is some evidence of an increased risk of cleft palate or cleft lip.

IV. **Preterm Labor (PTL)** is defined as regular uterine contractions accompanied by descent of the presenting part and progressive dilatation and effacement of the cervix occurring before 37 weeks from the first day of the LMP. PTL complicates only 8% to 10% of pregnancies but is responsible for more than 60% of all perinatal morbidity and mortality. Risk factors include occult maternal genitourinary tract infections, maternal smoking, high levels of stress, low socioeconomic status, maternal age younger than 18 years or older than 35 years, cervical dilatation >1 cm or cervical effacement >30% between 26 and 34 weeks' gestation, and uterine anomalies. Risk factors most likely are synergistic. Screening and treatment of bacterial vaginosis in high-risk women may decrease the incidence of preterm labor. (SOR **B**)

   A. **Diagnosis**. Early diagnosis is crucial, as tocolysis is most effective before 3 cm of cervical dilatation or 50% effacement. Symptoms suggestive of regular uterine contractions should be evaluated with serial examinations for cervical change and by external monitoring of uterine activity. Vaginal ultrasound to assess cervical length, along with fetal fibronectin measurements, may be helpful in predicting the likelihood of preterm birth.

B. Treatment. The risks of preterm delivery must outweigh the risks of tocolysis. Advancing gestational age clearly improves the preterm infant's prognosis until approximately 35 weeks, when delaying delivery has less effect overall. Survival increases to 90% at 29 weeks; mortality then decreases approximately 1% per week. The acuteness and severity of preterm labor suggest the type of treatment.

1. Uterine irritability without significant cervical change may benefit from rest at home, intake of fluids, and treatment of causative factors, such as urinary tract infection, if present.

2. Tocolytic therapy is indicated in preterm labor if no contraindications, such as severe preeclampsia or chorioamnionitis, exist. All tocolytics have potentially severe side effects for both mother and fetus. Choices include β-sympathomimetics, magnesium sulfate, nifedipine, and indomethacin.

3. Evaluation for possible triggers, particularly occult urinary tract infection, is indicated. Randomized controlled trials have found no clear benefit to the use of antibiotics in PTL with intact membranes on prolonging gestation or improving neonatal morbidity or mortality. (SOR **A**) Treatment with antenatal corticosteroids given before 34 weeks' gestation and >24 hours but <7 days prior to delivery has been shown to be of benefit in reducing the incidence and severity of respiratory distress syndrome and improves neonatal survival rates. (SOR **A**) In addition, use of betamethasone has been associated with a 50% decrease in the incidence of periventricular malacia. (SOR **B**)

V. Fetal Assessment and Postdates Pregnancy

A. Fetal assessment. Several methods have been developed to assess the well-being of the fetus when risk factors exist. Fetal assessment begins between 32 and 34 weeks' gestation or whenever the risk develops. Testing may begin as early as 26 to 28 weeks in particularly worrisome conditions. Major indications for antenatal testing include diabetes mellitus, hypertensive disorders, maternal substance abuse, third-trimester bleeding, IUGR, previously unexplained stillbirth, D (Rh) sensitization, oligohydramnios, multiple gestation, and decreased fetal movement as perceived by the mother. Fetal assessment techniques also are routinely applied when a pregnancy becomes postterm (42 weeks from the LMP). Testing is generally repeated weekly or biweekly until delivery. (SOR **C**)

1. **Fetal movement counts.** A quantitative method of counting fetal movements has been developed as a means of fetal assessment near term. The patient is asked to count fetal movements during a 2-hour period each day and report <10 movements during that period. A positive test (fewer than 10 movements) is an indication for additional fetal assessment. The advantages of this test are its low cost and maternal involvement. (SOR **C**)

2. **Fetal heart rate testing**

   a. The nonstress test (NST) is a noninvasive method based on the premise that in a healthy fetus, acceleration of the heart rate occurs during fetal movement. An external monitor is used to record the fetal heart rate while the mother reports fetal movement. A reactive or normal test has two or more accelerations of more than 15 beats per minute, each lasting for 15 seconds, in a 20-minute period and in the absence of decelerations. If fetal movement does not occur in 20 minutes, abdominal palpation or vibro-acoustic stimulation may be applied to awaken a sleeping fetus. A reactive NST accurately identifies a healthy fetus 98% of the time.

   Evaluation of a nonreactive NST should include extending the testing period to 60 to 90 minutes when possible. Nonreactive NSTs and variable decelerations on reactive NSTs should prompt additional evaluation. It must be noted that 15% of fetuses younger than 32 weeks may have a nonreactive NST in the absence of fetal compromise.

   b. The contraction stress test (CST) is a test of the fetal heart rate in response to uterine contractions. The uterus may be stimulated to contract through intermittent stimulation of one breast nipple or through intravenous infusion of low-dose oxytocin. A satisfactory test requires at least three contractions in 10 minutes. The test is interpreted as negative, or normal, if there are no decelerations and positive, or abnormal, if late decelerations follow 50% or more of contractions. A positive CST is highly suggestive of fetal distress and must be treated immediately with oxygen, positional changes, labor induction, or cesarean section. Equivocal results occur with intermittent late decelerations or significant variable decelerations and should be repeated in 24 hours.

3. An **amniotic fluid index** is used to complement fetal heart rate testing. Ultrasonography is used for estimating amniotic fluid volume, which is an indirect measure of placental function. The largest anteroposterior fluid depth in each of four quadrants of the uterus is measured. The sum should exceed 5 cm.

4. The **biophysical profile** (BPP) is a quantitative score that combines the NST with ultrasonic observation of the fetus for up to 30 minutes and measurement of the amniotic fluid index. A score of 2 is given **for each normal result** (fetal breathing movements, gross body movements, tone, amniotic fluid index, and NST) and 0 for an abnormal condition. A total score of 8 to 10 is reassuring, 6 is equivocal, and 4 or less is worrisome. An equivocal test should prompt delivery if at term or be repeated in 12 to 24 hours. A score of 4 or less should be a consideration for delivery regardless of gestational age or further evaluation. A combination of NST and amniotic fluid evaluation known as a modified BPP is considered comparable to the biophysical profile in assessing fetal well-being.

B. **Postterm pregnancy.** Defined as lasting longer than 42 weeks from the beginning of the LMP, approximately 3.5% to 12% of pregnancies are postdates. Prolonged pregnancy is one lasting longer than 41 weeks. Accurate dating is essential to avoid mislabeling a pregnancy as postterm. (SOR **A**)

1. Chronic uteroplacental insufficiency leading to fetal compromise occurs in up to 20% of postterm pregnancies. Additional complications include oligohydramnios, meconium passage, and macrosomia, which may contribute to a higher cesarean section rate.

2. **Evaluation.** Fetal assessment testing should be performed in all postterm pregnancies. Perinatal morbidity and mortality increase past 41 weeks; therefore, monitoring the pregnancy with antepartum testing is common practice. (SOR **C**)

3. **Management.** International randomized controlled clinical trials have shown a clear benefit to induction of labor at 41 to 42 weeks' gestation. The fetal mortality rate of 2 per 1000 at this gestational age is lowered to virtually zero, and cesarean rates are lowered. Elective induction with oxytocin, using prostaglandins for cervical ripening, is relatively safe and effective. Women with a favorable cervix are generally induced. (SOR **C**) Women with an unfavorable cervix may be managed expectantly or with induction. (SOR **A**) Delivery should be attempted if there is evidence of fetal compromise or oligohydramnios on testing. (SOR **A**) Sweeping (stripping) of the membranes reduces the need for other methods of induction, but may cause some discomfort for the patient. (SOR **A**)

VI. **Normal Labor and Delivery.** Signs of labor include passage of the mucus plug, bloody show (small amount of blood-tinged mucoid vaginal discharge), regular uterine contractions, and spontaneous rupture of membranes. In the general population, approximately 90% of women should be able to have a healthy birth outcome without medical intervention. The great majority of women deliver in the hospital utilizing family-centered birthing focusing on safety for the mother and child and fostering a positive experience for the woman, her partner, and family.

GENERAL REFERENCES

American Academy of Pediatrics and the American College of Obstetricians and Gynecologists: *Guidelines for Perinatal Care.* 5th ed. Elk Grove, IL: American Academy of Pediatrics; 2002.

Antenatal corticosteroid therapy for fetal maturation. ACOG Committee Opinion No. 273. American College of Obstetricians and Gynecologists. *Ostet Gynecol.* 2002;99:871-873.

Antepartum Fetal Surveillance. ACOG Practice Bulletin No. 9, October 1999. American College of Obstetricians and Gynecologists.

Assessment of Risk Factors for Preterm Birth. ACOG Practice Bulletin No. 31, October 2001. American College of Obstetricians and Gynecologists.

Briggs GG, Freeman RK, Yaffe SJ. *Drugs in Pregnancy and Lactation: A Reference Guide to Fetal and Neonatal Risk.* 6th ed. Baltimore, MD: Williams & Wilkins; 2001.

Centers for Disease Control and Prevention. Prevention of Group B streptococcal disease. *MMWR.* 2002; 51(No. RR-11):1-22.

Cochrane Pregnancy and Childbirth Group. Cochrane Database of Systematic Reviews (available in the Cochrane Library). www.cochrane.org. Accessed August 19, 2008.

Exercise during pregnancy and the postpartum period. ACOG Committee Opinion No. 267. American College of Obstetricians and Gynecologists. *Obstet Gynecol.* 2002;99:171-173.

Kirkham C et al. Evidence-based prenatal care: part I. General prenatal care and counseling issues. *Am Fam Phys.* 2005;71:1307-1316.

Muchowski K, Paladine H. An ounce of prevention: The evidence supporting periconception health care. *J Fam Pract.* 2004;53:126-133.

Nausea and Vomiting of Pregnancy. ACOG Practice Bulletin No. 52, April 2004. American College of Obstetricians and Gynecologists.

Obesity in pregnancy. ACOG Committee Opinion No. 315. American College of Obstetricians and Gynecologists. *Obstet Gynecol.* 2005;106:671-675.

Screening for Fetal Chromosomal Abnormalities. ACOG Technical Bulletin No. 77, January 2007. American College of Obstetricians and Gynecologists.

Smoking cessation during pregnancy. ACOG Committee Opinion No. 316.American College of Obstetricians and Gynecologists. *Obstet Gynecol.* 2005;106:883-888.

US Preventive Services Task Force. *Guide to Clinical Preventive Services: Report of the US Preventive Services Task Force.* 2006. Available through the Agency for Healthcare Research and Quality (http://www.ahrq.gov). Accessed August 19, 2008.

98   Postpartum Care

Jeannette E. South-Paul, MD

KEY POINTS

- Puerperal infections usually occur 2 to 5 days postpartum. Presenting symptoms include malaise, anorexia, abdominal pain, and fever. The most common puerperal infections are endometritis, perineal infections, and toxic shock syndrome. Intravenous antibiotics are used to treat these infections initially. First-line treatments are clindamycin, 2.4 to 2.7 g/d, divided four times daily; and gentamicin, 2 mg/kg loading dose followed by 1.5 mg/kg every 8 hours; or cefoxitin, 1 g (2 g if severe) every 8 hours. (SOR **C**)
- The most common nonpuerperal infections that can occur in the postpartum period are (1) urinary tract infections (UTIs) or pyelonephritis, which usually present with fever, dysuria, frequency, and urgency, and (2) mastitis, which usually presents with a sore, tender breast. Amoxicillin (500 mg orally three times daily for 10–14 days) is a good first choice for UTIs, while mastitis is usually treated with an anti-staphylococcal antibiotic like dicloxacillin, 500 mg orally four times daily for 10 days. (SOR **C**)
- Other common postpartum complications include thromboembolic disease, which requires heparin when deep disease is present; postpartum hemorrhage, which requires oxytocin, 10 U intramuscularly every 4 hours until bleeding stops; and postpartum depression, which requires supportive care or antidepressants.
- Discharge instructions should include daily rest, sitz baths, instructions on when to resume sexual activity, encouragement of breast-feeding (and continuation of prenatal vitamins if doing so), and when to return for the postpartum examination (6–8 weeks after birth). (SOR **C**)

I. Introduction

    A. **Definition.** The postpartum period, or puerperium, is that period of time that begins with the delivery of the placenta and ends with the resumption of ovulatory menstrual cycles, which, in nonlactating women, usually occurs 6 to 8 weeks after delivery.

    B. **Pathophysiology and epidemiological data**

        1. **Uterus.** The uterus decreases in size dramatically following delivery (involution); it weighs only approximately 500 g at the end of the first week and lies again in the true pelvis. This change is accompanied by a high level of uterine activity (contractions, afterpains) that diminishes smoothly and progressively after the first 2 hours postpartum. The placental implantation site sheds organized thrombi and obliterated arteries to prevent scar formation and preserve normal endometrial tissue.

2. **Cervix.** The cervical os admits two fingers for the first 4 to 6 days postpartum, but constricts thereafter and admits only a small banjo curette by the end of the second week.

3. **Vagina.** Large and smooth-walled following delivery, the vagina begins to develop rugae by the end of the fourth week. It regains its nonpregnant size by the end of the sixth to eighth week.

4. **Lochia.** The uterine discharge, which is bright red at delivery, changes within a few days to the reddish-brown lochia rubra, composed of blood and decidual and trophoblastic debris. Lochia serosa, a more serous combination of old blood, serum, leukocytes, and tissue debris, appears 1 week postpartum and last for a few days. Lochia alba, a whitish-yellow discharge that contains serum leukocytes, decidua, epithelial cells, mucus, and bacteria, then begins and continues until approximately 2 to 4 weeks postpartum. Lochia rubra that lasts >4 weeks suggests the presence of retained secundines or the formation of placental polyps, organized placental fragments.

5. **Urinary tract.** Passage of the infant through the pelvis traumatizes the bladder, and its wall may be edematous. Trauma or conduction analgesia may also cause the bladder to be insensitive to changes in intravesicular pressure, resulting in an impaired urge to urinate. Symptoms of urinary incontinence increase with parity. Practice of pelvic muscle exercise by primiparas has resulted in fewer urinary incontinence symptoms during late pregnancy and the puerperium. The glomerular filtration rate remains elevated during the first postpartum week. Urinary output, which often reaches 3 L in a 24-hour period, exceeds fluid intake. This output, combined with insensible losses, accounts for the approximately 12-lb weight loss seen during this period. The pregnancy-induced dilation of the ureters and renal pelves subsides to normal within 6 weeks.

6. **Abdominal wall.** The abdominal wall begins to resume a nonparous condition in approximately 6 to 7 weeks. The skin remains lax, but the muscles regain substantial tone with proper exercise.

7. **Cardiovascular changes.** Cardiac output decreases to nonpregnant levels within 2 to 3 weeks postpartum. Lower-extremity varicosities and pelvic varices regress during this period. Plasma volume decreases more rapidly than do cellular components initially, so that the hematocrit increases slightly during the first 72 hours postpartum.

8. **Weight change.** Weight gain during the first 20 weeks of pregnancy predicts postpartum retained weight. The influence of lactation on weight loss postpartum is unclear. Women lose approximately half of the average weight gain of pregnancy (25 lbs) in the first 2 weeks after delivery. The remainder is lost during the following weeks. Women should return to their nonparous weight in approximately 8 weeks.

9. **Breasts.** Milk production and engorgement begin within 3 days postpartum, following the decrease in estrogen and the increase in prolactin produced by suckling. Suckling is the single most important stimulus for the maintenance of milk production. A mother wishing to stop breast-feeding need only discontinue suckling. The accumulation of milk in the alveoli and major ducts leads to increased intra-alveolar and intraductal pressure, resulting in the cessation of milk formation. The historical practice of breast binding is thought to work by the same mechanism, but is being discouraged. Women who use breast-binding techniques postpartum seem to experience greater breast tenderness and breast leakage and require more analgesia than those who only use a firm bra. (SOR **C**)

10. **Hypothalamic–pituitary–ovarian function.** Forty percent of nonlactating women will resume menstruation within 6 weeks following delivery, 65% within 12 weeks, and 90% within 24 weeks. Approximately 50% of the first cycles are ovulatory. In nursing mothers, menstruation is resumed within 6 weeks in only 15% and within 12 weeks in only 45%. In 80% of these women, the first ovulatory cycle is preceded by one or more anovulatory cycles. Rapid decreases in blood levels of estrogen, progesterone, human placental lactogen, and insulin occur following delivery.

II. **Diagnosis and Treatment** (see Table 98–1 for a summary).
   A. **Abnormalities of the puerperium**
   1. **Puerperal infections.** *Puerperal infection* is defined as infection of the genital tract that sometimes extends to other organ systems. Onset is insidious and may occur 2 to 5 days postpartum. Nonspecific symptoms are malaise, anorexia, and fever. In many cases, a temperature of 38°C (100.4°F) or higher on any two of the first 10 days postpartum, exclusive of the first 24 hours, indicates a puerperal infection. Extragenital infections and noninfectious causes of fever must be excluded. The differential

TABLE 98–1. POSTPARTUM COMPLICATIONS REQUIRING TREATMENT

Complications	Symptoms	Etiology	Predisposing Factors	Treatment
Puerperal infection	2–5 d postpartum, $T > 100.4°$F, anorexia	Polymicrobial—anaerobes and aerobes; *Escherichia coli*; Group B streptococci	Prolonged ROM; malnutrition; hemorrhage/anemia; soft tissue trauma	Clindamycin 2.4–2.7 g/d in 3–4 doses + gentamicin 2 mg/kg load, then 1.5 mg/kg q 8 h IV OR ampicillin 2 g IV + sulbactam 1 g IV q 6 h OR cefoxitin or moxalactam
Endometritis/parametritis	Lethargy; $T >$ 100.4°F; lower abdominal pain	Polymicrobial	Prolonged labor and ROM; prior gynecologic infections; hematomas; devitalized tissue; maternal age younger than 17 years	Same as above
Urinary tract infections	Fever; abdominal pain; ± dysuria	Polymicrobial	Trauma-induced bladder hypotonicity; frequent catheterizations	Amoxicillin 500 mg po tid × 10–14 d
Deep vein thrombosis	Deep vein tenderness; Homan's sign; extremity swelling	Sluggish circulation; estrogen-induced hypercoagulability	Trauma to pelvic veins	Heparin 5000–10,000 U load to get PTT at 2 × normal or Enoxaparin 1 mg/kg SC bid followed by warfarin po to maintain INR 2.0–3.0
Superficial thrombophlebitis	Palpable cords in lower extremities; tenderness; skin warmth		High estrogen state	Elastic support stockings; walking; leg elevation at rest; moist local heat
Pelvic vein thrombosis (right ovarian syndrome)	Abdominal pain, fever, tender, sausage-shaped mass in right mid abdomen		High estrogen state	Heparin anticoagulation (as above)
Necrotizing fasciitis	3–5 d postpartum; symptoms as in other puerperal infections	Polymicrobial, especially anaerobes	Diabetes; immunocompromised state; status post C-section	Clindamycin 2.4 g/kg in 4 doses + gentamicin 1.5 mg/kg q 8 h IV; surgical debridement
Toxic shock syndrome	$T > 102°$F; macular erythematous rash, especially on palms and soles	*Staphylococcus aureus* exotoxin-1	Prolonged tampon use	Hospitalization; fluid; electrolytes; PRBCs; coagulation factors; oxacillin or nafcillin or methicillin 1 g IV q 4 h or vancomycin 100 mg q 6 h

INR, international normalized ratio; PRBCs, packed red blood cells; PTT, partial thromboplastin time; ROM, rupture of membranes; *T*, temperature.

diagnosis includes UTIs, mastitis, and thrombophlebitis, as well as other causes of fever unrelated to the postpartum state. Onset of fever after the 10th postpartum day is usually of a nonobstetric nature. Puerperal infections that are usually polymicrobial in origin are caused predominantly by anaerobes and sometimes by aerobes. *Escherichia coli* and group B streptococci are the most common causative agents, but there has been some reemergence of infections secondary to group A β-hemolytic streptococci that can result in tissue damage, toxin-mediated shock, and multiple organ failure. Multiple bacteria of low virulence, common in the genitourinary tract, may become pathogenic as a result of hematomas and devitalized tissue. Cultures are of limited usefulness, since the same organisms are identified in patients with or without infections. (SOR **A**)

a. **Predisposing factors**
   (1) **Antepartum.** Premature or prolonged rupture of membranes, malnourishment, and anemia increase the likelihood of puerperal infections.
   (2) **Intrapartum.** Soft tissue trauma, residual devitalized tissue, prolonged labor, and hemorrhage are also risk factors.
   (3) **Late-onset indolent metritis** has been attributed to antepartum *Chlamydia trachomatis* cervical infection, but this organism may not be isolated at the time these infections develop postpartum. (SOR **C**)

b. **Specific puerperal infections**
   (1) **Endometritis.** This term describes inflammatory involvement, especially leukocytic infiltration, of the superficial layers of the endometrium or decidual layer. When severe, endometritis may be accompanied by chills, extreme lethargy, lower abdominal pain, and fever. Temperature spikes to 40°C (104°F) usually indicate associated sepsis. It is not necessarily associated with significant uterine tenderness by abdominal or vaginal palpation. The prevalence of this type of infection, which is relatively uncommon following uncomplicated vaginal delivery, has decreased from 2.5% to 1.3% in the last 15 years. This prevalence approaches 6%, however, in high-risk women: those with protracted labor and prolonged rupture of membranes, prior history of gynecologic infections, hematomas or devitalized tissue, postpartum anemia, maternal age younger than 17 years, and where there is manual removal of the placenta. Prior to the common use of perioperative antimicrobials for women undergoing cesarean section, these women had an extraordinarily high risk of developing endometritis. The reported overall prevalence of postoperative uterine infection was 13% to 50%, depending on the socioeconomic group of the parturient.

   The polymicrobial cause of endometritis necessitates broad-spectrum therapy. A combination of clindamycin and gentamicin has been used traditionally. (SOR **C**) Clindamycin is administered intravenously in a dose of 2.4 to 2.7 g/d in three or four divided doses. Gentamicin is given in a loading dose of 2 mg/kg and then 1.5 mg/kg every 8 hours thereafter. Other treatment regimens have been evaluated recently, but the number of subjects studied has been small. Regimens reported to be as effective as clindamycin plus gentamicin include cefoxitin, moxalactam, cefoperazone, cefotaxime, piperacillin, cefotetan, and clindamycin plus aztreonam. (SOR **B**) Evidence now suggests that ampicillin (2 g) and sulbactam (1 g) intravenously every 6 hours is equally as effective as the clindamycin/gentamicin regimen for clinical cure, bacterial eradication, and incidence of adverse experiences. (SOR **A**) In all cases, intravenous therapy should be continued until the patient has been free of symptoms for approximately 48 hours.

   (2) **Group B streptococcal sepsis**. This is a major cause of puerperal infections usually presenting with fever within 12 hours of delivery, accompanied by tachycardia and endomyometritis. No localizing signs may be evident early in the course of the infection. **Group B streptococcal sepsis** positive mothers (typically distal vagina and anorectum cultured between 35 and 37 weeks gestation) are administered antibiotics intrapartum to produce a 30-fold risk reduction in the incidence of early-onset **group B streptococcal sepsis** infection. (SOR **A**) The Center for Disease Control and Prevention (CDC) and the American College of Obstetricians and Gynecologists (ACOG) endorsed recommendations indicate preference for Penicillin G rather than ampicillin because the

narrow spectrum of penicillin's activity makes selection of resistant organisms less likely. (SOR **B**)

(3) Parametritis. This infection involves the broad ligament adjacent to the uterus. Parametritis is usually associated with endometritis. In its most isolated mild form, it may follow cesarean section. Treatment is the same as for endometritis. (SOR **C**)

(4) Perineal infection. Such an infection is more likely in the presence of a small, unnoticed hematoma. Examination of the perineum reveals an edematous, erythematous lesion with purulent drainage. Sutures must be removed to enhance drainage.

(5) Mastitis (see Chapter 8).

2. Nonpuerperal complications

a. Urinary tract infections. The high incidence of UTIs during the postpartum period is usually attributed to trauma-induced hypotonicity of the bladder and frequent catheterization. Most patients with cystitis have had a negative result on initial screening culture and no urologic abnormalities. A 10- to 14-day course of antibiotics (amoxicillin, 500 mg orally three times daily for 10–14 days) is begun before cultures are ready (see Chapter 21). (SOR **C**) For a penicillin-allergic patient, refer to the alternative medications noted in Chapter 21, Table 21–1. Cystitis usually results in local symptoms without fever. In contrast, the symptoms of pyelonephritis are more severe: flank pain, shaking chills, and fever to 40°C (104°F) are frequent accompaniments.

b. Thrombophlebitis and thromboembolic disease. These conditions occur in fewer than 1% of all parturients, but occur significantly more often in the parturient than in the nonpregnant woman.

(1) Disorders of the deep veins in the postpartum period have been attributed to sluggish circulation, trauma to pelvic veins secondary to pressure from the fetal head, estrogen-induced hypercoagulability, and pelvic infection. Deep vein thrombophlebitis is characterized by fever, deep vein tenderness, Homan's sign, and extremity swelling secondary to venous obstruction. A useful, reliable diagnostic procedure is venography. (SOR **B**) The accuracy of Doppler ultrasonography depends on the skill of the technician (see Chapter 23).

(2) Superficial thrombophlebitis usually involves the saphenous system and is palpable on physical examination. Tenderness and increased skin warmth are also evident. Treatment methods include **elastic support stockings, walking, elevation of the legs at rest, a combination of analgesic drugs,** and **application of moist local heat** to the area. (SOR **C**) To prevent this form of thrombophlebitis, women should remain active and refrain from taking estrogens to suppress lactation or oral contraceptives, since these agents increase the risk of hypercoagulation. They should also avoid anti-inflammatory agents during pregnancy and lactation because of risk of premature closure of the fetal ductus arteriosus.

(3) *Right ovarian vein syndrome,* or **pelvic thrombophlebitis,** is the term used to describe thrombophlebitis occurring in the ovarian veins and other pelvic vessels. The patient often complains of abdominal pain and fever. If no evidence of pelvic abscess exists, and appropriate antibiotic therapy has resulted in no improvement in 72 hours in a patient with suspected endometritis, the diagnosis of ovarian vein syndrome should be considered. A sausage-shaped, tender mass may be palpated in the right midabdomen. Dramatic improvement usually results once **anticoagulation with heparin** is initiated, but defervescence may only occur after 4 to 5 days of heparin therapy, in doses similar to those used for the treatment of pulmonary embolism (SOR **C**) (see Chapter 23). Currently available imaging studies (computerized tomography scan and ultrasound) are poor in diagnosing this entity, so clinical suspicion is important.

(4) Massive pulmonary embolism is characterized by the sudden onset of pleuritic chest pain, cough (with or without hemoptysis), fever, apprehension, and tachycardia. Friction rub, signs of pleural effusion and atelectasis, hypotension, diaphoresis, electrocardiographic signs of right heart strain, and increasing central venous pressure may all be present in severe cases (see Chapter 20).

c. **Parametrial phlegmon.** A phlegmon, a three-dimensional mass that is palpable adjacent to the uterus on pelvic examination, develops most frequently when appropriate antimicrobial therapy has been delayed following evaluation of a postcesarean fever. A parametrial phlegmon is an intense area of induration within the leaves of the broad ligament occurring when endometritis and accompanying parametrial cellulitis follow cesarean delivery. The infection can be localized in the retroperitoneal area and presents with symptoms of peritonitis, such as an adynamic ileus. Treatment includes **bed rest, hydration with intravenous fluids, decompression of the bowel,** and **maintenance of electrolyte balance.** (SOR **C**) Clinical response occurs following intravenous antimicrobial therapy (the same antibiotics as are used for endometritis), although not usually until 5 to 7 days after initiation of treatment.

d. **Toxic shock syndrome.** Toxic shock syndrome toxin-1, an exotoxin produced by *Staphylococcus aureus,* causes toxic shock syndrome by provoking severe endothelial injury. Nearly 10% of pregnant women have been found to be colonized vaginally by *S. aureus,* and toxic shock syndrome has been reported in parturients. The syndrome most commonly occurs in young menstruating women who are using tampons. This severe, multisystem, acute febrile illness is characterized by a fever of 38.9°C (102°F) or higher; a macular erythematous rash, especially on the palms and the soles, that desquamates 1 to 2 weeks after onset of illness; hypotension, <90 mm Hg systolic, or orthostatic syncope; and involvement of three or more of the following organ systems: gastrointestinal, muscular, mucous membrane, renal, hepatic, hematologic, or central nervous.

Initial management includes hospitalization, fluid and electrolyte resuscitation (up to 12 L/d), and administration of packed red blood cells and coagulation factors as necessary. (SOR **A**) In addition to baseline laboratory studies, blood and vaginal cultures of *S. aureus* should be obtained promptly. Treatment with a β-lactamase-resistant antibiotic, such as nafcillin, oxacillin, or methicillin, is indicated; the dosage is 1 g intravenously every 4 hours. Vancomycin, 100 mg every 6 hours, is effective if the patient is allergic to penicillin. (SOR **A**)

e. **Necrotizing fasciitis.** This deep, soft tissue infection that involves muscle and fascia may develop adjacent to myofascial edges, including surgical incisions and other wounds. Such infections rarely develop during the postpartum period in healthy women, but are seen in diabetic and immunocompromised women. Symptoms most commonly occur 3 to 5 days following delivery. The microbes implicated in these perineal infections are similar to those causing other pelvic infections, but anaerobes predominate. A high index of suspicion is necessary with rapid surgical exploration if the diagnosis is probable. Therapy consists of **broad-spectrum antibiotics** (e.g., clindamycin, 2.4 g/kg in four divided doses) plus gentamicin (1.5 mg/kg every 8 hours), or others as noted above, as well as vigorous surgical **debridement**.

3. **Postpartum hemorrhage**

a. **Uterine atony.** This condition, which is the most common cause of postpartum hemorrhage, can result from excessive uterine stretching secondary to polyhydramnios, multiple gestation, multiparity, prolonged labor, and certain general anesthetic agents. Initial management includes **fundal massage, removal of any remaining placental fragments,** and **oxytocin** (10 U intramuscularly every 4 hours, or 10–40 U intravenously diluted in 1000 mL of 0.5 normal saline titrated intravenously) to control atony. (SOR **C**) Methylergonovine maleate (0.2 mg intramuscularly every 4 hours for 48 hours) may be used instead of oxytocin. Prostaglandin analogues can also be used alone or in combination with other uterotonic agents (carboprost tromethamine—0.25 mg IM every 15–90 minutes up to 8 doses; misoprostol—1000 μg, single dose via rectal, vaginal, or buccal routes). (SOR **C**)

b. **Lacerations.** Routine inspection of the cervix, vagina, and perineum immediately following delivery affords the opportunity for timely repair of extensions to the episiotomy or lacerations.

c. **Hematomas.** Perineal pain and noticeable mass suggest hematomas, which usually occur at the sites of lacerations or episiotomy repair. If managed within the first 24 hours after delivery with incision, drainage, and ligation of bleeding vessels, the cavity can be closed with a figure-of-eight suture. (SOR **C**)

      d. Less common causes of postpartum hemorrhage are placenta accreta, inverted uterus, coagulation defects (e.g., associated with amniotic fluid embolism or preeclampsia–eclampsia), retained placental fragments, or uterine rupture. Digital examination of the uterus and lower uterine segment upon delivery is necessary to detect uterine rupture, especially after a vaginal delivery following prior cesarean section.

  4. Postpartum emotional disorders

      a. "Baby blues," or **"postpartum blues."** This transient depression, which is encountered in 70% to 80% of women during the first week postpartum, usually on the second or third day following delivery, can be accompanied by tearfulness. This self-limited disorder usually resolves within 3 to 7 days. Twelve percent of women will present with clinically relevant depressive disorders within 6 weeks postpartum, but 90% of these cases are associated with a situational or long-standing problem. Postpartum depression, occurring between 2 weeks and 12 months postpartum, may relate to employment factors in the working parturient, such as work hours and duration of maternity leave, maternal fatigue, and quality of prenatal social support. If the symptoms are severe enough to interfere with the new mother's ability to cope with ordinary daily tasks and activities, counseling and pharmacotherapy are advisable (SOR **A**) (see Chapter 92). Individually based interventions are more effective than group-based interventions.

      b. Psychiatric disorders. If the patient exhibits excessive or no tearfulness, lack of interest in the baby, or excessive concern with the problems that will be encountered upon returning home that persist more than 24 hours while still in the hospital, or does not respond to counseling about problems developing subsequently, psychiatric evaluation is needed. Not only can major affective disorders appear during this time, but also the stress of gestation and parturition are nonspecific factors that may contribute to the development of various psychotic disorders.

III. Management Strategies

  A. Immunizations

      1. Nonisoimmunized D-negative women who deliver a D-positive infant should be given 300 mg of anti-D immune globulin (RhoGAM) shortly after delivery. (SOR **B**)

      2. The postpartum hospitalization period is also an appropriate time for vaccination of women not already immune to rubella. It is also appropriate to give a tetanus toxoid booster injection prior to discharge unless it is contraindicated. (SOR **C**)

  B. Discharge instructions

      1. Periods of rest during the day are advisable for the **first month postpartum.** All parturients, especially those who have been sedentary during pregnancy, become detrained during the third trimester and the postpartum period and should begin exercising at a baseline level. If vaginal bleeding increases upon resumption of exercise, parturients should stop for 2 to 3 days to allow further uterine involution and then resume activity. (SOR **A**) The parturient may gradually increase her activity and exercise level as soon as 2 weeks following an uncomplicated delivery. Only half of women seem to regain their usual level of energy by 6 weeks postpartum, however.

      2. Sitz baths, basins designed to fit over the toilet seat and be filled with warm water and 1 oz of Betadine solution, or tub baths for 30 minutes two to three times daily, are helpful for painful episiotomies or lacerations. (SOR **C**)

      3. Sexual intercourse

         a. For some time, **abstinence** has been recommended in the 6 weeks following delivery. The most common complaint is concern about dyspareunia during this period, which can be minimized by careful episiotomy. This period of discomfort can be shortened safely if no episiotomy is needed or if episiotomy repair is done meticulously so that healing occurs rapidly and comfortably. If tender areas in the episiotomy scar or in the vaginal wall persist after healing, a 1:1 steroid–lidocaine (1–2 mL of 1% Xylocaine without epinephrine and 1–2 mL of triamcinolone acetonide, 10 mg/mL) injection to the painful area can be used for relief. (SOR **C**)

         b. Otherwise, **sexual intercourse** can be resumed between the second and third postpartum weeks. The parturient can be encouraged to resume sexual activity when bleeding slows and when acceptable contraception has been provided. Contraception should be discussed and a method should be selected prior to discharge from the hospital (see Chapter 95). Intrauterine devices, diaphragms, sponges, and foams are not advised until after the puerperium. (SOR **C**)

4. **Breast-feeding**
   a. **Components of milk**
      (1) **Colostrum.** This liquid is secreted by the breasts for the first 5 days of parturition. It contains more protein, mostly globulin, and minerals and less sugar and fat than the more mature milk that is ultimately secreted. Host resistance factors, such as complement components, macrophages, lymphocytes, lactoferrin, lactoperoxidase, and lysozyme, as well as immunoglobulin, are present in colostrum and milk.
      (2) **Milk.** The major components are proteins (α-lactalbumin, β-lactoglobin, and casein), lactose, water, and fat. All vitamins except vitamin K are present in human milk in variable amounts. Iron is present in low concentrations, and iron levels in breast milk do not seem to be influenced by maternal iron stores. The predominant antibody present is secretory immunoglobulin A. These antibodies are thought to act locally within the infant's gastrointestinal tract.
   b. **Nursing**
      (1) **Advantages**
         (a) Accelerates involution of the uterus via oxytocin release.
         (b) **Gives ideal nourishment.** Breast milk meets the nutritional needs of the infant.
         (c) **Provides immunologic advantage.** In addition, breast-fed babies are less prone to respiratory and enteric infections than are bottle-fed babies.
         (d) **Contributes to bonding.** Nursing is generally well tolerated by infants.
         (e) **Delays ovulation**
      (2) **Disadvantages**
         (a) Privacy is needed for frequent feedings.
         (b) Contraindications include concurrent usage of certain drugs (e.g., chloramphenicol, streptomycin, metronidazole, sulfa drugs, antithyroid drugs, some anticancer agents, certain anticonvulsants, some diuretics, and radioactive agents). Women with certain maternal illnesses (e.g., active hepatitis A or B or tuberculosis) should not engage in breast-feeding. (SOR **A**)
         (c) Nursing can be an additional stressor in an already stressed mother.
   c. **Breast care.** Cleanliness and attention to fissures on the nipples are important. Water and mild soap can be used to cleanse the areolae before and after nursing. Lanolin-containing cream is recommended for nipple protection during the initial weeks of breast-feeding to deter chapping and cracking of the nipples. Should severe irritation of the nipples occur, a nipple shield can be used for 24 hours or more.
5. **Suppression of lactation.** Women who do not wish to breast-feed should avoid all breast stimulation, suckling, manipulation, and showers, and should use a firm bra (rather than breast binding), and analgesia for 1 week. Minor symptoms of tenderness and a sense of fullness are common. Otherwise, there are no risks or side effects. Neither parenteral Deladumone nor oral bromocriptine is currently recommended. Following the use of Deladumone, rebound symptoms are common; in 25% of cases, there is an associated risk of thromboembolism, and use of the medication rarely results in substantial decrease in lactation. (SOR **B**) Rebound symptoms affect approximately 25% of women using bromocriptine as well. Furthermore, additional risks include hypotension, nausea, headache, dizziness, strokes, and early ovulation. (SOR **A**)
6. **Postpartum examination.** The postpartum visit is usually scheduled for 6 to 8 weeks after delivery, since most of the systemic signs of pregnancy have resolved by this time. (SOR **C**) Recent research evaluating optimal timing of the postpartum examination demonstrates that scheduling the Pap smear at least 8 weeks following delivery, rather than at 4 to 6 weeks, results in an approximately 30% decrease in the number of abnormal smears requiring follow-up or colposcopic examination. (SOR **A**) Following normal labor and puerperium, the postpartum evaluation should consist of blood pressure and weight determinations, palpation of the thyroid gland, a breast examination, a pelvic examination with cytologic examination of the cervix, evaluation of rectal sphincter tone, examination of abdominal wall tone, and urinalysis. Routine postpartum hematocrits are unnecessary in clinically stable patients with an estimated blood loss of <500 cc.

GENERAL REFERENCES

Briggs GG, Wan SR. Drug therapy during labor and delivery, part 2. *Am J Health-Syst Pharm.* 2006; 63(12):1131-1139.

Dennis C. Psychosocial and psychological interventions for prevention of postnatal depression: systematic review. *BMJ* 2005; 331:15-22.

Swift K, Janke J. Breast binding . . . is it all that it's wrapped up to be? *J Obstet Gynecol Neonatal Nurs.* 2003; 32(3):332-339.

99　　Sexual Dysfunction

John G. Halvorsen, MD, MS

KEY POINTS

- Interference with their sexual response affects most people at some time in their sexual relationships.
- A simple question like, "How are things going for you sexually?" can help physicians to discover patients' sexual concerns. Patient surveys indicate that people are willing to talk with their physicians about their sexuality but hesitant to raise the subject themselves.
- Sexual dysfunction (e.g., erectile dysfunction in men and arousal disorder in women) may be the presenting sign or symptom of other serious underlying disorders (e.g., diabetes, hyperlipidemia, atherosclerosis, depression, tobacco, or drug abuse). Therefore, a thorough organic and psychological diagnostic evaluation performed by the primary physician is a necessary part of comprehensive management.
- Multiple treatment options can help to manage each one of the sexual dysfunctions.

I. **Introduction**
   A. **Definition.**
      The sexual dysfunctions represent disturbances in sexual desire and in the psychophysiologic changes that characterize the sexual response cycle.
   B. **Common Diagnoses.** The *Diagnostic and Statistical Manual of Mental Disorders,* 4th edition (DSM-IV-TR), classifies the dysfunctions according to the following system. All must be "persistent or recurrent," "cause marked distress or interpersonal difficulty," and not be "better accounted for by another Axis I disorder" or "due exclusively to the direct psychophysiologic effects of a substance (e.g., a drug of abuse, a medication) or a general medical condition." All disorders are further classified by subtype to indicate their onset (lifelong or acquired), the context (generalized or situational), and causative factors (caused by psychological factors or by combined factors) associated with each dysfunction.
      1. **Sexual desire disorders (SDDs)**
         a. **Hypoactive Sexual Desire Disorder (HSDD):** deficient (or absent) sexual fantasies and desire for sexual activity. In the National Health and Social Life Survey (NHSLS), a large, randomly chosen, representative national sample, 15% of men and 33% of women indicated that they lacked interest in sex for at least 1 of the past 12 months. Problems in a couple's relationship are the most common cause of SDD. A growing body of evidence now suggests that androgen deficiency may play a role in decreasing sexual motivation and desire in women.
         b. **Sexual Aversion Disorder:** extreme aversion to, and avoidance of, genital contact with a sexual partner. A rare desire disorder, sexual aversion is sometimes associated with vaginismus or dyspareunia. Patients commonly relate a history of sexual abuse accompanied by negative but unexpressed feelings about the partner relationship.
      2. **Sexual arousal disorders**
         a. **Male Erectile Disorder (ED):** inability to attain or maintain an adequate erection until sexual activity is completed.

Epidemiological surveys indicate that more than 10 million men in the United States experience ED. In a large cross-sectional, random sample survey of men aged 40 to 70 years, the prevalence of **minimal ED** was 17%; of **moderate ED**, 25%; and of **complete ED**, 10%. Multiple organic and psychogenic risk factors are implicated (Table 99–1).

  b. Female Sexual Arousal Disorder (FSAD): inability to attain or maintain an adequate lubrication—swelling response of sexual excitement until sexual activity is completed.

Estimates of arousal disorders in women range from 20% to 48%. Causative factors in women are less well known, but are presumed to include many of the same factors implicated in ED.

3. Orgasmic disorders

  a. Female Orgasmic Disorder (FOD): delayed or absent orgasm following normal sexual excitement.

Surveys suggest that **anorgasmia** affects 5% to 25% of women and that 20% to 48% report problems lubricating or reaching orgasm. Underlying psychogenic factors include fears of pregnancy, vaginal damage, or rejection by a sexual partner; hostility toward men; and guilt feelings associated with sexual impulses. Some women equate orgasm with losing control or with aggressive, destructive, or violent behavior. These women may express their associated fear through inhibited arousal or orgasm. Cultural expectations and societal restrictions on women may also contribute.

  b. Male Orgasmic Disorder (MOD): delayed or absent orgasm following normal sexual excitement.

Recent studies indicate a prevalence of 4% to 10%. Many men with this disorder were raised in rigid, puritanical families that considered sex sinful and the genitalia "dirty." These men also experience problems with closeness in relationships. Orgasmic disorders are more common in men with obsessive–compulsive personality disorders and in those with unexpressed hostility toward women. In addition to these psychosocial factors, many of the organic disorders and drugs listed in Table 99-1 can also interfere with male orgasm and ejaculation.

  c. Premature Ejaculation (PE): ejaculation with minimal stimulation before it is wanted, before, on, or shortly after penetration.

A total of 35% to 40% of men treated for sexual dysfunction experience PE. The community prevalence rate in one recent study was 36% to 38%. In the National Health and Social Life Survey, 28% of men reported climaxing too early.

Most men with PE ejaculate prior to or within 1 to 2 minutes after vaginal intromission. PE is more common in college-educated men and may relate to an excessive concern for their partner's satisfaction. It also relates to anxiety about the sex act, societal conditioning about men's sex roles, and stressful marriage relationships. Recent data indicate that men with PE come from families where other men experience rapid ejaculation and that this may result from disturbed or maladaptive serotonin receptors in specific brain loci. Other biological causes may include penile hypersensitivity, a hyperexcitable ejaculatory reflex, increased sexual arousability, and possible endocrinopathy.

4. Sexual pain disorders

  a. Dyspareunia: genital pain in either men or women associated with sexual intercourse.

As many as 30% of surgical procedures on a woman's genital tract result in temporary **dyspareunia**, and 30% to 40% of the women seen in sex therapy clinics for dyspareunia demonstrate pelvic disease. In the National Health and Social Life Survey, 5% of men and 15% of women reported dyspareunia in the past 12 months.

Many medical conditions may cause **dyspareunia in women**—inadequate vaginal lubrication, pelvic or urinary tract infections, vaginal or hymenal scar tissue, endometriosis, estrogen deprivation, allergic reactions, and gastrointestinal conditions. Provoked vestibulodynia (formerly termed vulvar vestibulitis) may be the most frequent form of chronic dyspareunia. At least 9% of women will experience this condition at some time. It appears to be caused by a reduced threshold for pain in the introital region that arises from centrally mediated mechanisms.

Structural abnormalities in the penis, Peyronie's disease, priapism, urethral stricture, prior genital surgery, or genital infections may cause **dyspareunia in men**.

TABLE 99–1. COMMON ORGANIC AND PSYCHOGENIC FACTORS ASSOCIATED WITH SEXUAL DYSFUNCTION

Organic Factors
1. **Chronic illness**
   a. Congenital illness or malformation
   b. Endocrine disease (e.g., diabetes mellitus; gonadal dysfunction; pituitary, adrenal, or thyroid disorders)
   c. Neurologic disorders (e.g., multiple sclerosis, spinal cord injury)
   d. Vaginal or pelvic pathology (e.g., vaginal atrophy, infections, endometriosis, childbirth injury)
   e. Genital trauma
   f. Cardiovascular and peripheral vascular disease
   g. Postsurgical complications (e.g., after prostatectomy, abdominal vascular surgery, sympathectomy, gynecologic procedures)
2. **Pregnancy (especially in the first and last trimesters)**
3. **Pharmacologic agents**

	Primarily Affects			
	Desire	Arousal	Orgasm	Hormones
a. Anticholinergics		+		
b. Antidepressants	+	+	+	
c. Antihistamines	+	+		
d. Antihypertensives	+	+	+	+
e. Antipsychotics	+	+	+	+
f. Anxiolytics	+		+	
g. Narcotics	+	+	+	+
h. Sedative–hypnotics	+	+	+	
i. Other drugs				
Cimetidine	+	+		+
Clofibrate	+	+		
Digitalis	+	+		
Ethinyl estradiol		+		+
Levodopa			+	
Lithium		+		
Ketoconazole	+	+		
Niacin		+		
Norethindrone	+	+		+
Phenytoin		+	+	
Primidone	+			
4. Drugs of abuse				
a. Alcohol	+	+	+	+
b. Amphetamines	+	+	+	
c. Cocaine		+	+	
d. Heroin	+	+	+	
e. Marijuana	+			
f. MDMA	+	+	+	
g. Methadone	+	+	+	
h. Phencyclidine (PCP)	+		+	
i. Tobacco		+		

Psychogenic Factors
1. **General psychogenic factors**
   a. Personal problems (e.g., depression, anxiety, diminished self-esteem, and intrapsychic conflict)
   b. Relationship problems (e.g., poor communication, unrealistic marital expectations, unresolved conflict, lost trust, poor relationship models, family system distress, sex role conflicts, and divergent sexual values)
   c. Psychosexual factors (e.g., prior sexual failure, chronic performance inconsistency, negative learning and attitudes about sex, prior sexual trauma, sexual performance anxiety, gender identity conflict, and paraphilias)
2. Remote vs. immediate factors
   a. Remote factors have historical origins (e.g., negative sexual learning in childhood, dysthymic depression, prior relationship failures)
   b. Immediate factors occur during sexual activity (e.g., sexual anxiety, denial of erotic feelings, ineffective sexual behaviors, failure to communicate desires and feelings)

Sexual Enactment Factors
Skill and knowledge deficits (e.g., inadequate penile stimulation, inadequate stimulation for vaginal lubrication, unfavorable pelvic position for intercourse)

MDMA, *S*-methoxy-3,4-methyleredioxy amphetamine.

Psychogenic theories for dyspareunia and vaginismus are similar and may involve a host of intrapsychic conflicts, faulty learning, or negative conditioning.

b. **Vaginismus:** involuntary muscular spasm of the outer third of the vagina that interferes with sexual intercourse.

Incidence estimates for **vaginismus** arising from sexual dysfunction clinics range widely, from 7.8% to 42%. It most often occurs in more educated women from higher socioeconomic groups.

Most vaginismus is psychogenic. Risk factors include sexual trauma (e.g., rape or incest), a strict religious background that associates sex with sin, unexpressed negative feelings toward a sexual partner or other important men, and phobia about the sexual response or intercourse.

5. **Sexual dysfunction caused by a general medical condition.**

This type of sexual dysfunction is fully explained by the direct physiologic effects of a defined medical condition.

6. **Substance-induced sexual dysfunction.**

This type of sexual dysfunction develops during or within 1 month of substance intoxication or when medication use is causally related.

II. Diagnosis

A. Symptoms

Physicians should include a brief query about sexual relationships during routine clinical encounters. They may bridge their conversation from the medical history to the sexual history with a statement such as, "Your sexual functioning is just as important to me as the rest of your body's functioning, so as a part of a complete history, I always ask a few questions about how things are going sexually."

General case-finding questions include queries such as "How are things going for you sexually?" "What questions or concerns do you have about your sexuality at this time?", or "How satisfying is your sex life for you?" Questions like these give patients "permission" to discuss their sexuality with the physician if they wish.

Specific questions that inquire into problems with various phases of the sexual response cycle are also appropriate.

1. **Present history**

Define the sexual problem better by collecting the following data: date and mode of onset; problem duration (lifelong, recent, and episodic); situational context (generalized to all encounters or only to specific ones); current sexual interactions of the couple, including frequency of intercourse or sex play, frequency that the patient and the partner would prefer, time of day for lovemaking, presence of fatigue during lovemaking, difficulties with privacy, verbal and nonverbal communication of desires, type and pleasurability of sex play that precedes intercourse, arousal level during intercourse, orgasm frequency, thoughts, visualizations, and fantasies during sex, pain felt during intercourse (this symptom itself must be pursued in more detail), any exacerbations or remissions of the problem; effects of any attempted treatment; the presence of any associated symptoms in other body systems; the level of personal and partner distress caused by the problem; and what the patient believes might be causing the difficulty.

2. **Sexual history**

Explore early experiences, emotional reactions, attitudes toward sexuality, sexual knowledge, frequency and types of past sexual practices, acceptance of cultural myths, the onset and development of the current sexual relationship, self-pleasuring practices and fantasies, homosexual experiences, any past negative sexual experiences (e.g., incest or sexual assault), personal body image, and sexual developmental history.

3. **Developmental and family history**

Discuss the family-of-origin's attitudes toward sexuality, parental modeling, religious influences, relationships with parents and siblings, family violence, and the level of function in the couple's families of origin.

4. **Nature of the current relationship**

Focus on the development and stability of the current relationship, changes in feeling toward the partner, the presence of unresolved conflict, loss of trust or fidelity, and communication problems (e.g., failures to listen and understand, hidden agendas, or using sex for power in the relationship).

5. **Current stressors**

Inquire about stresses that are both intrafamilial (e.g., death, illness, or problems with children) and extrafamilial (e.g., financial, occupational, or legal). Focus both on stresses and strains that normally occur as the individual and family progress through their life cycle stages and on stresses and strains that arise unexpectedly.

6. **Past medical history**

Identify any acute or chronic disease, injury, or surgery that could affect sexual functioning. Inquire specifically about those organic factors included in Table 99–1.

Many commonly used drugs may contribute to sexual dysfunction (Table 99–1). Drug effects vary by individual, depending on age, absorption, body weight, dosage, duration of use, rates of metabolism and excretion, presence of other drugs, underlying disorders, patient compliance, and suggestibility.

7. **Habits**

See Table 99–1 for the types of sexual dysfunctions associated with the common drugs of abuse.

8. **Questionnaires**

a. **The International Index of Erectile Function (IIEF)** is a 15-item inventory designed to assess erectile function, orgasmic function, sexual desire, intercourse satisfaction, and overall sexual satisfaction. It demonstrates test reliability, construct validity, and treatment responsiveness. A shortened 5-item version, the **IIEF-5**, is a useful screening instrument for ED, with a sensitivity of 98% and specificity of 88%.

b. **The Female Sexual Function Index** is a 19-item questionnaire designed to assess desire, subjective arousal, lubrication, orgasm, satisfaction, and pain in women. It demonstrates discriminant validity between normal women and those with FSAD, FOD, and HSDD.

These tools are brief, reliable, and valid measures that can help the busy physician to focus the history-taking process and to monitor treatment results.

B. **Signs**

A comprehensive physical examination will help to identify any concurrent acute or chronic illness and any associated physical conditions that could affect sexual functioning or treatment.

1. **Focus special attention on the following**

a. **General:** obesity, cachexia, vital signs, secondary sex characteristics, gynecomastia in men, and galactorrhea in women.

b. **Cardiovascular:** bruits (especially femoral), peripheral pulses, evidence of venous stasis, arterial insufficiency (especially in the lower extremities), and a pulsatile epigastric mass.

c. **Abdomin:** pain, tenderness, mass, guarding, tympany, and bowel activity.

d. **Neurologic:** gait, coordination, deep tendon reflexes, pathologic reflexes, sensation, motor strength, integrity of the sacral reflex arc (S_2–S_4) with perineal sensation, anal sphincter tone, and bulbocavernosus reflex (clinically present in 70% of normal men). Test penile temperature sensation with alcohol swabs and penile vibration perception threshold with a tuning fork placed sequentially on the glans and the midshaft.

2. **Male genitalia**

Observe the male genitalia for testicular size and consistency, penile size, malformations, and structural lesions. A normal flaccid adult penis is >6 cm in length and >3 cm in width.

Obtaining **penile blood pressure** measurements on any man with **ED** can help to diagnose arterial insufficiency. Place and inflate a 3-cm pediatric blood pressure cuff around the base of the penis and auscultate the central artery of the corpora cavernosa with a 9.5-MHz Doppler stethoscope as the cuff is deflated. The penile systolic pressure is the pressure at which one first hears the arterial pulse. The ratio between the penile systolic pressure and the brachial systolic pressure, the **penile brachial index**, should exceed 0.75. If it is below 0.60, significant penile vascular insufficiency likely exists. The **penile brachial index** is most predictive in patients with evidence for peripheral vascular disease but without other risk factors like diabetes or a pharmacologic agent that could affect erectile function. (SOR **Ⓒ**)

3. **Female pelvic examination**

Focus on the following:

a. **External genitalia:** dermatitis, vulvar inflammation, episiotomy or other scars, clitoral inflammation, and adhesions.

b. **Introitus:** hymenal rigidity, tags, or fibrosis; urethral carbuncle; Bartholin's gland inflammation and tenderness. Touching the vestibule, vulva, hymen, and minor vestibular glands with a cotton swab can help reproduce and localize pain associated with provoked vestibulodynia.

c. **Vagina:** spasm of the vaginal sphincter and adduction of the thighs with attempted vaginal examination, atrophy, discharge, inflammation, stenosis, relaxation of supporting ligaments, strength of pelvic muscles, and tenderness along the vaginal urethra or posterior bladder wall.

d. **Bimanual Examination:** cul-de-sac masses or tenderness; adnexal mass or tenderness; and position, size, mobility, and tenderness of the uterus.

e. **Rectovaginal Examination:** hemorrhoids, fissures, constipation, tenderness, and a stool specimen positive for occult blood.

C. **Laboratory tests**

1. **Evaluation for systemic disease**

   Baseline studies include a complete blood cell count, fasting blood sugar level, urinalysis, tests for sexually transmitted diseases, lipid profiles, and tests of thyroid, liver, and renal function.

2. **Evaluation for specific disorders**

   a. **Sexual desire disorders:** Obtain a morning **serum bioavailable testosterone** level in men with **SDD.** If levels are low or borderline, or if the low desire is associated with little or no masturbation history, obtain a **serum prolactin** level. Correlation between **sexual desire** and **levels of follicle-stimulating hormone (FSH), androstenedione, luteinizing hormone (LH),** and **estradiol is presently inconclusive.** In women in whom you suspect androgen insufficiency, obtain morning free and total testosterone levels between day 8 and 20 of the menstrual cycle. A level below the 25th percentile of the normal range for 20- to 40-year-old women may help to validate this diagnosis. (SOR **C**)

   b. **Female Sexual Arousal Disorder:** Experimental techniques for measuring nocturnal vaginal blood flow using a specially designed vaginal probe demonstrate that vaginal engorgement cycles occur in women during rapid eye movement (REM) sleep with the same frequency that erectile cycles occur in men.

   c. **Erectile Disorder:**

   (1) **Serum tests:** Obtain a morning **serum bioavailable testosterone** level to screen for hypogonadism. If the level is low, obtain **FSH, LH,** and **prolactin** levels. If FSH and LH are low and prolactin is normal, then the diagnosis is pituitary or hypothalamic failure. If FSH and LH are high and prolactin is normal, then the diagnosis is testicular failure. If FSH and LH are low, but prolactin is high, then there is a 25% to 40% chance that the patient has a pituitary adenoma. In this case request a **computerized tomographic** scan or **magnetic resonance imaging** scan of the sella turcica.

   (2) **Nocturnal penile tumescence (NPT) evaluation:** Because sleep eliminates the psychological factors that inhibit arousal, NPT evaluation helps to differentiate psychological from organic **ED.** Normally, three or four erections occur each night during rapid eye movement sleep with a total night erection time >90 minutes. Organic interference persists during sleep, disturbing erections. Psychogenic interference should not persist and erections will occur. Several techniques evaluate and quantify NPT.

   The **snap gauge** (Timm Medical Technologies, Eden Prairie, MN, USA) is a ring of opposing Velcro straps that are connected by three plastic strips. The man wraps the ring around the penis before sleep. During a normal rigid nocturnal erection, all bands break. By noting whether no, one, two, or three bands break, one can estimate the maximum erectile response during sleep. The three elements break at degrees of tension corresponding to intracorporeal pressures of approximately 80, 100, and 120 mm Hg. This is a useful screening tool, since it is inexpensive, is simple, and can be performed at home. False-negative results occur if it is not applied tightly enough. False positives occur if bands break while turning during sleep. This method only detects the maximal erectile event during sleep and does not measure erection duration, maximum number, or actual rigidity. Furthermore, one cannot correlate erections with rapid eye movement sleep cycles.

   More sophisticated tests, including the **RigiScan** (Timm Medical Technologies), the **NEVA System** (Urometrics, Inc., St. Paul, MN, USA), and **NPT monitoring** performed in a sleep laboratory are also available.

(3) **Pharmaco-penile duplex ultrasonographic scanning** provides high-resolution real-time ultrasonographic imaging and pulse Doppler analysis of the actual blood flow in the cavernous arteries before and after injection of a vasodilator. Normal vessels should double in size with an initial peak systolic flow velocity of 0.30 cm/s.

(4) **Pudendal angiography:** Selective internal pudendal angiograms can determine whether an arterial block exists that could be corrected by penile revascularization. This procedure is used most commonly in younger patients with clinical and noninvasive findings that suggest an arterial cause for their **ED** and who are candidates for reconstructive surgery.

(5) **Dynamic infusion cavernosometry and cavernosography** evaluate the veno-occlusive mechanisms of the corpus cavernosum. Through a butterfly needle inserted into the corpus cavernosum, the procedural physician first infuses a vasoactive agent (45–60 mg papaverine with 1–2.5 mg phentolamine or 20 μg of PGE_1), then heparinized saline and finally radiographic contrast. X-rays are taken to identify leaks in specific veins and to evaluate for glans or spongeosal leaks. These procedures are performed less frequently now since surgical procedures designed to correct venous leaks are less successful than anticipated.

(6) **Bulbocavernosus reflex latency tests** measure the integrity of the sacral reflex arc (S_2–S_4). When the glans penis is stimulated with a pinch or a squeeze, electromyographic needles in the bulbocavernosus muscle record muscle contraction and the time delay from stimulation to contraction. Longer times suggest a neurologic cause for **ED** and can help document suspected sacral nerve root, cauda equina, or conus medullaris lesions caused by multiple sclerosis, spinal cord trauma, spinal cord tumors, and herniated intervertebral disks.

(7) **Pudendal nerve somatosensory evoked potentials** record waveforms over the sacrum (conus medullaris) and the parietal cortex in response to dorsal penile nerve stimulation, and can therefore help localize neurologic lesions to peripheral, sacral, or suprasacral locations.

(8) **Vibration perception threshold** screens for abnormalities within the penile sensory afferent pathway. A portable handheld electromagnetic vibration device with a fixed vibration frequency and variable amplitude is placed against the penile shaft. A loss or decrease in sensation suggests a peripheral neuropathy.

(9) **Perineal electromyography** identifies problems in pudendal motor pathways that may relate to metabolic or toxic disorders such as diabetes and alcoholism.

(10) **Summary of evaluation for ED:** After conducting a comprehensive history, physical examination, and laboratory screening, one must form a "most probable" hypothesis for the man's **ED**. Is it psychological or organic? If it is organic, is the cause likely neurologic, vascular, endocrine, or a combination of these factors?

If one cannot separate psychological from organic factors, consider an **NPT evaluation**. If the hypothesis is "organic: neurologic or vascular," consider a therapeutic trial of one of the noninvasive agents used to treat **ED**. If the trial succeeds, continue therapy. If it fails, then consider further specific procedural evaluation for neurologic or vascular causes.

If the hypothesis is "organic: endocrine," then obtain a **serum bioavailable testosterone** level. If this is low, then obtain **FSH, LH**, and **prolactin** serum levels. If the serum testosterone is normal, revise the hypothesis and consider a therapeutic trial with a noninvasive agent.

d. **Sexual Pain Disorders:** Laboratory evaluation, guided by the clinical evaluation, helps to detect associated organic factors.

(1) **Office laboratory procedures** include saline and potassium hydroxide wet mounts of vaginal secretions to diagnose vaginitis or vaginosis; urinalysis, urine culture, and examination of prostatic secretions to diagnose associated genitourinary infections; and tests to diagnose chlamydial, herpes simplex, and gonococcal infections (see Chapters 21, 51, 61, and 64).

(2) **Colposcopy** may be useful in diagnosing specific vaginal or cervical disease such as human papillomavirus infections.

(3) **Pelvic ultrasonography** can help diagnose adnexal, uterine, or cul-de-sac problems.

(4) **Laparoscopy** can help diagnose, and in some cases treat, adnexal, or intraperitoneal disease.

(5) **Anoscopy or sigmoidoscopy** is used to identify associated colorectal problems (see Chapter 52).

III. Treatment

A. Therapeutic strategies. Physicians can relate to patients with a sexual problem at one of five levels.

1. Level 1: Case finding

Ask the initial sexual history question, but then refer to another professional for evaluation and treatment.

2. Level 2: Evaluate the chief complaint

Collect the basic sexual history during routine visits and provide basic education about normal anatomy, physiology, and sexual functioning. When patients raise sexual concerns, obtain a "history of present illness" with appropriate symptom pursuit and perform a focused physical examination. Refer to another professional if treatment involves more than reassurance or basic education.

3. Level 3: Comprehensive evaluation

Obtain a detailed sexual history that includes both the psychosocial and medical history. Perform a comprehensive physical examination and evaluate for organic causes with appropriate laboratory tests and diagnostic procedures.

4. Level 4: Manage organic problems and refer for psychosexual therapy

Treat any organic problems or coordinate care with another physician if a special procedure such as a penile implant is required. Continue to provide psychological support, but refer psychosexual therapy to a sexual therapist.

5. Level 5: Manage both organic and psychosexual therapy

6. Selecting a level of involvement.

Before primary physicians determine which role to play, they must ascertain their own interest in sexual concerns and the care they wish to provide. They must also build a professional referral network to provide care that is beyond their own competence or interest. Membership in or certification by one or more of the following organizations is one indication of a sexual therapist's competence: Society for Sex Therapy and Research; American Association for Sex Education, Counseling and Therapy; and Society for Scientific Study of Sex (SSSS).

B. Psychosexual therapy

1. Standard principles

Several basic principles undergird current psychosexual therapy.

a. People are responsible for their own sexuality.

b. Growth in sexual attitudes, performance, and feelings results from behavioral change.

c. Every person deserves sexual health.

d. Physiologic relaxation creates the foundation for sexual excitement.

e. Boundaries between the sexual and the nonsexual aspects of sexual dysfunction (e.g., career stress or marital problems) must exist.

2. Cognitive-behavioral therapy.

Cognitive-behavioral therapy that incorporates behavioral therapy into other treatments is the psychosexual treatment of choice for managing most sexual dysfunctions. Behavior therapists assume that sexual dysfunction is learned maladaptive behavior that causes patients to fear sexual interaction. During treatment, the therapist establishes a hierarchy of anxiety-provoking situations for the patient and then helps him or her to master the anxiety through systematic desensitization. This process inhibits the learned anxious response by encouraging antianxiety behaviors.

3. Masters and Johnson dual-sex therapy

Dual-sex therapy requires that a man–woman co-therapy team work with couples, acknowledging that men and women differ in sexual experiences and roles and establishing the therapeutic importance of gender fairness and balance. Few centers currently use dual-gender treatment teams, since other models are successful and less expensive.

4. Sensate focus

The original behavioral tasks developed by Masters and Johnson are termed "sensate focus" exercises, since they heighten sensory awareness to touch, sight, sound, and smell. As patients focus on their own sensations, they often relax and overcome barriers that impede natural physiologic responses. Partners first learn to enjoy touching, stroking, exploring, massaging, and fondling all the contours of each other's bodies except for their genitals. When both partners are adept and comfortable exchanging nongenital caresses, they add genital stroking exercises. Erogenous stroking progresses to vaginal penile containment, first without genital thrusting and then to full intercourse with orgasm. Couples learn to use fantasies to distract them from obsessive performance concerns and to communicate mutual needs verbally and nonverbally.

5. Hypnotherapy

Hypnotherapy begins with a series of nonhypnotic sessions to build a secure physician–patient relationship and to establish treatment goals. Therapy focuses on removing symptoms and altering attitudes. Patients begin to use relaxation techniques before a sexual encounter, and they also learn alternative ways to deal with anxiety-provoking sexual situations.

6. Group therapy

Group therapy can examine patients' intrapsychic and interpersonal problems within a strong support system that can counteract sexual myths, correct misconceptions, and provide accurate information about sexual anatomy, physiology, and varieties of behavior. Groups composed of sexually dysfunctional married couples are particularly effective in validating individual preferences and in enhancing self-esteem and self-acceptance.

7. Traditional couples therapy

Couples therapy is also important, since relationship problems that generate stress, fatigue, and dysphoria commonly underlie the sexual dysfunctions. Therapy helps the couple to develop communication skills, establish realistic relationship expectations, resolve conflict, and build trust.

C. Specific sexual therapy techniques

1. Directed self-stimulation

This is the most effective treatment program to date for primary orgasmic dysfunction in women. (SOR **B**) Beginning with basic education in sexual anatomy and physiology, women progress through the stages of tactile and visual self-exploration, manual stimulation to areas of pleasurable sensation, sexual fantasy and image development, sensate focus exercises alone and then with a partner, and finally sharing effective stimulation techniques with a partner.

2. The stop–start, or squeeze, technique

The stop–start technique of Semans and the squeeze technique modification of Masters and Johnson are used to treat **PE**. (SOR **B**) The technique begins as the couple embrace and caress one another until the man's penis is erect. He then lies on his back, his partner begins stimulating his penis, and he concentrates on his arousal sensations. Just before he reaches the point of imminent ejaculation, he tells his partner to stop stimulation. At this point, Masters and Johnson direct the woman to squeeze the penis firmly between her thumb and forefinger, under the corona of the glans. Most current therapists now suggest that the man apply the squeeze himself. When the woman applies the squeeze, it paradoxically suggests that control over erections is hers rather than the man's. With or without the squeeze, the couple wait for several minutes until arousal sensations dissipate. This process of stimulation and stopping repeats several times before the man ejaculates.

After four or five successful stimulation–stopping sessions, the couple tries the stop–start process with the penis in the vagina. The woman assumes the woman-superior position and the man glides her slowly up and down the shaft of his penis. As he again almost reaches the point of ejaculation, he ceases moving his partner until the need subsides. This process is also repeated several times before he ejaculates.

When the man can control ejaculation with this level of stimulation, his partner begins to stimulate his penis with vaginal thrusting until the man begins to feel the need to ejaculate. At this point, he tells her to stop stimulation until arousal wanes. This sequence is also repeated several times before he ejaculates.

The couple completes a start–stop sequence at least weekly until they learn to use it automatically during intercourse. Eventually, they use the method with other sexual positions. Most men, however, experience the greatest difficulty controlling ejaculation in the man-superior position. The couple-on-their-side often becomes the favored position for intercourse.

3. Systematic desensitization

Systematic desensitization treats both dyspareunia and vaginismus. (SOR **C**). The pelvic examination is the first step in the treatment process and must be conducted with care, reassurance, and proper education. The examination confirms the absence of pelvic disease, demonstrates that vaginal comfort is possible, confirms that vaginal events are under the woman's control, allows the woman to see the psychophysiologic components of the dysfunction (e.g., involuntary introital contractions can be seen with a mirror, allowing the woman to visualize the relationship between psychological conditioning and a physical event), and allows the physician to reassure the woman about her normality and to teach her specific techniques to help her overcome the disorder. During the examination, the physician also educates the partner in anatomy and psychosomatic physiology and ensures that he can observe the process of successful vaginal containment.

The first desensitization step after examination is to assure the woman that she is in complete control. When she says "Stop!," the examination stops. It may take several sessions to demonstrate painless vaginal insertion. The woman is given a handheld mirror to use throughout the examination so that the physician can teach vulvar and vaginal anatomy and so that she can visualize her own muscle contractions. She is taught to contract and relax her abdominal, medial thigh, and vaginal introital muscles sequentially. By identifying and contracting these muscles, she will have an easier time relaxing them.

The woman is then taught to "bear down and pull in" while contracting her introital muscles (Kegel exercises). When she can do this easily, the physician (with the patient's permission) places the tip of his or her index finger at the introitus and asks the woman to bear down and push the finger away. When this process is repeated several times, the fingertip will enter the vagina spontaneously. The woman often feels that instead of penetrating the vagina, the finger is "captured" by it. She learns that she can actively control what enters her vagina and that it can be painless.

When the woman comfortably contains the physician's fingertip, she repeats the same process first using her own fingertip and then her partner's. As she contracts and relaxes her vaginal muscles around a finger, she learns that she can control penetration and experience painless vaginal containment.

After the woman is comfortable with these exercises, she progresses through small steps to initiate intercourse. She inserts her partner's penis into her vagina after she is sufficiently aroused. Both partners must understand that the woman always controls the amount of contraction, relaxation, and penetration that occurs during intercourse and that she will not experience vaginal pain.

D. Hypoactive Sexual Desire Disorder

1. Testosterone

Testosterone does not benefit men with normal serum levels. In fact, it can compound the problem in men with **ED** who have normal levels by increasing sexual desire without concomitantly increasing arousal. (SOR **C**) In hypogonadal men with testosterone values <100 ng/dL, intramuscular testosterone enanthate or cipionate (100–200 mg every 2–4 weeks) is the standard treatment. (SOR **C**) Transdermal systems are also effective methods for replacing testosterone (Androderm, 2.5–7.5 mg/d, or Androgel, 50–100 mg/d). (SOR **A**) Oral agents are less effective and may cause hepatic disorders (e.g., cholestatic jaundice). (SOR **A**) Potential hazards of testosterone therapy include increased prostate-specific antigen levels and increased prostatic volume. These may increase the risk for prostatic cancer, and men should be screened for cancer at regular intervals.

Several well-designed studies demonstrate that transdermal testosterone in doses of 150 to 300 μg/d increased sexual desire and orgasm pleasure in postmenopausal and surgically menopausal women. (SOR **A**) A 2% testosterone vaginal cream along with sublingual and buccal preparations are now undergoing clinical trials. Androgens should only be prescribed with concurrent estrogen therapy. (SOR **B**)

2. Dopaminergic agent

Dopaminergic agents that have been associated with increased libido, include apomorphine (see Section III.F), bromocriptine, pergolide, levodopa, and cabergoline.

Bromocriptine mesylate (Parlodel) specifically treats hyperprolactinemia. Doses begin at 1.25 mg/d and increase by 1.25 mg every 3 to 7 days until the serum prolactin level is normal. (SOR **C**) The usual treatment dose is 2.5 mg twice daily.

3. **Antidepressants**

   Some studies indicate that antidepressants from several classes can increase libido. (SOR **B**) These agents include bupropion, nomifensine, trazodone, venlafaxine, and fenfluramine. See Chapter 92 on depression for dosing information.

E. **Sexual aversion**

   Psychosexual therapy that includes cognitive-behavioral techniques, desensitization, and resolving past abuses in combined individual and couples therapy is the most effective management strategy for sexual aversion. (SOR **C**)

F. **Erectile Disorder**

   1. **Systemic agents**

      a. **Testosterone** is used in hypogonadal men, as described for **HSDD.**

      b. **Sildenafil** is an orally active inhibitor of the type-V cyclic guanosine monophosphate-specific phosphodiesterase (PDE5), the predominant isoenzyme in the human corpus cavernosum. It increases levels of nitrous oxide, which relaxes the endothelial muscles, increasing blood flow into the corpora cavernosa. It effectively treats **ED** of organic, psychogenic, and mixed etiology. (SOR **A**) It enhances the erectile mechanism with sexual stimulation and does not work without stimulation. A man takes a single oral dose of 50 to 100 mg approximately an hour before intercourse. Sildenafil's activity begins in 30 minutes and lasts up to 4 hours. The most common adverse effects are headache (16%), flushing (10%), dyspepsia (7%), nasal congestion (4%), urinary tract infection (3%), visual effects (3%), and diarrhea (3%). Drug levels are increased by other drugs that are metabolized by or that inhibit the cytochrome P450 system. Sildenafil also potentiates the hypotensive effects of nitrates and is **absolutely contraindicated** in patients using organic nitrates in any form.

      Vardenafil and **tadalafil** are newer PDE5 inhibitors that are similar to sildenafil in pharmacologic action and effectiveness, but have some unique properties. Vardenafil has a high biochemical potency. It is well tolerated, with pharmacologic and adverse event profiles similar to sildenafil. A recent trial demonstrated that 60% of men who were nonresponders to sildenafil responded to vardenafil. (SOR **B**) It is administered in a dose of 10 to 20 mg taken 1 hour before intercourse.

      In comparison with the other PDE5 inhibitors, tadalafil has a slower onset of action, but its half-life is prolonged, resulting in a medication effect that lasts as long as 36 hours after administration. Its major unique adverse event is a 6% to 9% incidence of back pain that is usually mild and self-limited. Dosage is 10 to 20 mg 1 to 24 hours prior to intercourse.

      c. **Yohimbine** is an α-adrenoceptor antagonist that theoretically enhances penile erections by restricting penile venous outflow and by increasing libido through a central nervous system effect. The dosage is 6 mg orally three times daily. A recent systematic review of seven qualifying randomized controlled trials recommended it as an effective initial pharmacologic intervention. (SOR **A**) Some studies also indicated that it may be effective in treating selective serotonin reuptake inhibitor (SSRI)-induced sexual dysfunctions and that it may have a synergistic effect when administered with trazodone (100–200 mg at bedtime). (SOR **B**)

      d. **Phentolamine mesylate (Vasomax)** is an oral adrenergic receptor antagonist that causes erections by relaxing smooth muscle tissue and dilating arteries. It has been studied in men with minimal **ED** of broad-spectrum etiology. A man takes 20 to 80 mg approximately 15 minutes prior to intercourse. Side effects include headache, facial flushing, and nasal congestion. The drug appears safe and effective for treatment of mild **ED.** (SOR **B**)

      e. **Apomorphine** is believed to cause erections through its effect as a dopaminergic agonist that lowers the response threshold for erectile and ejaculatory reflexes. (SPR B) It has also been studied on men with minimal or insignificant organic disease. It is taken as a transbuccal tablet in dosage strengths of 2 mg, 4 mg, or 6 mg. The main adverse effect is nausea. Other observed adverse effects include persistent yawning, vomiting, and hypotension.

      f. **Naltrexone** is a long-acting opioid antagonist that reportedly promotes erectile function in doses of 25 to 50 mg/d. (SOR **C**) It may also act synergistically when combined with yohimbine.

2. Topical agents

   a. Nitroglycerine has a local effect on penile smooth muscle, causing relaxation and subsequent engorgement. (SOR **C**) Although controlled studies that support its effectiveness are sparse, men with mild vascular, neurologic, or mixed arousal dysfunction may benefit from a therapeutic trial with nitroglycerin before starting more invasive therapies. Men apply 0.5 to 1 inch of 2% ointment to the penile shaft just prior to intercourse, using a condom during intercourse to avoid mucosal absorption of the nitroglycerin and adverse systemic effects in their partners. A transdermal nitroglycerin patch applied 1 to 2 hours prior to intercourse also reportedly improves erections.

   b. Topical 2% Minoxidil solution applied to the glans has been demonstrated to produce erections in several studies. It may be even more effective than nitroglycerin. (SOR **C**)

   c. Topical Alprostadil combined with an absorption enhancer is now being studied in several clinical trials.

3. Intracavernosal injections

   Patients may inject **papaverine, PGE$_1$,** or various mixtures, into a corpus cavernosum with a 27-gauge needle to induce an erection. This technique is quite successful in men with neurogenic disorders, mild vascular problems, or combined neurogenic and vascular disorders, and in selected men with psychogenic causes for whom psychosexual treatment has failed. (SOR **A**) Therapy begins with a low dose of either papaverine or PGE$_1$, gradually titrating the dose to provide an adequate erection that lasts 1 to 2 hours. This usually requires 10 to 80 mg of papaverine or 10 to 40 μg of PGE$_1$.

   Bimix is a combination of papaverine 25 mg and phentolamine 0.8 mg/mL. Injections range from 1.0 to 1.5 mL. **Trimix** combines papaverine, PGE$_1$, and phentolamine.

   Injections are limited to three times per week and 10 times per month. Complications include priapism (0.33%), cavernous tissue fibrosis (2.8%), hematoma, cavernositis, pain, and changes in blood pressure (usually orthostatic hypotension). Erections that last more than 4 hours should be reversed by irrigating the corpora cavernosum with diluted phenylephrine.

   VIP 0.025 mg mixed with phentolamine 2.0 mg is an investigational agent that comes as a prefilled, ready-to-use autoinjector and demonstrates a reported overall efficacy of 80% and a 70% efficacy in men who failed other intracavernosal therapy. (SOR **B**) The most common adverse reaction is transient facial flushing (53%). The incidence of priapism, fibrosis, and pain occurs less frequently than with other injection therapies.

   Intracavernosal injections may be used to treat **PE** as well as **ED**. In the case of PE, they may allow sexual activity to continue despite the man's premature climax.

4. Intraurethral PGE$_1$

   Intraurethral therapy requires a man to insert a PGE$_1$ medicated pellet into his urethra with an applicator following urination. When absorbed through the mucosa, the PGE$_1$ relaxes smooth muscles and dilates arteries. Following insertion, the man must manually stimulate the penis for 10 seconds and then walk around for another 10 minutes to promote erection. The maximal response occurs in 20 to 25 minutes. Pellets are available in 125-, 250-, 500-, and 1000-μg dosage strengths. Adverse effects include penile pain (32%), urethral burning (12%), minor urethral bleeding (5%), testicular pain (5%), hypotension (3%), and dizziness (2%). (SOR **A**)

5. Combination therapy

   When monotherapy fails a trial of combined therapy may be successful. (SOR **B**) One study added sildenafil to intraurethral or intracavernosal alprostadil and reported a 47% to 100% success rate after monotherapy failure. Controlled trials are now investigating other combinations with sildenafil, including alprostadil, doxazosin, and apomorphine. Other combinations (e.g., mechanical pump with PDE5 inhibitor or intracavernosal or intraurethral alprostadil, PDE5 inhibitor with a topical agent) may also be successful, although these combinations have not yet been studied.

6. Penile prosthesis

   The penile prosthesis is the most reliable surgical option in the United States, with the inflatable prosthesis implanted most frequently. (SOR **A**) Manufacturers now provide reliable protheses consisting of cylinders that expand in both girth and length, a single scrotal pump, and an abdominal reservoir. To decrease the chance of mechanical failure in multicomponent devices and to mimic natural erection, self-contained inflatable devices have also been designed that include an inflation chamber, reservoir, and pump mechanism in a self-contained cylinder. Prosthesis implantation is relatively uncomplicated, but most devices require replacement after 48 to 60 months. Potential complications include mechanical failure (0%–3.2%), infection (1.9%–8.3%), erosion, penile gangrene, improper sizing, and silicone shedding.

7. **Mechanical agents**
   a. **Vacuum pump:** Penile vacuum pumps can also aid erections. (SOR **A**) The man places a lubricated cylinder over his penis, and using an attached handheld pump to withdraw air, he creates a vacuum that draws blood into the corpora cavernosum. When his penis is erect, he maintains engorgement by applying an elastic band around the penile base and removes the cylinder. Potential complications include penile edema, decreased penile sensation, impaired ejaculation, subcutaneous bleeding, and penile necrosis. These devices no longer require a physician's prescription.
   b. **Constriction rings** are usually packaged with the vacuum pump, but may be the only devices needed to manage erectile dysfunction in men with mild-to-moderate venous leakage and no arterial insufficiency. (SOR **C**) The **Soft Touch** ring (Mission Pharmacal Co., San Antonio, TX, USA) has the advantage of easy removal without entangling pubic hair, and the **Pressure Point** ring (Osbon, Augusta, GA, USA) includes a V-shaped ventral section to reduce urethral obstruction, thereby enhancing seminal flow.

G. **Female Sexual Arousal Disorder**
   1. **Comorbid conditions and underlying disease**.
      Treating comorbid conditions and underlying disease is the first step for managing **FSAD**. It rarely occurs as an isolated disorder, but frequently accompanies a concurrent condition that preceded the arousal problem. If genital pain, anorgasmia, or a chronic organic illness exist, those problems should be addressed and treated before attending specifically to arousal as a separate entity.
   2. **Systemic agents.**
      a. **Sildenafil** (50–100 mg) can increase blood flow to the clitoral corpus cavernosum. Clinical studies evaluating its effectiveness in treating **FSAD** ended in 2004, however, because evidence supporting it use was inconclusive.
      b. **Phentolamine Mesylate** as a 40 mg oral or vaginal solution enhanced vaginal blood flow and improved subjective arousal in one study. (SOR **B**)
      c. **Apomorphine** studies are ongoing in Europe.
   3. **Topical agents**
      Topical Alprostadil is currently being studied in clinical trials.
   4. **Mechanical agents**
      Eros Therapy (UroMetrics) is a small, handheld device composed of a soft plastic cup that is connected to a small vacuum pump. The woman places the cup over her clitoris and the pump creates a gentle vacuum that increases genital blood flow and subsequent clitoral engorgement. Increasing blood flow into the clitoris reportedly also increases vaginal lubrication and enhances the woman's ability to achieve orgasm. (SOR **B**)

H. **Female Orgasmic Disorder**
   1. **Psychosexual therapy**
      Sensate focus, systematic desensitization, and directed self-stimulation consistently show the highest rates of improvement for orgasmic dysfunction in many controlled treatment outcome studies. (SOR **B**)
   2. **Systemic agents**
      Bupropion in doses of 150 to 300 mg/d demonstrated significant improvement in orgasmic ability in one sample of nondepressed women. (SOR **B**)
   3. **Mechanical agents**
      Eros Therapy (discussed under Section III.G.3, treatment for **FSAD**) reportedly increases a woman's orgasmic capacity when used regularly (three or four times per week). (SOR **B**)

I. **Male Orgasmic Disorder**
   The most common cause for anorgasmia in men is using drugs that interfere with orgasm, especially antidepressants. Strategies for managing antidepressant-related sexual disorders (SDs) are discussed below in Section III.L, antidepressant-associated SDs. Psychosexual therapies, including self-stimulation exercises, can benefit some men. (SOR **C**)

J. Premature Ejaculation

1. Psychosexual therapy

The **start–stop–squeeze technique** (see Section III.C, specific sexual therapy techniques) was the standard therapy for **PE** before pharmacologic agents became available. It is now used most frequently in combination with pharmacologic agents (see the next section) for men who do not respond optimally to the drugs alone.

2. Systemic agents

a. **Clomipramine** at doses of 25 to 50 mg, taken 12 to 24 hours prior to intercourse, effectively prolonged intravaginal intercourse to at least 2 minutes in 70% of men with **PE** in one study. In another study, it prolonged ejaculatory latency from 2 to 8 minutes. The minimum time between drug ingestion and the maximum ejaculatory control is not yet known. The shortest studied interval was 4 to 6 hours (SOR **B**).

b. **Paroxetine** demonstrates increased ejaculatory latency when administered following several different protocols: as 20 mg 3 to 4 hours prior to intercourse as needed; as 10 mg once-daily chronic administration; and as 10 mg once daily with an additional 20 mg taken as needed 3 to 4 hours prior to intercourse. All methods increased ejaculatory latency, with the 10 mg/d plus 20 mg as needed protocol showing the greatest improvement. (SOR **B**) Another study demonstrated that one could achieve further benefit by adding 50 mg of sildenafil 1 h prior to intercourse to this last protocol. (SOR **B**)

c. **Sertraline** also delays ejaculation through its serotonergic effects. The usual dose is 50 to 100 mg taken 3 to 5 hours prior to sexual activity. The most common side effect is drowsiness.

d. **Fluoxetine** is also used to treat **PE** at doses of 20 to 60 mg.

e. **Dapoxetine** was heralded in clinical trials as the first drug to be FDA approved for PE. In published trials, 30 to 60 mg was taken 1 to 3 hours prior to intercourse and men reported a three- to fourfold increase in ejaculatory latency time. Although the initial application was not approved by the FDA, the manufacturer intends to continue to working toward approval.

f. **Tricyclic antidepressants** may help treat **PE** because they inhibit the cholinergic component of ejaculation. Men take a low initial dose (e.g., 25 mg of amitriptyline) 3 to 5 hours prior to sexual activity, increasing subsequent doses until they experience ejaculatory control, have side effects, or reach the maximal recommended dose. (SOR **B**)

g. **Thioridazine**, at standard antidepressant doses, may also benefit men with **PE**. (SOR **C**) It is the most potent anticholinergic and α-adrenergic blocking agent in its class and presumably delays ejaculation through these effects.

h. **Phenoxybenzamine** is an α-adrenergic blocker indicated for treating hypertension. Used by men with **PE** in daily doses of 20 to 30 mg, Phenoxybenzamine benefits ejaculation and erection with minimal side effects (SOR **C**). It is best used by men who do not wish to procreate, since Phenoxybenzamine inhibits seminal emission.

3. Topical agents

A **lidocaine–prilocaine cream (EMLA®)** can help to prevent **PE**. (SOR **B**) In clinical studies men applied 2.5 g to the glans and penile shaft 15 to 30 minutes before sexual contact, and then either covered the penis with a condom or wiped the cream off prior to intercourse. Analgesia reaches its maximum at 2 to 3 hours.

K. Dyspareunia and vaginismus

All physical causes should be treated in women who experience pain with intercourse. For persistent dyspareunia, and for vaginismus, programs of **systematic desensitization** (see Section III.C, specific sexual therapy techniques) are the most effective management. (SOR **C**)

L. Antidepressant-associated SD

Antidepressants commonly cause sexual dysfunction, with 40% to 70% of patients taking SSRIs reporting problems with sexual functioning. One must effectively manage these treatment-emergent dysfunctions so that patients will maintain therapeutic antidepressant treatment and thereby prevent relapse and recurrence of serious depression. Five treatment options are available to manage these troublesome side effects.

1. Prescribe drugs that counter the side effects

Various receptor agonists, partial agonists, or antagonist agents have been tried, but they lack well-designed placebo-controlled, double-blind studies to support their effectiveness. Limited studies with cyproheptadine, buspirone, amantadine, and granisetron do not demonstrate a response rate that significantly exceeds placebo.

2. **Select an antidepressant less likely to cause SD**

   When initiating antidepressant treatment, choose an agent such as nefazodone, mirtazapine, or bupropion that produces sexual dysfunction less frequently.

3. **Augment or substitute with another antidepressant**

   Bupropion is used most in this context, and prescribed in one of three ways: 75 to 150 mg as needed 1 to 2 hours prior to sexual activity, as daily add-on therapy in conjunction with an SSRI, or as an initial daily full dose add-on to relieve the SD, followed by a taper and discontinuation of the initial SSRI. (SOR **B**)

4. **Adaptation**

   Some patients develop spontaneous remission, or tolerance to treatment-emergent SD side effects. Controversy exists, however, about whether this occurs at a clinically significant rate. Since better management options exist, this wait-and-see approach has less support.

5. **Sildenafil**

   Evidence shows that sildenafil significantly improves ejaculation and orgasm in men with **ED** who are also taking SSRIs. (SOR **A**) Furthermore, depressed men with ED respond to sildenafil as well as any other subgroup of men. (SOR **A**) Study doses ranged from 25 to 200 mg taken 1 hour prior to anticipated sexual activity. Using sildenafil allows men to continue therapeutic doses of an effective antidepressant.

   In both open-label and double-blind, placebo-controlled studies, sildenafil, dosed at 50 to 100 mg prior to intercourse, also reversed treatment-emergent SD in women with an efficacy that compared to its use in men. (SOR **A**)

IV. Prognosis

A. Sexual desire disorders

The few published studies indicate that **SDDs** for both men and women resist sustained behavioral change. (SOR **B**) Following therapy, one study noted initial improvement that was sustained at 3 months but that had regressed to below pretherapy levels by 3 years. Prognosis is better if the problem is secondary, the partners are younger, the symptoms are present <1 year, the marital relationship is stable, the partners are emotionally calm and motivated toward intervention, both partners view each other as loving and attractive, both partners find pleasure in sexual behavior, neither partner has a conflict regarding sexual orientation or major psychopathology, and the couple complies with homework assignments during therapy.

B. Erectile Disorder

The natural history and prognosis of ED depend on many variables, most particularly the underlying problem. Most data on **psychosexual treatment** success were obtained before recent diagnostic advances permitted better differentiation between organic and psychogenic causes. Reported success rates range from 50% to 90%. (SOR **C**) Treatment success for **surgical implants** is 85% to 95% in achieving effective erections, with long-term patient satisfaction rates approaching 80% and partner satisfaction rates between 60% and 80%. (SOR **A**) Success with **intracavernosal injections** varies from 60% to 92%, but only 50% to 80% of men who start on self-injections continue to use them long term. (SOR **A**) Satisfaction with the **vacuum-constriction** device is 68% to 92%, with 60% of men who are able to apply it successfully continuing to use it long term (SOR **A**). Reported success rates with **intraurethral PGE$_1$** are approximately 40% (SOR **A**). Oral agents also vary in success. In a systematic review of randomized controlled studies, the pooled odds-ratio for treatment with yohimbine was 3.85, favoring treatment. (SOR **A**) From 70% to 85% of men using **sildenafil** and the other PDE5 inhibitors achieve erections firm enough for intercourse. (SOR **A**) Men with diabetes, and some of those with neurologic dysfunction, spinal cord injuries, prostatic surgery, and pelvic irradiation, report lower response rates, between 35% and 67%. (SOR **A**) In men with mild ED, **phentolamine** has a response rate of 37% at the 40-mg dose and 45% at the 80-mg level. (SOR **B**) Reported success with **apomorphine** in mild ED is 46% with 2 mg, 52% with 4 mg, and 60% with 6 mg. (SOR **B**)

C. Female Orgasmic Disorder

The natural history of untreated **FOD** is unknown. Women whose orgasmic disorder is primary respond rapidly to treatment with a high success rate when therapy focuses specifically on sexual matters. Women with secondary orgasmic disorders do better when traditional couples therapy is combined with sexual therapy. Masters and Johnson report success rates of 83% for primary disorders and 77% for secondary disorders using

dual-gender therapy. (^{SOR} **C**) **Directed self-stimulation** training to treat primary disorders is successful in helping women reach orgasm 90% of the time during self-stimulation and 75% of the time with a partner. (^{SOR} **C**) As new pharmacologic agents and Eros Therapy become integrated into treatment, these outcome figures may improve even more.

D. Male Orgasmic Disorder

Outcome studies on treatment for MOD are limited by its relative rarity. Reported success rates range from 46% to 82%. (^{SOR} **C**)

E. Premature Ejaculation

Masters and Johnson report 95% success rates with the **start–stop–squeeze technique.** (^{SOR} **C**) Others report rates around 60% (^{SOR} **C**). Long-term successes, however, are disappointing. In one study, men treated for PE showed immediate posttreatment gains in foreplay length, sexual relationship satisfaction, male acceptance, and intercourse duration. By 3 years posttreatment, however, frequency and desire for sexual contact, intercourse duration, and marital satisfaction all regressed, with marital satisfaction and intercourse duration dropping to pretreatment levels.

The best data on **pharmacologic management** are available for clomipramine, sertraline, fluoxetine, and paroxetine. Sexual satisfaction rates are reported at 53% for **clomipramine** along with a statistically significant increase in ejaculation latency time. (^{SOR} **B**) For **sertraline**, sexual satisfaction rates range from 42% to 87%, with significantly increased ejaculation latency. (^{SOR} **B**) The data on **fluoxetine's** success are variable. Some studies indicate a significant increase in ejaculation latency, but others suggest that it is no better than placebo. (^{SOR} **B**) When men use **paroxetine,** they report as much as a 75% improvement in the quality of their sexual activity. (^{SOR} **B**) When they **add sildenafil to paroxetine**, they can further prolong ejaculatory latency and the quality of overall sexual activity increases to 87.5%. (^{SOR} **B**) In the pilot sample used to study **topical lidocaine–prilocaine**, 80% graded the result as "excellent" or "better." (^{SOR} **B**)

F. Dyspareunia

Prognosis depends on the nature of any associated organic problems and the success with which they are treated. Women with a pure psychogenic basis for their problem report treatment success rates of around 95%. (^{SOR} **C**)

G. Vaginismus

Vaginismus is very amenable to treatment. In one group of women who were followed up for 4 years, 95% achieved and maintained sexual functioning. (^{SOR} **C**) A desire for childbearing, a husband-initiated consultation, and a couple's perception that the problem was psychogenic predicted successful outcomes. Unsuccessful outcomes were associated with a firm belief that the problem was organic, experience with a previous anatomic problem, abundant sexual misinformation, a negative attitude toward genitalia, fear of sexually transmitted disease, and negative parental attitudes toward sex.

GENERAL REFERENCES

Bachmann GA, Avci D. Evaluation and management of female sexual dysfunction. *The Endocrinologist.* 2004;14(6):337-345.

Basson R. Recent advances in women's sexual function and dysfunction. *Menopause.* 2004;11(6): 714-725.

Halvorsen JG: The clinical evaluation of common sexual concerns. *CNS Spectrums.* 2003;8(3): 217-224.

Lewis JH, Rosen R, Goldstein I. Erectile dysfunction: A panel's recommendations for management. *AJN.* 2003:103(10):48-57.

Meston CM, Frohlich PF. The neurobiology of sexual function. *Arch Gen Psychiatry.* 2000;57(11):1012-1030.

REFERENCES FOR QUESTIONNAIRES

Rosen RC, Riley A, Wagner G, et al. The International Index of Erectile Function (IIEF): A multidimensional scale for assessment of erectile dysfunction. *Urology.* 1997;49:822-830.

Rosen RC, Cappeleri JC, Smith MD, et al. Development and evaluation of an abridged, 5-item version of the International Index of Erectile Function (IIEF-5) as a diagnostic tool for erectile dysfunction. *Int J Impotence Res.* 1999; 11(6):319-326.

Rosen R, Brown C, Heiman J, et al. The female sexual function index (FSFI): A multidimensional self-report instrument for the assessment of female sexual function. *J Sex Marital Therapy.* 2000;26: 191-208.

SECTION V. Preventive Medicine & Health Promotion

100 Counseling for Behavioral Change

David Pole, MPH, Ryan M. Niemiec, PsyD, & Laura Frankenstein, MD

KEY POINTS

- To share advice successfully, providers must understand (1) what the patient's goals are, (2) what has worked and what hasn't worked for the patient in the past, and (3) what challenges the patient faces.
- Providers can develop skills to successfully share information in a way that helps patients understand how to incorporate medical management recommendations, successfully practice self-management, and incorporate prevention behaviors.
- Creating "Action Plans" with patients and cultivating their self-management skills enhances self-efficacy and positive outcomes.
- Providers need to use different approaches and communication based upon the patient's readiness for change.

I. **Introduction.** Providers should identify specific goals that enable patients to fully participate in preventing and treating their illness and/or maintaining wellness in their lives. Accomplishing improved health outcomes is dependent upon the interaction between a skilled and informed provider and an informed and activated patient. Patients do not always show up informed, activated, and with a high self-efficacy for engaging in health behaviors. The following techniques and guidelines are intended to provide a "tool kit" that enhances your ability to successfully counsel your patients on a variety of health behaviors.

II. **Components of an Effective Brief Intervention about Lifestyle Change (SOR Ⓐ)**
   A. Patient-focused: Whenever possible, frame the intervention to the patient's needs and interests.
   B. Health-connected: Review the rationale and projected impact of the intervention upon the patient's physical and/or mental health.
   C. Behavior-oriented: Focus on what the patient can "do" differently. Framing the intervention in terms of creating an "action plan" is helpful.
   D. Realistic: Consider what is within the patient's current capabilities of achieving. Make your interventions "bite-sized" and focus on "being successful at small steps."
   E. Controllable: Frame the intervention in terms of what the patient can readily control (e.g., walking 1 mile per day rather than losing 2 lbs/wk).
   F. Measurable: Track the progress the patient makes with the intervention, encourage patient self-monitoring.
   G. Practical: Apply the intervention to the patient's daily life and encourage them to begin to make changes immediately.

III. **The Mindset of the Practitioner**
   A. Consider the lifespan and context: This person has a life that has affected them to this point and there are numerous factors that can affect their present experience—culture, environment, emotions, beliefs, genetics, biology, spirituality, level of health literacy, etc.
   B. Stay in the present moment: Let go of personal concerns, your previous patient, or concerns about your next patient, and focus on the patient with whom you are meeting.
   C. Judge the behaviors and choices, not the person. It is not the patient who is flawed or "wrong," rather it is the choices and behaviors patients engage in that are flawed or problematic. Keep this adage on the forefront of your mind.
   D. Remember the positive: Despite their suffering and challenges at managing their condition, it is likely that there is more going right with each patient than wrong.
   E. Consider strengths: Each patient has strengths that can be tapped into to help them (e.g., creativity, hopefulness, teamwork, compassion, gratitude).

IV. **Stages of Change.** The Stages of Change model can be applied to virtually any change in lifestyle or behavior (e.g., smoking cessation, weight loss, healthy eating). Table 100–1

TABLE 100–1. THE STAGES OF CHANGE

Stage of Change	Description of Patient Intent	Provider Task
Precontemplation	No intention to change, may be unaware of the problem	Education about the health area
Contemplation	Aware of problem, but unwilling to make a change, may feel stuck or says will do in future	Cost–benefit analysis; Develop discrepancy between patient goals and behavior
Preparation	Planning to make change, usually within 1 mo	Brainstorm options; Assist in developing concrete action plan
Action	Involved in implementing/making a change	Encourage tracking/monitoring actions; Validate/provide feedback; Discuss/elicit social support
Maintenance	Has sustained change for a while, usually approximately 6 mo	Check progress; Trouble shoot slips/concerns of patient; Reinforce successes/build patient confidence
Addressing Relapse or Relapse Prevention	Patient behavior starts to slip, falls back to old behaviors	Judge choices, not the patient; Focus on past success, progress not perfection; Identify new skills or supports that reinforce health behavior

outlines the stage of change, what it represents for the patient, and the provider's tasks. (SOR **Ⓐ**)

A. **Determining stage or readiness for change.** Assess the patient's perceived importance of the issue and their confidence to engage in healthy/different behavior. The patient's rating of importance and confidence allows you to determine the level of intrinsic motivation and readiness for change. Ask the patient the following questions about a specific behavior:
   1. On a scale of 0 to 10, how important is it for you to ____ (quit smoking, exercise, disease management, etc.), in which 0 is not at all important and 10 is extremely important?
   2. On a scale of 0 to 10, how confident are you that if you decided to ____ (i.e., lose weight), that you could do it? 0 means you are not at all confident and 10 means you are extremely confident.
   3. Why did you rate it a ____ (i.e., 5)?
   4. What would it take to get your motivation or confidence to a 9 or 10?
   5. Utilize the patient answers to guide you in determining appropriate intervention, Table 100–1.

B. **Addressing precontemplation stage**
   1. Educate the patient about their condition and potential negative health outcomes.
   2. Educate the patient about the connection between their behaviors and the management of their condition/prevention of complications.
   3. Provide literacy level appropriate education materials regarding the health condition (see **Bibliotherapy and Handouts** section).
   4. Continue to ask about the behavior at each subsequent visit with the patient.

C. **Moving from contemplation to action**
   1. Use a Decisional Balance Sheet/Cost–Benefit of Change to help identify and highlight any conflict or ambivalence that the patient may be having about the change, for an example, see Table 100–2.
   2. Review patient statements and highlight conflict (e.g., I hear that quitting smoking feels like losing a friend, but that you are also very worried about your health).
   3. Acknowledge "cost" of change and determine patient's motivation/confidence to move toward "benefits" of change.

D. **Creating an action plan.** Encourage the patient to identify the following:
   1. Target behavior (exercise, medications, quit smoking, change diet, etc.).
   2. Specific goal within that behavior (I will begin walking for exercise).
   3. Quantity and frequency of the behavior (walk for 20 minutes, 3 days per week on Mondays, Wednesdays, and Fridays).
   4. Time of day the behavior will occur? (I will walk in the morning before work).
   5. Confidence in their action plan on a scale of 1 to 10.

TABLE 100–2. **EXAMPLE OF A DECISIONAL BALANCE FOR SMOKING CESSATION**

Continue to Smoke		Quit Smoking	
Cost	Benefits	Cost	Benefit
Worry about health	Helps with stress	More stress	Less hacking and cough in
Tired of smell	Been a "best friend"	Weight gain	the morning
Can't smoke	Enjoy smoking with	Lose my only pleasure	More energy
anywhere	friends	Withdrawal symptoms	Have more money
Social stigma			Better role model to kids
Get winded, cannot do			Get people off my back
some activities			

6. For additional information and suggestions on creating an Action Plan, go to www.improvingchroniccare.org (select Clinical Practice Change; select Steps for Improvement; select Self-Management Support).

E. Maintenance and relapse prevention

1. Ask about patient Action Plan and progress, review any tracking tools or log the patient has been keeping.
2. Make positive comments about any/all improvements in behavior.
3. Acknowledge and help patient see any links between behavior changes and health outcomes or clinical measures.
4. Slips and relapses occur naturally as part of behavior change. Judge the choices, not the individual, discuss and identify triggers for going off-track and also supports and barriers for maintaining the desired behavior
5. Ask questions to get patient reflecting upon choices and problem solving, avoid problem solving for the patient (suggestions and guided questions are OK). Identify resources and reinforce the positive steps the patient has taken in the past. Encourage tracking and monitoring progress to stay on track. Sample questions that help to get additional information from the patient:
   a. What happened?
   b. What's missing?
   c. What's next?

V. Understanding and addressing low health literacy (SOR **C**)

A. Definition: The capacities of individuals to obtain, process, understand, and apply health-related information to make informed health decisions. As of the 2003 National Assessment of Adult Literacy survey, more than one-third of your patients may have difficulty understanding and acting on the health information you provide—regardless of "grade level" they completed.

B. Chunk and Check (only give 2–3 points at a time, confirm level of understanding).

C. Use Teach-Back Techniques (have patient explain back key points to you).

D. Use plain language (living room discussion language or use terms the patient uses to describe their condition).

E. Speak more slowly (not louder).

F. Use pictures, diagrams, etc.

VI. Health Behavior-Specific Recommendations

A. **Tobacco use:** The effectiveness of clinician counseling in the prevention and cessation of tobacco use is well documented. (SOR **A**) Continue to ask the patient if they have considered quitting at each visit and provide information/education on smoking as it relates to their specific health condition. When the patient is ready to make a change, use the following strategies and encourage the patient to:

1. Set a specific "Quit Date."
2. Eliminate all smoking-related paraphernalia in the house and car.
3. Set up "No Smoking" signs in areas where they previously smoked.
4. Tell others they have quit and ask for specific support.
5. Make a list of the costs and impact of continued smoking and post it where it can be seen daily.
6. Make a list of the health and personal benefits of stopping smoking and keep it posted.
7. Practice a daily stress management activity (e.g., relaxation, self-hypnosis, or mindfulness meditation).

    8. Start or increase their level of daily exercise.

    9. Consider nicotine replacement therapy (e.g., gum, inhaler).

   10. Consider medication (e.g., Chantix, Zyban, etc.).

   11. For patients that are **ready to quit or initiate some behavior change** around tobacco use, there are self-help websites that can be recommended:

      a. American Academy of Family Practice—www.familydoc.org; then search the site for "stop smoking."

      b. American Lung Association—www.lungusa.org; scroll down to *Freedom From Smoking* program.

B. Nutrition: Nutrition and dietary patterns affect many chronic conditions as well as obesity. Take a complete dietary history; this may include interviewing the patient and requesting a food diary. The *My Pyramid* website has assessment tools and guidelines to access with dietary recommendations/eating plans www.mypyramid.gov. This site is excellent for diet/food assessments and for finding individualized recommendations.

    1. Adolescents and adult females need additional calcium.

    2. Pregnant women, infants and young children have unique dietary requirements.

C. Weight loss general recommendations:

    1. Involve registered dietitians and other trained staff (e.g., Diabetic Educator) when available.

    2. Recommend a balanced diet consisting of the *Food Guide Pyramid*'s five major food groups, which together meet nutritional requirements: (1) grains; (2) fruits; (3) vegetables; (4) dairy; and (5) meats and beans. (SOR **C**)

    3. Increase physical activity level and regular exercise beyond normal daily activity (goal is to increase up to an additional 1000 calories per week or 10,000 total steps per day). (SOR **A**)

    4. Identify easy ways to reduce fat calorie intake, trans-fats and saturated fats (CVD Risk; SOR **A**)

    5. Eat smaller meals more frequently that include fruits and vegetables. (SOR **B**)

    6. Practice a daily stress management activity (e.g. relaxation, self-hypnosis, focused breathing). (SOR **C**)

    7. Set a behavior-specific Action Plan and track their efforts. (SOR **A**)

D. Exercise: Advise all patients on the benefits of regular moderate aerobic exercise. Groups requiring additional attention due to age/gender/population specific risk include women, ethnic minorities, adults with lower educational attainment, and older adults. Recommendations for regular physical activity should be tailored to the health status and lifestyle of each patient (SOR **C**)

    1. Adults should accumulate 30 minutes or more of moderate-intensity physical activity over the course of most days of the week (including walking, gardening, dancing, etc.).

    2. Provide instructions on the safe performance of exercise. Those at increased risk of injury or medical complications should be advised about appropriate physical activity. Refer to disease-specific exercise guidelines and/or refer the patient to an accredited exercise specialist.

    3. Discuss the three components of F.I.T.—Frequency, Intensity, and Time.

    4. Standard cardiovascular warm-up and cool-down periods of 5 minutes each. Patients with heart disease or hypertension may require minimum of 7 to 10 minutes warm up/cool down.

    5. Recommend daily strengthening activities; stretching should be recommended following aerobic activity to prevent injuries.

    6. For older adults—Prescription Guidelines from AAFP. www.aafp.org/afp/20060801/437.html.

    7. For Diabetic Patients—See *Position Statement: Physical Activity/Exercise and Diabetes.* Diabetes Care. Vol. 27 Supplement 1, January 2004, S58-64.

E. Intentional injuries

    1. Suicide (SOR **C**)

      a. Be alert to suicidal ideation among patients at high risk as a result of recent divorce, separation, unemployment, depression, alcohol and other drug abuse, major medical illnesses, living alone, and recent bereavement. Adolescents are at particular risk for suicide; risk factors include declines in school performance or attendance, isolation or changes in peer relations, and excessive anger or fighting behavior. Older adults are also at excess suicide risk.

   b. Patients with suicidal ideations should be questioned about the extent of their plans (e.g., distribution of possessions, obtaining a weapon, and writing a suicide note). If suicidal intent is serious, clinicians should make immediate referrals to mental health professionals and consider possible hospitalization. Persons with suicidal thoughts should also be alerted to community resources such as local mental health agencies and crisis intervention centers.

  2. Violence (SOR Ⓒ)

    a. Both the history (discussion of previous violent experiences and current risk factors, such as weapons in the home and discord in the peer group and community) and the physical examination (detection of burns, bruises, and other traumatic injuries) can be used to identify victims of abuse or neglect. Clinicians who suspect violence among patients should refer both the victims and the perpetrators to mental health professionals and other community resources to prevent future episodes.

    b. Certain physical, behavioral, and medical signs indicate child neglect and abuse (see Chapter 91). Physicians must report probable cases of such abuse to local child protective service agencies. In addition, clinicians should be alert to risk signs for adolescent violence such as fighting, bullying, chronic victimization, weapon-carrying, history of domestic violence, and changes in peer relations.

F. Unintentional injuries

  1. Motor vehicle-related injuries. (SOR Ⓒ) Urge all patients to use federally approved occupant restraints (e.g., safety belts and child safety seats), to wear safety helmets when riding motorcycles and bicycles, roller skates, and ice skates (high risk of head injury with falls).

  2. Avoid driving or riding with a driver under the influence of alcohol or other psychoactive drugs.

  3. Counsel individuals at increased risk of motor vehicle injury, such as adolescents and young adults, alcohol and other drug users, and patients with any medical conditions that affect safe driving. These individuals should be encouraged to find transportation alternatives for social activities.

  4. Car seats for infants (SOR Ⓑ) (for full guidelines check American Academy of pediatrics at www.aap.org/family/carseatguide.htm)

    a. Always ask if the patient is using a car seat for their child.

    b. Never use a rear-facing car seat in the front seat of a vehicle with an air bag.

    c. All children younger than 13 are safer in the back seat.

    d. All infants should be in a rear-facing seat until they have reached 1 year old AND weigh at least 20 pounds, then can move to a front-facing car seat.

    e. Front-facing car seat or booster should be used until the child reaches 4'9" in height AND is between 8 and 12 years old

G. Environmental and household injuries. (SOR Ⓒ) Although passive interventions (e.g., child-resistant containers to prevent poisoning) are the most effective measures to control injuries, clinician counseling may help patients reduce their risks of household and environmental injuries (e.g., falls, drowning, fire, poisoning, suffocation, and firearm mishaps).

  1. Install smoke detectors and check monthly, change batteries annually.

  2. Lower temperature setting on hot-water heaters at 48.4°C (120°F).

  3. Encourage patients with **children in the home** to store all medications, toxic substances, matches, and firearms out of the reach of children and display emergency numbers prominently near telephones (e.g., the police department, the fire department, 911, the local Poison Control Center, etc.).

  4. Patients with pools should install four-sided fencing with self-latching and self-closing gates around swimming pools and spas.

  5. Recommend the installation of window guards on all windows not designated as emergency fire exits.

  6. Bicyclists and parents of children who ride bicycles/scooters should be made aware of the importance of wearing safety helmets and protective gear.

  7. To prevent falls among **older patients**, suggest modifications to their home environments, for example, tacking down carpets and arranging furniture so that pathways are not cluttered; lowering kitchen items to prevent over-reaching; testing their visual acuity periodically; and closely monitoring their use of drugs that can increase the risk of falls. Older patients should receive instructions on appropriate physical exercises to maintain and improve strength, flexibility, and mobility. Patients with medical conditions affecting mobility should receive special counseling on measures to prevent falls.

H. Sexual behavior
1. **Sexually transmitted infections (STIs)**
   a. Take a complete sexual and drug use history of all adolescent, adult, and older adult patients and offer STD screening according to recommended guidelines (see Chapter 102). Clinicians should discuss sexual behavior with respect, compassion, and confidentiality. Remember that seniors are also at high risk of infection and may not be aware of protective measures for safe sex.
   b. Sexually active patients should be counseled that the most effective strategy to prevent infection with human immunodeficiency virus (HIV) or other STIs is to abstain from sex or maintain a mutually monogamous sexual relationship with a partner known to be uninfected and use contraception. Patients should be counseled to engage in routine screening since many STIs are asymptomatic. Encourage patients to decrease the number of sexual partners and counsel on how to discuss infection status with their partners. Counsel women of childbearing age on the dangers of HIV and STD infection during pregnancy. (SOR **C**)
   c. Patients should be alerted that a nonreactive HIV test does not rule out infection if the sexual partner has engaged in sexual intercourse during the 6 months prior to testing. Safe (or "safer") sexual practices (e.g., massage, hugging, or dry kissing) should be encouraged.
   d. Counsel patients on the consistent and proper use of condoms (see Chapter 95).
   e. Intravenous drug users should be urged to participate in drug treatment programs, counsel against sharing and using un-sterilized drug paraphernalia, and direct them to community programs that make uncontaminated equipment available.
2. **Unintended pregnancy.** Discuss the efficacy, limitations, and proper use of available contraceptive techniques (see Chapter 95).

I. Dental disease
1. Counsel patients to visit a dentist regularly, to brush their teeth daily with fluoride-containing toothpaste, and to use dental floss daily to clean between teeth.
2. Young children should have their first dental visit by age 2. Children, particularly those younger than 6 years, should be taught to spit out rather than swallow toothpaste containing fluoride, to prevent dental fluorosis. Patients with dental abnormalities found through visual examination (e.g., nursing bottle tooth decay, crowding or misalignment of teeth, dental caries, or periodontal infections) should be referred to their dentist for further evaluation.
3. Patients should be advised to limit their intake of foods containing refined sugar, particularly between-meal snacks and/or keep a tooth brush and tooth paste available at work.
4. To reduce the risk of early childhood caries, infants should not be put to bed with a bottle. If a bedtime bottle is necessary, encourage to use only water.
5. Children living in areas with inadequate fluoride in their drinking water should be prescribed daily fluoride drops or tablets according to recommended guidelines. Clinicians prescribing fluoride supplements for children must know the concentration of fluoride in the child's drinking water.
6. Urge patients to reduce their risk of oral cancer by eliminating tobacco use and limiting alcoholic beverage consumption. All patients who smoke cigarettes, pipes, or cigars or who use spit tobacco should be counseled to stop, and those who do not use tobacco, especially adolescents and young adults, should be encouraged to resist pressure to start.

J. Alcohol and other drugs
1. The routine history for all adolescents and adults should include questions about the quantity, frequency, and other patterns of use of wine, beer, liquor, or other drugs. (SOR **B**) Questionnaires are available for more systematic detection of problem drinking.
2. Negotiate safe drinking amounts—Recommendations for healthy, nonpregnant women in standard drinks are no more than 7 drinks per week or 3 per occasion; recommendations for healthy men are no more than 14 drinks per week or 4 per occasion. For patients older than 65 years, recommend no more than 1 drink per day. For patients who drink over those amounts, an Action Plan to reduce or stop drinking should be developed. (SOR **B**) (Those patients with addictive personalities or a history of substance abuse should consume less than these amounts.)
3. There are **no documented safe levels** of alcohol intake during pregnancy. To reduce the risk of Alcohol Exposed Pregnancy (AEP) and Fetal Alcohol Spectrum Disorders

(FASD) in pregnant women, or those want to become pregnant should be counseled not to drink. (^{SOR} **B**) Women at risk of becoming pregnant, and who choose to drink, should be counseled on consistent and proper use of contraceptives. (^{SOR} **B**)

4. For additional information on AEP and FASD, visit the website for the Midwest Region Fetal Alcohol Syndrome Training Center at www.mrfastc.org or to order a FASD Prevention Tool Kit, to the American College of Obstetricians and Gynecologists website at www.acog.org and search for "FASD Prevention Tool Kit."

5. Provide substance-abusing patients with information about chemical dependence, the effects of the drug, and its effect on health. Intravenous drug users should be referred for treatment and warned against the use of contaminated or shared needles, which can transmit HIV, hepatitis B virus, and other organisms. Treatment plans should be tailored to the drug of abuse and the individual needs of the patient and his or her family (see Chapter 88).

K. Cancer self-examination. Although widely practiced, self-examinations have not been conclusively proved to be an effective maneuver for reducing cancer mortality. The teaching of self-examination is neither specifically recommended nor discouraged. (^{SOR} **C**)

1. The American Cancer Society (ACS) recommends that asymptomatic persons 20 to 39 with average risk should have a physical exam every 3 years to screen for cancers of testis, ovary, thyroid, oral cavity, and skin and every year for anyone aged 40 and older.

2. Counsel patients about frequency of screening for skin cancer (those at modestly increased risk should see a primary care physician annually); skin self-examination should be performed monthly.

3. Skin Cancer:
   a. To prevent skin cancer, advise all patients of effective techniques to reduce outdoor exposure to ultraviolet light.
   b. Patients with increased occupational or recreational exposure to sunlight as well as those who live in tropical climates should be counseled to regularly apply broad-spectrum sunscreen with UVA/UVB protection. They should also be advised to wear protective clothing, such as wide-brimmed hats and long-sleeved shirts and slacks, and to try to reduce outdoor activity between 10 AM and 3 PM.
   c. Remind parents to limit their children's exposure to ultraviolet light through similar measures.
   d. Use of tanning beds should be discouraged.
   e. Screen adults for precancerous lesions and/or refer to a dermatologist.

REFERENCES

American College of Sports Medicine Guidelines. *ACSM's Guidelines for Exercise Testing and Prescription.* 7th ed. Baltimore, MD: Lippincott, Williams and Wilkins; 2005.

American Diabetes Association. Position statement: physical activity/exercise and diabetes. *Diabetes Care.* 2004;27(Suppl 1):S58–64.

Miller W, Rollnick S. *Motivational Interviewing: Preparing People for Change.* New York, NY: Guilford Press; 2002.

U.S. Prevention Services Task Force (2007). *An Independent Panel of Experts in Primary Care and Prevention.* Web reference made October, 2007. Web publication of the Agency for Healthcare Research and Quality (ARHQ). Guide to Clinical Prevention Services, 2007. http://www.ahrq.gov/clinic/uspstfix.htm

BIBLIOTHERAPY AND HANDOUTS: MANY HELPFUL HANDOUTS CAN BE EASILY ACCESSED:

A. www.aafp.org American Academy of Family Physicians—select *Clinical Care; Patient ED*; then *Handouts.*

B. www.webmd.com Multiple health topics.

C. www.womenshealth.gov Women's Health information and resources.

D. www.kidshealth.com Youth health information for parents, kids and teens.

E. www.4girls.gov Girls Health website.

F. Health Literacy: www.nlm.nih.gov/medlineplus/tutorial.html Easy-To-Read Health Tutorials. www.ama-assn.org/ama/pub/category/8115.html AMA Understanding Health Literacy.

G. www.fda.gov/oc/seniors FDA Health information for seniors.

H. www.healthliteracy.worlded.org/teacher-2.htm Health and Literacy info and resources.

I. http://mypyramid.gov/ Steps to a Healthier You—nutrition and exercise info/tools.

J. www.eatright.org/ada/files/06_Referral_MNT.pdf Guidelines for Medical Nutrition Therapy.

K. www.eatright/org/nnn Find a Registered Dietitian in your area for Nutrition Educ/Therapy.

101   Immunizations

William E. Cayley, Jr., MD, MDiv

KEY POINTS
- Immunizations are among the most cost-effective preventive health measure, significantly reducing rates of infectious disease and now with the recent introduction of the HPV vaccine, cervical cancer.
- Every health visit is an opportunity to update immunization status. Immunizations should be given according to the current schedules on CDC's National Immunization Program's website. http://www.cdc.gov/nip/.
- Contraindications to vaccine usage should be checked in every patient. A full discussion of risks and benefits, including benefits to society, should be done with every patient or guardian to ensure informed consent.

I. Introduction.
A. Overview.
Immunizations have significantly reduced rates of infectious disease and are among the most cost-effective preventive health measures. (SOR **A**) Nevertheless, vaccine coverage of the general population is less than optimal because of missed opportunities and misconceptions by parents and clinicians.

B. Timing.
Every health care visit is an opportunity to update a patient's immunization status. Routine immunizations should be given according to the current schedules posted on the web site of the Centers for Disease Control and Prevention's (CDC) National Immunization Program (http://www.cdc.gov/nip/). Childhood schedules are updated annually, and schedules for adolescents and adults are revised as needed. Administering multiple vaccines at the same visit is both safe and effective. (SOR **A**) Inactivated vaccines can be given any time before or after other live or inactivated vaccines. Live vaccines not administered at the same time should be separated by at least 4 weeks. Interruptions or delays in a vaccination series do not require restarting that series since delays in dosing do not reduce final antibody response. If past records cannot be located, the patient should be considered nonimmune and started on the appropriate schedule of doses.

C. Administration.
Routes of administration are recommended by the manufacturer of each vaccine. Intramuscular (IM) injections are given at a 90-degree angle into the deep muscle mass of the anterolateral thigh (for infants) or the deltoid (for older children and adults). IM injections should not be given into the buttock, because of risk of injury to the sciatic nerve. Subcutaneous (SC) injections are administered at a 45-degree angle into the thigh of infants 12 months or younger, and into the upper-outer triceps of older patients. Intradermal (ID) injections are usually given on the volar aspect of the forearm, with the needle inserted parallel to the long axis of the arm with the bevel facing up so that the entire bevel penetrates the skin and the injected solution raises a small bleb. If two or more vaccinations are given, each should be given at a different anatomic site.

D. Safety.
Patients with a history of severe allergic response to a vaccine or one of its components should not receive further doses of that vaccine. Mild illnesses are not contraindications to vaccination, and research has generally demonstrated adequate antibody response to vaccinations given at the time of mild illness. Patients with more severe illness should be immunized once the acute phase of the illness is over, to avoid confusing effects of the illness with vaccine side effects. Live vaccines may pose some risk for immunosuppressed family members, and in this context an inactivated vaccine may be preferred. Since no vaccine is completely safe or completely effective, administration of vaccines requires an understanding of the risks and benefits involved—the benefits to the individual and to society at large, weighed against the risks to the individual.

II. Early Childhood Immunizations (Ages 0–6 Years).
Immunizations should be given according to the annually updated schedule published on the CDC web site.

TABLE 101–1. HEPATITIS B VACCINATION SCHEDULES*

	Maternal Hepatitis B Surface Antigen (HbsAg) Negative	Maternal HBsAg Unknown or Positive
Single antigen	Birth, 2 mo, 6 mo	Birth, 1 mo, 6 mo
PEDIARIX	Birth, 2 mo, 4 mo, 6 mo	Birth, 6 wk, 4 mo, 6 mo
COMVAX	Birth, 2 mo, 4 mo, 12–15 mo	Birth, 6 wk, 4 mo, 12–15 mo

*The first dose is always given with a single-antigen vaccine, and all infants of mothers whose HBsAg is positive or unknown should also receive 0.5 cc of hepatitis B immune globulin (HBIG) injected IM at another site.

A. Hepatitis B (HBV).
1. Overview.
Approximately 6000 people in the USA die each year of HBV-related liver disease, including cirrhosis and hepatocellular carcinoma. Universal immunization of infants against HBV is recommended (1) to protect children younger than 5 years, who are at higher risk of chronic disease if they become infected, and (2) to increase immunity among the general population. HBV vaccines are manufactured using recombinant DNA technology.
2. Timing and administration.
   a. First dose. Infants born to hepatitis B surface antigen (HBsAg) negative mothers should receive a dose of single-antigen HBV vaccine between birth and age 8 weeks. Infants born to HbsAg positive mothers should receive a first dose of HBV vaccine in the first 12 hours of life, along with 0.5 cc of hepatitis B immune globulin (HBIG) injected IM at another site. If the mother's HbsAg status is unknown, HBV vaccine should be given in the first 12 hours of life, the mother's HbsAg status should be tested, and HBIG should be given within 1 week of birth if the mother tests HbsAg positive.

   b. Series completion. The series is always started with a single-antigen HBV vaccine (0.5 cc IM for ages 0–19 years), and may be completed with a single-antigen vaccine or with a combination vaccine such as Pediarix (HBV-diphtheria–tetanus–acelluar pertussis [DtaP]-inactivated poliovirus vaccine [IPV]) or COMVAX (HBV–Hemophilus influenza type B [Hib]). For the recommended dosing schedules, see Table 101–1.

   c. Catch-up immunization. Older children not previously vaccinated against HBV should receive a complete series of three doses with a single-antigen HBV vaccine. There should be at least 1 month between doses 1 and 2, and 4 months between doses 2 and 3.
3. Cautions.
Local pain and a mildly elevated temperature are the most common reactions. There appears to be no association between HBV immunization and Guillain–Barré syndrome.

B. Diphtheria–tetanus–acellular pertussis (DTaP).
1. Overview.
Childhood vaccination against diphtheria, tetanus, and pertussis has been routine in the USA since the 1940s. The older DTP vaccine with inactivated whole-cell pertussis has been replaced by the newer DTaP using an acellular pertussis toxin. Immunity to pertussis wanes, with little protection after 5 to 10 years, but childhood DTaP vaccines should not be used for immunizing adults.
2. Timing and administration.
DTaP is administered by IM injection of 0.5 cc of vaccine, given at 2, 4, and 6 months. Booster doses are given at 15 to 18 months (or at least 6 months after the last dose), and again at 4 to 6 years. Patients who do not receive their fourth dose until after age 4 do not need a fifth dose.
3. Cautions.
Mild reactions (fever, drowsiness) or more severe reactions (high temperatures >105°F, or febrile seizures) are much less common after DTaP administration than with the older DTP vaccine. If encephalopathy, such as unresponsiveness or seizures, occurs within 7 days of DTaP administration and cannot be attributed to another cause, DT (diphtheria and tetanus toxoids alone) should be used for all subsequent immunizations. Stable neurologic conditions, or a family history of seizures, are not contraindications to pertussis immunization.

C. *Hemophilus influenzae* Type B (Hib).

1. **Overview.**
Before development of effective vaccinations, 1 in 200 children developed invasive *Hemophilus* disease before age 5, often leading to meningitis, hearing loss or mental retardation. Vaccines against *Hemophilus influenzae* type B have been 95% to 100% effective in preventing invasive Hib disease. Three Hib vaccines are available:

   a. *Hemophilus* b Diphtheria Protein Conjugate (HbOC).
   b. *Hemophilus* b Meningococcal Protein Conjugate (PRP-OMP).
   c. *Hemophilus* b Diphtheria Toxoid Conjugate (PRP-D).

2. **Timing and administration.**
Hib vaccines should not be given to infants younger than 6 weeks. The recommended schedule is a dose of Hib at 2, 4, and 6 months and a booster at 12 to 15 months. Children who have received PRP-OMP at 2 and 4 months do not require a dose at 6 months.

3. **Cautions.**
Adverse effects from Hib vaccination are rare, usually occur after the third dose if at all, and are usually limited to mild fever, or local redness, swelling, or warmth.

D. **Inactivated poliovirus vaccine (IPV).**

1. **Overview.**
Routine vaccination has led to control of polio in the Western Hemisphere. Since the live oral polio vaccine (OPV) carries a small but real risk of vaccine-associated paralytic polio, it has been replaced in the USA by the inactivated polio vaccine (IPV).

2. **Timing and administration.**
Recommended doses of IPV are at ages 2 months, 4 months, between 6 and 18 months, and between 4 and 6 years. The dose is 0.5 cc of vaccine administered SC.

3. **Cautions.**
No serious adverse events have been associated with the use of IPV.

E. **Measles–mumps–rubella (MMR).**

1. **Overview.**
MMR vaccination has reduced rates of measles, mumps, rubella ("german measles") and congenital rubella syndrome by 99% over the last century, although occasional outbreaks continue to occur among unimmunized persons. The MMR vaccine combines attenuated strains of all three viruses.

2. **Timing and administration.**
The first dose of MMR vaccine is given SC at 12 to 15 months of age, and the second dose at 4 to 6 years

3. **Cautions.**
Pain, redness, and local irritation may occur with all three vaccines. Rubella vaccine may rarely cause generalized lymphadenopathy in children or a transient arthralgia in young women, and mumps vaccine may rarely cause transient orchitis in young men. Egg allergy is not a contraindication to MMR vaccine, but the vaccine should not be given to persons with severe allergy to gelatin or neomycin. Patients with human immunodeficiency virus (HIV) may be given MMR unless they have low age-specific CD4 counts.

F. **Varicella-zoster virus (VZV).**

1. **Overview.**
The live attenuated VZV vaccine is 97% effective against moderate or severe varicella and at least 44% protective against any varicella for at least 7 years, and antibody response has been documented for up to 20 years. Approximately 1% of vaccinees per year develop mild, breakthrough infection that does not appear to be contagious.

2. **Timing and administration.**
Children with no history of chickenpox should be routinely vaccinated with a first 0.5 cc dose of VZV SC between 12 and 18 months of age, and a second dose between 4 and 6 years of age. Varicella-zoster immune globulin (VZIG) is indicated in varicella-susceptible individuals following significant exposure and in newborns of mothers with varicella that occurred in the interval from 5 days prior to 2 days following delivery.

3. **Cautions.**
The vaccine is contraindicated in immunosuppressed individuals. Transient zoster in recipients and transmission to susceptible contacts of vaccinees has been reported.

G. **Pneumococcal conjugate vaccine (PCV)**

1. **Overview.**
Streptococcus pneumoniae is a major cause of pediatric otitis media, pneumonia, meningitis, and bacteremia. Rates of disease are higher among children younger than

5 years and are highest in infants. The PCV contains antigens from seven serotypes of pneumococcus conjugated to a carrier protein, and is effective in reducing invasive disease and pneumonia .

2. Timing and administration.
PCV should be given as 0.5 cc IM to children at 2, 4, 6, and 12 to 15 months of age. Since the highest risk of invasive disease is in children younger than age 2, catch-up vaccination with PCV between ages 2 and 5 is recommended only for children with increased risk of disease because of HIV, sickle-cell disease, asplenia, or chronic illness.

3. Cautions. Local redness and tenderness at the injection site are the only reported adverse effects of PCV.

H. Hepatitis A (HAV).

1. Overview.
HAV is usually transmitted by the fecal-oral route. While acute disease is more common in adults, children generally have asymptomatic infection and so can be an important source of infection for older individuals. Hepatitis A immune globulin has been available for several years for inducing passive immunity, and since 1995 two inactivated-virus vaccines conferring active immunity against HAV have been available (Havrix and Vaqta).

2. Timing and administration.
Immunization against HAV is recommended for all children between 12 and 23 months of age, as well as older children who were not previously immunized. Both vaccines are given to individuals aged 12 months to 18 years as two doses of 0.5 cc IM, and to individuals older than 18 years at two doses of 1.0 cc IM. Doses must be separated by at least 6 months. Onset of immunity is in 15 to 30 days, and protection lasts for at least 10 years. No booster doses are recommended.

3. Cautions.
The only reported adverse effects from HAV vaccination are local warmth and soreness and occasional headache.

I. Influenza.

1. Overview.
Influenza virus is second only to respiratory syncytial virus (RSV) in causing hospitalizations among children with chronic illness. Even among healthy children younger than 2 years, influenza hospitalization rates are as high as 187 per 100 000 children. All children from 6 to 59 months old should be vaccinated annually with trivalent inactivated influenza vaccine (TIV). Children 5 years or older should also receive TIV annually if they have chronic metabolic, respiratory, or hematologic disease, or are receiving chronic aspirin therapy. The intranasal live attenuated influenza vaccine (LAIV) may only be used for healthy children 5 years or older.

2. Timing and administration.
Vaccination against influenza should ideally be done during October or November. Children aged 6 to 35 months receive 0.25 cc IM, and all those 3 years or older receive 0.5 cc IM. Anyone 8 years or younger receiving influenza immunization for the first time should receive two doses at least 4 weeks apart. The vaccine is not recommended for children younger than 6 months, though they may be protected from influenza by vaccination of household contacts.

3. Cautions.
Patients who are concerned about the influenza vaccine causing disease should be educated that the vaccine contains noninfectious killed virus. It cannot cause disease, but will not protect against coincident infection with other viruses. Local reactions of redness and tenderness are the most common adverse reactions, though anaphylactic reactions to residual egg protein from the virus culture process have rarely been reported.

J. Rotavirus.

1. Overview.
Rotavirus is responsible for one-third of the cases of childhood death from diarrheal disease worldwide, and over 550,000 hospitalizations annually in the USA. The virus is common, hardy, and highly contagious, thus even proper attention to hygiene and contact precautions may not prevent transmission. An earlier quadrivalent human-rhesus vaccine (RRV-TV) was removed from the market in 1999 after increased reports of intussusception. The newer oral Rotavirus vaccine is a live-virus vaccine that appears to be effective in reducing rates of disease with no increased rates of intussusception.

2. Timing and administration.
Immunization consists of 3 oral 2cc doses at age 2, 4 and 6 months. The vaccine series should not be started after age 12 weeks.

3. Cautions.
Approximately 2% to 3% of infants will experience mild vomiting or diarrhea after Rotavirus vaccination. The vaccine does not appear to increase the rate of intussusception. Because the vaccine is a live virus, it should not be given to children of mothers with HIV until it has been determined that the infant does not have HIV. The safety of using this vaccine for infants with other immunosuppressive conditions is currently unknown.

K. Menningococcal polysaccharide vaccine (MPSV4).
1. Overview.
Neisseria Meningitidis is the now most common cause of bacterial meningitis in children, with fatality rates up to 10% despite use of appropriate antibiotics. The MPSV4 vaccine protects against *N. Meningitidis* sero-types A, C, Y, and W-135. While it is up to 85% effective in school-age children, immunity declines after 3 years. At this time, childhood vaccination with MPSV4 is only recommended for children aged 2 to 10 years old with terminal complement deficiencies, or depressed or absent spleen function (e.g., caused by sickle cell disease or splenectomy).
2. Timing and administration.
MPSV4 is given to children age 2 to 10 years as a single 0.5 cc SC dose.
3. Cautions.
Local pain and redness, mild fever, fussiness, and headache may occur after administration of MPSV4, but there have been no severe side effects reported.

III. Late Childhood and Adolescent Immunizations (Ages 7–18).
Catch-up doses of certain vaccines are recommended from ages 7 to 10, and additional routine immunizations are recommended at age 11 or 12 years old. There are also specific vaccine recommendations for certain high-risk patients. Immunizations should be given according to the annually updated schedule published on the CDC website.
A. Tetanus–diphtheria–acellular pertussis (Tdap).
1. Overview.
The Tdap vaccine contains the same dose of Tetanus toxoid as the pediatric DTaP, but the dose of Diphtheria toxoid is much lower. Immunity to pertussis from childhood DTaP vaccination wanes with age and cases of adolescent pertussis have been increasing. Thus, the acellular pertussis component has been added to the recommended adolescent vaccinations and the Tdap vaccine has replaced the older recommendation for adolescent Td (Tetanus–Diphtheria) vaccination to extend the duration of protection from pertussis.
2. Timing and administration.
A single dose of Tdap 0.5 cc IM is recommended at age 11 or older for individuals who completed the primary pediatric series of immunizations. Adolescents who did not receive a primary series of vaccinations of tetanus toxoid vaccines should receive two doses of Td and one dose of Tdap.
3. Cautions.
Headache, injection site pain, myalgias, and fatigue are the most commonly reported adverse effects. Patients experiencing and Arthus hypersensitivity reaction or a temperature over 103°F after any dose of Tetanus toxoid should not receive further doses of Tetanus toxoid more frequently than every 10 years.
B. Human papilloma virus (HPV).
1. Overview.
Most HPV infections are asymptomatic, and 90% clear within 2 years. However, persistent HPV infection can cause cervical cancer in women and genital warts in both men and women. The quadrivalent vaccine against HPV types 6, 11, 16, and 18 was licensed in 2006 for females aged 9 to 26 years. Ideally, the series should be given before the onset of sexual activity. However, even for females who have begun sexual activity and been infected with HPV, the vaccine may provide some protection against further infection with other HPV serotypes.
2. Timing and administration.
Routine HPV vaccination is recommended for all females at age 11 or 12, with catch-up doses recommended for previously unimmunized females between ages 13 and 26. HPV vaccine is given as three 0.5cc IM doses. There should be 2 months between doses 1 and 2, and 4 months between doses 2 and 3.
3. Cautions.
Local pain, swelling, and redness are not unusual, and approximately 4% of patients may experience a mild fever. Severe adverse events have not been reported. It is important to realize that HPV vaccination will not eliminate the risk of cervical cancer

or the need for screening since the vaccine does not include all HPV types causing cancer. The long-term duration of immunity has not been definitively established.

C. Meningococcal conjugate vaccine (MCV4).

1. Overview.

The newer MCV4 vaccine provides longer-lasting immunity than the older MPSV4, but is only approved for individuals aged 11 to 55 years. Since crowded living conditions are a risk factor for meningococcal disease, MCV4 vaccination is recommended for college freshmen who will be living in dormitories and for military recruits.

2. Timing and administration.

MCV4 vaccination is given as a single 0.5 cc IM dose. It is recommended at age 11 or 12 years, or at high school entry (approximately age 15) for adolescents not previously immunized. MPSV4 may be used as an alternative if MCV4 is not available.

3. Cautions.

Mild fever and local pain, redness or swelling may occur after MCV4 vaccination, but there is minimal risk of severe side effects.

D. Catch-up immunizations.

1. Hepatitis B.

Adolsecents not previously vaccinated against HBV should receive a complete series of three doses with a single-antigen HBV vaccine. There should be at least 1 month between doses 1 and 2, and 4 months between doses 2 and 3.

2. Polio.

Any adolescent who has not already received a complete primary series of polio vaccine should be immunized. If previous doses were all IPV or all OPV and the third dose was after age 4, then a fourth dose is not needed. If previous doses were a combination of OPV and IPV, then a fourth dose is needed for series completion.

3. Measles–mumps–rubella.

Any adolescent not previously immunized should receive two doses of MMR vaccine at least 4 weeks apart.

4. Varicella-zoster virus.

Varicella immunization is recommended for all adolescents without a reliable history of immunity (such as documentation of prior age-appropriate vaccination, laboratory confirmation of immunity or of varicella disease, birth in the USA before 1980, or health-care provider diagnosis of chickenpox or zoster). Two doses of vaccine are given, spaced 3 months apart for those under 13 years and spaced 4 weeks apart for those 13 years or older.

E. Immunizations for high-risk groups.

Adolescents with certain health conditions may require additional protection from certain diseases.

1. Pneumococcal polysaccharide vaccine (PPV4).

In adolescents at increased risk of pneumococcal disease caused by heart disease or cardiomyopathy, diabetes mellitus, immunosuppression, or depressed or absent spleen function (e.g., caused by sickle cell disease or splenectomy), a single dose of the 23-valent pneumococcal polysaccharide vaccine (PPV) is administered as 0.5 cc SC and may be repeated once after at least 5 years if the risk of infection is particularly high.

2. Hepatitis A.

Adolescents living in communities at high risk for HAV should be vaccinated with two doses of HAVRIX or VAQTA as outlined above.

3. Influenza.

Annual influenza vaccination should be given to adolescents with asthma, diabetes, or other chronic metabolic disease, hemoglobinopathies, or immunosuppression because of medications or illness, or those on chronic aspirin therapy (because of the increased risk of Reye's syndrome associated with taking aspirin during influenza illness).

IV. Adult Immunizations.

While immunizations are ideally given at routine health maintenance visits, many adults seek medical care only for acute injury or illness and may not have had all recommended immunizations. Thus, episodes of acute care also are important times for assessing and updating immunization status. The adult immunization schedule is published on the CDC web site and is updated regularly. It lists vaccine recommendations by age group, and by medical condition.

A. Tetanus, diphtheria, and acellular pertussis (Tdap/Td).

Adults who have completed a primary series of pediatric Tetanus and Diphtheria vaccinations should continue to receive a tetanus booster every 10 years. Adult immunization against pertussis has recently been added to standard recommendations, to help reduce transmission from nonimmune and mildly infected adults to children and adolescents who are more vulnerable to pertussis. All adults should receive Tdap at the time of the next scheduled tetanus immunization, then continue with Tetanus–Diphtheria Td booster immunizations every 10 years. Those who have not completed a primary series should receive three doses of Tetanus toxoid (two doses Td, and one dose Tdap), with the second dose 4 weeks after the first, and the third dose 6 months after the second. During routine wound management, Tetanus toxoid administration is not required unless more than 10 years has elapsed since the last dose for clean, minor wounds. For contaminated or deep wounds, a booster is recommended if it has been longer than 5 years since the last dose or the immunization history is unclear. Tetanus immune globulin (250 IU intramuscularly) is also indicated for contaminated wounds in those with uncertain histories or with less than three primary Td doses.

B. Human papilloma virus.
Women who are 26 or younger who have not previously been vaccinated against HPV should be offered the HPV vaccine in three doses at the same intervals as recommended for adolescents.

C. Measles–mumps–rubella.
All persons born in 1957 or later who lack evidence of immunity to measles, mumps, or rubella or do not have documentation of having received MMR on or after their first birthday should receive a 0.5 cc SC dose of MMR. Persons born in 1956 or before are generally assumed to be immune. MMR or other live-virus vaccines should not be given during pregnancy. Any woman who is not pregnant and who has no history of MMR vaccination or evidence of immunity to rubella should be immunized with MMR or rubella vaccine (0.5 cc SC) and agree to avoid pregnancy for 3 months. Susceptible pregnant women should be immunized in the immediate postpartum period, with the same instructions.

D. Varicella zoster.
All adults without a reliable history of varicella immunity should be assumed susceptible and offered immunization with two 0.5 cc doses at least 4 weeks apart to decrease the risk of severe varicella, pneumonia, hepatitis, or encephalitis. A reliable history of varicella immunity includes documentation of prior age-appropriate vaccination, laboratory confirmation of immunity or of varicella disease, birth in the USA before 1980, or health-care provider diagnosis of chickenpox or zoster.

E. Influenza.
All adults 50 years or older should receive influenza vaccination annually in October or November. Annual influenza vaccination should also be given to residents of nursing homes or chronic-care facilities and to adults of any age with the following risk factors: asthma or other respiratory disorders, diabetes or other chronic metabolic disease, hemoglobinopathies, immunosuppression because of medications or illness, or chronic aspirin therapy. Pregnant women past 13 weeks' gestation should also be immunized. Influenza vaccine is 90% effective in preventing infection in young healthy adults, but only 30% to 40% effective in frail elderly or compromised adults. Health-care workers should be vaccinated annually to reduce the risk of transmitting influenza to susceptible individuals. Persons who contract influenza following immunization usually have a milder course and are less likely to have complications. Healthy nonpregnant adults who are not close contacts of immunocompromised individuals in special care units can receive LAIV or TIV. All individuals should only be given TIV.

F. Pneumococcus.
The 23-valent PPV should be given (0.5 cc SC) to all adults aged 65 or older because of their high risk of complications from pneumococcal disease. Anyone between ages 2 and 64 with chronic cardiovascular disease, chronic pulmonary disease (chronic obstructive pulmonary disease, but not asthma), diabetes mellitus, alcoholism, chronic liver disease, cerebrospinal fluid leaks, depressed or absent spleen function (e.g., caused by sickle cell disease or splenectomy), or immunosuppression, or anyone living in a chronic-care facility is also at risk of pneumococcal disease and should be vaccinated. One-time revaccination after an interval of 5 years is recommended for: (1) those under 65 who received the vaccine because of a high-risk medical condition (outlined above) who also have chronic immunodeficiency or immune suppression, and (2) for those aged 65 or older whose first dose was before age 65.

G. Immunizations for high-risk groups.
   1. Hepatitis B.
   HBV should be offered to persons with occupational risk (health-care workers and public service workers); persons with lifestyle risk (homosexual or bisexual men,

heterosexual persons with multiple partners or with any sexually transmitted disease, and injectable drug users); persons with hepatitis C or hemophilia and hemodialysis patients; and those with environmental risk factors (including household or sexual contacts of HBV carriers, prison inmates, and immigrants from HBV—endemic areas). All pregnant women should be screened prenatally for active HBV infection (HBsAg positive). HBV vaccine is administered as 1 cc IM, with a second dose given 1 month later and the third dose given at 6 months. Though not routinely recommended, booster doses of HBV vaccine and pre- and postimmunization serologic testing may be considered, based on the patient's risk factors. Postexposure prophylaxis using 0.06 cc/kg IM of HBIG, in addition to the HBV vaccine series, should be offered to persons with percutaneous or mucous-membrane exposure to blood or secretions known to be HBsAg positive, as soon as possible after exposure (within 72 hours).

2. **Hepatitis A.**
Immunization against HAV should be given to adults who live in endemic areas or travel internationally to countries with endemic HAV. Other groups at risk who should be immunized are men who have sex with men, users of illegal drugs, patients with clotting factor disorders, patients with chronic liver disease, and those with occupational exposure to HAV. Adult vaccination is given with 1.0 cc HAVRIX or VAQTA IM. Immediate postexposure protection against HAV can be achieved with immune serum globulin (ISG, 0.02–0.06 cc/kg IM). ISG should be given within 2 weeks of exposure to close household and sexual contacts of persons with HAV and to health-care workers and patients in centers with active cases of HAV. ISG affords protection against HAV for 3 to 6 months, depending on the dose given. The protective effect of HAV immunization takes 4 weeks to develop, but protection lasts for at least 10 years. For international travelers, it may be necessary to administer ISG at a different site, in addition to the vaccine, if travel is anticipated before 4 weeks has elapsed.

3. **Meningococcal vaccination.**
Meningococcal vaccination is recommended for college freshmen living in dormitories. Individuals should also be vaccinated if they are at increased risk of disease because of depressed or absent spleen function (e.g., caused by sickle cell disease or splenectomy), terminal complement component deficiencies, occupational exposure in a research or clinical setting, or travel to an endemic area (especially the "meningitis belt" of sub-Saharan Africa from Senegal to Ethiopia). MCV4 is recommended for anyone younger than 55 years, although MPSV4 is an acceptable alternative. MPSV4 should be used for all adults older than 55 years, and revaccination after 5 years may be considered for adults previously vaccinated with MPSV4 who remain at high risk for infection.

V. **Combination Vaccines.**
Combination vaccines allow adequate administration of recommended vaccines with fewer total injections, but only US Food and Drug Administration-licensed combination vaccines should be used. Combination vaccines are appropriate when any component vaccine is indicated and none of the component vaccines are contraindicated. Whenever possible, a vaccine series should be completed with all doses coming from the same manufacturer.

REFERENCES AND RESOURCES

Childhood and Adolescent Immunization Schedules. http://www.cdc.gov/nip/recs/child-schedule.htm. Accessed July 29, 2008.

General Recommendations on Immunization: Recommendations of the Advisory Committee on Immunization Practices (ACIP). MMWR 55(RR15);1-48. http://www.cdc.gov/mmwr/preview/mmwrhtml/rr5515a1.htm. Accessed July 29, 2008.

National Immunization Program of the Centers for Disease Control and Prevention. http://www.cdc.gov/nip

National Immunization Program's Adult Immunization Schedule. http://www.cdc.gov/vaccines/recs/schedules/adult-schedule.htm. Accessed July 29, 2008.

Shots Online (sponsored by the Group on Immunization Education of the Society of Teachers of Family Medicine). http://www.immunizationed.org/ImmunizationEDrog/ShotsOnline.aspx. Accessed July 29, 2008.

Zimmerman RK, Middleton DB, Burns IT, et al. Routine vaccines across the life span, 2007. *J Fam Pract.* 2007;56(2):S18-37, C1-3. http://www.jfponline.com/uploadedFiles/Journal_Site_Files/Journal_of_Family_Practice/supplement_archive/JFPSupp_Vaccines07_0207.pdf. Accessed July 29, 2008.

102   Screening Tests

Larry L. Dickey, MD, MPH

The strength of recommendations for this chapter is given using the rating system of the US Preventive Services Task Force (USPSTF). The meaning of the A, B, C, D, and I ratings are explained in Table 102–1. For screening tests that have not been rated by the USPSTF, strength of recommendations ratings are not given. The strength of recommendation ratings of other organizations for screening tests, if available, are not provided since the USPSTF is widely recognized as the leading authority in accessing the strength of scientific evidence for preventive services.

KEY POINTS

- The following screening tests and examinations should be considered for children and adults.
    - **A. Children**
        1. Body measurement
            - **a.** Head circumference (until age 2 years)
            - **b.** Height and weight
            - **c.** Blood pressure (beginning at age 3 years)
        2. Blood tests
            - **a.** Hypothyroidism (newborns)
            - **b.** Phenylketonuria (newborns)
            - **c.** Hemoglobinopathies (newborns)
            - **d.** Anemia (at 6–12 months of age and adolescent girls at risk)
            - **e.** Glucose (high risk)
            - **f.** Lead (high risk at 12 and 24 months)
            - **g.** Cholesterol (high risk, after age 2 years)

TABLE 102–1. U.S. PREVENTIVE SERVICES TASK FORCE (USPSTF) RATINGS: WHAT THE GRADES MEAN AND SUGGESTIONS FOR PRACTICE

Grade	Definition	Suggestions for Practice
A	The USPSTF recommends the service. There is high certainty that the net benefit is substantial.	Offer or provide this service.
B	The USPSTF recommends the service. There is high certainty that the net benefit is moderate or there is moderate certainty that the net benefit is moderate to substantial.	Offer or provide this service.
C	The USPSTF recommends against routinely providing the service. There may be considerations that support providing the service in an individual patient. There is at least moderate certainty that the net benefit is small.	Offer or provide this service only if other considerations support the offering or providing the service in an individual patient.
D	The USPSTF recommends against the service. There is moderate or high certainty that the service has no net benefit or that the harms outweigh the benefits.	Discourage the use of this service.
I Statement	The USPSTF concludes that the current evidence is insufficient to assess the balance of benefits and harms of the service. Evidence is lacking, of poor quality, or conflicting, and the balance of benefits and harms cannot be determined.	Read the clinical considerations section of USPSTF Recommendation Statement. If the service is offered, patients should understand the uncertainty about the balance of benefits and harms.

      3. Sensory screening
         a. Hearing* (newborns, children, and adolescents)
         b. Vision (amblyopia/strabismus until age 3–4 years, acuity beginning at age 3–4 years)
      4. Mental health screening
         a. Depression (high risk adolescents)
      5. Infectious diseases tests
         a. Hepatitis C (high risk)
         b. Human immunodeficiency virus (HIV) (high risk)
         c. Chlamydia/gonorrhea/syphilis (high risk adolescents)
         d. Tuberculosis (high risk)
      6. Cancer tests
         a. Testicular examination (boys beginning at age 15)
  B. Adults
      1. Body measurement
         a. Height and weight
         b. Blood pressure
         c. Bone density (women, beginning at age 60)
         d. Abdominal aortic ultrasound (men, smokers, age 65–75 years)
      2. Blood tests
         a. Cholesterol (men aged 35–65 years, women aged 45–65 years)
         b. Glucose (high risk)
         c. Thyroid (high risk)
      3. Sensory screenings
         a. Hearing (beginning at age 65)
         b. Vision (beginning at age 65)
         c. Glaucoma (high risk)
      4. Mental health screening
         a. Depression
      5. Infectious diseases tests
         a. Hepatitis C (high risk)
         b. HIV (high risk)
         c. Chlamydia/gonorrhea/syphilis (high risk)
         d. Tuberculosis (high risk)
      6. Cancer tests
         a. Breast examination and mammogram (women beginning at age 40)
         b. Cervical—Pap smear (women)
         c. Colorectal screening (stool guaiac cards, flexible sigmoidoscopy, barium enema, or colonoscopy beginning at age 50)
         d. Prostate examination and prostate-specific antigen (PSA) (men beginning at age 50)
         e. Skin examination
         f. Testicular examination (men)
         g. Thyroid examination

I. Body Measurement Screening
  A. Head circumference. The American Academy of Pediatrics (AAP) has recommended measurement of head circumference at every visit until a child is 2 years old. Other authorities have not made recommendations for or against this.
  B. Height and weight. Most major authorities have recommended regular measurement of height and weight at all ages (USPSTF I for obesity screening). For children and adolescents, these can be plotted using age-specific growth curve charts. For adults, standard height and weight charts can be used (Table 102–2) for assessing norms. Several authorities recommend periodic calculation and charting of body mass index (BMI = weight [kg]/height^2 [m]), since BMI is believed to be more reflective of total body fat than weight for height norms. According to the US Department of Agriculture, BMI of ≥ 25 constitutes overweight for adults, the point at which negative health consequences begin. The AAP classifies children with BMIs >95th percentile to be obese, and children with BMIs between the 85th and 95th percentiles to be at risk of being overweight.

TABLE 102–2. WEIGHT CHART FOR ADULT MEN AND WOMEN

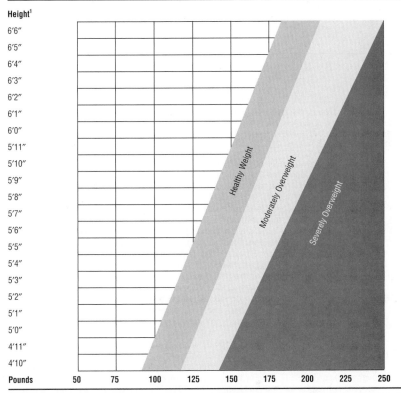

*The use of shading reflects the lack of consensus about exact cutoff points and emphasizes that disease risk varies with degree of overweight.

Note: To use this chart, find your height in feet and inches (*without shoes*) along the left side of the graph. Trace the line corresponding to your height across the figure until it intersects with the vertical line corresponding to your weight in pounds (*without clothes*). The point of intersection lies within a band that indicates whether your weight is healthy or is moderately or severely overweight. The higher weights apply mainly to men, who have more muscle and bone.

(Reprinted from US Department of Agriculture, US Department of Health and Human Services. *Nutrition and Your Health: Dietary Guidelines for Americans.* US Government Printing Office; 1995. *Home and Garden Bulletin* 232.)

C. Waist/hip measurement. Some authorities, such as the US Department of Agriculture and the US Department of Health and Human Services, have recommended measurement of waist and hip circumferences and calculation of waist/hip ratio (WHR) for adults. By some reports, this may be a more accurate predictor of negative health consequences than height/weight or BMI values. Upper limits of healthy WHR values are usually cited as 0.8 for women and 1.0 for men. According to the National Heart, Lung, and Blood Institute, an abdominal circumference of >40 inches for men and >35 inches for women constitutes abdominal obesity and should be considered a cardiovascular disease risk factor.

D. Blood pressure

1. Children and adolescents. The AAP and NHLBI recommend regular blood pressure screening of all children beginning at age 3 years. For children, values above the 95th percentile are considered elevated (Table 102–3). In 2003, the US Preventive Services Task Force found insufficient evidence to recommend for or against routine screening of children and adolescents, stating that evidence is poor that routine blood pressure measurement accurately identifies children and adolescents at increased risk for

TABLE 102–3. 95TH PERCENTILE OF BLOOD PRESSURE BY SELECTED AGES IN GIRLS AND BOYS, BY THE 50TH
AND 75TH HEIGHT PERCENTILES

Age (Years)	Girls' SBP/DPB		Boys' SBP/DBP	
	50th Percentile for Height	75th Percentile for Height	50th Percentile for Height	75th Percentile for Height
1	104/58	105/59	102/57	104/58
6	111/73	112/73	114/74	115/75
12	123/80	124/81	123/81	125/82
17	129/84	130/85	136/87	138/88

DBP, diastolic blood pressure; SBP, systolic blood pressure.
(Reprinted from National Institutes of Health. *The Sixth Report of the Joint National Committee on Prevention, Detection, Evaluation, and Treatment of High Blood Pressure.* US Department of Health and Human Services; 1997. NIH publication 98-4080.)

cardiovascular disease and that treatment of elevated blood pressure in children or adolescents decreases the incidence of cardiovascular disease (USPSTF I).

2. **Adults.** All authorities recommend regular routine screening of adults for elevated blood pressure (USPSTF A). The NHLBI recommends screening every 2 years for persons with systolic blood pressure <130 mm Hg and diastolic blood pressure <85 mm Hg, with more frequent screening for adults with higher pressures. The USPSTF has found insufficient evidence to recommend an optimal screening interval. For adults, systolic pressures ≥140 mm Hg and diastolic pressures ≥90 mm Hg are considered elevated. Elevated values should be confirmed on at least one or two additional visits before hypertension is diagnosed. The NHLBI classifies adult systolic pressures >120 mm Hg or diastolic pressures >80 mm Hg as "prehypertension," for which lifestyle modifications should be considered.

E. **Bone density.** The USPSTF recommends routine screening for normal-risk women age 65 or older and for high-risk women age 60 or older (USPSTF B). Although the optimal interval screening is not determined, intervals of at least 2 years may be necessary to detect changes. Other groups, such as the American Academy of Family Physicians, have recommended earlier screening beginning at age 60 for high-risk women.

F. **Abdominal aortic ultrasound.** The USPSTF recommends one-time screening for abdominal aortic aneurysm (AAA) by ultrasonography in men aged 65 to 75 who have ever smoked (USPSTF B). For this group, the moderate magnitude of net benefit from surgery outweighs the potential harms. The USPSTF has made no recommendation for or against screening for AAA in men aged 65 to 75 who have never smoked (USPSTF C) and recommends against screening for women (USPSTF D).

II. **Blood Test Screening**

A. **Cholesterol**

1. **Children and adolescents.** No major authority recommends routine cholesterol screening of children or adolescents. Several authorities, including the AAP, American Medical Association (AMA), and NHLBI, recommend total cholesterol screening of children older than 2 years and adolescents who have a parent with a total cholesterol level ≥240 mg/dL. These authorities also recommend lipoprotein analysis of children older than 2 years and adolescents who have a family history of premature cardiovascular disease (before age 55) in a parent or grandparent. The National Cholesterol Education Program (NCEP) recommends screening for at-risk children and adolescents every 5 years. The AMA states that during adolescence screening is needed only once if values are normal. The NCEP has classified cholesterol levels in children and adolescents as follows: acceptable (total <170 mg/dL, low-density lipoprotein [LDL] <110 mg/dL); borderline (total 170–199 mg/dL, LDL 110–129 mg/dL); and high (total = 200 mg/dL, LDL = 130 mg/dL). The USPSTF, in a recent review, found insufficient evidence to recommend for or against cholesterol screening for both normal-risk and high-risk children and adolescents (USPSTF I).

2. **Adults.** Recommendations vary regarding screening of adults. The most aggressive recommendations are those of the NCEP, which recommends screening all adults at least once every 5 years for total cholesterol and at the same time, if accurate results are available, for high-density lipoprotein (HDL) cholesterol. The USPSTF recommends screening for men aged 35 to 65 years and women aged 45 to 65 years (USPSTF A). The USPSTF does not recommend screening younger men and women

(USPSTF C) unless they are at high risk because of other coronary heart disease risk factors (USPSTF B) and found insufficient evidence to recommend screening for triglyceride (USPSTF I). The USPSTF states that the appropriate interval for screening is unknown. The NCEP has classified cholesterol level in adults without coronary artery disease as follows: desirable (total <200 mg/dL, LDL <130 mg/dL); borderline (total 200–239 mg/dL, LDL 130–159 mg/dL); and high (total ≥240 mg/dL, LDL ≥160 mg/dL). The NCEP considers HDL levels <35 mg/dL and ≥60 mg/dL to be positive and negative risk factors, respectively, for coronary artery disease.

B. Glucose

1. **Children and adolescents.** Because of the growing prevalence of type II diabetes in children and adolescents, the American Diabetes Association (ADA) recommends plasma glucose screening at a 2-year intervals for overweight children and adolescents (BMI >85th percentile) beginning at age 10 years with any two of the following risk factors: family history of type II diabetes in first- or second-degree relatives; belonging to a high-risk race/ethnic group (Native American, African American, Hispanic American, and Asian/South Pacific Islander); or having signs of insulin resistance or conditions associated with insulin resistance (acanthosis nigricans, hypertension, dyslipidemia, and polycystic ovary syndrome).

2. **Adults.** The USPSTF has found insufficient evidence to recommend routine plasma glucose screening of normal-risk adults and has recommended screening for adults with hypertension or hyperlipidemia (USPSTF B). The ADA recommends that screening be considered at 3-year intervals for those 45 years or older, particularly with a BMI >25 kg/m^2 and for people who are <45 years of age and are overweight if they have another risk factor for diabetes. According to the ADA testing should be considered at a younger age or be carried out more frequently in individuals who are overweight and have one or more of the other risk factors for type 2 diabetes.

C. Hemoglobin/hematocrit

1. **Children and adolescents.** The AAP recommends screening all children for anemia once between 9 and 12 months of age and annually during adolescence for menstruating teenagers. According to the Centers for Disease Control and Prevention (CDC), the cutoff points for defining anemia in children aged 6 months to 2 years are hemoglobin ≤11.0 g/dL and hematocrit ≤33.0%. The USPSTF has found insufficient evidence to recommend for or against screening for anemia in children (USPSTF I). The American College of Obstetricians and Gynecologists (ACOG) recommends screening of adolescents beginning at age 13 years at high risk because of Caribbean, Latin American, Asian, Mediterranean, or African ancestry or a history of excessive menstrual flow.

2. **Adults.** No major authority recommends routine screening of asymptomatic, nonpregnant adults for anemia. The ACOG recommends periodic screening of women with a history of excessive menstrual flow and women of Caribbean, Latin American, Asian, Mediterranean, or African ancestry. In nonpregnant women and adolescent girls older than 15 years, the cutpoints for anemia are hemoglobin ≤12 g/dL and hematocrit ≤36%.

D. Lead.

In 1997, the CDC recommended that state health officials develop plans for targeted blood lead level (BLL) screening of children based on assessments of the lead exposure and screening capacity in specific regions of the state. For targeted screening, the CDC recommends screening of children who reside in a zip code in which >27% of housing was built before 1950; receive services from public assistance programs for the poor, such as Medicaid or the Supplemental Food Program for Women, Infants, and Children; or whose parents answer "yes" or "don't know" to any of three question of a personal-risk questionnaire (Table 102–4). In areas where exposure to lead from older housing is unlikely, the CDC states that the personal-risk questionnaire could contain questions about other risk factors, such as parental occupation or use of lead-containing ceramic ware or traditional remedies. In the absence of a targeted screening plan or other formal guidance from state health officials, the CDC recommends universal screening of all children at age 1 and 2 years and of children 36 to 72 months of age not previously screened.

Diagnostic testing of venous blood should be performed for all patients with elevated BLLs >10 μg/dL at a follow-up interval based on degree of elevation of BLL (see Table 102–5). In 2006, the USPSTF revised its previous recommendation in favor of high-risk screening and found insufficient evidence to recommend routine screening for screening for high-risk children 1 to 5 years of age (USPSTF I) and recommended against screening of normal-risk children (USPSTF D).

TABLE 102–4. BASIC LEAD PERSONAL RISK PROFILE

1	Does your child live in or regularly visit a house that was built before 1950? This question could apply to a facility such as a home day-care center or the home of a babysitter or relative
2	Does your child live in or regularly visit a house built before 1978 with recent or ongoing renovations or remodeling (within the last 6 months)?
3	Does your child have a sibling or playmate who has or did have lead poisoning?

(Reprinted from Centers for Disease Control and Prevention. *Screening Young Children for Lead Poisoning: Guidance for State and Local Public Health Officials.* US Department of Health and Human Services; 1997.)

E. **Newborn screening.** The AAP and other authorities have recommended that newborn screening be performed according to each state's regulations. Using new tandem mass spectroscopy technology, several states have recently expanded required screening to 30 or more conditions. National authorities have made recommendations for the following important conditions:

1. **Hypothyroidism.** The AAP, American Thyroid Association (ATA), and USPSTF (USPSTF A) have recommended that all neonates be screened for congenital hypothyroidism between 2 and 6 days of life. Care should be taken to ensure that infants born at home, ill at birth, or transferred between hospitals in the first week of life are screened before 7 days of life.

2. **Phenylketonuria (PKU).** The AAFP and USPSTF (USPSTF A) have recommended that all infants be screened for PKU prior to discharge from the nursery. Premature infants and those with illnesses should be tested at or near 7 days of age. Infants tested before 24 hours of age should receive a repeat screening. According to the USPSTF, this should occur by the time the infant is 2 weeks of age.

3. **Hemoglobinopathies.** The Sickle Cell Disease Guideline Panel of the Agency for Health Care Policy and Research, US Public Health Service, has recommended universal screening of newborns for sickle cell disease. This recommendation has been endorsed by the AAP, American Nurses Association, and AMA. The USPSTF has also recommended neonatal screening for sickle hemoglobinopathies (USPSTF A), but it has stated that whether screening should be universal or targeted to high-risk groups should depend on the proportion of high-risk persons in the screening area. All screening must be accompanied by comprehensive counseling and treatment services.

F. **Thyroid function.** No authorities recommend screening of asymptomatic adults for thyroid dysfunctions. The ACOG recommends measurement of thyroid-stimulating hormone (TSH) levels adult women with a strong family history of thyroid disease or autoimmune disease. The USPSTF has found insufficient evidence for screening of asymptomatic persons, stating that although the yield of screening is greater in certain high-risk groups (e.g., postpartum women, people with Down syndrome, and the elderly), there is poor evidence that screening these groups leads to clinically important benefits (USPSTF I).

III. **Sensory Screening**

A. **Hearing**

1. **Children.** The Joint Committee on Infant Hearing (composed of the AAP, American Speech-Language-Hearing Association, American Academy of Otolaryngology—Head and Neck Surgery, and American Academy of Audiology) has endorsed universal screening of all neonates. These authorities recommend screening neonates for hearing impairment prior to hospital discharge, but not later than 3 months of age.

TABLE 102–5. SCHEDULE FOR DIAGNOSTIC TESTING OF A CHILD WITH AN ELEVATED BLOOD LEAD LEVEL ON A SCREENING TEST

If Result of Screening Test (μ/dL) Is:	Perform Diagnostic Test on Venous Blood Within:
10–19	3 mo
20–44	1 mo–1 wk*
45–59	48 h
60–69	24 h
≥70	Immediately as an emergency laboratory test

*The higher the screening blood lead level, the more urgent the need for a diagnostic test.
(Reprinted from Centers for Disease Control and Prevention. *Screening Young Children for Lead Poisoning: Guidance for State and Local Public Health Officials.* Washington, D.C.: US Department of Health and Human Services; 1997.)

The Joint Committee on Infant Hearing has identified recurrent or persistent otitis media with effusion for at least 3 months to be a risk factor requiring screening. The USPSTF has found insufficient evidence to recommend for or against universal screening of neonates (USPSTF I). The AAP has recommended routine screening of asymptomatic children with pure-tone audiometry at ages 3, 4, 5, 10, 12, 15, and 18 years.

   2. **Adults.** All major authorities recommend screening older adults for hearing impairment. The American Speech-Language-Hearing Association recommends using a hearing handicap questionnaire or pure-tone audiometry. The USPSTF recommends first questioning patients about hearing impairment and performing audiometry on those reporting abnormalities (USPSTF B). Patients found to have evidence of hearing loss by screening should be considered for referral to a specialist for comprehensive audiologic evaluation, especially if they feel handicapped by the hearing loss. Because approximately 10% of persons with hearing loss are amenable to medical or surgical treatment and because some patients are incorrectly identified as having hearing loss by screening, patients should not be referred directly to a hearing aid dealer. The primary care clinician should make sure that appropriate follow-up management is provided to all patients referred for audiologic evaluation. Patients may need considerable support and training to use their hearing aids effectively.

B. **Vision**

   1. **Children.** Recommendations regarding vision screening for children vary among authorities. The AAP has recommended questioning of parents regarding a child's vision at well-child visits, with the first objective test of visual acuity at age 3 years. If the child is uncooperative, this should be rescheduled 6 months later. Subsequent objective testing is recommended at 4, 5, 10, 12, 15, and 18 years of age. The USPSTF recommends screening to detect amblyopia, strabismus, and defects in visual acuity in children younger than 5 years (USPSTF B) and states that the choice of tests should be influenced by the child's age. During the first year of life, strabismus can be assessed by the cover test and the Hirschberg light reflex test. Screening children younger than 3 years for visual acuity typically requires testing by specially trained personnel. Newer automated techniques can be used to test these children. In children older than 3 years, stereopsis (the ability of both eyes to function together) can be assessed with the Random Dot E test or Titmus Fly Stereotest; visual acuity can be assessed by tests such as the HOTV chart, Lea symbols, or the tumbling E. The USPSTF has found insufficient evidence to recommend for or against routine visual acuity testing of schoolchildren (USPSTF I), because refractive errors of consequence present symptomatically and respond to corrective lenses without lasting effects.

   2. **Adults.** Recommendations for vision screening of adults vary considerably among authorities.

      a. **Visual acuity.** All major authorities recommend routine visual acuity screening for normal-risk adults beginning at age 65 (USPSTF B).

      b. **Eye examination.** The American Academy of Ophthalmology recommends screening for glaucoma as part of the comprehensive adult medical eye evaluation, starting at the age of 20, with a frequency depending on an individual's age and other risk factors for glaucoma: Primary care providers can perform the screening by measuring the intraocular pressure and evaluating the optic nerve if they have the appropriate skills and equipment. The Department of Veterans Affairs recommends that every veteran more than the age of 40 be screened for glaucoma in a primary care setting with a frequency depending on his or her age, ethnicity, and family history: The USPSTF has found insufficient evidence to recommend routine screening for glaucoma (USPSTF I), stating that it is unclear whether earlier detection and treatment of people with increased intraocular pressure or early primary open-angle glaucoma reduces impairment in vision-related function or quality of life.

         The National Eye Institute recommends comprehensive eye examinations every 2 years starting at age 60, with examinations beginning at age 40 for African Americans. All authorities recommend frequent, yearly, comprehensive eye examinations by eye care specialists for patients with diabetes mellitus.

IV. **Mental Health and Cognition**

   A. **Depression.** The USPSTF recommends screening adults for depression in clinical practices that have systems in place to assure accurate diagnosis, effective treatment, and follow-up (USPSTF B). The USPSTF found limited evidence on the accuracy and reliability of screening tests in children and adolescents and limited evidence on the effectiveness of therapy in children and adolescents identified in primary care settings (USPSTF I). Although formal screening tools (such as the Beck Depression Inventory or the Zung Self-Assessment Depression Scale) are available, the USPSTF states that asking two simple questions ("Over the past 2 weeks, have you felt down, depressed, or hopeless?" and "Over the past 2 weeks, have you felt little interest or pleasure in doing things?") may be as effective as using long instruments. The AAP recommends that pediatricians ask questions about depression in history-taking with adolescents, and the AMA recommends screening for depression in treating adolescents who may be at risk because of family problems, drug or alcohol use, or other risk factors.

B. Dementia. Although instruments such as the Mini-Mental State Examination are often used for screening older adults, the USPSTF has found insufficient evidence to recommend for or against routine screening of asymptomatic older adults for dementia (USPSTF I). The USPSTF recommends that clinicians assess cognitive function whenever cognitive impairment or deterioration is suspected.

V. Infectious Disease

A. Hepatitis C. In recognition of the heavy burden of disease caused by hepatitis C (1.8% of the US population infected, >US$600 million in medical and work-loss expenses annually), the CDC has recommended screening of high-risk populations. The US Preventive Services Task Force has found insufficient evidence to recommend screening of high-risk individuals because there is limited evidence that available treatments are effective in preventing cirrhosis in patients with asymptomatic HCV infection (USPSTF I) and has recommended against screening of the normal-risk population because of the potential adverse effects of unnecessary biopsies and labeling (USPSTF D).

B. Human immunodeficiency virus. All major authorities recommend that HIV screening be offered to patients at risk: those with another sexually transmitted disease (STD), homosexual and bisexual men; past or present injection drug users; persons with a history of prostitution or multiple sexual partners; persons whose past (or present) sexual partners are HIV-infected or injection drug users, or both; patients with a history of blood transfusion between 1978 and 1985; and persons born in, or with long-term residence in, a community in which HIV is prevalent (USPSTF A). The AMA also recommends offering testing and counseling to high-risk persons receiving family planning services or undergoing surgery. In 2006, the CDC recommended that all individuals between 13 and 64 yeas of age be screened for HIV regardless of recognized risk factors. In 2007, the USPSTF, after reviewing recent evidence, stated that it could make no recommendation for or against screening of individuals without risk factors (USPSTF C). Because of the high effectiveness of prenatal antiviral treatments, all major authorities recommend universal, voluntary HIV testing of all pregnant women (USPSTF A).

C. Other STDs

1. Chlamydia. The AAP and AMA have advocated screening all sexually active adolescents. The AAP recommends annual urine leukocyte esterase dipstick tests for all sexually active adolescents. The USPSTF recommends screening all sexually active females younger than 25 and other high-risk adult women for Chlamydia (USPSTF A). Chlamydia risk factors include a history of prior STDs, a new partner or multiple sex partners, inconsistent barrier contraceptive use, cervical ectopy, and being unmarried. The USPSTF has made no recommendation for screening women 25 or older who are not at high risk (USPSTF C) and has found insufficient evidence to recommend screening men (USPSTF I).

2. Gonorrhea. All major authorities recommend screening women at high risk for gonorrhea (USPSTF B). Women at risk include commercial sex workers, those with repeated episodes of gonorrhea, and women younger than age 25 with two or more sex partners in the last year. The USPSTF has found insufficient evidence to recommend for or against screening asymptomatic males at high risk for or gonorrhea (USPSTF I) and has recommended against screening individuals not at high risk for gonorrhea (USPSTF D). Although dipstick leukocyte testing is convenient and inexpensive, its positive predictive value has been found to be as low as 11% for chlamydia and 30% for gonorrhea. Thus, confirmation with more specific tests is required for all positive results.

3. Syphilis. All major authorities recommend that screening be performed for persons at high risk for infection (USPSTF A). These persons may include sexual partners of known syphilis cases, those with multiple sexual partners—especially in high-prevalence areas; prostitutes or those who trade sex for drugs, and males who engage in sex with other males. The USPSTF has recommended against the routine screening of normal-risk populations (USPSTF D). Because the causative agent of syphilis cannot be cultured, screening relies on serology. A nontreponemal test, either the VDRL or RPR, is recommended for initial screening. Because the specificity of these tests is limited, follow-up testing with a treponemal test, such as the FTA (fluorescent treponemal antibody), is required for positive results. Because the sensitivity of nontreponemal tests may be as low as 75% in primary syphilis, patients who have had recent contact with a person with a documented case of syphilis should be treated, even if serologic tests are negative.

D. Tuberculosis (TB). All major authorities recommend screening of persons at high risk for TB (USPSTF A). In general, authorities have not specified how often high-risk persons should be screened, although the AAP has recommended annual screening for children at risk. Populations at risk include (1) medically underserved, low-income populations, including those of African American, Hispanic, Asian, Native American, and Alaskan Native heritage; (2) foreign-born persons from high-prevalence countries (e.g., Asia, Africa, and Latin America); (3) persons in close contact with infectious TB cases (sharing accommodations as well as playing or working in the same enclosed area); (4) alcoholics and injection drug users; (5) residents of high-risk environments, including long-term care facilities, correctional institutions, and mental institutions; and (6) persons with medical conditions known to substantially increase the risk of TB, such as HIV infection, diabetes mellitus, and chronic renal failure.

The appropriate criterion for defining a positive skin-test reaction depends on the likelihood of TB exposure and the risk of TB if exposure has occurred. For persons with HIV infection, close contacts of infectious cases, and those with fibrotic lesions on chest radiograph, a reaction of ≥ 5 mm is considered positive. For other at-risk persons, including all infants and children younger than 4 years, a reaction of ≥ 10 mm is considered positive. Persons who are not likely to be infected with *Mycobacterium tuberculosis* should generally not be skin tested because the predictive value of a positive skin test in low-risk populations is poor. If a skin test is performed on a person who is not in a high-risk category or who is not exposed in a high-risk environment, a cutoff point of ≥ 15 mm is considered positive, although prophylaxis with isoniazid is not necessarily recommended for these persons.

In 2002, the FDA approved the use of a blood test, QuantiFERON-TB Test, for screening. Like skin testing, this test should not be used to screen normal-risk persons. Children (younger than 17 years), pregnant women, or persons with suspected tuberculosis should not be tested with this method. Positive test results should be confirmed with a skin test.

VI. Cancer Screening

A. Breast cancer

1. Clinical breast examination (CBE). Most major authorities recommend regular CBEs for women aged 50 years and older. The American Cancer Society and ACOG recommend annual breast examinations in this age range. The USPSTF has found insufficient evidence to recommend for against CBE for screening at any age (USPSTF I). The ACS recommends CBE every 3 years for women aged 20 to 39 years and annually thereafter. ACOG recommends CBE annually beginning at age 18. In performing the CBE, the examiner should be systematic, palpating every portion of the breast with the patient in both an upright and supine position. One of the best indicators of examiner accuracy is thought to be the amount of time spent.

2. Mammography and MRI. Most major authorities now recommend routine mammography for women aged 40 years and older. The ACS recommends annual mammography beginning at age 40. The USPSTF recommends mammography every 1 to 2 years for all women older than 40 years (USPSTF B). The ACOG and the National Cancer Institute recommend mammography every 1 to 2 years for women aged 40 to 49 years and annually thereafter. In 2007, the American College of Physicians recommended that clinicians base screening mammography decisions for women 40 to 49 years of age on benefits and harms of screening, as well as on a woman's preferences and breast cancer risk profile.

The clinician should keep in mind that the sensitivity of a mammogram is limited—approximately 90%. Thus, symptoms and positive physical findings should not be dismissed strictly on the basis of a negative mammogram result. The specificity is similarly limited; thus, women should be counseled against alarm based strictly on a positive mammogram result.

TABLE 102–6. RISK FACTORS FOR BRCA MUTATION TESTING

Askenazi Jewish
- First-degree relative with breast or cervical cancer
- Two second-degree relatives on the same side of the family with breast or ovarian cancer

Others:
- Two first relatives with breast cancer, one of whom received the diagnosis at age 50 years or younger
- A combination of ≥3 first- or second-degree relatives with breast cancer regardless of age at diagnosis;
- Both breast and ovarian cancer among first- or second-degree relatives
- A first-degree relative with bilateral breast cancer
- ≥2 first- or second-degree relatives with ovarian cancer
- A first- or second-degree relative with both breast and ovarian cancer
- A male relative with breast cancer

In 2007, the American Cancer Society issued recommendations that women with a 20% to 25% lifetime risk of breast cancer should receive MRI screening as an adjunct to mammography. Women at such high risk include those with BRCA genetic mutations, a strong family history or breast or ovarian cancer, and women who have treated for Hodgkin Disease with radiation. Evidence regarding when to start such dual screening is unclear, although ACS has stated that most women at such high risk should begin annual screening by 30 years of age.

3. **Genetic Testing.** In 2005, the USPSTF recommended that women whose family history is associated with an increased risk for deleterious mutations in *BRCA1* or *BRCA2* genes be referred for genetic counseling and evaluation for *BRCA* testing (USPSTF B). Women with a *BRCA1* or *BRCA2* mutation have a high risk (35%–84%) of developing breast cancer by 70 years of age. See Table 102–6 for risk factors indicating the need for BRCA testing. The USPSTF has recommended against genetic testing for women not at increased risk (USPSTF D).

B. **Cervical cancer.** All major authorities recommend routine Papanicolaou (Pap) smears for sexually active adolescent and adult women (USPSTF A). The USPSTF and ACS recommend beginning screening within 3 years of initiation of sexual activity or by age 21, depending on which comes first. The ACS recommends annual Pap smears (or every 2 years if the liquid-based cytology is used (until the age of 30. For women older than 30 this can be decreased to every 2 to 3 years (using either conventional or liquid-based cytology) if the last three annual Pap smears have been normal. The USPSTF recommends screening at least every 3 years and recommends against screening in women after age 65 if recent pap smears have been normal and they are not otherwise at risk for cervical cancer (USPSTF D). ACS recommendations suggest stopping cervical cancer screening at age 70 if 3 or more screenings have been normal and no screenings have been abnormal in the last 10 years. The USPSTF recommends screening in older women who have not been previously screened, when information about previous screening is unavailable, or when screening is unlikely to have occurred in the past (e.g., among women from countries without screening programs).

The use of an endocervical brush and wooden spatula provides the best yield of adequate samples, defined as containing endocervical cells. Although the presence of endocervical cells has not been demonstrated to result in improved clinical outcomes, it remains the accepted standard for adequacy of Pap smears. The USPSTF recommends against screening women who are without a cervix because of hysterectomy (USPSTF D) and found insufficient evidence to recommend the use of new screening technologies, such as liquid-based cytology, human papillomavirus (HPV) testing, and computerized rescreening (USPSTF I). The ACS states that the use of liquid-based cytology is acceptable and that with HPV testing the frequency of cervical cytology testing in women older than 30 years may be decreased to every 3 years.

C. **Colorectal cancer**
1. **Digital rectal examination.** Digital rectal examination is no longer recommended by major authorities as a modality for screening for colorectal cancer because of its poor sensitivity (<10%).
2. **Fecal occult blood testing.** All major authorities now recommend annual fecal occult blood testing for normal-risk persons beginning at age 50 (USPSTF A). Some authorities, such as the USPSTF and ACS, state that its use may be optional if sigmoidoscopy or colonoscopy is performed regularly. The sensitivity and specificity of fecal

occult blood testing are limited, resulting in many false-negative and false-positive results. The positive predictive value may be <10%. Those undergoing annual screening have a lifetime risk of approximately 40% of experiencing a false-positive result. The improved mortality attributed to screening may actually be partially because of the high rate of sigmoidoscopy and colonoscopy used to evaluate incidental false-positive fecal occult blood tests. Rehydration of samples with a few drops of water before development improves sensitivity but significantly decreases specificity. Clinicians should keep in mind that, because of limited sensitivity and the intermittent nature of colorectal cancer bleeding, cancer cannot be ruled out by repeated fecal occult blood testing after a positive result.

  3. **Sigmoidoscopy.** All major authorities now recommend sigmoidoscopy every 5 years as an acceptable screening tool for persons beginning at age 50 (USPSTF A). According to the USPSTF and ACS, this screening can be performed in addition to or in conjunction with annual fecal occult blood testing. The sensitivity of sigmoidoscopy is limited by the length of the scope, with approximately 40% of malignancies being beyond the reach of a 60-cm flexible scope. For this reason, some authorities recommend offering procedures that are able to examine the entire colon, such as colonoscopy and barium enema.

  4. **Colonoscopy.** Several authorities (ACS, American Gastroenterological Association [AGA], and USPSTF) recommend colonoscopy every 10 years—beginning at age 50 for normal-risk patients—as an alternative to fecal occult blood and sigmoidoscopy screening. The USPSTF stated that it is unclear whether the increased accuracy of colonoscopy compared with alternative screening methods offsets the procedure's additional complications, inconvenience, and costs.

  5. **Barium enema.** Several authorities (ACS, AGA, and USPSTF) have recommended a barium enema every 5 years—beginning at age 50 for normal-risk patients—as an alternative to other screening modalities. The USPSTF stated that there is no direct evidence that barium enema screening is effective in reducing mortality rates.

  6. **Virtual colonoscopy.** The development of new radiographic techniques now enables detailed "visualization" of the colon without endoscopy. However, this technique does not allow for concomitant biopsy and both the USPSTF and ACS have stated that the evidence is insufficient to recommend its use in routine screening.

D. Oral cancer. The ACS recommends periodic oral cavity examinations beginning at 20 years of age as part of a cancer-related check-up. The USPSTF states that there is insufficient evidence to recommend for or against screening examinations (USPSTF I), but states that clinicians should be alert to the possibility of oral cancer when treating patients who use tobacco or alcohol.

E. Ovarian cancer

  1. **Bimanual pelvic examination.** The USPSTF and ACOG do not recommend screening for ovarian cancer with bimanual pelvic examination. The ACS continues to recommend that bimanual examination be performed as a part of the routine gynecologic examination. The main limitation of pelvic examination for screening is its limited sensitivity, with many tumors becoming large in size before becoming detectable by examination.

  2. **Tumor markers.** No major authorities have recommended screening normal-risk women using tumor markers, such as CA-125 (USPSTF D). A National Institutes of Health consensus conference has recommended using annual CA-125 measurements and transvaginal ultrasonography to screen women at particularly high risk because of hereditary cancer syndrome. Because of limited specificity and low prevalence of the disease, the use of tumor makers for screening in normal-risk populations results in large numbers of false-positive results.

  3. **Ultrasonography.** No major authority currently recommends the use of ultrasonography to screen normal-risk women, largely because of its poor positive predictive value (USPSTF D). As previously described, some authorities have recommended its use in combination with tumor marker measurement to screen high-risk women.

  4. **Genetic testing.** The USPSTF has recommended that women at high risk for BRCA 1 or BRAC 2 (see Table 102–6) genetic mutations be counseled regarding genetic testing (USPSTF B). Women with *BRCA1* or *BRCA2* mutations are at a 10% to 50% risk of ovarian cancer by 70 years of age and may benefit from intensive screening or prophylactic surgery.

F. Prostate cancer. The ACS and American Urological Association (AUA) recommend offering annual digital rectal examination (DRE) and prostate-specific antigen (PSA) testing for normal-risk men beginning at age 50, and beginning at age 45 for men at high risk because of being African American or having a first-degree relative with a history of prostate cancer. The USPSTF found insufficient evidence to recommend for or against routine screening with DRE or PSA testing and, like other authorities, recommends that men be informed of the uncertain benefits and possible harms of prostate cancer screening (USPSTF I). The DRE has limited sensitivity (33%–69%) and positive predictive value (6%–33%) for detecting prostate cancer in asymptomatic men. The positive predictive value of PSA testing is estimated to be 10% to 35%, thus leading to many unnecessary biopsies. Efforts to refine PSA testing using age, prostate size based on ultrasound findings, and rates of change in PSA over time may lead to improvements in sensitivity and specificity. No major authority currently recommends using transrectal ultrasonography (TRUS) to screen for prostate cancer. Because TRUS cannot distinguish between benign and malignant nodules, its positive predictive value is lower than that of PSA testing.

G. **Skin cancer.** The ACS recommends skin examinations periodically beginning at 20 years of age. The ACOG states that skin examination may be a component of the annual examination adolescents and women at increased risk because of increased recreational or occupational exposure to sunlight, a family or personal history of skin cancer, or clinical evidence of precursor lesions. The USPSTF has found insufficient evidence to recommend for or against routine skin examinations by primary care clinicians, while recommending that they remain alert for skin lesions with malignant features, particularly in patients at risk (USPSTF I). Risk groups include fair-skinned men and women older than 65 years, patients with atypical moles, and those with >50 moles. Major characteristics that make a lesion suspicious for malignant melanoma may be remembered by the ABCDs: A, asymmetry; B, irregular borders; C, variation in color; and D, diameter greater than 6 mm.

H. **Testicular cancer.** The AUA recommends annual testicular examinations beginning at age 15. The ACS recommends examinations periodic examinations beginning at 20 years of age. The USPSTF recommends against routine screening (USPSTF D), stating that better evaluation of testicular problems may be more effective than widespread screening as a means of promoting early detection. A major factor against screening is the excellent prognosis of testicular cancer, regardless of how it is detected.

I. **Thyroid cancer.** The ACS recommends thyroid palpation periodically beginning at 20 years of age. The USPSTF has found inadequate evidence to recommend for or against routine screening by thyroid palpation (USPSTF I), while stating that screening of persons at high risk because of a history of external upper body radiation in infancy and childhood may be justified on other grounds, such as patient preference or anxiety.

REFERENCES

American Academy of Family Physicians, Commission on Science. *Summary of Recommendatons for Clinical Preventive Services.* Version 6.3, March, 2007. http://www.aafp.org/online/etc/medialib/ aafp_org/documents/clinical/clin_recs/cps.Par.0001.File.tmp/ Microsoft%20Word%20-%20Approved %20March%202007%20CPS.pdf. Accessed August 28, 2007.

American Academy of Pediatrics, Committee on Practice and Ambulatory Medicine: Recommendations for preventive pediatric health care. *Pediatrics.* 2000;105:645. http://www.aap.org/healthtopics/ commped.cfm. Accessed August 30, 2007.

American Cancer Society: *Guidelines for Early Detection of Cancer.* American Cancer Society. www.acs.org. Accessed August 23, 2007.

American College of Obstetricians and Gynecologists. Committee Opinion No. 280. The role of the generalist obstetrician–gynecologist in the early detection of ovarian cancer. *Gynecol Oncol.* 2002; 87(3):237-239.

American College of Obstetricians and Gynecologists: Routine Cancer Screening. ACOG Committee Opinion356, *Obstet Gynecol.* 2006; 108:1611-1613.

American College of Obstetricians and Gynecologists. Primary and Preventive Care: Periodic Assessments. Committee Opinion 357.*Obstet Gynecol.* 2006; 108:1615-1622.

American College of Physicians. Screening mammography for women 40 to 49 years of age: a clinical practice guideline from the American College of Physicians. *Ann Intern Med.* 2007; 146:511-515.

American Diabetes Association. Standards of Medical Care in Diabetes—2007. *Diabetes Care.* 2007;30: S4-41.

Centers for Disease Control and Prevention. Screening tests to detect *Chlamydia trachomatis* and *Neisseria gonorrhoeae* infections—2002. *MMWR.* 2002; 51:RR-15:1-27. http://www.cdc.gov/STD/ LabGuidelines.

US Department of Health and Human Services. *The Seventh Report of the Joint National Committee on Prevention, Detection, Evaluation, and Treatment of High Blood Pressure (JNC 7)*. http://www.nhlbi. nih.gov/guidelines/hypertension/index.htm. Accessed 20, 2007.

US Preventive Services Task Force. *US Preventive Task Force Recommendations*. http://www.ahrq. gov/clinic/uspstfix.htm#Recommendations; http://www.ahrq.gov/clinic/cps3dix.htm. Accessed August 23, 2007.

---

103 Chemoprophylaxis

Paul E. Lewis III, MD

KEY POINTS

- Age of household contacts and extent of exposure are the factors that determine need for meningitis prophylaxis.
- Aspirin has proven efficacy for primary and secondary prevention of myocardial infarction and ischemic stroke.
- Prophylaxis for endocarditis prior to dental procedures in now indicated in only a small subset of patients.
- All women of childbearing age capable of becoming pregnant should consume folic acid daily in order to reduce their risk of having a child with a neural tube defect.
- Patients who have had rheumatic fever need long term prophylaxis against group A strep.
- All pregnant women should be screened for Group B Streptococcal Disease (GBS) and those with a positive test need intrapartum prophylaxis.

I. **Definition.** Prophylaxis is derived from the Greek (*pro phulax*), which means "to put up a guard before it is necessary." Chemoprophylaxis is the use of a chemical or medication to prevent a disease. Chemoprophylaxis is widely utilized in modern medicine from preventing infectious diseases to treating chronic disease states.

II. **Bacterial Meningitis**

  A. **Pathogens**

   1. *Hemophilus influenzae*

     a. The mortality rate is approximately 5%, with 20% to 30% of survivors having neurologic sequelae.

     b. The risk of infection in a 1996 national study was 6% in children younger than 1 year, 2.1% in those younger than 4 years, and 0% in those older than 5 years.

     c. In the United States, the incidence is greatest in Native Americans, blacks, those in lower socioeconomic groups, and those with complement or immunoglobulin deficiencies.

       (1) The near universal administration of the *H. influenzae* type b vaccine has significantly reduced the incidence of this disease since 1987 and made the need for prophylaxis relatively rare.

   2. *Neisseria meningitidis*

     a. The mortality rate is approximately 10%, with children younger than 1 year of age having the greatest incidence.

     b. Vaccines against serotypes a and c have been developed, but just more than 50% of meningococcal infections in the United States are caused by type b, for which there is no vaccine.

     c. Meningococci are carried by 15% of contacts in their throats, but only 3% to 4% will carry a pathogenic strain. Eradication of this pharyngeal carriage and subsequent transmission is the goal of chemoprophylaxis.

  B. **Prophylaxis**

   1. *H. influenzae* type b meningitis

     a. **Criteria for prophylaxis**

       (1) There is no need to for prophylaxis in families with a child with *H. influenzae* meningitis if no one else in the environment is younger than 4 years. (SOR **C**)

      (2) If there is another child in the household younger than 4 years, the entire family (including the infected child) should receive prophylaxis. (SOR **C**)

      (3) Personnel of day-care centers **should receive prophylaxis** when two or more cases occur within 60 days. (SOR **C**)

      (4) Prophylaxis is not needed when all children in day care are older than 4 years.

      (5) Prophylaxis for day-care contacts >20 h/wk should be considered in a setting where children are younger than 4 years.

   b. Regimen. Rifampin, administered orally at 20 mg/kg/d in one dose for 4 days (maximum dose, 600 mg/d).

  2. *N. meningitidis* **meningitis**

   a. Criteria for prophylaxis

      (1) Household, day-care, and nursery school contacts. (SOR **B**).

      (2) Personnel who have had contact with oral secretions of the index case. (SOR **C**)

      (3) Prophylaxis is not indicated if exposure to the index case is brief. This includes most health-care workers unless they have been directly exposed to respiratory secretions via intubation, suctioning, or oral care. (SOR **C**)

      (4) **Travelers on an airplane seated next to the index patient for more than 8 hours. (**SOR **C**)

      (5) Protection is only temporary, as colonization rates rise quickly back to baseline by 6 to 12 months post prophylaxis.

   b. Regimen

      (1) Rifampin, administered orally every 12 hours at 5 mg/kg per dose in children younger than 1 year, 10 mg/kg per dose in children aged 1 to 12 years, and 600 mg in adults and children aged older than 12 years for a total of four doses (maximum 600 mg/d).

      (2) Ciprofloxacin, administered as a single oral 500-mg dose in adults, is equally as effective if rifampin is not tolerated.

      (3) Ceftriaxone, administered as a single intramuscular dose of 125 mg for children younger than 12 years and a dose of 250 mg for adults.

      (4) All three regimens have 90% to 95% efficacy in eradicating nasopharyngeal carriage of *N. meningitidis* and reduce transmission rate to zero. (SOR **B**)

      (5) Prophylaxis is most effective when used within 24 hours and may have some benefit up to 14 days later.

III. Cardiovascular Disease

  A. Primary prevention

   1. Large-scale meta-analysis clearly demonstrates that aspirin reduces the risk of a first myocardial infarction (MI) by at least one-third. (SOR **A**)

   2. Any recommendation to begin aspirin therapy should rely on the physician's clinical judgment after careful consideration of risk and patient preferences.

   3. The US Preventive Services Task Force "strongly recommends" that aspirin be considered in all patients whose Framingham 10-year risk score is 6% or greater (Tables 103–1 and 103–2). Other national organizations make very similar recommendations. (SOR **A**)

   4. Dosage recommendations in primary prevention. Doses of 75 to 160 mg/d are as effective as higher doses with a lower risk of gastrointestinal (GI) side effects. (SOR **B**)

   5. Aspirin also appears to reduce the severity of a new episode if its use was instituted prior to the event.

  B. Acute MI

   1. The Second International Study of Infarct Trial (ISIS-2) randomized patients on aspirin, intravenous streptokinase, both agents, or neither drug during an acute MI. Aspirin was demonstrated to provide a significant reduction in mortality at 5 weeks (23%), which was equivalent to intravenous streptokinase. The absolute mortality reduction was 24 vascular deaths prevented per 1000 patients treated. Aspirin was also demonstrated to significantly reduce the number of nonfatal MIs and strokes. There was no increase in risk of major bleeding/hemorrhage. Aspirin was by far the most cost-effective agent.

   2. Dosage recommendations for acute MI

    a. A loading dose of preferably 325 mg of uncoated aspirin should be administered within 24 hours of an acute MI. (SOR **A**)

    b. If the only preparation available is enteric-coated, then the tablet should be chewed or crushed.

TABLE 103–1. FRAMINGHAM POINT SCORES IN MEN*, †

Age (years)	Points
20–34	−9
35–39	−4
40–44	0
45–49	3
50–54	6
55–59	8
60–64	10
65–69	11
70–74	12
75–79	13

Total cholesterol mg/dL (mmol/L)	Age 20–39	Age 40–49	Age 50–59	Age 60–69	Age 70–79
<160 (3.4)	0	0	0	0	0
160–199 (3.4–5.15)	4	3	2	1	0
200–239 (5.17–6.18)	7	5	3	1	0
240–279 (6.2–7.21)	9	6	4	2	1
≥280	11	8	5	3	1

	Age 20–39	Age 40–49	Age 50–59	Age 60–69	Age 70–79
Nonsmoker	0	0	0	0	0
Smoker	8	5	3	1	1

HDL cholesterol mg/dL (mmol/L)	Points
≥60 (1.55)	−1
50–59 (1.29–1.53)	0
40–49 (1.03–1.27)	1
<40 (1.03)	2

Systolic blood pressure (mm Hg)	Untreated	Treated
<120	0	0
120–129	0	1
130–139	1	2
140–159	1	2
≥160	2	3

Point total	10-year risk (%)	Point total	10-year risk (%)
0	1	10	6
1	1	11	8
2	1	12	10
3	1	13	12
4	1	14	16
5	2	15	20
6	2	16	25
7	3	≥17	≥30
8	4		
9	5		

*The point total is determined in each category and the 10-year risk determined in the bottom row.
†These risk estimates for the development of coronary heart disease do not account for all important cardiovascular risk factors. Not included are diabetes mellitus, which is considered a coronary heart disease equivalent, alcohol intake, and the serum C-reactive protein concentration.
HDL, high-density lipoprotein.
(Adapted from Adult Treatment Panel III at http://www.nhlbi.nih.gov/.)

TABLE 103–2. FRAMINGHAM POINT SCORES IN WOMEN[*,†]

Age (years)	Points
20–34	−7
35–39	−3
40–44	0
45–49	3
50–54	6
55–59	8
60–64	10
65–69	12
70–74	14
75–79	16

Total cholesterol mg/dL (mmol/L)	Age 20–39	Age 40–49	Age 50–59	Age 60–69	Age 70–79
<160 (3.4)	0	0	0	0	0
160–199 (3.4–5.15)	4	3	2	1	1
200–239 (5.17–6.18)	8	6	4	2	1
240–279 (6.2–7.21)	11	8	5	3	2
≥280 (7.24)	13	10	7	4	2

	Age 20–39	Age 40–49	Age 50–59	Age 60–69	Age 70–79
Nonsmoker	0	0	0	0	0
Smoker	9	7	4	2	1

HDL cholesterol mg/dL (mmol/L)	Points
≥60	−1
50–59 (1.29–1.53)	0
40–49 (1.03–1.27)	1
<40 (1.03)	2

Systolic blood pressure (mm Hg)	Untreated	Treated
<120	0	0
120–129	1	3
130–139	2	4
140–159	3	5
≥160	4	6

Point Total	10-year risk (%)	Point total	10-year risk (%)
<9	<1	18	6
9	1	19	8
10	1	20	11
11	1	21	14
12	1	22	17
13	2	23	22
14	2	24	27
15	3	≥25	≥30
16	4		
17	5		

[*]The point total is determined in each category and the 10-year risk determined in the bottom row.
[†]These risk estimates for the development of coronary heart disease do not account for all important cardiovascular risk factors. Not included are diabetes mellitus, which is considered a coronary heart disease equivalent, alcohol intake, and the serum C-reactive protein concentration.
HDL, high-density lipoprotein.
(Adapted from Adult Treatment Panel III at http://www.nhlbi.nih.gov/.)

      c. Therapy should be continued at a dose of 75 to 162 mg (enteric-coated) indefinitely. (SOR **A**)
3. Several clinical trials have established the efficacy of aspirin therapy in non-ST segment elevation coronary syndromes, in non-Q-wave MIs, and in unstable angina. Aspirin significantly reduced the risk of an acute MI or death at 5, 30, and 90 days and at 1 year of treatment when used in these settings.
4. **Recommendations for aspirin in non-MI coronary syndromes**
    a. Aspirin should be considered for all patients with new-onset angina, angina at rest, or crescendo angina. (SOR **A**)
    b. Patient with GI distress may tolerate a lower dose of aspirin or can take clopidogrel or ticlopidine.

C. Acute stroke
1. The International Stroke Trial (IST) demonstrated that aspirin-treated patients had significant reductions in the 14-day recurrence of ischemic stroke (2.8% versus 3.9%) and in the combined outcome of nonfatal stroke or death (11.3% versus 12.4%) when administered within 48 hours of the onset of symptoms compared to subcutaneous heparin or no treatment.
2. The Chinese Acute Stroke Trial (CAST) demonstrated a 14% reduction in total mortality at 4 weeks in the aspirin group compared to placebo.
3. These two trials demonstrate that aspirin therapy is crucial in the acute stroke setting, with an overall reduction of 13 deaths or significant residual impairment per 1000 patients treated at a 6-month follow-up.
4. **Recommendations in acute stroke**
    a. Aspirin should be administered to all patients with acute ischemic stroke if no contraindication exists. (SOR **A**)
    b. Dosing should fall between 162.5 and 325 mg based on current literature. Enteric-coated preparations should be chewed or crushed initially. (SOR **A**)
    c. Therapy should continue indefinitely and the risk–benefit ratio must be examined individually.
    d. Other antiplatelet drugs including clopidogrel, ticlopidine, or the combinations of aspirin and dipyridamole may be equally effective after the acute event for those who cannot tolerate aspirin, but aspirin should be used initially. (SOR **B**) (See Chapter 86 for dosages.)

D. Atrial fibrillation (AF)
1. **Aspirin**
    a. Several trials have attempted to demonstrate the efficacy of aspirin in the prevention of thromboembolic events in patients with AF, with conflicting results.
    b. Meta-analysis of the trials (including the AFASAK trial and the SPAF-I trial) reveals that although there is modest benefit of aspirin, this benefit varies widely with age and risk.
    c. Aspirin should be considered for primary prevention only in the patient with no additional risk factors for thromboembolism. Risk factors include a prior embolic event, left ventricular dysfunction, valvular heart disease, especially mitral stenosis, hypertension, age >60 years, and diabetes. (SOR **A**)
2. **Warfarin**
    a. Meta-analysis of five primary stroke prevention trials clearly demonstrates that anticoagulation with warfarin significantly reduces the risk of stroke in patients with AF when compared to aspirin or placebo. Overall, treating 100 patients with warfarin will prevent nearly three strokes per year.
    b. Trials evaluating the additive effect of warfarin plus aspirin therapy demonstrate that the combination is **not** beneficial. (SOR **A**)
    c. Indications for warfarin therapy in atrial fibrillation
      (1) Warfarin should be administered to patients with AF who are at higher risk of thromboembolism. The International Normalized Ratio (INR) should be maintained at 2.0 to 3.0. (SOR **A**)
      (2) For patients with mechanical heart valves, the target INR should be at least 2.5. (SOR **B**)

E. Diabetes mellitus
1. The Antithrombotic Trialist's Collaboration analyzed nine trials evaluating aspirin as a preventive agent in diabetic patients. Based on these data, aspirin is recommended for all patients with type 2 diabetes mellitus at increased cardiovascular risk. This includes

age older than 40 years, family history of CVD, hypertension, smoking, dyslipidemia, or albuminuria.

IV. Bacterial Endocarditis

A. Pathophysiology

1. Infective endocarditis (IE) is a localized infection consisting of fibrin, platelets, and microorganisms that adhere to the cardiac valves. The pathogenesis of IE initiates with a bacteremia.
2. Procedures that result in transient bacteremia include invasive oral and dental surgery where the mucosa is penetrated or traumatized. Invasive genitourinary or GI procedures are less likely to cause a significant bacteremia.
3. Without appropriate treatment, the mortality rate approaches 100%.
4. Clinical manifestations include fever, cardiac murmurs, anemia, splenomegaly, petechiae, pyuria, and peripheral emboli.
5. The causative organisms for native valves are *Streptococcus viridans* and other streptococci (60%), *Staphylococcus aureus* (25%), enterococci (10%), and other gram-negative organisms (5%). For prosthetic valves beyond 2 months of placement, *S. viridans* and other streptococci account for 30% of cases; coagulase-negative staphylococci, 20%; *Staph. aureus,* 15%; and enterococci and gram-negative organisms, 10%.

B. Prophylaxis

1. In April 2007, the American Heart Association released new guidelines for the prevention of endocarditis. Prophylaxis is now recommended prior to dental procedures only in patients with the following cardiac conditions, (SOR **C**):
   a. Patients with prosthetic cardiac valve(s).
   b. Patients with a history of previous infectious endocarditis.
   c. Patients with congenital heart disease (CHD).
      (1) Unrepaired cyanotic CHD, including palliative shunts and conduits.
      (2) Completely repaired CHD for six months after the procedure.
      (3) Repaired CHD with residual defects.
   d. Cardiac transplantation recipients who develop cardiac valvulopathy.
2. Administration of antibiotics solely to prevent endocarditis is not recommended for patients who undergo a genitourinary or gastrointestinal tract procedure. (SOR **B**)
3. The importance of excellent oral hygiene for those patients at risk for IE cannot be underestimated. This includes brushing and flossing regularly, using oral antiseptics, providing atraumatic care for acneiform pustules, avoiding nail biting, and careful gum care. (SOR **C**)
4. Amoxicillin is the antibiotic of choice for endocarditis prophylaxis, with other options for patients who are penicillin-allergic or cannot tolerate oral medications (Table 103–3).

V. Neural Tube Defects (NTDs)

A. Studies reveal that 20% of women whose pregnancies ended in miscarriages and up to 30% of women with recurrent miscarriages had an inadequate folate level. Several

TABLE 103–3. **PROPHYLACTIC REGIMENS FOR DENTAL, ORAL, RESPIRATORY TRACT, OR ESOPHAGEAL PROCEDURES**

Situation	Agent	Regimen: single dose 30–60 min before procedure*
Standard general prophylaxis	Amoxicillin	Adults: 2.0 g; children: 50 mg/kg orally
Unable to take oral medications	Ampicillin	Adults: 2.0 g IM or IV; children: 50 mg/kg IM or IV
Allergic to penicillin	Clindamycin	Adults: 600 mg; children: 20 mg/kg orally Adults: 2.0 g;
	or	children: 50 mg/kg orally
	Cephalexin[†]	Adults: 500 mg; children: 15 mg/kg orally
	or	
	Azithromycin or clarithromycin	
Allergic to penicillin and unable to take oral medications	Cephazolin[†] *or*	Adults: 1.0 g; children: 25 mg/kg IM or IV within 30 min before procedure
	Clindamycin	Adults: 600 mg; children: 20 mg/kg IV within 30 min before procedure

*Total children's dose should not exceed adult dose.
[†] Cephalosporins should not be used in individuals with immediate-type hypersensitivity reaction (urticaria, angioedema, or anaphylaxis) to penicillins.
IM, intramuscular; IV, intravenous.

studies suggest that consumption of folic acid decreases the incidence of NTDs in the fetuses of pregnant women when taken during the first 6 weeks after conception. These studies include trials of folate supplementation, dietary consumption of folate, and folate concentrations in serum and red blood cells.

B. Recommendations for folate supplementation

1. The US Public Health Service and The Food and Nutrition Board of the Institute of Medicine recommend that all women of childbearing age capable of becoming pregnant consume 0.4 mg of folic acid per day in order to reduce their risk of having a child with NTD, since nearly half of all pregnancies are unplanned. (SOR **B**)

2. Many experts recommend doses far higher than this (800 μg/d) for women trying to conceive. All women should consume 0.6 mg of folate per day during pregnancy and 0.5 mg of folate per day during lactation. (SOR **A**)

3. Women who have delivered a child with an NTD should consume 4 mg/d of folate 1 month prior to conception and for the first 3 months of pregnancy. The minimal effective folate dose is unknown. (SOR **B**)

C. The US Food and Drug Administration decided in 1993 to fortify staple foods by adding 1.4 mg folic acid/kg of cereal grain. Folic acid consumption may mask the hematologic manifestations of pernicious anemia in the elderly. Folate doses should be kept under 1 mg/d in those with low vitamin B_{12} levels, particularly those with achlorhydria and gastric atrophy lacking intrinsic factor.

D. Moderate increases in folate supply should also lower serum homocysteine in patients heterozygous for the gene for homocystinuria. Elevated homocysteine levels appear to be a strong independent risk factor for coronary vascular disease.

VI. Rheumatic Fever

A. Rheumatic fever is a **complication of group A β-hemolytic streptococcal infection** of the upper respiratory tract that is most frequently observed in children aged 5 to 13 years.

B. Diagnosis is based on meeting the **Jones criteria:** two major criteria or one major and two minor criteria plus evidence of a preceding streptococcal infection.

C. Prophylaxis

1. The goal of prophylaxis against group A strep is to prevent a **recurrence** of acute rheumatic fever. Recurrence rates decrease with increasing age, but recurrences have been documented as late as the fifth or sixth decade.

2. **Recommendations for treatment duration**
   a. Patients who have had rheumatic fever with carditis and residual heart disease need prophylaxis for at least 10 years beyond the last episode and until age 40 years or perhaps for life. (SOR **C**)
   b. Patients who have had rheumatic fever with carditis, but without residual heart disease need prophylaxis for at least 10 years since the last episode or well into adulthood, whichever is longer. (SOR **C**)
   c. Patients who have had rheumatic fever without carditis need prophylaxis for at least 5 years since the last episode or until age 21, whichever is longer. (SOR **C**)

3. **Recommended regimen**
   a. Benzathine penicillin G (1 200 000 U intramuscularly every 3–4 weeks).
   b. Penicillin V (250 mg by mouth twice daily).
   c. Sulfadiazine (500 mg/day orally if <60 lbs; 1 g/d orally if >60 lbs).
   d. Erythromycin (250 mg by mouth twice daily).

4. A possible alternative to long-term prophylaxis in the future may be a streptococcal vaccine that would eliminate primary rheumatic fever by eliminating the causative organism.

VII. Group B Streptococcal Disease (GBS).
GBS is a Gram-positive bacterium that colonizes the human GI tract and genitourinary tract. It is the most frequently encountered bacterial pathogen in neonates, and prevention of GBS transmission during vaginal delivery is crucial.

A. History of intrapartum antibiotic prophylaxis (IAP)

1. Two approaches to IAP existed prior to 2002. The first was risk factor based and the second was screening based.

2. A 1999 study raised questions about the inconsistency of these two strategies. Infants born to women whose physicians used the risk factor–based approach were 50% more likely to have early-onset GBS disease.

B. Revised 2002 IAP Screening Guidelines

1. All pregnant women should be screened for GBS colonization with swabs of both the lower vagina and the rectum at 35 to 37 weeks' gestation. (SOR **A**)

   2. Patients with GBS bacteriuria in the current pregnancy or with a positive GBS infant in a previous pregnancy should receive IAP regardless. (SOR **B**)
C. Patients recommended for IAP
   1. Pregnant women with a positive GBS screen unless a planned cesarean section is performed in the absence of labor or rupture of membranes. (SOR **A**)
   2. Pregnant women who have had a prior infant with GBS disease. (SOR **B**)
   3. Women with GBS bacteriuria during the current pregnancy. (SOR **B**)
   4. Pregnant women whose culture status is unknown and who also have delivery at <37 weeks, rupture >18 hours, or temperature spike to >100.4°F. (SOR **A**)
D. Regimen
   1. Penicillin G (5 million units intravenously initial dose, then 2.5 million units every 4 hours). (SOR **A**)
   2. Ampicillin (2 g intravenously initial dose, then 1 g every 4 hours). Penicillin has a narrower spectrum and is preferred. (SOR **A**)
   3. Cefazolin (2 g initial dose, then 1 g every 8 hours). (SOR **C**)
   4. If a patient has an anaphylaxis risk to penicillins, the physician may give clindamycin (900 mg intravenously every 8 hours) or erythromycin (500 mg intravenously every 6 hours). (SOR **C**)

REFERENCES

Bilukha OO, Rosenstein N. Prevention and control of meningococcal disease. Recommendations of the Advisory Committee on Immunization Practices. *MMWR. Recomm Rep.* 2005;54(RR-7):1-21.

Braunwald E, Antman EM, Beasley JW, et al. ACC/AHA 2002 Guideline update for the management of patients with unstable angina and non-ST segment elevation myocardial infarction summary article. A report of the American College of Cardiology/American Heart Association task force on practice guidelines. *J Am Coll Cardiol.* 2002;40:1366-1374.

Fuster V, Ryden LE, Cannom DS, et al. ACC/AHA/ESC 2006 Guidelines for the management of patients with atrial fibrillation. *J Am Coll Cardiol.* 2006;48:e149-e246.

Lauer MS. Clinical practice. Aspirin for the primary prevention of coronary events. *N Engl J Med.* 2002;346:1468-1474.

Pearson TA, Blair SN, Daniels SR, et al. AHA guidelines for the primary prevention of cardiovascular disease and stroke: 2002 Update: consensus panel guide to comprehensive risk reduction for adult patients without coronary or other atherosclerotic vascular diseases. American Heart Association Science Advisory and Coordinating Committee. *Circulation.* 2002;106:388-391.

Sandercock P, Gubitz G, Foley P, Counsell C. Antiplatelet therapy for acute ischaemic stroke. *Cochrane Database System. Rev.* 2003;2:CD000029. doi: 10.1002/14651858.CD000029.

Smith SC, Jr., Allen J, Blair SN, et al. AHA/ACC guidelines for secondary prevention for patients with coronary and other atherosclerotic vascular disease: 2006 update endorsed by the National Heart, Lung, and Blood Institute. *J Am Coll Cardiol.* 2006;47:2130-2139.

Wilson W, Taubert KA, Gewitz M, et al. Prevention of infective endocarditis. guidelines from the American Heart Association: a guideline from the American Heart Association Rheumatic Fever, Endocarditis, and Kawasaki Disease Committee, Council on Cardiovascular Disease in the young, and the Council on Clinical Cardiology, Council on Cardiovascular Surgery and Anesthesia, and the Quality of Care and Outcomes Research Interdisciplinary Working Group. *Circulation.* 2007;116:1736-1754.

---

104   Travel Medicine

Mark K. Huntington, MD, PhD

KEY POINTS

A. Know your traveler!
   1. Age, gender, chronic illnesses, or pregnancy.
   2. Destination, duration, modes of travel.
   3. High-risk activities or behaviors.
B. Nonpharmacologic measures
   1. Arthropod bite prevention. The following measures can afford nearly 100% protection from ticks and mosquitoes (SOR **B**):

- Limiting the amount of exposed skin,
- Proper coverage of exposed areas of skin with 30% to 35% DEET
- Use of permethrin-impregnated clothing and bednets

2. **Food and water precautions. (SOR C)**
   - "Boil it, peel it, cook it, or forget it."
   - Avoid unpasteurized milk
   - Avoid reheated foods (especially from street vendors). Food should be served and eaten piping hot.
   - Consume seafood with caution.
   - Drink bottled, boiled, carbonated, or treated water only.

3. **Sunscreen.** Use Sun Protection Factor (SPF) of 15 or greater. Use of clothing (long sleeves, hats, etc.) to protect from the sun is even more effective.

C. **Vaccinations.** CDC's National Immunization Program @ (http://www.cdc.gov/nip/) and Table 104-2 (SOR A)

D. **Pharmacological measures**
   1. **Malarial chemoprophylaxis.** See Table 104–3 and 104–4. (SOR A)
   2. **Travelers diarrhea.** See Table 104-5 (SOR A)
   3. **Motion sickness and jet lag.** See Tables 104–6 and 104–7. (SOR B)

E. **Geopolitical issues.** Keep abreast of current events. The State Department webpage (www.travel.state.gov) aids in keeping up-to-date on destination-specific events, customs, and other hazards.

F. **Staying current.** The Centers for Disease Control and Prevention (http://www.cdc.gov/travel) and the World Health Organization (www.who.int) web sites offer current information.

G. **Posttravel illness**
   - Fever in a returning traveler is malaria until proven otherwise. (SOR B)
   - Persistent diarrhea isn't necessarily of an infectious etiology.

I. **Introduction.** In 2006, 842 million people traveled internationally. Despite economic downturns, terrorism, and regional conflicts, and emerging diseases, international travel is increasing. Travel medicine, also known as emporiatrics, addresses the travel-specific health concerns of these people.

A. **The pretravel visit.** The clinic visit should be as far in advance of travel as possible, to ensure adequate time for vaccinations. A clinic visit just days prior to travel, while not ideal, can still be beneficial.

B. **Vaccinations for travel**
   1. **Routine vaccinations.** All routine and childhood vaccinations should be current according to established guidelines. An accelerated vaccination schedule can be used to catch-up children who are delinquent prior to travel (see Chapter 101 and http://www.cdc.gov/nip/), and there are additional deviations from guidelines that may be considered before embarking on travel (Table 104–1).
   2. **Travel-specific vaccinations.** These are summarized on Table 104–1. Careful review of travel plans is required to ensure adequate protection without administering unnecessary vaccinations, some of which are quite expensive and have potential for adverse effects. The CDC website, www.cdc.gov/travel, is a valuable source for this information.

C. **Medications for travel**
   1. **Malaria.** Malarial prophylaxis is absolutely critical. Local resistance patterns should be considered prior to prescribing prophylaxis (Table 104–2). Table 104–3 gives dosage instructions. For travelers with prolonged travel to areas endemic with *Plasmodium vivax* or *ovale*, terminal prophylaxis with primaquine may be needed. The most deadly malaria is *Plasmodium falciparum*. People traveling to areas where *P. falciparum* malaria is endemic, who will be unable to access medical care within 24 hours, should be proactively prescribed emergency antimalarial treatment, in addition to their prophylactic medication.
   2. **Travelers' diarrhea (TD)**
      a. **Prophylaxis.** The CDC does not recommend prophylactic antibiotics for TD in most travelers. Nevertheless, some may elect to take prophylactic antibiotics, particularly if even a portion of a lost day to illness would be catastrophic (e.g., diplomats, athletes, business people, etc). Ciprofloxacin (500 mg/d), norfloxacin (400 mg/d),

TABLE 104–1. RECOMMENDATIONS FOR THE PREVENTION OF VACCINE-PREVENTABLE DISEASES IN TRAVELERS

Vaccinations (Earliest Effective Date)	Indication	Administration	Booster Requirements	Contraindications*	Miscellaneous Comments
Cholera Whole-cell-B subunit vaccine Dukoral (7 d after last dose)	Consider for long-term travel to cholera-endemic areas or areas with active cholera outbreak	Two doses (ages >6 y) or three doses (age 2–6 y) at intervals of 7–42 d.	Every 3 mo for ages >2 y to insure enterotoxic E. coli (ETEC) protection, otherwise every 2 y for age >6 y and every 6 mo for ages 2–6 y.	Not approved in pregnancy but risk is remote and theoretical; benefits may outweigh risk.	The risk for the average traveler is so remote (2 per million travelers) that cholera vaccination is of questionable benefit. Long-term travelers to cholera-endemic areas, or travelers to areas with an active cholera outbreak *may* benefit from this vaccine. Effective against ETEC travelers' diarrhea after two doses. Not available in the United States. Contact manufacturers for availability: www.travellersdiarrhea.com
Hepatitis A† vaccine (1 mo after first dose)	All travelers, including children to endemic areas	Two doses, 6–24 mo apart	None		If the vaccine is not administered at least 1 mo prior to travel, immune globulin prophylaxis prior to travel is recommended. Although hepatitis A vaccine is approved for children older than 2 y, data suggest it is safe and efficacious in children as young as 1 y. Children who do not receive the vaccine should receive immune globulin prior to travel.
Hepatitis A immune globulin (Immediately effective)	Travelers to areas with high hepatitis A endemicity or who have a contraindication to hepatitis A vaccine or did not receive the vaccine prior to 1 mo pre-travel	Short-term (1–2 mo) coverage: 0.02 mg/kg IM Long-term (3–6 mo) coverage: 0.06 mg/kg IM	Booster dependent on initial dose given and length of continued stay. Booster not needed if hepatitis A vaccine given just prior to travel.		
Hepatitis B (2 wk after second dose)	All travelers	3 doses at 0, 1 mo, and 6–12 mo	None		

796

Hib (*Haemophilus influenzae*, type b)	All travelers < 5 y of age and previously unvaccinated asplenic travelers	Single dose in splenectomized people > 5 y. Accelerated program available for infant travelers (see chapter 101.)	NA	
Influenza*,‡ (2 wk)	All travelers	Annually	Egg allergy	In tropical regions, influenza is a perennial disease, and the peak incidence in one hemisphere is opposite the other. Vaccines from the northern and southern hemispheres are not necessarily the same, so vaccination with one vaccine does not necessarily confer immunity in the opposite hemisphere. Inter-hemispheric travelers should take these seasonal differences into consideration and consider vaccination upon arrival at their destination. Travelers in situations where multinational groups (perhaps from the opposite hemisphere) gather in close quarters (eg, cruise vacations and international conventions) should also consider vaccination. While not a substitute for vaccination, prophylactic medications such as amantadine, zanamivir, or oseltamivir can be prescribed if influenza vaccine is unavailable.

(*continued*)

TABLE 104–1. CONTINUED

Vaccinations (Earliest Effective Date)	Indication	Administration	Booster Requirements	Contraindications *	Miscellaneous Comments
Japanese encephalitis (after 2 doses)	Travelers for > 1 mo to endemic rural areas of eastern Asia including the Indian subcontinent	3 doses on d 0, 7, and 14–30.	Every 3 y	Hypersensitivity reactions have occurred as late as 10 d postvaccination (after any dose in series). Delay of travel recommended for at least 10 d if traveling to area with poor medical access	Endemic to rural Southeast Asia, most travelers are at low risk for this disease. Those traveling in rural areas for more than 1 mo should consider this vaccination series.
Meningococcal (10 d)	Travelers to Saudi Arabia Travelers to sub-Saharan Africa, especially those with asplenia, should consider vaccination.	Single injection	Every 3 y		Entry into Saudi Arabia for the Hajj, Umra, or seasonal work requires proof of quadrivalent (A, C, W-135, Y) meningococcal vaccination more than 10 d but less than 3 y prior to arrival. The quadrivalent vaccine is poorly immunogenic in young children, but is still recommended in children traveling to high-risk areas. A monovalent conjugate vaccine to serogroup C is available in Canada, Australia, and Europe and is highly effective in people of all ages, but not against the predominant serotype in sub-Saharan Africa (serogroup A). There is no effective vaccine for serogroup B, a common serogroup in the Western Hemisphere and Europe.

Vaccine				
Measles–mumps–rubella (MMR)	All travelers over 6 mo of age. Normally first given between ages 12 and 15 mo, children aged 6 and 12 mo traveling to the developing world may benefit from an early MMR or monovalent measles vaccine.	Booster >4 wk after first dose.	Known allergy to neomycin, gelatin. **Allergy to eggs is not a contraindication.** CD4+ count <200 cell/μL	If an MMR is given prior to the first birthday, the routine MMR vaccine schedule must be restarted at age 12–15 mo.
Pneumococcal disease* (2 wk)	Age > 65 y, persons with chronic diseases, and asplenic travelers	5-y booster in some populations		
Polio (inactivated poliomyelitis vaccine [IPV]* or oral polio vaccine (OPV) [4 wk])	All travelers	Single dose administered by injection (IPV) or orally (OPV) prior to travel to an endemic area	Known reaction to formaldehyde. OPV contraindicated in immunosuppressed individuals	In addition to childhood immunizations, a single IPV booster is recommended once as an adult before travel to endemic areas
Rabies* (1 wk after final dose) Human Diploid Cell Vaccine (HDCV) 1-cc IM dose or 0.1-cc intradermal dose. Purified Chick Embryo Cell (PCEC). 1 cc IM only Rabies Vaccine Absorbed (RVA) 1 cc IM only	Preexposure prophylaxis is recommended for high-risk travelers including animal handlers, trekkers, cyclists, veterinarians, spelunkers, field biologists, children, and missionaries	Series of 3 injections at 0, 7, and 21–28 d for preexposure prophylaxis	2–3 y depending on risk of exposure. Preexposure vaccination does not eliminate need for postexposure management	Preexposure vaccines should never be given in the gluteal muscle because of decreased efficacy with this route Concomitant dosing of HDCV with chloroquine or mefloquine can dampen the immune response and should not be given within 1 wk of them Preexposure rabies vaccination does simplify the postbite rabies regimen but does not eliminate the need for prompt medical care.

(continued)

TABLE 104-1. CONTINUED

Vaccinations (Earliest Effective Date)	Indication	Administration	Booster Requirements	Contraindications *	Miscellaneous Comments
Tetanus–diphtheria (Td), and tetanus–diphtheria–pertussis (DTaP, DTP, Tdp)	All travelers	For those 7 y or older or who have not received the full tetanus–diphtheria series should receive a 3-dose series of Td. First two doses, 4–8 wk apart and the third dose 6–12 mo after the second. If last dose cannot be insured, the third dose can be administered 4–8 wk after the second.	At ages 11–12 y if it had been at least 5 y since last pediatric dose. Every 10 y for all others.	High fevers can occur in children who receive the DTP formulations. For these children, DTaP should be used. Children with some neurologic disorders may not be able to take the pertussis component. For these individuals, the DT formulation is recommended.	All children <7-y old should be vaccinated with DTaP according to routine immunization schedule.
Tick-borne encephalitis * (2 wk after second dose)	High-risk travelers to rural areas of Europe	Series of 3 IM injections at 0 d, 4–12 wk, and 9–12 mo	3 y	Sensitivity to thiomersal	Not available in the United States, but is available in Canada and Europe. Disease can be acquired by tick bite and by consuming unpasteurized milk.
Tuberculosis (BCG) (4 wk)	Consider for infants <6 mo of age and high-risk health care workers	One dose, intradermally	None	Severely immunocompromised	Rarely administered in the United States, BCG should be considered in very young children and health care workers who will have prolonged exposure to populations with high tuberculosis endemicity.

Vaccine	Indications	Schedule	Contraindications/Precautions	Comments
Typhoid fever[*] (1 wk)	Recommended for high-risk areas if duration of stay is over 1 mo Parenteral age >2 y Oral age >6 y	Parenteral, one dose IM. Oral, 4 doses on d 1, 3, 5, and 7.	Parenteral—2 y Oral—6 y. (Stop proguanil, mefloquine, and antibiotics 1 wk before and after administration of oral vaccine.)	Parenteral vaccine more likely to cause a systemic reaction	Breast-feeding may confer passive immunity.
Yellow fever (10 d)	Sub-Saharan Africa and tropical South America	Single injection	10 y	Egg allergy Immunocompromise Never use in infants younger than 6 mo due to an increased risk of postvaccine encephalitis. Only use in children from 6 to 9 mo of *age if traveling to an area with an active yellow fever outbreak.* Pregnancy	Closely regulated. Available only through an approved yellow fever vaccination center. Administration must be properly recorded on the International Certificate of Vaccination (Form PHS-731) for entry into some countries. The certificate is valid 10 d after immunization. For those individuals in whom yellow fever vaccination is contraindicated, a waiver letter on a physician's letterhead should be given and an official stamp placed on the bottom of the waiver letter.

*Hypersensitivity can occur with any vaccine. Previous hypersensitivity is a contraindication to further vaccination.

†Immunoglobulin recommended for children younger than 2 years. Hepatitis A vaccine is approved for children older than 1 year in Europe.

‡Because of seasonal variations between hemispheres, may need to receive vaccination at destination. Indicated for travel at any time to tropical areas.

TABLE 104–2. MALARIAL RESISTANCE AND PROPHYLACTIC DRUG CHOICE

Geographic Resistance/Susceptibility	Drug Choices in Order of Preference
Chloroquine-susceptible areas	Chloroquine, doxycycline, mefloquine, atovaquone–proguanil
Chloroquine-resistant areas	Mefloquine, doxycycline, atovaquone–proguanil
Mefloquine-resistant areas	Doxycycline, atovaquone–proguanil

      ofloxacin (400 mg/d), levofloxacin (500 mg/d), and Pepto-Bismol (2 tablets four times daily) are all reasonable choices. (SOR **C**)

    b. Treatment of TD. Most TD is self-limited. Antibiotics can hasten recovery in most cases. (SOR **B**) Dosages can be found in Table 104–4. Maintaining adequate hydration is critical, particularly for children. (SOR **A**)

  3. Symptomatic medications
    Travelers should be instructed to bring any over-the-counter medications that they might occasionally use. Examples include acetaminophen, ibuprofen, topical antibiotics and antifungals, antihistamines, etc. Not all medicines readily available in the United States are available abroad, and those that are may have unfamiliar trademarks and even generic names.

II. Illness and Injury Prevention

  A. Arthropod bite prevention

    1. N,N-diethyl-3-methylbenzamide (DEET) is the most used, most effective, and best-studied insect repellent on the world market; used as directed, its safety profile is unmatched. (SOR **A**) Plant-based repellents (Bite Blocker, Skin-so-Soft, and citronella) are much less effective. DEET is available in 5% to 100% concentrations; higher concentrations afford longer protection times between applications. Extended-release preparations allow longer durations of action at lower the concentrations. For the vast majority of travelers, including pregnant women and children, a concentration of 30% to 35% provides adequate protection. Reapply every 4 hours, more often when perspiring heavily or after swimming. When applying sunscreen and insect repellent together, the sunscreen should be applied first. While the *Anopheles* and *Culex* species of mosquitoes are nighttime feeders, *Aedes* species, responsible for yellow and dengue fevers, are daytime feeders. Round-the-clock protection is necessary in endemic areas.

    2. Permethrin is a contact insecticide that is applied to clothing. Combined with DEET, permethrin can afford nearly 100% protection from ticks and mosquitoes. (SOR **A**) Insecticidal effects linger through several launderings.

    3. Other measures. Using permethrin-impregnated mosquito netting for sleeping, having air-conditioned sleeping quarters, spraying sleeping quarters with insecticide for flying insects (e.g., Raid), wearing light-colored clothing, and avoiding colognes and perfumes can further reduce the risk of arthropod bites.

    4. Special note of caution. A variety of insect vectors of disease such as the tsetse fly, sandfly, and black fly are not well repelled by DEET. Barrier protection against their bite is essential, and having a high index of suspicion for vector-borne disease after travel in endemic areas is vital.

  B. Food and drinking water safety. TD and other food-borne illnesses are the most common causes of morbidity among travelers to developing countries.

    1. Water. Avoid consuming tap water in developing countries. Water that has been brought to boil or properly treated with water purification systems or halogen additives (chlorine or iodine) may be safe. Using ice in beverages and using tap water to brush teeth are common lapses (SOR **C**)

    2. Vegetables and fruits. Raw, unpeeled vegetables, and salads should be avoided. (SOR **B**) Melons and other fruit should be closely inspected for puncture marks as unscrupulous vendors often inject fruit with water to increase the weight.

    3. Dairy products. Unpasteurized dairy products should be avoided. (SOR **C**)

    4. Seafood. Fish and shellfish can harbor both pathogens and toxins. Proper cooking eliminates most pathogens, but not the toxins.

      a. Shellfish poisoning. The four most common are paralytic, diarrheic, amnesic, and neurotoxic. These toxins are tasteless and odorless and can be found in fresh shellfish. These toxins are heat-stable and are not neutralized by cooking. Dinoflagellate toxins released during red and brown algae blooms cause these poisonings. Governmental authorities may issue shellfish warnings in response

TABLE 104–3. MALARIA CHEMOPROPHYLAXIS DRUG DOSAGES

Drug	Adult Dosing	Pediatric Dosing/Concerns	Pregnancy/Lactation Concerns	Side Effects, Precautions, and Miscellaneous Concerns
Chloroquine (Aralen)	500 mg *weekly* beginning 12 wk before travel and continuing 4 wk after return	5 mg/kg up to adult dose. Liquid formulation available in some countries. May require pharmacy compounding.	Safe in pregnancy and lactation. Concentrations in breast milk are not protective for infant.	Usually minor: itching, skin eruptions, headache. Contraindicated in patients with severe hepatic insufficiency. The therapeutic window is fairly narrow. Fatal overdoses of young children have been reported at doses as little as 300 mg. Accurate dosing in young children is critical.
Mefloquine (Lariam)	250 mg *weekly* beginning 1–2 wk before travel and continuing 4 wk after return	<15 kg: 5 mg/kg weekly (will require pharmacy compounding into liquid form for accurate dosing) 15–19 kg: ¼ tablet weekly 20–30 kg: ½ tablet weekly 31–45 kg: ¾ tablet weekly >45 kg: adult dose	Safe in second and third trimesters.	25%–40% will experience mild side effects (nausea, headaches) Neuropsychiatric side effects uncommon in prophylactic dosages. Contraindicated in patients with epilepsy, serious psychiatric illness, or cardiac conduction disturbance. Concomittant use with beta-blockers increases risk of cardiac arrest.
Atovaquone-proguanil (Malarone)	250 mg/100 mg *daily* beginning 1–2 d before travel and stopping 1 wk after return.	<11 kg: not recommended at this time 11–20 kg: 1 pediatric tablet (62.5/25) po daily 21–30 kg: 2 pediatric tablets po daily 31–40 kg: 3 pediatric tablets po daily >40 kg: 1 adult tablet po daily	First trimester usage unstudied. Concentrations in breast milk are not protective for nursing infant.	Contraindicated in patients with severe renal insufficiency (creatinine clearance <30 mL/min)
Doxycycline (Vibramycin and others)	100 mg po *daily* beginning 1–2 d before travel and continuing for 4 wk after return	>8 y: 2 mg/kg/d up to adult dose. Contraindicated in children 8 y old and younger.	Contraindicated in pregnancy and lactation	A photo sensitizer. Increases risk for sunburn. Recommend sunscreen.
Primaquine (Palum)	26.3 mg po *daily* for 14 d after departure *from an endemic area* for those with prolonged exposure to *P. vivax* and *P. ovale*	0.5 mg/kg up to adult dose	Contraindicated in pregnancy .	Contraindicated in G6PD deficiency.

803

TABLE 104–4. TREATMENT OF TRAVELERS' DIARRHEA (TD)

Drug	Adult Dosing	Pediatric Dosing/Concerns	Pregnancy/Lactation Concerns	Side Effects, Precautions, and Miscellaneous Concerns
Azithromycin (Zithromax)	200 mg/d for 3 d	10 mg/kg/d × 3 d after onset of diarrhea	May use in pregnancy.	
Bismuth subsalicylate (e.g., Pepto-Bismol)	524 mg (2 tablets or 30 cc) qid	**9–12 y:** 1 tablet or 15 cc qid **6–8 y:** $^2/_3$ tablet or 10 cc qid **3–6 y:** $^1/_3$ tablet or 5 cc qid Not recommended for children < 3 y	Should avoid during last half of pregnancy	Not recommended for travel longer than 3 wk. Contraindicated in aspirin allergy, renal insufficiency, or gout.
Ciprofloxacin (Cipro)	500 mg po bid for 3 d	15–20 mg/kg/dose bid up to adult dose. Some experts recommend for severe TD/dysentery.	Relative contraindication in pregnancy. Some experts recommend for severe TD/dysentery.	Relative contraindication in childhood and in pregnancy due to studies showing arthropathy in immature animals.
Levofloxacin (Levaquin)	500 mg po qd for 3 d	Not recommended	Relative contraindication in pregnancy	
Loperamide (Imodium)	4 mg followed by 2 mg for each unformed stool. Maximum of 16 mg/d	**30–45 kg:** $^1/_2$ adult dose Maximum 6 mg/d **22–29 kg:** $^1/_4$ adult dose. Maximum 4 mg/d **<22 kg or <6 ys old:** not recommended	May use in pregnancy.	Avoid use with serious illness such as fever or bloody diarrhea, as this may worsen/prolong illness.
Rifaximin (Xifaxan)	200 mg po tid for 3 d	Not recommended	Not absorbed systemically, may be used in pregnancy/lactation	Not for use in bloody diarrhea, severe or systemic symptoms.
Trimethoprim/sulfamethoxazole (Bactrim)	160/800 mg po bid for 3 d	>2 mo: 10 mg/kg/d divided BID up to adult dose	Safe in pregnancy	Resistance is increasingly a problem.

to algae blooms, but many developing countries do not reliably survey for these conditions. Contacting local officials and tour and hotel operators regarding this risk is recommended.

b. Ciguatera poisoning. Produced by dinoflagellates, this toxin is concentrated in large, predaceous fish such as barracuda, red snapper, grouper, amberjack, and mackerel. This toxin is odorless, tasteless, and heat-stable and can be found in freshly caught fish. Symptoms are gastroenteritis followed by symptoms such as dysthesias, the sensation of loose teeth, temperature reversal (cold feeling hot and vice versa), and weakness.

c. Scombroid poisoning. Scombroid toxin is produced by a bacterial overgrowth in improperly refrigerated fish, particularly tuna, mackerel, mahi-mahi, amberjack, bluefish, and herring. Fish unrefrigerated for more than 2 hours should be avoided.

d. Fugu poisoning. Puffer fish is a delicacy in Japan. If improperly prepared, this delicacy can harbor tetrodotoxin, which has a 60% case fatality rate.

C. Unintentional injuries during travel. Nearly one quarter of overseas fatalities are because of accidents; the most common causes are motor vehicle accidents and drowning. The most common nonfatal injuries were falls and water recreation-related injuries. Alcohol consumption correlates with an increased risk of injury and death while traveling. Travelers should bring personal protective gear such as helmets if they intend to ride bicycles or motorbikes. They should become familiar with road conditions and laws and customs of the road. If travelers are going to be participating in water-based recreation during their travel, encourage them to know the area well before engaging in these activities, particularly higher-risk activities like scuba diving.

D. Deep vein thromboses. Deep vein thromboses and pulmonary emboli associated with long airline flights are rare, but there appears to be an increased risk in those with hypercoagulable states. These travelers should stretch and walk frequently about the plane, taking into consideration flying conditions and air turbulence. Compression stockings may offer some protective benefit in these patients. Aspirin has not been shown to reduce the risk of thromboembolic events in travelers, but is a low-risk intervention. Low-molecular-weight heparin is unstudied for this indication.

E. Motion sickness. Motion sickness (air sickness, seasickness) is thought to be caused by an asynchrony between the sight and vestibular senses. The symptoms include fatigue, headache, nausea, and vomiting. Several medications have been shown to be effective in preventing or reducing the symptoms of motion sickness (see Table 104–5).

Nonpharmacologic methods of preventing motion sickness (acupressure bracelets, ginger) have not been shown to be effective in clinical trials. Motion sickness can be reduced by sitting in the front seat of the car or over the wings in an aircraft.

F. Jet lag. Rapidly crossing multiple time zones disrupts a traveler's normal sleep-wake cycle. This effect increases as more time zones are crossed and is particularly troublesome for travelers traveling in an easterly direction. Adjustment to a new time zone usually requires 1 day for every time zone crossed. Strategies to reduce jet lag are summarized in Table 104–6.

Several trials have demonstrated the effectiveness of melatonin in reducing the symptoms of jet lag. The benefit is greater the more time zones are crossed and for eastward flights. Many pretravel, en route, and posttravel melatonin-dosing regimens have been described—some can be quite complicated. Melatonin is an unregulated substance, and formulations vary considerably. A simplified dosing regimen is 5 mg en route taken at the destination bedtime and 5 mg orally nightly for 3 to 5 nights posttravel. Short-acting agents such as zolpidem (Ambien) and benzodiazepines can be used in a similar manner.

G. Sun protection. Sun exposure has short- and long-term consequences, including sunburn, photo-aging, and skin cancer. Wearing protective clothing and hats, avoiding exposure during the time of day when the sun's rays most intense (10:00 AM to 3:00 PM), and applying sufficient sunscreen reduce the untoward consequences of sun exposure. (SOR **B**) The sun protection factor (SPF) determines a sunscreen's strength. While a sunscreen with a sun protection factor of 15, when applied as directed, can afford more than 90% protection, most people apply sunscreen much more sparingly and less frequently than recommended. Recommending a higher sun protection factor can partially compensate for this deficiency.

H. Sexually transmitted disease (STD) prevention. Up to 15% of international travelers will report at least one new sexual encounter during their travels. Human

TABLE 104–5. **MOTION SICKNESS PROPHYLAXIS**

Drug	Dosages	Side Effects	Additional Comments
Scopolamine hydrobromide (Transderm Sc p, Scopace)	1.5 mg transdermal patch behind ear q 3 d 0.4 mg tablet po, 1–2 tabs po q 8 h	Dry mouth (66%), drowsiness (33%)	Tablets better suited for shorter outings. Patch costs 10× more than tablets. Patch is effective 6–8 h after it is placed. Oral forms are effective within 1–2 h. Efficacy may be enhanced and drowsiness reduced by concurrent use of sympathomimetics such as ephedrine, D-amphetamine, and methylphenidate
Promethazine (Phenergan) 25-, 12.5-mg tablets, 12.5-mg/5-cc elixir	25 mg po q 6–18 h; 1 mg/kg/dose for children	Less dry mouth and more drowsiness compared to scopolamine	Usual dosing interval is 12 h
Dimenhydrinate (Dramamine)	50–100 mg po q 6–8 h (12 y and older); 25–50 mg po q 6–8 h (6–12 y old); 12.5–25 mg q 6–8 h (2–6 years old)		Most effective over-the-counter medication. Chewable tablet formulations available.
Cyclizine (Marezine)	50 mg po q 4–6 h	Less sedation compared with other antihistamines	
Meclizine (Antivert, Bonine) 12.5-, 25-, 50-mg tablets	25–50 mg po daily (12 y and older)		Pregnancy category B. Chewable tablet formulations available.

immunodeficiency virus (HIV) and hepatitis B infection rates are very high in some countries, particularly among prostitutes. Abstinence should be strongly encouraged. Latex condoms, consistently and correctly used, may afford some protection to those unwilling to abstain. (SOR **A**) Pretravel hepatitis B vaccination and a posttravel examination to screen for STDs of these travelers should be recommended.

III. Special Travelers
  A. Pregnant travelers
    1. **Air travel.** Many women travel well into their third trimester. Commercial air travel generally does not pose a significant risk to the pregnant patient or her fetus. (SOR **B**) Decreased Pao$_2$ present at the standard cabin altitude of 5000 to 8000 ft (1500–2500 m) has little, if any, effect on fetal oxygenation because of a favorable fetal hemoglobin disassociation curve. Pregnancy does confer an increased risk of thromboembolism, so it is recommended that the pregnant traveler should walk about frequently while traveling, flying conditions, and turbulence permitting. Each airline has defined policies regarding the pregnant traveler. US domestic and intra-European travel is usually

TABLE 104–6. **STRATEGIES FOR LESSENING JET-LAG SYMPTOMS**

Direction of Travel	Pretravel Bedtime Adjustments	Wakefulness During Flight	Bright Light Exposure at Destination	Vigorous Exercise at Destination
Eastward	Go to bed 1 h earlier each night for three nights prior to departure	Try to sleep on plane. Avoid caffeinated beverages.	Bright light in early morning—avoid sunglasses for first few days.	Mid-morning exercise
Westward	Go to bed 1 h later each night for three nights prior to departure.	Try to stay awake during flight. Drink caffeinated beverages.	Bright light in late afternoon—avoid sunglasses for first few days.	Late afternoon exercise

allowed up until the 36th week in uncomplicated pregnancies. Air travel across great distances, particularly transoceanic travel, is permitted up until the 32nd week of uncomplicated pregnancies. Many airlines require medical authorization before permitting travel by pregnant women beyond 28 weeks' gestation. Pregnant travelers should carry a copy or summary of the prenatal record. Blood type and due date are particularly important data to carry.

2. **Vaccines in pregnancy.** Most vaccines are safe in pregnancy. Measles–mumps–rubella, varicella, and yellow fever are the notable exceptions and should be avoided until the postpartum period. Other live viral/bacterial vaccines (oral typhoid, oral polio, and Japanese encephalitis virus vaccine) have relative contraindications but can be given if travel to areas with active outbreaks or high levels of endemicity cannot be avoided and the vaccine's benefit outweighs any perceived risks. (SOR **Ⓑ**) Indications for killed, inactivated, or split-virus vaccines are not altered by pregnancy.

3. **TD and food-borne illnesses in pregnancy.** While quinolones are contraindicated in pregnancy, many experts believe that these medications should not be withheld from the pregnant patient for cases of *severe* TD (dehydration or dysentery). Azithromycin, cefixime, furazolidone, and trimethoprim sulfamethoxazole (TMP-SMX) are also reasonable choices. Hepatitis E, which is not vaccine-preventable, is usually contracted from contaminated food or water. This infection carries a 17% to 33% case fatality rate in the pregnant patient. Strict food and water discipline is critical for the pregnant traveler.

4. **Malaria and the pregnant traveler.** Malaria can be catastrophic to the pregnant patient and her fetus. Maternal mortality can approach 10%. Recreational travel to malarious areas during pregnancy should be avoided if at all possible. In the event that travel to malarious areas is unavoidable, malarial prophylaxis and arthropod vector control is paramount. Chloroquine and mefloquine are safe throughout pregnancy. Travel to mefloquine-resistant areas should be avoided during pregnancy because no proven safe prophylaxis exists at this time. Doxycycline has a relative contraindication during pregnancy; there is little evidence of a class effect in this regard. Data on the safety of atovaquone-proguanil (Malarone) are incomplete at this time and cannot be formally recommended for use in the pregnant traveler. Primaquine is contraindicated during pregnancy because the glucose-6-phospate dehydrogenase (G6PD) status of the fetus is unknown. In cases where primaquine terminal prophylaxis is necessary, chloroquine should be continued until delivery (even if it requires months of treatment after return). Primaquine can then begin in the postpartum period. DEET and permethrin, used as directed, are safe in pregnancy.

5. **Miscellaneous travel hazards in pregnancy.** Scuba diving and water skiing are contraindicated during pregnancy. Acetazolamide for high-altitude illness prophylaxis is not recommended during the first trimester. Nifedipine and dexamethasone are safe throughout pregnancy.

B. **The pediatric traveler**
1. **Air travel.** The CDC recommends that children younger than 6 weeks old should avoid air travel, WHO places the cutoff at 1 week. There are no prospective or case–control studies substantiating either of these recommendations. Most US carriers have no lower age restrictions for air travel. Nevertheless, contacting the airline well in advance of travel is recommended. Ear pain during ascent and descent has been reported in as many as 15% of pediatric air travelers. Bottle-feeding, nursing, and decongestants have been advocated to ameliorate these symptoms, but multiple small studies have shown little, if any, benefit.

2. **Vaccinations in childhood.** See Section I.B above, Chapter 101 and the web site of the CDC's National Immunization Program (http://www.cdc.gov/nip/).

3. **Malarial chemoprophylaxis in childhood.** Children are at increased risk of mortality from *P. falciparum* malaria. Chloroquine and mefloquine, in appropriate doses, are safe for all ages. Overdoses of these medications can be fatal, so proper compounding of suspensions and accurate dosing are *critical*. When a mosquito-free microenvironment can be assured (e.g., permethrin-impregnated netting over a bassinet, stroller, playpen or car seat, combined with DEET), one may defer chemoprophylaxis.

4. **TD in childhood.** Quinolones are the most effective treatment for TD in all age groups, including children, see Table 104–4 for dosage. Quinolone use has caused long bone arthropathy in skeletally immature experimental animals, but clinical use of long-term quinolones in children with cystic fibrosis has not demonstrated this risk. Azithromycin,

cefixime, furazolidone, and TMP-SMX can also be used, but quinolones should be considered first-line treatment in cases of children with severe TD with dehydration or dysentery (bloody diarrhea with high fever). Vigorous rehydration of children with TD is essential. WHO recommends rehydration with reconstituted prepackaged WHO Oral Rehydration Salts in the following amounts:

a. Children younger than 2 years: 1/4 to 1/2 cup (50–100 mL) after each loose stool.

b. Children 2 to 10 years: 1/2 to 1 cup (100–200 mL) after each loose stool.

c. Older children and adults: unlimited amount. (As a substitute to the prepackaged WHO Oral Rehydration Salts: 6 level tsp of sugar plus 1 level tsp of salt and 1 level tsp of baking soda in 1 L/quart of safe drinking water can be used.)

C. Travelers with chronic diseases

1. General considerations. Prescribed medications should be hand-carried and in sufficient quantity to last the duration of the trip. A reserve supply of medications should be packed in a separate, checked bag. Medications should be in their original containers and labeled with generic names. A letter on official letterhead from the physician explaining dosages and indications of medications, particularly scheduled medications and diabetic needles and syringes, may avert legal problems at some international borders and assist with replacement, if needed.

2. Immunosuppressed travelers. The risk of infectious disease is increased in the immunocompromised traveler, including those with diabetes, transplant patients, chemotherapy patients, those with rheumatological disorders, and those who are infected with HIV.

a. TD in the immunocompromised traveler. Antibiotics are not routinely recommended to prevent TD in immunocompromised travelers. However, certain circumstances where any time lost because of illness may be considered critical or where the risk of illness would significantly compromise the traveler's health may warrant the use of daily prophylactic antibiotics such as ciprofloxacin 500 mg a day. HIV-positive travelers on TMP-SMX prophylaxis for pneumocystis pneumonia may also experience some benefit in the prevention of TD, but it should not be prescribed for TD to those not currently taking it, as it does have potential side effects and may lead to resistance when it is needed for other reasons. Acute treatment plans as outlined in Table 104–4 are also effective in this group, but may need to be extended for 7 days.

b. Immunizations in the immunocompromised traveler

(1) HIV-positive travelers. Vaccine immunogenicity may be decreased in HIV-positive patients with CD4$^+$ peripheral cell count <300 cells/μL. Generally, live vaccines should be avoided in the severely immunocompromised traveler, defined as the presence of opportunistic infections or a CD4$^+$ peripheral cell count <200 cells/μL. Inactivated vaccines should be used in place of live vaccines wherever possible (e.g., poliomyelitis, typhoid, and cholera). Measles and yellow fever vaccines should only be given to those with CD4$^+$ peripheral cell count >200 cells/μL. Killed vaccines are generally considered safe.

(2) Other immunocompromised travelers. Travelers who have recently received high-dose steroids for >14 days should delay vaccination 2 weeks after the completion of high-dose steroid therapy. Similarly, many cancer patients undergoing radiation or chemotherapy may also be immunosuppressed and should avoid vaccinations during this time. Cancer patients who are not actively being treated may be vaccinated. Travelers with leukemia who have been in remission for 3 months or transplant patients no longer needing immunosuppression may also be vaccinated.

c. Travel restrictions for the HIV-positive patient. In most countries, travelers staying <1 month are not required to show proof of being HIV-negative. For travelers wishing to stay >1 month, many countries require HIV testing, and most who are HIV-positive will be denied entry. Some countries will deny entry to travelers carrying antiretroviral medications. HIV-positive travelers should consult the US State Department web site (http://www.travel.state.gov/HIVtestingreq.html) for further information. Since regulations change frequently, contacting the consulate of the country in question prior to travel planning is also recommended.

3. The diabetic traveler. It is critical that the diabetic traveler carry adequate medications and monitoring supplies on the trip. This equipment and medication (including glucagon) should be hand-carried during travel. Insulin can be stored at room temperature for up to 30 days without losing effectiveness. Nevertheless, exposure of insulin to sunlight and temperature extremes should be avoided.

Travel across time zones can shorten or lengthen the "24-hour day," changing insulin and meal requirements. Travel in an easterly direction shortens the day and may decrease insulin and meal requirements. Conversely, westward travel lengthens the day and can increase insulin and meal requirements. Frequent blood glucose monitoring is essential. Having ready access to snack foods is recommended. Coordinating premeal insulin dosing with unpredictable meal times during air-travel can be simplified by using short-acting insulins .

Insulin concentrations may vary from the standard U100 concentration prescribed in North America: U80 and U40 concentrations with corresponding syringes can be found in other countries. Mixing syringes with different concentrations of insulin increase the chances of overdosing or underdosing. Bringing adequate diabetic supplies can minimize this risk.

Severe TD can predispose the diabetic traveler to wildly fluctuating blood glucoses and adverse sequelae such as diabetic ketoacidosis; it should be aggressively treated.

4. **Travelers with cardiovascular disease.** A recent report determined that approximately two-thirds of in-flight fatalities on US carriers are because of cardiac disease. Hypobaric hypoxemia (decreased pressure of oxygen at altitude) can increase the risk of cardiac events.

   Special considerations for air travelers with cardiac disease include the following:
   a. Those with compensated congestive heart failure, stable angina, or a sea-level PaO_2 <70 mm Hg should arrange for in-flight oxygen. (SOR **❻**)
   b. Carrying a recent copy of electrocardiogram (ECG) results is recommended (with and without magnet ECG for pacemakers).
   c. A wallet card documenting pacemaker/AICD placement can speed transit through airport security.

   Cardiovascular contraindications to air travel are summarized in Table 104–7.

5. **Travelers with pulmonary disease.** As with travelers with cardiac disease, those with pulmonary disease are also susceptible to the hypobaric hypoxemia of air travel. A PaO_2 >70 mm Hg at room air does not usually require supplemental oxygen at altitude. If a pretravel arterial blood gas measurement is not feasible, a traveler who can walk up a flight of stairs or walk 50 m at a brisk pace without becoming severely dyspneic will usually tolerate flight without supplemental oxygen. A more sophisticated test, the high altitude simulation test (HAST), in which 15% FIO_2 is inhaled to mimic the partial pressure of oxygen at altitude, can be used to assess the pulmonary status prior to air travel.

   If in-flight supplemental oxygen is required, special arrangements must be made:
   a. Filled personal oxygen bottles are not permitted on commercial aircraft. Personal O_2 bottles must be purged and transported as checked luggage.
   b. In-flight oxygen can be arranged through each airline. It is recommended that the traveler contact the airline well in advance of travel. Most airlines will require a letter or prescription from a physician.

TABLE 104–7. CARDIOVASCULAR CONTRAINDICATIONS TO AIR TRAVEL

(1) Uncomplicated myocardial infarction within 2–3 wk
(2) Complicated myocardial infarction within 6 wk
(3) Unstable angina
(4) Decompensated congestive heart failure
(5) Uncontrolled hypertension
(6) Coronary artery bypass grafting within 10–14 d
(7) Stroke within 2 wk
(8) Uncontrolled ventricular or supraventricular tachycardia
(9) Eisenmenger syndrome
(10) Severe symptomatic valvular heart disease

(Reproduced with permission from Aerospace Medical Association MGTF: *Medical Guidelines for Airline Travel.* 2nd ed. Aviat Space Environ Med. 2003;74(5, Section II):A1.)

    c. If supplemental oxygen is needed during layovers, arrangements for oxygen must be made with venders in that particular locale. The airline usually does not provide this service.

        Pulmonary contraindications to air travel include severe, labile, uncontrolled asthma, and individuals with a pneumothorax. For individuals at high risk of pneumothorax (e.g., bullous emphysema), preflight end-expiratory chest radiographs should be performed.

IV. Health care abroad.

  A. Obtaining care

    Consular officers at embassies can assist in locating appropriate medical services, but the costs of care and, if necessary, air evacuation, are usually the traveler's financial responsibilities. Lists of English-speaking health-care providers by country can be obtained from the following sources:

    1. Office of Overseas Citizens Services, Room 4811, 2201 C Street, N.W., Washington, DC 20520. Indicate country or region of interest when you write.

    2. International Association for Medical Assistance to Travelers (IAMAT), (519) 836-0102.

    3. International Society of Travel Medicine, www.istm.org (directory of clinics and providers).

        Travelers should carry the name, phone number, and e-mail address of their personal physician for consultation if needed.

  B. Affording care

    1. Medical insurance. If the traveler's insurance plan provides for international coverage, it is important to bring an insurance card as proof of coverage and a claim form. Many insurance plans do not provide coverage at the point of service, and the traveler may be responsible for payment even before services are rendered. Some plans will offer partial or complete reimbursement upon return, so it is critical to save all receipts. **Medicare does not cover health expenses incurred outside of the United States.** Seniors may want to contact the American Association of Retired Persons about a Medicare supplement that provides international coverage.

    2. Evacuation insurance. Since medical care in most of the developing world is substandard by Western standards, the most prudent thing in the event of severe illness or injury may be air evacuation. Evacuation can be prohibitively expensive. Evacuation insurance is strongly recommended.

    3. Sources. Medical and evacuation insurance can be purchased at a reasonable cost through a travel agent or online. See the US State Department web site at www.travel.state.gov/medical.html for a list of private insurance and air evacuation companies. Most policies include both medical and evacuation coverages.

V. Special Activities

  A. Travel to high-altitude destinations. Altitude illness can occur in travelers who travel to high-altitude destinations. These illnesses include acute mountain sickness (AMS), high-altitude cerebral edema (HACE), high-altitude pulmonary edema (HAPE), high-altitude retinal hemorrhage (HARH), and high-altitude seizures (HAS). HACE and HAPE can be life threatening. The risk of occurrence is dependent on rate of ascent, sleeping altitude, the traveler's home altitude, and other aspects of individual physiology. AMS, the most common and least severe type of high-altitude illness, occurs in roughly one quarter of travelers to elevations of 7000 to 9000 ft (1850–2750 m) and >40% of travelers to elevations of 10,000 ft (3000 m). The incidence of HACE and HAPE is 0.1% to 4.0%. AMS and HACE are likely the same disease process at different points along a continuum—HACE being a very severe form of AMS. Most cases of HARH are asymptomatic and resolve spontaneously in 2 to 8 weeks. It has been suggested that HARH is an indication of the progression of AMS toward HACE; patients with AMS should be evaluated for HARH and advised against further ascent. Macular involvement may result in permanent visual damage, symptomatic HARH should prompt a descent. HAS is a recently recognized manifestation of altitude sickness. Though rare, they appear to be associated with central or obstructive sleep apnea. It is critical that travelers are aware of symptoms of high-altitude illness so immediate corrective action can be taken. Table 104–8 summarizes the symptoms, signs, prevention, and treatment of high-altitude illnesses.

  B. Freshwater activities

    1. Schistosomiasis prevention. Travelers to endemic areas (Africa, tropical South America, South and Southeast Asia, and the eastern Caribbean) should be cautioned

TABLE 104–8. SUMMARY OF SYMPTOMS/SIGNS, PROPHYLAXIS, AND TREATMENT FOR HIGH-ALTITUDE ILLNESSES

	Symptoms/Signs	Prophylaxis	Treatment
Acute mountain sickness (AMS)*	• Headache (most common) • Nausea • Difficulty sleeping • Fatigue • Anorexia	• Gradual ascent (<300 m/daily) at elevations >3000 m with rest day every 2–3 d. • Sleeping altitudes most critical. Climb high but sleep low. • Acetazolamide 250 mg po bid starting 1 d prior to ascent • Dexamethasone 4 mg po bid starting 1 d prior to ascent • Gingko biloba 120 mg po bid starting 5 d prior to ascent	• Rest • Avoid further ascent until symptoms resolve • Descent for severe AMS • Antiemetics • Oxygen • Acetazolamide 250 mg po bid–tid • Dexamethasone 4 mg po/IM q 6 h
High altitude cerebral edema (HACE)*	• Ataxia—inability to walk heel-to-toe (tandem walk test) • Altered level of consciousness ± • Symptoms of AMS	• Avoid hypothermia • Keep well hydrated • Avoid sedatives/narcotics that result in hypoventilation during sleep	• Immediate descent to lower altitude • Oxygen • Acetazolamide or dexamethasone in doses noted above • Portable hyperbaric chamber
High altitude pulmonary edema* (HAPE)	• Dyspnea on exertion • Cough • Blood-tinged sputum • Often coexists with AMS/HACE • Crackles, especially RML early on	• Gradual ascent, avoidance of hypothermia, hydration, and avoidance of sedatives and narcotics • Nifedipine SR 20 mg po tid • Salmeterol MDI 1–2 puffs bid • Persons with prior history of HAPE are at extremely high risk of recurrence (66% recurrence in one study). Avoidance of rapid altitude increases in these individuals should be strongly encouraged. • Risk is increased in patients with patent foramen ovale.	• Immediate descent • Reduce exertion • Oxygen • Continuous positive airway pressure • Portable hyperbaric chamber • Nifedipine 10 mg po followed by 20–30 mg SR bid–qd • Inhaled β-adrenergic agonists may be helpful
High-altitude retinal hemorrhage (HARH)	• Usually asymptomatic • May have visual disturbances	• Similar to HACE	• Patients with symptomatic HARH should not continue to ascent. • Upon return from altitude, most HARH spontaneously resolve in 2–8 wk
High-altitude seizure (HAS)	• New-onset seizure at altitude	• Travelers with history of central apnea or obstructive sleep apnea should consider avoiding high altitude. • Gradual ascent (<300 m/d) at elevations >3000 m with rest day every 2–3 d. • Sleeping altitudes most critical. Climb high but sleep low. • CPAP may help	• Anti-seizure medication (treat as any other seizure). • Oxygen • Descent

(*Data from Basnyat B, Murdoch DR. High-altitude illness. *Lancet.* 2003;361:1967-1974.)

against swimming in fresh water because of risk of acquiring this disease. Precise areas of endemicity can be found at the CDC and WHO web sites.

2. **Leptospirosis prevention.** Activities such as kayaking, canoeing, whitewater rafting, or swimming in endemic or epidemic areas increase one's risk for acquiring this potentially fatal disease, particularly in Latin America and Southeast Asia. Recent heavy rains and flooding increase the risk of this disease. For at-risk travelers, doxycycline prophylaxis (200 mg orally weekly beginning 1 to 2 days prior to activity and continuing for the duration of the activity) can be protective. Combining this use of doxycycline with its use for malaria prophylaxis would be an example of elegant prescribing, two-for-one!

3. **Scuba diving.** Scuba diving is generally well regulated in developed countries. Many popular dive sites in underdeveloped countries may not be as well regulated, and instruction/supervision of novice divers may be rudimentary at best. Obtaining education and certification by a reputable instructor prior to travel and diving with experienced divers, is strongly recommended.

   Air travel after diving increases the risk of decompression sickness. A minimum surface interval of 12 hours prior to air travel after a single dive is recommended before flying. For repetitive dives in a single day, a longer surface interval (at least 17 hours) prior to flying is recommended.

   The Divers Alert Network (www.diversalertnetwork.org) is a reputable resource for medical concerns associated with diving.

VI. **Geopolitical concerns**

Accidents and infections are not the only threats to a health trip. Geopolitical issues represent a significant consideration for the would-be traveler.

Since the 9/11 attacks, no one is unaware of the hazard posed by terrorist elements. An attentiveness to one's surroundings, including checking with one's embassy/consulate or www.state.gov for official "alert levels," can decrease one's risk of becoming a victim of terrorism-induced ill-health.

Transnational terrorists are not the only risks. At any given time, regions of our planet are war zones. In some places, defacto governments have been established by rebel forces who may not recognize visas issued by the official government (and vice versa). In other places, criminal elements may present a grave risk to travelers. Other areas of instability may deteriorate into civil war in relatively short order. Wars, declare or undeclared, can rapidly render a traveler unhealthy! Checking the Travel Advisories and Consular Information Sheets at www.state.gov can aid the traveler in monitoring the pulse of their intended destination.

Official policies may inhibit travel. For example, passports bearing entry stamps for Israel are denied entry to most Arab nations. Similar situations exist between a significant number of states; the Consular Information Sheets can provide valuable direction in this regard. Travelers with dual citizenship should be aware that they may be subject to both governments' laws and requirements, including military conscription. The one nation may not be able to intervene on behalf of its citizen who is detained in another nation of which that individual is also a citizen.

VII. **Travel After-Care.** Between 20% and 70% of travelers to developing countries will have an illness or injury associated with their travel. Of these travelers, 1% to 5% will seek medical care during travel or shortly after return. Travelers, particularly those to developing nations, are advised to seek medical attention upon return in the following situations:

A. **Fever**

Fever in a returning traveler is malaria until proven otherwise. (SOR **C**) This is the most commonly missed diagnosis: the average time of presentation-to-diagnosis for malaria is nearly a week in North America, which is inexcusable.

Fever with severe retrobulbar pain is strongly suggestive of dengue fever; if accompanied by petichaie, ecchymoses, and shock, dengue hemorrhagic syndrome or other hemorrhagic fevers must be considered.

Other febrile illnesses that may rapidly lead to death and must be considered include meningococcemia, leptospirosis, African trypanosomiasis, arboviral encephalitides, rickettsial disease, and typhoid. Many other causes of fever that are not immediately life threatening may be acquired abroad. A full discourse on each of these is beyond the scope of this chapter and the reader is referred to the "general references" listed in the bibliography. Additionally, a useful web tool for determining the etiology of a fever in an otherwise healthy, nonpregnant adult traveler can be found at www.fevertravel.ch.

B. Persistent diarrhea or vomiting.

Nearly half of travelers develop diarrhea; though usually self-limiting, in 10% it persists more than 2 weeks, and for some it lasts a month or more.

In evaluating persistent diarrhea, it is important to be aware of associated signs and symptoms. Arthralgias may be associated with *Campylobacter, Shigella, Samonella,* and *Yersinia* infections. Fevers, bleeding, and severe pain are suggestive of invasive causes of diarrhea such as *Campylobacter, Clostridium, Entamoeba, Escherichia coli* O157:H7, *Listeria, Aeromonas, Vibrio,* and *Yersina*. Explosive, malabsorptive diarrhea is suggestive of *Giardia* or tropical sprue; eosinophilia is seen with the parasitic worms.

Laboratory evaluation of those with diarrhea lasting more than a week is warranted. Fecal leukocytes and occult stool hemoglobin are indicative of invasive diarrhea. Routine stool culture typically includes only Samonella, Shigella, and Campylobacter, so it is important to alert the laboratory if clinical suspicions suggest other organisms. Microscopic examination for ova and parasite may be helpful; three samples collected at 24- to 48-hour intervals is necessary to have adequate sensitivity, and cryptosporidia must be specified if suspected, as special staining techniques are employed. Both stool and serum enzyme-linked immunosorbent assay testing is available for many pathogens. Rarely, endoscopic visualization of the colon may be useful.

Bear in mind that there exist prolonged yet self-limitting postinfectious irritable bowel and postinfectious malabsorptive syndromes, which affects a quarter of patients following acute infectious gastroenteritis. Failure to recognize this results in fear of "occult" infectious processes and excessive (and expensive) testing that is of no benefit to the patient.

C. Jaundice

Jaundice, with or without other symptoms, following a trip to the tropics requires evaluation. The most common cause of jaundice is infectious hepatitis. Hepatitis A is food borne, and is not rare among unvaccinated travelers. Travelers who have had sexual encounters or other body fluid exposures while abroad are at significant risk for the development of hepatitis B. Serology for acute viral hepatitis is indicated in the workup of jaundice in returning travelers.

Parasitic infections may also cause jaundice or other hepatobiliary symptoms. The liver and biliary flukes are naturally found in the relevant anatomical sites, and *Ascaris* or other roundworms may occasionally be found there. Stool ova or serological testing may be employed in the diagnosis of these organisms.

Excessive hemolysis, such as that encountered in malaria or its treatment may present with jaundice. Mefloquine and atovaquone/proguanil are known to elevate transaminase levels, and of course primaquine causes severe hemolysis in patients with G6PD deficiency. The underlying cause must be identified and addressed.

Other infectious causes may range from leptospirosis to yellow fever. An assortment of noninfectious causes of liver toxicity, including things such as aflotoxin, hepatotoxic herbal remedies, or industrial toxins, may be encountered while traveling in developing nations and should also be included in the differential diagnosis.

D. Newly acquired skin disorders.

The most common skin disorder presented by returning travelers in a 1995 study was cutaneous larval migrans, a puriritic creeping eruption. Caused by zoonotic nematodes, these respond well to ivermectin (12 mg single dose). A dozen years later, a similar study found that infectious cellulitis was number one, followed closely by scabies (the latter of which is also treated with ivermectin at a similar dose of 0.2 mg/kg). In this later report, "pruritis of unknown origin" was a close third!

The characteristics of the rash can direct the diagnostic directions undertaken. Ulcers may be because of leishmaniasis, anthrax, or leprosy, as well as other more common things such as venous stasis. Onchocerciasis, leprosy, myiasis, scabies, pinta, insect bites, and phytodermatitis are among the causes of maculopapular rashes. Diffuse rashes are suggestive of rickettsial infections (e.g., the spotted fevers), typhoid, multiple insect bites, drug reactions, or viral conditions ranging from measles to the hemorrhagic fevers. Appropriately obtained biopsies, cultures, and serologies are of great value in reaching the diagnosis.

REFERENCES

General References

Centers for Disease Control and Prevention. *Yellow Book 2008;* Atlanta: CDC; 2008. (Has information on vaccinations (routine and travel-related), travelers' diarrhea; precautions in consuming water and dairy products abroad; and air travel for pediatric travelers).

Cook GC, Zumla A: *Manson's Tropical Diseases.* Edinburgh: Saunders/Elsevier; 2003.

Jong EC, McMullen R. *The Travel and Tropical Medicine Manual.* 3rd ed. Philadelphia: Saunders; 2003.

Strickland GT. *Hunter's Tropical Medicine and Emerging Infectious Diseases.* Philadelphia: Saunders; 2000.

World Health Organization. *International Travel and Health*; Geneva: WHO; 2008. (Has information on vaccinations (routine and travel-related), travelers' diarrhea; fever onset from fly bite in trypanoso-miasis; precautions in consuming water and dairy products abroad; precautions in consuming food and water in pregnant patients; and air travel for pediatric travelers).

World Tourism Organization. http://www.world-tourism.org/. Accessed July 18, 2008.

High-Altitude Illness and Diving

Basnyat B, Murdoch DR. High-altitude illness. *Lancet* (June 7). 2003;361:1967-1974.

Divers Alert Network. http://www.diversalertnetwork.org. Accessed July 18, 2008.

Maa E, Roach R, Patz M, et al. High altitude seizures: the epidemiology of an acute symptomatic seizure. *Abstract, International Hypoxia Symposium 2007: Hypoxia and the Circulation*, February 27–March 4, Chateau Lake Louise, Alberta, Canada.

Tingay TG, Tsimnadis P, Basnyat B. A blurred view from Everest. *Lancet.* 2003;362:1978.

Illness and Injury Prevention

Barbier HM, Diaz JH. Prevention and treatment of toxic seafoodborne diseases in travelers. *J Travel Med.* 2003;10(01):29-37.

Castelli F, Saleri N, Tomasoni LR, et al. Prevention and treatment of Travelers' Diarrhea. *Digestion.* 2006; 73(suppl. 1):109-118.

Chen LH, Wilson ME, Schlagenhauf P. Prevention of malaria in long-term travelers. J Am Med Assoc. 2006;296:2234-2244.

Fradin MS. Mosquitoes and mosquito repellents: a clinician's guide. *Ann Intern Med.* 1998;128:931-940.

Matteelli A, Carosi G. Sexually transmitted diseases in travelers. *Clin Infect Dis.* 2001;32:1063-1067.

Scurr J. Frequency and prevention of symptomless deep venous thrombosis in long-haul flights: a randomised trial. *Lancet.* 2001;357:1485-1489.

Jet Lag and Motion Sickness

Herxheimer A, Petrie K. Melatonin for the prevention and treatment of jet lag (Cochrane Review). *Cochrane Database Syst Rev.* 2003;2:CD001520.

Sherman CR. Motion sickness: review of causes and preventive strategies. *J Travel Med.* 2002;9(05):251-256.

Skin Diseases

Ansart S, Perez L, Jaureguiberry S, et al. Spectrum of dermatoses in 165 travelers returning from the tropics with skin diseases. *Am J Trop Med Hyg.* 2007;76:184-186.

Caumes E, Carriere J, Guermonprez G, et al. Dermatoses associated with travel to tropical countries: a prospective study of the diagnosis and management of 269 patients presenting to a tropical disease unit. *Clin Infect Dis.* 1995;20:542-548.

Travelers with Special Needs

Aerospace Medical Association MGTF: Medical Guidelines for Airline Travel. 2nd ed. *Aviat Space Environ Med.* 2003;74(5, Suppl.):A1-19.

American College of Obstetrics and Gynecology Committee on Obstetric Practice: Committee Opinion Number 282: Immunization during pregnancy. *Obstet Gynecol.* 2003;101(1):207-212.

Castelli F, Patroni A. The human immunodeficiency virus-infected traveler. *Clin Infect Dis.* 2000;31: 1403-1408.

Stauffer WM, Kamat D. Traveling with infants and children. Part II: immunizations. *J Travel Med.* 2002;9(2):82-90.

Stauffer WM, Kamat D, Magill AJ. Traveling with infants and children. Part IV: insect avoidance and malarial prevention. *J Travel Med.* 2003;10(4):225-240.

Stauffer WM, Konop RJ, Kamat D. Traveling with infants and young children. Part I: anticipatory guid-ance: travel preparation and preventive health advice. *J Travel Med.* 2001;8(5):254-259.

Stauffer WM, Konop RJ, Kamat D. Traveling with infants and young children. Part III: travelers' diarrhea. *J Travel Med.* 2002;9(3):141-150.

Teichman PG, Donchin Y, Kot RJ. International aeromedical evacuation: *N Engl J Med*. 2007;356: 262-270.

Vaccinations

CDC's National Immunization Program http://www.cdc.gov/vaccines. Accessed July 18, 2008.
Duke T, Mgone CS. Measles: not just another viral exanthem. *Lancet*. 2003;361:763.
Pollard AJ, Shlim DR. Epidemic meningococcal disease and travel. *J Travel Med*. 2002;9(1):29-33.
LoRe V, Gluckman SJ. Travel immunizations. *Am Fam Physician*. 2004;70:89-99.
Ryan ET, Calderwood SB. Cholera vaccines. *J Travel Med*. 2001;8(2):82-91.
Watson D, Ashley R. Pretravel health advice for asplenic individuals. *J Travel Med*. 2003;10(2):117-121.
U.S. State Department travel site http://www.travel.state.gov. Accessed July 18, 2008.

---

105   Preoperative Evaluation

Sarah R. Edmonson, MD, MS

KEY POINTS

- The purpose of the preoperative evaluation is to identify and manage risk, not to guarantee a problem-free surgery.
- The most common complications of surgery are infectious, cardiac, and pulmonary problems.
- Preoperative testing should be customized to the findings of the history and physical examination. No test is recommended for every patient.
- The final important step in a preoperative evaluation is communication of your findings to both the patient and the consulting surgeon. The operative plan should include measures to decrease the patient's operative risk as much as possible.
- Figure 105–1 shows a suggested algorithm for approaching the preoperative evaluation.

I. Introduction
A. Role of the primary care physician
1. The primary care physician is frequently asked to perform a preoperative evaluation on surgical patients. When this consultation is made, the implicit task is to identify and quantify the patient's risk for adverse outcome from the surgical procedure.
2. The preoperative evaluation cannot "clear" the patient for surgery, as all surgeries involve some level of risk. Rather, this evaluation allows the patient to balance the need for surgery against the risk of adverse outcome, in order to make an informed decision.
3. The consultation also allows the surgeon and primary care physician to work together to minimize the known risks before, during, and after the procedure.
4. The efficacy of preoperative evaluation has not been well demonstrated in the literature. Nonetheless, preoperative evaluation is recommended by most organizations, because operative risks are identified and controlled in the outpatient setting, hospital stays are shorter, and fewer surgeries are cancelled or postponed. (SOR **C**)

B. Timing.
1. The ideal timing for the preoperative assessment is several weeks before the procedure. This timing allows the provider time to evaluate problems and initiate therapy without having to postpone a scheduled surgery.
2. The Joint Commission on Accreditation of Healthcare Organizations requires all surgical patients to have a medical history and physical examination within 30 days of surgery. (SOR **C**)

C. Outcomes.
1. Overall, between 15% and 20% of surgeries cause at least one complication. The most common types of adverse outcomes are summarized in Table 105–1.

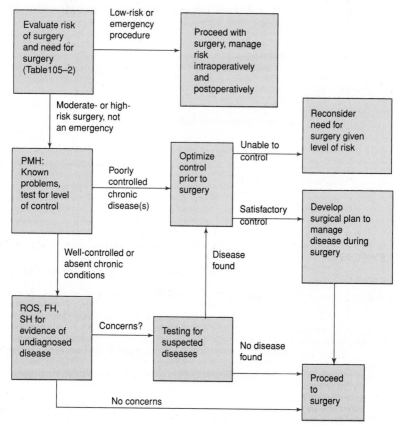

FIGURE 105–1. Preoperative evaluation algorithm. FH, family history; PMH, previous medical history; ROS, review of systems; SH, social history.

TABLE 105–1. POTENTIAL SURGICAL COMPLICATIONS

Category	Examples
Infectious	Wound infections, pneumonia, urinary tract infections, bacterial endocarditis, and frank systemic sepsis.
Cardiac	Myocardial infarction, cardiac arrest, pulmonary edema, and complications of congestive heart failure
Pulmonary	Pneumonia, atelectasis, bronchitis, respiratory failure with unplanned intubation, inability to wean from the respirator, and pulmonary embolus
Thrombosis	Peripheral venous thromboembolism, cardiac or pulmonary thromboses, and renal or mesenteric arterial thrombosis
Adverse reaction to anesthesia	Malignant hyperthermia and drug or materials (e.g., latex) allergy including anaphylaxis
Gastrointestinal	Gastritis, peptic ulcer disease, postoperative constipation, ileus, or hyperemesis
Psychological	Postoperative delirium. Exacerbation of latent psychiatric disease.
Social	Financial or professional ramifications of missed work and possibly altered body function. Increased burden on caregivers.

2. Prospective studies to determine if preoperative evaluation reduces the rate of complications have not been published. However, preoperative evaluation can help the physician predict and manage complications, whether or not they are avoidable.

3. Surgical morbidity and mortality rates vary depending on the type of surgery, the anatomical location of the procedure, and the condition of the patient.

4. The most common adverse outcomes of surgery are infection, cardiac events, and pulmonary problems.

   a. Cardiac events are uncommon in children; in adults, they are the events that are most likely to be lethal.

   b. Pulmonary problems are most frequently seen after abdominal or thoracic surgery and among obese patients; they are the most common adverse events for children.

   c. Diagnosis of postoperative venous thromboembolism can be difficult as more than half of cases are asymptomatic.

II. **Preoperative Assessment Algorithm (SOR Ⓑ)**

   A. The algorithm is summarized in Figure 105–1.

   B. **Consider urgency of surgery.** If the risk of delaying surgery outweighs the benefits of preoperative evaluation, then the patient must obviously proceed to surgery. Such situations are innately high risk for the patient, regardless of underlying medical condition. Surgery for acute trauma often falls into this category, as do surgeries for rupture of intraperitoneal organs such as spleen, bowel, or bladder. In general, preoperative evaluations are requested for procedures which are elective or at least able to be deferred.

   C. **Evaluate** risk of surgery (Table 105–2). As a general rule, the preoperative workup should be more thorough for patients undergoing high-risk surgeries.

   1. A high-risk surgery is defined as one in which the risk of cardiopulmonary complications is >5%.

   2. The literature about surgical risk is difficult to assess, because of constant improvements in surgical and anesthesiology techniques. Thus, results may be inaccurate for all but the most recent publications.

   3. However, intrathoracic, intraperitoneal, vascular, and orthopedic surgeries are usually considered high risk.

   4. Potentially prolonged surgery, or surgery involving large loss of blood or fluid shift should also be considered high risk.

   5. Lower-risk surgeries include superficial dermatologic procedures and ophthalmology surgeries.

   D. Check status of known chronic conditions

   1. Perform testing and examination as appropriate to establish whether chronic conditions are as well controlled as possible.

   2. When practical, optimize control before proceeding to surgery.

   E. Scrutinize review of systems, family and social history, and physical examination findings for evidence of undiagnosed disease. As with known chronic conditions, new conditions identified at the preoperative evaluation should be worked up and stabilized prior to surgery whenever possible.

III. **Specific Inquiries**

   A. **Previous surgical experience.** Patients who have had bleeding complications, anesthesia reactions (such as malignant hyperthermia), or other adverse responses to surgery should have their previous history investigated carefully. This history should strongly

TABLE 105–2. **RISK OF CERTAIN SURGERIES**

High-risk surgeries	High anticipated blood loss
	Aortic or peripheral vascular surgery
Moderate-risk surgeries	Abdominal or thoracic surgery
	Head and neck surgery
	Carotid endarterectomy
	Orthopedic surgery
	Prostate surgery
Low-risk surgeries	Breast surgery
	Cataract surgery
	Superficial dermatologic surgery
	Endoscopy

TABLE 105–3. **PATIENT RISK FACTORS FOR CARDIOVASCULAR DISEASE**

Hypertension, particularly uncontrolled
History of stroke
Diabetes mellitus
Advanced age
Previous abnormal electrocardiogram
Nonsinus cardiac rhythm (asymptomatic)
Tobacco use
Hyperlipidemia
Obesity
Family history of heart disease, particularly in male first-degree relatives who
　　develop heart disease when younger than 50 years and female first-degree
　　relatives younger than 60 years

influence the perioperative care plan. For example, work-up of a patient with prior bleeding complications may show a clotting disorder, which can be treated with preoperative supplementation of clotting factor or fresh frozen plasma immediately before surgery.

B. **Cardiac evaluation.** Because of the high morbidity and mortality associated with perioperative cardiac problems, every patient should have a careful cardiac evaluation.
　　1. When and how to evaluate:
　　　　a. Well-known **preoperative algorithms** can be used to evaluate cardiac risk. These include Goldman's risk index, Detsky's risk index, the American Society of Anesthesiology's preoperative guideline, the Lee Risk Index, the American College of Physicians guideline, and the American College of Cardiology/American Heart Association (ACC/AHA) guideline. Comparative studies have not established the superiority of any one of these guidelines, and all may be cumbersome in the clinical setting.
　　　　b. The use and weighting of risk factors for cardiac disease varies depending on the guideline used. Overall, factors that have been shown to predispose a patient to coronary artery disease are summarized in Table 105–3; the presence of three or more risk factors indicates a need for additional cardiac evaluation.
　　　　c. Functional capacity: Cardiac risk may also be predicted by the intensity of physical effort that the patient is capable of regularly performing. (SOR Ⓐ)
　　　　　　(1) Typically functional capacity is measured in METs (metabolic equivalents of oxygen consumption) according to the Duke Activity Status Index, Table 105–4.
　　　　　　(2) A patient who is able to perform moderate intensity activity (>4 MET equivalent) is unlikely to have significant coronary artery disease.
　　　　　　(3) Poor functional capacity correlates highly with coronary artery disease and may require further preoperative work-up. Intermediate functional capacity should be considered for evaluation, particularly if one or more risk factors are also present.

TABLE 105–4. **DUKE ACTIVITY STATUS INDEX**

Functional Class	METs	Activity
I	7.5–8	Heavy housework
		Strenuous sports
		Can run a short distance
II	4.5–5.5	Climb one flight of stairs
		Sexual relations
		Light yardwork
III	2.5–3.5	Light housework
		Walk two level blocks
		Self-care (dressing, bathing)
IV	1.75	Walk short distances indoors

METs, metabolic equivalents of oxygen consumption.
(Reproduced with permission from Hlatky MA, et al. A brief self-administered questionnaire to determine functional capacity (the Duke Activity Status Index). *Am J Cardiol.* 1989;64:651-654.)

(4) Functional capacity cannot be evaluated in a number of patients because of noncardiac factors that limit exercise. For example, a patient with mobility impairment because of osteoarthritis cannot run, but may have intact coronary vasculature. When functional capacity is unknown, it is advisable to err on the side of caution.

d. Certain surgical procedures are associated with a higher risk of perioperative myocardial infarction (Table 105–2). The physician threshold for cardiac testing should be lower for the patient preparing to undergo a high-risk surgery.

2. A summary of the ACC/AHA guideline is shown in Figure 105–2. According to the AHA algorithm, the initial evaluation should divide the patients into the following groups (SOR **C**):

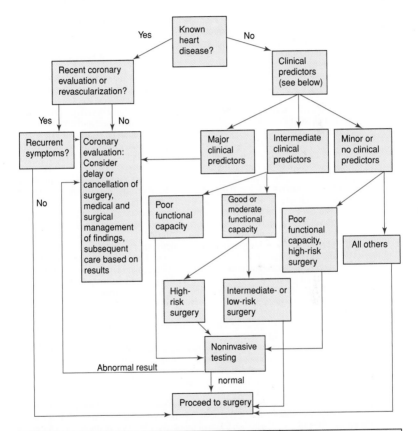

Major Clinical Predictors	Intermediate Clinical Predictors	Minor Clinical Predictors
Unstable coronary syndromes	Mild angina pectoris	Advanced age
Decompensated CHF	Prior myocardial infarction	Abnormal electrocardiogram
Significant arrhythmias	Compensated CHF	Rhythm other than sinus
Severe valvular disease	Diabetes mellitus	Low functional capacity
	Renal insufficiency	History of stroke
		Uncontrolled hypertension

FIGURE 105–2. American College of Cardiology/American Heart Association guidelines for preoperative cardiac evaluation (summarized). CHF, congestive heart failure.

a. High risk: Patients with clearly established, uncontrolled disease such as unstable coronary disease, myocardial infarction within the past 6 weeks, decompensated congestive heart failure, significant arrhythmia, or severe valvular disease should defer surgery until better control is achieved.

   (1) If the patient has had a recent myocardial infarction, he or she is at high risk for another attack during or after surgery, and the operation should be deferred whenever possible. As the risk for recurrent myocardial infarction decreases after 6 weeks, the patient should be re-evaluated at that time. (SOR **B**)

   (2) People with clinically important coronary artery disease should defer noncardiac procedures until 6 months after revascularization, when possible. (SOR **B**)

   (3) Patients who have undergone cardiac revascularization in the past 6 months should defer surgery or have repeat evaluation of their coronary arteries prior to surgery. (SOR **B**)

   (4) Even under optimal medical management, patients with congestive heart failure, previous myocardial infarction, or coronary artery obstruction that is not amenable to repair are at higher risk of perioperative cardiac events. This risk has to be balanced against the benefits of surgery on a case-by-case basis. (SOR **C**)

   (5) Assessment of left ventricular function (such as echocardiogram) does not change the management patients with congestive heart failure, and is not recommended. (SOR **A**)

b. Patients with intermediate risk, including those with stable or mild coronary artery disease, heart failure, renal insufficiency, or patients with signs and symptoms consistent with previously undiagnosed heart disease, such as exertional chest pain, dyspnea, and poor functional capacity, should receive additional testing to better define their level of disease. Patients who have multiple cardiac risk factors (Table 105–3) should also be evaluated for cardiac disease. (SOR **C**)

   (1) Insufficient date exists to determine whether preoperative EKG is predictive of intraoperative cardiac risk; consequently, more detailed studies are recommended to clarify risk in intermediate-risk patients. (SOR **B**)

   (2) If the review of systems reveals symptoms consistent with angina or anginal equivalent, the patient should undergo noninvasive (stress) testing to clarify the likelihood of coronary artery disease. (SOR **C**)

   (3) Patients with ongoing or recurrent symptoms that have been previously established to be angina should have evaluation of their coronary arteries (catheterization or angiography) prior to surgery, to determine whether revascularization should be performed before elective surgery is scheduled. (SOR **C**)

c. Low risk: Patients who have no concerning history or symptoms and who have fewer than two risk factors are at low risk for heart disease and can proceed to surgery.

   (1) Some experts suggest screening EKG in asymptomatic patients older than 55 years. (SOR **C**)

   (2) Asymptomatic patients who have had a normal stress test in the past 2 years, bypass surgery in the past 5 years, or angioplasty in the past 5 years are unlikely to have developed significant new disease. These patients may proceed to surgery without further cardiac work-up. (SOR **B**)

3. Perioperative management

   a. In known coronary artery disease, perioperative beta-blocker therapy reduces risk (SOR **A**); beta-blockade has not been found to be advantageous in lower-risk patients. (SOR **B**) Administer an initial dose of atenolol intravenously 30 minutes before the procedure. After the procedure, order either atenolol 5 mg intravenously every 12 hours, or 50 to 100 mg orally once daily up to a maximum of 7 days. This therapy is contraindicated in patients with hypotension, active congestive heart failure, bronchospasm, bradycardia, or third-degree heart block.

   b. Alpha2-agonists may be a reasonable alternative to beta-blockers in patients who cannot take them. (SOR **B**)

   c. Calcium channel blockers and nitrates have not been shown to influence perioperative cardiac risk. (SOR **A**)

   d. Statin use is also associated with improved perioperative outcomes in high-risk patients, but randomized trial data is lacking. (SOR **B**)

    e. Arrhythmias generally indicate some level of underlying cardiac damage. Perioperative management of the arrhythmia involves addressing any hemodynamic instability caused by the arrhythmia, and managing any thrombogenic potential generated by the arrhythmia. For arrhythmias that increase the risk of thrombosis (such as atrial fibrillation), postoperative prophylaxis against pulmonary embolus or deep venous thrombosis can be used. See Section IV.F.5 for details.

        Valvular disease can cause both hemodynamic instability and increased risk for bacterial endocarditis. All patients with valvular disease should receive antibiotic prophylaxis before and during the procedure (see Chapter 103 for more information).

C. Pulmonary evaluation
1. Pulmonary complications of surgery are most common in surgeries that are anatomically close to the diaphragm.
2. Preexisting respiratory disease such as asthma, chronic obstructive pulmonary disease (COPD), pulmonary fibrotic diseases such as sarcoidosis, pneumonia, tuberculosis, or other pulmonary conditions increase the chance of bad outcomes.
3. Smoking, obesity, dyspnea, and a history of cough are risk factors for pulmonary problems after surgery.
4. Evaluation
    a. Chest X-ray is indicated for evaluation of physical examination abnormalities or reported symptoms of dyspnea or cough. Radiography may also be helpful for clarifying the status of previously diagnosed problems. Routine baseline chest x-rays in all patients undergoing surgery has been shown to be unhelpful.
    b. Pulmonary function testing is useful for evaluation of patients with suspected asthma or COPD. This testing may also be useful for demonstrating the status of these problems prior to surgery. (SOR **B**)
    c. Arterial blood gases are rarely useful in the preoperative patient. (SOR **B**) Patients whose pulmonary function is diminished enough to affect blood oxygenation are at inherently high surgical risk; these patients should be easily identifiable from the history and physical alone.
5. Pulmonary medication, including steroids, should be continued perioperatively. Patients with severe COPD or asthma may benefit from a course of prophylactic steroid therapy prior to surgery. (SOR **C**) Nasogastric decompression may reduce the risk of pulmonary complications after abdominal surgery. (SOR **A**)
6. **High-risk patients can be taught to perform incentive spirometry before, during, and after the procedure to minimize the chances of pulmonary complications.** (SOR **B**)

D. Diabetes mellitus may increase the risk of cardiac events as well as perioperative infection.
1. Perioperatively, the blood sugar should be maintained as close to euglycemia as possible, avoiding both hyper and hypoglycemia. (SOR **B**) The best regimen for accomplishing this has not been established.
2. Patients with previously diagnosed diabetes should be evaluated for current diabetic control and presence of secondary organ damage. If not recently done, testing including hemoglobin A_{1C}, urine microalbumin levels, and renal function testing should be performed. In addition, diabetic patients should be considered high risk for cardiac disease and evaluated as such. (SOR **A**)
3. All patients undergoing surgery should be screened for the signs and symptoms of diabetes mellitus, including polyuria, thirst, weight loss, blurring vision, acanthosis nigricans, and truncal obesity. All patients older than 50 years, patients with a family history of diabetes, or patients whose history or physical suggests any possibility of diabetes mellitus should have a fasting blood glucose test performed. (SOR **C**)
4. New or uncontrolled diabetes mellitus should be brought into good glycemic control prior to surgery. (SOR **C**)

E. Additional conditions that affect perioperative risk.
1. **Immunocompromise.** Certain patients are at high risk for infectious complications, including patients with genetic immune deficiencies, rheumatologic disease requiring immunosuppressive therapy, HIV, and diabetes mellitus, as well as chemotherapy recipients. In addition, patients with asplenia and valvular heart disease are at increased risk of catastrophic bacterial infection. These patients should be considered

for prophylactic antibiotic therapy during the procedure and should be closely monitored throughout the operative period. (SOR **⊙**)

2. **Anemia.** Anemia may result from a number of causes and can be particularly dangerous when the proposed surgery is likely to result in significant blood loss. Review of systems may reveal fatigue, syncope, or cold intolerance, and examination may reveal pallor, pale mucus membranes, rapid pulse, or a functional heart murmur. A hemoglobin level should be checked in any patient with a history of anemia or a suggestive history or physical examination; hemoglobin may also be a useful test prior to surgeries that often cause significant bleeding. (SOR **⊙**) Any finding of anemia warrants work-up to determine the cause prior to surgery. Transfusion may be necessary prior to any surgery that cannot be deferred. The optimal hemoglobin level is unclear and probably varies by patient and by procedure.

3. **Malnutrition.** Individuals with protein-calorie malnutrition or specific vitamin or mineral deficiencies have a much higher rate of postoperative complications. Weight loss, edema, fatigue, syncope, pallor, dental disease, financial or social deprivation, anemia, or frequent illness can be warning signs of malnutrition. Laboratory tests to evaluate malnutrition should include a blood count, albumin level, and specific vitamin assays. Supplements and hyperalimentation prior to and immediately after the procedure are helpful. For surgeries that require a fasting patient, enteral or parenteral nutrition may be chosen to sustain the malnourished patient. (SOR **⊙**)

4. **Peripheral vascular disease.** In general, the risk of peripheral vascular disease closely parallels that of ischemic cardiac disease. Thus, the presence of one should promote evaluation for both, and all patients with claudication symptoms or abnormal peripheral pulses should receive both peripheral vascular and cardiac evaluation. Noninvasive peripheral arterial evaluation may include Doppler or Duplex scanning, high-resolution computerized tomography, or magnetic resonance angiography (MRA). If the testing shows evidence of peripheral vascular disease, the postoperative plan should include prevention of pressure ulcers. (SOR **⊙**)

5. **Hypercoagulable or hypocoagulable state.** The patient should be questioned about a personal or family history of hypercoagulable conditions as well as rheumatologic disease. At-risk patients should receive perioperative prophylaxis against venous thromboembolism including subcutaneous heparin (5000 U subcutaneously every 8 hours) or low-molecular-weight heparin (such as enoxaparin, 40 mg subcutaneously once daily), and intermittent limb compression. There is no indication for routine checking of coagulation studies. (SOR **⑧**)

6. **Peptic ulcer disease.** Most postoperative gastrointestinal complications are new-onset, so all patients should be monitored closely. However, patients who have a prior history of peptic ulcer, or who are experiencing symptoms of dyspepsia or reflux, should receive prophylactic therapy in the preoperative and perioperative periods. (SOR **⑧**)

7. **Renal or hepatic failure.** Patients with end-stage liver or kidney disease face unique surgical challenges. Maintenance of blood pressure and fluid balance is more difficult in such patients, and many medications are metabolized at different rates in these patients. In addition, patients with renal failure often have disrupted hematopoiesis and concurrent anemia. Liver failure leads to decreased synthesis of important proteins including clotting factors. Prior to end-stage disease, the physiologic stress of surgery may worsen the organ's function either temporarily or permanently. Patients with significant renal disease should consider preparation for dialysis prior to surgery, including placement of long-term or permanent venous access. Patients with significant liver failure should not undergo surgery except in life-threatening situations.

8. **Psychiatric disease.** Symptomatic control should be evaluated in all patients with known psychiatric disease. In addition, all patients should be monitored for signs of active psychiatric disease, and their social support system assessed. Patients with evidence of or predisposition for psychiatric disturbance should delay surgery until acute problems are controlled and should be monitored during and after surgery for exacerbation. (SOR **⊙**)

9. Lifestyle risks
   a. **Drug or alcohol use/abuse.** Patients who abuse alcohol or drugs must be evaluated for use-associated organ damage such as alcoholic hepatitis. In addition,

the perioperative period presents risks for withdrawal symptoms. Ideally, the addicted patient should undergo medically monitored detoxification prior to surgery (see Chapter 88). If a history of intravenous drug use is elicited, testing for HIV and hepatitis C is warranted.

  b. **Cigarette smoking.** Smokers have a higher risk of cardiovascular and pulmonary disease and should be evaluated carefully for those problems. In addition, smokers should be advised that smoking cessation at least 8 weeks before surgery can improve their mucociliary capacity considerably and thus decrease their chances of postoperative pneumonia. Fewer than 8 weeks of smoking cessation has not been associated with an improvement in operative morbidity or mortality.

  c. **Sexual behavior.** Brief questioning about sexual behavior will uncover female patients at risk for pregnancy and will help identify patients at risk for HIV. A urine pregnancy test should be performed in all sexually active, premenopausal women. (SOR **C**)

10. **Medications.** Certain medications can increase the patient's perioperative risk. Anticoagulant therapy such as warfarin or platelet aggregation inhibitors should be stopped 1 week before surgery. For some patients, the risk of even short-term discontinuation of anticoagulants exceeds the risk of surgery. These patients can be started on intravenous unfractionated heparin, titrated to maintain an activated partial thromboplastin time level of 55 to 85 seconds, or given a low-molecular-weight heparin subcutaneously, at a typical dose of 1 mg/kg body weight. Heparin can be discontinued several hours before the procedure to minimize intraoperative bleeding complications. Over-the-counter anti-inflammatories or some herbal remedies also cause a predisposition for excess bleeding, and the patient may not think to mention these products without specific prompting.

IV. Special Cases

  A. **Children.** Children are far less likely to have coronary artery disease but are at higher risk of having undiagnosed pulmonary, immunologic, anatomic, or genetic abnormalities. The preoperative history should include the prenatal and birth history and a history of recent infections. Upper respiratory infections or pneumonia should be allowed to completely resolve prior to surgery. (SOR **C**)

  B. **Patients who are unable to give a history.** Evaluation of functional capacity and current symptoms is impossible if a patient is unconscious or incapable of communicating with the physician. In this case, a careful physical examination becomes the only tool the primary care physician has to identify risks. In this situation, a lower threshold for ordering predictive tests should be employed. (SOR **C**)

  C. **Pregnancy.** Except in life-threatening situations, surgery should be avoided in all pregnant women. (SOR **B**)

  D. **Elderly patients.** The likelihood of serious medical problems increases with age, and thus the perception arises that older patients are at higher risk during surgery. In fact, healthy geriatric patients do not have a higher surgical morbidity. These patients should be carefully evaluated for medical problems or social support issues, but can expect to undergo surgery quite successfully. Because of the high prevalence of dementia, the primary care examiner should perform a mental status examination on every geriatric patient. (SOR **C**)

V. The Perioperative Plan

  A. **Communication of results to surgeon.** The primary care consultation to the surgeon should include the following:

  1. A listing of the patient's known risk factors and medical conditions.
  2. Appraisal of how these factors will affect the patient's overall surgical risk.
  3. Suggestions for controlling, minimizing, or eliminating risks discovered in the preoperative evaluation.

  B. **Patient counseling.** The primary care physician should discuss the risks and benefits of surgery clearly with the patient. The patient should understand:

  1. That all surgery may include unanticipated complications.
  2. Any factors that create particularly high risk for this patient.
  3. Your suggestions to the patient for minimizing risk.
  4. Your suggestion for long-term follow-up of any medical problems found in the examination.

REFERENCES

Eagle KA, Berger PB, Calkins H, et al. *ACC/AHA Guideline Update on Perioperative Cardiovascular Evaluation for Noncardiac Surgery: A report of the American College of Cardiology/American Heart Association Task Force on Practice Guidelines (Committee to Update the 1996 Guidelines on Perioperative Cardiovascular Evaluation for Noncardiac Surgery).* Bethesda, MD: American College of Cariology Foundation; 2002. Available at http:/www.acc.org/clinical/guidelines/perio/dirIndex.htm.

Fleisher LA, Beckman JA, Brown KA, et al. ACC/AHA 2006 Guideline update on perioperative cardiovascular evaluation on noncardiac surgery: focused update on perioperative beta-blocker therapy. A report of the Americal College of Cardiology/American Heart Association Task Force. *J Am Coll Cardiol.* 2006;47:2343-2355.

Flood C, Fleisher LA. Preparation of the cardiac patient for noncardiac surgery. *Am Fam Physician.* 2007;75:656-665.

Institute for Clinical Systems Improvement (ICSI). *Preoperative Evaluation.* Bloomington, MN: Institute for Clinical Systems Improvement (ICSI); 2006.

Kapoor AS. Strength of evidence for perioperative use of statins to reduce cardiovascular risk: systematic review of controlled studies. *BMJ.* 2006;333:1149.

Lawrence VA, Cornell JE, Smetana GW, et al. Strategies to reduce postoperative pulmonary complications after noncardiothoracic surgery: Systematic review of the American College of Physicians. *Ann Intern Med.* 2006;144:596-608.

Smiley DD, Umpierrez GE. Perioperative glucose control in the diabetic or nondiabetic patient. *Southern Med J.* 2006;99:580-589.

Index